COMPREHENSIVE RESPIRATORY NURSING

A Decision Making Approach

LAUREL D. KERSTEN, RN, PhD (cand)

Clinical Specialist/Nurse Researcher
Nursing Services
University of California, Davis, Medical Center
Sacramento, California

1989

W.B. SAUNDERS COMPANY
Harcourt Brace Jovanovich, Inc.
Philadelphia London Toronto Montreal Sydney Tokyo

W. B. SAUNDERS COMPANY
Harcourt Brace Jovanovich, Inc.

The Curtis Center
Independence Square West
Philadelphia, PA 19106

Library of Congress Cataloging-in-Publication Data

Kersten, Laurel D.

Comprehensive respiratory nursing.

Includes index.

1. Respiratory disease nursing. I. Title. [DNLM: 1. Decision Making—nurses' instruction. 2. Respiratory Tract Diseases—nursing. WY 163 K41c]

RC735.5.K47 1989 610.73′692 87–28387

ISBN 0–7216–5395–2

Editor: Michael Brown
Developmental Editor: David Prout
Designer: W. B. Saunders Staff
Production Manager: Bill Preston
Manuscript Editor: Mary Anne Folcher
Illustrator: Sharon Iwanczuk
Illustration Coordinator: Peg Shaw
Indexer: Julie Schwager
Cover: Capnogram tracing of a patient on mechanical ventilation.

Comprehensive Respiratory Nursing ISBN 0–7216–5395–2

Last digit is the print number: 9 8 7 6 5 4 3 2 1

FOR ANDREA VICTORIA,
My understanding daughter
Who gave me the "bright idea"
And lived with this project
From start to finish.

Preface

This book establishes a collaborative theory base for decision-making in respiratory nursing care of mainly the adult patient. It is intended for the nurse who wishes to refine respiratory decision-making skills.

Though the provision of a collaborative theory base is the book's main purpose, it was not the original one. The original purpose was to publish a textbook for graduate nursing students that emphasized a broad multidisciplinary knowledge framework, comprehensive respiratory assessment skills, and refined clinical decision-making skills. These criteria were formed based on several personal observations. In my role as a clinical specialist, I have always been astounded at how little the critical care nurse knows of chronic care, how little the rehabilitation nurse knows of acute care, and how much more optimal the level of respiratory care could be if both types of nurses had a common knowledge base in respiratory care. In my role as an educator, I have observed that many nurses tend to place an acceptable label on a respiratory problem, without going through the mental decision-making processes needed to formulate a specific respiratory diagnosis, which in turn naturally leads to correct intervention. From a research-oriented administrative perspective, I have observed that development of a valid and reliable taxonomy of respiratory diagnoses may help the development of an equitable system for placing a financial charge on respiratory care provided. When charge is based on nursing diagnosis in addition to medical diagnosis and patient acuity, the respiratory patient may lose the reputation as a "financial loser" in our present fixed-priced, health care delivery system.

Because of persisting incongruities between nursing theory and practice, the aforementioned described criteria for writing this book were met while simultaneously establishing a theory base for collaborative practice. The rationale for the theory base is further explained in the Introduction.

In retrospect, this conceptual and integrated approach to respiratory care has become as much if not more important than the content itself because of implications for other nursing subspecialties struggling with implementation of nursing diagnoses in the clinical setting. I believe that changing the way the nurse thinks about nursing care will promote excellence at the clinical level, provide a new and more fruitful set of questions at the research level, and narrow the gap between theory and practice.

Organization

The book is divided into six parts, based on the nursing process. The first three parts, *Structure and Function of the Respiratory System*, *Pulmonary Pathophysiology*, and *Basic Assessment Parameters*, establish a respiratory assessment theory base. Parts 4 and 5, *Basic Interventions* and *Specialized Interventions*, establish a respiratory intervention theory base. In these parts, an assessment approach to care is emphasized to facilitate data collection and interpretation during both the assessment and intervention steps of the nursing process.

Part 6, *Clinical Application*, shows the nurse how to use the respiratory theory base established in Parts 1 through 5 to make clinical decisions. Emphasis is on the *process* of decision-making for the patient with acute and chronic respiratory problems.

Each part has an introduction followed by a glossary of respiratory and decision-making terms. The glossary orients the reader to the terminology and content in each section and serves as a quick-reference guide in clinical and educational settings.

Each chapter begins with a general outline, followed by learning objectives to orient the reader to key concepts and to guide further study.

The text uses the terms *respiratory* and *pulmonary* in various explanations. For clarification, the term *pulmonary* refers to lung function, whereas the term *respiratory* refers to the lungs and other organs that directly or indirectly contribute to gas exchange.

To clarify other terms, *Appendix I* at the end of this book lists abbreviations for the many pulmonary terms and symbols used throughout this text and in the clinical setting. When it is used with the Index, the reader can locate information on the respiratory topics in the text.

LAUREL D. KERSTEN

Acknowledgments

This book took seven years to write. Because it evolved over many years and in association with numerous practice settings throughout California, it is difficult to remember and fully acknowledge all persons involved.

My greatest appreciation goes to my family and close friends. They provided continuous support as I juggled family responsibilities, clinical practice, and doctoral studies, while working nearly continuously on this manuscript.

The initial research for this book began in 1978 while teaching graduate students in the School of Nursing at the University of California, Los Angeles. At that time, I consolidated past experiences from a variety of acute, ambulatory, and home care settings and developed courses and seminars in respiratory nursing care. The lectures on respiratory assessment served as frameworks for the basic assessment parameters in this book. Stimulating discussions with students and faculty on the controversial topic of nursing diagnosis helped me to begin to develop a collaborative approach to respiratory decision-making.

I am in debt to my professors, particularly Wesley Bjur, Ph.D. in the School of Public Administration, University of Southern California, for guidance in the areas of theory building and heuristics. By temporarily stepping out of nursing and viewing the world from a different discipline, I was better able to understand the issues and controversies of nursing diagnosis in clinical decision-making. New insights relating to the development of a collaborative theory base provided direction for this book's conceptual framework as well as for later research on the subject.

Two clinicians faithfully read manuscript in extremely rough form during the first four years of the project: Constance Hyman, R.N., M.N. formerly from the American Association of Critical Care Nurses and Oscar Scherer, M.D., Director of Pulmonary Medicine at Herrick Hospital and Health Center, Berkeley, California, and Associate Clinical Professor of Medicine, University of California at San Francisco. Their constructive criticism, attention to clinical detail, and insistence on my taking a firmer stand on issues are largely responsible for the depth of discussions in this book.

Other health professionals who reviewed manuscript or facilitated research in some other way include the following:

Linda Anderson, R.N., M.N.
Respiratory Clinical Nurse Specialist
Redwood City, California

Shirley Bell, Ed.D.
Assistant Professor
College of Nursing
Arizona State University
Tempe, Arizona

Bonnie Burkhart, R.N.C., F.N.P.
Sharp HealthCare
San Diego, California

Erick Burkhart, R.C.P.T.
Sharp Memorial Hospital
San Diego, California

Stanley M. Cassan, M.D.
Pulmonologist
Associate Clinical Professor
UCLA School of Medicine
Los Angeles, California

Donna Carosella, R.N., B.S.
Clinical Nurse
Richmond, Virginia

Maria Chow, R.P.T.
Casa Colina Hospital for Rehabilitative Medicine
Pomona, California

Diane Czlonka, R.N., M.S.
Pulmonary Clinical Nurse Specialist
Sinai Hospital of Detroit
Detroit, Michigan

Linda Fahr, R.N., M.N.
Pulmonary Clinical Nurse Specialist
Visiting Nurse Association
Instructor
Oregon Health Sciences University School of Nursing
Portland, Oregon

Marita Florini, R.N., M.D., F.N.P.C.
Endwell, New York

Marsha D.M. Fowler, Ph.D., M.S.(N.), R.N.
Associate Professor
School of Nursing and Graduate School of Theology
Azusa Pacific University
Azusa, California

Linda Hasara, R.N., B.S.N.
Clinical Nurse
UCLA Hospital
Center for the Health Sciences
Los Angeles, California

Richard Hyman, M.D.
Cardiologist
Beverly Hills, California

Heino Kemnitz, C.P.T.
University of California, Davis, Medical Center
Sacramento, California

Ann Cohlan Keren-zvi, R.N., M.N.
Respiratory Clinical Nurse Specialist
Arleta, California

Susan Oshiro, R.N., M.N., C.C.R.N.
Clinical Nurse Specialist
Straub Clinic & Hospital
Honolulu, Hawaii

Joseph Perloff, M.D.
Professor of Medicine
Division of Cardiology
UCLA School of Medicine
Los Angeles, California

Valerie Sheba, R.N., B.S.N.
Clinical Nurse
UCLA Hospital
Center for the Health Sciences
Los Angeles, California

Debbie Thompson, R.N.
Clinical Nurse
UCLA Hospital
Center for the Health Sciences
Los Angeles, California

William Volz, R.N., R.R.T.
University of California, Davis, Medical Center
Sacramento, California

Irwin Ziment, M.D.
Professor and Chief
Department of Medicine
Olive View Medical Center
UCLA School of Medicine
Los Angeles, California

In 1984, I thought the book was completed. However, reviews from the publisher indicated a need to reorganize chapters, expand critical care content, and clarify my "unconventional" approach to care as well as the relevance of the collaborative theory base. Though originally considered a setback, the reviews were priceless. They precipitated further refinement of the manuscript and delayed publication to a time when nursing leaders, such as Lynda Carpenito, formally recognized the need to interface nursing diagnoses with collaborative problems. Clinicians and academicians are now ready to consider a different but complimentary approach to care. I am grateful to the following reviewers for their comments:

Pamela J. Becker, M.S.N., R.N.
Barnes Hospital
Pulmonary Clinical Nurse Specialist

Shirley K. Bell, B.S.N., M.S.N., Ed.D.
Assistant Professor
College of Nursing
The Ohio State University

Patricia Dettenmeier, R.N., M.S.N., C.C.R.N.
Pulmonary Specialist
St. Louis University Medical Center

Lauren D. Edwards, M.S., R.N.
Former Instructor
Department of Medical Nursing
Rush Presbyterian-St.Luke's Medical Center

Ellen Elpern, R.N., M.S.N.
Pulmonary Medicine
Rush Presbyterian-St.Luke's Medical Center

Phyllis Goodrich, R.N., M.S.N., C.S.
Educational Coordinator/Instructor
Critical Care Nursing Program/Units
Sequoia Hospital District

Nancy Holloway, R.N., M.S.N., C.C.R.N.

Gwendolyn J. McDonald, R.N., M.S.

Ann Neureuter, M.S.N., R.N.
Pulmonary Medicine Department
Berkshire Medical Center

Margaret Nield, R.N., M.S.
Doctoral Candidate
University of Illinois, Chicago

Anne G. Perry, R.N., M.S.N.
Associate Professor of Nursing
School of Nursing
St. Louis University Medical Center

Carolyn E. Sabo, Ed.D., R.N.

Catherine A. Spearing, B.S.N., M.S.N., C.S.
Hospital of the University of Maryland

Karen York, R.N.; M.S.N.

Health professionals with whom I worked kept me as close as possible to the cutting edge of respiratory care practices. In particular, I thank the nursing, medical, and respiratory therapy staffs from the following health agencies: Critical Care Division, UCLA Hospital; Lung Institute, City of Hope National Medical Center, Duarte, California; and the Hospital and Clinics of the University of California, Davis, Medical Center. In addition, I thank the California Research and Medical Education Fund of the American Lung Association for grants supporting my doctoral work. Studies in administrative theory and decision-making later influenced the final reorganization of the book and provided direction for future research.

Stephen Beebee, a free-lance artist, provided initial art services. Most of the photography was made possible by the medical illustration departments at UCLA, City of Hope National Medical Center, and UCDMC. In addition, countless respiratory products companies graciously supplied photographs included to enhance the nurse's understanding of advanced respiratory technology.

Finally, I thank the editors at W. B. Saunders Company, particulary Michael Brown, Nursing Editor, and Katherine Pitcoff, former Nursing Editor, for their understanding and support throughout this project. Though pressed with publication deadlines, they respected my seemingly overindulgent attention to detail and patiently waited for the end product, resisting the temptation to publish an incomplete work.

Contents

Part Two

Part Three

Introduction
The Theory Base for Collaborative Nursing Practice

Most nurses providing respiratory care are in collaborative practice with physicians and other health team members. In spite of ongoing collaboration in clinical practice and the American Nurses Association's code that includes collaboration (1985), a specific theory base for such practice has not been established. This book provides a theory base for collaborative practice that serves as a conceptual and practical framework for decision-making in respiratory nursing care.

A persistent complaint of practicing nurses who attempt to apply standard nursing diagnoses to clinical situations is that the broad and imprecise diagnostic categories are relatively useless. Nursing theorists have acknowledged this problem (see Kritek, 1986). Though they point out the uselessness for developing diagnostic labels in a conceptual vacuum and the need for developing collaborative diagnoses, progress in the area of collaborative diagnoses has been extremely slow. Current nursing diagnoses for decision-making processes remain conceptually designed for the nurse in independent practice, not the respiratory nurse who is almost always in collaborative practice with other health team members.

In light of this practice problem, this introduction also focuses on the decision-making theory and the process of decision-making. It clarifies the state of the art of nursing diagnosis and explains the need for more specific respiratory diagnoses and refined assessment skills in collaborative practice. Perhaps once theorists and clinicians better understand this need, nursing diagnosis and collaborative diagnosis will not be seen as incommensurable, as mistakenly assumed by some health care professionals. The reader can better appreciate how the collaborative approach in this book reflects reality in the clinical setting and complements rather than conflicts with existing nursing literature in respiratory care.

Collaborative Theory—What is It?

Collaborative theory is defined as those statements that account for or characterize the phenomenon of collaborative practice. The statements form a body of knowledge that is shared with other health team members caring for the patient. *Collaborative practice* is the joint determination of relationships among health team members whose sole purpose is to integrate their care practices into a comprehensive approach to meet patient and family needs (England, 1986).

In the conceptual representation in Figure 1, collaborative theory results from the blending of discipline-specific knowledge frameworks with decision-making theory. Nurses use nursing, medical, and other knowledge frameworks for interpreting clinical findings, making a respiratory diagnosis, and providing appropriate respiratory nursing care. The amount of theory extracted from the knowledge frameworks depends on each clinician's personal, institutional, professional, and legal scope of practice. Furthermore, all decisions are shaped by a set of shared assumptions that stress principles, values, and commitments about the way optimal respiratory care should be given. These assumptions are unstated and untestable and in nursing are sometimes referred to as propositions. Though they guide decision-making as part of a paradigm or world view, they are not formally recognized by health care professionals themselves (Newton-Smith, 1981).

Assumptions That Guide Collaborative Practice

The assumptions that guide collaborative practice are summarized as follows:

- The focus of decision-making is on health problems.
- Decision-making is shared among patient, family, and health team members.
- The goals of care are to reduce illness, optimize wellness, and provide comprehensive and continuing care.
- Collaboration among health team members increases the potential for healing the whole person and reduces the costs of care.
- The patient has a right to health care at a reasonable cost.

KNOWLEDGE FRAMEWORKS	DECISION-MAKING THEORY
• Medicine • Nursing • Pharmacy • Respiratory Therapy • Physical Therapy • Occupational Therapy • Social Services • Others	• Information Processing Theory

↓

COLLABORATIVE THEORY

↓

COLLABORATIVE PRACTICE

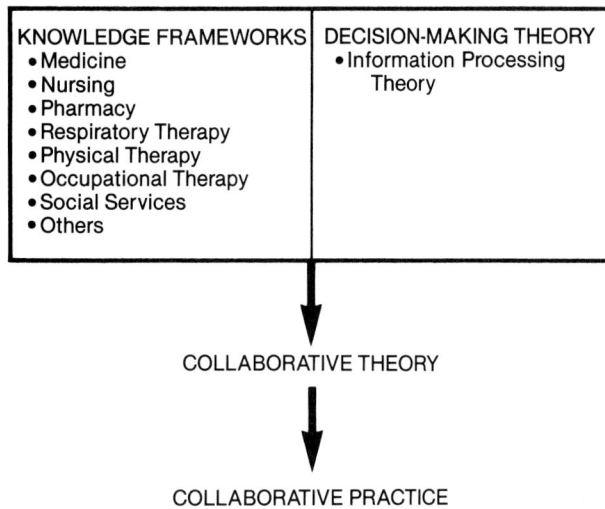

Figure 1. The making of collaborative theory—the blending of discipline-specific knowledge frameworks with decision-making theory. The nurse uses collaborative theory for collaborative practice with other health professionals.

HEALTH PROBLEMS—THE FOCUS OF DECISION-MAKING

In collaborative practice, the focus of decision-making is on health problems. Labels among different disciplines and settings may vary. However, comprehensive and continuing care cannot occur without at least the mental identification of specific respiratory problems.

The concept of health problems is not new to nursing, as evidenced by problem-oriented charting and nursing diagnosis literature. However, the concept has not been consistently applied to educational or clinical settings. For example, the traditional approach to teaching respiratory nursing care is to focus on a prototype disease, such as adult respiratory distress syndrome (ARDS) or chronic obstructive pulmonary disease (COPD). The educator teaches the pathophysiology, etiologic factors, and appropriate medical and nursing interventions that will either cure the disease or at least reduce signs and symptoms. Sometimes interventions are introduced by the educator under the topics of health problems or nursing diagnoses associated with medical diagnoses. However, emphasis is typically on the naming of appropriate interventions, rather than on the identification and assessment of health problems in individual patient situations.

This focus on diseases rather than on health problems impedes the development of respiratory nursing care because it reinforces the nurse's tendency to emphasize intervention at the expense of assessment during decision-making. In past years, nurses have defined their roles primarily in terms of interventions, treatments, or tasks, and only secondarily in terms of assessment, planning, and evaluation (Price, 1980). Aspinall (1976) has documented the low performance of nurses in diagnoses of respiratory problems and attributes this to their action orientation. When the nurse intuitively decides, for example, that the ventilator dependent patient needs suctioning, observation leads directly to action, without diagnosis of the specific problem. The crucial step of hypothesis testing that leads to correct diagnosis is entirely omitted. The result is that the patient receives treatment that is not necessarily indicated and may be detrimental to health.

SHARED DECISION-MAKING

Another assumption that guides the use of collaborative theory relates to shared decision-making and the interdependent nature of relationships among health team members.

In collaborative practice, decision-making is shared among patient, family, and health team members, as represented graphically in Figure 2. The nurse has a collegial rather than a subservient relationship to the physician. Similarly, the patient is an equal partner in the decision-making process.

Shared decision-making represents a major shift away from the traditional medical model. In the traditional model, the physician is at the top of the chain of command, exercising dictatorial authority over the nurse, ancillary personnel, and ultimately the patient at the bottom of the hierarchy.

Shared decision-making assumes interdependence among health care professionals in theory, practice, or both. For example, in spite of discipline-specific expertise and accountability and in spite of different roles in individual practice settings, a physician, nurse, and

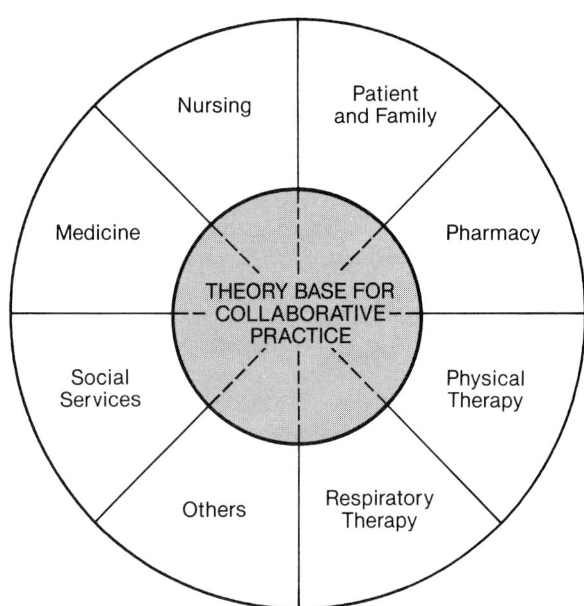

Figure 2. The relationship of nursing and other disciplines to the theory base for collaborative practice. In this conceptualization, health team members, patient and family are equal members in clinical decision-making. The nurse utilizes both nursing and collaborative theory.

respiratory therapist must all be able to diagnose a patient's oxygenation problem. The home health care nurse must know how to give respiratory therapy treatments because (1) home respiratory therapy services are not usually reimbursed by third-party payers and (2) the nurse is accountable for the assessment aspects of therapy, even when a respiratory therapist gives the treatment.

The changing nature of professional interdependence reflects the nature of the collaborative theory base represented in Figure 2. The lines between disciplines are dotted to represent the changing and as yet ill-defined nature of the collaborative theory base in clinical practice (Carnevali, 1983). This ambiguity explains the paucity of clear definitions for collaborative theory in the nursing literature. In addition, it explains why this text often uses the terms health problem and nursing diagnosis interchangeably whenever assessment and intervention fall within the nurse's area of accountability.

The solid lines between the disciplines in Figure 2 serve to preserve nursing, medicine, and other disciplines as separate entities with a unique perspective, body of knowledge, and skill for making decisions. Though respiratory nursing draws heavily from the collaborative theory base, the reader is reminded that some aspects, such as counseling on smoking cessation or avoidance of inhaled lung irritants, may fall within the scope of independent nursing practice and, hence, may not require shared decision-making.

From another perspective, however, whatever represents independent nursing practice may quickly become collaborative in nature. For example, when counseling on smoking cessation eventually focuses on the use of nicotine-containing chewing gum (Nicorette), a medically prescribed drug, the nurse must share decision-making with the physician to provide appropriate advice.

Moreover, though collaborative theory represents shared knowledge, it still remains within the realm of nursing. Its adaptation to the nursing milieu occurs as the nurse utilizes it within practice models (see England, 1986) and the broad scope of nursing practice (see Fawcett, 1983).

GOALS OF RESPIRATORY CARE

The goals of respiratory care are to reduce illness, optimize wellness, and provide comprehensive and continuing care. This assumption provides the rationale for the extensive and varied theory base required to deal with the complex and multiple problems of the respiratory patient. In addition, it accounts for the emphasis on acute, chronic, and preventive aspects of care.

Because of changes in our current health care delivery system relating to shorter hospital stays and to the provision of more intensive care at home, a knowledge of both acute and chronic care is essential. The critical care nurse must be prepared to address not only the patient's acute needs but also the patient's self-care needs within a limited period of time. When self-care needs are met, the patient is more likely to learn to cope adaptively to the limitations of respiratory disease before hospital discharge, in spite of inadequate financial coverage for home care follow-up.

Similarly, at the other end of the health care continuum, knowledge of both acute and chronic care prepares the home health nurse to practice both intensive and rehabilitative therapy. The need to practice intensive nursing care in the home will undoubtedly increase in the future, as respiratory patients are discharged earlier, in a more unstable condition and, sometimes, on long-term mechanical ventilation.

This book's emphasis on comprehensive respiratory skills hopefully will eliminate the current acute-chronic dichotomy that exists in the current literature and fragments the continuity of care among practice settings. When this dichotomy is eliminated, collaboration among nurses and other health care professionals is facilitated; the patient's transfer between settings goes more smoothly; and the patient's need for hospital readmission is greatly reduced.

COLLABORATION—A HOLISTIC AND COST-EFFECTIVE APPROACH

Collaboration among health team members increases the potential for healing the whole person and reduces the costs of care. Costs may relate to patient, family, health team members, or society.

The most obvious reduction is in the financial cost. A collaborative approach is more cost effective than nursing care without a collborative approach, because it facilitates the constant exchange of information about the health status of a patient and family as well as the constant decision-making, as the patient moves through the health care continuum. The ongoing nature of decision-making results in better decision-making and more appropriate interventions, which in turn result in decreased need for professional services and decreased cost to patient, family, and society.

Other reductions relate to the human suffering averted, because of more appropriate decision-making and less time and energy necessary for the encoding and decoding of messages among team members. The last benefit is associated with enhanced communication because all team members use standardized respiratory terminology when discussing patient situations.

Because of the confusion over the meaning of medical versus nursing terms, this text uses standard respiratory terminology for diagnostic labels. In addition to enhancing interdisciplinary communication, this approach encourages close working relationships among health care professionals who have the demanding and sometimes thankless task of providing respiratory care.

HEALTH CARE—A RIGHT OR PRIVILEGE?

The last assumption about collaborative practice is that the patient has a right to health care at a reasonable cost. This assumption holds true at the clinical practice level. However, due to increasing medical costs and budgetary restraints, controversy at institutional and governmental levels exists over whether health care is a privilege or a right.

Decision-Making Theory

Utilization of theory from discipline-specific knowledge frameworks requires decision-making theory. *Decision-making* refers to clinical judgments about the health status of a respiratory patient and the patient's family. *Decision-making theory* is defined as the statements about how the clinician recalls knowledge from memory and chooses between alternatives in individual patient situations. This theory is process-oriented and represents a separate body of knowledge, as shown in Figure 1. Before approaching the patient, the nurse must know how to collect and interpret data, how to rule in or rule out a health problem, and when and how to intervene appropriately. Without this knowledge, an inappropriate decision may result in inappropriate therapy, disease exacerbation, unnecessary patient suffering, and patient reluctance to reenter the health care delivery system for follow-up treatment.

In both the collaborative practice and the nursing discipline, decision-making theory is based on the information processing theory described by Newell and Simon (1972). Application of theory is in relation to the nursing process, the problem solving model advocated in nursing today.

The Nursing Process

Respiratory content in this book is presented in relation to the nursing process. The five components of the nursing process are *data collection, diagnosis (problem definition), planning of the intervention, implementation of the intervention*, and *evaluation of the intervention* (Bloch, 1974; American Nurses Association, 1973) (Figure 3).

Collectively, the term *assessment* refers to the first two components of the nursing process—data collection and diagnosis. The term *intervention* refers to the last three steps—its planning, implementation, and evaluation. These categories provide a framework for the delivery of respiratory care and, hence, the organization of this book. However, the boundaries between assessment and intervention are not clear, and the components of the nursing process are not always sequential in clinical practice. In fact, the respiratory nurse frequently alternates between assessment and intervention to monitor patient progress and diagnose new problems. This "switching back and forth" is reflected in how the content of this book is presented. Elements of intervention may appear in assessment chapters and vice versa.

The Definition of Nursing Diagnosis

Comprehensive respiratory care depends on the nurse's ability to identify health problems or nursing diagnoses. *Health problem* is a broad term, and Bloch (1974) defines it as a "deficit or potential deficit in the health status of an individual, family, or community that is believed to be in need of correction."

The definition of *nursing diagnosis* is not yet firmly established because of the controversy surrounding the domain of nursing practice. The following historical perspective of the development of the nursing diagnosis definition helps to explain persistent implementation problems in collaborative practice.

Experts have been working on the identification and validation of nursing diagnoses since 1950. In 1973, the North American Nursing Diagnosis Association (NANDA), an organization of nurses from the United States and Canada, was formed to identify, develop, and classify diagnostic concepts. To elucidate nursing diagnoses, this group used retrospective identification of health conditions encountered by nurses in clinical practice. An alphabetic classification of 30 diagnostic categories and 100 subcategories was delineated by the 150 nurse participants who attended the NANDA sponsored First National Conference for Classification Of Nursing Diagnoses. Nursing diagnoses were defined as "health problems or health states diagnosed by nurses and treated by nursing intervention" (Gebbie and Lavin, 1975).

The definition of nursing diagnosis has changed at least twice since 1973. Throughout the late 1970s, nurses referred to a nursing diagnosis as an "actual or potential health problem which nurses, by virtue of their education and experience, are capable and licensed to treat" (Gordon, 1976). This definition supported the belief that a clinical diagnosis is a nursing one only if the nurse performs *independent* nursing action to alleviate the problem. An independent action is one that does not require a physician's order. With this guideline, theoretically, a nurse may not diagnose hypoxemia (i.e., low oxygen tension in arterial blood), because he or she cannot legally prescribe oxygen, the appropriate therapy. Nevertheless, in clinical practice, nurses routinely monitor for the problem of hypoxemia, because the assessment component of the nursing process as opposed to the intervention component *is* an independent nursing action. Moreover, in some cases, failure to diagnose hypoxemia and intervene with oxygen may be grounds for a malpractice suit. In

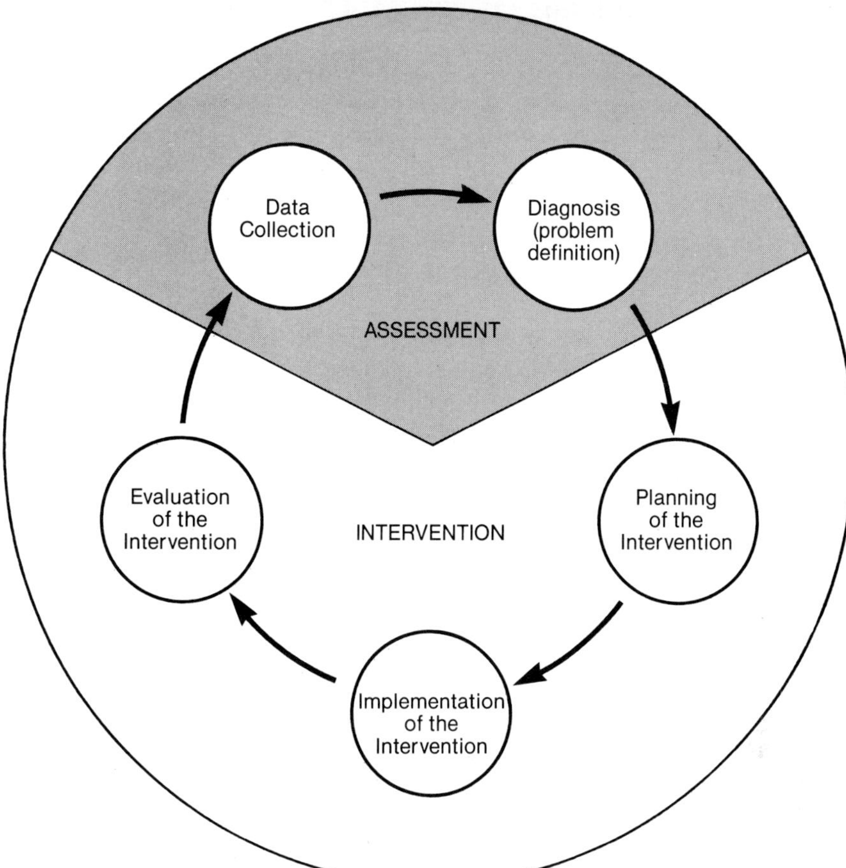

Figure 3. Components of the nursing process. Assessment is shaded for emphasis because it is the key to comprehensive respiratory care.

reality, the nurse is accountable for actions that are not classified as independent.

This focus on independent nursing action leads to a split of clinical diagnoses into biophysically medical diagnoses and psychosocially oriented nursing diagnoses, without regard for collaborative diagnoses shared by all health team members.

In 1984, the current nursing diagnosis definition was published in the Proceedings of the Fifth National Conference on the Classification of Nursing Diagnoses (Shoemaker, 1984). It reads as follows:

> ". . . a nursing diagnosis is a clinical judgment about an individual, family, or community that is derived through a deliberate, systematic process of data collection and analysis. It provides the basis for prescriptions for definitive therapy for which the nurse is accountable. It is expressed concisely and includes the etiology of the condition when known."

This definition has two important implications for respiratory nursing care. First, note that it emphasizes the delibrate, systematic process of data collection necessary to make a diagnosis. Deliberateness is key; for example, in an initial nursing assessment, the nurse must know what information to retrieve before assessing the respiratory patient. A strong theory base for respiratory assessment and intervention is mandatory before the nurse can apply the diagnostic reasoning process to identify and classify information gathered in the clinical setting, and this book provides such a theory base.

Second, note that the scope of nursing diagnosis has been broadened to the nurse's area of accountability. Though this approach theoretically provides for collaborative practice, controversy still exists about what is an acceptable nursing diagnosis, and experts have not formally addressed the area of collaborative diagnosis. This omission has caused implementation problems for many nurses caring for respiratory patients. Up to 90% of their time is devoted to collaborative practice, e.g., carrying out the physician's orders and following established respiratory protocols, while as little as 10% is devoted to independent nursing practice. While these nurses regularly make biophysical respiratory diagnoses in hospital, clinic, and home settings, they have no accepted framework for labelling them or writing them in the chart for documentation.

Current Nursing Diagnoses

A list of current nursing diagnostic categories is presented in Chapter 31. The health problems are described by concept labels, such as impairment of skin integrity or altered self-concept. Conceptual definitions are "as varied as the views of nursing itself,'" e.g., Dorothea Orem's self-care agency deficits, Dorothy Johnson's dysfunctional behavioral systems, and Marjorie Gordon's dysfunctional health patterns (Gordon, 1985). Variations in labelling reflect the lack of consensus regarding the conceptual domain of health conditions described by nursing diagnoses.

RESPIRATORY DIAGNOSES

Current respiratory diagnoses that apply to the adult are limited to a few broad categories as follows: *alteration in respiratory function* (Carpenito, 1984), *ineffective airway clearance, ineffective breathing pattern,* and *impaired gas exchange.* The last three NANDA diagnoses are summarized in Table 1. Though NANDA definitions are most frequently referred to, other definitions and adaptations exist in nursing literature (Gordon, 1985; Carpenito, 1984).

Keep in mind that respiratory and other types of diagnoses are not yet standardized in nursing; they are tentative. As broad prescientific abstractions, they have been approved by a consensual process rather than by a scientific authentication process. They have been developed deductively (i.e., from general to specific) in accordance with broad national classification guidelines.

Implementation Problems. The nature of current respiratory diagnoses has created implementation problems. Because their limited number makes differential diagnoses nearly impossible, nurses tend to overlook or incompletely assess key respiratory problems. Because of the broad scope of diagnoses, nurses evaluating the same patient may make different diagnoses. Subcategories with critical defining characteristics have not been developed to facilitate the type of decision-making required in respiratory care, as described in the next section.

In addition, the varied nursing language used to describe categories has caused considerable confusion over the meaning of respiratory diagnoses. As with other nursing diagnoses, respiratory diagnoses must be rephrased in common medical language to facilitate comprehension among other health team members. For example, physicians and respiratory therapists will

Table 1. RESPIRATORY NURSING DIAGNOSES ACCEPTED BY THE NORTH AMERICAN NURSING DIAGNOSIS ASSOCIATION (NANDA)*

Diagnosis	Definition	Defining Characteristics	Related Factors
Ineffective airway clearance	A state in which an individual is unable to clear secretions or obstructions from the respiratory tract to maintain airway patency.	Abnormal breath sounds Rales (crackles) Rhonchi (wheezes) Changes in rate or depth of respiration Tachypnea Cough, effective or ineffective, with or without sputum Cyanosis Dyspnea	Fatigue/decreased energy Tracheobronchial Infection Obstruction Secretion Perceptual/cognitive impairment Trauma
Ineffective breathing pattern	The state in which an individual's inhalation and/or exhalation pattern does not enable adequate pulmonary inflation or emptying.	Dyspnea Shortness of breath Tachypnea Fremitus Abnormal arterial blood gas values Cyanosis Cough Nasal flaring Respiratory depth changes Assumption of three-point position Pursed-lip breathing/prolonged expiratory phase Increased anteroposterior diameter Use of accessory muscles Altered chest excursion	Neuromuscular impairment Pain Musculoskeletal impairment Perception/cognitive impairment Anxiety Decreased energy/fatigue
Impaired gas exchange	The state in which the individual experiences a decreased passage of oxygen, and/or carbon dioxide between the alveoli of the lungs and the vascular system	Confusion Somnolence Restlessness Irritability Inability to move secretions Hypercapnea Hypoxia	Ventilation perfusion imbalance

*Data from McLane, A. (ed.). Classification of nursing diagnoses—Proceedings of the Seventh Conference, North American Nursing Diagnosis Association. St. Louis, C.V. Mosby Co., 1987.

not understand the exact meaning of the "ineffective airway clearance" diagnosis. The patient may have mucus in the airway, aspiration of a foreign object, bronchospasm, or some other respiratory problem requiring different treatment. The problem of encoding and decoding information among the disciplines remains relatively neglected, partially because of nursing's effort to firmly establish itself as a scientific discipline separate from medicine and allied sciences.

Though research is in progress to validate existing respiratory diagnoses and solve implementation problems, study results have been inconclusive (McDonald, 1985; York, 1985; Hurley, 1986). Also, the reliability and validity of findings are limited by convenience sampling, small sample size, limited clinical expertise of the subjects, and other research design problems.

In spite of design problems, research has provided valuable insight into how clinical nurses view nursing diagnosis. For example, in the study by York, nurses believed that etiologies and defining characteristics were identified by NANDA and must, therefore, all be appropriate. This tendency to support "acceptable" diagnoses, even though they have been validated by consensual rather than by scientific processes, has become a major barrier to innovative theory development on the topic.

Respiratory Decision-Making. In addition to implementation problems described previously, another reason for the limited applicability of respiratory diagnoses pertains to the complex and difficult nature of respiratory decision-making itself.

Respiratory diagnosis is difficult for many nurses because pulmonary patients tend to have mixed chest pathology and multiple problems of biophysical and psychosocial causation. Assessment requires a relatively high level of abstraction because of the large collection of data that must be considered before making a decision. Moreover, biophysical, psychosocial, and sociocultural problems are so intermeshed that one cannot assess one problem without considering related problems at the same time. Hence, to maintain a holistic approach to care, the nurse initiates the diagnostic process at the beginning of data collection and continues the diagnostic process throughout the entire nursing process, until the patient no longer needs respiratory care.

Incremental and Categorical Decisions. Another important reason why respiratory diagnosis is difficult pertains to the type of decision-making in respiratory care. Decision-making tends to be incremental rather than categorical. An *incremental decision* is variable or reversible. It depends on data assessed at the moment and is usually associated with a series of mental decision-making processes that eventually leads to correct diagnosis and intervention. The decision is a complex one, requiring intuition and a substantial knowledge base. Moreover, it creates a greater memory load than the systematic nature of general to specific approaches to decision-making.

In contrast, a *categorical decision* is made based on the presence of a few defining criteria, regardless of other data. It is a relatively simple decision because the nurse systematically applies one or two decision rules (Sowell, 1980).

To understand the difference between an incremental and a categorical decision, consider a nurse reviewing recent laboratory blood gas results in the absence of a physician. The results from two patients appear to be abnormal. In the first case, the patient's oxygen tension of arterial blood ($Pa{O_2}$) is 40 mmHg. Immediately, the nurse diagnoses hypoxemia and applies oxygen, without gathering more data. The decision to label the problem as hypoxemia was categorical because the nurse knows that a $Pa{O_2}$ below 60 mm Hg defines hypoxemia (in her institution). Similarly, the decision to apply oxygen immediately was also categorical, because the nurse knows that a patient with a greatly reduced $Pa{O_2}$ will always require at least some oxygen, regardless of other clinical signs and symptoms.

In the second case, the patient's $Pa{O_2}$ is 55 mmHg. Again, the nurse diagnoses hypoxemia because the $Pa{O_2}$ is below 60 mmHg (i.e., categorical decision). However, she is unable to decide whether oxygen is indicated, without quickly gathering more data, such as the patient's normal resting $Pa{O_2}$, age, medical diagnosis, mental status, and chest assessment findings. If she decides that oxygen is needed, the question then arises as to how much to give. In chronic obstructive pulmonary disease (COPD), too much oxygen may cause physical decompensation. If other signs of hypoxemia develop, the nurse may (1) add oxygen in small amounts, (2) continue to try to reach the physician, and (3) observe carefully the response to therapy. In this situation, decisions relating to intervention are incremental because the nurse never knows with certainty whether the patient's condition will improve with a given amount of oxygen. A series of decisions and actions is required. Most important, these decisions are considered part of a theory based contingency plan as opposed to a final prescription.

Moreover, in this last situation, as interventions are carried out, final outcome is crucial. Interventions are labelled appropriate, if the patient's condition improves. If, however, the patient's condition deteriorates, and the nurse misdiagnoses the problem and fails to give required oxygen, she may be sued for negligence or malpractice. Hence, even though incremental diagnoses require a high level of abstraction, the professional nurse is legally required to assess and intervene appropriately.

New Directions For Respiratory Nursing Care

The mastery of incremental decision-making depends on the development of refined respiratory assessment skills. This book's emphasis on assessment provides a new direction for respiratory nursing care.

Assessment—The Key to Comprehensive Care. Assessment is emphasized in this book for several reasons. First, assessment is the most crucial component of the nursing process. Though it is represented by a specific area in Figure 2, assessment is not static. It is not restricted to a specific time period or event, but assessment occurs throughout the nursing process, as demonstrated in the clinical application part of this book.

Second, most nurses lack the diagnostic skills needed to make data-based nursing decisions.

As discussed further in Chapter 31, acute care nurses often receive low scores in carrying out procedures, such as tracheal suctioning, because they fail to learn or retain the concepts and principles underlying complex procedures (Grossback-Landis and McLane, 1979). Similarly, at the other end of the health care continuum, community health nurses have more difficulty with diagnosis and evaluation than any other component of the nursing process. They can more easily treat a problem, but have difficulty labelling it (Dalton, 1979). Diagnosis is clearly the weakest link in the nursing process.

Third, assessment skills prepare the nurse to advance from the novice to expert stages of professional development. It is the expert who has the ability to zero in on an accurate region of a problem, without the wasteful consideration of a large range of alternative diagnoses and solutions (Benner, 1984). The expert nurse also can process the constant flow of patient data that may overwhelm the novice nurse in clinical practice.

Last, assessment is emphasized because it promotes a comprehensive approach to care, a characteristic feature of the collaborative theory base described earlier in this introduction.

Once nurses and other professionals develop expert assessment skills, perhaps then will the pulmonary patient and individual at risk to develop pulmonary disease have better chances of receiving comprehensive and continuing health care.

Theory Development—The Key to Solving Respiratory Diagnosis Implementation Problems. Problems in the implementation of respiratory nursing diagnosis point out a need for theorists, researchers, and clinicians to return to the following first step in theory development: the period of specifying, defining, and classifying concepts in described phenomena (Jacox, 1974). This step in respiratory nursing remains incompletely developed.

In response to this need for theory building, this text examines what nurses think and do to deliver comprehensive and continuing respiratory care. In the process, it provides a theory base for specific and clinically relevant diagnostic subcategories, such as hypoxemia. This descriptive approach is intended to encourage experts to proceed inductively (from specific to general) in the development of nursing diagnoses. Only then will clinicians successfully complement the deductive approach of theorists who are establishing the frameworks for assessment and intervention in nursing practice.

REFERENCES

American Nurses Association. Code for Nurses with Interpretive Statements. Kansas City, American Nurses Association, 1985.

American Nurses Association. Standards of Nursing Practice. Kansas City, American Nurses Association, 1973.

Aspinall, M. Nursing diagnosis—the weak link. *Nursing outlook,* 24(7):433–437, 1976.

Benner, P. From Novice to Expert—Excellence and Power in Clinical Nursing Practice. Menlo Park, California, Addison-Wesley Publishing Co., 1984.

Bloch, D. Some crucial terms in nursing—what do they really mean? *Nursing outlook,* 22(11):689–694, 1974.

Bruce, J. and Snyder, M. The right and responsibility to diagnose. *American journal of nursing* 82(4):645–646, 1982.

Burchell, R., Thomas, D., and Smith, H. Some considerations for implementing collaborative practice. *American journal of medicine,* 74(1):9–13, 1983.

Carnevali, D. Nursing Care Planning: Diagnosis and Management. Philadelphia, J. B. Lippincott Co., 1983.

Carpenito, L. Handbook of Nursing Diagnosis. Philadelphia, J. B. Lippincott Co., 1984.

Dalton, J. Nursing diagnosis in a community health setting. *Nursing clinics of north america,* 14(3):525–531, 1979.

England, D. Collaboration in Nursing. Rockville, Maryland, Aspen Systems Corp., 1986.

Fawcett, J. Hallmarks of Success in Nursing Theory Development. In Advances in Nursing Theory Development (Chinn, P.- ed.). Rockville, Maryland, Aspen Systems Corp., 1983.

Gebbie, K. and Lavin M. (eds.). Classification of Nursing Diagnoses—Proceedings of the First National Conference. St. Louis, C.V. Mosby Co., 1975.

Gordon, M. Nursing Diagnosis. Annual Review of Nursing Research, vol. 3. (Werley, H. and Fitzpatrick, J.- eds.). New York, Springer Publishing Co., 1985.

Gordon, M. Nursing Diagnosis—Process and Application. New York, McGraw-Hill Book Co., 1982.

Gordon, M. Nursing diagnoses and the diagnostic process. *American journal of nursing,* 76(8):1298–1300, 1976.

Grossbach-Landis, E. and McLane, A. Tracheal suctioning: a tool for evaluation and learning needs assessment. *Nursing research,* 28(4):237–242, 1979.

Hurley, M. (ed.). Classification of Nursing Diagnoses—Proceedings of the Sixth Conference, North American Nursing Diagnosis Association. St. Louis, C.V. Mosby Co., 1986.

Jacox, A. Theory construction in nursing. *Nursing research,* 23(1):4–13, 1974.

Johnson, D. State of the Art of Theory Development in Nursing. Theory Development: what, why, how? (no. 15-1708). New York, National League for Nursing, 1978.

Kersten, L. Heuristics for decision-making in respiratory nursing care—are we ready for it? (Unpublished paper.) School of Public Administration, University of Southern California, 1986.

Kritek, P. Diagnostics: the struggle to classify our diagnoses. *American journal of nursing,* 86(6):722–723, 1986.

McDonald, B. Validation of three respiratory nursing diagnoses. *Nursing clinics of north america,* 20(4):697–710, 1985.

Newell, A. and Simon, H. Human Problem Solving. Englewood Cliffs, New Jersey, Prentice Hall, 1972.

Newton-Smith, W. The Rationality of Science. Boston, Routledge & Kegan Paul, Inc. 1981.

Price, M. Nursing diagnosis: making a concept come alive. *American journal of nursing,* 80(4):668–671, 1980.

Shoemaker, J. Essential Features of a Nursing Diagnosis. In Classification of Nursing Diagnoses—Proceedings of the Fifth National Conference. (Kim, M., McFarland, G., and McLane, A.-eds.). St. Louis, C.V. Mosby Co., 1984.

Sowell, T. Knowledge and Decisions. New York, Basic Books, Inc., 1980.

York, K. Clinical validation of two respiratory nursing diagnoses and their defining characteristics. *Nursing clinics of north america,* 20(4):657–667, 1985.

STRUCTURE AND FUNCTION OF THE RESPIRATORY SYSTEM

Part One

The theory base for decision-making in respiratory nursing care begins with the structure and function of the respiratory system described in Chapters 1 to 6. This base serves as a description of patient wellness, the goal of respiratory care.

A brief *overview of the respiratory system* is given in Chapter 1. Specific structures are described in Chapter 2, beginning at the airway in the *upper respiratory tract* and ending at the microscopic level of the alveolar-capillary membrane in the *lower respiratory tract.*

The main function of gas exchange occurs at the alveolar-capillary membrane by a process called *diffusion.* Basic principles of *gas diffusion and oxygenation* are presented in Chapter 3.

Once gases are exchanged at the alveolar-capillary membrane, oxygenated blood continues through the *pulmonary circulation* (Chapter 4) to the left side of the heart and finally to the peripheral tissues of the body.

Though gas exchange depends upon properly functioning transport systems for both air (gas) and blood, perhaps the most crucial variable is the proper matching of ventilation to perfusion (blood flow) within the lungs. Chapter 5 introduces *lung ventilation and ventilation/perfusion (V/Q) ratios.*

Chapter 6 discusses how the respiratory system moves the lungs and chest wall during breathing (*mechanics of breathing*), and how it regulates gas exchange to achieve dynamic equilibrium (*control of breathing*).

The content in these chapters in written in considerable detail. The reason for the detail is two-fold. First, it forms an essential theory base for clinical applications, particularly in those chapters presenting pathophysiology and assessment parameters as well as for clinical applications in each nurse's practice setting. (The chapters are relatively short to facilitate quick reference.)

Second, detail is necessary to understand how the respiratory system's architectural design and adaptive capacities allow it to adapt effectively and efficiently to actual or potential respiratory problems. For example, if the mucociliary transport system fails to clear inhaled dust, defense cells called macrophages are readily available to engulf particles that reach distal areas of the lower respiratory tract (see Chapter 2). If a mucus plug obstructs a large airway, distal collateral air channels manage to prevent complete lung collapse. Most important, if a patient's lung ventilation does not maintain normal gas exchange, $PaCO_2$ rises and PaO_2 falls, which in turn triggers special receptors (chemoreceptors) in the body. The result is hyperventilation to maintain normal gas exchange. These are only some of the adaptive responses or feedback mechanisms that are discused in Part One. Clearly, the normal adult respiratory system is well equipped to deal with the strenuous requirements of the activities of daily living.

Commonly used terms to describe pulmonary pathophysiology and related respiratory problems are listed in the following glossary.

Glossary of Commonly Used Terms in Structure and Function of the Respiratory System

accessory muscles of breathing—muscles used during active breathing, e.g., sternocleidomastoid, scalene, internal intercostal, and abdominal.

acinus (acinar unit)—basic unit of the lung consisting of all structures distal to the terminal bronchiole.

airway resistance—pressure difference or driving pressure between the alveoli and the mouth necessary to produce a unit of flow. Airway resistance is the major component of total resistance to breathing in the respiratory system.

alveolar-capillary membrane—membrane between alveoli and pulmonary capillaries consisting of two parts, as follows: (1) a "thin side" called the *air-blood barrier,* where most gas exchange occurs and (2) a "thick side" with its alveolar interstitial space.

alveolar hyperventilation—increase in lung ventilation causing a decrease in Pa_{CO_2}.
alveolar hypoventilation—decrease in lung ventilation causing an increase in Pa_{CO_2}.
alveolus—the smallest and most distal structure in the terminal respiratory unit where gas exchange takes place in the lung.
anatomic shunt (normal)—unoxygenated venous blood from the bronchial circulation that mixes with arterialized blood within the pulmonary veins.
apex of the lung—top portion of the upper lobe.
base of the lung—bottom portion of the lung that rests on the diaphragm.
bony thorax—chest cage consisting of 12 pairs of ribs and their cartilages, 12 thoracic vertebrae and intervertebral discs, and the sternum.
bronchial circulation—circulatory system that provides nutrient blood to conducting airways, terminal respiratory units, and surrounding structures.
bronchiole—small airway in conductive zone of the lung.
bronchopulmonary segment—subunit of a lung lobe.
bronchus—large airway, e.g., right or left main stem bronchus, secondary bronchus.
CaO_2—total oxygen content in arterial blood.
carina—site where the trachea divides into right and left main stem bronchi.
chemoreceptors—receptors that respond to changes in chemical composition of surrounding body fluid and send appropriate feedback to medullary centers to alter respiration.
cilia—hair-like projections on the tracheobronchial surface lining.
collateral channels—pores or openings between alveoli (Kohn's pores) or between alveoli and airways (Lambert's canals) that help keep the lung expanded.
compliance—distensibility of the lungs, chest wall, or both. Lung compliance is increased in emphysema and decreased in interstitial fibrosis.
conducting airways—tracheobronchial tree.
control of breathing—neural, mechanical, and chemical activation and regulation of breathing.
costophrenic sulci (costodiaphragmatic recesses)—pleural space where costal and diaphragmatic parietal pleural are in direct contact with each other. Size varies with depth of respiration.
diffusion (gas)—gas movement by random molecular motion in response to a pressure gradient.
fissure—division between lung lobes.
fractional concentration (gas)—percent concentration of a gas divided by 100. In decimal form, e.g., 40% O_2 concentration = FIO_2 0.40.
frequency (f)—respiratory rate per minute.
hilum—clinically defined as the root of the lung at the level of T_4 or T_5.
hypoxemia—insufficient amount of oxygen in arterial blood, i.e., less than 80 mmHg for a normal adult.
hypoxia—insufficient amount of oxygen in body tissues.
humidification—saturation of dry air with water vapor (PH_2O = 47 mmHg).
interstitial space—connective tissue located in the "thick side" of the alveolar-capillary membrane (alveolar interstitial space). Peribronchial and perivascular interstitial spaces are potential spaces that may drain excess fluid from the alveolar interstitial space.
interstitium—connective tissue or "skeleton of the lungs." This tissue forms interstitial spaces and provides mechanical support for airways, alveoli, and capillaries.
laminar airflow—pattern of airflow with a parabolic velocity profile and low resistance.
larynx—commonly called the "voice box." Connects the pharynx with the trachea and consists of nine cartilages united by muscles and ligaments.
lobes—major portions of lung separated by fissures.
lower respiratory tract—the trachea, bronchi, bronchioles, and terminal respiratory units with alveoli.
macrophage—phagocytic cell on the alveolar surface that digests foreign particles or carries them to the mucociliary escalator for transport towards the mouth.
mast cell—mucosal or submucosal cell in the conductive zone involved in allergic reactions.
mechanical receptors—receptors in the lungs, airways, and chest wall. Receptor stimulation triggers reflexes between brain and receptor organ to change depth and rate of respiration.
mechanics of breathing—how the lung is supported, inflated, and deflated.
mediastinum—partition between the lungs that houses the heart, aorta, thymus, vagus and phrenic nerves, esophagus, trachea, and numerous other vessels.
minute ventilation (minute volume of ventilation) (V_E)—total amount of exhaled gas per minute, i.e., tidal volume (V_T) multiplied by respiratory rate (f).
mucociliary escalator—mucus and cilia along conducting airways. The rapidly beating cilia propel mucus and foreign particles towards the mouth, thus protecting the respiratory system from foreign particles and infection.
oxyhemoglobin dissociation curve—S-shaped curve that describes the equilibrium relationship between the partial pressure of oxygen in plasma and the saturation of hemoglobin with oxygen.
Pa_{CO_2}—partial pressure of carbon dioxide in arterial blood.
Pa_{O_2}—partial pressure of oxygen in arterial blood.
parenchyma—lung tissue that consists primarily of alveoli.
partial pressure (tension)—pressure that a gas exerts alone or mixed with other gases. Expressed in mmHg or torr.
perfusion—blood flow.
pharynx—musculomembranous tube extending from the nose (nasopharynx) to the mouth (oropharynx) and larynx (laryngopharynx).

pleura—lining of the lung consisting of two thin contiguous layers: (1) inside *visceral* pleura and (2) outside *parietal* pleura.
pleural pressure—pressure in the pleural space.
pleural space—potential space between visceral and parietal pleurae.
phrenic nerve—nerve originating in the cervical plexus and innervating right or left hemidiaphragm.
pneumotaxic center—respiratory center in the pons of the brain that stimulates inspiration.
pulmonary circulation—circulation of blood through the lungs.
pulmonary vascular resistance—resistance to blood flow through the pulmonary system. Alterations occur in response to drug therapy (e.g., vasoconstrictor and vasodilator agents) or to changes in $Pa{O_2}$, $Pa{CO_2}$, blood volume, blood viscosity, and other parameters.
respiration—exchange of oxygen for carbon dioxide at the alveolar level in the lungs (external respiration) or at the tissue or cellular level (internal respiration).
respiratory exchange ratio (R)—ratio of carbon dioxide produced to oxygen consumed per minute. R equals RQ in equilibrium states.
respiratory quotient (RQ)—molar ratio of CO_2 production to O_2 consumption. Normal RQ is about 0.80 at rest.
$Sa{O_2}$—saturation of arterial blood with oxygen.
sternal angle (angle of Louis)—junction of the manubrium with the body of the sternum.
sternum—breastbone consisting of three parts: (1) manubrium, (2) body, and (3) xiphoid process.
suprasternal notch—concavity superior to the manubrium.
surfactant—a phospholipid substance that lowers alveolar surface tension and helps prevent alveolar collapse.
terminal respiratory unit—acinus or acinar unit.
tidal volume (V_T)—volume of gas inhaled or exhaled during normal quiet breathing.
turbulent airflow—pattern of airflow with disorganized streamlines and high resistance.
Type I cell (squamous pneumocyte)—flat squamous cell that lines 95% of the alveolar surface.
Type II cell (granular pneumocyte)—alveolar cell believed to be the chief producer of surfactant.
upper respiratory tract—nasal cavity, pharynx, larynx, and other structures superior to vocal cords.
V_D/V_T—ratio of dead space to tidal volume, normally equals 0.33.
ventilation—movement of gas volumes in and out of the lungs.
V/Q—ventilation/perfusion ratio: a major determinant of oxygenation in the body.

Overview of the Respiratory System

1

Main Objectives

1. Locate the upper and lower respiratory tracts on an unlabelled diagram of the respiratory system.
2. Define and state the function of the alveolus.
3. Describe the structure of the lungs, with attention to
   a. location of the lobes
   b. minor and major fissures
   c. visceral and parietal pleura
   d. hilum
   e. right and left hemidiaphragms
4. Describe diaphragmatic movement and alterations in pleural recesses during respiration.
5. Define and describe the general structure, contents, and anatomical boundaries of the mediastinum.
6. Locate the following structures of the bony thorax on an unlabelled diagram:
   a. suprasternal notch
   b. manubrium
   c. body of the sternum
   d. xiphoid process
   e. sternal angle
   f. costal angle
   g. true ribs
   h. false ribs
   i. second intercostal space
   j. spinous process of T_4
7. Describe the passage of venous and arterial blood through pulmonary and systemic circulatory systems.
8. Name at least four functions of the respiratory system.
9. Name and discuss the chief function of the respiratory system. Explain the difference between external respiration and internal respiration as well as the interrelationship of the respiratory exchange ratio (R) with the respiratory quotient (RQ).
10. Explain the clinical relevance of at least one nonrespiratory function.

This chapter provides an overview of the structure and function of the respiratory system. The first part introduces basic structures, emphasizing the gross anatomy necessary to understand the upper and lower respiratory tracts (see Chapter 2), the mechanics of breathing (see Chapter 6), the pulmonary circulation (see Chapter 4), and the anatomic landmarks used in physical assessment and chest roentgenology (see Chapters 12 and 15). Respiration, the chief function of the respiratory system, as well as other functions that facilitate the maintenance of body equilibrium, is included at the end of this chapter.

Basic Structure

UPPER AND LOWER RESPIRATORY TRACTS

The respiratory system is divided into two parts, as follows: (1) the *upper respiratory tract* and (2) the *lower respiratory tract* (Fig. 1–1). The upper respiratory tract conducts gas to and from the lungs, which are located in the lower respiratory tract.

The lower respiratory tract conducts gas to and from the upper airway and the numerous alveoli in the lungs. The *alveolus* or *air sac* is the most distal structure in the lower respiratory tract (Fig. 1–2). This air sac is the site of respiration or gas exchange between its air space and adjacent pulmonary capillaries.

LUNGS WITHIN THE CHEST CAGE

The lung is the chief organ of respiration. It is a paired organ that acts as a unit within the chest cage or *bony thorax*.

The lungs consist of two cone-shaped masses of spongy tissue, pinkish in color at birth and grayish with a mottled pattern at adulthood (Fig. 1–3). The grayish color is from years of inhaling dust and soot present in the atmosphere.

The right lung is thicker and wider than the left lung. Also, it is slightly shorter than the left because the diaphragm is higher on the right side to accommodate the liver which is housed below it. The left lung is thinner and longer than the right lung. It is narrower because the heart extends into the left thorax and takes up space.

The rounded top portion of the lung is referred to as the *apex*. (There are two *apices*.) The broad concave inferior portion of the lung resting on the convex surface of the diaphragm is the *base* of the lung. The *costal surface* of the lung lies against the rib cage and follows the ribs all the way around the chest to the spinal column. The *mediastinal (medial) surface* faces inwards and exhibits a deep concavity to accommodate

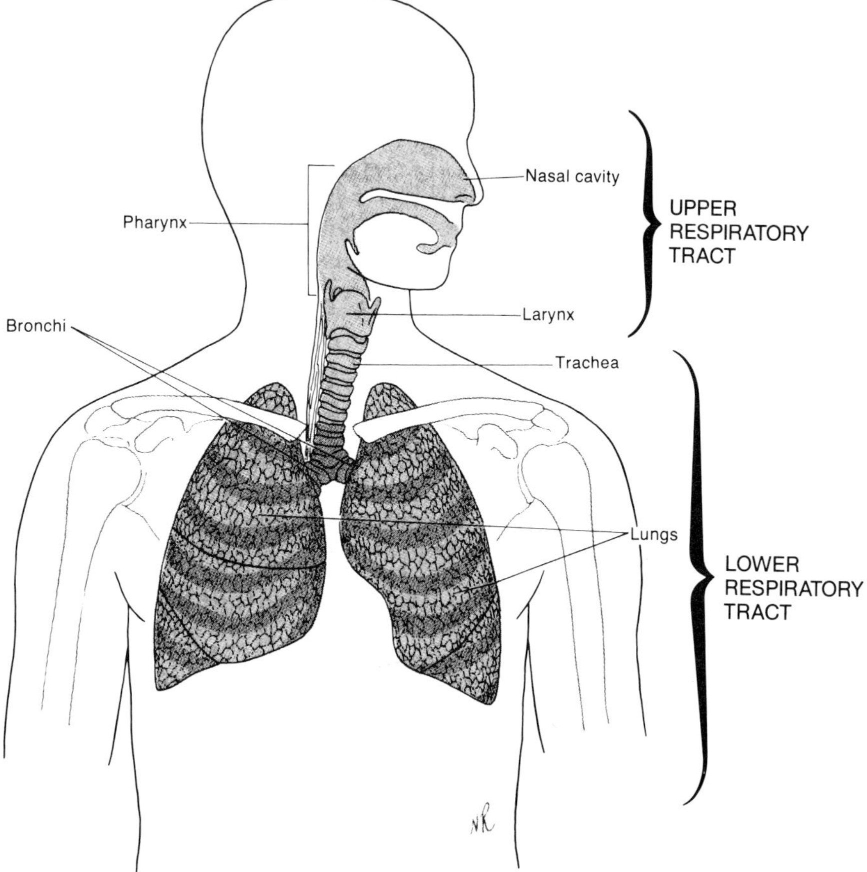

Figure 1–1. Main components of the upper and lower respiratory tracts. The former includes the nasal cavity, pharynx, and larynx; the latter includes the trachea, bronchi, and lungs. (Reproduced by permission from Tortora, G.: Principles of Human Anatomy, 3rd ed. New York, Harper & Row Publishers Inc., 1983.)

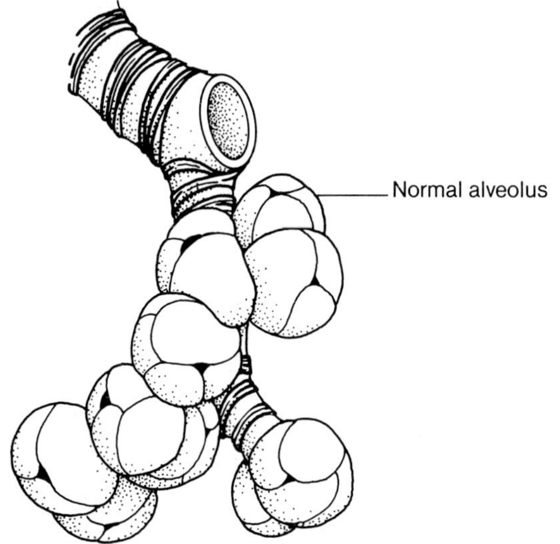

Figure 1–2. Alveoli or air sacs at the end of the conducting airways in the lower respiratory tract. (Reproduced and adapted by permission from Eli Lilly and Company, Indianapolis, Indiana, 1984.)

the heart. The notch or impression for the heart is called the *cardiac notch.*

Note in the anterior view of Figure 1–3 that the right lung is divided into three lobes—right *upper, middle,* and *lower.* The left lung is divided into two lobes—left *upper* and *lower.*

Fissures

Fissures are potential spaces that divide the lobes of the lungs. The *minor fissure,* also called the *horizontal fissure,* separates the right middle lobe from the right upper lobe (Fig. 1–4A). The fissure lies at about the level of the fourth rib. The left lung does not have a minor fissure because it has no middle lobe.

Each lung has a *major fissure,* also called an *oblique fissure.* It extends from about T3 or T4 (third or fourth thoracic vertebra) into the posterior chest downward and forward to about the level of the sixth rib in the anterior chest (Fig. 1–4B). In the right lung, the major fissure separates the upper and middle lobes from the

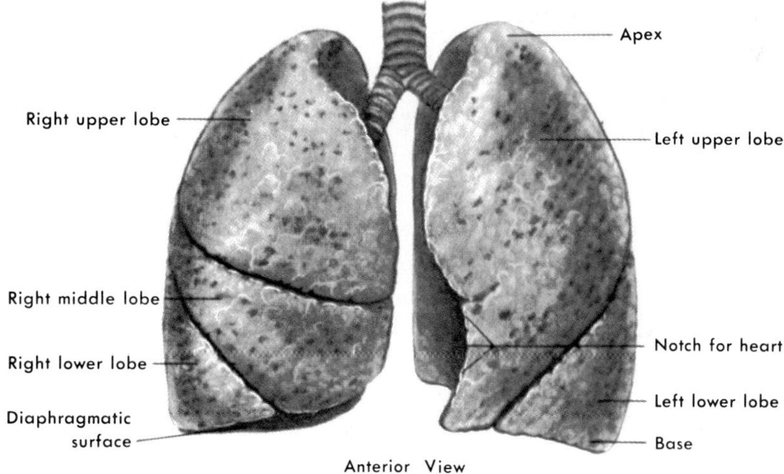

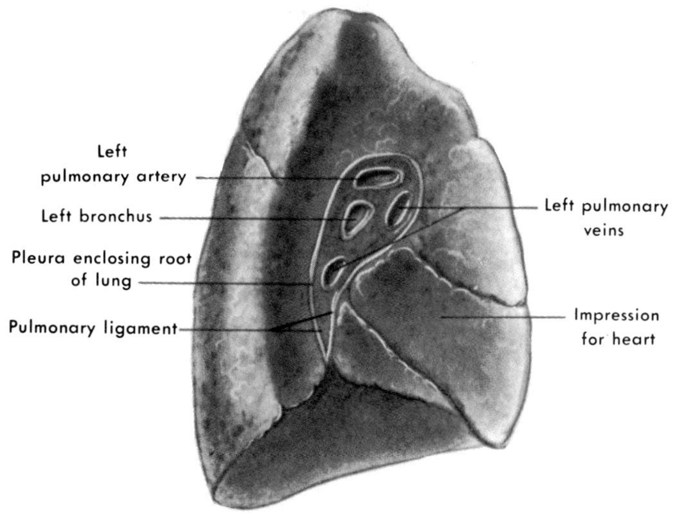

Figure 1–3. Anterior view and medial surface of the lungs. (Reproduced by permission from Dienhart, C.: Basic Human Anatomy and Physiology, 3rd ed. Philadelphia, W.B. Saunders Co., 1979.)

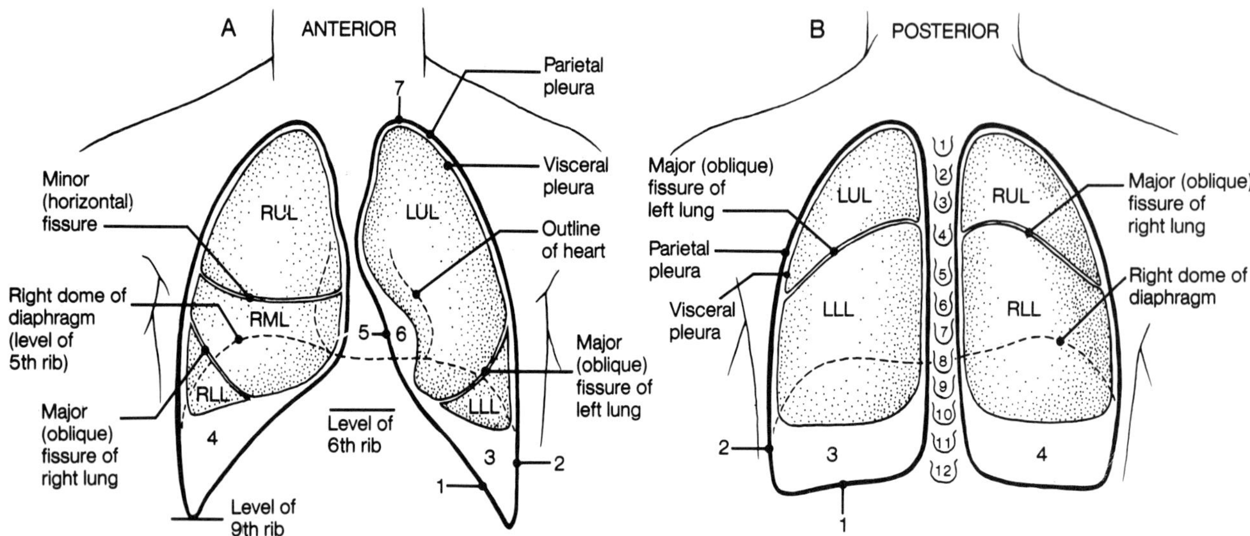

Figure 1–4. Pleurae and fissures of the lungs:
A, Anterior view
1. Diaphragmatic (parietal) pleura
2. Costal (parietal) pleura
3. *Left* costodiaphragmatic recess (costophrenic sulcus)
4. *Right* costodiaphragmatic recess (costophrenic sulcus)
5. Mediastinal pleura
6. Costomediastinal recess
7. Dome or cupola of the pleura (cervical pleura)

B, Posterior view
1. Diaphragmatic (parietal) pleura
2. Costal (parietal) pleura
3. Left costodiaphragmatic recess (costophrenic sulcus)
4. Right costodiaphragmatic recess (costophrenic sulcus)

(RUL = right upper lobe; RML = right median lobe; RLL = right lower lobe; LUL = left upper lobe; LLL = left lower lobe.)

posteriorly located lower lobe. In the left lung, this fissure separates the upper lobe from the lower lobe.

PLEURA

Each lung is lined with two thin layers of serous membrane, collectively called the *pleura*. The inner layer, the *visceral pleura*, is a smooth glistening membrane that covers the surfaces of each lung as well as the fissures between lobes. It is inseparably connected to the lung.

The outer layer, the *parietal pleura*, is labelled according to the region it touches or covers. The portion that lies against the ribs and chest wall is called the *costal pleura*. The *diaphragmatic pleura* covers most of the diaphragm, whereas the *mediastinal pleura* is reflected over mediastinal structures occupying the middle of the thorax. The *cervical pleura* extends into the neck to about 1 to 1.5 in (2.5 to 4 cm) above the medial third of the clavicle, where it forms the *dome* or *cupola of the pleura* over the lung apex.

Together the visceral and parietal pleurae have a smooth and polished appearance. Their approximating surfaces are moistened by minimal amounts (10 to 20 ml) of serous fluid that allow them to slide against each other with minimal friction, remaining in constant contact with each other during all phases of respiration.

The potential space between visceral and parietal layers is termed the *pleural cavity* or *pleural space*. It is exaggerated in Figure 1–5 to show its location. Normally, it is not apparent unless the lung collapses or unless air or fluid collects between the visceral and parietal layers.

At the *root of the lung*, the mediastinal parietal pleura becomes continuous with the visceral pleura (Fig. 1–6). Hence, the pleura is actually one continuous sheet, with both inside and outside layers. This arrangement has been likened to pushing a fist into an inflated balloon (Fig. 1–7). The inner wall of the balloon (next to the fist) and the outer wall are continuous at the wrist, just as the visceral and parietal layers are continuous at the root of the lung. The space between the balloon's inner and outer layers is analogous to the pleural space with air in it, in this case. The fist represents a lung within a pleural sac. This analogy helps one understand the statement that each lung (fist) lies freely within a pleural sac. The lung's only attachment to other thoracic structures is via its root and pulmonary ligament.

Each lung is attached to the mediastinum via its *root*, composed of the pulmonary veins, pulmonary

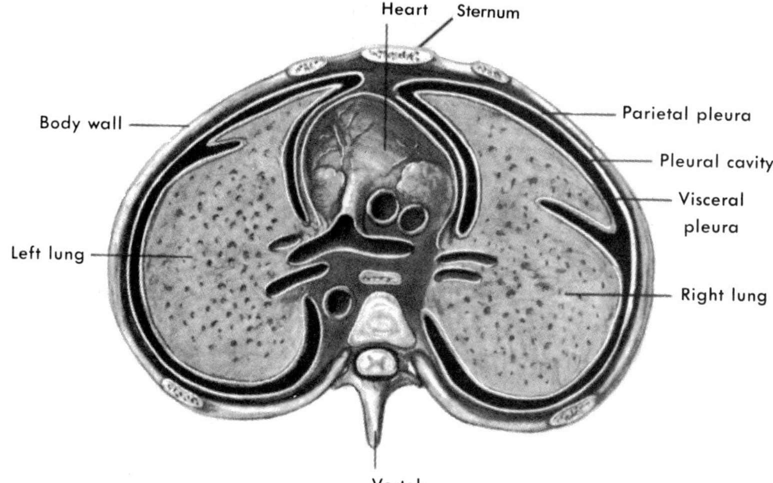

Figure 1–5. Cross section of the thorax as viewed from above, showing the relationship of the lungs and pleurae. (Reproduced by permission from Dienhart, C.: Basic Human Anatomy and Physiology, 3rd ed. Philadelphia, W.B. Saunders Co., 1979.)

artery, bronchus, nerves, and lymph nodes. Anatomists call the vertical slit through which these structures enter and exit the lung the *hilum* or *hilus*. Many clinicians describe the hilum or hilus more generally as the root of the lung at the level of T4 or T5 or more specifically as the depression or recess where structures enter and exit the lung. There are two *hila*, one for each lung root.

Close examination of the root of the lung and surrounding pleurae in Figure 1–3 reveals that the root is in the shape of an upside-down pear. The mediastinal

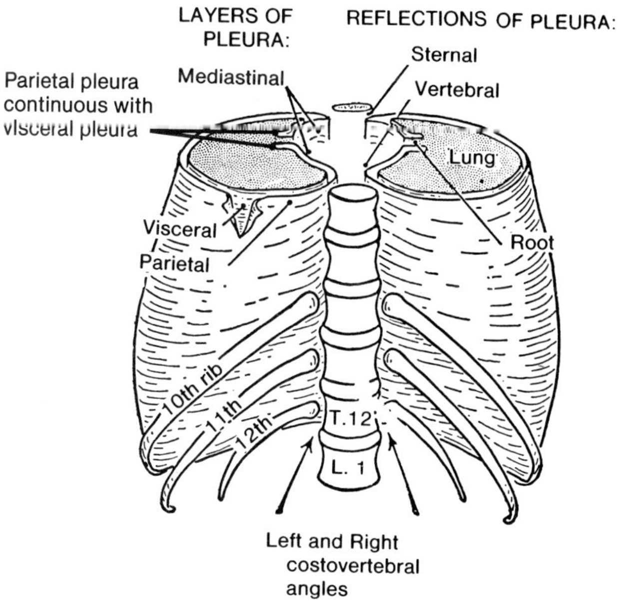

Figure 1–6. The (mediastinal) parietal pleura becomes continuous with the visceral pleura at the root of the lungs. Anteriorly (behind the sternum), the mediastinal pleura is continuous with the costal pleura at the *sternal reflection*. Posteriorly, these layers are continuous at the *vertebral reflection* (anterior to the heads of ribs 1 to 12). (Reproduced by permission from Moore, K.: Clinically Oriented Anatomy, 2nd ed. Baltimore, Williams & Wilkins, 1980.)

pleura enclosing the lung's root is continuous with the *pulmonary ligament*. This ligament descends as a stalk of a pear from the root to the base of the lung. The stalk portion forms a thin, free border more medial to where the pulmonary ligament is labelled in Figure 1–3.

Pleura during Respiration

Figure 1–4 assists in review of the position of the lungs with their inseparable visceral covering in relation to the parietal pleura at expiration. The diaphragm is represented by the dotted line at the level of the fifth rib anteriorly and T8 posteriorly. Although it is one continuous muscle, it is often referred to as the *right* and the *left hemidiaphragm* because each half has its own convex *dome*, as illustrated.

During a full inspiration, the right and left lungs

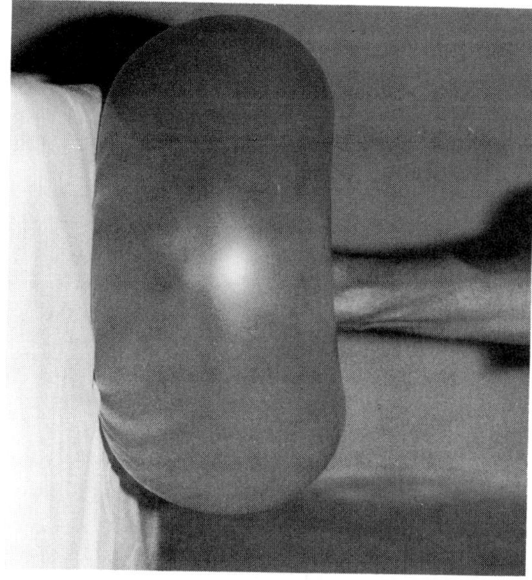

Figure 1–7. A fist pushed into an inflated balloon is analogous to a lung lying freely within a pleural sac.

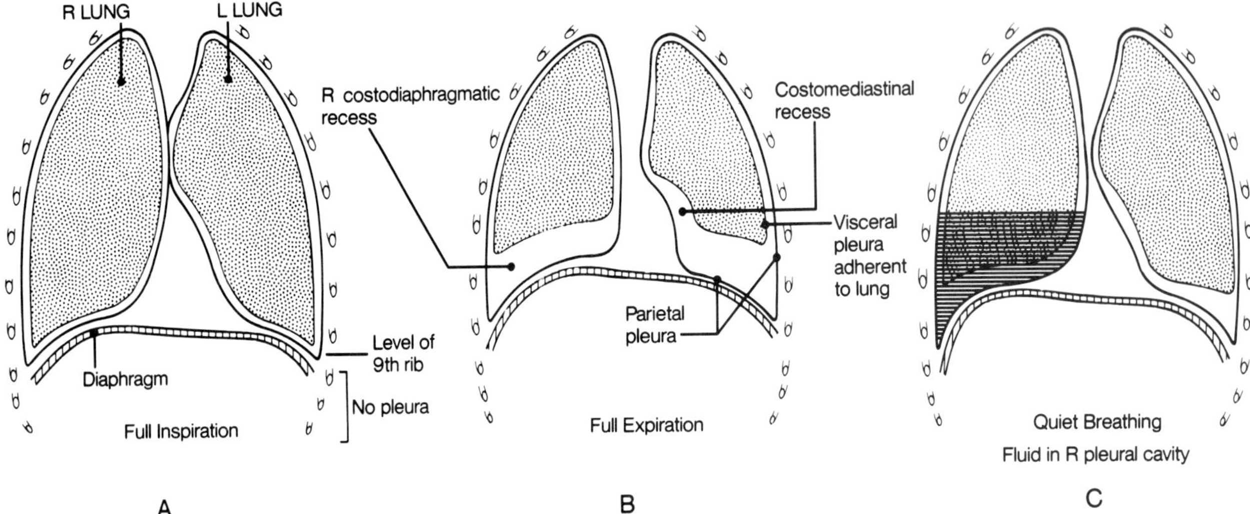

Figure 1–8. Coronal sections of the thorax and lungs during different phases of breathing. *A*, At the end of a *full inspiration*, parietal and visceral pleurae remain in continuous apposition. Recesses are absent. *B*, At the end of a *full expiration*, the lungs retreat, and two surfaces of parietal pleurae directly touch each other. Recesses form. *C*, During *quiet breathing*, recesses are always present, varying only slightly in size. The area with horizontal bars represents fluid in the pleural cavity, filling the right costodiaphragmatic recess, and is called a right pleural effusion.

extend medially, and their sternal pleural reflections approximate each other, sometimes overlapping slightly between the second and fourth ribs. The lungs completely fill the pleural cavities. Parietal and visceral pleura are in continuous apposition (Fig. 1–8A).

During full expiration or quiet breathing, three pleural recesses form, as follows: the *right* and *left costodiaphragmatic recesses*, also called the *costophrenic sulci*, and the *costomediastinal recess* (see numbers 3, 4, and 6 in Fig. 1–4A). The costophrenic sulci are formed as the lungs with their adherent visceral layers retreat superiorly during expiration, leaving costal and diaphragmatic parietal pleurae in direct contact with each other. The costomediastinal recess is formed by the heart, as the lingular segments of the left lung retreat laterally during expiration, leaving costal and mediastinal parietal pleurae in direct contact with each other.

In essence, these recesses are sites where lung no longer fills the pleural cavity. They vary in size depending on the depth of respirations. The recesses are absent or nearly absent at full inspiration (Fig. 1–8A) and are largest at the end of full expiration (Fig. 1–8B). During quiet breathing, the lower limit of the lung with its visceral covering is always about 5 cm above the lower limits of the parietal pleura—the lung seldom extends to its limit inferiorly.

The location of these recesses is clinically significant because, in disease states, excess fluid in the pleural space tends to collect in dependent recesses. Note the excess fluid in the right pleural cavity in Figure 1–8C.

MEDIASTINUM

The mediastinum is technically defined as the partition between the two pleural sacs that contain the lungs. In Figure 1–5, it lies in the middle of the thorax between the sternum and vertebrae and the right and left lungs. (It is unlabelled.) The mediastinum's superior limit is the *thoracic inlet*, a kidney-shaped passageway between the superior border of the manubrium (top part of the sternum) and the first thoracic vertebrae. The trachea and esophagus descend into the thorax through this inlet. The mediastinum's inferior border is the diaphragm or the muscle that forms the floor of the entire thoracic cavity.

The mediastinum is divided into *anterior*, *middle*, *posterior*, *superior*, and *inferior compartments*, as illustrated in Figure 1–9. Knowledge of the locations of these compartments is particularly important in chest roentgenology.

The contents of the mediastinum include the heart, with its pericardial covering; aorta; thymus; vagus and phrenic nerves; esophagus; trachea; and numerous other vessels.

BONY THORAX

The lungs and mediastinum are housed within a chest cage or an osseocartilaginous framework called the *bony thorax*. This thorax consists of 12 pairs of ribs and their cartilages, 12 thoracic vertebrae and intervertebral discs, and the sternum (Fig. 1–10). The scapula and clavicles are included because they serve as important attachments for some respiratory muscles and are used as landmarks in physical assessment.

In the anterior view of the bony thorax, the apices of the lungs extend about 1 in above the clavicles. The bases lie at about the level of the sixth rib and are well protected by the framework.

The sternum consists of three parts; the *manubrium*, the *body*, and the *xiphoid process*. The superior mar-

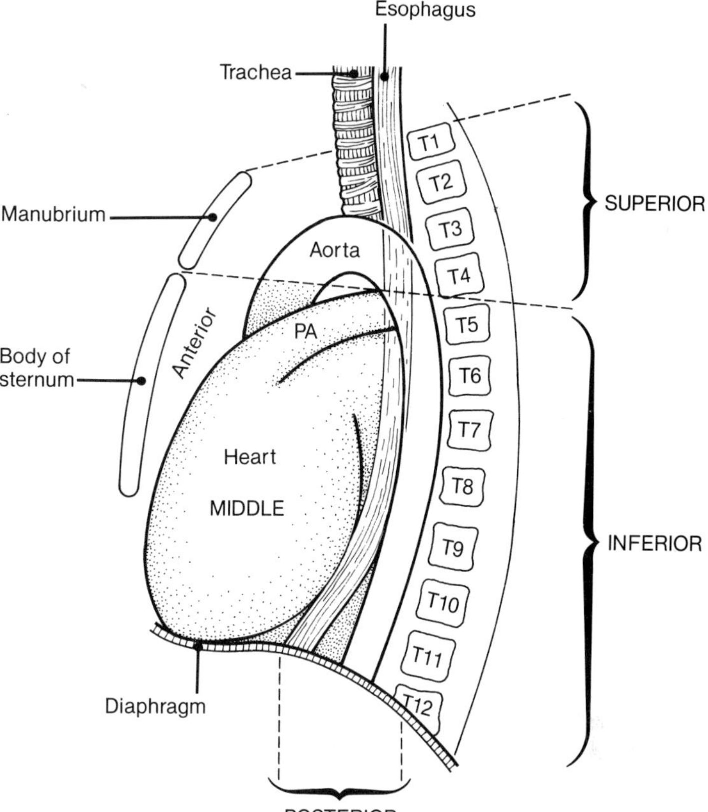

Figure 1–9. Left lateral view of the mediastinal compartments. The *superior (anterior) compartment* lies between the sternum and the heart's pericardium (covering). The *middle compartment* lies between the anterior and posterior pericardium (dotted area). The *posterior compartment* is situated between the posterior pericardium and the anterior aspect of the vertebral column; it includes the descending aorta as well as the esophagus situated just posterior to the heart. (PA = main pulmonary artery.) (Typology from Williams, P. and Warwick, R. Gray's Anatomy, 3th ed. Philadelphia, W.B. Saunders Co., 1980.)

gin of the manubrium is slightly concave, forming the *suprasternal notch*. The junction of the manubrium with the body of the sternum is called the *sternal angle* or *angle of Louis*.

Ribs one through seven are called *true ribs* because they connect directly to the sternum via their costal cartilages. Ribs eight through ten are called *false ribs* because each cartilage attaches to the rib above it rather than directly to the sternum. The roughly 45-degree angle that the costal cartilages form with the xiphoid process is termed the *costal angle*. Ribs 11 and 12 in the posterior chest area are called *floating ribs* because they have no direct skeletal attachments. The spaces between ribs are called *intercostal spaces* (ICS).

The scapula covers the lateral aspect of the thorax posteriorly and approximately over ribs two through seven. The spinous process of each vertebra lies at the level of the rib below. For example, the spinous process of T1 lies directly over the second thoracic vertebra at the level of the second rib.

PULMONARY CIRCULATION

The pulmonary circulation is a system of blood vessels within the lungs. Its chief function is to receive venous blood from the right side of the heart, to pass this blood by the alveoli for oxygenation and carbon dioxide (CO_2) removal, and to then drain the oxygenated blood into the left side of the heart (Fig. 1–11). After oxygenation, arterial blood is pumped through the systemic circulation for use by body tissues. Venous blood returns to the pulmonary circulation via the right atrium and right ventricle of the heart.

The total volume of blood in the lungs is estimated to be 295 ml/m^2 body surface or about 10% of total circulating blood volume. Two lungs of a man of average size contain about 500 ml of blood. The pulmonary capillaries contain only about 75 ml of blood at rest and up to 20% more of this amount during exercise (Murray, 1986).

Functions of the Respiratory System

The respiratory system has many respiratory and nonrespiratory functions. Most functions are related to gas exchange, blood reservoir maintenance, particle filtration, fluid exchange, and lung metabolism.

GAS EXCHANGE

The chief function of the respiratory system is to provide for gas exchange, i.e., the intake of oxygen

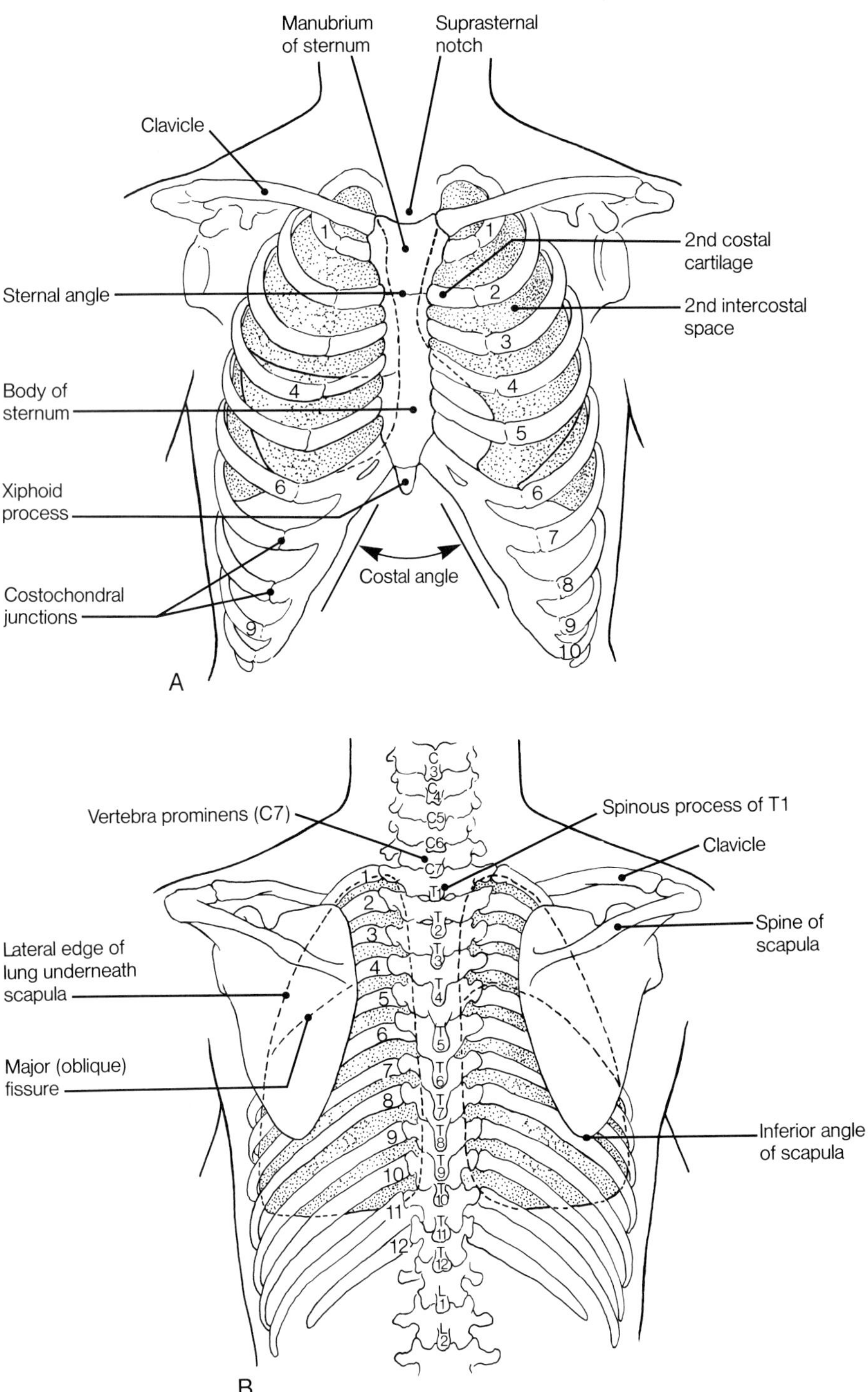

Figure 1–10. The lungs in the bony thorax. The dotted lines mark fissures and borders of the lungs underneath bone. *A*, Anterior view. *B*, Posterior view.

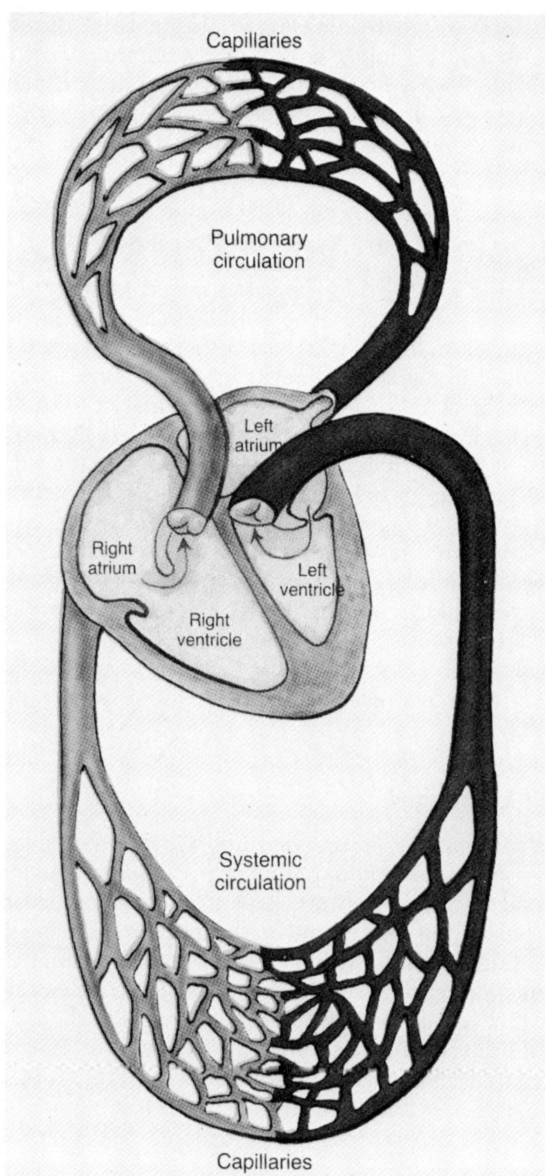

Figure 1–11. Schematic showing the relationship between pulmonary and systemic circulation. Note that the pulmonary veins and systemic arteries are shaded dark gray to denote their higher level of blood oxygenation. (Reproduced and adapted by permission from Jacob, S., et al.: Structure and Function in Man. Philadelphia, W.B. Saunders Co., 1982.)

(O_2) (the life giving substance essential to cell metabolism) and the elimination of CO_2 (the body's chief waste product).

External Respiration. Respiration or exchange of O_2 for CO_2 occurs at two levels. First, *external respiration* occurs at the alveolar level in the lungs. By a process called *diffusion*, gas moves from an area of higher pressure to an area of lower pressure. Accordingly, O_2 in the lungs moves out of alveoli and into adjacent capillaries, because the pressure (tension) of O_2 in alveoli is lower than that in capillaries. From the pulmonary capillaries, O_2 is transported to body tissues by the systemic circulation, as previously mentioned. Simultaneously, CO_2 diffuses from pulmonary capillaries and into alveoli to be exhaled through the nose and mouth.

This external gas exchange system is evaluated by measurement of the *respiratory exchange ratio* (R), i.e., the ratio of CO_2 produced to O_2 consumed per minute. The formula may be written as follows:

$$R = \frac{CO_2 \text{ produced}}{O_2 \text{ consumed}}$$

The normal respiratory exchange ratio is 0.80, as shown next.

$$R = \frac{200 \text{ ml/min } CO_2 \text{ produced}}{250 \text{ ml/min } O_2 \text{ consumed}} = 0.8$$

Internal Respiration. Respiration at the tissue or cellular level is called *internal respiration.* It involves the chemical combustion of foodstuffs and O_2 to form CO_2 and water and to produce energy. Some of the energy is lost as heat, and the rest is used for cellular needs during activities of daily living.

The internal gas exchange system is evaluated by the metabolic *respiratory quotient* (RQ) defined as the *molar* ratio of CO_2 production to O_2 consumption. The normal value for RQ equals 0.80 to 0.85 at rest (Slonim and Hamilton, 1987). This value is relatively constant during steady and unsteady states. It changes when dietary intake consists of one major foodstuff rather than a mixture of carbohydrate, fat, and protein. Each of these major foodstuffs produces a different RQ. The RQ for fat is low—about 0.70. For protein, it is slightly less than 0.80. When only glucose (carbohydrate) is available (e.g., continuous intravenous infusion of dextrose in water), the increased CO_2 production is largely responsible for raising the RQ to 1.00, as shown in the following equation:

$$C_6H_{12}O_6 + 6\ O_2 \longrightarrow 6\ CO_2 + 6\ H_2O + \text{energy}$$

$$R = \frac{CO_2 \text{ produced}}{O_2 \text{ consumed}} = \frac{6\ CO_2}{6\ O_2} = 1.00$$

In this last situation, healthy persons usually adapt to the extra load of CO_2 by excreting it via the lungs. A patient with severe respiratory disease, however, has a limited ability to do so because of lung dysfunction.

Another circumstance that causes a change in the respiratory quotient is exercise. Early in the course of exercise, a higher proportion of carbohydrate is burned, causing an increased value for RQ. After prolonged heavy exercise, a high proportion of fat is burned, producing a low value for RQ (below 0.80).

The so described external and internal gas exchange systems are interrelated. Their measurements—the respiratory exchange ratio (external) and the metabolic respiratory quotient (internal)—both equal 0.80 during steady states or homeostases. They balance each other in the following ways: (1) the CO_2 produced at the tissue level is balanced by the CO_2 elimination at the lungs and (2) similarly, tissue oxygen consumption is balanced by the transfer of more O_2 from the lungs to the pulmonary and systemic circulatory systems and, ultimately, to the peripheral body tissues.

Clinical Application. In the clinical setting, R and RQ are assumed to be equal. They may vary when acute disease alters CO_2 elimination and O_2 uptake, but R and RQ promptly become equal again after a new steady state is achieved. Because both R and RQ typically reflect cellular metabolism, clinicians tend to use the two terms interchangeably.

For a ratio determination, measurements are made at the mouth while the patient breathes through a closed system. Calculations are made from the clinical formula summarized in the box.

*CALCULATION OF THE RESPIRATORY EXCHANGE RATIO (OR RESPIRATORY QUOTIENT)**

$$R = \frac{\dot{V}CO_2 \text{ volume of } CO_2 \text{ exhaled per minute}}{\dot{V}O_2 \text{ volume of } O_2 \text{ consumed per minute}}$$

$$\dot{V}CO_2 = \dot{V}_E \times FE_{O2}$$

$$\dot{V}O_2 = \dot{V}_E \times (FIO_2 - FE_{O2})$$

$$= \frac{200 \text{ ml/min } CO_2 \text{ produced}}{250 \text{ ml/min } O_2 \text{ consumed}}$$

$$= 0.8$$

(Normal)

*(See Appendix I for pulmonary symbols)

The calculated ratio helps in the evaluation of metabolic needs and in the determination of optimal proportions of foodstuffs for each patient. Also, R is used in various blood gas formulas, such as measurement of intrapulmonary shunting described in this book (see Chapter 13). However, because the technique for ratio measurement is not simple, clinicians may only estimate rather than actually calculate the respiratory exchange ratio, or they may assume it is 1.0 to make calculations easier.

OTHER FUNCTIONS

The respiratory system has several other functions in addition to gas exchange.

Blood Reservoir

The blood volume in the pulmonary circulation and right atrium of the heart serves as a reservoir for the left ventricle whenever cardiac output falls. In addition, when the lungs and the rest of the body are overloaded with fluid, this reservoir system expands and increases its capacity to accommodate excess fluid without significantly raising pulmonary vascular pressures.

Filter to Protect the Systemic Circulation

Located strategically between mixed venous blood and systemic arterial blood, pulmonary vessels trap fine particles that might have otherwise entered the systemic circulation and occluded either peripheral or more central vessels, such as the coronary or cerebral arteries. Fine particles enter venous blood by natural processes; by trauma; and by some therapeutic measures, such as intravenous administration of drugs or fluids. Particles may include gas bubbles, small fibrin or blood clots, fat cells, agglutinated red blood cells, aggregates of platelets or white blood cells, and other pieces of cellular debris. Once captured, these particles are disposed of by the lung's defense system, which involves special lytic enzymes, macrophage cells, and lymphatic channels (described subsequently).

Fluid Exchange

When water is introduced into airways and alveoli, it passes rapidly into pulmonary capillary blood. In normal lungs, alveoli are kept free of water because the balance of vessel and tissue pressures favors the retention of fluid within vessels and the pulling of excess water from alveoli and into blood. In essence, pressure relationships in the lungs, as well as the nature of the substance inhaled, ingested, or injected, determine the nature, rate, and extent of fluid exchange in the lung.

Metabolic Functions

From one perspective, the lung may be considered to have a passive role in respiration, since the respiratory muscles provide mechanical force for ventilation and the heart pumps blood through the pulmonary circulation. However, the lung is a metabolically active organ, particularly when lung disease is present. The normal lung's contribution to whole body oxygen consumption is only about 1% of total oxygen expenditure at rest (Murray, 1986).

The lung uses oxygen for a variety of metabolic purposes, as discussed in the following sections.

Maintenance of Lung Metabolism. The lung provides the metabolic requirements for about 40 different cell types. Though most O_2 is supplied through the blood stream, distal lung tissue and small airways obtain adequate O_2 for their metabolic needs directly from inspired air.

Surfactant Synthesis. The lung synthesizes *surfactant*, a substance that lowers surface tension during expiration and prevents lung collapse.

Table 1–1. HORMONES IN THE LUNGS*

Hormone	Known or Suspected Sites of Lung Production	Effect of Hormonal Release
Adrenocorticotropic hormone	Pulmonary endocrine cells (?)	Possible role in regulation of steroids
Arachidonic acid metabolites		
Prostaglandins	Alvelolar macrophages, endothelium, fibroblasts, smooth muscle, Type II cells, platelets	Constriction or dilatation of airways and blood vessels; Platelet aggregation or antiaggregation
Leukotrienes	Mast cells, basophils, neutrophils	Constriction of airways and blood vessels
Histamine	Mast cells	Constriction of airways and blood vessels
Serotonin, various peptides	Pulmonary endocrine cells, nerves	Variable

*Data consolidated from Becker, K. and Gazdar, A.: The Endocrine Lung in Health and Disease. Philadelphia, W. B. Saunders Co., 1984.

Protein and Connective Tissue Syntheses. The lung contains a large number of diverse proteins. Many participate in energy production, such as *enzymes of glucose metabolism* (e.g., lactic dehydrogenase) or lipid metabolism (e.g., phospholipases). Connective tissue proteins, such as *collagen* and *elastin*, serve to support the lung and maintain its elastic nature.

Endocrine Functions. The role of the lungs as endocrine organs is incompletely understood. However, substantial research is in progress to more thoroughly understand hormonal events in normal and pathologic situations.

The main hormones in the lungs are listed in Table 1–1. Of those listed, arachidonic acid metabolites are perhaps most important because of their roles in asthma and other clinical conditions. Two groups of metabolites, the leukotrienes and prostaglandins, are representative of two complicated metabolic pathways that are simplified in Figure 1–12. The *prostaglandins* are released from the lungs during anaphylaxis, inflammation, lack of oxygen in tissue, pulmonary edema, and mechanical stimulation. The *leukotrienes* (notably LTC_4, LTD_4, and LTE_4) and possibly selected prostaglandins are believed responsible for airway constriction in asthma. Abnormal concentrations of leukotrienes are found in other pulmonary diseases as well, such as cystic fibrosis and pulmonary hypertension. However, clinical implications are unclear.

Currently, both pathways of arachidonic acid metabolism shown in Figure 1–12 are under investigation, in hope of developing more selective antiasthma medications and other medications for pulmonary patients.

Transformation of Biochemical Substances. The lungs are strategically located to degrade or modify circulating blood substances and, thereby, to influence indirectly other body systems. For example, *angiotensin-converting enzyme* resides on the lumenal surface of the pulmonary endothelium and acts on two circulating peptides to regulate systemic blood pressure.

One peptide is called *bradykinin*. It is a potent endogenous vasodilator that is believed to play a role in inflammatory responses and neonatal circulatory adjustments.

The other circulating peptide is *angiotensin I*. It is transformed rapidly in the lungs to the more potent systemic pressor *angiotensin II*.

Conclusion

This chapter provides an overview of the structure and function of the respiratory system.

The content related to structure has provided a clearly defined body of knowledge necessary for understanding chest pathophysiology and chest assessment techniques (see Part Two and Part Three). Similarly, the content related to the respiratory system's gas exchange function serves as a firm foundation for understanding why, for example, a pulmonary patient retaining CO_2 may require mechanical lung ventilation, limited carbohydrate food intake, or both during acute illness.

Moreover, this chapter suggests that nonrespiratory functions are just as important as gas exchange functions. For example, the lung's filtering function has a clinical implication for the nurse; a few small bubbles infusing through an intravenous line may be insignificant because of the lung's filtering function. However,

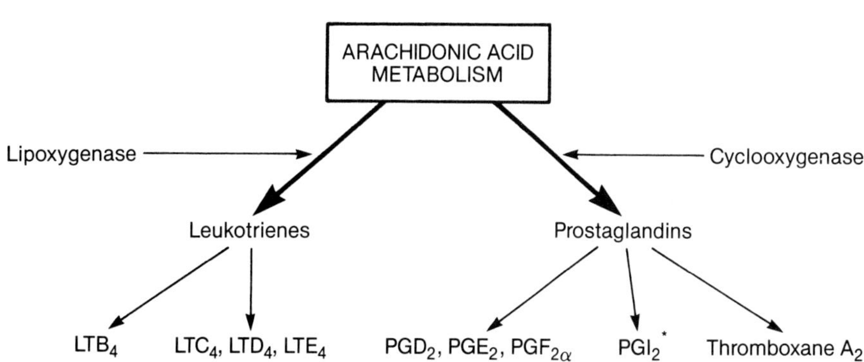

Figure 1–12. Pathways of arachidonic acid metabolism in the lungs. Arachidonic acid is converted into active substances (e.g., various leukotrienes and prostaglandins) via the two following pathways: (1) the lipoxygenase pathway and (2) the cyclooxygenase pathway. Each pathway is named after the catalytic enzyme involved in the initial reaction. (LT = leukotriene; PG = prostaglandin; PGI_2 = prostacyclin.)

many clinical implications of metabolic and other non-respiratory functions are still unclear because they remain incompletely understood.

REFERENCES

Becker, K. and Gazdar, A.: *The Endocrine Lung in Health and Disease.* Philadelphia, W. B. Saunders Co., 1984.

Comroe, J.: *Physiology of Respiration—An Introductory Text,* 2nd ed. Chicago, Year Book Medical Publishers, Inc., 1974.

Dienhart, C.: *Basic Human Anatomy and Physiology,* 3rd ed. Philadelphia, W. B. Saunders Co., 1979.

Harper, R.: *A Guide to Respiratory Care—Physiology and Clinical Applications.* Philadelphia, J. B. Lippincott Co., 1982.

Jacob, S., Francone, C. A., and Lossow, W.: *Structure and Function in Man.* Philadelphia, W. B. Saunders Co., 1982.

Moore, K.: *Clinically Oriented Anatomy,* 2nd ed. Baltimore, Williams & Wilkins, 1985.

Murray, J.: *The Normal Lung: The Basis for Diagnosis and Treatment of Pulmonary Disease,* 2nd ed. Philadelphia, W. B. Saunders Co., 1986.

Netter, F.: *The CIBA Collection of Medical Illustrations, vol 7: Respiratory System.* New York, CIBA Pharmaceutical Co., 1979.

Slonim, N. and Hamilton, L.: *Respiratory Physiology,* 5th ed. St. Louis, C. V. Mosby Co., 1987.

Tortora, G.: *Principles of Human Anatomy,* 3rd ed. New York, Harper & Row Publishers, Inc., 1983.

Williams, P. and Warwick, R.: *Gray's Anatomy,* 36th ed. Philadelphia, W. B. Saunders Co., 1980.

Upper and Lower Respiratory Tracts

2

Main Objectives

1. Locate the following on unlabelled diagrams of the upper respiratory tract:
   a. right and left nasal cavities
   b. superior, middle, and inferior conchae (turbinates)
   c. adenoids and palatine tonsils (faucial tonsils)
   d. maxillary, frontal, ethmoid, and sphenoid paranasal sinuses
   e. nasopharynx, oropharynx, and laryngopharynx
   f. larynx, thyroid cartilage, cricoid cartilage, epiglottis, glottis, and vocal cords.
2. Name and describe the three functions of the nasal cavity.
3. Identify and explain the clinical significance of four upper airway reflexes.
4. Define the following lower respiratory tract terms: airway generation, conductive zone, transitional and respiratory zones, cilia, mucociliary escalator, terminal respiratory unit (acinus), alveolus, parenchyma, lobule, interlobular septa, lung interstitium, and surfactant.
5. Locate the following on an unlabelled diagram:
   a. carina
   b. trachea
   c. right and left main stem bronchi, intermediate bronchus
   d. key bronchopulmonary segments for the upper lobes (anterior, apical or apical posterior, superior and inferior lingular), right middle lobe (medial and lateral), and lower lobes (superior, posterior, lateral).
6. Name and describe the three histologic layers of the trachea and main bronchi.
7. Explain the clinical significance of the following alveolar structures: alveolar space, Type II cells (granular pneumocytes), alveolar macrophage, Kohn's pores, and other collateral channels, and thick and thin sides of the alveolar-capillary membrane.

8. **Compare and contrast the alveolar interstitial space with the peribronchial/perivascular interstitial spaces.**

This chapter discusses upper and lower respiratory tracts in detail. The *upper respiratory tract* includes primarily the nasal cavity, pharynx, and larynx, as illustrated in Figure 1–1. The *lower respiratory tract* includes the trachea, bronchi, other conducting airways, and terminal respiratory units with their alveoli. The division between these two respiratory tracts is at the vocal cords (or sometimes at the lower border of the cricoid cartilage).

The Upper Respiratory Tract

The upper respiratory tract extends from the nasal cavity to the vocal cords within the larynx.

NASAL CAVITY

Structure

Upon inhalation, air first passes through two openings called *nostrils* or *external nares*. These nares lead to right and left *nasal cavities*, which are divided by a vertical partition called the *nasal septum* (Fig. 2–1 and Fig. 2–2).

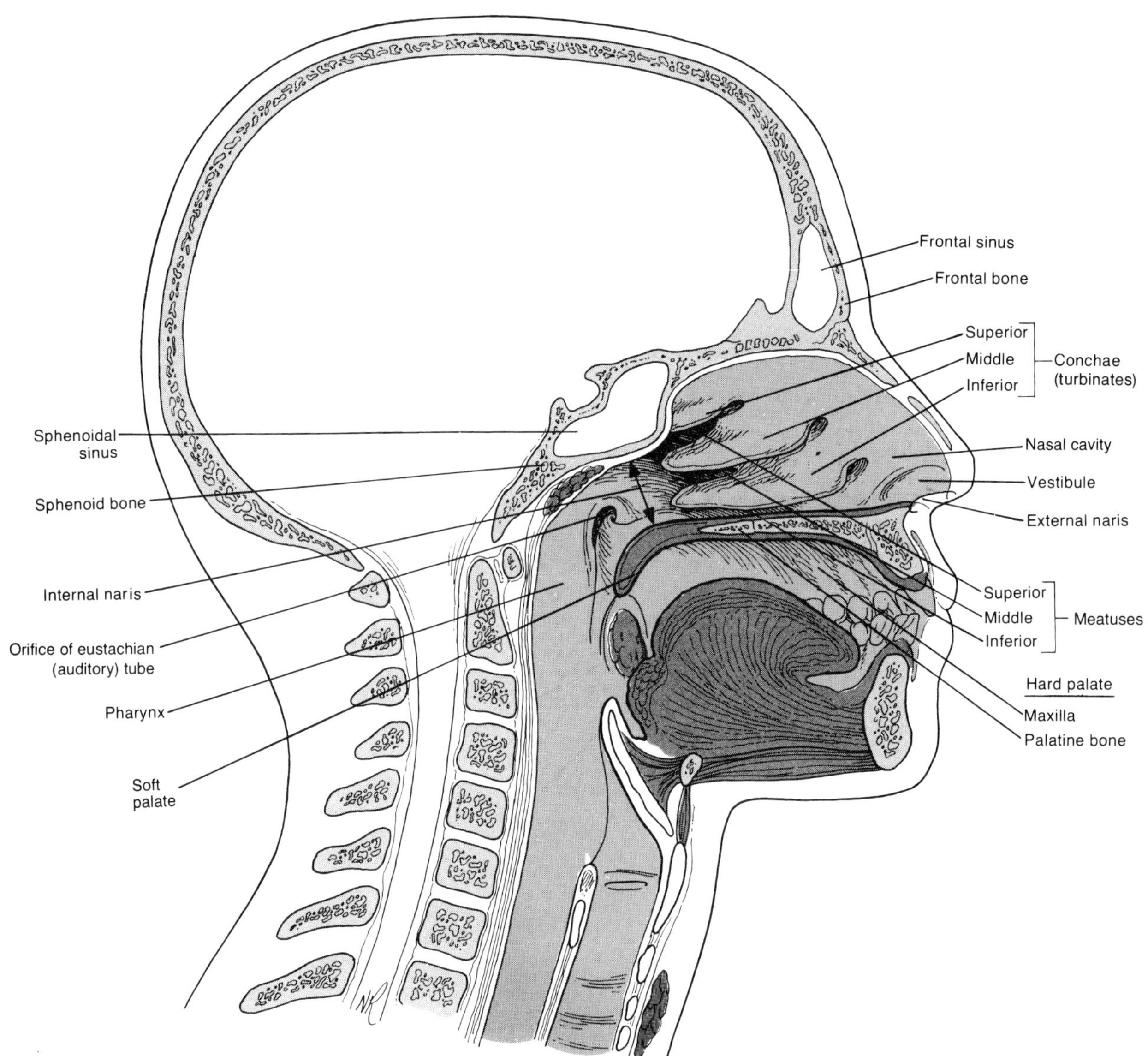

Figure 2–1. Sagittal section of the right nasal cavity. (Reproduced by permission from Tortora, G.: Principles of Human Anatomy, 3rd ed. New York, Harper & Row Publishers, Inc., 1983.)

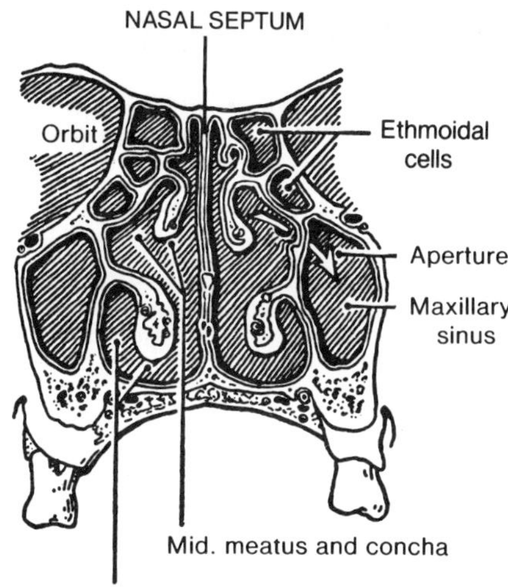

Figure 2–2. Coronal section of right and left nasal cavities separated by the nasal septum. Note the relationship of the nasal cavities to the paranasal sinuses. (Reproduced by permission from Moore, K.: Clinically Oriented Anatomy, 2nd ed. Baltimore, Williams & Wilkins, 1985.)

Cartilage rather than bone makes up most of the anterior portion of the septum. Normally, the vertical orientation of the septum keeps the two wedge-shaped nasal cavities symmetrical and the nasal passages patent. If this septum becomes deviated owing to some minor accident (often unknown to either the patient or physician), the patient must use the opposite nasal cavity or the mouth for breathing. In such a patient, the clinician may not be able to pass a suction catheter, nasal airway, or endotracheal tube down the obstructed cavity during an emergency.

As air enters the external nares, it passes through the *vestibule*, a hair-covered area that filters out large dust particles. Air then passes through a series of grove-like passageways called *meatus*, more specifically, the *superior*, *middle*, and *inferior*. These meatus are formed from the three shelf-like projections of the *superior*, *middle*, and *inferior conchae* or *turbinates* that extend out of the lateral wall of each nasal cavity. As air whirls around the meatus and turbinates, it is warmed, humidified, filtered, and conducted posteriorly through the internal nares and into the pharynx.

Functions

The nasal cavity has five main functions, as follows: air conduction, olfaction, filtration, temperature control and humidification, and voice resonance.

Air Conduction. The general conduction of air through nasal passages is described previously. The narrowest portion of airway in the nose is in the *anterior naris*, a name that refers to airway between the nostril and nasal turbinate. Here, air passes the vestibule and must make a sight directional bend to pass through the meatus. This bend marks a constricted area where air flow becomes turbulent and high inspiratory air flow becomes reduced. The constriction is largely responsible for the high nasal resistance to air flow at rest, nearly *half* of the total resistance to respiratory air flow. During rapid breathing, the nostrils tend to collapse, limiting the degree of nasal breathing possible and necessitating the augmentation of the nasal airway by low-resistance oropharyngeal breathing.

Filtration. The nose acts as a filter, cleansing freshly inhaled air of dusts, bacteria, and other particulate matter. Most particles larger than 10 μm impact in the nasal cavity and do not reach the lower airways. Many impact on the stratified squamous epithelium in the anterior nares. They become trapped by thick nasal hairs called vibrissae and are removed by nose blowing or sneezing. Other particles impact more posteriorly and are swept backward over the mucus-lined, pseudostratified ciliated columnar epithelium to the nasopharynx where they are swallowed. Murray (1986) reports that the mucous layer of the main nasal passages is cleared about every 10 to 15 minutes, and the rate of movement of particles on the mucosal surface is 4.8 mm/min.

Temperature Control and Humidification. Inspired air is quickly brought to body temperature (37°C) and fully saturated with water vapor (PH_2O 47 mmHG), as it passes over the nasopharyngeal mucosa. To control for temperature, the mucosa can absorb heat if incoming air is too hot. More typically, since room temperature is usually lower than body temperature, cool air is warmed via dilatation of the rich venous plexus beneath the epithelium of the lower nasal turbinates. At the same time, humidification occurs from transudation of moisture from the epithelial lining and to a lesser extent from secretions of mucous glands and cells. The body loses about 250 ml of water each day in expired air by this process and much more during rapid breathing.

Changing from nasal to mouth breathing shifts the main site of temperature control and humidification from the nose to the pharynx and larynx. Normal individuals adapt to this shift. Even a stable ambulatory patient with total laryngectomy breathes directly in and out of the trachea with no apparent adverse effects, after an initial adjustment period. However, when respiratory disease is present or when the upper airway is by-passed with an endotracheal tube or tracheostomy cannula, the airway's temperature control, humidification, and filtering mechanisms can easily become overtaxed. Inadequate warming and humidification result in drying of tracheal and bronchial mucous membranes and cessation of ciliary action on epithelial surfaces, predisposing the individual to infection.

Olfaction. Receptors for the sense of smell are located in the olfactory epithelium. This epithelium is a yellowish brown area, extending from the middle of the roof of the nasal cavity about 8 to 10 mm downward on each side of the nasal septum and onto the surface of the superior turbinate.

Voice Resonance. The nasal cavity, in addition to

the larynx, pharynx, paranasal sinuses, and mouth cavity, contributes to voice resonance.

PARANASAL SINUSES

The paranasal sinuses are air-filled spaces lined with ciliated epithelium similar to that of the nasal cavity but containing fewer and smaller glands. Commonly asymmetrical in shape, they are paired and include the *maxillary, frontal, ethmoid,* and *sphenoid* sinuses (Fig. 2–3). All sinuses drain into the nasal cavity in a meatus or near a turbinate. The function of these sinuses is as follows: (1) to lighten the bones of the skull; (2) to provide mucus for the nasal cavity, and (3) to act as resonant chambers in the production of sound.

Sinusitis is inflammation of the sinuses. An individual with a rhinovirus (common cold) or a chronic respiratory disease (bronchial asthma, bronchiectasis) may have sinusitis or a sinus infection, involving usually frontal or maxillary sinuses. Sinus infections are likely to begin in the anterior ethmoid sinuses because these sinuses are closest to the inspired air stream. Infection of the sphenoid sinus (located posteriorly to the eye in the sphenoid bone) can cause vision impairment because of its proximity to the optic nerve.

PHARYNX

The pharynx or throat is a 5-in long musculomembranous tube with two main functions. First, it serves as a common passageway for air to the trachea and food to the esophagus. Second, it plays an important part in the formation of sound, particularly in the creation of vowel sounds. The pharynx is divided into the three following sections: *nasopharynx, oropharynx,* and *laryngopharynx* (Fig. 2–4).

Nasopharynx

The uppermost section, the nasopharynx, extends from the internal nares to the soft palate. It contains two important structures: the orifices of the two auditory (eustachian) tubes and the pharyngeal tonsils (adenoids). The *auditory tube* connects the pharynx with the middle ear and allows the equalization of pressure between the two structures during swallowing. Occlusion of this tube's orifice by mucosal edema, tenacious secretions, excessive adenoid tissue, or endotracheal or nasogastric tube, can cause the buildup of negative pressure in the middle ear and mastoid air cells, drawing the tympanic membrane inwards and causing ear malfunction. In addition, ear infections due to the transmission of microorganisms from the

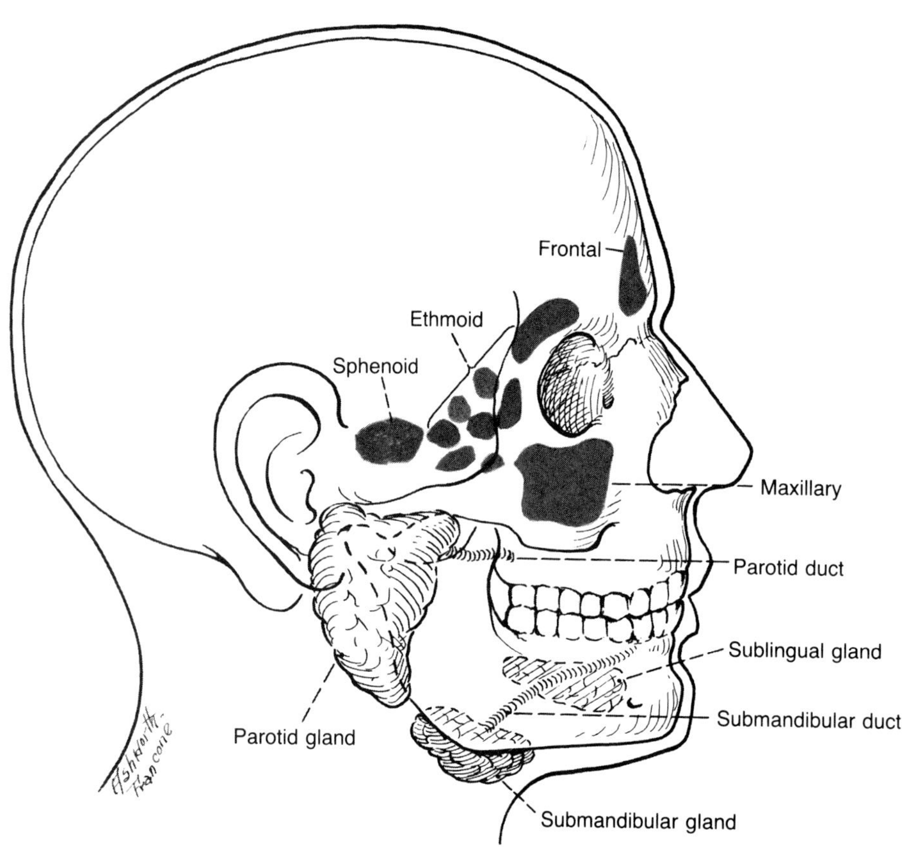

Figure 2–3. Lateral view of head showing sinuses and salivary glands. (Reproduced by permission from Jacob, S., et al.: Structure and Function in Man, 5th ed. Philadelphia, W. B. Saunders Co., 1982.)

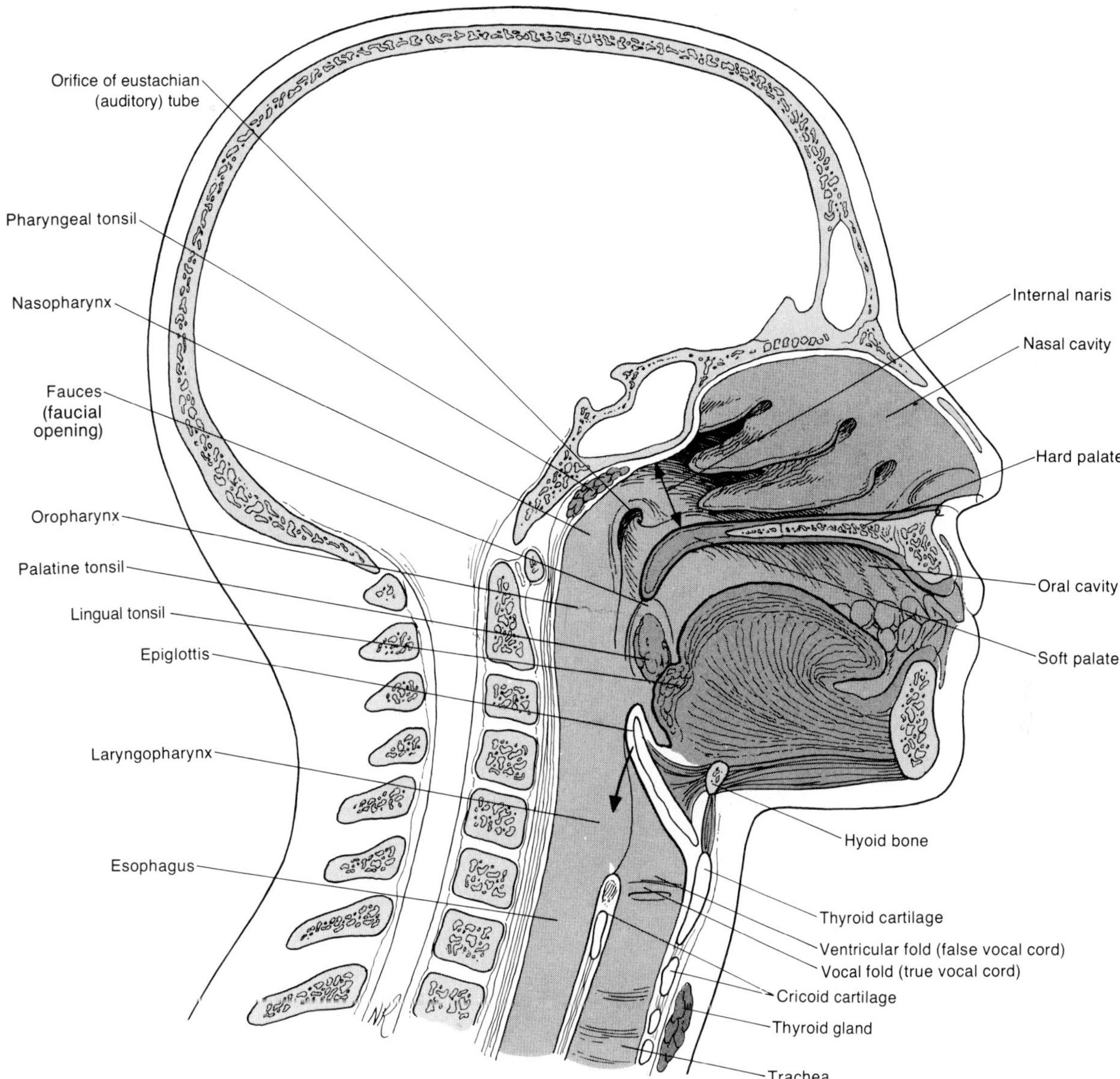

Figure 2–4. Sagittal section of the head and neck. (Reproduced by permission from Tortora, G.: Principles of Human Anatomy, 3rd ed. New York, Harper & Row Publishers, Inc., 1983.)

nasopharynx through the auditory tubes to the ears are common complications of respiratory disease, specifically upper respiratory tract infections.

The *adenoids* are located at the superior posterior wall of the pharynx. They are part of a ring of lymphatic tissue that includes the palatine and lingual tonsils in the oropharynx. All of these structures tend to be enlarged in children and are believed to play important roles in the development of immunity. When enlarged, adenoids may obstruct nasal passages and limit air flow, especially when inflamed; inflammation of the tonsils (tonsillitis) is also present. Adenoids may become easily traumatized during nasal intubation, causing significant bleeding.

Oropharynx

The oropharynx is located behind the oral cavity and extends from the soft palate down to the hyoid bone. It serves as a common passageway for both air and food. The presence of food initiates a swallowing reflex, which propels the food posteriorly into the esophagus and simultaneously closes a valve (epiglottis) in the larynx to prevent aspiration of the food into the anteriorly located trachea.

The *lingual tonsil* is located in the oropharynx at the base of the tongue. This tonsil consists of a collection of numerous, slightly raised nodules embedded in submucous tissue along the tongue's posterior surface.

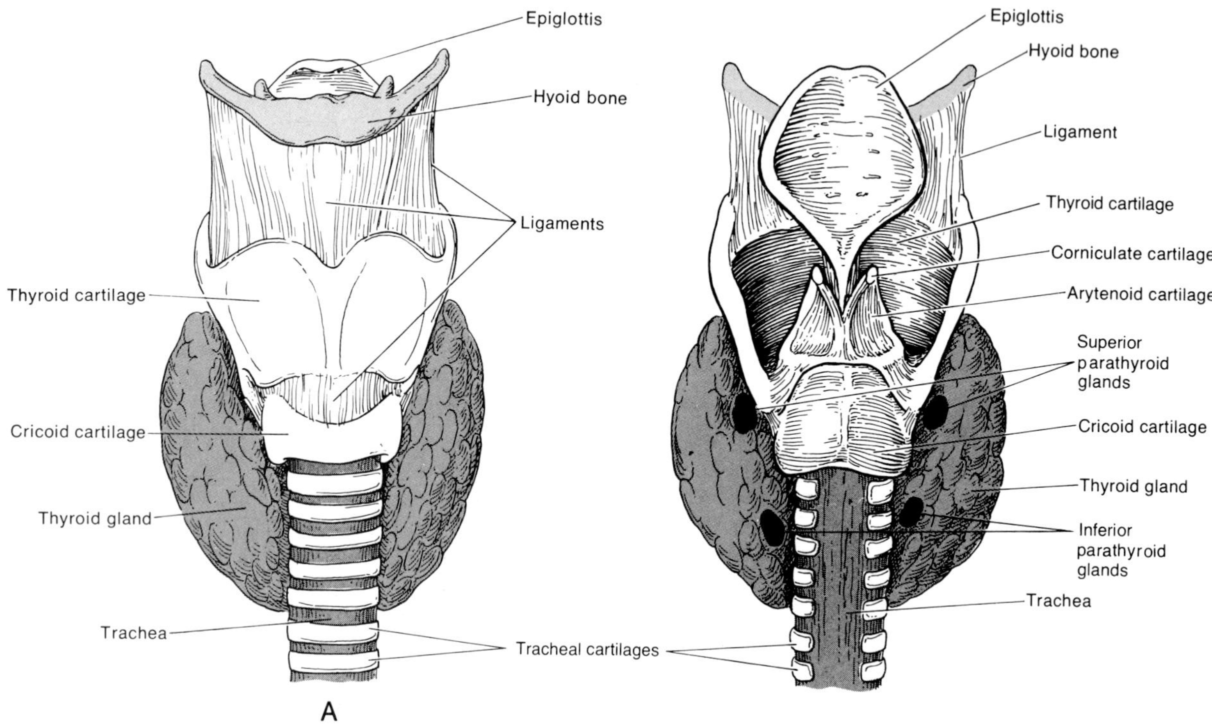

Figure 2–5. The larynx. Anterior view *A*, and posterior view *B*. (Reproduced by permission from Tortora, G.: Principles of Human Anatomy, 3rd ed. New York, Harper & Row Publishers, Inc., 1983.)

Laterally, the two *palatine tonsils*, also called the *faucial tonsils* or commonly just "the tonsils," are arranged one on each side of the pharynx, extending into the *fauces* or *faucial opening*. Repeated enlargement of the palatine tonsils in children used to be a common indication for surgical removal (tonsillectomy). Now, tonsillectomy is indicated for repeated tonsillitis in adults and is performed in children only in urgent situations, such as upper airway obstruction.

The *tongue* is another important oropharyngeal structure that can obstruct the airway, by falling back against the posterior pharyngeal wall. Airway obstruction by this mechanism is most likely to occur in the supine unconscious or comatose patient.

Laryngopharynx

This lowest portion of the pharynx extends from the hyoid bone down to the esophagus posteriorly and to the larynx anteriorly. Similar to the oropharynx, it

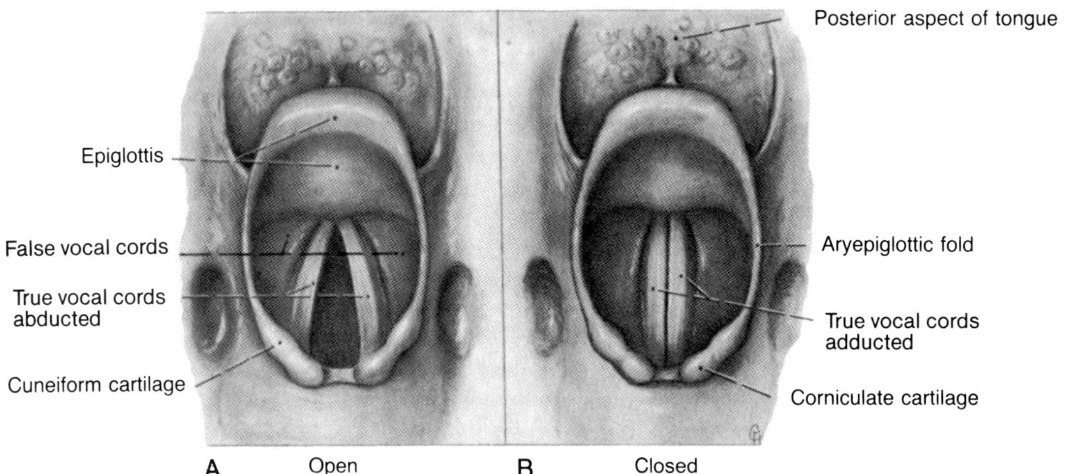

Figure 2–6. Superior view of vocal cords. *A*, Open. *B*, Closed. (Reproduced by permission from Jacob, S., et al.: Structure and Function in Man, 5th ed. Philadelphia, W. B. Saunders Co., 1982.)

Table 2–1. STRUCTURES OF THE LARYNX*

Structure	Description	Significance
Unpaired Cartilages		
Thyroid	Largest laryngeal cartilage Shaped like the bow of a ship Forward prominence, called the "Adam's apple," more protuberant in males	Houses the vocal cords
Cricoid	Located inferiorly to the thyroid cartilage Shaped like a signet ring with the signet facing posteriorly Only complete ring of cartilage in the airway Narrowest site in a child's airway	In child, an uncuffed rather than a cuffed endotracheal tube is used for endotracheal intubation. If its size is just smaller than the cricoid, a significant air leak around the tube does not occur.
Epiglottis	Large leaf-shaped piece of cartilage lying on top of the larynx "Stem" attached to the superior border of the thyroid cartilage "Leaf" portion acts as a trap door, closing off the larynx to liquids and food during swallowing.	Prevents aspiration of food or vomitus
Paired Cartilages		
Arytenoid	Pyramidal-shaped cartilages attached to the superior portion of the cricoid cartilage (see Fig. 2–5B). They also attach to pharyngeal muscles and posterior ends of the vocal cords.	Provides leverage for opening and closing the vocal cords. Dislocation is occasionally observed during endotracheal intubation. Trauma to the vocal cords and any of these paired cartilages may potentially occur with faulty technique during endotracheal intubation and suctioning procedures.
Corniculate	Small cone-shaped elastic cartilages sitting on top of the arytenoid cartilages.	
Cuneiform	Small rod-shaped cartilages located in the mucous membrane folds (aryepiglottic fold) next to and in front of the corniculate cartilages.	
Other Key Structures		
Glottis	The V-shaped air passageway between vocal cords	Vocal cords mark the narrowest point in the adult's airway.
Vocal cords	Mucous membranous folds are arranged in two pairs, as follows: (1) a lower pair called *true vocal cords* or *vocal folds*. They border the glottis and are lined underneath by elastic ligaments. (2) An upper pair called *false vocal cords* or *ventricular folds*, located laterally next to the true vocal cords.	During coughing, vocal cord closure allows the initial trapping of air in the lungs. With abdominal muscle contraction against a fixed diaphragm, the cords remain closed, allowing the further buildup of intrathoracic pressures to as much as 100 mmHg. As the cords open, the high airway pressures generate the high expiratory flow rates necessary for productive coughing.
	Vocal cords remain approximated anteriorly (Fig. 2–6A) and open and close posteriorly, altering the V-shaped glottic aperture (Fig. 2–6B).	When air is directed against the vocal cords, they vibrate and produce sound. Laryngeal muscle contraction and relaxation alters cord tension and shape to produce different pitches and sounds.
Musculature	*Extrinsic* muscles support and connect the larynx with surrounding muscles and ligaments	Function to move the larynx as a unit.
	Intrinsic muscles join together the cartilages of the larynx	Function to open and close the glottis during inspiration and expiration, close the laryngeal aperture and glottis during swallowing, and alter vocal cord tension to produce sound.
Branches of the vagus nerve	*Recurrent laryngeal nerve* is the chief motor nerve that supplies the laryngeal musculature. *Superior laryngeal nerve* is the main sensory nerve.	Injury of the recurrent laryngeal nerve during surgery of the thyroid gland causes hoarseness or inability to speak. Polyps or tumors can press on this nerve and cause vocal cord paralysis.
Recesses	Recesses are dead-end spaces in the larynx, e.g., *valleculae*, located anteriorly between the epiglottis and base of the tongue, and *pyriform sinus*, located laterally between the larynx and pharyngeal wall.	Food, aspirated foreign bodies, catheters, or tubes may lodge in one of the recesses.
Epithelial lining	Anterior surface and upper half of the posterior surface of the epiglottis as well as the vocal cords are lined with *stratified squamous epithelium.*	This durable lining is suitable for phonation and other functions involving frequent approximations of tissues.
	At the base of the epiglottis, *ciliated epithelium* reappears and continues down the larynx, trachea, and bronchi.	The cilia beat towards the mouth and move particles, microorganisms, and mucus from the lungs towards the exterior of the body.

*See Figure 2–5.

serves both respiratory and digestive tracts and is lined by stratified squamous epithelium, a lining that can take the wear and tear of passing foodstuffs.

LARYNX

The larynx is commonly called the "voice box" because its chief function is phonation. Connecting the pharynx with the trachea, it lies in the midline of the neck anterior to the fourth through sixth cervical vertebrae. The larynx consists of nine cartilages (three paired and three unpaired) united by muscles and ligaments. These and other main structures of the larynx are summarized in Table 2–1 and illustrated in Figure 2–5 and Figure 2–6.

UPPER AIRWAY REFLEXES

Upper respiratory tract airways and secretions (saliva, expectorated mucus) have floras that are considered contaminated when compared with the sterile environment of the lower respiratory tract. Aspiration of secretions or foreign objects beyond the vocal cords and into the trachea can cause aspiration pneumonia in addition to airway obstruction. The pharynx, larynx, and trachea have reflexes that form the body's first line of defense in the protection of the lower respiratory tract from contamination as well as airway obstruction. These reflexes are grouped and presented next, within the typology according to Trout (1976). This typology presents main reflexes according to anatomic location.

1. The *pharyngeal reflex* has a sensory supply via the ninth cranial nerve (glossopharyngeal) and a motor innervation via the tenth cranial nerve (vagus). This reflex is responsible for gagging and swallowing.

2. The *laryngeal reflex* is a *vagovagal* reflex because both afferent and efferent components are part of the vagus nerve. Triggered by food, liquid, or particulate matter, this reflex commonly causes only coughing. Triggered by tissue trauma or infection, it may cause apposition of the vocal cords (laryngospasm) and associated closure of the epiglottis.

3. The *tracheal reflex* is also another vagovagal reflex. Stimulation of this reflex by local irritation or foreign bodies results in coughing (see Chapter 6).

4. The *carinal reflex*, another vagovagal reflex, causes coughing with irritation of the carina (located at the base of the trachea).

This typology has an important clinical application. With neurological impairment and gradual loss of consciousness, these reflexes become dysfunctional from the top down, e.g., first, pharyngeal, then laryngeal, and so forth; they recover in reverse order. Hence if any one reflex is absent, others below it may also be absent. For example, if a patient cannot swallow a small quantity of water, he or she may not be able to cough voluntarily or with stimulation from a suction catheter in the trachea.

The Lower Respiratory Tract

The lower respiratory tract is anatomically divided into two parts and is often labelled with different names; each name may reflect a different shade of meaning, depending on the source. This text, however, uses the following two categories because of their functional orientation:

1. *Conducting airways* (also called tracheobronchial tree).

2. *Terminal respiratory units* (also called *acinar units* or *acini* because of their grape-like or berry-like appearance, as acinus means berry in Latin; *parenchyma* (Shapiro et al, 1985); and *primary lobules*, a rarely used possibly outdated anatomical term).

The alveolar-capillary membrane and interstitial space are presented in a subsequent section on the lower respiratory tract because of their intimate structural and functional relationships to alveoli within terminal respiratory units.

LUNG ZONES

Conducting airways and terminal respiratory units lie within three zones of the lung, as follows: (1) conducting, (2) transitional, and (3) respiratory (Fig. 2–7).

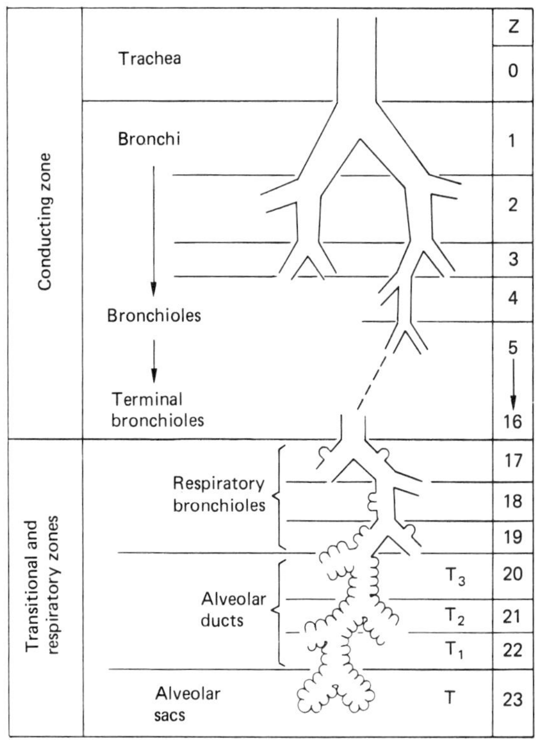

Figure 2–7. Airway generations in the human lung. (Reproduced by permission from Weibel, E.: Design and structure of the human lung. In Fishman, A. (ed.): Assessment of Pulmonary Function. New York, McGraw-Hill Book Co., 1980.)

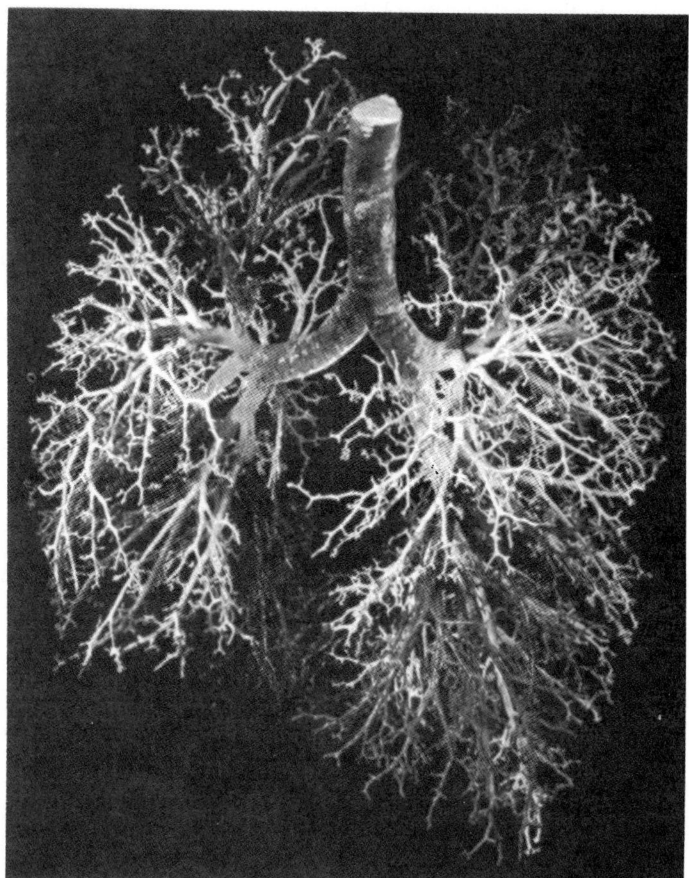

Figure 2–8. Cast of the airways of a human lung. The alveoli have been pruned away, but the conducting airways from the trachea to the terminal bronchioles can be seen. (Reproduced by permission from West, J.: Respiratory Physiology—The Essentials, 3rd ed. Baltimore, Williams & Wilkins, 1985.)

The *conducting zone* conducts air from the trachea through two main stem bronchi (primary bronchi), many secondary bronchi, and numerous bronchioles (small airways). Finally, it reaches the terminal bronchioles. Normally, the conducting zone contains 150 ml of air called the *anatomic dead space* because the air never reaches alveoli for gas exchange.

The *transitional zone* of the lung lies distal to the terminal bronchioles (see Fig. 2–7). This zone is partially lined with alveoli for gas exchange, whereas the more distal *respiratory zone* is completely lined with alveoli.

Each level of airway branching in the three lung zones represents an airway generation (abbreviated z), beginning with the main stem bronchi (z = 1) and ending with the dead-end alveolar sacs at about z = 23 in the respiratory zone.

CONDUCTING AIRWAYS

The conducting zone consists of numerous generations of conducting airways that branch in all directions (Fig. 2–8).

Special Features

Airway diameter progressively decreases with each successive airway generation. It is smallest at the lung periphery. What is unique is that a progressive *decrease* in *individual* airway diameter is accompanied by a progressive *increase* in the *total* cross-sectional areas of airway lumens. This increase is especially pronounced in small airways distal to the origin of bronchioles, as shown in Figure 2–9. This conceptual drawing compares small airways with large airways. Weibel (1973) indicates that total airway cross-section nearly doubles with each generation beyond z-16. This anatomic feature helps explain why resistance to airflow is much *less* in small airways compared with larger airways, such as the trachea and bronchi. In addition, the increase in cross-sectional area promotes the transfer of gases in alveolar sacs.

Two other features are important to keep in mind in regard to the conducting airways. First, although

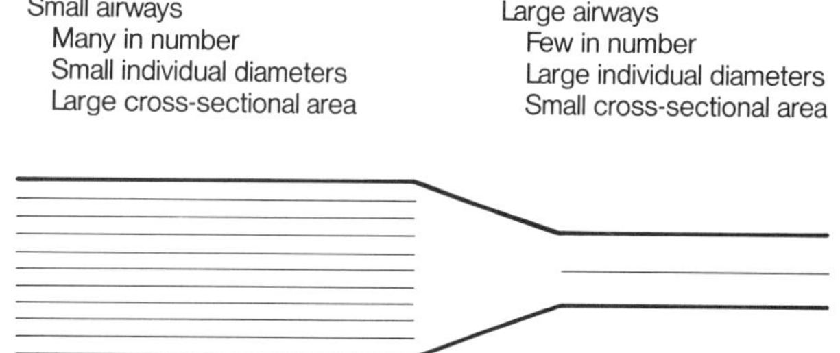

Figure 2–9. Conceptual drawing of small airways compared with large airways.

the numbers of generations in the lungs remain relatively stable among individuals, the patterns of branchings can vary greatly. Second, the length and nature of pathways to different terminal respiratory units in the same lung can vary greatly. On the one hand, pathways may be short and more irregular in central regions of the lungs. On the other hand, they tend to be longer and straighter to distal areas of the lung, with larger cross-sectional areas. This feature helps explain why many infective droplets tend to be deposited in the lung periphery rather than in more central locations.

Major Airways

Trachea. The trachea (z = 0) or "windpipe" is a tubular passageway about 12 cm (4.5 in) in length and 2.5 cm (1 in) in diameter. Located in front of the esophagus, it extends from the cricoid cartilage of the larynx to about the level of the fifth thoracic vertebra, where it divides at the *carina* into right and left main bronchi (Fig. 2–10A).

The tracheal walls are composed of 16 to 20 C-shaped hyaline cartilages connected together by a fibroelastic membrane. These cartilaginous rings vary somewhat in width and thickess *within* individuals and in general shape *among* individuals. The rings give the trachea its rigid structure. The noncartilaginous, open segment of the C-shaped structure points posteriorly towards the esophagus (Fig. 2–11). Here, smooth muscle (musculus trachealis) is embedded in the fibroelastic membrane, allowing the esophagus to expand into the trachea during swallowing and the airway to narrow during coughing. The latter action serves to increase the velocity of expiratory air flow and to create a shearing force during coughing for dislodging material lying on mucosal surfaces.

Right and Left Main Stem Bronchi. The right main stem bronchus (primary bronchi or z = 1) leads to the right lung, and the left main stem bronchus leads to the left lung. The right one is shorter (2.5 cm in length) and wider than the left one (5 cm in length). The right main stem bronchus sometimes appears as an extension of the trachea, as it forms about a 25-

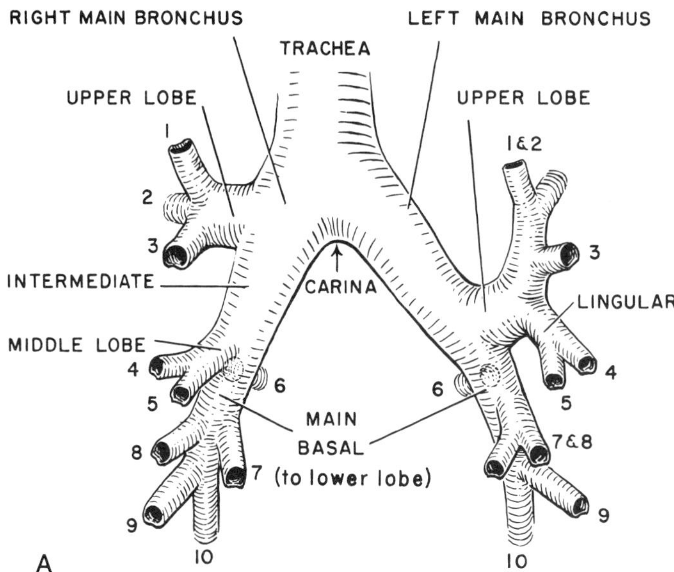

Figure 2–10. Major airways, lobes, and bronchopulmonary segments of the lungs.

A, The trachea leading to the right and left main stem bronchi and, finally, to segmental bronchi (numbered as listed).

Right Lung	Left Lung
Upper lobe	Upper lobe
1. apical	1&2. apical posterior
2. posterior	3. anterior
3. anterior	4. superior lingular
Middle lobe	5. inferior lingular
4. lateral	Lower lobe
5. medial	6. superior
Lower lobe	7&8. anteromedial basal
6. superior	9. lateral basal
7. medial basal	10. posterior basal
8. anterior basal	
9. lateral basal	
10. posterior basal	

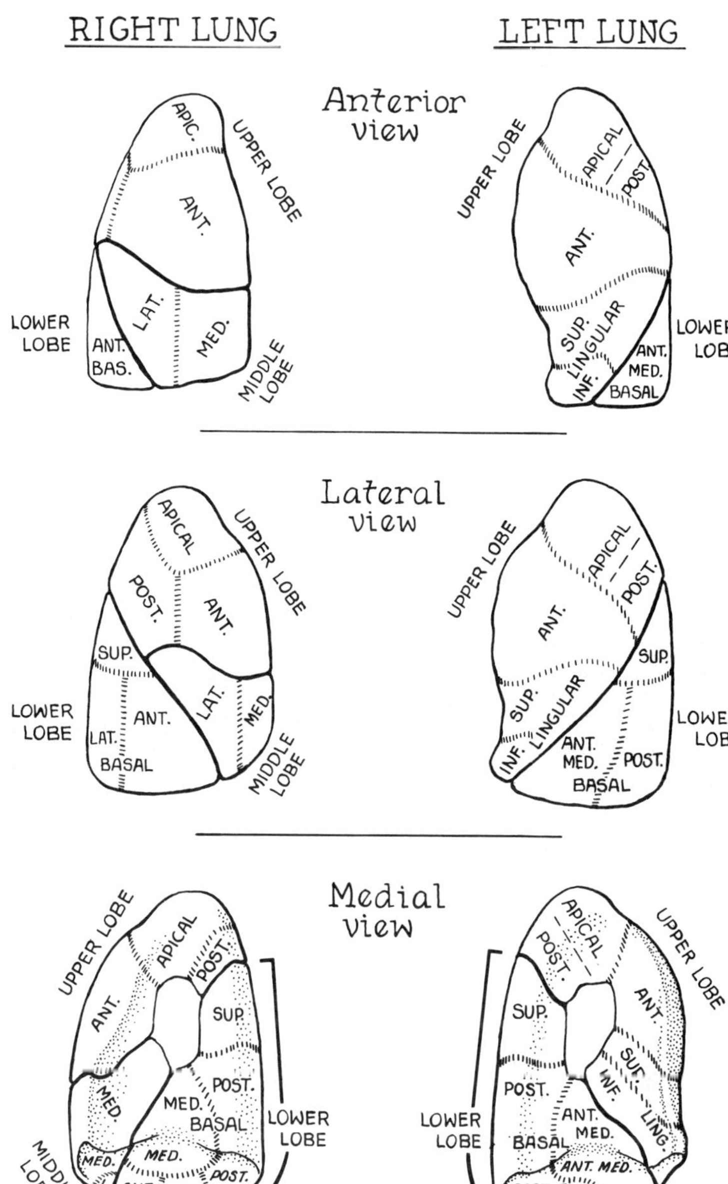

Figure 2–10 *Continued B*, Bronchopulmonary segments of right and left lungs. (Reproduced with permission from Johnson, J., et al.: Surgery of the Chest, 4th ed. Copyright © 1970 by Year Book Medical Publishers, Inc. Chicago.)

degree angle with the vertical axis. The left main stem bronchus forms a larger angle of about 40 to 60 degrees. These angles vary from person to person, depending on body build.

In spite of variations among individuals, however, the right main stem bronchus almost always has a more vertical orientation compared with the left bronchus within the same individual. In the clinical setting, this fact accounts for the more frequent passage of suction catheter tips into the right rather than left bronchus for aspiration of pulmonary secretions. In addition, it is the cause of the more frequent aspiration of food and foreign bodies into the right rather than the left lung.

Lobar and Segmental Bronchi. The right main stem bronchus divides into three branches on the right that serve the upper, middle, and lower lobes of the right lung. The left main bronchus divides into only two lobar bronchi that serve the upper and lower lobes on that side. Each lobar bronchus, in turn, gives rise to *segmental bronchi*. Those bronchi are named according to the *bronchopulmonary segment* each bronchus supplies (see Fig. 2–10).

Knowledge of lobar and segmental bronchi is important in the application of various respiratory therapy procedures, such as postural drainage (see Chapter 19). The secondary bronchi are $z = 2$ and the tertiary bronchi are $z = 3$. Note in Figure 2–10A that the general arrangement of bronchi in the right and left lungs is similar, with one major exception. In the right

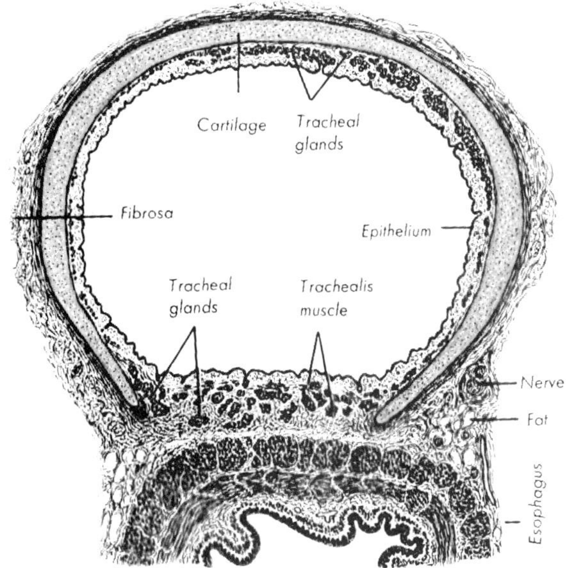

Figure 2–11. Transverse section through midregion of trachea and adjacent part of esophagus. The section is through a cartilage ring of a woman 35 years old. (×5) (Reproduced by permission from Copenhaver, W. M., et al.: Bailey's Textbook of Microscopic Anatomy, 18th ed. Baltimore, Williams & Wilkins, 1984.)

lung, the intermediate bronchus gives rise to middle lobe and lower lobe (main basal) bronchi. No middle lobe bronchus exists in the left lung because the left lung does not have a middle lobe. Its lingular segments are comparable to the right lung's middle lobe. With this fact in mind, note that the lingular segmental bronchi originate from the upper lobe bronchus rather than the main stem bronchus.

Histological Features of Conducting Airways

Conducting airways are not passive structures. They expand and contract with inspiration and expiration; they secrete substances, mucus being the major one; and they actively respond to neurohumoral and chemical stimuli. Knowledge of the histologic features of the conducting airways and terminal respiratory units serve as a basis for understanding these capacities. The following discussion presents the basic histology of the conducting zone in particular.

Histological Layers. The walls of the trachea and main bronchi have three main histological layers: mucosa, submucosa, and adventitia (Fig. 2–12 and Table 2–2).

Mucosa. This layer is lined with ciliated pseudostratified columnar epithelium that extends down from the

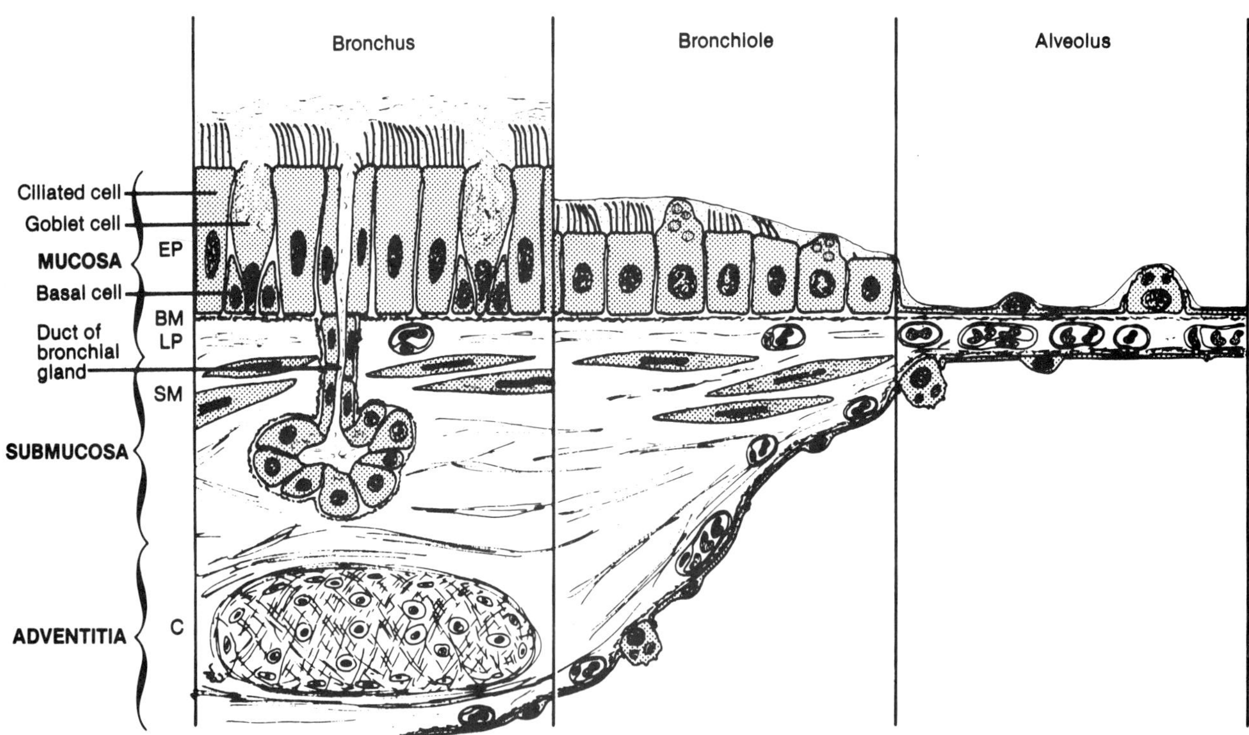

Figure 2–12. Histologic changes in airway wall structure at bronchial, bronchiolar, and alveolar levels. EP = epithelium; BM = basement membrane; LP = lamina propria; SM = smooth muscle fibers; C = cartilage. (Reproduced and adapted by permission from Weibel, E. and Burri, P.: Funktionelle aspekte der lungenmorphologie. Aktuelle probleme der roentgendiagnostik, vol. 2. In Fuchs, W. and Voegeli, E. (eds.). Bern, Huber, 1973.)

Table 2–2. MAIN HISTOLOGICAL FEATURES OF CONDUCTING AIRWAYS AND TERMINAL RESPIRATORY UNITS

	Conducting Airways				Terminal Respiratory Units (Acinar Units)		
*Generation Numbers (Z)**	*0*	*1* *Conducting Zone*	*5*	*16*	*17* *Transitional Zone*	*20* *Respiratory Zone*	*23*
Histological Feature	TRACHEA	BRONCHI	BRONCHIOLES	TERMINAL BRONCHIOLES	RESPIRATORY BRONCHIOLES	ALVEOLAR DUCTS	ALVEOLAR SACS
Epithelium	ciliated pseudostratified columnar →		ciliated simple columnar →		ciliated and nonciliated simple cuboidal →		
					←	simple squamous lining alveoli →	
Goblet cells	← numerous →			absent (present here only in smokers)— replaced by nonciliated Clara cells →			
Smooth muscle	posterior muscle band connects end of C-shaped cartilage rings →	becomes a separate layer beyond main bronchi →		most prominent here —	thinner —	muscle fibers in alveolar ducts →	absent
Bronchial glands	← most numerous in medium-sized bronchi →		absent				
Cartilage	thick C- or U-shaped rings —	irregular plates and islands →	absent				
Connective tissue	separates trachea from esophagus →	forms a sheath around cartilaginous airways and adjacent vessels →	ensheaths smooth muscle layer and is firmly and directly attached to adjacent lung parenchyma →			forms a delicate lattice in alveolar septa →	

*See airway generations in Figure 2–7.

upper airways. It has three main cell types, as follows: (1) *ciliated cells* that line the mucosal surface; (2) *goblet cells* that rest on a basement membrane and secrete mucus onto mucosal surfaces; and (3) *basal cells* that are not known to have a special function but can differentiate and replace superficial ciliated and goblet cells. The epithelium rests on a thick layer of loose connective tissue (lamina propria) that contains significant amounts of elastic and reticular fibers and lymphoid cells.

Submucosa. This loose connective tissue layer contains *bronchial glands*, sometimes called *submucosal* or *seromucous glands.* These sac-like structures are lined with serous, mucous, and other cells. Innervated by parasympathetic nerve fibers, they secrete seromucous substances that are evacuated via long ducts projecting through the mucosa to the mucosal surface. *Mast cells,* important in the pathogenesis of asthma, are found in the submucosa as well as the adventitia. Sometimes these cells migrate to the mucosa.

Adventitia. This layer is composed of cartilage and dense connective tissue. It serves as a protective *fibrous coat* around the airway.

Changes in Histologic Layers. The aforementioned histologic arrangement varies as airways become progressively smaller. The bronchial wall gradually thins out to simple squamous epithelium at the alveolar level, as illustrated in Figure 2–12. Important airway changes responsible for this thinning process are summarized next and diagrammed in Table 2–2.

1. Tracheal C-shaped cartilages become irregular plates and islands in lobar bronchi and disappear completely in bronchioles, where airway caliber decreases to 1 mm (Fig. 2–13).

2. Bronchial glands disappear along with cartilage, making goblet cells the sole producers of mucus at the bronchiolar level in the conducting zone of the lung.

3. Smooth muscle forms an oblique crisscross pattern around airways, such that muscle contraction results primarily in narrowing of the lumen.

4. The mucosae of bronchioles normally have longitudinal folds due to the absence of cartilage and the proportional increase in muscle and elastic fiber at this level. With smooth muscle contraction, these pliable mucosal folds press inwards, significantly narrowing the lumen and obstructing the airflow in the presence of respiratory disease, e.g., asthma (Fig. 2–13C).

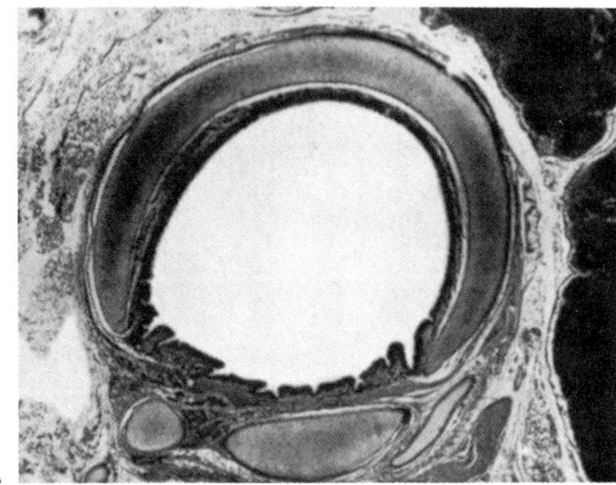

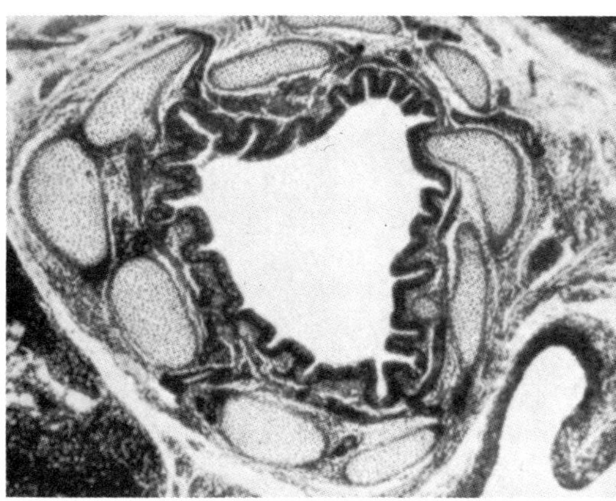

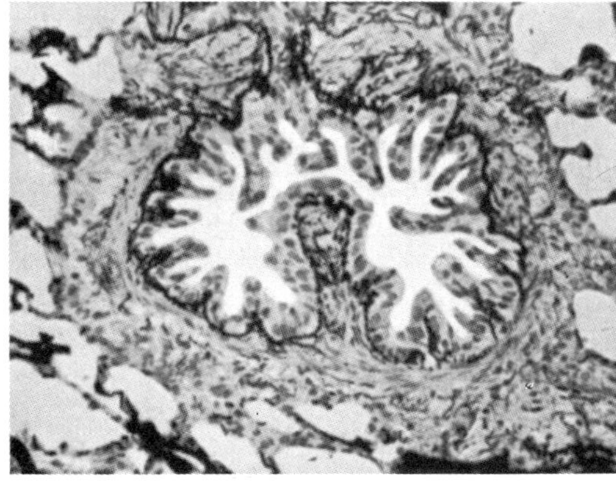

Figure 2–13. Cross section of large and small bronchi. *A,* C-shaped cartilage in a *main stem bronchus* (×20). *B,* Several plaques or islands of cartilage in the wall of a *lobar bronchus* (×40). *C,* Absence of cartilage in a partly bronchoconstricted *small bronchiole* of a rat (×180). (*A* and *B* reproduced by permission from Towers, B.: The muscle-cartilage relationship in the extrapulmonary bronchi. J. Anat., 87:337–344, 1953, and Cambridge University Press. *C* reproduced by permission from Comroe, J.: Physiology of Respiration, 2nd ed. Chicago, Year Book Medical Publishers, Inc., 1974. Courtesy of Dr. Sorokin.)

Tracheobronchial Surface Lining

Cilia and mucus compose the most superficial histologic layer in the conducting zone of the lung. Together, they line tracheobronchial epithelial surfaces and serve as a major defense mechanism of the lower respiratory tract, as described subsequently.

Cilia. The conducting zone of the lung as well as most of the upper airway is lined with numerous hair-like cilia, arising from ciliated cells. Their length and large numbers (about 200/ciliated cell) make lumenal surfaces look like "shag rugs" under the electron microscope (Fig. 2–14). These cilia are constantly active and beat at a very high rate, measured at about 14 beats/sec for nasal, tracheal and lobar airways, and about 10 beats/sec for more peripheral subsegmental airways (Rutland et al, 1982).

Mucus. Cilia are completely covered with an unin

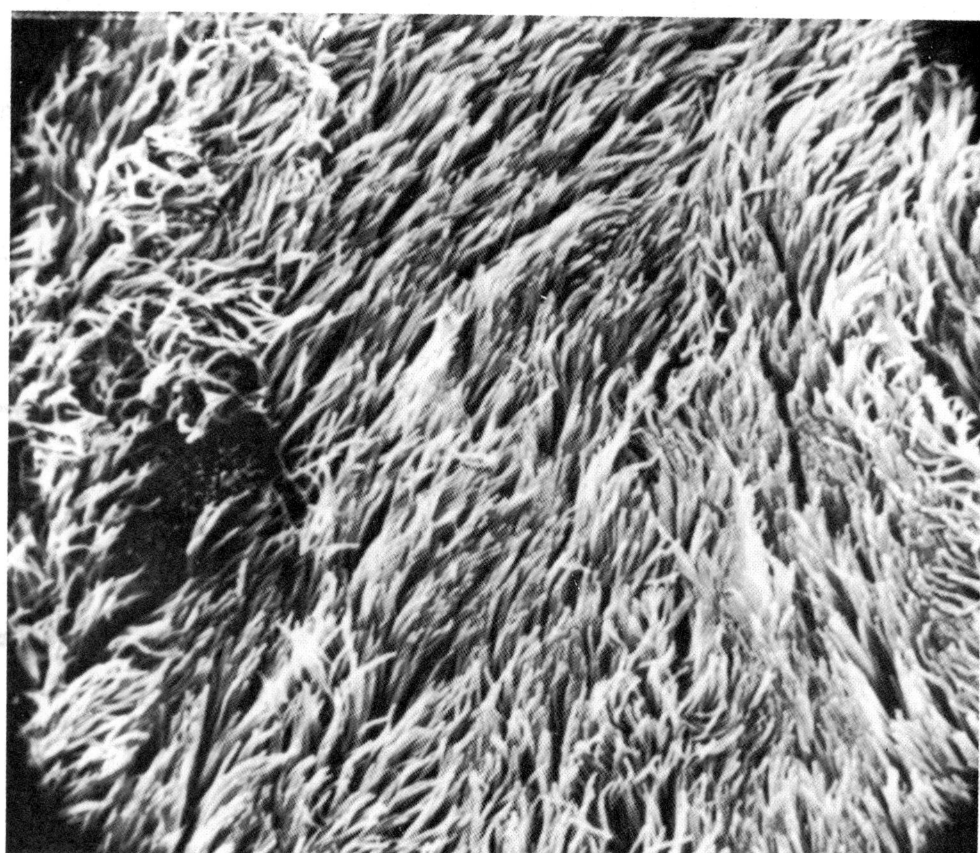

Figure 2–14. Scanning electron photomicrograph of *ciliated epithelium* from a healthy adult bronchiole. Several cells with numerous cilia surround a nonciliated cell on the left-hand side of the photomicrograph. (Reproduced by permission from Hinshaw H. and Murray, J.: Diseases of the Chest, 4th ed. Philadelphia, W. B. Saunders Co., 1980.)

terrupted blanket of mucus secreted by the goblet cells and bronchial glands beneath mucosal surfaces. Bronchial glands, the chief source of mucus in bronchi, produce about 100 ml of secretions per day to maintain this blanket. The mucus that constitutes this blanket consists of 95% water, 2% glycoprotein, 1% carbohydrate, a trace of lipid and deoxyribonucleic acid (DNA), cellular debris, and other foreign particles (Shapiro et al, 1985). The composition and the associated physical properties can change greatly in the presence of pulmonary and cardiac disease.

Mucous-lined epithelial surfaces are actually composed of two layers, as follows: (1) an inner liquid *sol layer* and (2) an outer viscous *gel layer* (Fig. 2–15). The latter is nonabsorbent to water, serves to protect the sol layer from drying up, and traps and carries particles along its sticky surface.

Mucociliary Escalator. Within the sol layer, the rapidly beating cilia demonstrate a characteristic biphasic stroke—a fast forward flick followed by a slow backward movement. The fast forward flick extends the cilia so that their tips just strike the innermost portion of the gel layer (see Fig. 2–15). During the slow backward movement, cilia fold back on themselves, sinking towards the bottom of the sol layer. Because this biphasic stroke creates a forward wave of surface motion with little backward pull, mucus and other particles stuck within the mucosal surface are continuously propelled towards the mouth at an average rate of 2.15 cm/min (compared with 0.48 cm/min in nasal passages). In the upper airway, secretions are either swallowed, expectorated, or expelled by blowing the nose.

Because mucus and particles stuck to it are constantly propelled forward towards the mouth, this important defense mechanism is often referred to as the *mucociliary escalator.* Dysfunction of this mechanism is responsible for many of the physiologic problems associated with respiratory disease, such as mucus retention and chest infection.

TERMINAL RESPIRATORY UNITS (ACINAR UNITS)

The *terminal respiratory unit (TRU), acinar unit,* or *acinus* is considered the basic unit of the lung just as the nephron is considered the basic unit of the kidney. The TRU consists of all structures distal to the terminal bronchiole (Fig. 2–16).

The following description traces the pathway that

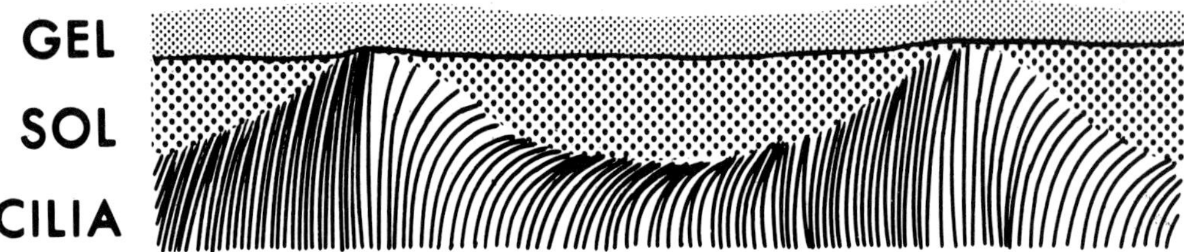

Figure 2–15. Schematic respresentation of the mucociliary escalator. (Reproduced by permission from Hinshaw, H. and Murray, J.: Diseases of the Chest, 4th ed. Philadelphia, W. B. Saunders Co., 1980. Modified from Hilding, A. C.: Trans. Am. Acad. Ophthal. Otolaryngol. 65:475, 1961.)

gas must travel to reach the *alveolus,* the most distal structure within the TRU. When air enters the TRU, it first passes through two to five generations or orders of *respiratory bronchioles,* the last one leading to two to five orders of short alveolar ducts. Then, the last alveolar duct empties through an *atrium* into one to three, dead-end, dome-shaped *alveolar sacs.* Each curvature within the wall of the labelled alveolar sac in Figure 2–16 represents an alveolus. Alveoli completely line alveolar sacs and extend proximally to the alveolar ducts (six to eight alveoli line each duct in cross-sectional view) and to distal generations of respiratory bronchioles.

Most important, it is the alveolus that gives the TRU its gas exchange function. Structures that are completely alveolarized make up the respiratory zone of the lung, consisting of alveolar ducts, alveolar sacs, and alveoli. Because respiratory bronchioles are only partially alveolarized, they compose the transitional zone of the lung, a zone with both air conduction and gas exchange as primary functions.

Other Lung Units and Terminology Problems

The TRU defines lung tissue in terms of conducting airways or bronchial tree. Two other terms—*parenchyma* and *lobule*—define the lung somewhat differently. It is useful to define these terms because practitioners tend to confuse them and one then is given an appreciation of other gross aspects of the lung and the TRU not yet mentioned.

Parenchyma. The word parenchyma comes from a Greek word meaning "visceral flesh." Webster's Third New International Dictionary defines it as "the essential and distinctive tissue of an organ." Some sources equate the term parenchyma with TRU, as defined in this text. Others use parenchyma interchangeably with the term acinus and define it as a unit in which *all* airways participate in gas exchange (Weibel, 1973). Theoretically, this usage eliminates most if not all first-order respiratory bronchioles, since they lie within the transitional zone of the lung. While experts continue to debate this definitional problem, many pulmonary clinicians continue to use the word parenchyma with its general, visceral flesh meaning.

A close look at lung parenchyma through an electron microscope gives one an appreciation of the three-dimensional nature of the TRU within the lung. First, review the TRU structures in Figure 2–17. Then, study the more detailed electron micrograph of human lung parenchyma in Figure 2–18. Note that in reality, TRUs are not well defined. They are not unidirectional—they appear to be traveling in all directions. The way they interdigitate has been likened to a three-dimensional jigsaw puzzle. Alveoli are back to back, separated from each other by thin walls (septa). As previously mentioned, alveoli do in fact completely line the alveolar duct, as shown in the middle of the micrograph. This micrograph describes the essence of the lung very well.

Lobule. Whereas the TRU is described as the basic structural unit of the lung, the *lobule* (secondary lobule) is often mentioned as the primary *functional* unit of the lung. Actually, the *primary lobule,* another possibly outdated term, is considered to be the functional unit of the lung. It is defined as lung parenchyma supplied by a first-order alveolar duct, including accompanying vessels and nerves. This unit cannot be visualized radiologically and has little if any practical

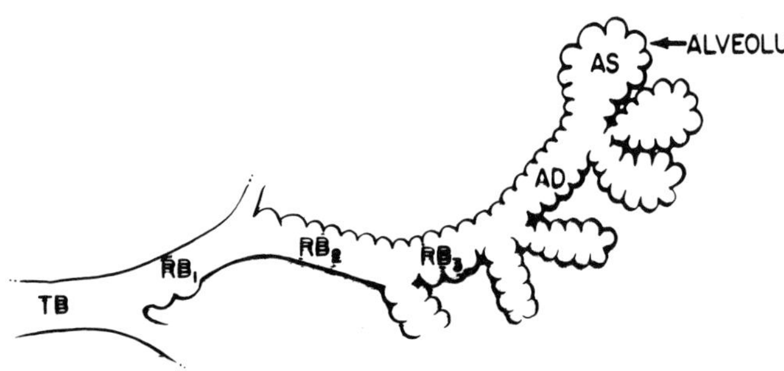

Figure 2–16. A terminal respiratory unit (acinar unit). TB = terminal bronchiole; RB = respiratory bronchiole; AD = alveolar duct; AS = alveolar sac. (Reproduced by permission from Thurlbeck, W.: Chronic Obstructive Lung Disease. In Sommers, S. (ed.): Pathology Annual. New York, Appleton-Century-Crofts, 1968.)

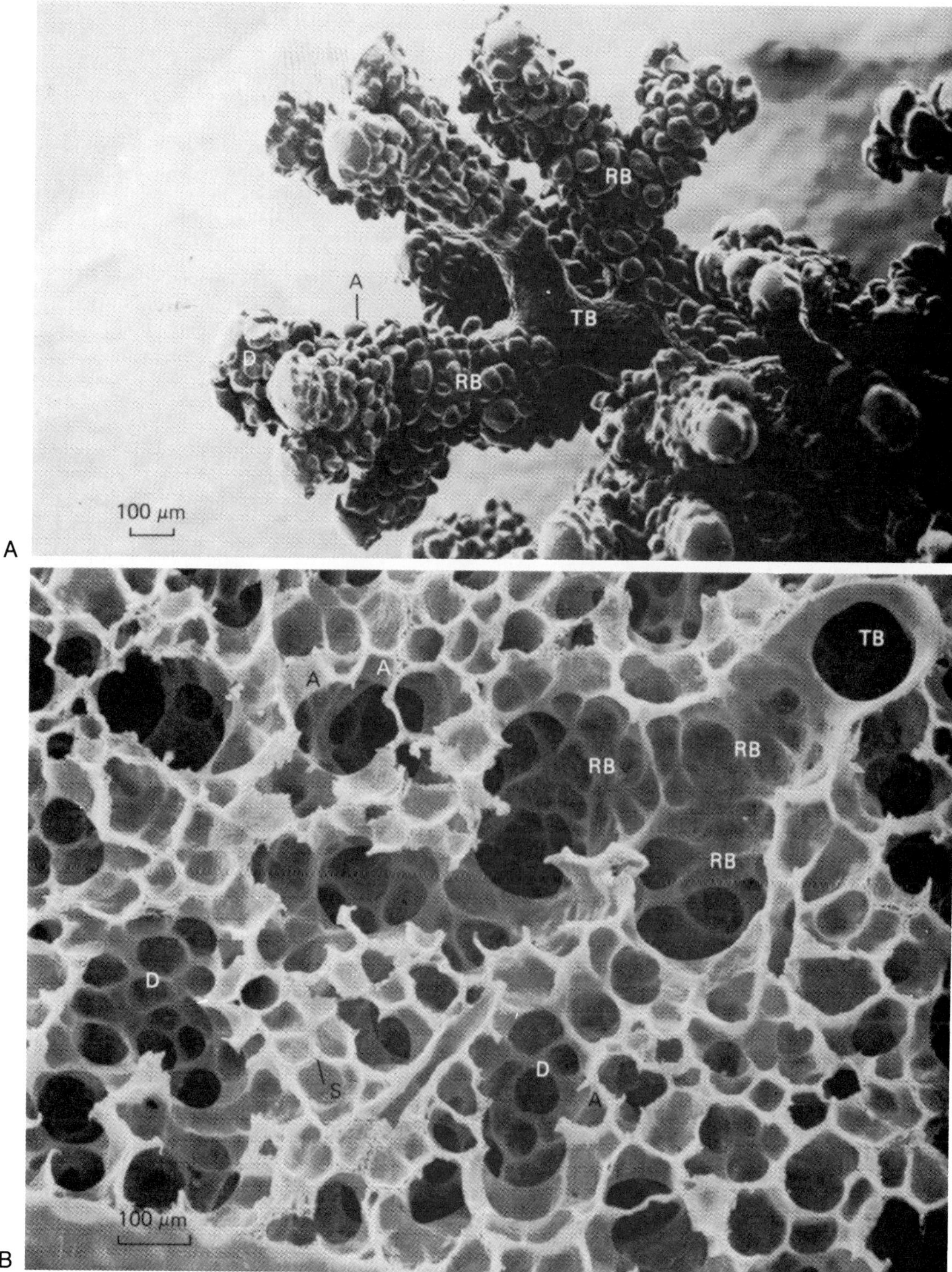

Figure 2–17. Scanning electron micrographs of airway branches peripheral to terminal bronchiole. *A*, In silicone-rubber cast of cat lung. *B*, In whole-tissue preparation of air-filled, perfusion-fixed rabbit lung. Note that branching can be followed from terminal bronchiole to alveolar ducts. A = alveolus; D = alveolar duct; RB = respiratory bronchiole; TB = terminal bronchiole; S = alveolar septum. (Reproduced by permission from Weibel, E.: Design and Structure of the Human Lung. In *Assessment of Pulmonary Function.* (Fishman, A., ed.) New York, McGraw-Hill Book Co., 1980.)

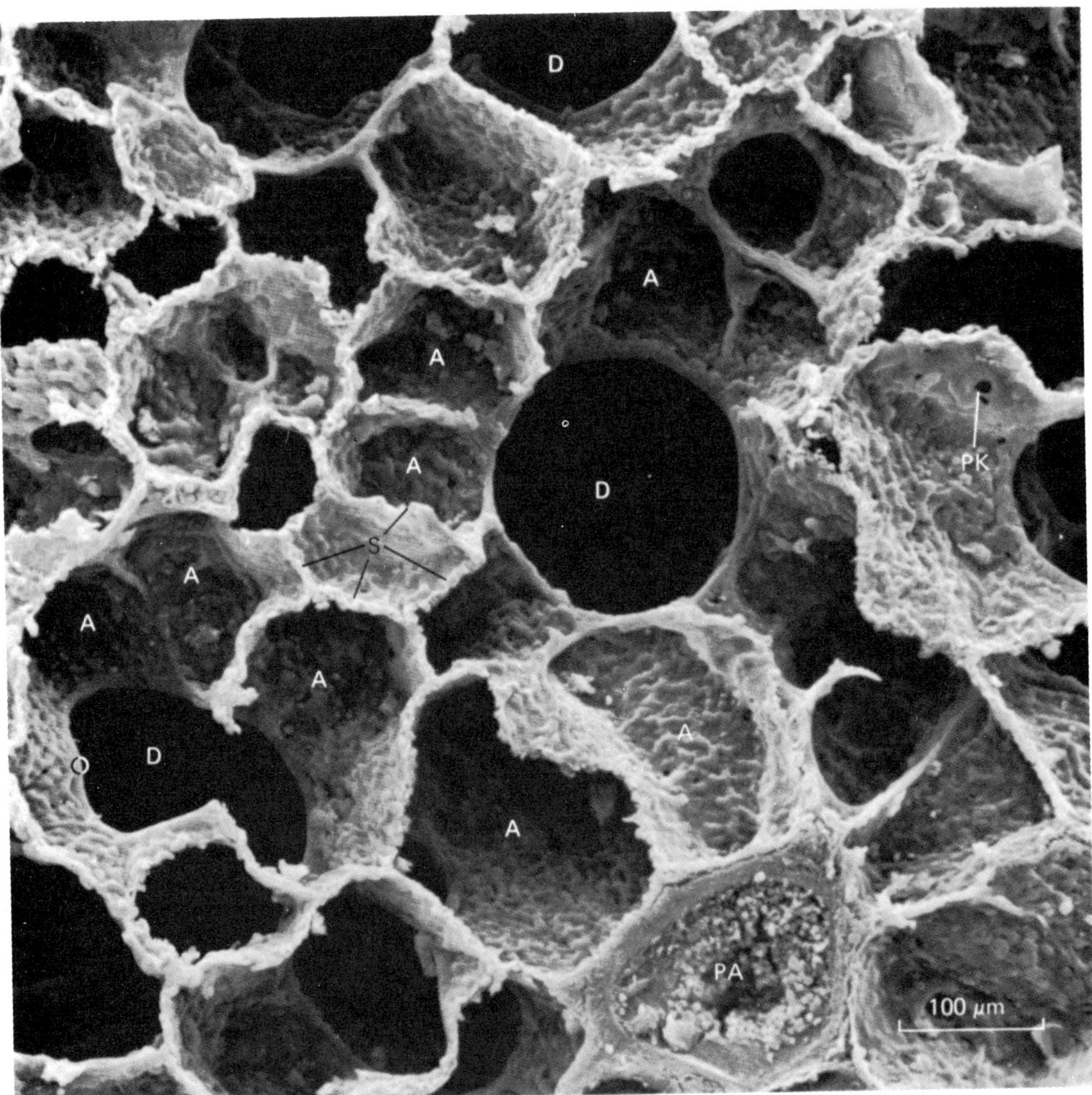

Figure 2–18. Scanning electron micrograph of human lung parenchyma. Alveolar ducts (D) are surrounded by alveoli (A) that are separated by thin septa (S). Note small branch of pulmonary artery (PA). PK = interalveolar pore of Kohn. (Reproduced by permission from Weibel, E.: Design and Structure of the Human Lung. In *Assessment of Pulmonary Function.* (Fishman, A., ed.) New York, McGraw-Hill Book Co., 1980.)

significance. About 30 to 50 primary lobules make up a secondary lobule, the number varying with the size of the secondary lobules. Because the lobule's structural and functional aspects have few practical applications in the clinical setting, it is considered an outdated term. Nevertheless, lobule is mentioned here for clarification of terms. Also, certain aspects about the lobule help one understand the structure and function of the lung as well as the radiological assessment.

The lobule consists of a cluster of three to five terminal bronchioles and their TRUs and is considered the smallest discrete portion of lung surrounded by connective tissue septum. It is roughly 1 to 2 cm in size and pyramidal in shape, with the apex of the pyramid pointing towards the center of the lung (Fig. 2–19).

In contrast to lobes, which are the only lung portions *completely* encased by connective tissue, the *interlobular septa* that separate adjacent lobules are incomplete in places. Because of this feature, lobules exist in discrete form only on the lung surface. They become difficult to define towards the center of the lung.

Lobules are considered important functional units of the lung because pulmonary vessels show a characteristic relationship to them. Whereas pulmonary arteries follow major airways towards the lung periphery, pulmonary veins (with adjacent lymphatic channels) take a different course and follow interlobular septa towards the center of the lung, collecting blood from

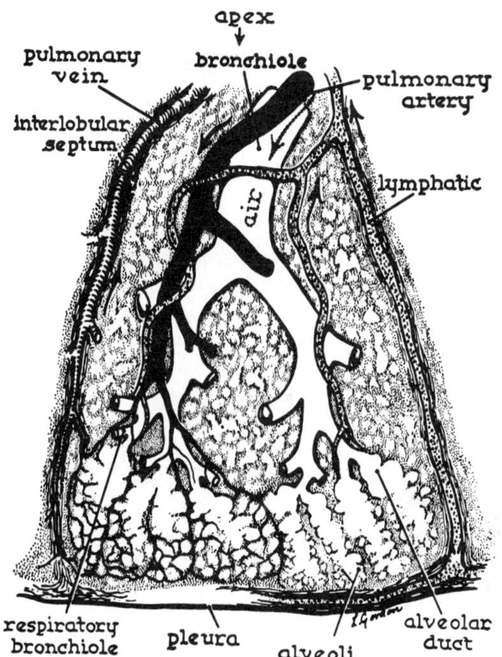

Figure 2–19. Diagram of a lobule of the lung with its base abutting on the pleura. The sizes of the bronchioles and air passages, as well as those of the blood vessels and lymphatics, have been exaggerated for clarity. To make it easier to follow the course of the blood vessels and lymphatics, the former have been omitted from the *right side,* and the latter from the *left side.* (Reproduced by permission from Ham, A. and Cormack, D.: Histology, 8th ed. Philadelphia, J. B. Lippincott Co., 1979.)

adjacent lobules and TRUs along the way (see Fig. 4–5B and Chapter 4). From this particular perspective, the lobule is important for its provision of venous and lymphatic drainage.

Two other aspects are of significance. First, the lobule's interlobular septa are part of the lung *interstitium,* which provides crucial mechanical support for the lung during breathing, as described subsequently. Second and of radiologic importance, interlobular septa have certain patterns. They are more numerous over certain areas of the lung, e.g., lateral and anterior surfaces of the lower lobe; they are virtually nonexistent over other areas, e.g., along interlobar fissures, posterior and mediastinal aspects of the lung; and they are poorly developed in the central portion of the lung. On the chest x-ray, the presence or absence of septa in various lung regions helps to diagnose the presence or absence of cardiopulmonary disease.

Histologic Features of Alveoli

Since the TRU as a unit has been presented and contrasted with other lung units, histologic features of alveoli lining its respiratory zone are discussed.

Alveoli are extremely small structures only 200 to 300 μm in diameter. The lungs of one person contain about 300 million alveoli, and values as high as 500 million have been found. Specifics about the structure and function of alveoli are discussed subsequently.

Alveolar Space. The lumen or air space of an alveolus is referred to as the *alveolar space* (AS) (Fig. 2–20). Many chest diseases become manifest on chest x-ray films primarily within this space and hence are called *alveolar diseases,* e.g., alveolar pulmonary edema.

Type I and Type II Cells. The alveolar epithelium is composed of two main cell types, as follows: *Type I cells,* also called *squamous pneumocytes;* and *Type II cells,* also called *granular pneumocytes.*

Most of the alveolar surface is lined with Type I cells. They are flat squamous cells with cytoplasmic extensions that cover about 95% of the alveolar surface. Type II cells are usually situated in the angles or corners of alveoli. Although quantitative analyses have shown that they occur in equal or greater numbers compared with Type I cells, they cover less than 5% of the alveolar surface because of their irregular, cuboidal shape and more vertical orientation (see Fig. 2–20) (Weibel, 1973, and Murray, 1985).

Surfactant. Type II cells are believed to be the chief producers of *surfactant,* a phospholipid film made primarily of the compound *dipalmitoyl-lecithin.* This substance has the amazing property of progressively lowering the surface tension, as the surface area becomes smaller. In the lung, it lowers alveolar surface tension during expiration, a time when surface resistive forces are greatest. This action prevents alveoli from continuing to contract and collapse, as they become smaller. In contrast during inspiration, the increase in alveolar surface area prompts surfactant to produce a higher surface tension. This action helps to limit expansion and promote reduction in volume. These changes in surfactant surface tension during respiration promote alveolar and lung mechanical stability. Normal lung function depends on the continuous production and secretion of this vital substance. Surfactant deficiency has been suggested as a cause of alveolar collapse in many respiratory disorders and is associated with a number of factors, e.g., the cardiopulmonary by-pass machine, the prolonged inhalation of 100% oxygen, and adult and infant respiratory distress syndromes.

The Alveolar Macrophage and Macrophage Transport. Macrophages are phagocytic cells that line alveolar extracellular surfaces (Fig. 2–21). They are important cells because of their chief role in the clearance of particles from TRUs that settle on alveolar surfaces. Foreign particles, small enough to reach TRUs, are about 2 μm in diameter, although tiny particles 0.5 μm in diameter are also retained in great numbers because they more easily diffuse to distal sites before impaction. When the load of particles or dust is light, macrophages eliminate most by digestion, transportation along the alveolar surface to the beginning of the mucociliary escalator, or both. From there, the macrophages and their particles are propelled to the oropharynx and swallowed. Sometimes, the macrophages

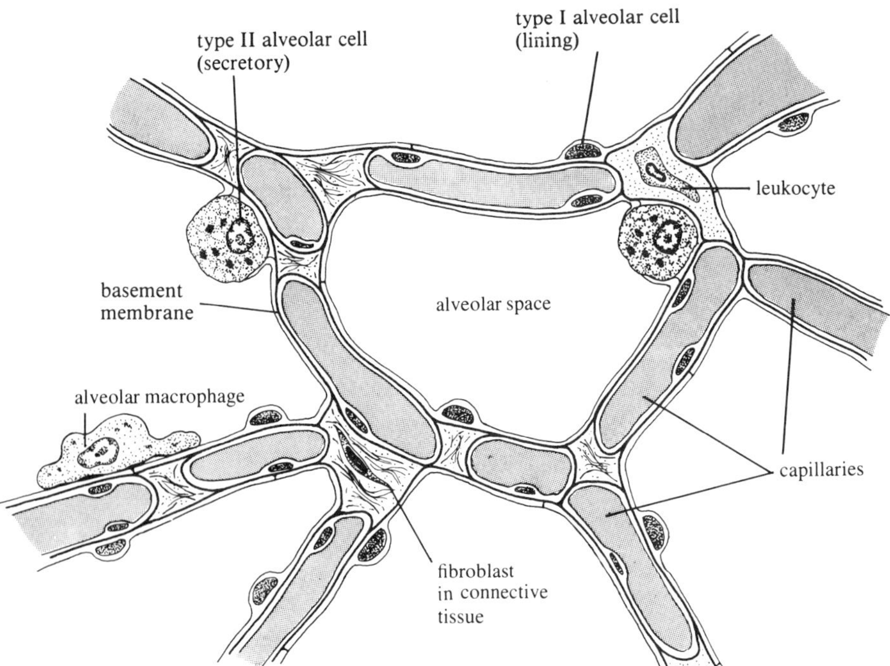

Figure 2–20. An electron microscopic representation of the walls of several alveoli, showing the alveolar membrane, capillaries, and associated cells. (Reproduced by permission from Borysenko, M. and Beringer, T.: Functional Histology, 2nd ed. Boston, Little, Brown & Co., 1979.)

take a "short cut" and pass through interalveolar septa to larger bronchioles. When particulate load is heavy, macrophages become overwhelmed and particles enter adjacent lymphatic channels and sometimes reach the blood stream. Dysfunction of this so-called *macrophage transport system* is believed to contribute to the pathogenesis of pulmonary infections (Murray, 1985).

Kohn's Pores. Alveolar surfaces are interrupted in places by interalveolar pores or openings called *Kohn's pores* (see Fig. 2–21). The diameter of these pores varies from 3 to 13 μm, and the width is about 2 μm, the thickness of the alveolar septum (between capillaries). Although the pores are often occluded by extracellular surface-lining material, they are believed to provide collateral channels for gas movement between contiguous alveoli. This collateral movement of gas helps to equilibrate air pressure within lobules and to guard against alveolar collapse. However, this type of movement also provides a vehicle for the spread of infection throughout the lung parenchyma.

Other Collateral Channels. Alveoli may communicate directly with respiratory bronchioles, terminal bronchioles, or possibly larger airways through intercommunicating channels called *Lambert's canals.* Kohn's pores, Lambert's canals, and other postulated channels are believed to be responsible for significant *collateral air drift* or alveolar ventilation other than

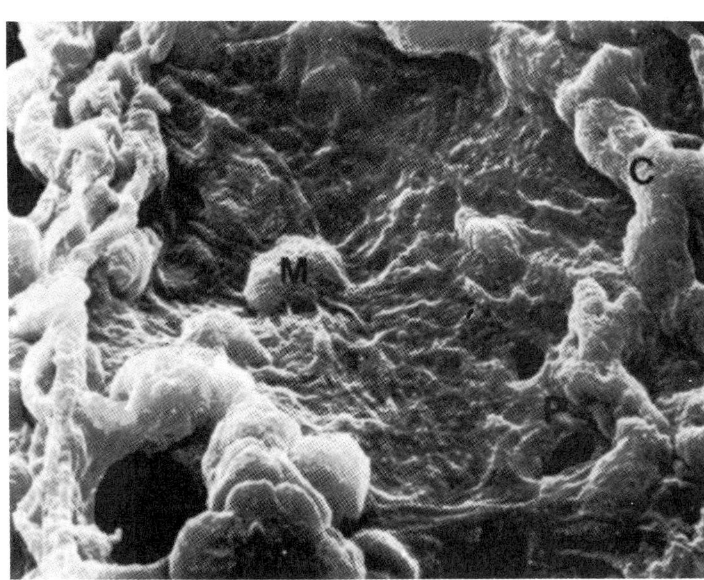

Figure 2–21. Surface of an alveolus. Note surrounding capillaries (C), a macrophage (M), and alveolar pores (P). (Scanning electron microscope, ×3650.) (Courtesy of Dr. Nai San Wang, McGill University, Montreal. Reproduced by permission from Fraser, R. and Paré, J.: Diagnosis of Diseases of the Chest, 4th ed. Philadelphia, W. B. Saunders Co., 1977.)

by established airway connections. However, little is known about the number, location, and extent of these channels or about the extent to which they actually contribute to alveolar ventilation in the human lung.

Capillaries in Interalveolar Septa. Many structures and substances lie within the walls or *septa* between alveoli, such as connective tissue, fluid, leukocytes, and wandering macrophages. However, an alveolar cross-sectional view proves that, unquestionably, the pulmonary capillary is the predominant structure (see Fig. 2–20). Each capillary consists of a tubular sheath of endothelial cells with plasma and red blood cells (erythrocytes) within its lumen. These structures form a dense network in alveolar septa, often bulging from beneath epithelial surfaces into alveolar spaces (see Fig. 2–21). Contact of alveolar surfaces with capillary surfaces forms the *alveolar-capillary membrane.*

ALVEOLAR-CAPILLARY MEMBRANE

One basic structural feature of the lung is the extraordinary reduction of tissue mass to a thin sheet—the alveolar-capillary membrane—so that air and blood come into intimate and extensive contact. Yet while tissue mass is reduced, the surface area of this thin membrane is immense; consider these figures. At the end of maximum inspiration, lung volume consists of 80% air, 10% blood, and only 10% tissue. This small amount of tissue is spread over 100 to 200 m^2, the size of a tennis court (Weibel, 1973). Murray (1985) reports that alveolar surface area is about 80 m^2, and 85% to 95% of this is in contact with pulmonary capillaries. This architectural design facilitates gas exchange, particularly when the body's demand for oxygen is high.

Thin Side or Air-Blood Barrier

The alveolar-capillary membrane is divided into two regions, as follows: (1) a "thin" side and (2) a "thick" side of the interalveolar septum (Fig. 2–22). The thin side is where the capillary surface bulges into the alveolar space and where alveolar and capillary basement membranes become fused into one thin layer. Although gas exchange occurs through many different layers here (Table 2–3), the distance is small (about 0.5 μ) and the pathway direct. These features explain why this thin side, formally called the *air-blood barrier*, is the primary site for gas exchange in the lung.

Thick Side with the Interstitial Space

The thick side of the alveolar-capillary membrane is where the alveolar basement membrane and the capillary basement membrane are separated by the interstitial space (see Fig. 2–22 and Table 2–3). The interstitial space of interalveolar septa is made of connective tissue, mostly *elastic fibers, collagen fibrils*, and *fibroblasts* and is drained by lymphatic channels. Because this space dramatically increases the distance and density through which gases must travel to penetrate the alveolar capillary membrane, the thick side is not conducive to gas exchange. It is known as the primary site for liquid and solute exchange in the lung, although some gas exchange may take place here as well.

THE INTERSTITIAL SPACE—WHERE IS IT ANYWAY?

Students may have difficulty understanding exactly where the interstitial space is located, especially when it is omitted or unlabelled in simplified medical illustrations. From an anatomical viewpoint, confusion is understandable because interstitial connective tissue forms more of a meshwork rather than a continuous sheet of tissue. Capillaries wind back and forth through the interstitial space of the interalveolar septum, forming a thin side at one site and a thick side at another.

Furthermore, the interstitial space as described connects directly with a more centrally located peribronchial/perivascular connective tissue sheath with its own adjacent interstitial spaces. Each bronchus travels peripherally within a sheath or sleeve of connective tissue that encloses the bronchus, its adjacent pulmonary artery, its lymphatics, and the (potential) interstitial space.

Whenever extra fluid accumulates in the *alveolar interstitial space*, an elimination or a reduction in the amount of fluid present takes place in two ways. First, fluid is drained by the lymphatic circulation, as shown on the left side of Figure 2–23. Though lymphatics are not generally found at the level of the air-blood barrier or interalveolar septa, they are in very close proximity. Pulmonary capillaries are at most 1 mm away from the nearest lymphatic.

Second, excess fluid in the alveolar interstitial space is believed to rapidly drain along connective tissue fibers into *peribronchial/perivascular interstitial spaces.* One must remember that the perivascular/peribronchial interstitial spaces, unlike alveolar interstitial spaces, are normally *potential* spaces until fluid seeps within septa and around airways and arteries,

Table 2–3. THIN AND THICK SIDES OF THE INTERALVEOLAR SEPTUM*

Thin Side (Air-Blood Barrier) for Gas Exchange	Thick Side for Fluid Exchange
alveolar space	alveolar space
↓	↓
surfactant lining	surfactant lining
alveolar epithelium	alveolar epithelium
basement membrane (fused)	alveolar basement membrane
capillary endothelium	↓
capillary plasma	interstitial space
erythrocyte (RBC)	↓
	capillary basement membrane
	capillary plasma
	erythrocyte (RBC)

*See Figure 2–22.

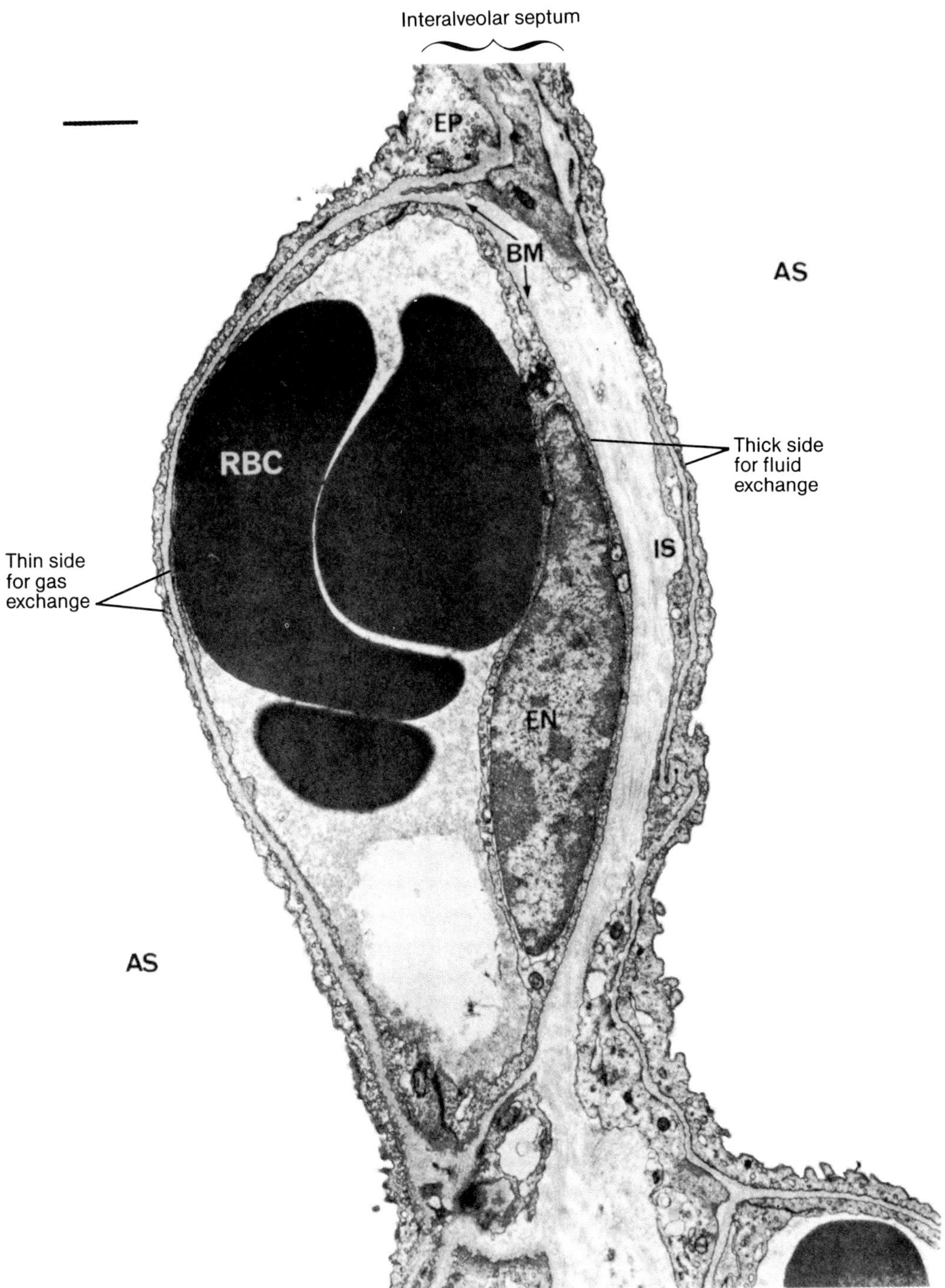

Figure 2–22. Cross-sectional, electron microscopic view of the interalveolar septum between two alveolar spaces (AS). A capillary containing red blood cells (RBCs) is suspended in the middle of the septum. On the left side of the photomicrograph, the basement membranes (BM) of the alveolar epithelium (EP) and capillary endothelium (EN) appear fused, forming a "thin side" or the *air-blood barrier*. On the right side, the basement membranes are separated by the interstitial space (IS), forming the "thick side" of the septum or the *alveolar-capillary membrane*. (Horizontal bar = 1 μm; ×11,000.) (Reproduced by permission from Hinshaw, H. and Murray, J.: Diseases of the Chest, 4th ed. Philadelphia, W. B. Saunders Co., 1980. Courtesy of Dr. Ewald Weibel.)

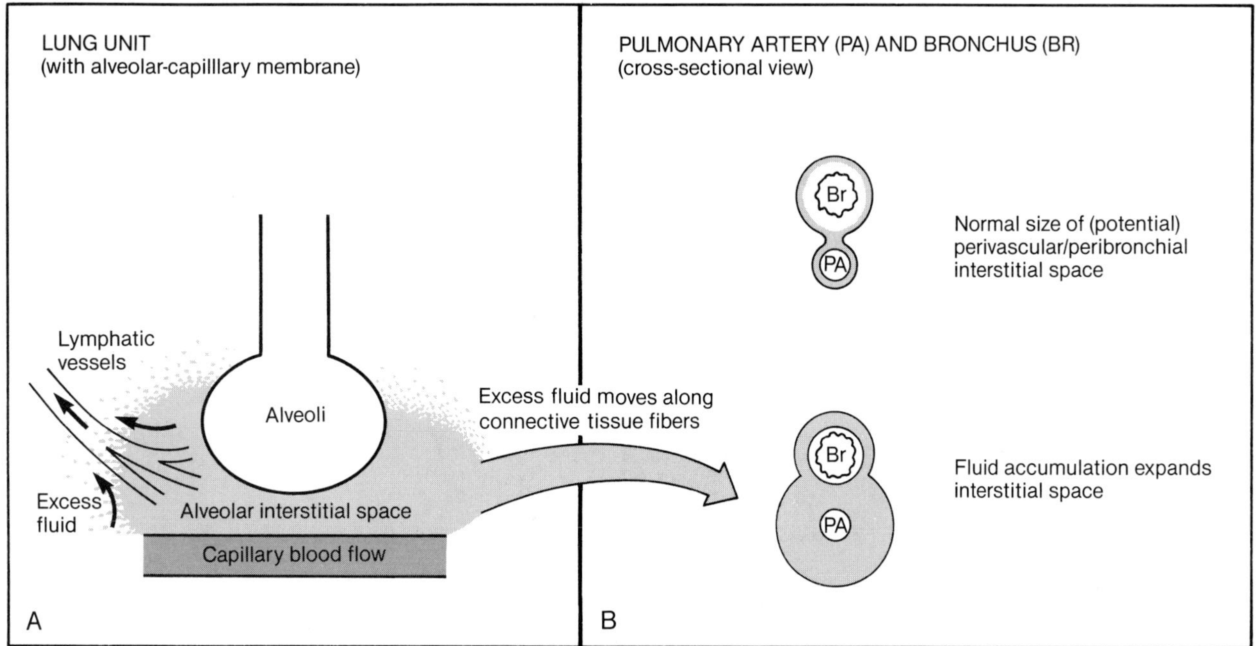

Figure 2–23. Conceptualization of the alveolar interstitial space and perivascular/peribronchial interstitial spaces. Excess fluid in the lung moves from the *alveolar* interstitial space into the lymphatic circulation *(A)* and to the centrally located *perivascular/peribronchial* interstitial space *(B)*. (CT = connective tissue.) (Adapted with permission from Staub, N.: The pathophysiology of pulmonary edema. Human Pathol. 1:419–413, 1970.)

creating an actual space with fluid, as illustrated in the lower right of Figure 2–23.

Hence, the interstitial space is actually found in many different locations in the lung, and probably no one simple illustration can accurately portray its location, size, and extent. Simple conceptual illustrations, such as the lung unit in Figure 2–23, however, are presented in this text. These may include a labelled or an unlabelled interstitial space to simplify the illustration or to emphasize other physiological concepts in addition to exchange. When viewing these and other illustrations, the reader must constantly keep in mind that the alveolar interstitial space is actually absent or minimal on the thin side of the alveolar-capillary membrane where most gas exchange takes place. Also, capillary blood flow almost completely surrounds each alveolus, even though it is illustrated at the base of the lung unit for the purpose of simplification.

Conclusion

This chapter has presented upper and lower respiratory tracts in detail, starting at the nasal cavity, moving downward to the conducting airways, and ending at the alveolus, alveolar-capillary membrane, and adjacent interstitial space.

The emphasis on detailed description and pulmonary terminology serves two purposes. First, it clarifies common terms, such as interstitial space, bronchiole, and collateral channel in the lung, so that the true nature of these and other structures is fully appreciated by the nurse in clinical, educational, and research settings. Second, the explanations prepare the nurse for further understanding of the details of the lung's gas exchange function (see Chapter 3) as well as the pathophysiology of disorders affecting the upper and lower respiratory tracts (see Part Two).

REFERENCES

Bloom, W. and Fawcett, D.: *A Textbook of Histology*, 10th ed. Philadelphia, W. B. Saunders Co., 1975.

Borysenko, M. and Beringer, T.: *Functional Histology*, 2nd ed. Boston, Little, Brown & Co., 1984.

Comroe, J.: *Physiology of Respiration—An Introductory Text*, 2nd ed. Chicago, Year Book Medical Publishers, Inc., 1974.

Fishman, A.: *Assessment of Pulmonary Function*. New York, McGraw-Hill Book Co., 1980.

Fraser, R. and Paré, J.: *Diagnosis of Diseases of the Chest, vol. 1*, 2nd ed. Philadelphia, W. B. Saunders Co., 1977.

Gail, D. and Lenfant, J.: State of the art—cells of the lung: biology and clinical implications. *American Review of Respiratory Disease*, 127(3):366–387, 1983.

Ham, A. and Cormack, D.: *Histology*, 8th ed. Philadelphia, J. B. Lippincott Co., 1979.

Hinshaw, H. and Murray, J.: *Diseases of the Chest*, 4th ed. Philadelphia, W. B. Saunders Co., 1980.

Jacob, S., Francone, C., and Lossow, W.: *Structure and Function in Man*, 5th ed. Philadelphia, W. B. Saunders Co., 1982.

Janson-Bjerklie, S.: Defense mechanisms: protecting the healthy lung. *Heart and Lung*, 12(6):643–649, 1983.

Johnson, J., et al.: *Surgery of the Chest*, 4th ed. Chicago, Year Book Medical Publishers, Inc., 1970.

Kelly, D.: *Bailey's Textbook of Microscopic Anatomy*, 18th ed. Baltimore, Williams & Wilkins, 1984.

Moore, K.: *Clinically Oriented Anatomy,* 2nd ed. Baltimore, Williams & Wilkins, 1985.

Murray, J.: *The Normal Lung: The Basis for Diagnosis and Treatment of Pulmonary Disease,* 2nd ed. Philadelphia, W. B. Saunders Co., 1986.

Rutland, J., Griffin, W., and Cole, P.: Human ciliary beat frequency in epithelium from intrathoracic and extrathoracic airways. *American Review of Respiratory Disease,* 125(1):100, 1982.

Shapiro, B., Harrison, R., et al.: *Clinical Application of Respiratory Care,* 3rd ed. Chicago, Year Book Medical Publishers, Inc., 1985.

Staub, N.: Lung structure and function—1982. *Basics of Respiratory Disease,* 10(3), 1982.

Staub, N.: The pathophysiology of pulmonary edema. *Human Pathology,* 1(3):419–431, 1970.

Thurlbeck, W.: Chronic obstructive lung disease. In *Pathology Annual: Nineteen Sixty-Eight.* (Sommers, S., ed.). New York, Appleton-Century-Crofts, 1968.

Tortora, G.: *Principles of Human Anatomy,* 3rd ed. San Francisco, Harper & Row, Publishers, Inc., 1983.

Towers, B.: The muscle-cartilage relationship in the extrapulmonary bronchi. *Journal of Anatomy,* 87(4):377–344, 1953.

Trout, C.: Artificial airways: tubes and trachs. *Respiratory Care,* 21(6):513–519, 1976.

Waldhausen, J. and Pierce, W.: *Johnson's Surgery of the Chest,* 5th ed. Chicago, Year Book Medical Publishers, Inc., 1985.

Weibel, E. and Burri, P.: *Funktionelle aspekte der lungenmorphologie. Aktuelle probleme der roentgendiagnostik, vol.* 2 (Fuchs, W. and Voegeli, E., eds.). Bern, Switz., Huber, 1973.

West, J.: *Respiratory Physiology—The Essentials,* 3rd ed. Baltimore, Williams & Wilkins, 1985.

Gas Diffusion and Oxygenation

3

Main Objectives

1. **Explain how oxygen and carbon dioxide diffuse across the alveolar-capillary membrane or air-blood barrier.**
2. **State how Dalton's law applies to the partial pressures of gases in the atmosphere.**
3. **Calculate the partial pressures of atmospheric gases at the mouth and in the trachea.**
4. **Name five factors that affect gas diffusion.**
5. **State normal ranges for PaO_2 at sea level. Describe how age and altitude alter normal PaO_2.**
6. **Define the following terms: PaO_2, PAO_2, PvO_2, FIO_2, SaO_2, P_{50}, and CaO_2.**
7. **Calculate and state the significance of the total blood oxygen content (CaO_2) for a patient with PaO_2 100 mmHg, SaO_2 100% and hemoglobin 15 gm %.**
8. **Compare and contrast the two forms of oxygen, dissolved oxygen and oxyhemoglobin, in the blood.**
9. **Identify and explain the clinical significance of the oxyhemoglobin dissociation curve's critical zone.**
10. **Explain why administration of 100% oxygen concentration to a patient with a PaO_2 95 mmHg will not significantly increase oxygen saturation.**
11. **Explain the clinical significance of right and left shifts of the oxyhemoglobin dissociation curve.**
12. **Define hypoxemia. State the main physiologic cause of hypoxemia in the pulmonary patient.**
13. **Define hypoxia and state the four types.**

This chapter discusses basic principles of gas diffusion and oxygenation. More detailed principles related to diffusion (e.g., clinical measurement of diffusion) and oxygen (O_2) and carbon dioxide (CO_2) transport are presented in the chapters on blood gases and pulmonary function tests (see Chapter 13 and Chapter 14).

Basic Principles of Gas Diffusion

O_2 and CO_2 move back and forth across the alveolar-capillary membrane by gas diffusion. Diffusion is defined as the *process by which matter moves from one place to another as a result of random molecular motion.* The overall direction of molecular movement is from an area of high pressure to an area of lower pressure.

Both mass flow and diffusion explain how air reaches the alveoli and the air-blood barrier (Fig. 3–1). Mass flow occurs predominantly in large airways. Towards the periphery of the lung, gas diffusion becomes increasingly important as the vehicle for gas conduction because of the small structure of the terminal respiratory units (TRUs) and because of the sizable amount of stagnant residual air remaining in the lungs at the end of expiration.

Diffusion is explained in terms of partial pressures of gases and pressure gradients in the lung.

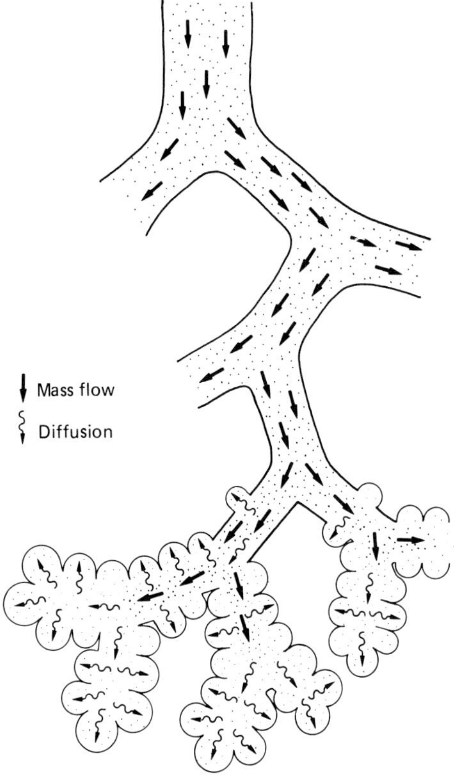

Figure 3–1. Oxygen molecules reach alveoli by combined mass airflow and molecular diffusion; the importance of diffusion increases toward the periphery. (Reproduced by permission from Weibel, E.: Design and Structure of the Human Lung. In Fishman, A.: Assessment of Pulmonary Function. New York, McGraw-Hill Book Co., 1980.)

PARTIAL PRESSURES OF GASES

Partial pressures of gases help explain the diffusion of gases in gas mixtures.

A *partial pressure* or *tension* of a gas (P) is defined as its pressure, whether the gas is alone or in a mixture with other gases. The value is not affected by the presence of other gases because each gas in a mixture acts independently, as if it alone occupied the given space. It is determined by the frequency of random collisions of molecules against the sides of the given container or space. Molecular collisions, in turn, depend on the *number of molecules* in the container, the *volume* of the container, and the *temperature.*

Several gas laws and their corresponding mathematical equations govern the behavior of a gas when variables such as mass, volume, or temperature change. Of these, *Dalton's law,* known as the law of partial pressures, is central to understanding the derivation of partial pressures of gases in the atmosphere and in the lung. Dalton's law states

> The total pressure exerted by a mixture of gases is equal to the sum of individual gas partial pressures that each gas would exert if it alone occupied the volume in question.

It is expressed in the following equation for total pressure for a given volume (PV), as follows:

$$PV = V\,(P_1 + P_2 + P_3 + \ldots + P_n)$$

Application of this law to total atmospheric pressure or barometric pressure yields this statement:

> Barometric pressure is equal to the sum of the individual partial pressures of oxygen, nitrogen, carbon dioxide, and water vapor, the main components of air.

In equation form as follows:

$$P_B = PO_2 + PN_2 + PCO_2 + PH_2O$$

The value for P_B equals 760 mmHg (also called torr) at sea level. In other words, gas molecules that constitute the earth's atmosphere have a weight. This weight presses down on the earth's surface with a force sufficient to support a column of mercury *760 mm* high at sea level. This value varies as high and low pressure areas move across the face of the earth, changing regional weather; the value decreases with high altitude.

Composition of Inspired Air

Figure 3–2 summarizes the changing partial pressures of air at sea level on its way to alveoli. The fractional concentrations (see Percent of Total Gas) of the aforementioned gases that make up P_B are listed. In studying these figures, note that most of the atmosphere is composed of nitrogen—78.1% to 79%. The value for nitrogen varies from source to source, because many physiologists interpret the term nitrogen to mean *any* nonabsorbable or "inert" gas rather than

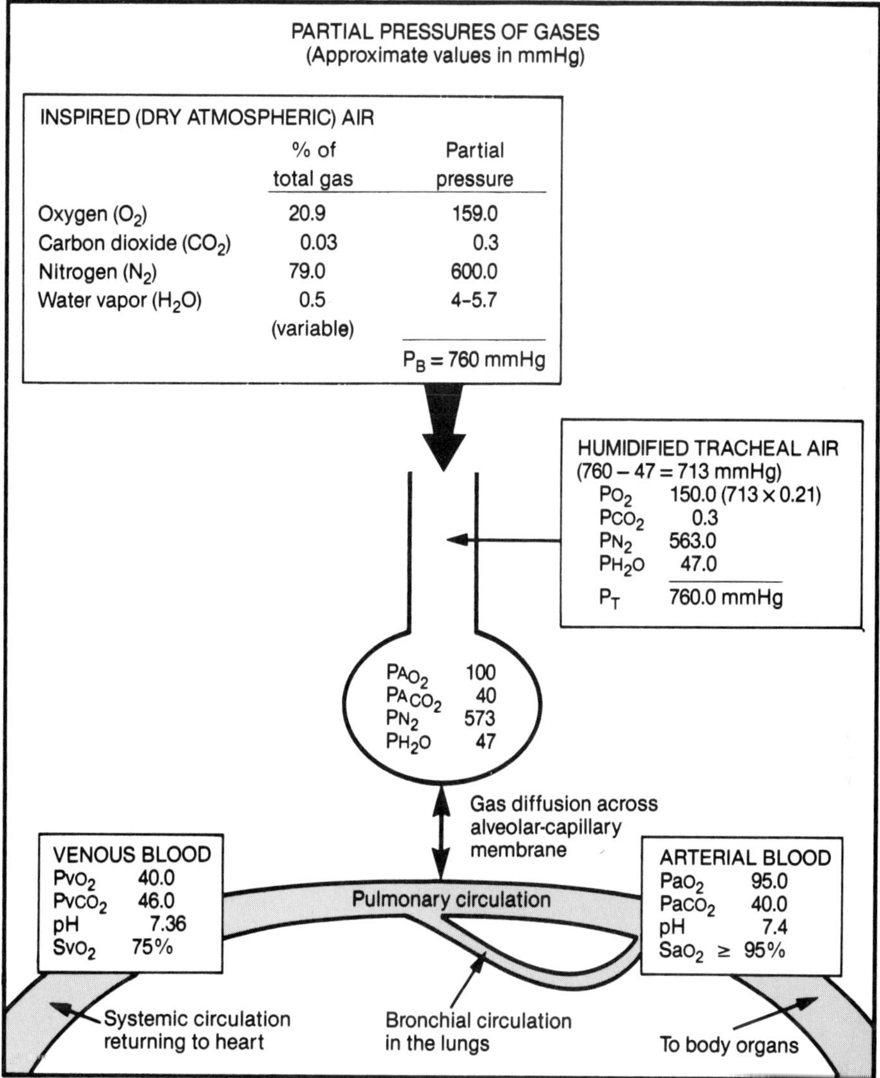

Figure 3–2. Partial pressures of gases. Approximate values are in mmHg at sea level under BTPS conditions (body temperature of 37°C, ambient pressure, and saturated with water vapor).

just the element nitrogen. The atmosphere contains very small amounts of nonabsorbable gases, such as argon, neon, krypton, and ozone, which may vary slightly in quantity from time to time (e.g., ozone) or place to place. Slonim and Hamilton (1987) report considerable evidence that inert gases are not inert in high concentrations or chronic exposures.

Other gas concentrations in the atmosphere include 21% O_2, only 0.3% CO_2, and 0.5% water vapor, a value that varies with the weather and changing quantities of water vapor.

Calculation of Partial Pressures

With application of Dalton's law, the fractional concentration of a gas multiplied by the total gas pressure (P_B) gives the partial pressure of the gas. For inspired O_2, fractional concentration × P_B = pressure of gas.

$$Po_2 = 0.209\ (0.21) \times 760 \text{ mmHg} = 159 \text{ mmHg}$$

Partial pressures for the other atmospheric gases are calculated in the same manner.

Tracheal Partial Pressures

The trachea adds water vapor (humidity) to inspired air, which alters calculations somewhat. Taking up space in the trachea, water vapor exerts a partial pressure of *47 mmHg*. This value may vary somewhat depending on the body temperature (Table 3–1) and the health of the body's temperature control and humidification functions in the nasotracheobronchial epithelium. For most practical purposes, however, this value is assumed to remain constant at 47 mmHg. Before partial pressure calculations are begun, 47 must be subtracted from 760 (760–47 = 713). Now the equation for O_2 looks like the following:

$$Po_2 = 0.21 \times 713 = 150 \text{ mmHg}$$

PN_2 and Pco_2 are calculated in the same way. The product for Pco_2 (0.21 mmHg), however, is only a rough approximation—it is slightly lower than the actual tracheal Pco_2 (0.31 mmHg), due to the mixing of tracheal inspired air with CO_2-rich air in airways at the end of expiration.

Table 3–1. RELATIONSHIP BETWEEN TEMPERATURE AND WATER VAPOR PRESSURE (PH_2O)

Temperature °C	PH_2O mmHg
25	23.76
26	25.21
27	26.74
28	28.35
29	30.04
30	31.82
31	33.70
32	35.66
33	37.73
34	39.90
35	42.18
36	44.56
37	47.07
38	49.69
39	52.44
40	55.32

The shaded box contains normal values.

Alveolar Partial Pressures

The partial pressures of alveolar gases (PA), specifically PA_{O_2} and PA_{CO_2}, cannot be calculated because of the numerous and changing variables affecting alveolar ventilation and pulmonary capillary blood flow through the lungs. Because of this restraint, one has no choice but to memorize two key values for PA estimation: PA_{O_2} equilibrates at around *100 mmHg*, and PA_{CO_2} at *40 mmHg*. These values for healthy persons breathing room air are rules of thumb.

Values for nitrogen and water vapor remain stable at 573 mmHg and 47 mmHg, respectively, at the alveolar level as well as in venous and arterial blood.

PRESSURE GRADIENTS

Gas diffusion across the alveolar-capillary membrane occurs in response to a *pressure gradient.* When partial pressures on both sides of a semipermeable membrane are equal, a pressure gradient is absent and gases are said to be in a state of *dynamic equilibrium.* A pressure gradient develops when partial pressure on one side becomes higher than that on the other side of the membrane. As a rule, a *gas moves from the area of higher pressure across the membrane to the area of lower pressure,* until pressures on both sides are equal.

Each gas moves in response to its own pressure gradient regardless of the partial pressures of other gases. Hence, the movement of oxygen in the lungs is from the alveoli, where PA_{O_2} equals 100 mmHg, into the pulmonary circulation, where partial pressure of venous oxygen (PvO_2) equals only 40 mmHg. In contrast, CO_2 moves *from* venous blood ($PvCO_2$ = 46 mmHg) and *into* alveoli (PA_{CO_2} = 40 mmHg), the region with the lower partial pressure.

Pressure gradients largely determine the rate and extent of gas diffusion—the larger the pressure gradient, the faster the diffusion of gases across the alveolar capillary membrane. Rate of diffusion slows as pressures move towards equalization. Other factors affecting gas diffusion include the following: (1) *molecular weight*—heavy molecules are less diffusible than lighter ones; (2) *solubility*—CO_2 diffuses about 20 times faster than O_2 because it is more soluble; (3) *rate of blood flow past acinar units*—decreased cardiac output increases gas contact time and promotes diffusion; (4) *surface area available for gas exchange;* and (5) other factors (see Chapter 14).

Discrepancy between Alveolar and Arterial PO_2

In Figure 3–2, alveolar and arterial PO_2 equilibrate at 40 mmHg. However, arterial PO_2 (95 mmHg) is slightly less than alveolar PO_2 (100 mmHg). The explanation for this small discrepancy relates to the normal 2% shunt of oxygenated blood through the lung's bronchial circulation (see Chapter 4). This blood returns to the left side of the heart unoxygenated. For all practical purposes, arterial and alveolar PO_2 are assumed to be equal in healthy persons.

Basic Principles of Oxygenation

Basic principles of oxygenation are best explained in relation to the PO_2 (mmHg), SO_2 (%) (percent hemoglobin oxygen saturation), *and* oxyhemoglobin dissociation curve. PO_2 and SO_2 measurements are the most commonly used parameters for assessing the adequacy of oxygenation in the body.

In the explanation to follow, as well as in the clinical situation, remember that the small "a" in PaO_2 (or any gas tension measurement) stands for *arterial* blood. The small capital "A" in PA_{O_2} indicates *alveolar* gas. The small "v" in PvO_2 indicates *venous* blood, whereas the "$\bar{v}$" in $P\bar{v}O_2$ indicates *mixed venous* blood drawn from an indwelling central catheter in the pulmonary artery. When PO_2 appears without a defining letter, arterial blood is usually assumed.

PaO_2 MEASUREMENT

The normal laboratory value for arterial PO_2 is about 100 mmHg. In the clinical setting, the normal range for PaO_2 varies depending on factors including the patient's age, the diagnosis, and the elevation above sea level. Because of these factors and individual variations, it is easier and perhaps more useful for the nurse to remember these general normal ranges for PaO_2.

NORMAL RANGES FOR Pao_2*

Adult and child	80–100 mmHg
Newborn infant	40–70 mmHg
Aged 60 to 80 years	60–80 mmHg

The following formulas may be used for more precise determination of normal Pao_2 in the adult (Bates et al, 1971).

NORMAL Pao_2 IN THE ADULT

Upright Pao_2 (mmHg) = 104.2 − 0.27 × age (years)

Supine Pao_2 (mmHg) = 103.5 − 0.42 × age (years)

For normal adults and children, *hypoxemia* is defined as *arterial Po_2 of less than 80 mmHg.* Note that hypoxemia refers to a lack or an insufficient amount of O_2 in arterial blood. It must not be confused with the term *hypoxia,* defined as the lack of O_2 in body tissues.

Several factors, including age, history, and altitude, are important to consider in the assessment of hypoxemia.

Age. A young adult is hypoxemic at a Pao_2 of 70 mmHg, but this value is within the acceptable range for a 70-year-old adult. The aging process produces a gradual decline in lung function.

History. Previous arterial blood gas (ABG) results help determine normal ABG values for each person. For example, a teenager may be clinically diagnosed as hypoxemic with a Pao_2 of 88 mmHg, if this value represents a drop from a previously determined normal value of 97 mmHg.

Altitude. Elevations above sea level affect normal Pao_2 ranges (Table 3–2). In cities located 1 mi (5280 ft) above sea level, such as Denver, Colorado and Albuquerque, New Mexico, inspired atmospheric PO_2 is about 130 mmHg instead of 150 mmHg. An individual is normally not considered to have impairment of O_2 transfer; however, technically and actually, one is hypoxemic with a Pao_2 of 75 mmHg and an Sao_2 of 94% at this elevation.

During initial assessment, baseline ABG values, including Pao_2, with the patient breathing room air help the physician make a medical diagnosis and determine treatment. O_2 is never withheld from a patient who is hypoxemic or in respiratory distress. As a general guideline, the nurse routinely notifies the physician whenever Pao_2 falls below 80 mmHg.

Looking at FIo_2 helps assess hypoxemia. FIo_2 stands for *fractional concentration of inspired oxygen* and is always written in decimal form. An FIo_2 of 0.40 is the same as an O_2 concentration of 40%. As an example of the importance of FIo_2, consider a patient who maintains a Pao_2 of 80 mmHg, while FIo_2 gradually increases to 0.80. The patient is not technically hypoxemic, but O_2 transport is becoming progressively more impaired because a higher FIo_2 is required to maintain the same Pao_2. As another example, the patient with a Pao_2 of 70 mmHg and FIo_2 of 0.50 is more hypoxemic than the patient with the same Pao_2 but lower FIo_2 of 0.35.

Table 3–2. EFFECTS OF ALTITUDE ON ATMOSPHERIC, ALVEOLAR, AND ARTERIAL OXYGEN TENSIONS IN HEALTHY YOUNG ADULTS

Altitude (Feet)	Barometric Pressure (mmHg)	Atmospheric Oxygen Pressure (mmHg)	Alveolar Oxygen Pressure (mmHg)	Arterial* Blood Oxygen Pressure (mmHg)
0	760	159	110	96
1000	733	153	104	91
2000	707	148	99	87
3000	687	142	94	83
4000	656	137	89	79
5000	631	132	85	75
6000	604	126	80	71
8000	564	116	69	63

*Values for normal older individuals may be 10 to 15 mm lower than these listed.

(Reprinted by permission from Fulmer, J. and Snider, G.: ACCP-NHLBI Conference on Oxygen Therapy. *Chest,* 86(2):240, 1984.)

Most important regardless of the situation, when Pao_2 falls below *60 mmHg,* a serious oxygenation problem exists that requires O_2 administration. The O_2-hemoglobin dissociation curve (described subsequently) explains why values below 60 mmHg in particular are so dangerous.

OXYGEN TRANSPORT

Basic principles of O_2 transport help explain what the oxyhemoglobin dissociation curve is and its relation to the Sao_2 measurement.

O_2 transport pertains to the delivery of O_2 to body tissues. Figure 3–3A illustrates the *loading* of O_2 onto hemoglobin molecules to prepare for blood transport. The illustration to the right (Fig. 3–3) illustrates the *unloading* of O_2 at the tissue level, where cellular metabolism takes place. Note that blood carries O_2 in the two following forms: (1) *dissolved O_2* or O_2 dissolved in plasma (aqueous form) and (2) *oxyhemoglobin* or O_2 in chemical combination with hemoglobin in red blood cells. These two forms constitute what is known as *total O_2 content* in arterial blood, or simply *total blood O_2 content* (Cao_2).

Dissolved Oxygen

Under normal physiological conditions, O_2 dissolved in plasma makes up less than 1% of the total blood O_2 content.

CALCULATION OF TOTAL BLOOD OXYGEN CONTENT (CaO_2)

volumes percent (vol%) = milliliters of O_2 per 100 ml blood

grams per cent (gm%) = grams of hemoglobin per 100 ml blood

BTPS conditions = body temperature, ambient pressure, saturated with water vapor

STEP 1—CALCULATION OF DISSOLVED O_2 IN BLOOD PLASMA

a. For each 100 ml of blood at BTPS, 0.003 ml of O_2 can be dissolved for each 1 mmHg of O_2 tension. This is the solubility coefficient for O_2 and blood.

b. For an individual with a normal PaO_2 of 100 mmHg

$$\underset{\text{(solubility coefficient)}}{0.003 \text{ ml } O_2/100 \text{ ml blood/mmHg}} \times \underset{(PaO_2)}{100 \text{ mmHg}} =$$

$$\frac{0.3 \text{ ml } O_2}{100 \text{ ml blood}} \text{ or } 0.30 \text{ vol\%}$$

STEP 2—CALCULATION OF O_2 ATTACHED TO HEMOGLOBIN

a. At BTPS (body conditions), 1 gm of hemoglobin fully saturated with O_2 can carry 1.34 ml of O_2. (Because of varying *in vivo* conditions, this value varies. Some authorities use 1.36 or 1.39, the theoretically ideal value.)

b. When hemoglobin equals 15 mg%, PaO_2 equals 100 mmHg, and SaO_2 equals 100%, as follows:

$$\underset{(Hgb)}{15} \times \underset{(1.34)}{1.34} \times \underset{(SaO_2)}{1.00} = 20.10 \text{ vol\%}$$

STEP 3—O_2 DISSOLVED IN PLASMA PLUS O_2 ATTACHED TO HEMOGLOBIN EQUALS TOTAL BLOOD O_2 CONTENT

$$0.30 \text{ vol\%} + 20.10 \text{ vol\%} = 20.40 \text{ vol\%}$$

Note O_2 dissolved in plasma is less than 1% (0.015%) of total blood O_2 content.

This small amount is directly proportional to the partial pressure of alveolar oxygen (PAO_2). Since PaO_2 is assumed to be about equal to PAO_2, O_2 dissolved in plasma is clinically determined by the measurement of PaO_2.

Even though PaO_2 reflects less than 1% of total blood O_2 content, it is a crucial measurement for two reasons. First, along with PA_{O_2}, it can be used to determine the PA_{O_2}-Pa_{O_2} pressure gradient. This gradient is the difference in mmHg between alveolar PO_2 and arterial PO_2. Its clinical use as a measurement reflecting the adequacy of O_2 transfer into the blood is described in Chapter 13. Second, as a blood plasma measurement, PaO_2 determines the *availability* of O_2 for chemical combination with hemoglobin in adjacent red blood cells. In this respect, blood plasma holds an important intermediate position between acinar units receiving inspired O_2 and red blood cells transporting O_2 to body tissues in the form of oxyhemoglobin.

One further point about dissolved O_2 in blood plasma—the only way to increase the amount present is to increase PA_{O_2}. This is done simply by adjustment of FIO_2 up to 1.0 (100% O_2 concentration). In large medical centers, hyperbaric chambers are used, which do the same thing, except they produce even greater increases in PA_{O_2} through the use of high atmospheric pressures. The high PA_{O_2} increases the amount of dissolved O_2 in plasma so that it constitutes a larger fraction of total blood O_2 content, provided hemoglobin is already fully saturated with O_2. O_2 transport is facilitated, and O_2 becomes readily available to tissues.

Oxygen Combined with Hemoglobin and SaO_2 (%)

The hemoglobin in red blood cells acts as a magnet, pulling O_2 from dissolved plasma and causing it to attach or *load* onto molecular attachment sites. (Each molecule of hemoglobin contains four attachment sites.) At rest, more than 95% of O_2 delivered to body tissues is transported in combination with hemoglobin as oxyhemoglobin. This value can exceed 99% during exercise.

Unlike dissolved O_2, the amount of O_2 combined with hemoglobin is *not* directly proportional to the partial pressure of O_2. In other words, an increase or decrease in PaO_2 does not necessarily cause a proportional increase or decrease in the percent hemoglobin that is saturated with O_2. Changes in values yield an S-shaped rather than a linear curve, as illustrated in Figure 3–4.

The *% saturation of hemoglobin with O_2* may be abbreviated *% HbO_2 saturation, % O_2 saturation,* or *SaO_2(%)* in the clinical setting. SaO_2 is defined as the amount of hemoglobin actually combined with O_2 divided by the total amount of hemoglobin available. The formula is written as follows:

$$\% \text{ } HbO_2 \text{ saturation} = \frac{\text{Hb combined with } O_2}{\text{total hemoglobin}} \times 100\%$$

THE NORMAL OXYHEMOGLOBIN DISSOCIATION CURVE

The normal oxyhemoglobin dissociation curve in Figure 3–4 illustrates that normal arterial blood has a

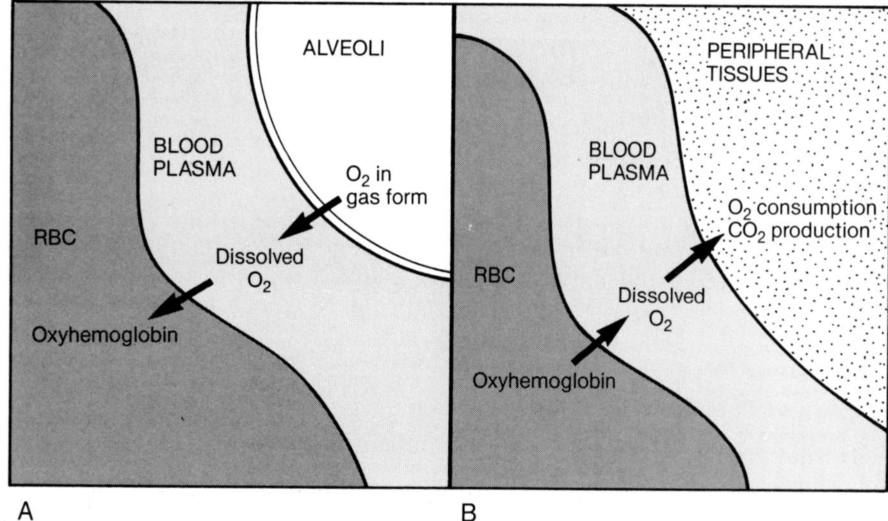

Figure 3–3. Oxygen transport from the lungs to body tissues.

A, **Loading** of oxygen for blood transport:

Oxygen moves into pulmonary capillaries to the red blood cell (RBC) and attaches to hemoglobin to form *oxyhemoglobin.*

B, **Unloading** of oxygen for cell metabolism:

In systemic capillaries, oxygen moves into tissues for cell metabolism.

PaO_2 of 97 mmHg and an O_2 saturation of 97%. Mixed venous blood has a $P\bar{v}O_2$ of 40% and an O_2 saturation of 75%.

In addition, the curve shows the location of P_{50}. The measurement P_{50} is defined as the *PaO_2 at which 50% of the hemoglobin is saturated under the following standard laboratory conditions: T = 37°C, $PaCO_2$ = 40 mmHg, and pH = 7.40.* The normal adult has a P_{50} of 27 mmHg—this means hemoglobin is 50% saturated with O_2 at a PaO_2 of 27 mmHg. This measurement is useful as an index of the position of the oxyhemoglobin dissociation curve under standard conditions. Moreover, it may be employed clinically to detect variant forms of the hemoglobin molecule that have different oxygen-combining properties.

The Curve's Flat Portion

Figure 3–5 shows that the flattest portion of the dissociation curve lies at the top of the curve *above* a PaO_2 of 60 to 70 mmHg. Here, *great changes in PaO_2 yield small changes in O_2 saturation.* For example, if PaO_2 drops from 100 mmHg (point a) to 80 mmHg (point b), O_2 saturation will fall from about 99% to 96%, which is only a 3% change. Hemoglobin is still well saturated with O_2, and the person is in no

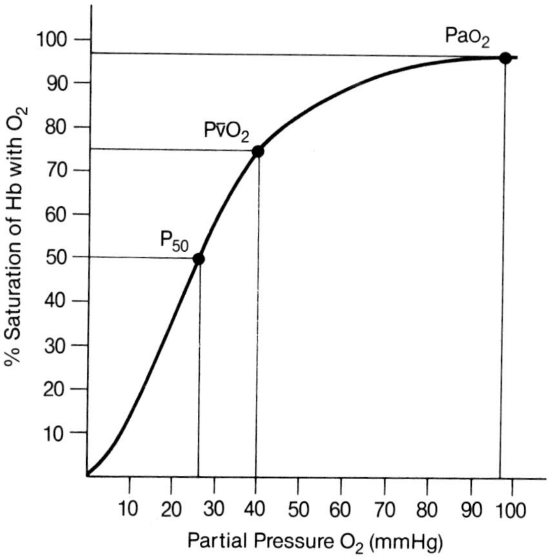

Figure 3–4. The normal oxyhemoglobin dissociation curve.

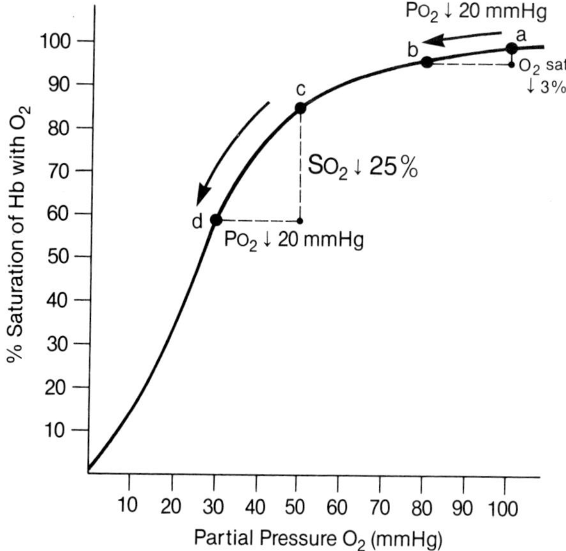

Figure 3–5. The flat and steep portions of the oxyhemoglobin dissociation curve (see text). (Hb = hemoglobin.)

immediate danger. Study the curve carefully until you understand this point.

The Curve's Steep Portion

In contrast, the steepest portion of the curve lies *below* 60 mmHg, between 10 and 50 mmHg. Here, the same 20 mmHg drop in Pa_{O_2} produces a much larger drop in O_2 saturation. A fall in Pa_{O_2} from 50 mmHg (point c) to 30 mmHg (point d) causes O_2 saturation to fall from 85% to about 60%, a 25% difference.

Important Points

In clinical practice, it is essential to remember the following: *A Pa_{O_2} of less than 60 mmHg lies in the oxyhemoglobin dissociation curve's critical zone* (Fig. 3–6). Here, small changes in Pa_{O_2} are important because they produce large changes in O_2 saturation.

For example, a decrease in Pa_{O_2} by only a few mmHg—from 55 to 51—results in a significant drop in O_2 saturation. By the same token, a small increase in Pa_{O_2}—from 51 to 55 mmHg—can produce a significant increase in O_2 saturation and O_2 delivery to body tissues. Hence, when the patient's Pa_{O_2} lies in the critical zone, O_2 therapy and other interventions are usually necessary to increase Pa_{O_2} to a level greater than 60 mmHg.

In this discussion of the oxyhemoglobin dissociation curve, emphasis has been placed on the role of partial pressures in determining the movement of oxygen; therefore, it is very useful to remember the following:

1. *At the top of the curve* where Pa_{O_2} is high, hemoglobin clings to O_2 but limits further O_2 uptake because it is already saturated. *Application:* Under normal circumstances, giving 100% O_2 to a patient with an already high Pa_{O_2} (e.g., 95 mmHg) will not significantly increase O_2 saturation because the hemoglobin molecule is already saturated.

2. *At the bottom of the curve,* hemoglobin readily gives up O_2 to blood plasma where it becomes available to tissue cells with a very low Pa_{O_2} (less than 10 mmHg). At the same time, the desaturated hemoglobin will readily take up O_2 as it becomes available. *Application:* Giving 100% O_2 to the patient with cardiopulmonary arrest and a low Pa_{O_2} provides a continuous supply of O_2 to O_2-deprived body tissues.

SHIFTS OF THE OXYHEMOGLOBIN DISSOCIATION CURVE

Certain conditions change hemoglobin's affinity for O_2, as illustrated by the shifts in the position of the normal dissociation curve.

Right Shift

A shift of the dissociation curve to the right implies a decrease in hemoglobin affinity for O_2. This *decrease*

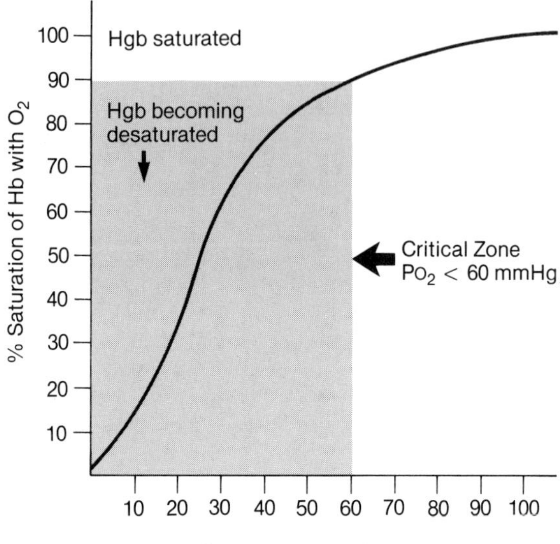

Figure 3–6. The critical zone of the oxyhemoglobin dissociation curve. (Hgb = hemoglobin.)

in affinity is most useful at the tissue level, where hemoglobin readily releases O_2 to blood plasma.

In the curve to the right of the normal dissociation curve in Figure 3–7, the letter R marks the new point at which hemoglobin is 70% saturated with O_2. Comparison of point N on the normal curve with point R leads to the following generalization:

> When the normal curve shifts to the right, a higher Pa_{O_2} is required to maintain the same O_2 saturation.

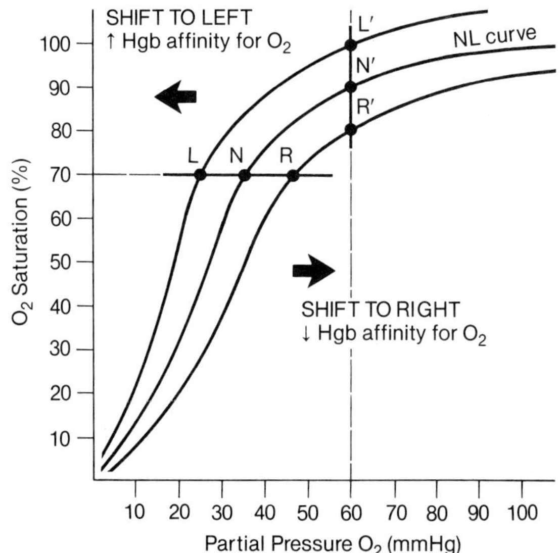

Figure 3–7. Right and left shifts of the oxyhemoglobin dissociation curve. (Hgb = hemoglobin; NL = normal.)

From another perspective, as follows:

Maintenance of the same PaO_2 results in a lower O_2 saturation.

This concept is illustrated in Figure 3–7 by the vertical shift from point N′ on the normal curve to R′.

In this way, the right shift always favors the release of O_2 to peripheral tissues, and it usually arises out of the body's increased need for O_2. When a right shift occurs at the bottom of the curve (e.g., PaO_2 = 30 mmHg) where low tissue PO_2 already favors the unloading of O_2, the effect is magnified because the need for O_2 is great.

A shift of the curve to the *extreme* right results in decreased oxyhemoglobin as well as decreased total blood O_2 content. In this case, lung PO_2 determines oxyhemoglobin saturation. More specifically, the loading of hemoglobin with O_2 in the lungs rather than O_2 unloading at the tissue level becomes the crucial factor in the determination of how much O_2 reaches body tissues. In other words, regardless of how easily O_2 dissociates from hemoglobin molecules, it cannot be unloaded in peripheral tissues, if an inadequate O_2 supply exists.

Left Shift

A shift of the dissociation curve to the left implies an increase in hemoglobin affinity for O_2. An *increased affinity* causes hemoglobin to cling to O_2.

In the curve to the left of the normal curve in Figure 3–7, comparison of point N with point L leads to the following generalization:

When the normal curve shifts to the left, a lower PaO_2 or less O_2 is needed to maintain the same O_2 saturation (70%, in this case).

From another perspective, as follows:

For any given PaO_2, a shift to the left always results in increased O_2 saturation.

This last concept is illustrated by the vertical shift from point N′ on the normal curve to point L′.

On one hand, a left shift is beneficial to the patient because it increases oxyhemoglobin and O_2 transport by the blood. On the other hand, it can have a damaging effect on the body. As hemoglobin affinity for O_2 becomes stronger, hemoglobin molecules become more and more reluctant to give up O_2 to tissues. As a result, peripheral tissues can become extremely hypoxic (O_2 starved).

Table 3–3. CONDITIONS THAT SHIFT THE OXYHEMOGLOBIN DISSOCIATION CURVE

Left Shift Increased Hemoglobin Affinity for Oxygen—O_2 Moves from Tissues to Blood	Right Shift Decreased Hemoglobin Affinity for Oxygen—O_2 Moves from Blood to Tissues
Hypometabolism Hypothermia, hypothyroidism	Hypermetabolism Fever, hyperthyroidism, exercise, excess growth hormone, excess testosterone
Alkalemia (↑ pH)	Acidemia (↓ pH)
Alveolar hyperventilation (↓ $PaCO_2$)	Alveolar hypoventilation (↑ $PaCO_2$)
Residence at high altitude	
High-affinity abnormal hemoglobins	Low-affinity abnormal hemoglobins
Fetal hemoglobin	
Decreased 2, 3-DPG* Stored bank blood, septic shock, hypophosphatemia	Increased 2, 3-DPG* Chronic hypoxemia, anemia, cyanotic congenital heart disease, low cardiac output conditions, hyperphosphatemia
Carbon monoxide poisoning	

*2, 3-DPG (diphosphoglycerate) is a metabolite of glucose that facilitates the dissociation of O_2 from hemoglobin by competing with O_2 for hemoglobin attachment sites.

Conditions Causing Right or Left Shifts

Table 3–3 lists main conditions causing right or left shift of the oxyhemoglobin dissociation curve. Emphasis must be placed on the fact that *small shifts to the right or left are adaptive.* In the case of fever, the curve's right shift facilitates the transfer of O_2 to tissues. It permits the release of O_2 in regions of high metabolism where there is high O_2 consumption and high CO_2 production. However, *sudden severe shifts in the curve are life-threatening.* A severe acid base disorder or sudden increase in $PaCO_2$, for example, will decrease total blood O_2 content and limit the amount of O_2 available to O_2-starved tissues. This type of situation requires immediate medical intervention.

IMPORTANCE OF TOTAL BLOOD O_2 CONTENT (CaO_2)

Whereas pressure gradients determine the movement of gases between systemic capillary blood and tissues as well as between pulmonary capillary blood and alveoli, it is the total blood O_2 content that determines the amount of O_2 transported to tissues. Since over 95% of total blood O_2 content is in the form of oxyhemoglobin, the amount of hemoglobin in the body largely determines the amount of O_2 transported to tissues.

When blood hemoglobin is above the normal level of 15 g/dl, as in *polycythemia,* more hemoglobin is available for O_2 attachment, and more O_2 can be carried for each unit of blood. O_2 transport to tissues is favored. When blood hemoglobin is below normal, as in *anemia,* less hemoglobin is available for the attachment and transport of O_2. The amount of O_2 transported to tissues is limited. Anemia is a cause of hypoxia, as mentioned subsequently.

Physiologic Causes of Hypoxemia and Hypoxia

While the previous section explains oxygenation in relation to the oxyhemoglobin dissociation curve, this section provides an overview of specific pulmonary and extrapulmonary causes of hypoxemia and hypoxia in the clinical setting.

The physiologic causes of hypoxemia are summarized in the box. Of the four pulmonary causes, a ventilation/perfusion abnormality is the main cause in the majority of pulmonary disorders discussed in this text. The abnormality relates to the mismatching of ventilation to blood flow (perfusion) in the lung, as explained in Chapter 5 and Chapter 13.

Hypoxia, also called *anoxia,* has been defined as the tissue (rather than the arterial) lack of O_2. Hypoxia can occur from either severe pulmonary disease or from extrapulmonary disease, affecting gas exchange at the tissue level.

The four main types of hypoxia are (1) hypoxemic hypoxia, (2) circulatory hypoxia, (3) anemic hypoxia, and (4) histotoxic hypoxia.

Hypoxemic Hypoxia. Hypoxemic hypoxia is hypoxia from a low Pa_{O_2}. It occurs in pulmonary disease when hypoxemia becomes so severe, peripheral tissues do not receive an adequate supply of O_2.

Circulatory Hypoxia. Circulatory hypoxia is hypoxia from inadequate capillary circulation. In the case of reduced cardiac output, the decrease must be severe and accompanied by a decrease in Pa_{O_2} to produce hypoxia. In circulatory insufficiency due to local vascular obstruction (e.g., arteriosclerotic disease), hypoxia is often manifested during periods of increased tissue O_2 demand, as in exercise. Though tissue P_{O_2} is reduced, Pa_{O_2} remains normal.

Anemic Hypoxia. Anemic hypoxia occurs from a low hemoglobin and hematocrit values. It is rarely accompanied by hypoxemia. Other disorders, such as carbon monoxide poisoning, do not fall under this category but are similar in nature because they too cause hypoxia by reducing the blood's ability to carry O_2.

Histotoxic Hypoxia. Histotoxic hypoxia occurs when a toxic substance, such as cyanide, interferes with the ability of tissues to utilize available O_2. In cyanide poisoning, O_2 consumption in peripheral tissues remains low even though oxygen concentrations in both venous and arterial blood remain relatively high (West, 1985).

PHYSIOLOGIC CAUSES OF HYPOXEMIA

PULMONARY CAUSES

1. Alveolar hypoventilation
2. Right to left intrapulmonary shunting
   a. Increased absolute shunt—anatomic and capillary
   b. Venous admixture
3. Diffusion defect
4. Ventilation/perfusion abnormality

EXTRAPULMONARY CAUSES

1. Breathing less than 21% oxygen (low $P_{A_{O_2}}$), as follows: high altitude, smoke-filled rooms, poorly ventilated underground mines.
2. Inadequate blood transport of oxygen
   a. Reduced ability of blood to carry O_2, as follows: anemia, carbon monoxide poisoning, methemoglobinemia.
   b. Decreased cardiac output
   c. Circulatory insufficiency, as follows: atherosclerosis, vasospasm, thrombosis, emboli.
3. Inadequate tissue oxygenation
   a. Tissue edema
   b. Poisoning of cellular systems, as follows: carbon monoxide or cyanide poisoning.
   c. Inadequate release of O_2 from hemoglobin, as follows: abnormal blood hemoglobins, decreased total O_2 content from low $P_{A_{O_2}}$ or decreased cardiac output.
   d. Abnormal tissue demand for O_2, as follows: increased metabolic rate.

Conclusion

This chapter presents the basic principles of gas diffusion and oxygenation, with emphasis on the relevance of the oxyhemoglobin dissociation curve to respiratory nursing care. In addition, it provides an overview of the physiologic causes of hypoxemia and hypoxia, the main oxygenation problems in respiratory care.

Though this content is intended to prepare the reader for the study of blood gas assessment parameters in Chapter 13, most of the information is applicable to both assessment and intervention phases of decision-making. For example, the onset of a fever (39°C) in a dyspneic patient should cause the nurse to intervene promptly, e.g., inform the physician, obtain an Sa_{O_2} value to document or rule out possible hypoxemia, treat the fever, give O_2 as ordered, and so forth. In this case, prompt decision-making is crucial, since fever is a hypermetabolic condition causing a right shift of the oxyhemoglobin dissociation curve; an increased unloading of O_2 to O_2-starved tissues; and, hence, a tendency towards blood O_2 desaturation.

REFERENCES

Bates, D., Macklem, P., and Christie, R.: *Respiratory Function in Disease.* Philadelphia, W. B. Saunders Co., 1971.

Braun, H., Cheney, F., and Loehnen, C.: *Introduction to Respiratory Physiology,* 2nd ed. Boston, Little, Brown & Co., 1980.

Fishman, A.: *Assessment of Pulmonary Function.* New York, McGraw-Hill Book Co., 1980.

Fulmer, J. and Snider, G.: ACCP-NHLBI Conference on Oxygen Therapy. *Chest,* 86(2): 240, 1984.

Murray, J.: *The Normal Lung: The Basis for Diagnosis and Treatment of Pulmonary Disease,* 2nd ed. Philadelphia, W. B. Saunders Co., 1986.

Shapiro, B., Harrison, R., and Walton, J.: *Clinical Application of Blood Gases,* 3rd ed. Chicago, Year Book Medical Publishers, Inc., 1982.

Slonim, N. and Hamilton, L.: *Respiratory Physiology,* 5th ed. St. Louis, C. V. Mosby Co., 1987.

West, J.: *Respiratory Physiology—the Essentials,* 3rd ed. Baltimore, Williams & Wilkins, 1985.

Pulmonary Circulation

4

Main Objectives

1. Describe the pathway of blood flow through the heart and pulmonary circulation.
2. Describe differences and similarities between systemic and pulmonary circulations.
3. Define the following terms: cardiac output, transmural pressure, driving pressure, mean pulmonary artery pressure, pulmonary vascular resistance, systemic vascular resistance, capillary hydrostatic pressure, and capillary serum oncotic (osmotic) pressure.
4. Name at least five factors that affect pulmonary vascular resistance.
5. Explain how increased pressure in the lungs (e.g., from mechanical ventilation) affects alveolar vessels and venous return to the right side of the heart.
6. Describe the relationship between the bronchial circulation and the normal anatomic shunt.
7. State the two functions of the lymphatic circulation.
8. Identify the general location of the main lymphatic channels and lymph nodes along the tracheobronchial tree.
9. Name two factors in Starling's equation that determine fluid balance in the lung.

Chapter 1 introduced only one type of pulmonary circulation; however, the respiratory system actually has three types of pulmonary circulation, as follows: (1) the main *pulmonary circulation* that conducts blood through the lungs, (2) the connecting *bronchial circulation* within the lungs, and (3) the *lymphatic circulation*.

Pulmonary Circulation

The term pulmonary circulation most commonly refers to the system of vessels that receives deoxygenated blood from the right side of the heart, passes it

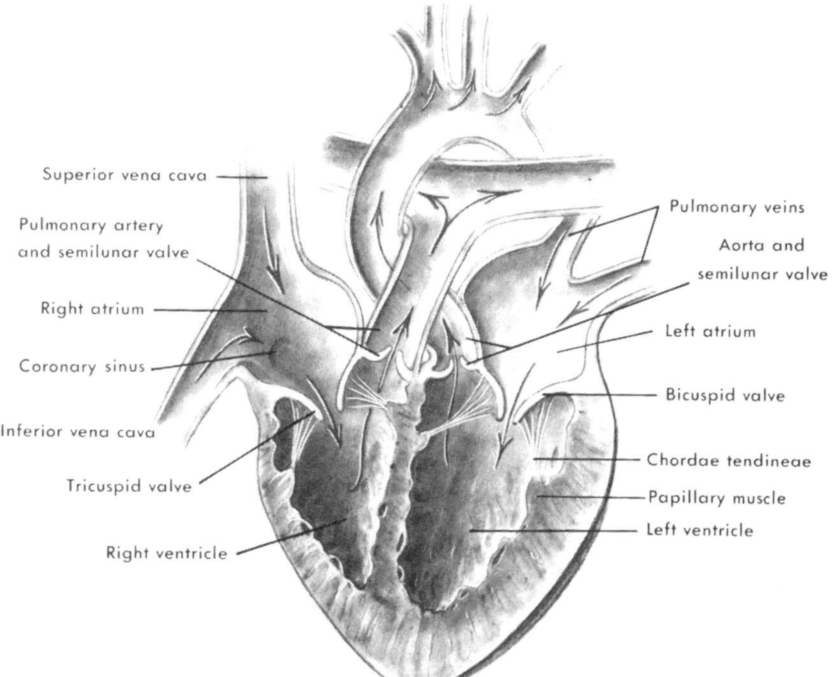

Figure 4–1. Diagram of the heart showing chambers, valves, and direction of blood flow. (Reproduced by permission from Dienhart, C. M.: Basic Human Anatomy and Physiology, 3rd ed. Philadelphia, W. B. Saunders Co., 1979.)

by the air-blood barrier, and returns it fully oxygenated to the heart's left side.

PATHWAY OF BLOOD FLOW (Fig. 4–1)

To reach the pulmonary circulation, blood must first pass through the right side of the heart. The right atrium collects blood from the three following veins: (1) *superior vena cava*, which drains the upper portions of the body; (2) *inferior vena cava*, which drains the lower portions of the body; and (3) *coronary sinus*, which drains blood from vessels supplying the walls of the heart. The right atrium pumps blood past the tricuspid valve and into the right ventricle.

To pass through the lungs, blood is pumped from the right ventricle, through the pulmonic valve, and into the *main pulmonary artery*, also called the *pulmonary trunk*. This vessel passes upwards, backwards, and to the left, where it divides into two branches, as follows: (1) the *right pulmonary artery* running to the right lung and (2) the *left pulmonary artery* running to the left lung (Fig. 4–2). The pulmonary arteries follow the bronchi down the centers of the secondary lobules as far as the terminal bronchioles. At this level, *arterioles* (small arteries) branch into *capillaries* in the walls of alveoli. Each capillary has a diameter of about 10 microns, just large enough for one red blood cell to pass through it at a time. Each RBC spends about 1 second in the dense network of capillaries termed the *pulmonary capillary bed*.

After gas exchange occurs at the air-blood barrier, small *venules* running between lobules collect oxygenated blood, uniting to form four large *veins*. These veins drain into the left atrium (Fig. 4–3).

To reach the systemic circulation, blood is pumped from the left atrium, through the mitral valve, and into the left ventricle. Then, this muscular chamber pumps blood through the aortic valve into the aorta and subsequently to other arteries of the systemic circulation.

PULMONARY VERSUS SYSTEMIC CIRCULATIONS

The pulmonary circulation is very similar to the systemic circulation. It has a pump that produces a pulsatile pressure; it has a distributing system (arteries and arterioles), an exchange system (capillary bed), and a collecting system (venules and veins). However, the pulmonary circulation possesses several unique features that account for the efficiency with which it carries out its functions.

The box on pages 55 and 56 contains a glossary of vascular terms used to describe the pulmonary circulation. Many of these terms are clinical measurements employed to quantify the effectiveness of *blood transport*, the pulmonary circulation's chief function. This glossary prepares the reader for a review of the contents of Table 4–1 and an understanding of the respiratory applications of hemodynamic monitoring (see Chapter 29). Table 4–1 compares pulmonary and systemic circulations, with emphases on variables that reveal unique features of the pulmonary circulation. Many of these features are discussed in further detail in subsequent chapters on chest pathophysiology (see Chapter 9).

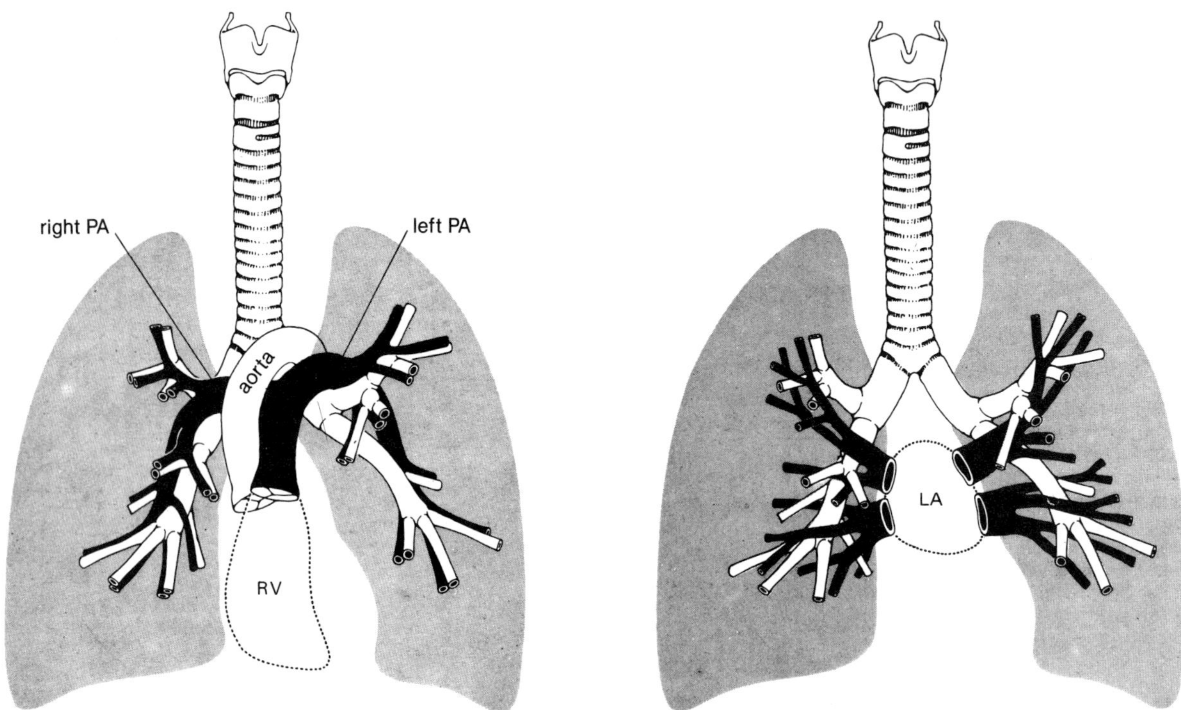

Figure 4–2 Figure 4–3

Figure 4–2. Main brainches of the pulmonary artery in relation to the bronchi. RV = right ventricle; PA = pulmonary artery. (Reproduced by permission from Weibel, E. In Fishman, A.: Assessment of Pulmonary Function. New York, McGraw-Hill Book Co., 1980.)

Figure 4–3. Two main stems of pulmonary veins penetrate into lungs on each side. LA = left atrium. (Reproduced by permission from Weibel, E. In Fishman A.: Assessment of Pulmonary Function. New York, McGraw-Hill Book Co., 1980.)

Table 4–1. COMPARISON OF PULMONARY AND SYSTEMIC CIRCULATORY SYSTEMS

Variable	Pulmonary Circulation	Systemic Circulation
Vessel contents	Arteries contain *unoxygenated* blood Veins contain *oxygenated* blood	Arteries contain oxygenated blood Veins contain unoxygenated blood
Blood volume	500 ml or 10% of total circulating volume	6 to 8 L including pulmonary circulation
Nature of vessel walls	Thin and distensible Little smooth muscle	Thick and less distensible abundant smooth muscle around arterioles
Arterial pressure	Pulmonary artery	Systemic artery
systolic/diastolic	25/8, 15 mmHg (low)	120/80, 100 mmHg (high)
mean		
Vascular resistance*		
at rest (sitting)	PVR = 1.43 mmHg/L/min (low)	SVR = 13.5 mmHg/L/min (high)
with exercise	PVR = 0.62 mmHg/L/min (low)	SVR = 6.9 mmHg/L/min (high)
Initial response to lack of oxygen	Vasoconstriction	Vasodilatation

*Data from Murray, J.: The Normal Lung: The Basis for Diagnosis and Treatment of Pulmonary Disease, 2nd ed. Philadelphia, W. B. Saunders Co., 1986.

PULMONARY VASCULAR PRESSURE AND OTHER MEASUREMENTS

INTRAVASCULAR OR INTRALUMENAL PRESSURE
Blood pressure in the lumen of a blood vessel. Pulmonary arteries = 15 mmHg, capillaries = 8 to 10 mmHg, and veins = 5 to 6 mmHg.

EXTRAVASCULAR PRESSURE
Pressure of tissue surrounding a vessel. It is equal to intrathoracic pressure, a reflection of pleural pressure (for tissue near pulmonary arteries and veins); alveolar pressure (for tissue next to alveoli); or some pressure in between (for tissue near arterioles, capillaries, and venules).

TRANSMURAL PRESSURE
Difference between intravascular pressure and extravascular pressure.

DRIVING PRESSURE (ΔP)
Difference between pressures at one point in a vessel and another point downstream. For the pulmonary circulation

$$\begin{aligned} \Delta P &= \text{input pressure} - \text{output pressure} \\ &= 15 \text{ mmHg (pulmonary artery pressure)} - 5 \text{ mmHg (left atrial pressure)} \\ &= 10 \text{ mmHg (normal value)} \end{aligned}$$

PULMONARY BLOOD FLOW
Dependent upon right ventricular output and the relationship among flow, pressure, and resistance.

$$\text{blood flow} = \frac{\text{mean blood pressure}}{\text{resistance to flow}}$$

Normally assumed to be equal to cardiac output (left ventricular output). *Instantaneous pulmonary blood flow* may be measured using the body plethysmograph in the pulmonary function laboratory.

CARDIAC OUTPUT (Q)
Expressed in the following equation:

$$Q = \underset{\text{(mls of blood ejected per heart beat)}}{\text{stroke volume}} \times \underset{\text{(beats per min)}}{\text{heart rate}} = \underset{\text{(normal value)}}{5 \text{ to } 8 \text{ L/min}}$$

May reach 25 to 30 L/min during strenuous exercise. Measured in the clinical setting by direct Fick's method or indicator dilution method.

PULMONARY VASCULAR RESISTANCE (PVR)
Defined as resistance to blood flow through the pulmonary circulation and considered a measure of right ventricular afterload, the resistance against which the right ventricle must pump. Most resistance to blood flow normally occurs in arterioles and capillaries—venules and veins offer little resistance. Alterations in PVR occur in two ways, as follows: (1) *actively* by contraction or relaxation of smooth muscle of vessel walls in response to neural stimuli (actually produces little to no effect), humoral stimuli (e.g., vasoconstrictors or vasodilators), or chemical stimuli (e.g., lack of oxygen or excess carbon dioxide); and (2) *passively* by changes in the caliber of pulmonary vessels secondary to changing *mechanical conditions* within the lung (e.g., blood volume; lung inflation or deflation; and pulmonary artery, interstitial, or transpulmonary pressures) or secondary to *hemodynamic events in the systemic circulation* (e.g., blood volume, blood viscosity, and left atrial pressure).
PVR is calculated from this equation as with airway resistance and resistance in any vascular system:

$$\text{Resistance (R)} = \frac{\text{driving pressure } (\Delta P)}{\text{blood flow (Q)}}$$

In the clinical setting, PVR is calculated from measurements taken via a catheter in the pulmonary artery (see Chapter 29). The equation is as follows:

$$\text{Normal PVR} = \frac{\text{mean pulmonary artery pressure (PAP)} - \text{left atrial pressure (LAP or pulmonary capillary wedge pressure)}}{\text{cardiac output (Q)}}$$

$$\begin{aligned} &= \text{about } 0.1 \text{ mmHg/ml/sec or } 1.0 \text{ mmHg/L/min} \\ &= 80 \text{ dynes/sec/cm}^{-5} \end{aligned}$$

(mmHg/L/min multiplied by 80 equals dynes/sec/cm^{-5})

OR

= less than 60 dynes/sec/cm^{-5} (young adults)
= less than 80 to 100 dynes/sec/cm^{-5} (elderly)

SYSTEMIC VASCULAR RESISTANCE (SVR)
Defined as resistance to blood flow through the systemic circulation and considered a measure of left ventricular afterload, the resistance against which the left ventricle must pump. Normal SVR = 800 to 1200 dynes/sec/cm^{-5}.

CAPILLARY HYDROSTATIC PRESSURE
Fluid or intravascular pressure that tends to force fluid out of capillaries. Normally 8 to 10 mmHg.

CAPILLARY SERUM ONCOTIC PRESSURE
Also called *colloid osmotic pressure*; pressure related to protein (mostly albumin), which tends to retain fluid within capillaries. Normally 25 to 30 mmHg. It is the balance between capillary (and interstitial) hydrostatic and oncotic pressures that causes most fluid to be retained in capillaries. (Slight filtration of fluid from capillaries to interstitial spaces normally occurs.)

LOW PRESSURE SYSTEM

Perhaps the most distinguishing features of the pulmonary circulation are its low pressures. The pressure within the pulmonary artery is about 25/8 mmHg, with a mean pressure of 15 mmHg. The pressure within capillaries is about 8 to 10 mmHg, although the exact pressure has never been determined in the human lung. The low pressure of the system is due to its *low* resistance to blood flow (pulmonary vascular resistance) and the distensibility of its vessels. Pulmonary vessels are shorter, thinner, more distensible, and contain less smooth muscle than systemic vessels. Because of the low pressure, small changes in extravascular pressure produce greater effects on the dimensions of pulmonary vessels than on systemic vessels. High vessel distensibility allows blood volume in the lungs to change with relatively little change in pressure.

ALVEOLAR VESSELS

Another distinguishing feature is the presence of *alveolar vessels,* defined as capillaries within alveolar septa that are exposed to alveolar pressure. In contrast, *extra-alveolar vessels* in the lung are vessels exposed to other extravascular pressures described in the preceding glossary.

Alveolar vessels are particularly sensitive to changes in alveolar pressure induced by respiration or by artificial ventilation with a ventilator. When positive alveolar pressure is excessive, it compresses alveolar septa, pinching shut capillaries and flattening them, ultimately decreasing pulmonary blood flow. Simultaneously, the increased pressure in the lungs is transmitted through the right side of the heart, increasing right atrial pressure and reducing the pressure gradient promoting venous return. In this way, both the pinching shut of alveolar vessels as well as the transmission of increased pressures to the right atrium contribute to the resulting fall in cardiac output.

By the same vessel closure mechanism, alveolar vessels in upper regions of the normal lung are usually narrowed because pressure in adjacent alveoli is higher, owing to the effects of gravity. The resulting decrease in pulmonary blood flow, however, is a regional effect and is compensated for by increased blood flow in other parts of the lungs, as described in Chapter 5.

Bronchial Circulation

The lung has another circulatory system that connects with the pulmonary circulation deep within lung tissue called the *bronchial circulation*. It is relatively small in size, receiving only 1% to 2% of the total cardiac output.

The primary function of the bronchial circulation is the provision of a continuous supply of nutrient blood to conducting airways and terminal respiratory units (TRUs) so that the lung can carry out its many functions. Also, through various anastomoses with other vessels, it supplies nutrient blood to the trachea, vagi, and other mediastinal structures.

Pathway of Blood Flow. Bronchial arteries are the vessels that deliver blood to the lung parenchyma. They vary markedly in number and origin in the human lung. Each lung possesses at least one bronchial artery, arising from the proximal portion of the thoracic aorta, from one of its two intercostal arteries, or from some other artery in close proximity.

Bronchial arteries follow airways into the lung parenchyma. Along the way, they branch elaborately and rejoin to form networks around bronchi and in bronchial submucosa. When the vessels reach the end of conducting airways and the beginning of TRUs, they anastomose with pulmonary artery capillaries from the pulmonary circulation.

Blood returns to the heart via the following drainage systems (Fig. 4–4):

1. *Proximally,* near main stem bronchi, blood travels

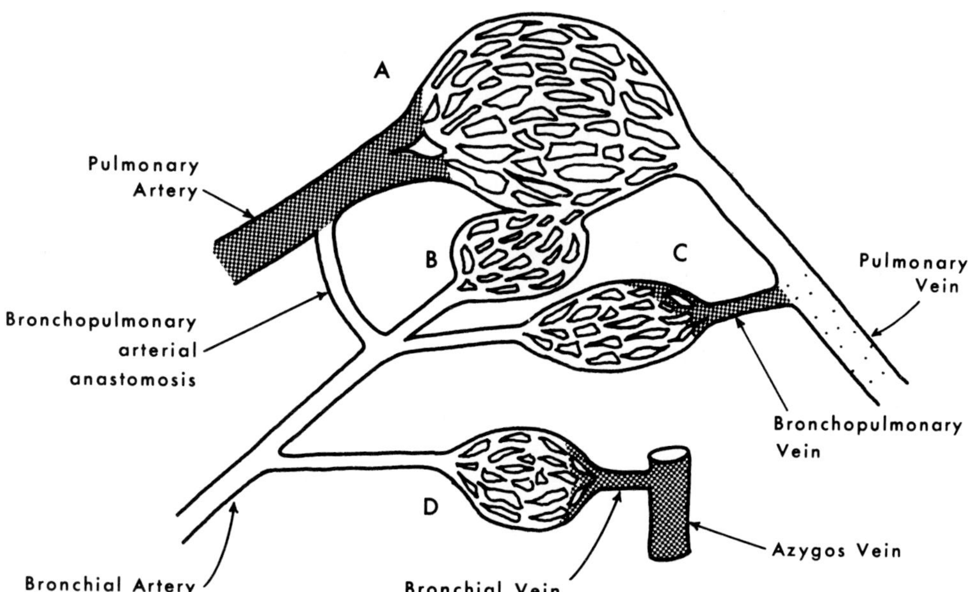

Figure 4–4. Schematic representation of relationships between pulmonary and bronchial circulations. In the *pulmonary circulation* (top network), the pulmonary artery supplies the pulmonary capillary bed. Blood returns to the left atrium through pulmonary veins. In the *bronchial circulation*, the bronchial artery supplies two drainage systems as follows: (1) the proximal system (A) drains into the bronchial vein, azygos vein, superior vena cava, and right atrium and (2) the distal system drains terminal bronchioles that anastomose the pulmonary capillaries (B). Also, the distal system drains another bronchial capillary network (C) via the bronchopulmonary vein. The networks in the distal system return blood to the left atrium through the pulmonary veins. Network D represents the bronchial capillary supply to lobar and segmental bronchi; these vessels form true bronchial veins that drain into the azygos, hemiazygos, or intercostal veins. The shaded areas represent blood of low O_2 content. (Reproduced by permission from Murray, J.: The Normal Lung: The Basis for Diagnosis and Treatment of Pulmonary Disease, 2nd ed. Philadelphia, W. B. Saunders Co, 1986.)

via true bronchial veins (Fig. 4–4A) into azygos veins, eventually the superior vena cava, and then the right atrium. It is estimated that about 25% to 33% of the bronchial arterial supply returns to the heart via bronchial veins.

2. *Distally*, bronchial venous drainage around terminal bronchioles flows through the aforementioned anastomoses with alveolar capillaries (Fig. 4–4B) and returns to the left atrium via the pulmonary veins. Similarly, another bronchial capillary network (Fig. 4–4C) drains into pulmonary veins.

The mixing of bronchial venous blood with arterialized blood from the pulmonary circulation accounts for the small amount of unoxygenated blood within pulmonary veins. About 65% to 75% of the bronchial circulation flows into the pulmonary veins. This amount is termed the *normal anatomic shunt* and represents about 2% to 5% of total cardiac output.

Importance of Bronchial Circulation. Though small in size, the importance of the bronchial circulation cannot be overestimated. It is thought to have a nutritional role in the fetus and neonate as well as in the child and adult. Many diseases significantly alter its structure and function, e.g., congenital cardiac anomalies and chronic inflammatory or neoplastic disease. Most important, blood flow between bronchial and pulmonary circulations is normally in a balanced state because of anastomoses. Hence, when disease produces decreased blood flow from the pulmonary circulation to localized lung tissue (e.g., tissue distal to an obstructed vessel), the bronchial circulation increases blood flow to that part of the lung via its collateral channels. Conversely, when blood flow to the bronchial circulation decreases, the pulmonary circulation will increase its blood supply to tissues formerly supplied by bronchial vessels. This reciprocal relationship facilitates adaptation whenever structures of either circulatory system become impaired by disease.

Lymphatic Circulation

The lung has another circulatory system—the lymphatic circulation. It consists of a system of thin-walled lymphatic vessels resembling veins with *lymph nodes* or small rounded collections of lymphatic tissue at various intervals (Fig. 4–5).

The lymphatic circulation has two primary functions.

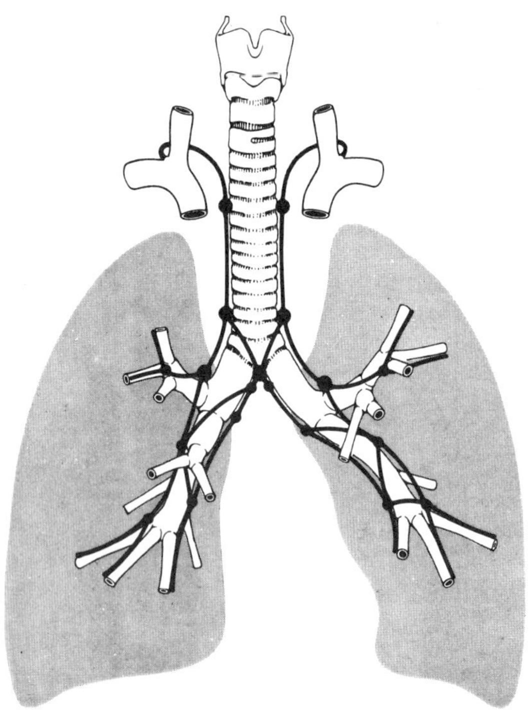

Figure 4–5. Schematic diagram of the distribution of lymph nodes and main lymphatic channels along the bronchial tree. (Reproduced by permission from Weibel, E. In Fishman, A.: Assessment of Pulmonary Function. New York, McGraw-Hill Book Co., 1980.)

First, it drains excess fluid from interstitial spaces as well as any protein molecules that leak out of blood vessels. The composition of the drainage or *lymph* is identical or nearly identical to that of interstitial fluid. Second, it provides an exit route for inhaled particles or microorganisms that manage to reach alveolar surfaces.

The lung has two sets of lymphatic vessels. First, *superficial vessels* form a continuous network (or a pleural network) around the lung, dipping into the lung parenchyma and returning to the surface of the lung at times. Although it is possible for lymph to flow around the entire lung via these superficial vessels, the general flow of lymph is *inwards* towards the center of the lung via *deep vessels.* Deep vessels have two routes, as illustrated and described in Figure 4–6.

Emphasis must be placed on the complexity and variability of the lymphtic drainage patterns described. Drainage routes can vary considerably from person to person, and the routes normally occur through a maze of interconnecting mediastinal, paratracheal, and subdiaphragmatic lymph nodes and channels.

Lymph flow through these various routes is slow—only a few ml/hour—although flow can greatly increase if capillary pressures become higher over a long period of time. In the presence of an acute increase in fluid in the lungs (e.g., pulmonary edema), it is believed that lymph flow can rise at least sevenfold to tenfold.

Lung-fluid Balance

Figure 4–7 shows the movement of fluid and proteins out of the pulmonary capillary and through the interstitial space to the lymph vessel. In this fluid balance arrangement, the amount of interstitial fluid available for lymphatic drainage is largely determined by Starling's equation, shown in the box. This equation

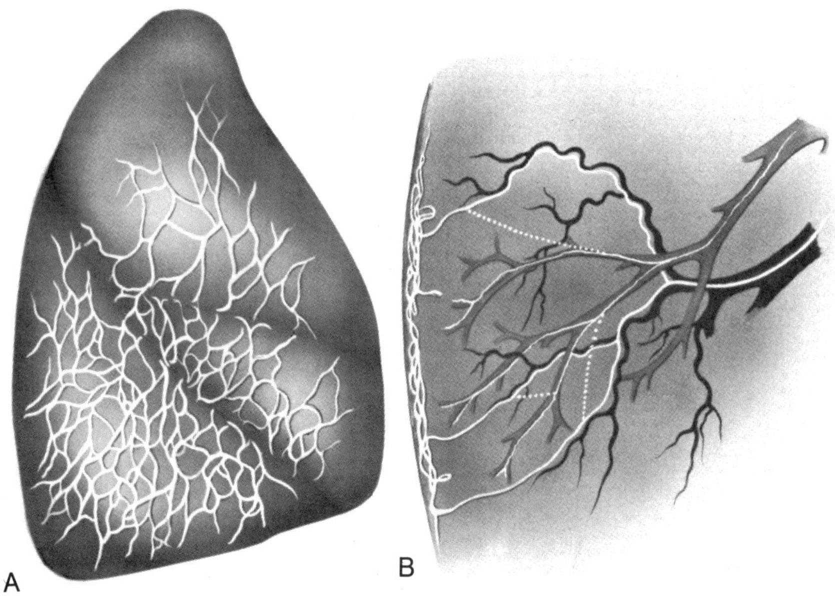

Figure 4–6. Lymphatic drainage of the lungs and its lining (pleura). *A, Superficial vessels* are more numerous over the lower half of the lung than over the upper half. *B, Deep vessels* follow one of two routes as follows: (1) superficial vessels enter the lung at interlobular septa and follow venous vessels (dark-shaded vessels) inward and (2) lymphatic channels in the lung parenchyma extend inward along the connective tissue sheath around bronchi and arteries (light-shaded vessels). Other lymphatics (dotted lines) connect peribronchial and perivenous lymphatics. (Reproduced by permission from Fraser, R. and Paré, J.: Diagnosis of Diseases of the Chest, vol. 1, 2nd ed. Philadelphia, W. B. Saunders Co., 1977.)

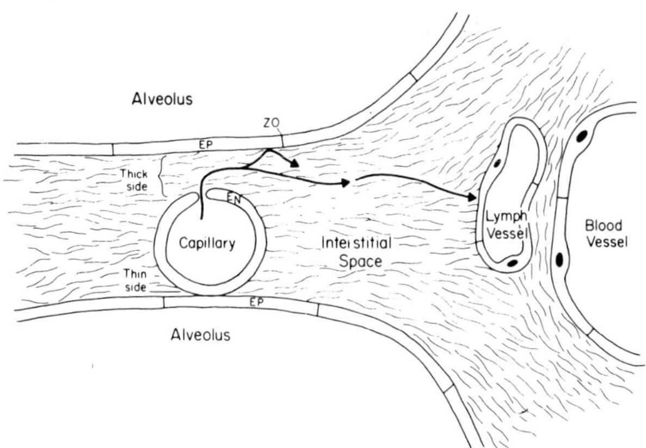

Figure 4–7. Movement of fluid and proteins out of the pulmonary capillary and towards the lymph vessel. Fluid movement occurs at the thick side of the interalveolar septum, as described in Chapter 2. The normal "leaky" capillary endothelium (EN) has a relatively large intercellular junction compared with the tight alveolar junction labelled ZO (zonulae occludens). EP = epithelium. (Reproduced by permission from Nieman, G.: Current concepts of lung-filled balance. Resp. Care 30:1062–1076, 1985.)

determines fluid balance in the lungs. It states that the direction of fluid flow (Q_f) across a membrane is related to capillary hydrostatic pressure, which determines fluid filtration, and plasma colloid osmotic pressure, which determines fluid absorption into interstitial spaces.

STARLING'S EQUATION TO DETERMINE LUNG-FLUID BALANCE

EQUATION

$$Q_f = K_f[(P_c - P_i) - \sigma(\pi_c - \pi_i)]$$

DEFINITION OF TERMS

Q_f = direction of fluid flow across a membrane (or transcapillary flow)
K_f = endothelial filtration coefficient (describes the permeability of the endothelium to fluid)
P_c = capillary hydrostatic pressure
P_i = interstitial hydrostatic pressure
σ = coefficient for endothelial permeability to protein (describes the degree to which the endothelium acts as a physical barrier to protein movement)
π = capillary osmotic pressure
π_i = interstitial space osmotic pressure

In the normal lung, the balance of forces in Starling's equation results in a small net pressure gradient favoring filtration and drainage by lymphatics. Furthermore, whereas capillaries have relatively high permeability to fluid and plasma proteins, the alveolar epithelium remains relatively impermeable, as shown in Figure 4–7. This relationship prevents the flooding of fluid into alveolar spaces.

In cardiopulmonary disease, a high pulmonary capillary pressure (e.g., in left ventricular failure) or a highly permeable alveolar-capillary membrane (e.g., in adult respiratory distress syndrome) will upset the balance of forces affecting lung-fluid balance. Fluid rapidly moves into interstitial, alveolar or both types of spaces, impairing gas exchange and placing an excessive fluid load on the lymphatic circulation. Nieman (1985) provides a more detailed explanation of the complex relationships between fluid filtered by pulmonary capillaries and that drained by lymphatics.

Conclusion

This chapter explains pulmonary, bronchial, and lymphatic circulations of the lungs. In addition, it introduces Starling's equation and its role in the maintenance of normal lung-fluid balance.

Information in this chapter helps the nurse understand numerous clinical applications (e.g., why blood pressure falls with application of positive pressure to the lungs, as in mechanical ventilation). The contents assist the nurse in understanding reasons for checking the right rather than the left cardiac silhouette on the chest x-ray for signs of early right ventricular failure (see Chapter 15). This chapter also facilitates comprehension of hemodynamic monitoring (see Chapter 29)

REFERENCES

Brigham, K. and Newman, J.: The pulmonary circulation. *Basics of Respiratory Disease,* 8(1): 1979.

Fishman, A.: *Assessment of Pulmonary Function.* New York, McGraw-Hill Book Co., 1980.

Fraser, R. and Paré, J.: *Diagnosis of Diseases of the Chest, vol. 1,* 2nd ed. Philadelphia, W. B. Saunders Co., 1977.

Jacobs, S., Francone, C., and Lossow, W.: *Structure and Function in Man,* 5th ed. Philadelphia, W. B. Saunders Co., 1982.

Murray, J.: *The Normal Lung: The Basis for Diagnosis and Treatment of Pulmonary Disease,* 2nd ed. Philadelphia, W. B. Saunders Co., 1986.

Nieman, G.: Current concepts of lung-fluid balance. *Respiratory Care,* 30(12): 1062–1076, 1985.

Staub, N.: Lung structure and function—1982. *Basics of Respiratory Disease,* 10(3), 1982.

West, J.: *Respiratory Physiology—The Essentials,* 3rd ed. Baltimore, Williams & Wilkins, 1985.

Lung Ventilation and Ventilation/ Perfusion (V/Q) Ratios

5

Main Objectives

1. **Define the following terms: tidal volume, vital capacity, residual volume, minute ventilation, total lung ventilation, alveolar hypoventilation, alveolar hyperventilation, shunt-producing disorders, and dead space–producing disorders.**
2. **Explain why minute ventilation is never used as the sole monitoring parameter in a clinical setting.**
3. **Name the best and most practical measurement of alveolar ventilation.**
4. **Define the following types of dead space ventilation: anatomical, alveolar, physiological, and mechanical.**
5. **State the clinical significance of the ratio of dead space to tidal volume (V_D/V_T).**
6. **Explain the relationship between minute ventilation, V_D/V_T and $PaCO_2$.**
7. **In the upright lung, explain why basilar regions are better ventilated and better perfused compared with apical regions.**
8. **Explain why the V/Q ratio is the most important determinant of normal gas exchange.**
9. **Identify and describe the two main types of mismatching of ventilation to perfusion, giving one clinical example for each type.**
10. **Discuss the effect of V/Q abnormality on gas exchange.**

This chapter discusses lung ventilation, lung perfusion, and ventilation/perfusion (V/Q) ratios. Of these three concepts, the last is perhaps most important because V/Q explains why some patients readily adapt to lung disease and why others become extremely hypoxemic, with onset of the same type and extent of lung disease.

Lung Ventilation

Lung ventilation is the movement of gas volumes in and out of the conducting airways and terminal respiratory units of the lungs.

Knowledge of basic lung volumes and capacities facilitates comprehension of other concepts discussed, such as minute ventilation, total lung ventilation, and regional differences in lung ventilation.

BASIC LUNG VOLUMES AND CAPACITIES

Air in a person's lungs is divided into subdivisions called *lung volumes.* Combinations of lung volumes are called *lung capacities.* Basic lung volumes and capacities are presented in Figure 5–1 and discussed further in Chapter 14 in relation to pulmonary function tests.

The two most commonly referred to measurements in the clinical setting are tidal volume and vital capacity. *Tidal volume* (V_T) is the *volume of air exhaled with each normal breath at rest. Vital capacity* (VC) is the *volume of air exhaled after a maximal inspiration.* Both of these volumes are measured with a monitoring device called a *spirometer* or *respirometer.* Though a decrease in both V_T and VC may signal the onset of moderate to severe pulmonary disease, a complete pulmonary function test is needed to determine the exact nature and severity of the abnormality.

The volume of air left in the lungs after a vital capacity breathing maneuver is called the *residual volume* (RV). The *total lung capacity* (TLC) consists of vital capacity and residual volume, as shown in Figure 5 1. Functional residual capacity (FRC) is similar to residual volume, except it represents air in the lungs at the end of a normal rather than a maximal expiration.

RV, TLC, and FRC are not routine monitoring parameters because their measurement involves the use of sophisticated equipment in the pulmonary function laboratory. As part of the complete pulmonary function test, these parameters are most useful in the diagnosis and evaluation of subacute or chronic pulmonary disease.

MINUTE VENTILATION

Minute ventilation, also called *minute volume of ventilation,* is a basic parameter used to assess overall lung ventilation and mechanics of breathing. It is usually abbreviated $\dot{V}_E$ and defined as the *total expired volume of air (gas mixture) per minute.* (Note that a dot over any letter stands for per minute.)

In the clinical setting, minute ventilation is calculated by multiplying V_T by respiratory rate or frequency (f) in breaths per minute. Normal respiratory rate is 8 to 20 breaths/min, depending on the level of wakefulness. Normal $\dot{V}_E$ is about 5 to 10 L/min and for an average healthy adult is calculated as follows:

$$\begin{array}{ccccc} V_T & \times & f & = & \dot{V}_E \\ 0.5\text{ L (500 ml)} & \times & 12\text{ breaths/min} & = & 6\text{ L/min} \end{array}$$

To determine $\dot{V}_E$ the clinician may multiple a patient's average V_T at rest by respiratory rate counted over a 1 minute time period. A more precise method is to use the spirometer to measure cumulative exhaled tidal volumes for 1 minute. To simplify monitoring, many mechanical ventilators have attached or built-in spirometers as well as the capacity to display digitally changing $\dot{V}_E$ values.

Perhaps the most important point to remember about $\dot{V}_E$ is that it is a general rather than a specific monitoring parameter. Though an increase or decrease in value may indicate a corresponding increase or decrease in lung ventilation and possible respiratory dysfunction, $\dot{V}_E$ may remain insensitive to changes in lung ventilation at the alveolar level. Consider the following calculations:

$$\textit{Patient A}\ V_T\ (500\text{ ml}) \times f\ 12 = \dot{V}_E\ 6\text{ L/min}$$
$$\textit{Patient B}\ V_T\ (250\text{ ml}) \times f\ 24 = \dot{V}_E\ 6\text{ L/min}$$

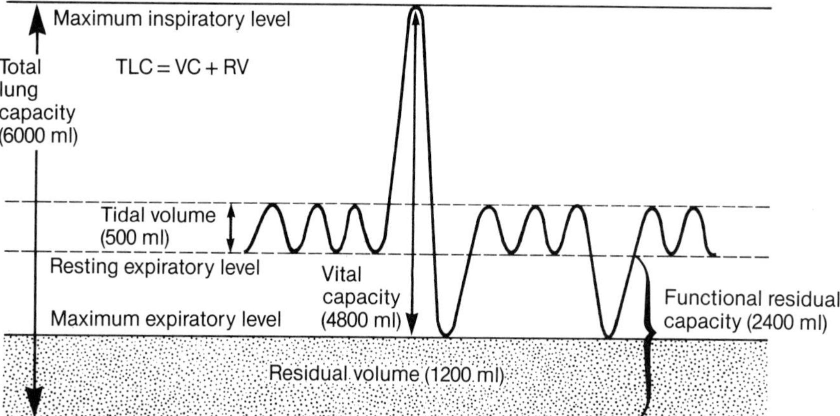

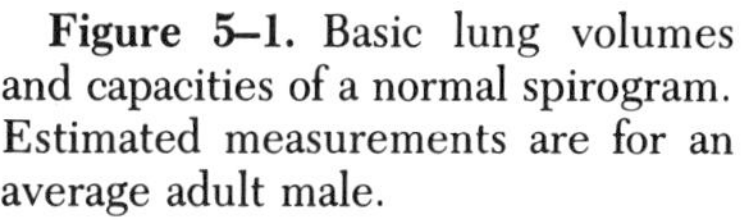
Figure 5–1. Basic lung volumes and capacities of a normal spirogram. Estimated measurements are for an average adult male.

Although both patients have a normal V_E, patient B can be expected to have ventilatory or gas exchange problems. The low V_T and high f represent shallow and rapid breathing. When tidal volume is drastically reduced, as in this case, inadequate lung expansion and alveolar collapse are likely.

Because $\dot{V}_E$ may remain grossly insensitive to changes in alveolar ventilation, it is always considered along with other assessment data, including separate measurements of V_T and f, blood gas and pulmonary function data, and chest assessment findings. Nevertheless, in the absence of more specific assessment parameters, $\dot{V}_E$ is a relatively simple and cost-effective way to monitor changes in total lung ventilation.

TOTAL LUNG VENTILATION—ALVEOLAR AND DEAD SPACE VENTILATION

Total lung ventilation (V) is defined physiologically as the sum of alveolar ventilation (V_A) and dead space ventilation (V_D). The formula is written, as follows:

$$V = V_A + V_D$$

Alveolar Ventilation (V_A)

This value is defined as the volume of inspired air that reaches the alveolar level and participates in gas exchange. Arterial PCO_2 is the best and most practical measurement of V_A.

Normal V_A is defined as the level of V_A that produces a normal $PaCO_2$ level (about 40 mmHg).

Alveolar hypoventilation refers to a decrease in ventilation below the level necessary to maintain a normal $PaCO_2$. The decrease in V_A allows CO_2 to accumulate in the lungs, producing a *high* $PaCO_2$, as follows:

$$\downarrow V_A \rightarrow \uparrow PaCO_2$$

Alveolar hyperventilation refers to an increase in ventilation above the level necessary to maintain a normal $PaCO_2$. The increase in V_A promotes the rapid elimination of CO_2 from the lungs, producing a *low* $PaCO_2$, as follows:

$$\uparrow V_A \rightarrow \downarrow PaCO_2$$

Dead Space Ventilation (V_D)

V_D is the volume of inspired air that does not participate in gas exchange. The four different types of dead space are *anatomic, alveolar, physiologic,* and *mechanical.*

Anatomic Dead Space (VD_{ANAT}). This concept is introduced in Chapter 2, and VD_{ANAT} is the volume of air in the conductive zone of the lung, from the nose and mouth down to the terminal respiratory bronchioles. About one third of each V_T is composed of VD_{ANAT}. In the adult, it totals 150 ml or about 1 ml/lb (2 ml/kg) of ideal body weight. Though this resting value may be higher for individuals with large body builds and lower for individuals with small body builds, it remains constant unless cardiopulmonary disease develops.

The most common cause of increased VD_{ANAT} is a rapid shallow breathing pattern. Because of small V_Ts,

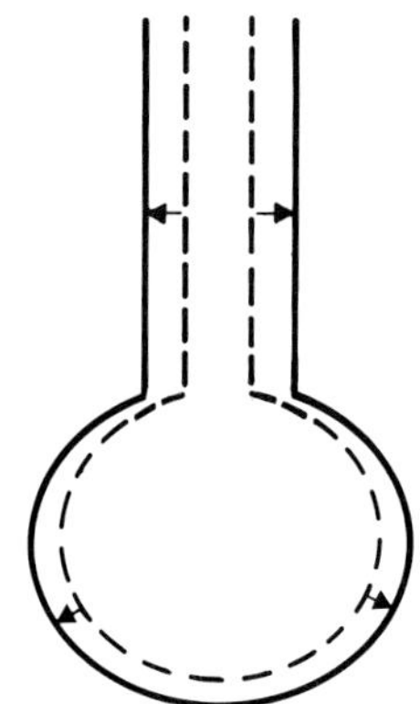

A Increased VDANAT
INCREASE IN AIRWAY VOLUME
As in: Large tidal volumes from exercise
or pulmonary disease
Positive pressure breathing
Bronchiectasis
Lung hyperinflation
Old age

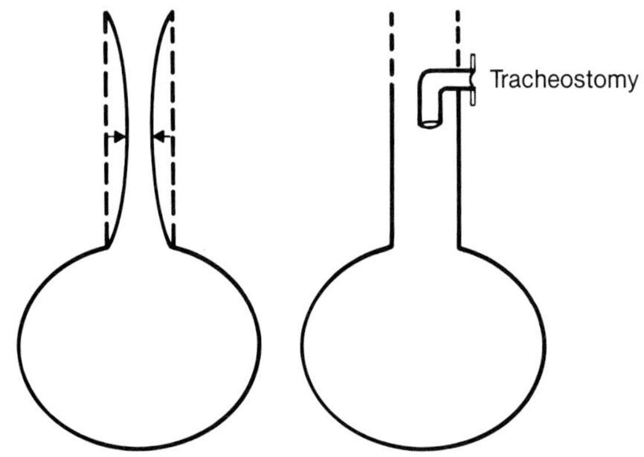

Figure 5–2. Mechanisms of increased and decreased anatomic dead space (VD_{ANAT}).

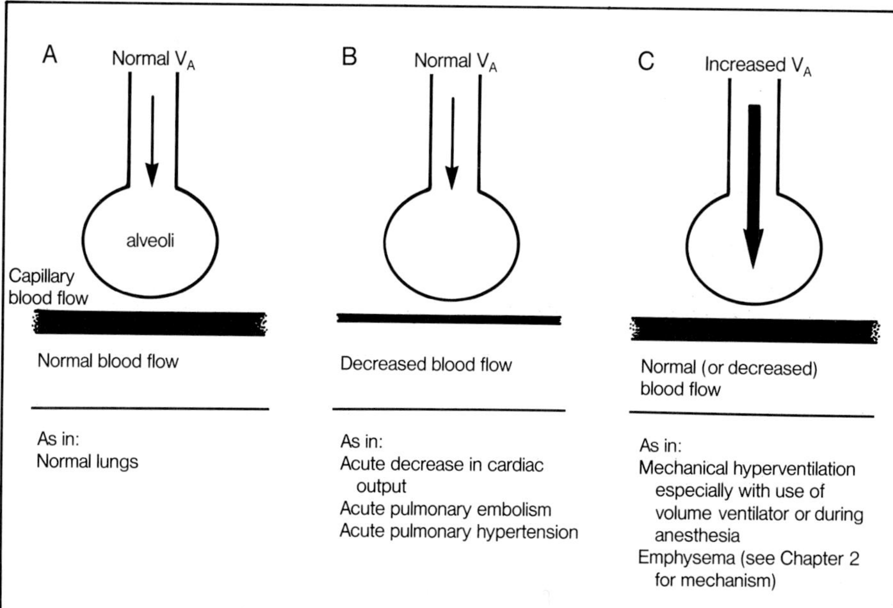

Figure 5–3. Mechanisms of normal (A) and increased (B, C) alveolar dead space (VD_{ALV}). V_A = alveolar ventilation.

a proportionally smaller amount of each volume reaches alveoli for gas exchange, resulting in a proportionally larger amount of CO_2-rich gas in lower airways at the end of exhalation. The extra volume of CO_2-rich gas increases VD_{ANAT}. Although a further increase in respiratory rate helps maintain $\dot{V}_E$ it also greatly increases VD_{ANAT} providing V_T remains small.

In addition to rapid shallow breathing, increased VD_{ANAT} results from general airway dilatations or conditions that increase airway caliber and volume on each breath (Fig. 5–2A).

Lowered VD_{ANAT} results from conditions that decrease the volume of conducting airways. Examples include the surgical removal of lung tissue (e.g., pneumonectomy), tracheal by-pass (e.g., insertion of a tracheostomy tube), and airway obstruction or bronchoconstriction due to pulmonary disease (Fig. 5–2B).

Alveolar Dead Space (VD_{ALV}). This value is defined as the volume of gas in acinar units that does *not* participate in gas exchange. In other words, it is the volume of inspired gas which is not useful or effective in arterializing venous blood (Forester et al, 1986).

Figure 5–3 compares a normal lung unit (Fig. 5–3A) with two dead space–producing situations (Fig. 5–3B and Fig. 5–3C). Keep in mind that these three situations represent ventilation and perfusion relationships for healthy or diseased regions of the lung or for the lungs as a whole. Regional changes in ventilation and perfusion may be more drastic than the last two illustrations portray.

In Figure 5–3A, normal alveolar ventilation is matched with normal capillary blood flow. All alveolar air participates in gas exchange. VD_{ALV} is absent or minimal. (In reality, minimal amounts of alveolar air do not exchange with capillary blood, owing to normally varying capillary blood flow.)

In Figure 5–3B, alveoli are ventilated but underperfused. A portion of each breath does *not* participate in gas exchange because of inadequate contact with capillary blood. VD_{ALV} is the nonparticipating portion of alveolar air.

In Figure 5–3C, ventilation is in excess of perfusion. The lung has two responses to this situation. First, all of the extra alveolar air may participate in gas exchange because capillary blood flow is high enough and readily available. PO_2 levels in arterial blood may actually improve owing to the increase in alveolar ventilation. However, when ventilation is far in excess of perfusion, a portion of inspired gas entering alveoli is wasted—it is exhaled without giving up O_2 to venous blood. Ventilation far in excess of what the lungs normally require constitutes *wasted ventilation*. In this case, the wasted ventilation is the VD_{ALV}.

The two aforementioned dead space situations are sometimes labelled differently, owing to slightly varying terminology among various sources of medical literature. Some medical sources might label Figure 5–3B as true *alveolar dead space* and the wasted ventilation in Figure 5–3C as *deadspace effect* (Shapiro et al, 1982).

Most important, because deadspace situations are highly variable and unpredictable, a patient's findings may represent a variation of alveolar dead space or deadspace effect or move back and forth between the two, depending on compensatory mechanisms, stage of disease, and varying regional changes in ventilation and perfusion.

Physiologic Dead Space (V_D). This value is the sum of anatomic and alveolar dead space, as follows:

$$V_D = VD_{ANAT} + VD_{ALV}$$

It represents the total volume in the conducting airways and alveoli *not* participating in gas exchange.

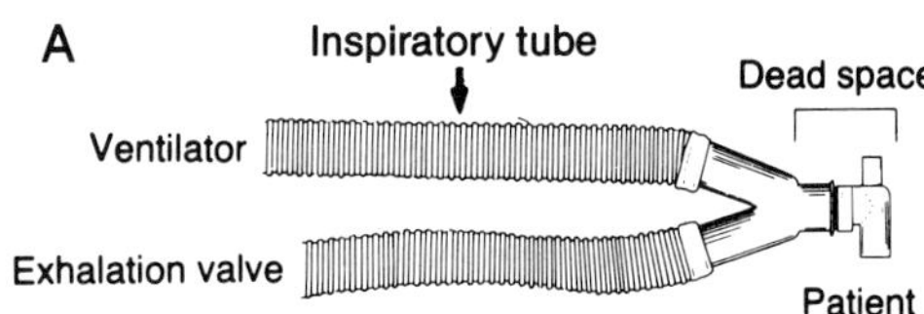

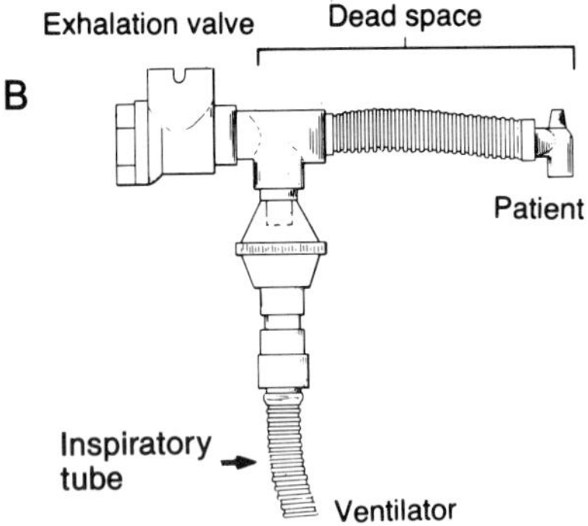

Figure 5–4. Mechanical (apparatus) dead space. *A*, Minimal dead space. *B*, Maximal desired dead space under normal circumstances. (Reproduced and adapted by permission from Pierce, A.: Acute Respiratory Failure. In Pulmonary Medicine, 2nd ed. Philadelphia, J. B. Lippincott Co., 1982.)

V_D is determined by measuring the partial pressure of CO_2 in expired gas ($P\bar{E}CO_2$) collected during a 3-minute period of quiet breathing. At the same time, a sample of arterial blood is taken to determine $PaCO_2$. V_D is then calculated, using the following formula:

$$V_D = \frac{PaCO_2 - P\bar{E}CO_2}{PaCO_2} \times V_T$$

Mechanical (Apparatus) Dead Space. This term refers to dead space external to the patient in the breathing circuit of a ventilator. More specifically, it is the volume of tubing filled with exhaled gas at the end of exhalation that is rebreathed during the next inspiration. For the patient on mechanical ventilation, mechanical dead space is kept to a minimum, as shown in Figure 5–4A. For patients on mechanical ventilation (positive pressure) and those receiving intermittent positive pressure breathing (IPPB) treatments, no more than one 5- to 6-in long flex tube is added to the mouthpiece or ventilator connector (see Fig. 5–4B). (A flex tube usually equals 50 to 60 ml of dead space.) Under normal circumstances, the dead space volume between the patient and exhalation valve of a breathing circuit is kept at approximately 75 to 100 ml (Guenter and Welch, 1982). In the critical care setting, however, one or more flex tubes may be added to or subtracted from a ventilator's breathing circuit in an effort to normalize the patient's $PaCO_2$.

Dead Space Tidal Volume Ratio (V_D/V_T)

Dead space is most commonly measured and expressed as the *ratio of dead space to tidal volume* (V_D/V_T). This ratio is sometimes estimated by substituting VD_{ANAT} for V_D. Figure 5–5 shows that for a 150-lb or 75-kg adult

$$\frac{V_D}{V_T} = \frac{150 \text{ ml}}{450 \text{ ml}} = 0.33$$

The main problem with substitution of VD_{ANAT} for V_D is that it does not take into consideration alveolar dead space ventilation. In the absence of cardiopulmonary disease, alveolar dead space is minimal. As a result, V_D is only slightly larger than VD_{ANAT} and V_D/V_T remains in the range of 0.30 to 0.35. Values for VD_{ANAT} and V_D differ appreciably when VD_{ALV} ventilation is elevated from diffuse pulmonary disease.

As a general rule, V_D/V_T must be *less than 0.55* for effective alveolar ventilation and adequate oxygenation of venous blood. An elevated V_D/V_T ratio suggests a decrease in blood flow to ventilated alveoli or a decrease in functioning capillaries in contact with ventilated alveoli. This measure is particularly useful in the early diagnosis of pulmonary vascular disease when the patient still has normal alveolar ventilation.

V_D and V_D/V_T are not routinely measured because V_D is technically more complicated to measure except in a fully equipped, pulmonary function laboratory. In most cases, a $PaCO_2$ measurement suffices to assess lung ventilation and to determine whether alveolar ventilation is reduced in spite of a normal $\dot{V}_E$.

RELATIONSHIP BETWEEN $\dot{V}_E$, V_D/V_T, and $PaCO_2$

The graph in Figure 5–6 serves as a summary of this discussion of lung ventilation. The graph shows the relationships among $\dot{V}_D$, V_D, V_T, and $PaCO_2$. The most important point to remember is as follows: if V_D/V_T

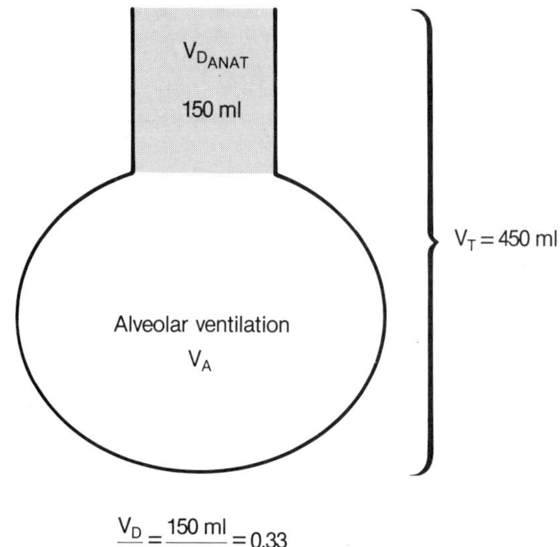

$$\frac{V_D}{V_T} = \frac{150 \text{ ml}}{450 \text{ ml}} = 0.33$$

Figure 5–5. Anatomic dead space and the V_D/V_T ratio.

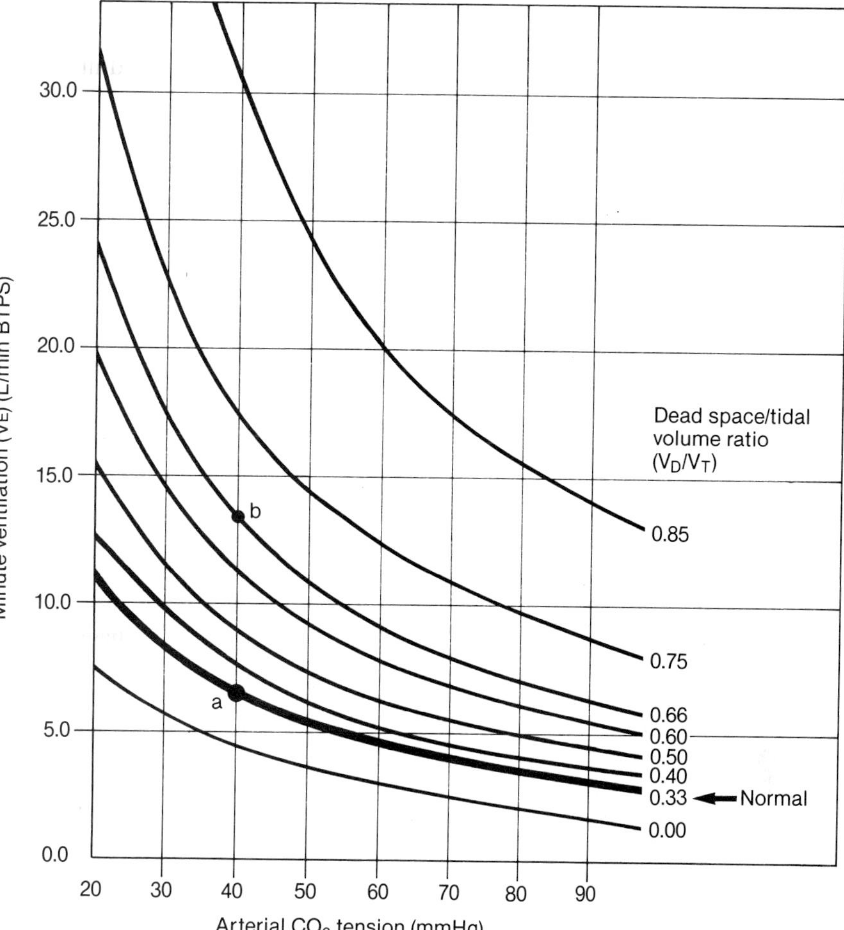

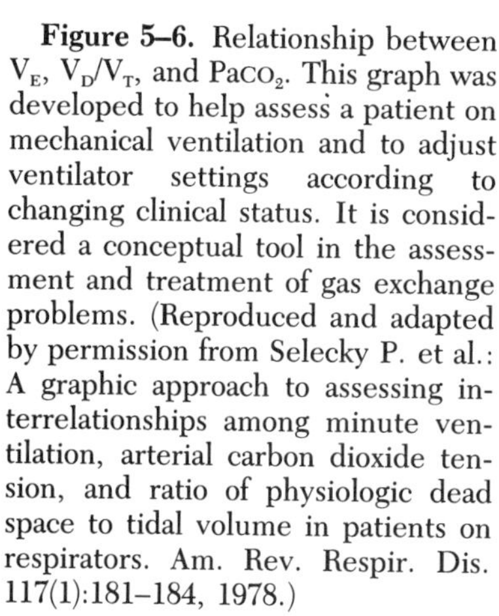
Figure 5–6. Relationship between V_E, V_D/V_T, and $PaCO_2$. This graph was developed to help assess a patient on mechanical ventilation and to adjust ventilator settings according to changing clinical status. It is considered a conceptual tool in the assessment and treatment of gas exchange problems. (Reproduced and adapted by permission from Selecky P. et al.: A graphic approach to assessing interrelationships among minute ventilation, arterial carbon dioxide tension, and ratio of physiologic dead space to tidal volume in patients on respirators. Am. Rev. Respir. Dis. 117(1):181–184, 1978.)

increases from its normal value to 0.33 (point a) to 0.66 (point b), more minute ventilation will be required to maintain the normal $PaCO_2$ of 40 mmHg. Similarly, if the patient's condition improves, and V_D/V_T decreases to 0.33, less $\dot{V}_E$ is needed to achieve normal alveolar ventilation.

REGIONAL DIFFERENCES IN LUNG VENTILATION

All regions of the normal lung are ventilated to different degrees.

In the upright position, the apex receives more gas per breath than the base of the lung. The reason for this finding pertains to normal differences in pleural pressure. Because of the weight of the lung, pleural pressure in the apex is more subatmospheric than that in the base (Fig. 5–7). The large negative pressure keeps the apical alveoli expanded to a relatively large resting volume. In contrast, the alveoli in the lung base have a smaller resting volume due to the compression of tissue from the lung's weight and the less negative pressure to keep the alveoli expanded.

The small alveolar volume in the lung base has a physiological advantage. Basilar alveoli are more capable of fully emptying with each breath and, as a result, have a larger *change in volume*/min than apical alveoli. Hence, alveolar ventilation is actually smaller in the apex, becoming progressively larger towards the lung base.

Body Position Changes

The aforementioned relationship is maintained when body position changes. Regardless of position, dependent areas are always better ventilated than uppermost areas. In lateral and supine positions, dependent lung regions are better ventilated than uppermost anteriorly located lung regions, assuming airways and alveoli are not pathologically blocked.

Low Lung Volumes

Exactly the opposite distribution of ventilation occurs normally at low lung volumes. Alveoli in the lung apices are better ventilated than alveoli in the lung bases (Fig. 5–7). Pleural pressures are again responsible for changes in lung ventilation. After a full expiration to residual volume, pleural pressure actually

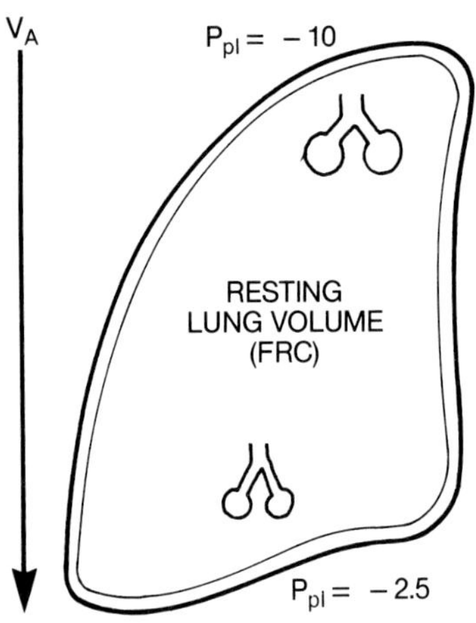

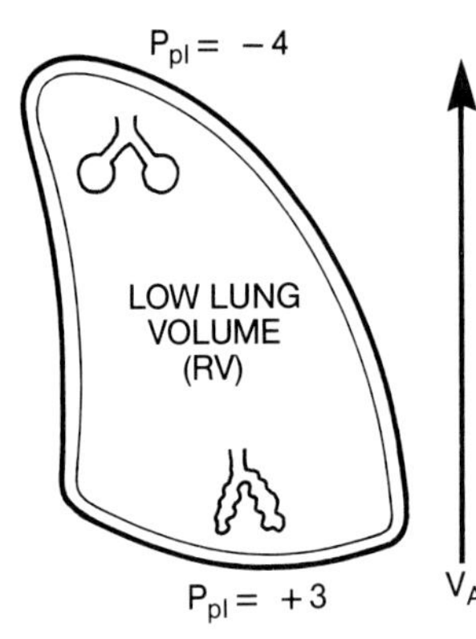

Figure 5–7. Regional changes in ventilation at resting lung volume (left) and at low lung volume or full expiration (right). FRC = functional residual capacity, and RV = residual volume. P_{pl} = pleural pressure.

exceeds airway pressure. *Airway closure* occurs, probably in the region of the respiratory bronchioles, before all the gas is squeezed out of terminal respiratory units (TRUs) (West, 1985). Hence, apical regions of the lung are better ventilated than basilar regions. After a full expiration, inspired air preferentially enters the apex before expanding partially collapsed TRUs in the lung base.

Lung Perfusion

Previously presented text explains the ventilation component of the ventilation/perfusion ratio, and this section explains the important aspects of lung perfusion.

REGIONAL DIFFERENCES IN PERFUSION

Regional differences in perfusion occur as a result of varying pulmonary arterial, venous, and alveolar pressure relationships, as described next.

Pulmonary arterial pressures vary markedly throughout the lung, owing to gravitational or *hydrostatic* effects. To understand this concept, consider the upright lung as a continuous vertical column of blood 30-cm high. Gravity causes the pressure at the bottom (lung base) of the column to exceed that at the top (lung apex) by a hydrostatic pressure gradient of 30 cm H_2O or 23 mmHg. This is a large pressure gradient for a low pressure system such as the pulmonary circulation.

As a result of this hydrostatic gradient, continuous blood flow is absent at the very top of the lung (zone 1 in Figure 5–8), and it does not begin until pulmonary arterial pressure becomes greater than alveolar pressure (zone 2 of the lung). Zone 1 is actually more theoretical, because blood flow is not normally, totally absent in the apices. Since pulmonary artery pressure is pulsatile, in late cardiac diastole, if pressure in the main pulmonary artery decreases below 11 cmH_2O, blood flow will stop briefly in the uppermost portion of the lung (Staub, 1982). (The distance from the main pulmonary artery to the top of the lung is about 11 cm.) Portions of lung are most likely to enter into zone 1 whenever vascular pressures become extremely low, e.g., from hemorrhagic shock and positive pressure breathing.

Note in Figure 5–8 that blood flow in the lung increases almost linearly from zone 1 at the apex through zone 3 near the base. The increase occurs because changing hydrostatic pressure gradients alter pulmonary *arterial*, *venous*, and *alveolar* pressure relationships, as summarized in the left-hand column of the illustration. The pressure gradients between the bold-faced pressures govern the flow and distribution of blood in the lung.

In lung zone 4, blood flow decreases slightly, but it is still greater than blood flow in the top half of the lung. Here, unlike the other zones, hydrostatic pressure is only one factor altering pressure relationships. Other factors are responsible for the vascular narrowing and increased resistance to blood flow characteristic of this lung zone. The vascular narrowing is thought to be due to increasing interstitial pressures and other local factors.

Supine Position

The unequal blood flow in different lung regions can be attenuated by decreasing the height of the lung, thus decreasing hydrostatic pressure gradients. Moving from upright to the supine position reduces the height of the lung and makes the lung more evenly perfused—blood flow increases in the apices, while basal flow remains virtually unchanged. However, blood flow in posterior dependent areas remains higher than in anterior areas.

Exercise

One other way to reduce regional differences in perfusion throughout the lung is to increase pulmonary

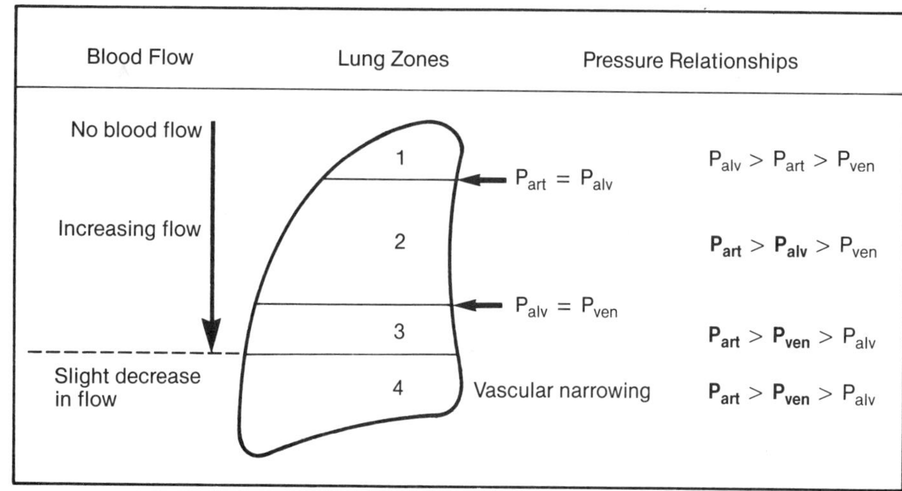

Figure 5–8. Regional changes in pulmonary blood flow due to changing pressure relationships. P_{alv} = alveolar pressure, P_{art} = pulmonary arterial pressure, and P_{ven} = pulmonary venous pressure.

Lung zone 1—Alveolar pressure is greatest, producing absent to minimal blood flow.

Lung zone 2—Resistance to blood flow is determined by the pressure difference from pulmonary artery to alveoli. P_{ven} exerts no effect in this region.

Lung zones 3 and 4—Resistance to blood flow is determined by the pressure difference from pulmonary artery to pulmonary vein. (After Murray, J.: The Normal Lung: The Basis for Diagnosis and Treatment of Pulmonary Disease, 2nd ed. Philadelphia, W. B. Saunders Co., 1986, and West, J.: Respiratory Physiology—The Essentials, 3rd ed. Baltimore, The Williams & Wilkins Co., 1985.)

artery pressure so that more blood flow reaches apical areas. This normally occurs during mild exercise.

Ventilation/Perfusion Ratios

In different lung regions, alveolar ventilation compared with perfusion in L/min is called the *ventilation/perfusion ratio (V/Q)*. The adequacy of gas exchange largely depends on normal V/Q ratios, maintained by the proper *matching* of ventilation to perfusion in different regions of the lungs. Other factors are also responsible for normal gas exchange, such as total perfusion, reflected by cardiac output, and total ventilation, reflected by alveolar ventilation and arterial PCO_2. However, the matching of ventilation to perfusion is the most important determinant of normal oxygenation in the body. In pulmonary disease, the *mismatching* of ventilation to perfusion (described subsequently) is responsible for most instances of impaired gas exchange. Hence, a basic understanding of V/Q ratios is essential.

REGIONAL DIFFERENCES IN V/Q RATIOS

Normally, *in apical lung regions*, alveolar ventilation far exceeds capillary blood flow, resulting in a high V/Q ratio (Fig. 5–9). At the other end of the spectrum, in lung bases, blood flow or perfusion is in excess of alveolar ventilation. This results in a low V/Q ratio.

The illustration in Figure 5–10 summarizes the pattern for regional V/Q ratios in the upright lung. The V/Q ratio at the top of the lung is exceedingly high because lung ventilation decreases very slowly up the lung, whereas perfusion decreases much more rapidly.

Regional V/Q ratios contribute to normal alveolar PO_2 and PCO_2 in different regions of the lung (Fig. 5–11). *In apical regions,* O_2 uptake by capillaries is low because of the minimal blood flow there. Hence, alveolar PO_2 remains amazingly high (about 132 mmHg), and alveolar PCO_2 low. (An interesting clinical application is that this O_2-rich environment promotes the growth of certain organisms in apical regions, notably *Mycobacterium tuberculosis.*) *Near the lung bases,* the situation is exactly the opposite, except alveolar PO_2 and PCO_2 values are not as extreme and remain closer to the normal PaO_2 of 100 mmHg and normal $PaCO_2$ of 40 mmHg. Alveolar PO_2 is slightly on the low side of normal, and alveolar PCO_2 is slightly on the high side.

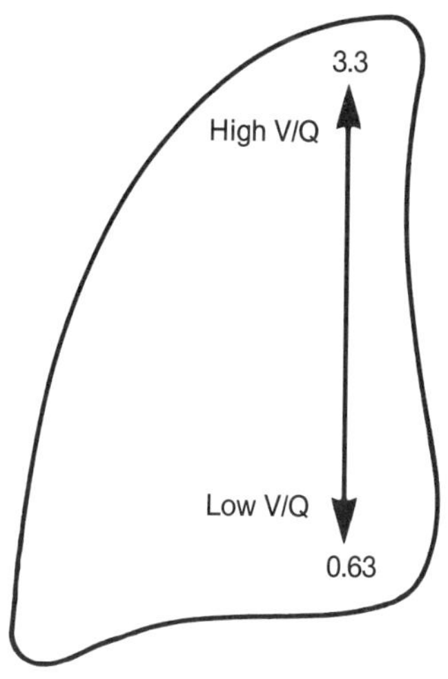

Figure 5–9. Regional changes in the normal ventilation/perfusion (V/Q) ratio.

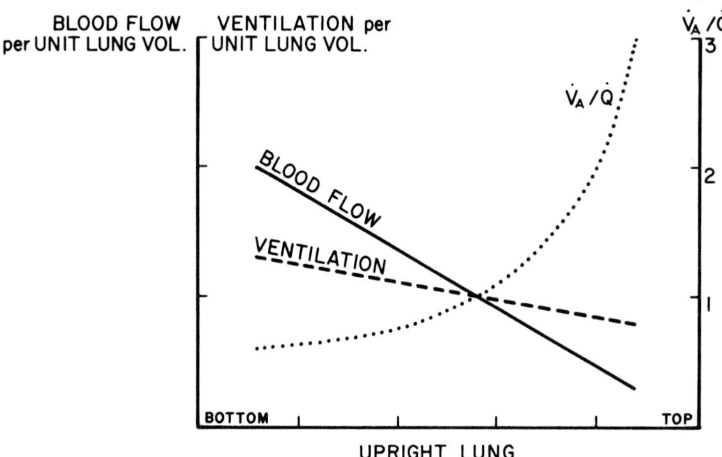

Figure 5–10. Summary of regional blood flow and ventilation in the upright lung. Both blood flow and ventilation decrease from bottom to top, but ventilation decreases at a slower rate. The result is a greatly elevated V/Q ratio at the top of the lungs (3.0), where alveoli are relatively overventilated in relation to their perfusion. The ratio is low at the bottom of the lungs, where alveoli are relatively underventilated. (Reproduced by permission from Cherniack, R., et al.: Respiration in Health and Disease, 3rd ed. Philadelphia, W. B. Saunders Co., 1983.)

MATCHING OF VENTILATION TO PERFUSION

In the ideal lung unit, a given quantity of blood bypassing an alveolus is matched by an equal quantity of alveolar gas. The V/Q ratio approximates 1:1. This arrangement permits optimal CO_2 elimination and O_2 uptake at the alveolar-capillary membrane.

This concept of the ideal lung unit helps in understanding the meaning of the V/Q ratio and the importance of relative proportions rather than absolute numbers for ventilation and perfusion. Otherwise, the concept is without clinical application and may be considered irrelevant. Ratios are normally not the same everywhere but vary widely among different lung regions, as described. Also, it is not the V/Q ratio for the lungs as a whole that determines gas exchange; rather, the important factor is *the matching of ventilation to perfusion between lung units or lung regions.* In healthy lungs, high V/Q regions compensate for low V/Q regions to promote normal gas exchange.

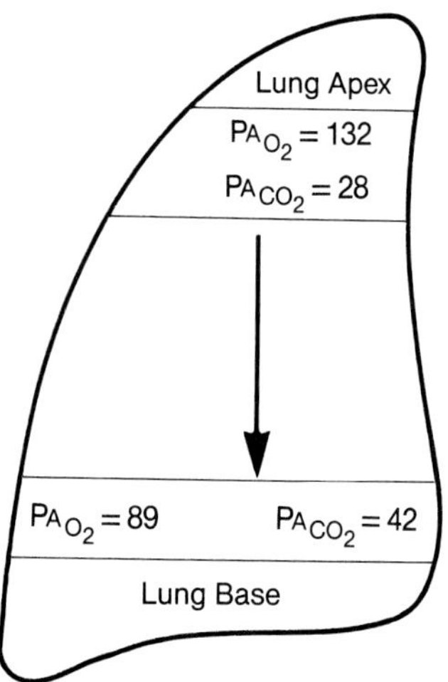

Figure 5–11. Regional differences in alveolar P_{O_2} (PA_{O_2}) and alveolar P_{CO_2} (PA_{CO_2}) down the normal lung.

MISMATCHING OF VENTILATION TO PERFUSION

Figure 5–12 compares normal and abnormal V/Q ratios. In normal lung function (Fig. 5–12a), the matching of ventilation to perfusion produces a normal V/Q ratio within or between different lung regions. In respiratory disease, the mismatching of ventilation to perfusion produces an *abnormal V/Q ratio,* also called a *ventilation-perfusion abnormality.* The two types of mismatching are (1) *perfusion in excess of ventilation* and (2) *ventilation in excess of perfusion.* Examples of these types are shown in Figure 5–12B and Figure 5–12C.

In Figure 5–12B, perfusion is in excess of ventilation because a mucus plug is obstructing distal airways, significantly reducing alveolar ventilation, and a *low V/Q ratio* results. It is characteristic of *shunt-producing disorders,* such as pneumonia and atelectasis.

In Figure 5–12C, acute cardiogenic shock drastically reduces and in some cases eliminates perfusion to fully ventilated alveoli; a *high V/Q ratio* results. In another example, a blood clot may obstruct pulmonary blood flow (as in pulmonary infarction), causing alveolar ventilation to remain normal to increased. A high V/Q ratio is characteristic of *dead space–producing disorders.*

IMPORTANT CONCEPTS OF V/Q ABNORMALITY

The effect of V/Q abnormality on gas exchange is a complicated and clinically relevant topic, and this section of the chapter summarizes important related concepts. These concepts are explored further in the chapters elucidating pathophysiology and blood gas analysis (see Part Two and Chapter 13).

1. Respiratory patients will maintain adequate gas exchange if V and Q are reduced proportionately in some regions of the lungs and increased proportionately in other regions. In other words, although in-

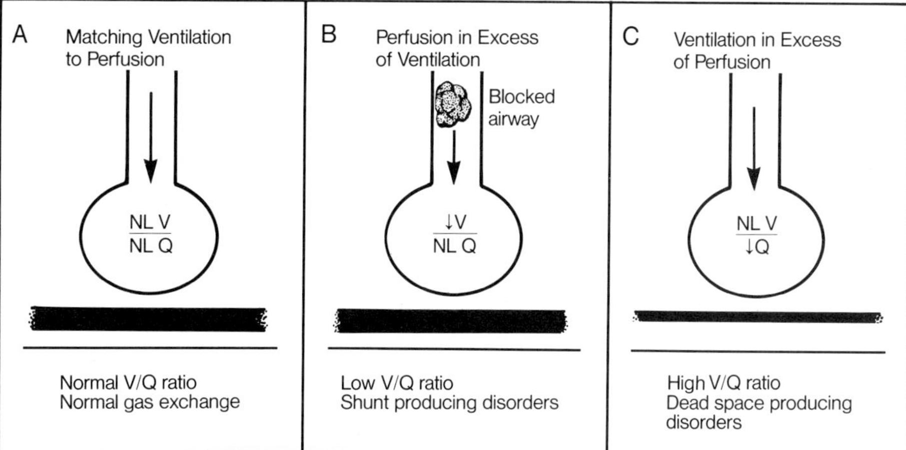

Figure 5–12. Normal and abnormal ventilation/perfusion (V/Q) ratios.

spired air and perfusion may not be uniformly distributed throughout the lung because of disease, as long as they are distributed in the same pattern, gas exchange and hence arterial blood gas measurements remain normal.

2. Even when mismatching occurs, as in mild lung disease, compensatory mechanisms may redistribute ventilation and perfusion within the lungs to once again create matching and normal gas exchange.

3. The degree of V/Q mismatching greatly influences O_2 exchange in the body. *Patients with diseases with very low V/Q ratios typically present with low $Pa{O_2}$s.* Hypoxemia occurs because low V/Q areas cannot be compensated for by high V/Q areas, since blood from the latter areas is already fully saturated with O_2 (see Chapter 13).

4. With regard to CO_2 exchange, *total* alveolar ventilation (V_A) rather than regional V/Q ratios is the most important factor to consider. For example, when lung disease increases $Pa{CO_2}$, a patient increases ventilation to bring $Pa{CO_2}$ down towards normal.

5. *Oxygenation is a problem in dead space–producing diseases, when mismatching is great and when low V/Q regions contribute significantly to the drop in $Pa{O_2}$.* Consider the case of pulmonary infarction, as follows: compensatory hyperventilation increases ventilation to all lung regions, resulting in high V/Q ratios in healthy and diseased regions. On one hand, in healthy regions, the increased ventilation is wasted because blood flow is normal and quite sufficient for gas exchange. This high V/Q ratio does not contribute to hypoxemia. On the other hand, in infarcted regions, absent perfusion with increased alveolar ventilation contributes to hypoxemia in two ways. First, infarcted regions may become completely nonfunctional, as alveolar ventilation is shunted to healthier alveolar-capillary units. This is a compensatory mechanism to avoid further V/Q mismatching in diseased regions. Second, when perfusion becomes absent, blood is similarly diverted to other lung regions. It is the increased blood flow to other healthy and partially diseased lung regions that increases the number of low V/Q regions, thus causing severe hypoxemia in the clinical setting. Furthermore, when the patient already has significant V/Q mismatching from underlying chronic lung disease, hypoxemia from acute pulmonary infarction is likely to be even more severe.

6. The presence of a V/Q abnormality is determined indirectly from a number of parameters, such as blood pressure, cardiac output, arterial blood gas analysis, minute ventilation, V_D and V_D/V_T, and intrapulmonary shunt (see Chapter 13).

7. The patient with a normal $\dot{V}_D$ and normal cardiac output may have extensive regional V/Q mismatching and hence abnormal gas exchange. (Remember, $\dot{V}_E$ does not always reflect $\dot{V}_A$).

8. Both V_A and Q decrease in the patient with alveolar hypoventilation and cardiogenic shock. Though the overall V/Q ratio for the lungs as a whole may remain equal, extensive regional mismatching occurs because what little perfusion remains goes entirely to the lung bases. Also, airway edema further reduces ventilation and low V/Q ratios in this location. The mismatching impairs gas exchange.

Conclusion

This chapter discusses lung ventilation, lung perfusion, and V/Q ratios, emphasizing the lung's adaptive ability to appropriately match ventilation to perfusion and to avoid gas exchange problems in health and during pulmonary disease.

The content of this chapter helps the nurse begin to understand why *lung ventilation and V/Q ratios* are often considered the most important components of the respiratory system and why respiratory patients are more apt to develop severe gas exchange problems, compared with persons with normal lungs. In addition, the content in this chapter and in Chapter 13 helps to explain why nursing interventions aimed at the maintenance of normal lung ventilation and normal V/Q ratios always take precedence over interventions that are necessary but less crucial, for the moment. For example, the intervention of switching from a face mask to a standard nasal cannula that provides O_2 during a patient's meals achieves the goal of maintaining normal V/Q ratios in the lungs and hence normal gas exchange at *all* times. Though it is a simple and sometimes overlooked intervention, it should take precedence over any routine monitoring that may be conveniently delayed for a few moments.

REFERENCES

Ayers, L., Whipp, B., and Ziment, E.: *A Guide to the Interpretation of Pulmonary Function Tests.* New York, Projects in Health, Inc., 1974.

Cherniack, R., Cherniack, L., and Naimark, A.: *Respiration in Health and Disease,* 3rd ed. Philadelphia, W. B. Saunders Co., 1983.

Forester, R., II, Dubois, A., Briscoe, W., and Fisher, A. *The Lung—Physiologic Basis of Pulmonary Function Tests,* 3rd ed. Chicago, Year Book Medical Publishers, Inc., 1986.

Guenter, C. and Welch, M.: *Pulmonary Medicine.* Philadelphia, J. B. Lippincott Co., 1982.

Pierce, A.: Acute respiratory failure. In *Pulmonary Medicine,* 2nd ed. Philadelphia, J. B. Lippincott Co., 1982.

Selecky, P., et al: A graphic approach to assessing interrelationships among minute ventilation, arterial carbon dioxide tension, and ratio of physiologic dead space to tidal volume in patients on respirators. *American Review of Respiratory Disease,* 117(1): 181–184, 1978.

Shapiro, B., Harrison, R., and Walton, J.: *Clinical Application of Blood Gases,* 3rd ed. Chicago, Year Book Medical Publishers, Inc., 1982.

Staub, N.: Lung Structure and Function—1982. *Basics of Respiratory Disease,* 10(3), 1982.

West, J.: *Respiratory Physiology—The Essentials,* 3rd ed. Baltimore, Williams & Wilkins, 1985.

West, J.: *Ventilation/Blood Flow and Gas Exchange,* 3rd ed. Oxford, Blackwell Scientific Publications, 1977.

Mechanics and Control of Breathing

6

Main Objectives

1. Name the respiratory muscles involved in quiet and active breathing.
   a. Identify the main breathing muscle.
   b. Explain how respiratory muscle groups complement each other to avoid respiratory muscle fatigue.
2. Describe the elastic properties of the lungs and chest wall that account for the equilibrium position of the lungs within the chest cage as well as for lung inflation and deflation.
3. Name and explain alveolar and pleural pressure changes during quiet breathing.
4. Define and state the significance of the following terms: transpulmonary pressure, transmural (airway) pressure, laminar flow, and turbulent airflow.
5. Describe the physiologic basis for low airway resistance in peripheral airways in the lungs. Explain why this feature may be considered advantageous *or* disadvantageous for the individual with respiratory disease.
6. Describe how these three respiratory centers in the brain control breathing: medullary, apneustic, and pneumotaxic.
7. Name the nerves that innervate the diaphragm and the intercostal muscles of the chest.
8. List four mechanical receptors in the lungs. Explain how they alter the depth and rate of respiration.
9. Discuss how central and peripheral chemoreceptors control breathing.
10. State one clinically relevant aspect of mechanics or control of breathing that is incompletely understood at this time.

This last chapter in Part One, Structure and Function of the Respiratory System, discusses the mechanics and control of breathing, two integrated components that regulate breathing on a moment-to-moment basis. *Mechanics of breathing* refers to how the lung is supported and how it is inflated and deflated during breathing; *control of breathing* refers to nervous and chemical activation and regulation of breathing.

Mechanics of Breathing

Mechanics of breathing is discussed presently from several different perspectives. For example, the descriptions of structural features of respiratory muscles show how these muscles are specially designed to do the work of breathing. Sections on the elastic and mechanical properties of the lungs and chest wall demonstrate how the lung is supported during inflation and deflation. Because respiratory interventions strive to help the patient keep resistance in the respiratory system to a minimum, the topics of pressures and resistances during breathing are covered in considerable detail.

RESPIRATORY MUSCLES

The respiratory muscles are responsible for the expansion of the chest and the filling of the lungs with air (Fig. 6–1).

Different muscles are used during quiet and active breathing. Though main muscles and muscle groups are presented subsequently, further detailed descriptions are also presented in Table 6–1 and Table 6–2, with frequent reference to the supplementary illustrations that enhance comprehension.

Quiet Breathing

Inspiration is an active process brought about by active contraction of the *diaphragm*, the main breathing muscle (Fig. 6–2). This muscle performs about 80% of the work of breathing. The rest of the work of breathing is performed by the *external intercostals* and *parasternal intercartilaginous intercostals*. Some accessory muscles (e.g., scalene muscles of the neck) may contribute to inspiratory movements of the chest, but their main role is during active breathing (described subsequently).

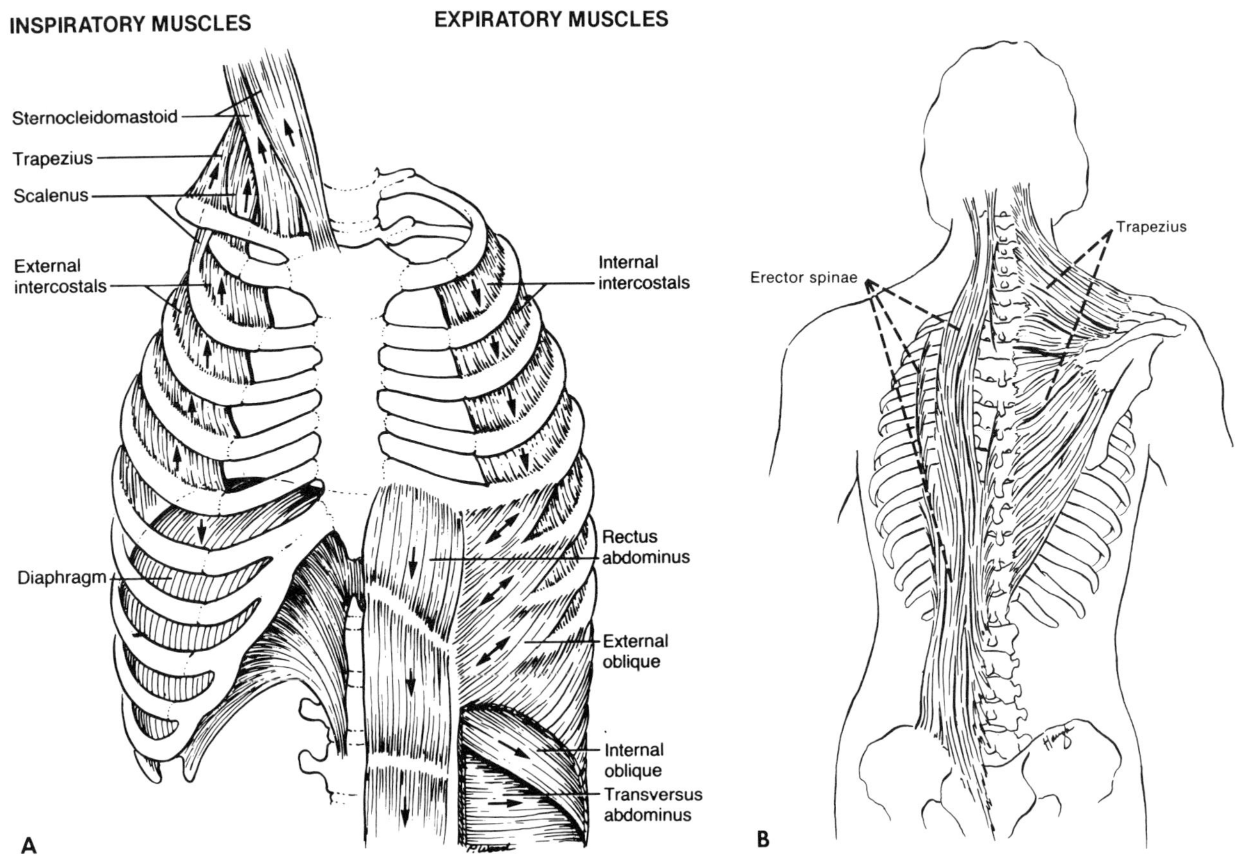

Figure 6–1. Muscles of respiration. *A*, Inspiratory and expiratory muscles. The parasternal intercartilaginous, an inspiratory muscle, is not shown in the drawing, but it is located in the blank spaces between the sternum and external intercostals, connecting costal cartilages. Arrows indicate the direction of muscular action (see Table 6–1 for further explanation). *B*, Posterior view of respiratory muscles. (*A* reproduced by permission from Luce, J. and Culver, B.: Respiratory muscle function in health and disease. Chest 81(1):82–90, 1982; *B* reproduced by permission from Frownfelter, D.: Chest physical therapy and pulmonary rehabilitation—an interdisciplinary approach. Chicago, Year Book Medical Publishers, Inc., 1978.)

Table 6–1. RESPIRATORY MUSCLES USED DURING QUIET BREATHING

Respiratory Muscle	Description of Muscle and Effects of Contraction
Diaphragm	Muscle origin has three portions (see Fig. 6–2). 1. *sternal* portion—two muscle slips to the xiphoid process 2. *costal* portion—muscle fibers along the inner surfaces of the lower costal cartilages and ribs, which interdigitate with the transverse abdominis muscle 3. *lumbar* portion—crura muscles and arcuate ligaments connect diaphragm to the twelfth rib. The muscle fibers of the diaphragm converge into a *central tendon.* This tendon is roughly triangular in shape with the apex directed towards the xiphoid process; it is located immediately below the pericardium, with which it is partially intermeshed.
Effects of contraction:	Pulls the central tendon downwards and forwards; this action has two effects, as follows. 1. It pulls the dome of the diaphragm downwards, pushing before it the abdominal viscera and displacing the abdominal wall outwards. This increases the vertical length of the lungs and chest cage (see Fig. 6–3). 2. It elongates the heart on inspiration, since the diaphragm is connected to the heart via the central tendon. Because of its rib attachments and dome shape, the diaphragm lifts the rib cage upwards and outwards (see Fig. 6–4). This action increases the transverse diameter of the lower rib cage. Normally creates a pressure gradient across the diaphragm of 10–20 cmH_2O. Exerts an expiratory action at high lung volumes, e.g., normally during deep breathing and when the dome is flattened by disease. In these cases, the diaphragm exerts a high negative pleural pressure, which "sucks in" the lower chest and may decrease the transverse diameter.
External intercostals	Each muscle connects the inferior border of the rib above with the superior border of the rib below (see Fig. 6–1A). Becomes continuous with a membrane that connects the muscle to the sternum.
Effects of contraction:	These muscles raise the ribs during inspiration by swinging them outwards and upwards similar to a bucket handle. This so-called *bucket handle movement* greatly elevates the mid-portion of each rib owing to front-to-back rotation at each rib's costovertebral joint, thereby increasing transverse diameter of the chest. Although ribs two to ten are involved in this movement, it is most pronounced where the radius of rib curvature is greatest (lower ribs), as shown in Figure 6–5. Raising the ribs has another effect. Movement at each rib's costovertebral joint about a side-to-side axis raises the sternal end of each rib. The sternum is thrust forward, thus increasing anteroposterior (AP) diameter (see superior view of the third rib, Figure 6–5). The raising and lowering of each rib at its sternal end during inspiration and expiration has been likened to the movement of a pump handle. Hence, it has been termed *pump-handle movement.* Upper ribs two through six are mainly involved in this movement. With the bucket-handle movement of the lower ribs (seven to twelve), AP diameter decreases slightly, as shown by the superior view of the ninth rib in Figure 6–5.
Parasternal intercartilaginous (anterior portion of the internal intercostals)	Connects costal cartilages together. Each muscle extends from the sternum laterally to the more superficial external intercostals, where it becomes continuous with the rest of the internal intercostal muscles.
Effects of contraction:	Helps the external intercostals elevate the ribs. Exerts muscle tension that prevents intercostal space bulging or collapse during respiration. (All intercostal muscles contribute to this effect.)

In contrast to inspiration, an active process, expiration is a passive process not requiring active muscular work. The lungs and chest wall contract down or recoil to their original positions with the release of energy stored in elastic tissues from the previous lung inflation. Although expiration is usually passive, sometimes expiratory muscles contract to help regulate breathing during activities such as speaking and singing.

Details on how inspiratory muscles increase the size of the chest cage are presented in Table 6–1 and Table 6–2. Basically, the chest cage enlarges as measured in three diameters: *anterior-posterior* (external intercostals and accessory muscles); *transverse* (bucket-handle effect of lower ribs); and *vertical* (downward movement of diaphragm). These diameters increase to a greater degree during active breathing to permit greater lung inflation.

Active Breathing

Active breathing refers to breathing during maximal normal deep breathing, forced breathing maneuvers,

Table 6–2. ACCESSORY MUSCLES USED DURING ACTIVE BREATHING DESCRIPTION OF MUSCLES AND EFFECTS OF CONTRACTION

Accessory Muscle(s)	
Sternocleidomastoid	A strong neck muscle that arises from the manubrium and medial part of the clavicle and inserts behind the ear into the mastoid process. **Effects of contraction:** Helps to elevate the sternum during inspiration thus increasing anteroposterior (AP) diameter.
Scalene (scalenus)	**Effets of contraction:** Anterior, medial, and posterior scalenes attach to transverse processes of the lower five cervical vertebrae and inferiorly to the upper surfaces of the first two ribs. **Effects of contraction:** Elevates the first two ribs during active inspiration, thereby increasing AP diameter. Stabilizes the chest cage so that external intercostal muscle contraction can elevate the remaining ribs.
Internal intercostals	Each muscle connects the superior border of the rib below with the inferior border of the rib above. Extends from its anterior parasternal and intercartilaginous portion, around the chest to the vertebrae. **Effects of contraction:** Pulls the ribs downward and inward.
Abdominal	*Rectus abdominis* arises from the pubic crest and inserts into the xiphoid process and costal margin of the fifth, sixth, and seventh costal cartilages. *External oblique* (obliquus externus abdominis) forms an oblique muscle mass from the fifth costal cartilage to the twelfth rib. *Internal oblique* (obliquus internus abdominis) originates from the thoracolumbar fascia, the iliac crest, and the inguinal ligament and inserts into the lower borders of the last three ribs. It lies beneath the external oblique muscle. *Transversus abdominis* lies beneath the internal oblique muscle. It runs transversely and has many attachments, including the inner surface of the lower six costal cartilages and the xiphoid processes. **Effects of contraction:** These abdominal muscles compress the abdomen when the chest cage and pelvis are fixed. During forced exhalation or coughing, they help to force the diaphragm upwards and to empty the lungs of air. The external oblique muscle assists the internal intercostals to depress and compress the lower part of the thorax (see Fig. 6–3 for chest movements during forced exhalation).
Shoulder and back	*Trapezius*—a diamond-shaped muscle mass extending from the head, down the back, and out to the shoulder (see Fig. 6–1B). *Pectoralis minor*—a small muscle beneath the pectoralis major muscle. It connects the third, fourth, and fifth ribs to the scapula. **Effects of contraction:** The trapezius muscle elevates the shoulder (e.g., shrugging) and stabilizes the scapula so that the serratus anterior and pectoralis minor muscles can elevate the ribs during active breathing. *Pectoralis major*—a large muscle in the upper part of the anterior chest that connects the clavicle, sternum, and second to sixth ribs with the humerus. **Effects of contraction:** During forced inspiration, this muscle draws the ribs towards the arms (when the arms are fixed). This action increases thoracic diameter. *Serratus anterior*—a sheet of muscle extending from the outer surfaces of the first eight to nine ribs, laterally and backwards to the scapula. **Effects of contraction:** During active breathing, this muscle may help to elevate the ribs (when the scapula is fixed). *Erector spinae*—long muscles extending down the back from the sacrum to the skull, inserting into various ribs and vertebrae on the way up (see Fig. 6–1B). **Effects of contraction:** During a deep or forced inspiration, erector spinae muscles extend the vertebral column and allow further elevation of the ribs.

and respiratory distress. It is the action of *accessory muscles* that augments inspiratory and expiratory movements of the chest to make quiet breathing active. Accessory muscles include the *internal intercostals* and various *neck*, *abdominal*, and *shoulder and back* muscles described in Table 6–2. Shoulder and neck muscles are recruited at very high levels of inspiratory activity, as in severe physical exertion in health or marked respiratory distress or breathlessness in cardiopulmonary disease.

Respiratory Muscle Groups

Researchers are grouping respiratory muscles differently based on new findings on respiratory muscle actions and interactions. For example, Luce and Culver (1982) have identified three muscle groups: (1) the *diaphragm*, (2) *intercostal and accessory muscles*, and (3) *the abdominal muscles*. Each group has an inspiratory and expiratory function. Moreover, these groups seem to complement and support each other. While

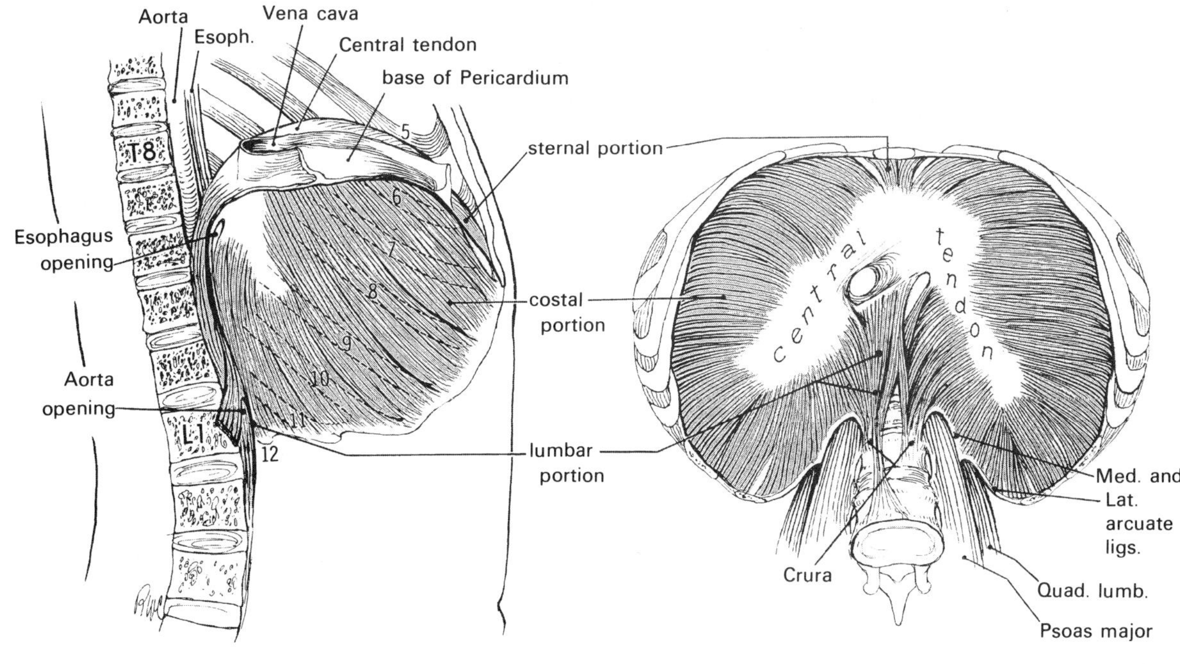

Figure 6–2. Lateral and inferior views of the diaphragm. (Reproduced by permission from Kendall, F. and Wadsworth, G. Muscles—Testing and Function, 3rd ed. Baltimore, Williams & Wilkins, 1983.)

the diaphragm contracts, the other muscles stabilize the chest wall and convert diaphragmatic contraction into intrathoracic pressure and volume changes (Fig. 6–3). During abnormal breathing patterns, muscle groups seem to work together, alternating their levels of activity to prevent total exhaustion by any one muscle group. During acute or severe illness, however, muscles can easily become overworked and fatigued. Patients so affected may require mechanical ventilation or muscle relaxation techniques to relieve the muscle fatigue and, eventually, respiratory muscle training to build up endurance and work efficiency once the acute illness has stabilized. Because of the development of new interventions aimed at reducing respiratory muscle fatigue and achieving a muscle training effect, knowledge of and familiarity with respiratory muscles are likely to become increasingly more important for the nurse in the clinical setting.

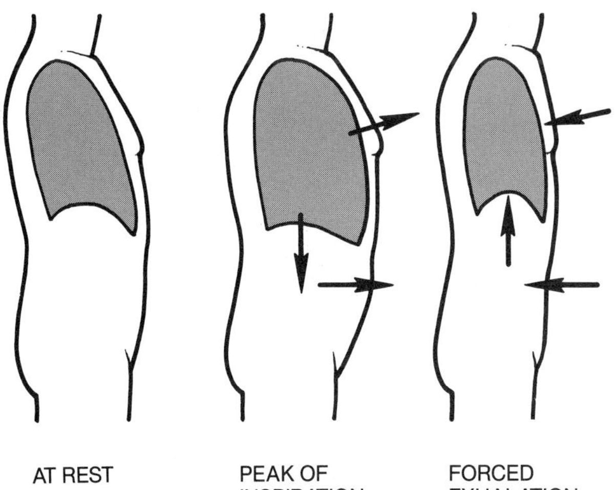

Figure 6–3. Normal movements of the lungs and chest wall. (Redrawn and adapted by permission from Luce, J. and Culver, B.: Respiratory muscle function in health and disease. Chest 81(1):82–90, 1982.)

Upper Airway Muscles

The role of upper airway muscles as muscles of respiration is not understood at this time. These muscles appear to have a role in maintaining nasal and oropharyngeal airway patency. Certain disorders result from inadequate or ineffective nervous activation of upper airway muscles during sleep, as in sudden infant death syndrome and obstructive sleep apnea in the adult. When nervous activation is present, it may not be coordinated with efforts of the chest wall muscles (Strohl, 1981).

ELASTIC PROPERTIES OF THE LUNGS AND CHEST WALL

While respiratory muscles perform the work of breathing, lung and chest wall expansion and contraction (Fig. 6–3 to Fig. 6–5) are possible largely due to the elastic behavior of their tissues. *Elasticity* or *elastic recoil* refers to the return of tissue to resting position after stretching.

The chest wall's elastic recoil is such that if it existed as a separate unit, as in Figure 6–6A, it would move

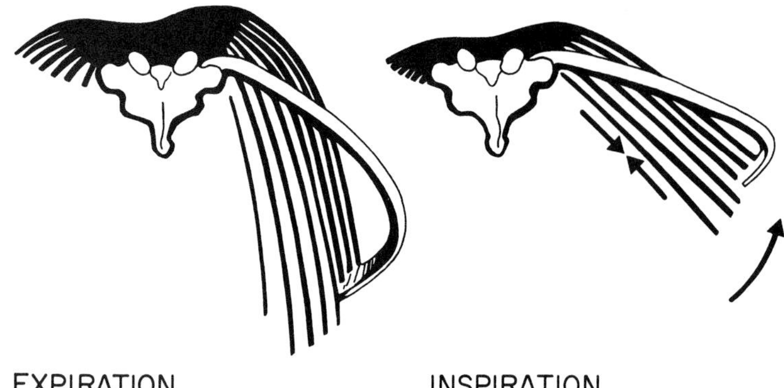

Figure 6–4. Contraction of the dome-shaped diaphragm during inspiration results in elevation of the ribs with a consequent increase in transverse diameter of the chest. (Reproduced by permission from Cherniack, R. et al.: Respiration in Health and Disease, 3rd ed. Philadelphia, W. B. Saunders Co., 1983.)

outwards. The chest wall would expand to about 70% of the lung's total lung capacity (TLC). In contrast, if the lungs were removed from the chest to eliminate the influence of the chest wall, as in Figure 6–6B, they would recoil *inwards* and collapse to an airless state. At the end of a normal expiration, these two forces oppose each other—the inward movement of the lungs and outward movement of the chest wall generate a subatmospheric pressure of about 5 cmH_2O in the pleural space, as illustrated in Fig. 6–6C. This position is the equilibrium resting position of the lungs and chest wall.

Lung Elasticity and Compliance

Lung elasticity is primarily due to elastin fibers within alveolar walls and surrounding bronchioles and pulmonary capillaries. These fibers may become stretched to about twice their resting length. The less stretchable collagen fibers within the lung contribute less to elasticity and probably act to limit expansion at high lung volumes. Together, elastin and collagen fibers act, when stretched during lung inflation, as a nylon stocking does. Stretching seems to involve more of an unfolding and geometric rearrangement of fibers and only a slight elongation of individual fibers (Weibel, 1980).

Elastin and collagen fibers determine lung distensibility or *compliance*, defined as *volume change per unit of pressure change*. Lung compliance changes in health and disease as a result of alterations in these fibers. The normal aging process and pulmonary diseases characterized by tissue destruction (e.g., emphysema) cause an increase in compliance—lung tissue becomes more distensible, and the lungs are easier to inflate. In contrast, other diseases (e.g., interstitial

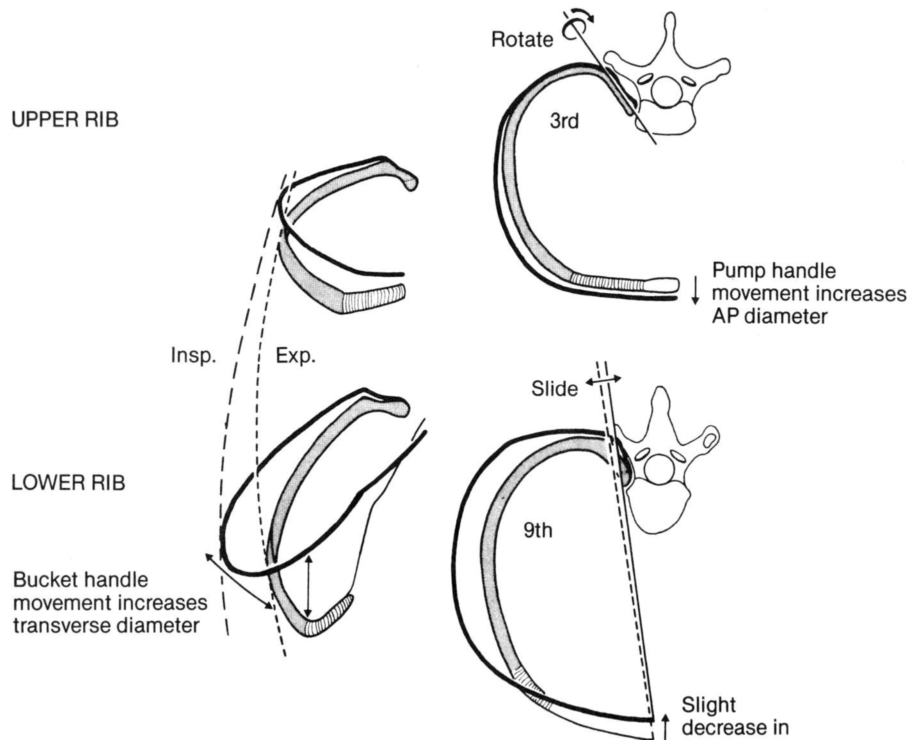

Figure 6–5. Anteroposterior (AP) view (on the left) and superior view (on the right) of upper and lower ribs during inspiration and expiration (see Table 6–1 for explanation). (Reproduced and adapted by permission from Cherniack, R. et al.: Respiration in Health and Disease, 3rd ed. Philadelphia, W. B. Saunders Co., 1983.)

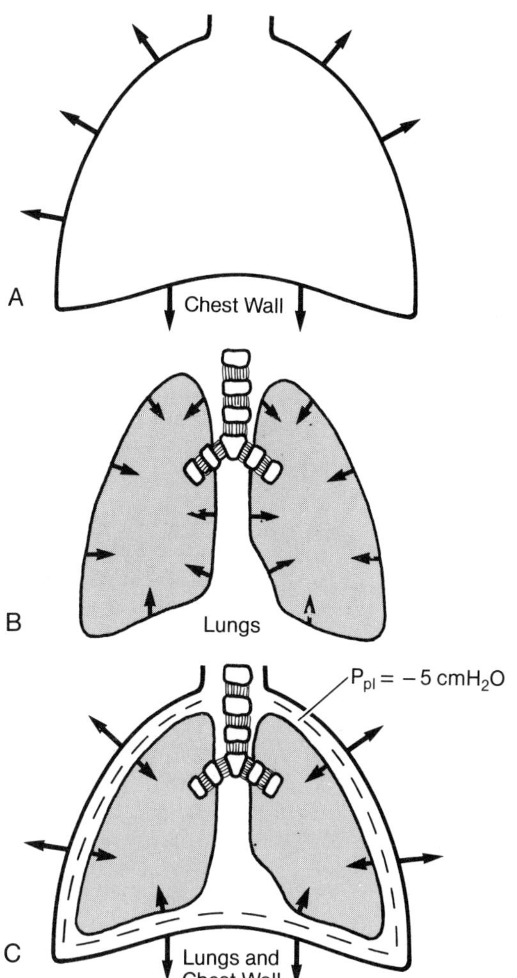

Figure 6–6. Elastic forces of the lungs and chest wall. *A*, Chest wall. *B*, Lungs. *C*, Lungs and chest wall. P_{pl} = pleural pressure.

fibrosis) cause a decrease in compliance—lung tissue becomes stiffer or less distensible, and the lungs are more difficult to inflate. The concept of compliance is discussed further in Chapter 8 in relation to restrictive pulmonary disease.

MECHANICAL SUPPORT FOR THE LUNGS—LUNG INTERSTITIUM

The elastin and collagen fibers described form an extensive network of connective tissue known as the lung's *interstitium.* More specifically, the interstitium is composed of connective tissue forming the interstitial spaces of the lung (described previously). The interstitium has been described as the "skeleton of the lungs," because its fibers provide crucial mechanical support for airways, alveoli, and capillaries (Shapiro and Musallam, 1977). This network provides channels for the transmission of chest wall movements into lung tissue. Without the interstitium, the lung could not achieve the mechanics necessary for respiration.

The Fibrous Network

The lung is supported by a fibrous network consisting of interstitium attached to pleural connective tis- There are two fiber systems, as follows: central and peripheral (Fig. 6–7).

Central Fiber System. Fibers along central airways travel peripherally within the peribronchial/perivascular connective tissue sheath. At the bronchiolar level, they become firmly anchored to adjacent lung parenchyma. They continue down to the entrance of alveoli, where they form a delicate lattice in alveolar septa (Fig. 6–7B). (Review connective tissue changes in Table 2–2).

Peripheral Fiber System. From the other direction, fibers in the lung periphery (by the pleura) travel *into*

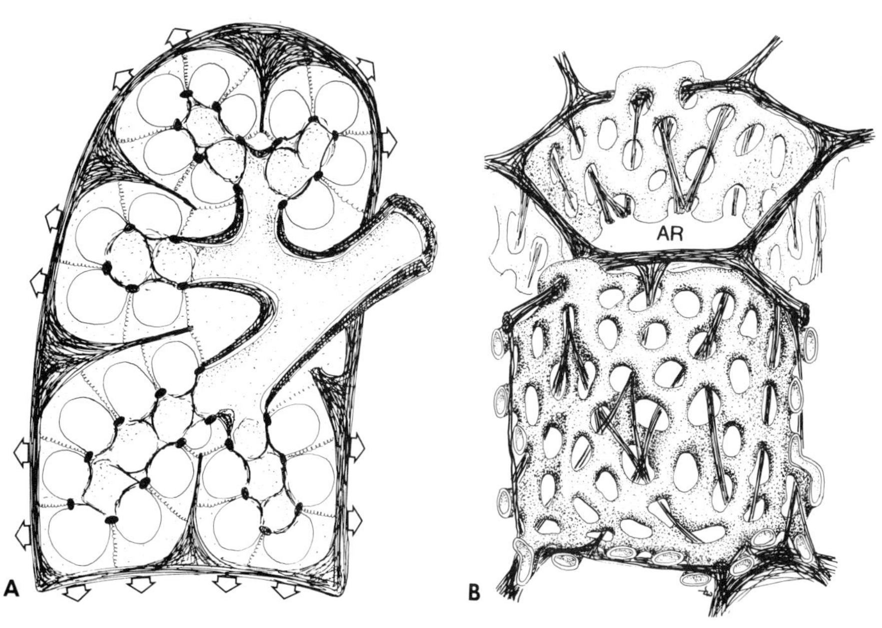

Figure 6–7. Schematic representation of the lung's fibrous network. *A*, Dense fibers course radially in an axial fiber system along central airways and pulmonary arteries, extending into alveolar entrance rings. Peripheral fibers extend from the pleura into lung parenchyma. Central and peripheral fiber systems are connected by fine fibers in alveolar septa (represented by springs). *B*, Fine connective tissue fibers interlace with the capillary network in the alveolar septum. Connective tissue is particularly thick around alveolar mouths, forming the so-called *alveolar entrance ring* (AR). (Reproduced by permission from Weibel, E. and Gil, J.: Structure-function relationships at the alveolar level. In West, J. (ed.). Lung Biology in Health and Disease, vol. 3. Bio-engineering Aspects of the Lung. New York, Marcel Dekker, Inc., 1977.)

the lung and lung parenchyma, following the course of the pulmonary veins and interlobular septa. These fibers connect with central fibers via fine fibers in alveolar septa.

This meeting of central and peripheral fibers at the alveolar level is of functional significance during respiration. *During inspiration,* respiratory movements of the chest and diaphragm are transmitted deep into lung tissue along the peripheral fiber system. With alveoli anchored by the central fiber system, these movements can exert substantial tugging on alveolar septal fibers. This tugging or mechanical pull along with surfactant changes effects an increase in alveolar volume. Simultaneously, the mechanical pull exerts traction on adjacent airways, widening lumens and decreasing resistance to airflow.

During expiration, the recoil of stretched elastin fibers and the contraction of the spirally arranged peribronchial smooth muscle fibers return airways and alveoli to resting volume.

Importance of the Interstitium

It is important to remember that the interstitium is a separate entity because of its mechanical function as well as its fluid exchange function, since fluid exchange involves interstitial spaces. Moreover, the interstitium also acts as the chief pathological site for ***interstitial lung disease,*** e.g., interstitial fibrosis and interstitial pulmonary edema. Such diseases can grossly alter mechanics of breathing.

PRESSURE CHANGES DURING BREATHING

Changes in pulmonary pressures determine airflow through the tracheobronchial tree and the *degree* of lung inflation and deflation. Main pressures used to describe pressure changes in mechanics of breathing are summarized in the box.

Airflow during breathing occurs as follows: at the end of expiration, pleural pressure is about −5 cm H_2O. This represents the equilibrium resting position of the lungs within the chest cage, as described. Pressure at the mouth and alveolar pressure are both zero. Airflow is absent (Fig. 6–8A).

During inspiration, contraction of inspiratory muscles causes the chest cage to enlarge and the pleural pressure to become more and more subatmospheric (Fig. 6–8B). As pleural pressure is transmitted across the lung, alveolar pressure also becomes subatmospheric (−1 or −2 cmH_2O). This negative alveolar pressure is necessary to overcome airway resistance that hinders airflow into the lungs. Negative pressure "sucks" air into the lungs until alveolar pressure again reaches zero (see Fig. 6–8C). At this point, airflow ceases.

During expiration, the elastic recoil of the lung generates *positive* alveolar pressure (P_{ALV} = +1 or +2 cmH_2O). This produces a driving pressure that results in airflow out of the lung until alveolar pressure equals mouth pressure (see Fig. 6–8A). Simultaneously, pleural pressure rises to −5 cmH_2O.

The following points summarize pressure changes during breathing:

1. During quiet breathing, alveolar pressure varies between −1 or −2 and +1 or +2. These pressures as well as pleural pressures vary slightly from person to person, depending on the depth of respiration and

PULMONARY PRESSURES AFFECTING AIRFLOW

mouth pressure (P_m)—pressure measured at the mouth. Equal to atmospheric pressure and designated as zero (0) pressure.

airway pressure (P_{aw})—pressure in airways.

alveolar pressure (P_{ALV})—pressure in alveoli.

pleural pressure (P_{pl})—pressure in the potential space between visceral and parietal pleurae.

body surface pressure (P_{bs})—pressure at the external surface of the chest. Normally equal to atmospheric pressure.

pressure difference, pressure drop, or **driving pressure (ΔP)**—difference between pressures at one point in an airway and another point located more distally.

transairway pressure (P_{taw})—the drop in pressure within airways from the mouth to alveolar level.

transpulmonary pressure (P_{tp})—pressure difference across lung tissue from the mouth (or alveoli) to the pleural space. Considered a measure of elastic recoil of the lung.

transthoracic pressure (P_w) or **chest wall pressure** (P_{cw})—pressure difference from the pleural space and the external surface of the chest (P_{bs}). Considered a measure of the elastic recoil of the chest wall.

transmural pressure (P_{tm})—difference between the pressure within the airway and pressure surrounding the airway. This pressure gradient is lowest at the end of expiration when airway caliber is reduced, and highest at the peak of inspiration when airway pressure is greatest. Changes in lung compliance alter transmural pressure and affect airway caliber and, hence, airflow to alveoli.

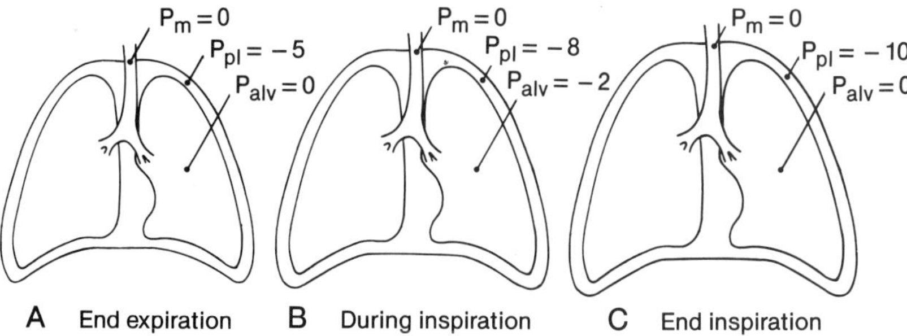

Figure 6–8. Pleural and alveolar pressure changes during quiet breathing. P_n = pressure at the mouth, P_{pl} = pleural pressure, and P_{alv} = alveolar pressure. (Reproduced by permission from Fishman, A.: Assessment of Pulmonary Function. New York, McGraw-Hill Book Co., 1980.)

the effort required for breathing. The −2 to +2 cmH_2O range translates to about −1.5 to +1.5 mmHg. Centimeters of water are converted to millimeters of mercury by dividing cmH_2O by 1.36. (Conversely, millimeters of mercury are converted to centimeters of water by multiplying mmHg by 1.36.) This text uses cmH_2O because it has more clinical applications, e.g., chest tube setups described in Chapter 30.

2. Pleural pressure varies between −5 and −10 cmH_2O. During inspiration, negative pleural pressure always leads or precedes negative alveolar pressure.

3. Maximal inspiratory effort may reduce pleural pressure to as far as −60 cmH_2O.

4. In contrast, forced expiratory maneuvers generate extremely high positive pleural and alveolar pressures in the range of +20 to +40 cmH_2O.

5. It is the change in transpulmonary pressure ($P_{ALV} - P_{pl}$) that effects a change in the volume of air in the lungs.

RESISTANCE TO AIRFLOW

Driving pressures in conducting airways and terminal respiratory units must be great enough to overcome resistance to airflow, before air will enter the lungs. Resistance to airflow is a major consideration in the assessment of a patient's mechanics of breathing.

The work of breathing is directed towards overcoming two resistances, as follows: (1) elastic recoil of the lung or *elastic resistance* and (2) *nonelastic resistance.* The latter is composed of *airway resistance* and *tissue resistance.* Tissue resistance is the frictional resistance of lung tissues to displacement during breathing. It is frequently omitted in discussions on resistance within the respiratory system because it is not measured in the clinical setting, and the value constitutes only 10% to 20% of the total nonelastic resistance.

AIRWAY RESISTANCE

Airway resistance (R_{aw}) contributes the most to nonelastic resistance. It is defined as driving pressure divided by flowrate or

$$R_{aw} = \frac{\Delta P\ (P_m - P_{ALV})}{\text{flow rate}} \text{ or } \frac{\Delta P}{F}$$

Driving pressure is the pressure difference between alveoli and the mouth necessary to move air in and out of the lungs (transairway pressure). Flowrate is the volume of gas delivered in a given amount of time (e.g., L/min).

In the formula, the magnitude of the driving pressure is crucial. On the one hand, consider the normal situation in which flowrate remains constant and driving pressure remains small—only 1 or 2 cmH_2O. The physiological outcome is low airway resistance. Little pressure is needed to deliver a given volume of air to the lungs. Clinically, the patient has no problem maintaining a normal breathing pattern, normal respiratory rate, and normal minute ventilation, signs of normal mechanics of breathing.

On the other hand, pulmonary disease may greatly alter transairway pressure, producing abnormally high or low airway resistance and abnormal mechanics of breathing. For example, if a mucus plug partially obstructs a major airway, flow rate becomes reduced. Air cannot reach alveoli because of the airway obstruction. To achieve an adequate flow rate, the patient generates greater negative pleural and alveolar pressures on inspiration, and more positive pressures on exhalation, to move air past the obstruction. The physiological outcome is a larger driving pressure (since P_m remains at zero) and a dramatic increase in airway resistance. Clinically, the patient develops abnormal mechanics of breathing. He uses accessory muscles of breathing. Simultaneously, he increases both respiratory rate and minute ventilation in an effort to generate a driving pressure large enough to overcome airway resistance, to adequately ventilate the lungs, and to maintain normal gas exchange.

Because increased airway resistance may produce grossly abnormal mechanics of breathing, ultimately resulting in impaired gas exchange, *an important goal of respiratory intervention is to keep airway resistance to a minimum level.* As the R_{aw} formula points out, low airway resistance minimizes the driving pressure necessary for ventilation and reduces the respiratory muscles' work of breathing, allowing the patient to readily adapt to respiratory dysfunction, without developing respiratory muscle fatigue.

Distribution of Airway Resistance

In the normal lung, the largest fraction of airway resistance is in the upper respiratory tract where the airway is curved, more irregular, and variable in size. Weibel (1980) reports that the nose constitutes up to 50% of total airway resistance to quiet breathing. During quiet *mouth* breathing, the mouth, pharynx, larynx, and trachea constitute 20% to 30% of the airway resistance. This amount increases to 50% when breathing rate and depth increase, as during vigorous exercise.

A clinically significant fact to remember about the distribution of airway resistance is that central airways (from the nose to about z = 7) have a relatively small cross-sectional area, and they account for a large percentage of total airway resistance—about 80% to 90%.

In contrast, small peripheral airways, particularly those less than 2 mm in diameter, have a relatively large cross-sectional area. They represent a relatively *small* percentage of total airway resistance—only 10% to 20%. Because small airways and nearby alveoli contribute little to total airway resistance, they make up what is known as the *silent zone* of the lung (Fig. 6–9). When pathology selectively alters peripheral airways (e.g., mild asthma) or alveoli (e.g., mild emphysema), airway resistance never increases beyond 20% of total airway resistance. Individuals with such pathology may be totally asymptomatic. If they are symptomatic, they are less so than individuals with pathology affecting more centrally located airways (e.g., tumor in a main bronchus, severe asthma, and severe emphysema).

Determinants of Airway Resistance

Many factors determine airway resistance in health and disease. The three main determinants are, as follows: (1) airway caliber and length, (2) rate of airflow, and (3) pattern of airflow.

Airway Caliber and Length. Essentially, an increase in airway caliber reduces airway resistance, as during lung inflation; a decrease in caliber increases it, as during lung deflation. During quiet breathing, however, this variation in airway resistance is slight and offset by airway lengthening and shortening during inspiration and expiration.

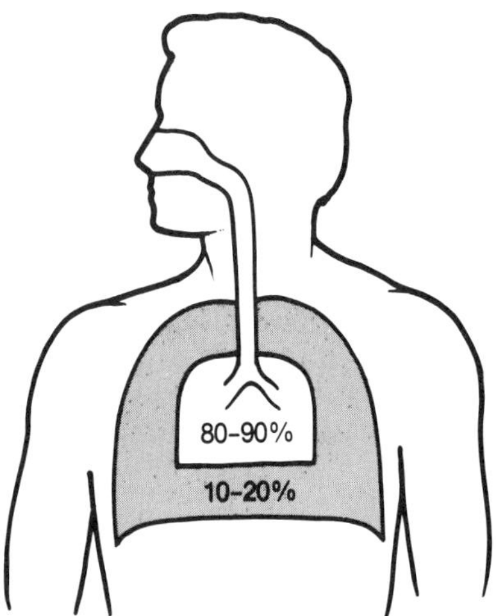

Figure 6–9. Airway resistance in central and peripheral airways. The shaded portion is the *silent zone* of the lung, where airway resistance is lowest (% = percent of total airway resistance in the respiratory system).

In airway diseases, *mucosal edema, hypertrophy and hyperplasia of mucous glands, mucus,* or *hypertrophy of smooth muscle* may decrease airway caliber and grossly increase airway resistance. Also, diseases affecting the surrounding lung parenchyma may narrow airways. For example, the loss of structural support around airways from tissue destruction (e.g., emphysema) decreases transmural pressure and favors airway collapse, especially during expiration when transmural pressure is normally low and airway caliber is normally reduced.

Length also affects airway resistance, although it has less of an effect compared with airway caliber. Basically, *short airways* produce *less* resistance to airflow than long airways. In the clinical setting, long lengths of tubing attached to breathing circuits of mechanical ventilators may increase airway or tube resistance to such a degree that airflow to alveoli becomes significantly reduced. For this reason, tubing lengths are always kept to a minimum.

Other respiratory interventions may alter airway caliber, length, or both. For example, insertion of an artificial airway, such as a tracheostomy, will decrease both airway caliber and length in addition to anatomical dead space. The result may be a drastic reduction in airway resistance and work of breathing for the patient.

Rate of Airflow. An extremely *high flow rate,* as in rapid breathing, *increases* airway resistance because it produces air turbulence. A *low flow rate,* as in slow breathing, *decreases* airway resistance, but it may be inadequate to ventilate the lung. The optimal flow rate is somewhere between these high and low levels and may vary in different individuals, depending on the nature and extent of disease and the mechanics necessary to ventilate the lung. Essentially, an optimal flow rate is one that produces the most laminar flow and, at the same time, adequate ventilation of the lung. Rate of airflow is significant because of the *pattern of airflow* it produces. Different patterns characteristically increase or decrease rate of airflow, as described next.

Patterns of Airflow. Laminar flow and turbulent flow are the two basic airflow patterns. Transitional flow is a mix of these two basic patterns (Fig. 6–10).

Laminar Flow. This pattern is characterized by parallel streamlines capable of sliding over one another as they traverse the airway. The velocity profile is parabolic—streamlines in the center of the airway travel faster than those at the sides (Fig. 6–10). In this pattern, resistance to airflow depends on the length (l) and radius (r) of the airway and the viscosity of the gas (n) according to *Poiseuille's equation,* as follows:

$$R_{aw} = \frac{8\ nl}{\pi r^4}$$

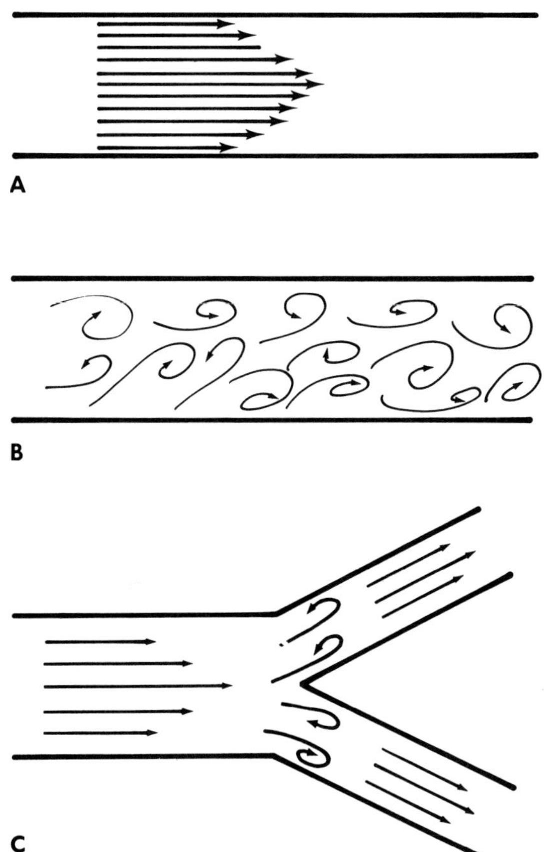

Figure 6–10. Patterns of airflow. *A*, Laminar flow. *B*, Turbulent flow. *C*, Transitional flow. (Reproduced by permission from Fishman, A.: Assessment of Pulmonary Function. New York, McGraw-Hill Book Co., 1980.)

This equation indicates that doubling the length of a tube or an airway only doubles airway resistance. However, if the radius of the airway is halved by airway pathology, for example, resistance increases sixteenfold! (Note that r in the denominator is to the fourth power.) Large driving pressures will be needed to overcome this huge increase in airway resistance and maintain a given flow rate.

Clinical Application of Poiseuille's Equation. Insertion of an endotracheal tube with a small radius creates far more airway resistance than a tube that is the correct radius but is too long. According to Poiseuille's equation, a small tube that decreases airway radius by half will increase airway resistance by sixteen. This situation requires a change to a larger tube size. A tube that is 2 inches too long increases airway resistance by a small fraction. Nevertheless, the extra airway resistance is easily eliminated by cutting off the endotracheal tube close to the patient's lips.

Though laminar flow remains a goal of respiratory therapy, it normally occurs only in small peripheral airways. Here, airflow is slow and resistance is low because airways have enormous cross-sectional areas, as previously described.

Turbulent Flow. This pattern is characterized by the complete disorganization of streamlines (see Fig. 6–10B). Because gas molecules move laterally, collide with each other, and change velocities, pressure-flow relationships change constantly. Gas movement is uneven, and airflow is not proportional to driving pressure, as in laminar flow.

Turbulent flow is most likely to occur when flow rate is high, tube diameter small, gas viscosity low, and gas density high. This pattern is the characteristic pattern of airflow in the trachea. Moreover, since airflow is especially dependent on gas density in turbulent regions, a physician sometimes will attempt to reduce airway resistance in large airways by ordering a breathing mixture that is less dense than air, e.g., a mixture of helium and O_2.

Transitional Flow. Airflow is *transitional* in most of the tracheobronchial tree, although pure turbulence may occur in the trachea at high flow rates, especially at the peak of exercise. Transitional flow occurs at lower flow rates during expiration, particularly at airway branchings. Here, the parabolic velocity profile becomes blunted. The straight streamlines move away from the sides of the airway, creating minor *eddy formations*, represented by the curved arrows in Figure 6–10C. Airflow velocity in transitional flow is slower than in laminar flow but faster than in the turbulent pattern.

Airflow Patterns in Perspective. The aforementioned basic airflow patterns are based on pressure-flow relationships in *rigid* tubes, the model used for the tracheobronchial tree. Although this simplification facilitates comprehension, airways are actually a system of irregular branching tubes; they are not entirely rigid nor perfectly circular as metal pipes. Hence, while the goal of respiratory interventions is to produce a more laminar flow, the ideal laminar flow is difficult, if not impossible, to obtain in central lung regions in particular. As previously mentioned, the clinician can only strive for optimal flow rate, in reality more of a general or conceptual goal rather than a measurable one.

Condition of Airways. The last main determinant of airway resistance is the condition of airways. It largely determines whether airflow remains more laminar, transitional, or turbulent. Disease (bronchiectasis) may exacerbate normal airway irregularity. More common, airway irregularities occur along with processes that cause a decrease in airway caliber (described previously). Airflow streamlines become more frequently interrupted, and eddy formation predominates. Air turbulence and airway resistance increase dramatically.

Control of Breathing

Control of breathing may be divided into three interrelated categories: *neural, mechanical,* and *chemical.* Associated physiological processes direct respiratory muscle activity and effect adjustments in breathing pattern, so that respiratory muscles perform a minimum amount of work for any given level of ventilation. Such control mechanisms allow the respiratory and other body systems to work together and to adapt to changing conditions during health. In addition, these mechanisms allow alterations to compensate for any respiratory problem that might arise in the clinical setting.

NEURAL CONTROL

Breathing is coordinated by the respiratory centers in the brain stem, the *medullary respiratory center* and the *apneustic* and *pneumotaxic centers.* These centers are not discrete structures but rather poorly defined collections of neurons with complex, interrelated, and incompletely understood functions. Impulses from the brain stem are involuntary and produce the automatic process of breathing. Within certain limits, however, the *cerebral cortex* of the brain can override the brain stem activity to produce voluntary breathing, such as voluntary hyperventilation and breath holding.

Medullary Respiratory Center

The interaction between the *inspiratory* and *expiratory components* of the medullary respiratory center results in the rhythmic inspiratory and expiratory phases of respiration. These components maintain their inherent rhythmicity by inhibiting each other reciprocally—when the inspiratory component stimulates inspiration, the expiratory component is temporarily inhibited (Fig. 6–11).

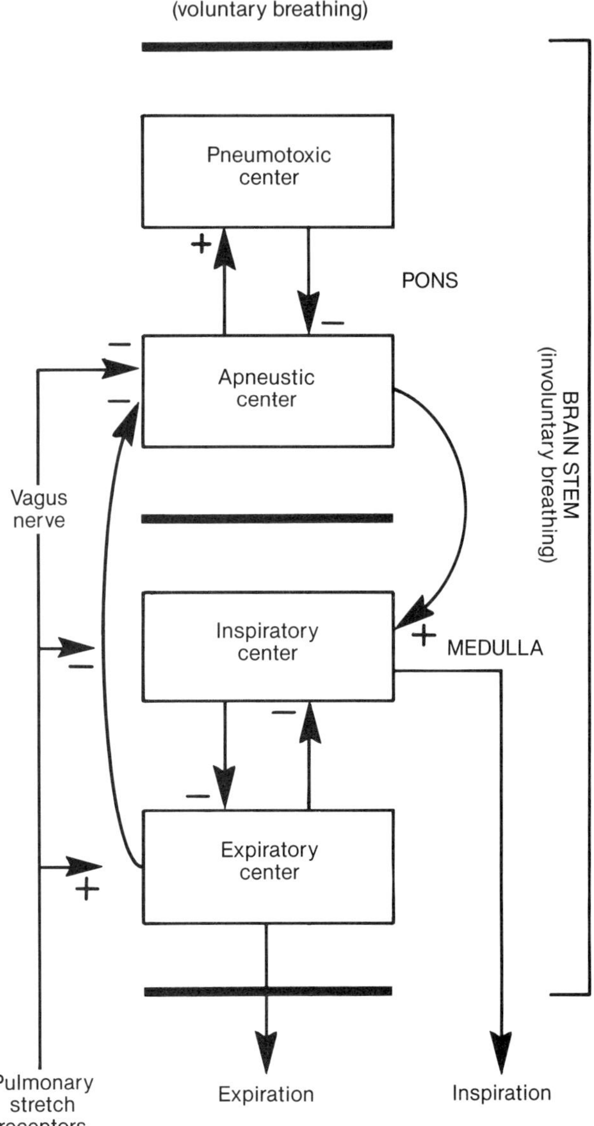

Figure 6–11. Neural control of breathing. (Adapted from Asperheim, M. and Eisenhauer, L.: The Pharmacologic Basis of Patient Care, 4th ed. Philadelphia, W. B. Saunders Co., 1981.)

Apneustic and Pneumotaxic Centers

Located in the pons just anterior to the medulla, these centers affect the activity of the medullary respiratory center. The *apneustic center* stimulates inspiration, even when the brain stem is severed just above this center. This center is inhibited by vagus nerve stimulation, by the pneumotaxic center, or by the expiratory center in the medulla (Asperheim and Eisenhauer, 1981). The *pneumotaxic center* is thought to inhibit inspiration by inhibiting the apneustic center and possibly by directly inhibiting the inspiratory component of the medullary center. In this way, it regulates respiratory rate.

Nervous Stimulation of Main Effector Muscles

Rhythmic neural stimulation from the medulla descends within the spinal cord and innervates the thoracic cage via two sets of nerves. First, high *cervical spinal nerves* join together to form the *phrenic nerve* and exit the spinal cord at level C3–C5. Innervating the two hemidiaphragms, the right and left phrenic nerves coordinate abdominal breathing. Second, *intercostal nerves* exit from the thoracic region and innervate the intercostal muscles, those responsible for movement of the mid and upper sections of the thoracic cage.

One can see that the medulla's role in breathing is crucial. As the central controller of respiration, it coordinates respiratory muscle activity through appropriate nervous activity. Without properly functioning nervous control, breathing becomes uncoordinated—the thoracic muscles may try to initiate inspiration while the abdominal muscles are still completing exhalation.

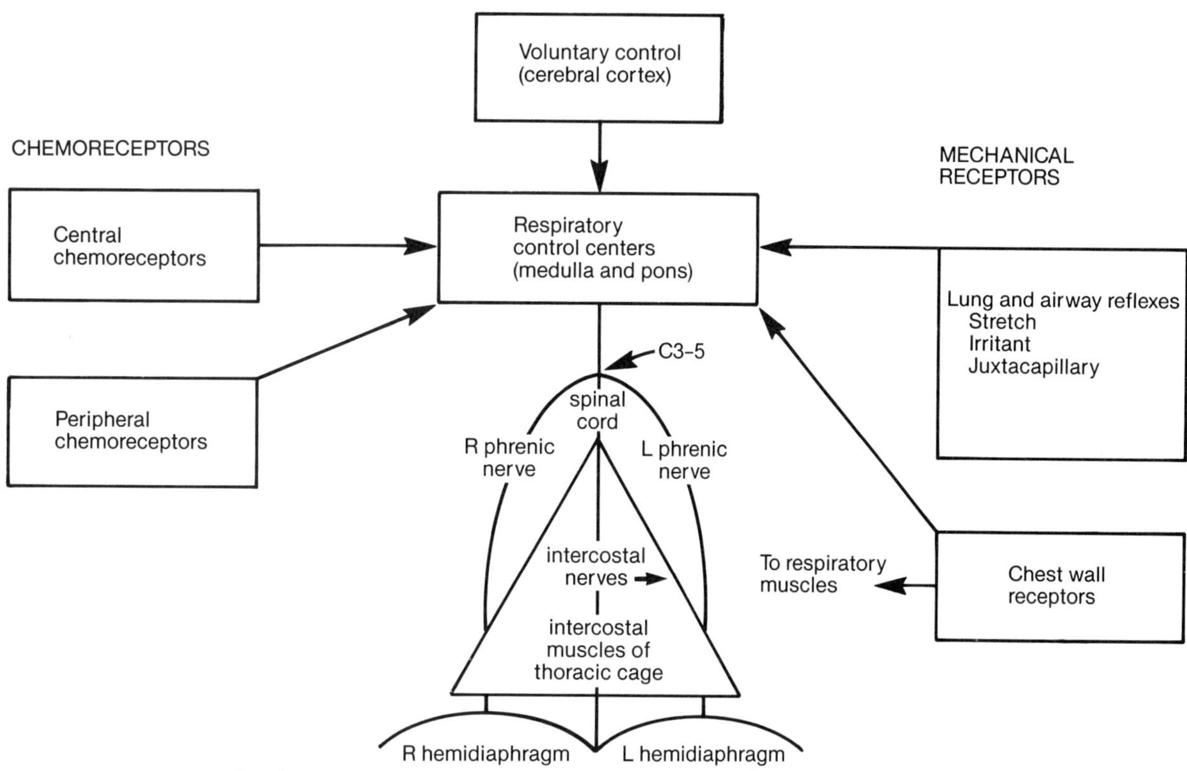

Figure 6–12. Neural and chemical stimulation of respiratory muscles. Adapted from Pavlin, E. and Hornbein, T.: The control of breathing. Basics of Respiratory Disease, 7(2):1–6, 1978.)

MECHANICAL CONTROL

Signals from *mechanical* receptors in the lungs, airways, and chest wall alter the tension of their respective receptor organs and trigger reflexes. These reflexes modify the complex activities of the medulla and pons, ultimately producing changes in depth and rate of respiration. Most reflexes are mediated by the vagus nerve. Main reflexes are defined next (Fig. 6–12).

Pulmonary stretch receptors are located within bronchial and bronchiolar smooth muscle and in smooth muscle around the trachea. *Lung distention* stimulates these stretch receptors, which in turn stimulate the medullary center to inhibit further inspiration and inflation. This so-called *Hering-Breuer reflex* decreases depth of respiration by prolongation of the expiratory component of the medullary center. Although this reflex is thought to prevent overdistention of the lung, West (1985) indicates this reflex is largely inactive in adults, unless tidal volume exceeds 1 L, as in exercise. In newborn babies and animals, it is responsible for shortening the inspiratory phase of respiration.

Irritant receptors are located in airway epithelium from the trachea down to respiratory bronchioles and seem to be more active in certain locations, e.g., the carina. The receptors are stimulated by lung irritants (e.g., cigarette smoke, noxious gases, inhaled dusts, and cold air), collapse of bronchial walls, and airway narrowing due to asthma. The effect of receptor stimulation is reflex hyperventilation and coughing, when the tracheobronchial tree is exposed to sudden mechanical deformation or noxious chemical stimuli.

Juxtacapillary or J receptors are located in alveolar walls close to capillaries. They are stimulated by alveolar wall distortion, as in engorged pulmonary capillaries and increased interstitial fluid volume. Also, J receptors are thought to play a role in the sensation of shortness of breath in interstitial lung disease. Stimulation produces rapid, shallow breathing, and intense stimulation may cause cessation of breathing.

Chest wall receptors are located in the wall of the thorax. These receptors are believed to be responsible for the sensation of dyspnea. In the presence of disease, receptor input about the position of the chest wall produces changes in intercostal muscle activity and modification of breathing pattern. For example, with intercostal muscle contraction during acute airway obstruction, chest wall receptor stimulation produces a reflex increase in inspiratory effort. This response is capable of producing normal alveolar ventilation (Pavlin and Hornbein, 1978).

CHEMICAL CONTROL

The body has central and peripheral *chemoreceptors* that respond to changes in the chemical composition of surrounding body fluid. Chemical changes alter the rhythmic inspiratory and expiratory phases of respiration established by the respiratory centers in the brain.

Central Chemoreceptors

These receptors are located near the ventral surface of the medulla near the exit of the ninth and tenth cranial nerves. They respond to changes in hydrogen ion (H^+) concentration in brain extracellular fluid—an increase in H^+ stimulates ventilation and a decrease inhibits it.

Although local blood flow and cell metabolism near these receptors alter H^+, the *amount of CO_2 in cerebrospinal fluid* (CSF) is the chief factor governing central chemoreceptor activity. Molecular CO_2 readily diffuses across the blood-brain barrier into CSF. Other ions, such as H^+ and bicarbonate (HCO_3^-), do not readily cross the blood-brain barrier. When blood is high in bicarbonate ions, 36 to 48 hours are necessary for these ions to cross the barrier. When $Paco_2$ rises, CO_2 readily diffuses into CSF, and H^+ ions are liberated from cerebral blood vessels. The extra supply of H^+ decreases blood and CSF pH (see Chapter 13 for discussion of pH). This stimulates the central chemoreceptors and produces a compensatory hyperventilation, which in turn eliminates the extra CO_2 from the body.

The central chemoreceptors are important receptors exerting minute-by-minute control of breathing. An acute change in CSF chemical composition affects ventilation more than the same degree of change in arterial blood. Because of its different composition—it is more acidic and contains less protein than blood—CSF is less able to adapt to chemical changes.

Peripheral Chemoreceptors

These receptors are located peripherally in the *aortic bodies* above and below the aortic arch and in the *carotid bodies* at the bifurcation of the common carotid arteries. In humans, the carotid rather than the aortic bodies are more active in the control of breathing.

Peripheral chemoreceptors respond to chemical changes in arterial blood. The following chemical changes all stimulate breathing and lung ventilation: (1) decreased Pao_2, (2) *excess H^+* (decreased blood pH), and *increased $Paco_2$* (in the carotid bodies only). The greater the drop in Pao_2 below normal, the greater the increase in respiratory rate. In response to changes in $Paco_2$, peripheral chemoreceptors contribute only 20% of the total ventilatory response; most of the ventilatory response is attributed to central chemoreceptor activity. Most important, chemical changes sensed by peripheral chemoreceptors act synergistically. For example, the increase in chemoreceptor activity as a result of the lack of O_2 is potentiated by a stimultaneous increase in $Paco_2$ or decrease in blood pH.

OTHER FACTORS

The rhythmicity of normal breathing may be altered by other nervous and physical factors. *Peripheral nerve receptors* may send impulses up the spinal cord to the brain, which trigger changes in respiratory rate and depth. The sensations of cold, pain, and pressure to the skin have this effect. Other factors include *passive movements of joints, emotional states,* such as anxiety or anger, and various activities that normally interrupt breathing, such as sneezing, coughing, glottic closure with swallowing, gagging, and vomiting.

Conclusion

This chapter discusses the basic concepts of mechanics and control of breathing. Though these concepts represent separate components of the respiratory system, they function in an integrated fashion to regulate breathing on a moment-to-moment basis, in response to changing metabolic needs. For example, when a patient's Pao_2 decreases, the body adapts by utilizing compensatory mechanisms to normalize the Pao_2. Peripheral chemoreceptors act on the brain stem, ultimately bringing about nervous stimulation of phrenic and intercostal nerves. This nervous stimulation effects appropriate contraction of respiratory muscles to increase respiratory rate and tidal volume that, in turn, increase alveolar ventilation and return Pao_2 to normal. In the chain reaction, nervous, chemical, and mechanical factors initiate and regulate the body's response, while the respiratory muscles actually do the work involved in changing the breathing pattern.

In addition to pointing out the integration of the components of the respiratory system, this chapter suggests that our theoretical and clinical knowledge of many normal and abnormal lung functions is extremely limited. The case of the respiratory muscles is a prime example. Though we know that, theoretically, fatigued muscles should be rested to avoid physical decompensation and weakened muscles should be trained to improve endurance, researchers have yet to identify the exact boundary between muscle fatigue and muscle weakness (Marini, 1986). Since the clinical boundary between muscle fatigue and weakness also remains obscure, the development of refined clinical decision-making skills has become crucial in the identification of patients who may be physically decompensating from interventions, such as those related to respiratory muscle training (see Chapter 20) and weaning from mechanical ventilation (see Chapter 28).

REFERENCES

Asperheim, M. and Eisenhauer, L.: *The Pharmacologic Basis of Patient Care,* 4th ed. Philadelphia, W. B. Saunders Co., 1981.

Cherniack, R., Cherniack, L., and Naimark, A.: *Respiration in Health and Disease,* 3rd ed. Philadelphia, W. B. Saunders Co., 1983.

Fishman, A.: *Assessment of Pulmonary Function.* New York, McGraw-Hill Book Co., 1980.

Frownfelter, D.: *Chest Physical Therapy and Pulmonary Rehabilitation—An Interdisciplinary Approach.* Chicago, Year Book Medical Publishers, Inc., 1978.

Hedemark, L. and Kronenberg, R.: Chemical regulation of respiration—normal variations and abnormal responses. *Chest,* 82(4):488–493, 1982.

Kendall, F. and Wadsworth, G.: *Muscles—Testing and Function,* 3rd ed. Baltimore, Williams & Wilkins, 1983.

Luce, J. and Culver, B.: Respiratory muscle function in health and disease. *Chest,* 81(1):82–90, 1982.

Marini, J.: Exertion during ventilator support: how much and how important? *Respiratory Care,* 31(5):385–387, 1986.

Pavlin, E. and Hornbein, T.: The control of breathing. *Basics of Respiratory Disease,* 7(2), 1978.

Schapiro, R. and Musallam, J.: A radiologic approach to disorders involving the interstitium of the lung. *Heart & Lung,* 6(4):635, 1977.

Strohl, K.: Upper airway muscles of respiration (editorial). *American Review of Respiratory Disease,* 124(3):211–212, 1981.

Weibel, E.: Design and structure of the human lung. In *Assessment of Pulmonary Function* (Fishman, A., ed.). New York, McGraw-Hill Book Co., 1980.

Weibel, E. and Gil J.: Structure-function relationships at the Alveolar Level. In *Lung Biology in Health and Disease, vol. 3: Bioengineering Aspects of the Lung.* (West, J., ed.). New York, Dekker, 1977.

West, J.: *Respiratory Physiology—The Essentials,* 3rd ed. Baltimore, Williams & Wilkins, 1985.

Wojciechowski, W.: *Respiratory Care Sciences—An Integrated Approach.* New York, John Wiley & Sons Inc., 1985.

PULMONARY PATHOPHYSIOLOGY

Part Two

In spite of the body's amazing ability to adapt, these responses may not be sufficient for the maintenance of normal lung function and normal gas exchange. The following three chapters describe pulmonary pathophysiology—how respiratory disease alters the structure and function of the respiratory system.

Respiratory diseases are divided into obstructive and restrictive categories based on pathology and pulmonary function abnormality. Chapter 7 introduces *obstructive pulmonary disease,* with emphases on three common diseases, as follows: asthma, bronchitis, and emphysema. Chapter 8 provides an overview of *restrictive pulmonary disease* and introduces the conglomeration of pathologically dissimilar diseases that make up this category.

In addition to detailed pathophysiology, Chapter 7 and Chapter 8 introduce main signs and symptoms, general progression of disease, and basic goals and interventions for the prototype diseases in obstructive and restrictive categories. This basic content prepares the reader for the more detailed content on clinical manifestations and interventions discussed throughout the remainder of the book.

Pathologic changes characteristic of obstructive and restrictive diseases may lead to *pulmonary heart disease,* also known as *cor pulmonale.* Chapter 4 discusses this topic in considerable detail to clarify the physiologic chain of events leading to end-stage pulmonary disease and also to explain how treatment of problems related to the primary pulmonary disease (e.g., airway obstruction and hypoxemia) stop or slow down the progression of the underlying disease and impending cor pulmonale.

Pathophysiology is emphasized in this section of the book for two reasons. First, it provides a theory base for biophysical respiratory problems. The nurse is responsible for the identification of common problems, such as bronchospasm, whether in a patient with asthma, heart failure, or adult respiratory distress syndrome. A detailed knowledge of respiratory problems prevents reliance on medical diagnosis and intervention as a model for decision-making in respiratory nursing care. As suggested in the introduction, the reliance on medical diagnosis or the practice of taking a cookbook approach to care may lead to inappropriate interventions, especially since patients with the same pulmonary disease may have different respiratory problems.

Second, pathophysiology is emphasized because it prepares the nurse to begin respiratory assessment, the actual gathering of data for problem identification (discussed in Part Three).

Terms commonly used to describe pulmonary pathophysiology and related respiratory problems are listed in the following glossary:

Glossary of Commonly Used Terms in Pulmonary Pathophysiology

Acquired immune deficiency syndrome (**AIDS**)—an immunologic disease characterized by a deficiency of helper T-lymphocytes and a decrease in the helper:suppressor T-cell ratio. Patients with advanced disease are susceptible to opportunistic pulmonary infections and malignancies and have poor prognoses for survival.

Adult respiratory distress syndrome (**ARDS**)—a life-threatening acute syndrome associated with a heterogeneous group of disorders, including gram-negative sepsis, pneumonia, fat emboli, and high concentrations of oxygen. The basic pathology is injury of alveolar-capillary units, followed by "capillary leak" and alveolar flooding.

air trapping—incomplete emptying of alveoli during

expiration owing to loss of tissue elasticity (emphysema), bronchospasm (asthma), or upper airway obstruction (aspiration of foreign object).

airway hyperreactivity—increased responsiveness of airways to lung irritants and potential allergens.

allergen—substance to which an individual has a specific hypersensitivity.

antigen—substance that induces antibody formation.

asthmatic bronchitis—combination of asthma and bronchitis, e.g., chronic asthma with superimposed acute bronchitis.

atelectasis—lung collapse due to airway obstruction, abnormal breathing pattern, or compression of lung tissue.

blue bloater—patient with advanced chronic bronchitis who looks cyanotic and plethoric.

bronchial asthma—reversible disease with multiple etiologic factors characterized by airway hyperreactivity, and narrowing.

bronchiectasis—defined anatomically as abnormal dilatation of the bronchi, and associated with repeated bronchial infections.

bronchiolitis—inflammation of the bronchioles.

bronchoconstriction—airway narrowing from bronchospasm, inflammation, mechanical obstruction, or any other cause.

bronchodilatation—enlargement in airway diameter during normal breathing on inspiration or as the result of therapy (e.g., relaxation training, pulmonary medications).

bronchospasm—bronchoconstriction associated with asthma.

bulla—hole in the lung greater than 1 to 2 cm in diameter on the chest x-ray. A pathologic feature of emphysema.

chronic airflow limitation—pulmonary function term for chronic reduction in expiratory airflow (e.g., obstructive defect).

chronic bronchitis—known clinically as cough or sputum production on most days for at least 3 months of the year for 2 successive years.

chronic obstructive pulmonary disease (COPD)—chronic obstructive diseases of the lower airways, including bronchial asthma, chronic bronchitis, emphysema, bronchiolitis, bronchiectasis, and cystic fibrosis. Some pulmonologists may restrict use of the term to emphysema and chronic bronchitis.

cor pulmonale—pulmonary heart disease or enlargement of the right ventricle from hypertrophy, dilatation, or both secondary to disorders that affect the structure or function of the lungs.

cystic fibrosis (mucoviscidosis)—an inherited disease involving generalized dysfunction of exocrine glands, resulting in pancreatic insufficiency; COPD; abnormally high sweat electrolyte levels; and, in some cases, cirrhosis of the liver.

dynamic compression of airways—airways narrowing due to changes in transmural pressure during breathing.

elastic recoil—the tissue's ability to return to resting position after stretching.

emphysema—irreversible disease associated with smoking and an inherited enzyme deficiency (alpha$_1$-antitrypsin). Characterized by destruction of alveolar septa and enlargement of air spaces.

extrapulmonary restriction—decrease in lung volume due to processes peripheral to the visceral pleura, e.g., chest wall or pleural diseases.

fibrosis—scarring.

granuloma—granular tumor usually composed of lymphoid or epitheloid cells. A characteristic of granulomatous diseases such as tuberculosis.

hay fever—allergic sensitization of the upper respiratory tract manifested by rhinitis, sneezing, burning eyes, and itchy nose.

hyperinflation—overinflation of the lungs at rest due to air trapping.

hypoxic vasoconstriction—constriction of pulmonary arterioles in response to a low PAO_2 producing local tissue hypoxia and acidosis.

Immunoglobulin E (IgE)—a sensitizing antibody (reagin) produced by plasma cells and lymphoid tissue in response to an antigen. A high level of IgE indicates an allergic reaction.

interstitial fibrosis (diffuse)—heterogeneous group of restrictive diseases characterized by thickening or fibrosis of the alveolar interstitium.

intrathoracic—any location within the thorax that is normally subject to changing pleural and alveolar pressures during breathing.

lesion—any abnormal change in the structure of an organ due to injury or disease.

mechanical obstruction—narrowing from a lesion at the site.

mediator substances—cellular substances, such as histamine and the leukotrienes. When released into bronchial tissue, they mediate the hypersensitivity reaction in asthma.

mucoviscidosis—(see cystic fibrosis).

neoplasm—tumor or growth.

obstructive disease—chest disease characterized by increased resistance to air flow due to lumenal obstruction, intrinsic airway narrowing, or peribronchial obstruction.

parenchymal disease—disease located in the parenchyma distal to conducting airways.

pink puffer—patient with advanced emphysema who is ruddy in complexion, short of breath, and cachectic.

pleural effusion—fluid in the pleural space.

pneumoconiosis—occupational lung disease caused by retention of inhaled dust in the work place.

pneumonia (pneumonitis)—inflammation of the lung parenchyma due to infection, radiation, smoke inhalation, aspiration of gastric contents, and other causes.

pneumothorax—gas in the pleural space causing lung collapse.

polycythemia—increased red blood cell count; value over 55 per cent is predictive of heart failure and suggests a need for oxygen therapy.

pulmonary edema—abnormal increase in the amount of extravascular fluid in the lungs.

pulmonary embolism—plugging of pulmonary vessels with an embolus, such as blood clots, tumors, fragments, air bubbles, or fat droplets.

pulmonary hypertension—prolonged increase in pulmonary artery pressures at rest or during exercise; systolic pressure over 30 mmHg; mean pressure over 18 mmHg.

pulmonary restriction—decrease in lung volume due to pathology within the lung.

radial traction—tissue elasticity around airways that pulls the walls of airways outward, thus preventing airway collapse.

recruitment—the opening of previously closed alveoli or pulmonary vessels; a compensatory mechanism to increase lung ventilation or perfusion.

restrictive disease—any disorder that limits lung expansion and produces a decreased total lung capacity (TLC) on the pulmonary function test.

right ventricular failure—inability of the right ventricle (RV) to sustain an increased RV workload. As the RV fails, it dilates (acute cor pulmonale), and fluid backs up to the right atrium and systemic venous system.

sleep apnea syndrome—30 or more apneic episodes lasting at least 10 seconds and observed during 7 hours of nocturnal sleep. Associated with a broad range of disorders, including obesity, Ondine's curse, and sudden infant death syndrome.

tracheal stenosis—narrowing of the trachea due to disease or as a complication of endotracheal intubation or tracheostomy.

upper airway obstruction—obstruction located in the conducting airways (from the mouth to the tracheal carina).

Obstructive Pulmonary Disease

7

Main Objectives

1. Define the following terms: Chronic obstructive pulmonary disease (COPD), chronic airflow limitation, bronchial asthma, airway hyperreactivity (hyperresponsiveness), chronic bronchitis, emphysema, bronchiolitis, bronchiectasis, and cystic fibrosis.
2. Define and describe the three pathologic processes causing obstructive disease.
3. Differentiate between upper airway obstruction and obstructive disease of the lower airways.
4. Explain the rationale for the identification of individual obstructive components in a patient with mixed chest pathology.
5. For the main obstructive diseases—acute and chronic upper airway obstruction, bronchial asthma, chronic bronchitis, emphysema, and cystic fibrosis
   a. Identify patients who may already have disease or those who are at increased risk to develop disease.
   b. Name at least three pathologic features that characterize the disease.
   c. List the main signs and symptoms.
   d. Describe the general progression of disease.
6. Name six triggers (etiological factors) that provoke bronchospasm in asthma.
7. Name the main physiological events of the allergic

reaction in asthma (type I, immediate hypersensitivity reaction).

8. **Compare and contrast the main pathophysiologies of bronchial asthma, chronic bronchitis, and emphysema.**

The primary purpose of this chapter is to review basic pathophysiology of obstructive pulmonary disease. The content provides a firm foundation for understanding chest pathology, clinical manifestations, and associated respiratory problems discussed in subsequent chapters of this book.

A thorough understanding of obstructive pulmonary disease is essential in nursing for several reasons. First, the main pulmonary disease, *chronic obstructive pulmonary disease* (COPD), is increasing in prevalence in the general population, presumably owing to the prevalence of cigarette smoking and the growing problems associated with air pollution in many work settings and various geographic regions of the country.

Second, nursing is playing a greater role in the identification of individuals with COPD or other obstructive disease as well as of those at increased risk for developing the disease. Identification may involve the careful monitoring of the acutely ill patient to detect subtle signs of airway obstruction, or it may involve the periodic or continuous monitoring of the home or clinic patient who would remain unable to adjust to chronic illness without support from a knowledgeable and competent nurse. In other situations, nurses may be required to screen outpatient populations for the presence of pulmonary disease. This screening can be a difficult task because of the lack of specific objective indicators for *early* COPD and because of the broad spectra of possible pulmonary diseases and disease presentations in different individuals.

Third, one or more *chronic* obstructive pulmonary diseases commonly exist in the patient hospitalized for an acute problem, such as acute respiratory failure. When underlying chronic disease exists, patient problems tend to be numerous and diverse, involving many pathophysiological variables, many of which are responsible for or contribute to psychosocial problems. Moreover, problems tend to be complex because the COPD patient, in particular, rarely presents with a "pure" form of disease—two obstructive processes may coexist in the same patient, each requiring a slightly different approach to treatment. To complicate matters, when disease is disabling, treatment also tends to be complex. It may require enormous amounts of time, energy, money, and expertise to implement. Coordination of care involves the *constant* reassessment of the patient as he or she moves through the health care continuum. This process requires use of a *firm* knowledge base of the pathogenesis of obstructive diseases to sort through the array of pathophysiological variables considered in the identification of acute and chronic problems.

Fourth, because of growing consumer demand for smoking cessation, air pollution control, and self care programs, health team members are focusing more on preventive and rehabilitative aspects of care. Most pulmonary rehabilitation programs focus on patients with obstructive rather than restrictive diseases. To participate in health teaching and to implement techniques designed to treat obstructive pathological processes, the nurse needs a thorough knowledge of obstructive disease.

Last, knowledge of obstructive disease helps the nurse realize that obstructive processes are common in restrictive diseases as well. For example, although pneumonia is a restrictive pulmonary disease, when mucus plugs up airways, airway obstruction occurs. Interventions focus on relief of airway obstruction as well as on treatment of the underlying restrictive disease.

Definition and Main Pathologic Processes

An obstructive disease is defined as a chest disease characterized by *increased resistance to airflow* primarily from one or more of the following pathological processes: (1) *lumenal obstruction* (from inside the airway); (2) *intrinsic airway narrowing* (from within the wall of the airway); and (3) *peribronchial obstruction* (from outside the airway). Figure 7–1 illustrates these processes.

LUMENAL OBSTRUCTION

Lumenal obstruction occurs when something inside the airway causes occlusion of the lumen. Occlusion or obstruction may be partial or complete, depending on the nature and severity of disease. Retained secretions from bronchitis, pulmonary edema, and pneumonia may cause lumenal obstruction. Aspiration of a small foreign object or presence of a tumor or thick mucus plug may cause complete or intermittent obstruction in a localized area of lung.

INTRINSIC AIRWAY NARROWING

Intrinsic airway narrowing occurs when a disorder within the wall of the airway causes airway narrowing. A classic example is contraction of bronchial smooth muscle producing bronchospasm, as in asthma. In bronchitis and asthma, airway edema and inflammation also narrow the size of airways. Other causes of intrinsic airway narrowing are tracheal stenosis, tumors within the wall of the airway, laryngospasm, and peribronchial fibrosis.

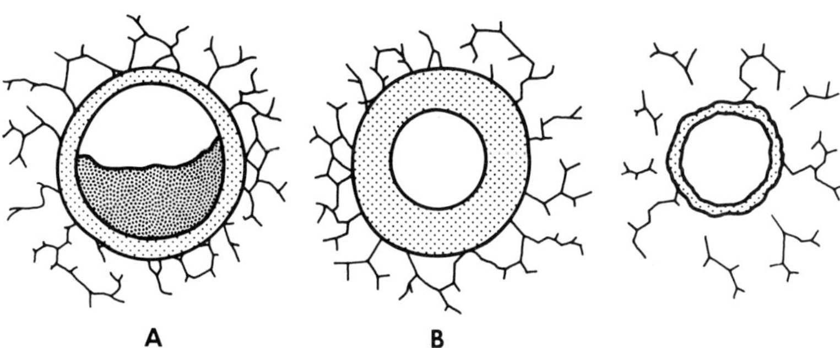

Figure 7–1. Pathologic processes causing airway obstruction. *A*, Lumenal obstruction, e.g., from excess secretions. *B*, Intrinsic airway narrowing, e.g., from bronchospasm. *C*, Peribronchial obstruction, e.g., from loss of radial traction due to destruction of surrounding lung tissue. (Reproduced by permission from West, J.: Pulmonary Pathophysiology: The Essentials, 2nd ed. Baltimore, Williams & Wilkins, 1982.)

PERIBRONCHIAL OBSTRUCTION

Peribronchial obstruction is airway obstruction occurring from outside the airway in the peribronchial region. Obstruction of a bronchus may occur from compression by a nearby enlarged lymph node or tumor. Peribronchial edema from interstitial pulmonary edema also can cause airway narrowing. If the pleural space fills the air and fluid as in pneumothorax and pleural effusion, respectively, compression of underlying lung tissue can cause the same problem. Last, with the destruction of lung tissue, as in emphysema, airways tend to narrow and collapse owing to the lack of normal supporting tissues around airways. Normally, the elasticity of supporting lung tissue provides a kind of radial traction pulling the walls of airways outward. This effect keeps airways open. If disease destroys this elastic supporting tissue, producing what is known as the *loss of radial traction*, then airways collapse inward and cause airway obstruction.

Most important, not only do these three processes help to define various obstructive pulmonary diseases, but they also represent obstructive processes found in restrictive diseases, such as pneumonia, pulmonary edema, and atelectasis. In such cases, one states that the individuals with primary restrictive diseases have developed *obstructive components*. Identification of an obstructive component is important because immediate treatment with additional medications and other forms of respiratory therapy may be required to relieve airway obstruction.

Classification of Disease

Obstructive (and restrictive) diseases are divided into *acute* and *chronic* forms based on the need for medical treatment and the duration of signs and symptoms. On the one hand, *acute disease* is characterized by the need for *immediate* medical attention and usually a relatively short duration of signs and symptoms, e.g., acute upper airway obstruction. *Chronic disease*, on the other hand, is characterized by a long history (usually years) of signs and symptoms, e.g., chronic obstructive pulmonary disease.

Pulmonary diseases are further classified according to severity into *mild*, *moderate*, and *severe* based on pulmonary function test results (see Table 14–6).

Obstructive diseases are divided anatomically into *diseases of the upper airways* and *diseases of the lower airways*. The upper airways include the portion of the conducting system from the mouth to the tracheal carina. The lower airways involve airways and lung tissue beyond the tracheal carina. In the case of lower airway obstruction, the obstruction can occur in a localized area of one lung or diffusely throughout both right and left lungs.

Obstructive Disease of the Upper Airways

Upper airway obstruction occurs in *acute* and *chronic* forms; the area of pathology can be *intrathoracic* or *extrathoracic* in location.

ACUTE FORMS

Acute upper airway obstruction (acute UAO) is readily recognizable because the patient usually demonstrates overt signs of respiratory distress and rapid physical deterioration unless prompt treatment is initiated to relieve the obstruction.

CHRONIC FORM

The chronic form is more subtle. Although signs and symptoms are relatively mild, considerable narrowing or weakening of the airway wall may exist owing to chronic disease. A precipitating factor, such as a common cold, may worsen airway narrowing, placing the individual at increased risk to develop acute UAO and complete airway occlusion. Furthermore, the nurse's familiarity with the chronic form of disease is important because it is often misdiagnosed as asthma or chronic bronchitis, owing to similar clinical manifestations. In this case, misinterpretation of findings sometimes leads to inappropriate interventions.

Importance of the Patient's Age

Whether acute or chronic, UAO is always more critical in infants and children because they have proportionally smaller airways than adults. Also, infants and children tend to be more susceptible to inflammation of the upper respiratory tract, which causes further airway narrowing. In normal adults, a small change in airway diameter produces little to no change in airway resistance and work of breathing. In children, however, a small decrease in airway diameter, particularly in the normally narrowed glottic and subglottic regions, produces a considerable increase in airway resistance and work of breathing. Hence, complete obstruction is more likely in infants and children than in adults.

Young boys may be less able than young girls to ventilate the lungs when upper or lower airway obstruction is present. Normal, young boys 3 to 6 years of age have lower airflow rates than girls of the same age. The reason is unknown, but it may pertain to the postulation that airways in young girls may be larger than those in young boys (Taussig et al, 1981).

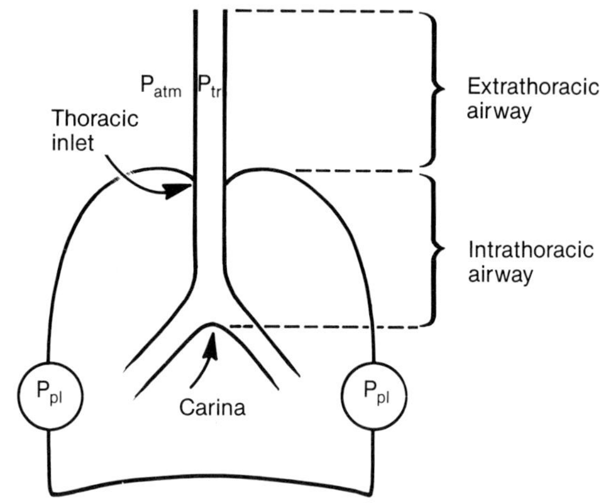

Figure 7–2. Pressures affecting transmural pressure and airway caliber of upper airways. P_{pl} = pleural pressure, P_{tr} = tracheal pressure, and P_{atm} = atmospheric pressure.

LOCATION OF UPPER AIRWAY LESIONS

A *lesion* is defined as any abnormal change in the structure of an organ due to injury or disease. Pathology that causes upper airway obstruction is often referred to as an *upper airway lesion.*

Upper airway lesions may be *intrathoracic* or *extrathoracic* in location. The particular location of a lesion is important because the aforementioned two sites are subject to different pulmonary pressures and transmural pressures, which tend to either collapse or open the airway during inspiration and expiration. The collapsing or opening of the airway is the physiological basis for the absence or presence of lung sounds in upper airway obstruction.

An *intrathoracic* upper airway lesion is located in or adjacent to the trachea somewhere between the carina and thoracic inlet (or suprasternal notch). Since the lesion is located within the chest, it is subject to changes in pleural pressure (P_{pl}), as illustrated in Figure 7–2. An *extrathoracic* lesion is located more superiorly in the trachea above the suprasternal notch or in the larynx, pharynx, nose, or mouth. It is subjected to atmospheric pressure (P_{atm}).

Determination of intrathoracic versus extrathoracic location is made by means of a specialized pulmonary function test (flow-volume loop) ordered by the physician. This test senses and records changes in airway caliber during respiration. Not only do test results help the physician determine the location of the obstructive lesion, they also provide other diagnostic information about the nature and severity of the causative disease (see Chapter 14).

ACUTE UPPER AIRWAY OBSTRUCTION

Causes of the *acute* form of UAO are listed in Table 7–1, along with examples of associated disorders and situations in the clinical setting.

Infection is a major cause of disease. Acute infection of the tracheobronchial tree is observed in *laryngotracheobronchitis,* also known as *childhood croup.* Croup is usually viral in etiology and affects the subglottic region of the upper airway as well as the bronchi and bronchioles. It occurs most frequently in children 6 months to 3 years of age. *Acute epiglottitis,* seen in adults and in children between 18 months and 8 years of age, is an acute fulminant infection of the epiglottis, aryepiglottic folds, and surrounding tissue caused by a bacterial microbe, usually *Haemophilus influenzae,* type B (Loughlin and Taussig, 1979). It is a medical emergency and requires immediate and definitive therapy to prevent complete airway obstruction. *Pharyngeal abscesses* can also cause acute airway obstruction. An acute retropharyngeal abscess may extend from the retropharyngeal space into the mediastinum, causing an acute mediastinal abscess as well. *Laryngeal diphtheria* is a rare cause of upper airway infection, but the nurse may see it in patients living in locations with poor immunization programs.

Other causes of acute airway obstruction are laryngeal edema from a variety of causes, including acute allergic (anaphylactic) reactions; retropharyngeal hemorrhage; aspiration of foreign bodies; and faulty placement of an endotracheal tube.

Mechanical obstruction of the oropharynx may occur in the acute care setting in a patient with excessive secretions or blocked airway from displacement of the tongue against the pharyngeal wall. Examples of those who are likely to experience obstruction in this manner are comatose or semicomatose patients who are not

Table 7–1. MAIN CAUSES OF ACUTE UPPER AIRWAY OBSTRUCTION

Cause	Associated Disorders/ Situations
Infection	Acute epiglottitis Acute retropharyngeal abscess Laryngotracheitis Laryngeal diphtheria
Laryngeal edema (noninfectious)	Trauma Inhalation of irritant noxious gases Inherited angioneurotic edema Acute anaphylactic reaction (from inhalants, bee stings, drugs) Postendotracheal tube extubation
Retropharyngeal hemorrhage	Neck surgery Trauma Diagnostic procedures (e.g., carotid angiography) Erosion of an artery from infection
Foreign bodies	Children—aspiration of small objects, usually peanuts, coins, plastic bullets, screws Adults—food aspiration, usually meat, and bones Pharyngeal muscle dysfunction
Faulty placement of endotracheal tubes	Intubation of right (rarely left) main bronchus; tube cuff occludes orifice of left main bronchus
Mechanical obstruction of oropharynx	Excessive oral secretions Seizures Gross obesity Cardiac arrest Loss of consciousness

intubated; cardiac arrest victims; patients with convulsive seizures; and critically ill, grossly obese individuals. Obese individuals tend to have ventilatory problems and anatomical predispositions to upper airway obstruction in the recumbent position. The short stocky neck is difficult to keep extended so that the airway remains patent.

CHRONIC UPPER AIRWAY OBSTRUCTION

Chronic upper airway obstruction is caused by a wide variety of disorders, as listed in the box. The majority of these disorders are recognized more frequently in children and are congenital, as in obstruction from (1) *craniofacial malformations*; (2) *congenital subglottic stenosis*, defined as narrowing of the subglottic region of the larynx; and (3) *laryngomalacia*, a condition produced by an underdeveloped epiglottis and redundant aryepiglottic folds. The last disorder has a variety of names, including congenital laryngeal stridor, floppy epiglottis, and benign stridor. It is the most common cause of chronic stridor in the newborn. The stridor is a high-pitched crowing sound that is intermittent and often disappears with sleep. By the time the child is 2 years of age, stridor usually has disappeared completely.

Acquired disorders include *trauma* to the thorax, neck, and throat and *tracheal stenosis*, defined as narrowing of the trachea. Tracheal stenosis may occur as a complication of endotracheal intubation or tracheostomy. If a tracheostomy tube is in place, stenosis may occur in the three following places: (1) at the level of the stoma, where the tube enters the trachea (the most common); (2) at the level of the inflated cuff; and (3) where the tip of the tube touches the tracheal wall (rarely). Contact of the tube or cuff against the airway produces local inflammation, progressing to mucosal ulceration and pressure necrosis, as blood supply to surrounding tissues is compromised. Underlying cartilaginous rings may become exposed, then softened, split, fragmented, and destroyed in severe cases. Once the tube is removed, tissue fibrosis occurs at the site resulting in stenosis. Intubated patients at increased risk to develop tracheal stenoses are those who undergo prolonged periods of intubation, those who have endotracheal tubes with high pressure rather than low pressure cuffs, and those who are debilitated and have increased susceptibility to inflammation.

MAIN DISORDERS ASSOCIATED WITH CHRONIC UPPER AIRWAY OBSTRUCTION

Congenital abnormalities
Allergy
Tracheal stenosis
Tracheomalacia
Neoplasms, cysts
Foreign body aspiration
Subglottic stenosis
(congenital or acquired)
Vocal cord paralysis
Enlarged tonsils and adenoids
Obstructive sleep apnea syndrome

Tracheomalacia is a condition characterized by weakness of the tracheal walls and supporting cartilages, predisposing the patient to tracheal collapse during expiration. Tracheomalacia may develop as a complication of endotracheal intubation, causing permanent tracheal stenosis in severe cases or transient stenosis due to focal kinking or buckling of the trachea during forced expiration or coughing. The condition is associated with a deficiency of cartilage from tissue trauma, inflammation, mechanical changes, or malignancy; it may represent a developmental or congenital defect.

Some acquired lesions associated with chronic UAO are associated with *sleep disturbances,* more specifically *sleep apnea* (periods of no breathing) (see Chapter 12). In essence, the upper airway becomes obstructed from the collapse of pharyngeal soft tissue and from the posterior displacement of the tongue, as in gross obesity and some craniofacial anomalies. In children, hypertrophied (enlarged) tonsils and adenoids may occlude the airway at night. Partial obstruction results in slow, shallow breathing unnoticed by the sleeping individual. Alteration in the soundness or pattern of sleep typically results in signs and symptoms of sleep deprivation during the day. The exact mechanisms of obstruction have not been well defined (see Chapter 8 for discussion of sleep apnea syndrome).

Other forms of chronic airway obstruction result from allergy, aspiration of foreign bodies, unilateral or bilateral vocal cord paralysis, cysts, and neoplasms (tumors). Papillomas causing *papillomatosis* are the most common laryngeal tumors in children and are occasionally found in adults. These epithelioid tumors are usually benign, in single or multiple form, and sometimes extend down the tracheobronchial tree to obstruct airways in the lungs. Cancerous tumors rarely occur in the trachea as a primary site compared with the more frequent cancerous tumors of the larynx and bronchi. The commonest primary cancer of the trachea is squamous cell carcinoma.

PATHOPHYSIOLOGY

Signs and symptoms of UAO are attributed to airway narrowing from *mechanical obstruction* at the lesion site and from *dynamic compression* of airways. The latter term is defined as *airway narrowing due to changes in transmural pressure during respiration.* The presence and extent of dynamic compression during different phases of respiration depends on whether the lesion is intrathoracic or extrathoracic in location—pressure relationships (and transmural pressures) differ in intrathoracic and extrathoracic locations. Dynamic compression also depends on whether the lesion is of the "stiff" *fixed type* or of the soft, pliable, *variable type* (see Chapter 14).

Inspiratory stridor is the classic finding in a patient with acute or chronic *extrathoracic* UAO. *Stridor* is defined as a harsh whistling or high-pitched crowing sound caused by partial obstruction of the upper airway from edema, inflammation, or a mass. If the lesion is *intrathoracic* in location, then the stridor (and wheezing from lower airways, if present) is predominant during the *expiratory* phase of respiration when the airway is narrowest.

The pitch of this loud vibrating sound depends on the degree of the obstruction and the mass of the vibrating structures. Higher pitched noises generally result from greater narrowing of airways. Low-pitched stridor may result from supraglottic obstruction.

In an adult, airway narrowing and stridor is primarily from mechanical obstruction as opposed to dynamic compression of airways because the trachea is well supported with cartilage. Children with extremely compliant tracheas and individuals with tracheas weakened by disease (e.g., tracheomalacia) are more likely to develop additional narrowing from dynamic compression of airways. They are the patients most likely to develop stridor and severe ventilatory problems in the presence of UAO.

Specific pathophysiological features of UAO vary depending on the nature of the particular disorder, but certain generalizations can be made regarding the effects of complete and partial obstruction on lung ventilation. Figure 7–3A shows that complete obstruction results in the absence of lung ventilation, a situation that is incompatible with life. Not only is alveolar ventilation absent, but the perfusion component of the V/Q ratio also drops, as the oxygen-starved heart fails to maintain cardiac output. In partial UAO (Fig. 7–3B) alveolar ventilation is decreased, but air is distributed evenly throughout the lung, unlike localized obstructions in the lower airways (Fig. 7–3C).

When partial UAO occurs, the patient attempts to breathe deeper and faster to keep the lungs adequately ventilated. Compensatory mechanisms are successful in the case of mild disease. With moderate to severe obstruction, the lung becomes underventilated. The alveolar hypoventilation predisposes the patient to lower respiratory tract complications, such as atelectasis and pneumonia, and creates an oxygenation problem. During physical exercise or during crying episodes in children, lung ventilation becomes reduced even more because the rapid deep breathing increases airflow past the site of obstruction. On the one hand,

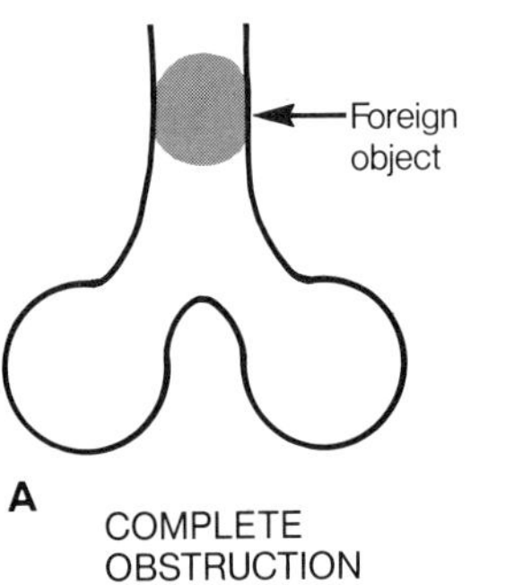

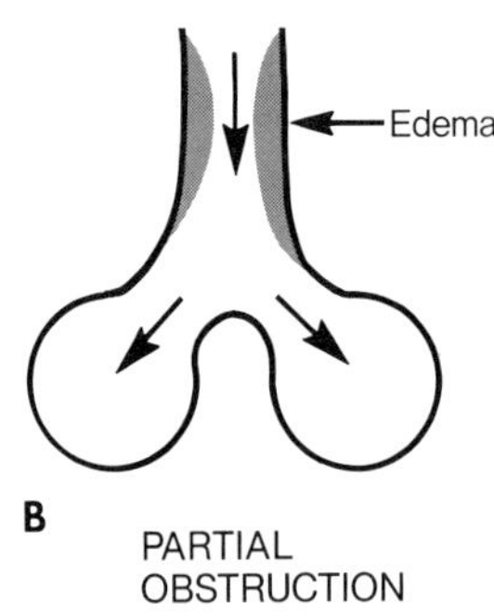

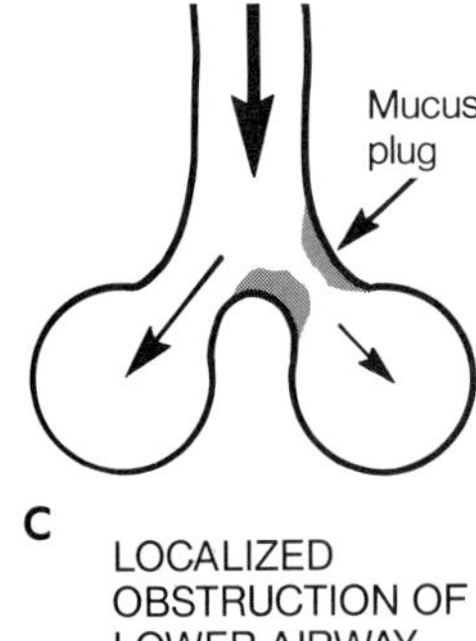

Figure 7–3. Complete and partial upper airway obstruction contrasted with localized obstruction of the lower airway. *A,* Complete obstruction. *B,* Partial obstruction. *C,* Localized obstruction of lower airway.

Table 7–2. MAIN SIGNS AND SYMPTOMS OF UPPER AIRWAY OBSTRUCTION

Acute	Chronic
Sudden onset of shortness of breath (SOB)	SOB—first with exercise, then at rest
Stridor	Stridor
Voice change	Voice change
Fever and cough (upper respiratory tract infection)	Nonproductive cough
Feeling of suffocation; clutching of throat	Snoring during sleep

the increased airflow produces air turbulence, which in turn increases airway resistance and work of breathing. The patient becomes short of breath. On the other hand, slow deep breathing decreases air turbulence, airway resistance, and work of breathing. Slow deep breathing promotes lung ventilation, and the more relaxed patient may be able to eliminate shortness of breath completely. Herein lies the physiological basis for encouraging slow deep breathing during episodes of acute obstruction.

MAIN SIGNS AND SYMPTOMS/ PROGRESSION OF DISEASE

Main signs and symptoms of acute and chronic airway obstruction are presented in Table 7–2.

Acute Obstruction

The cardinal symptom of acute obstruction is the *sudden onset of shortness of breath* (SOB) or a *feeling of suffocation.* The other signs and symptoms may or may not be present depending on the nature and severity of the disorder. In the case of the sudden aspiration of food or a foreign object, the first manifestations of a completely or almost completely obstructed airway are typically those of the individual clutching the throat, the so-called distress signal of choking, and the inability or difficulty in talking or coughing.

Untreated, acute UAO becomes worse in minutes, hours, or a few days if the onset is more gradual. Careful observation of the patient is necessary when signs and symptoms appear because respiratory distress may rapidly worsen and lead to sudden cessation of breathing (respiratory arrest). With the worsening of signs and symptoms, an experienced physician performs a tracheotomy, a surgical incision between the second and third tracheal cartilaginous rings, and a tracheostomy tube is inserted to establish an airway. In some cases, depending on the nature and location of the obstruction, the physician might be able to carefully pass an endotracheal tube past the obstruction and into the trachea, using a laryngoscope or a bronchoscope. If the patient cannot be intubated or if a tracheostomy is impossible at the moment, a temporary opening is made between the thyroid and cricoid cartilages by excising the cricothyroid membrane (Fig. 7–4). The procedure is called a *cricothyroidotomy.* A hollow tube of some kind is temporarily inserted for emergency ventilation, oxygen is provided, and a tracheostomy is scheduled as soon as possible.

Chronic Obstruction

Shortness of breath is the patient's usual presenting complaint in chronic UAO. It appears first with exercise and then at rest.

Obstruction becomes gradually worse over a period of weeks, months, and years. Many disorders are treatable. For example, obese individuals with obstructive sleep apnea can lose weight, or use a special breathing device called a nasal continuous positive airway pressure mask at night to keep the upper airway open. In tracheal stenosis, the upper airway can be by-passed with insertion of a tracheostomy tube. An alternative to tracheostomy is surgical removal of the stricture and end-to-end anastomosis of healthy trachea. Craniofacial anomalies may be treated with corrective surgical procedures, and enlarged tonsils and adenoids can be removed surgically, if necessary. In some cases, intervention may be unnecessary. Some developmental forms of disease may be outgrown by children, as in laryngomalacia.

Sometimes, the afflicted individual does not seek medical attention or, more commonly, the chronic obstructive process, e.g., some tumors, continues to progress in spite of treatment. The course of disease is often marked by episodes of *acute* UAO precipitated by respiratory tract infections. If the individual survives these exacerbations, advanced pulmonary disease develops (see Chapter 4).

GOALS AND INTERVENTIONS

Goals for treatment and basic interventions for both acute and chronic UAO are summarized in the box.

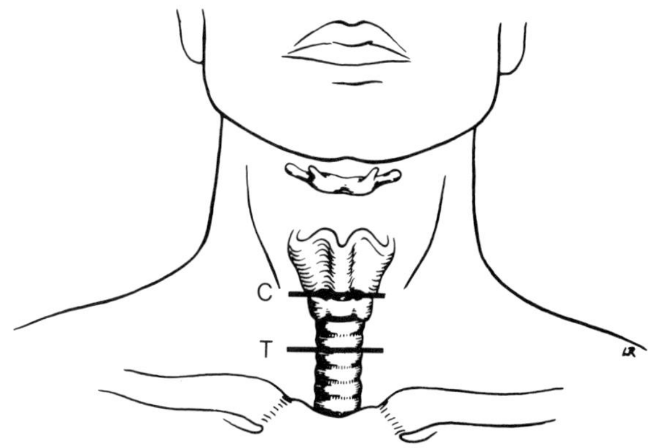

Figure 7–4. Location of surgical incisions for tracheostomy (T) and cricothyroidotomy (C) over the cricothyroid membrane. (Reproduced by permission from McCullough, D.: Surgical management of acute upper airway obstruction. Semin. Resp. Med. 2:1, 1980.)

GOALS AND INTERVENTIONS FOR UPPER AIRWAY OBSTRUCTION (UAO)

GOALS

Eliminate upper airway obstruction
Reduce tissue inflammation
Maintain normal oxygenation and ventilation

INTERVENTIONS (ACUTE UAO)

Monitor closely in an intensive care unit. Keep a muscle relaxant (e.g., succinylcholine), a 14-gauge needle (for cricothyroid puncture), and a tracheostomy tray at bedside for emergency use.

Pulmonary medications include racemic epinephrine by aerosol; intravenous corticosteroids (of uncertain benefit); and bronchodilator, if bronchospasm is present.

Avoid physical stimulation but do not sedate (e.g., in cases of inflammation obstruction).

Establish a patent airway, as described in Chapter 24 (e.g., in cases of aspiration of foreign object).

Keep the head of the bed elevated.

Treat the primary cause of the obstruction (e.g., administer antibiotics for infection).

Oxygen or helium-oxygen mixture by face mask (the low density gas mixture decreases airway resistance).

Tracheostomy or cricothyroidotomy

INTERVENTIONS (CHRONIC UAO)

Treat the primary cause of the obstruction
Oxygen
Tracheostomy
Self-care education

Most of the interventions listed are discussed in detail elsewhere in this book.

Obstructive Diseases of the Lower Airways

The vast majority of adults with obstructive disease have chronic disease of the *lower* airways commonly called *chronic obstructive pulmonary disease* (COPD).

Historically, the term COPD refers to all chronic obstructive pulmonary diseases in general, especially bronchial asthma, chronic bronchitis, and emphysema.

In the recent past, leading authorities in pulmonary disease have critically evaluated the use of the word "obstructive" in COPD. Petty and Scoggin (1979) and Soffer (1980), at the 22nd Aspen Lung Conference on the topic of COPD, concluded that use of this word is misleading and conceptually incorrect. Petty and Scoggin explain that the term obstruction suggests primary involvement of the conducting airways. In emphysema, the loss of lung elasticity seems to be the major factor limiting expiratory airflow rather than the airway obstruction per se. Hence, the "state of the art" now favors the term "chronic airflow limitation" which refers to all disorders in which expiratory airflow is reduced or delayed. Primary chest diseases with chronic airflow limitation are bronchial asthma, chronic bronchitis, emphysema, and cystic fibrosis.

Though experts agree that the term chronic airflow limitation is more precise, in actual practice many physicians, nurses, and others continue to include all the aforementioned diseases under the nonspecific and noncommittal category of COPD. Furthermore, they may use other terms for COPD, such as *chronic obstructive lung disease* (COLD) or *chronic airways obstruction* (CAO).

For precision, clarity, and consistency with regard to recent definitions, health professionals should use the term COPD to refer to only the entities of chronic bronchitis and emphysema. Bronchial asthma should be considered a disease entity separate from chronic bronchitis and emphysema—its pathophysiology is completely different. The goals of therapy as well as the approach to the patient in the clinical setting are different.

Yet, in the midst of new terms that have come and gone over past years, the nonspecific COPD category remains the most common to describe the broad spectrum of obstructive disease. Health professionals in the nurse's practice setting may be *firmly* entrenched with its usage, even though they know it is conceptually misleading. In light of this situation, to insist on new terms when professionals still use old ones may be inviting unnecessary confusion that may not make a difference in the care given. Therefore, while the new terminology is preferable, this text uses the more common meaning of the term COPD, unless discussion specifically contrasts the entity COPD (bronchitis and emphysema) with asthma. In some places, COPD is used interchangeably with chronic airflow limitation; the last term is used to emphasize pulmonary function aspects.

OVERVIEW OF MAIN DISEASES—PURE AND MIXED FORMS

Main obstructive diseases of the lower airways include bronchial asthma, chronic bronchitis, emphysema, bronchiolitis, bronchiectasis, and cystic fibrosis.

Of these diseases, the first three—bronchial asthma, chronic bronchitis, and emphysema—are most important to understand for three reasons. First, a thorough knowledge of the pathophysiologies of these diseases is necessary to understand bronchiectasis, cystic fibrosis (an extremely complex disease), and other chest diseases discussed in other chapters.

Second, each of these diseases may occur in a "pure"

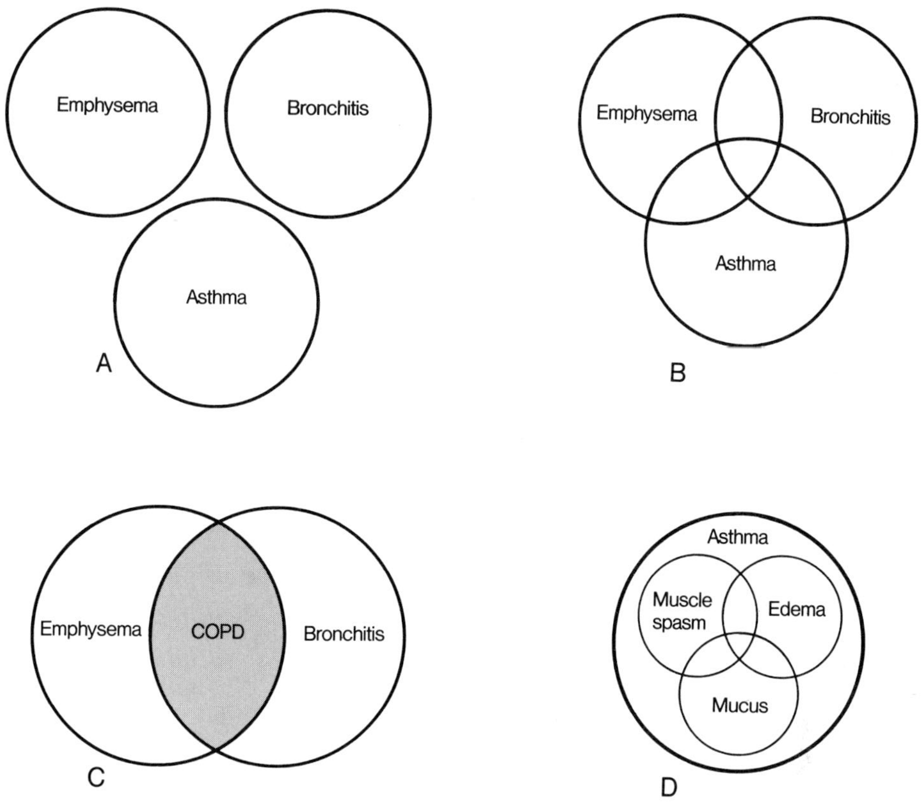

Figure 7–5. Conceptual representations of asthma, emphysema, and chronic bronchitis. *A*, Pure forms. *B*, Mixed forms. *C*, Emphysema and bronchitis—a common clinical presentation termed chronic obstructive pulmonary disease (COPD) (shaded area) by many pulmonologists. *D*, Pure asthma with various combinations of pathologic features.

or "mixed" form, as shown conceptually in Figure 7–5. They may occur alone (Fig. 7–5A), but they more commonly occur in combination with each other (Fig. 7–5B) or in combination with another obstructive process, e.g., bronchitis and bronchiectasis, as in cystic fibrosis. Though any combination of asthma, bronchitis, and emphysema is possible, common clinical presentations include emphysema and bronchitis (Fig. 7–5C) (correctly termed COPD, as previously explained) and pure asthma (Fig. 7–5D), as seen in young children and adults. In the asthma representation (see Fig. 7–5D), the diagram illustrates the point that pathological processes in asthma (and many other obstructive diseases) vary among individuals. For example, some asthmatics manifest only muscle spasm (e.g., wheezing), whereas others manifest all three pathological processes, e.g., wheezing, sputum production, and signs of airway edema.

When two or more diseases coexist, the patient is said to have "mixed chest pathology." In the case of asthma and bronchitis, the individual is said to have "mixed chest pathology with an asthmatic component and a bronchitic component." The primary disease is the component that produces more signs and symptoms.

Another reason why asthma, bronchitis, and emphysema are important to understand relates to their relationship to restrictive pulmonary disease (see Chapter 8). These diseases represent common obstructive processes that accompany or are superimposed on many restrictive diseases. In the hospital, a patient with restrictive disease may present with an acute asthmatic or bronchitic component requiring immediate medical treatment. In the industrial setting, the worker who smokes cigarettes commonly manifests signs and symptoms of an obstructive process (e.g., bronchitis) long before signs and symptoms of an accompanying chronic restrictive disease (e.g., asbestosis) become evident.

Though mixed chest pathology is often the case, the following descriptions of asthma, bronchitis, and emphysema emphasize the pure forms. This approach allows the nurse to more easily identify the components of mixed chest pathology. In addition, the planning of interventions that are specific to the identified components is facilitated.

BRONCHIAL ASTHMA

Bronchial asthma is a disease characterized by hyperreactivity of airways to various stimuli causing widespread airway narrowing. It is known as a *reversible* lung disease because airway narrowing changes in severity either spontaneously or as a result of therapy.

Since asthma frequently appears in the form of an allergic reaction, it must be differentiated from *hay fever*. Hay fever is allergic sensitization of the upper respiratory tract (URT). It is a *local* allergic reaction affecting the URT mucous membranes and producing URT signs and symptoms of rhinitis, sneezing, burning eyes, itchy nose, and absence of fever. Asthma is a more general allergic reaction affecting the lower respiratory tract (the trachea and airways in the lungs), producing pulmonary rather than URT symptoms.

This reversible chest disease may be newly diagnosed in children or adults, but it has been known as a disease in children because of its high incidence (up to 12%) (Fraser and Paré, 1979). The incidence is only about 1% in the general population. Asthma occurs more frequently in boys under the age of 14 years, in men over the age of 45 years, and in women between the ages of 15 and 45 years. About 30% of children with hay fever develop asthma. Most children completely outgrow asthma.

Pathologic Features

The three main pathological features of asthma are as follows:

1. *Muscle spasm*—hypertrophied smooth muscle around the airway contracts.
2. *Swelling of the mucosa*— edema is the cause.
3. *Thick secretions*—mucous glands increase in number, hypertrophy, and secrete thick, tenacious mucus that commonly is heavily infiltrated with eosinophils, a type of leukocyte.

All of these processes contribute to bronchoconstriction (airway narrowing) and associated wheezing in the patient, regardless of the initial stimulus to the asthmatic attack. Bronchoconstriction occurring in this manner is more specifically referred to as *bronchospasm*. To appreciate the extent of bronchoconstriction possible in asthma, observe the illustrated normal bronchiole in Figure 7–6, comparing its airway lumen (cross-sectional view) with the airway lumen of the diseased bronchiole in Figure 7–7.

Asthma Triggers

An asthma trigger is an etiologic factor responsible for asthma. Common triggers include allergy, infection, drugs, and others as listed in the box (Leff, 1982).

An allergic reaction may be triggered by food, food or drug preservatives (e.g., metabisulfites), or food additives (e.g., monosodium glutamate and dyes such as tartrazine); it may be triggered by exposure to dust, smog, or numerous environmental factors discussed in Chapter 10.

As an asthma trigger, infection is usually viral rather than bacterial in origin. Common causative viruses are rhinovirus (common cold) and influenza virus type A.

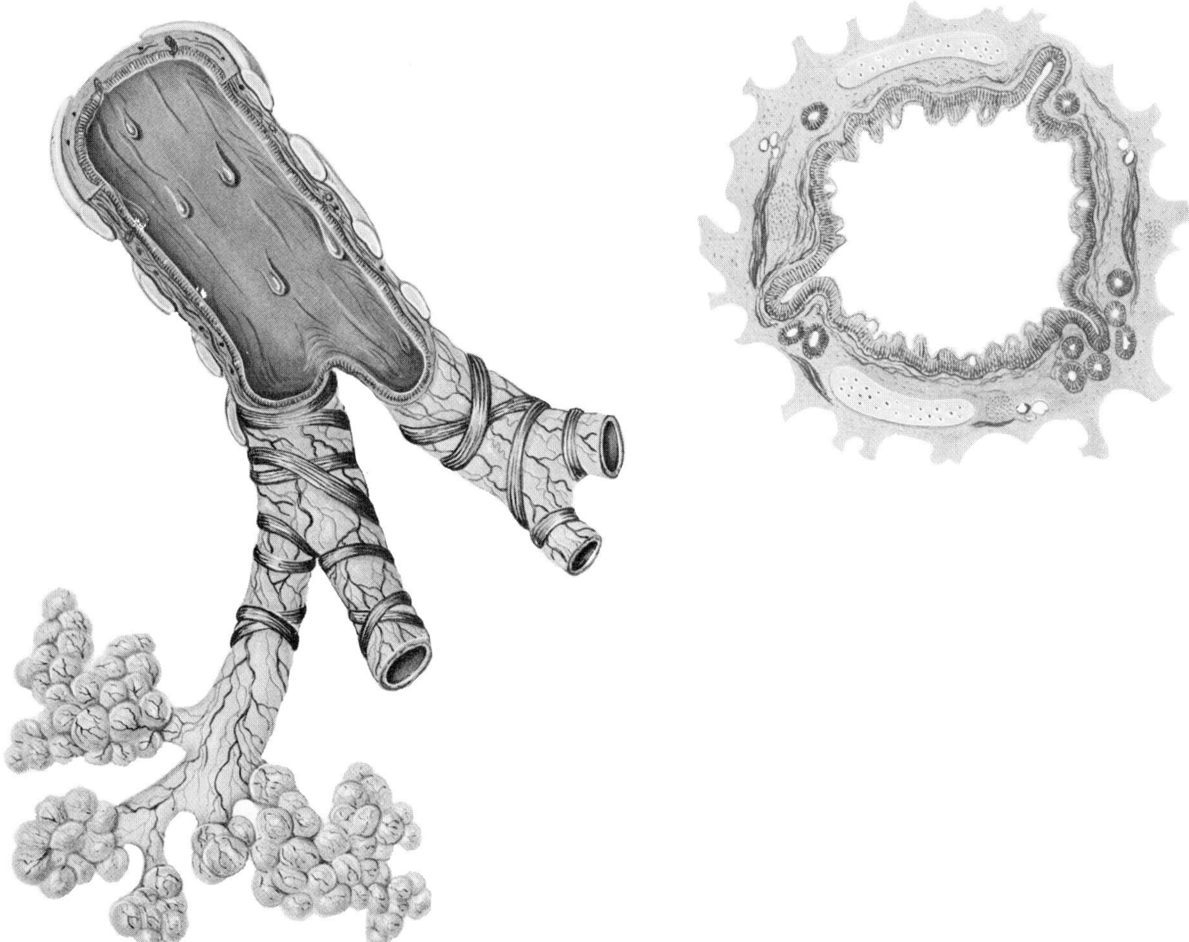

Figure 7–6. A normal bronchiole. (Reproduced by permission from American College of Chest Physicians, 1974.)

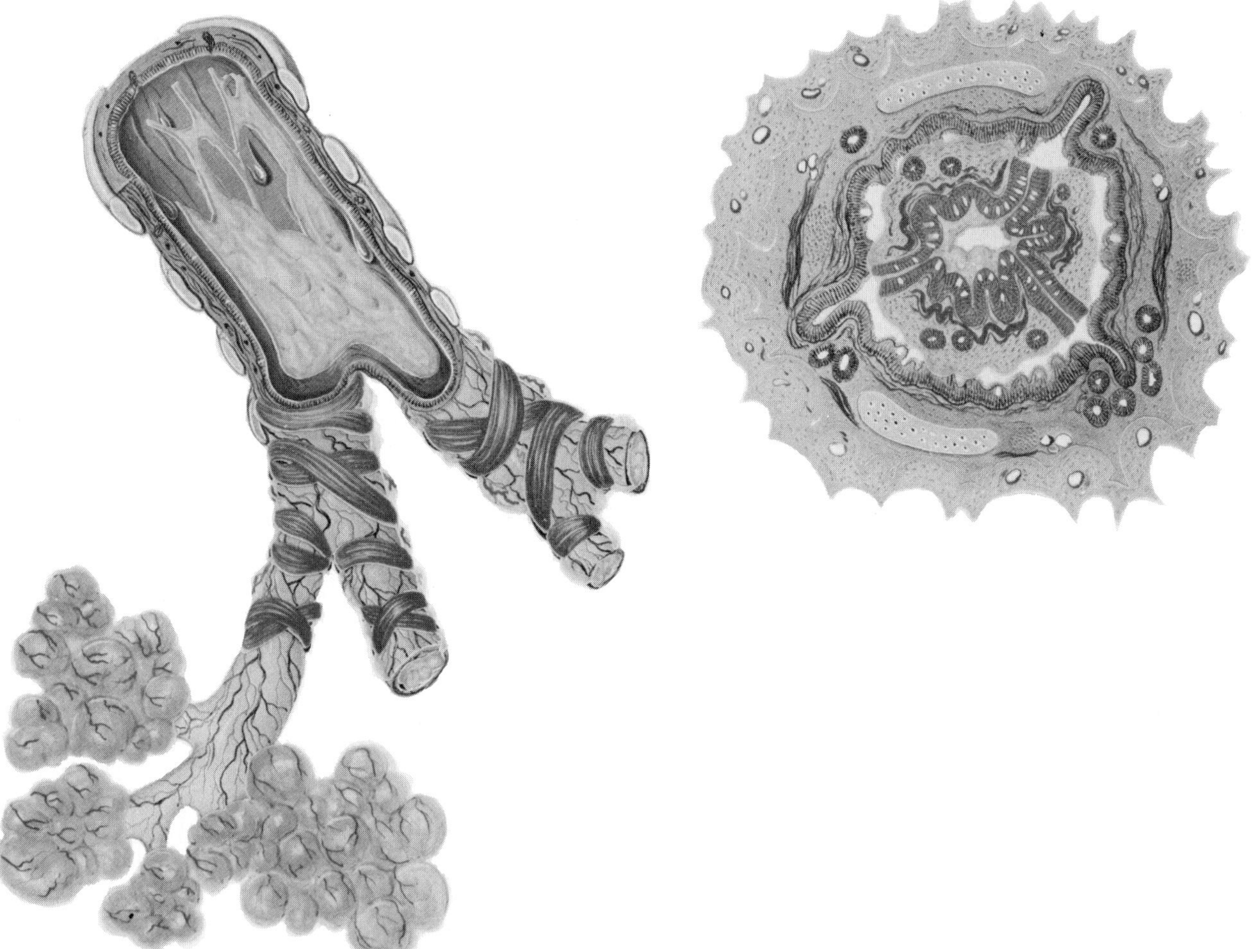

Figure 7–7. Bronchial asthma. (Reproduced by permission from American College of Chest Physicians, 1974.)

MAIN ASTHMA TRIGGERS

ALLERGY
Release of mediators

INFECTION
Viral

AUTONOMIC NERVOUS SYSTEM IMBALANCE
Stimulation of irritant receptors
Dominance of parasympathetic nervous system
Mediator-autonomic nervous system interactions

PHARMACOLOGIC FACTORS
Beta-adrenergic blockade, e.g., propranolol
Prostaglandin inhibitors, e.g., aspirin
Alcohol
Anticholinesterase drugs

PSYCHOLOGIC FACTORS

EXERCISE

In the presence of autonomic nervous system imbalance, stimulation of lung irritant receptors may cause bronchospasm. Gastroesophageal reflux is another trigger. Though it is incompletely understood, bronchospasm probably is related to reflex parasympathetic nervous system stimulation, in response to the reflux of acid into the esophagus at night (Nelson, 1984).

Pharmacologic factors, notably drugs, may cause an allergy (e.g., from penicillin) or a nonimmunological hypersensitivity reaction (e.g., from aspirin). Aspirin-induced bronchospasm in patients with asthma, rhinosinusitis, and nasal polyps is found in 20% to 44% of all asthmatics (Simon, 1986). In addition, an aspirin-sensitive person tends to have a similar intolerance to nonsteroidal anti-inflammatory drugs.

Psychologic factors include panic reactions, anxiety and depression dependency, anger, and denial (Spector, 1986). Though any kind of emotional upset may trigger bronchospasm, little evidence exists to suggest that emotional upset is the sole factor responsible for asthma.

Exercise is another common trigger. In addition, airway cooling, as a consequence of body cooling, has been identified as a trigger for asthmatic attacks at night (Chen and Chai, 1982).

Table 7–3. THE ALLERGIC REACTION IN ASTHMA COMPARED WITH THE NORMAL IMMUNOLOGIC RESPONSE

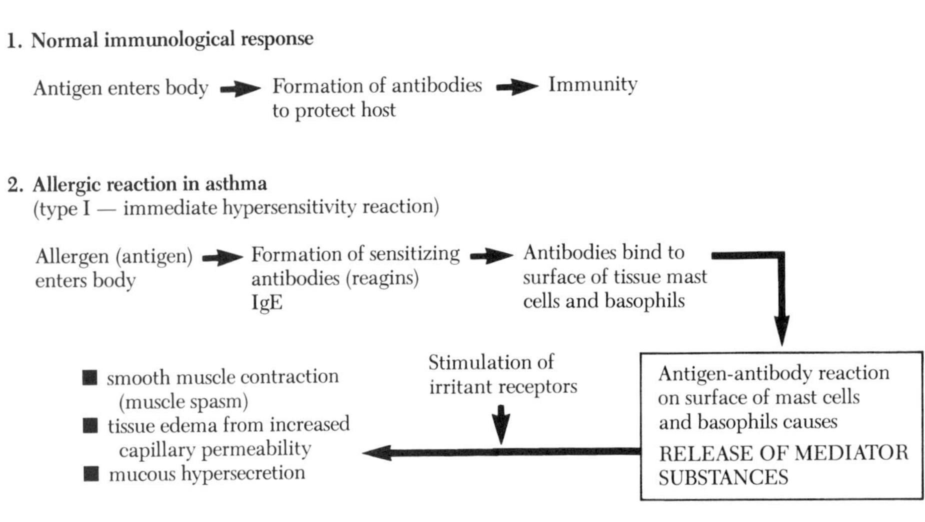
1. Normal immunological response
Antigen enters body
Formation of antibodies to protect host
Immunity
2. Allergic reaction in asthma
(type I — immediate hypersensitivity reaction)
Allergen (antigen) enters body
Formation of sensitizing antibodies (reagins) IgE
Antibodies bind to surface of tissue mast cells and basophils
Antigen-antibody reaction on surface of mast cells and basophils causes RELEASE OF MEDIATOR SUBSTANCES
Stimulation of irritant receptors
smooth muscle contraction (muscle spasm)
tissue edema from increased capillary permeability
mucous hypersecretion

Asthma is divided into two major types, extrinsic and intrinsic. These types and their corresponding triggers are discussed next.

Extrinsic Asthma

Extrinsic asthma is the allergic form of the disease. An asthmatic episode is attributed to an immunological response to exposure to an *allergen*, a substance to which an individual has a specific hypersensitivity. This form of asthma occurs in individuals with family or personal histories of atopy (pronounced at′ ō pē) or allergic reactions manifested by asthma, hay fever, and inflammatory wheals of the skin.

Normal Immunological Response. The allergic reaction causing bronchoconstriction in extrinsic asthma is not completely understood as yet. To understand the recent hypothesis of the body's immunological response to allergens, one must review the normal individual's response to an antigen. An *antigen* is a substance that induces the formation of antibodies in the body, whereas an *antibody* is a protein substance developed in response to an antigen. Table 7–3 shows that immunity develops if the host successfully forms antibodies to protect against adverse effects of foreign antigens entering the body. Subsequent contact with the antigen has little if any effect on the host's health.

Allergic (Hypersensitivity) Reaction. In asthma, an allergic or hypersensitivity reaction occurs as described next. Since the individual has had an allergic response to a specific antigen in the past, the antigen is called an allergen. Contact with an allergen via an inhalation (e.g., fumes and pollen from plants), an ingestion (e.g., drugs and food), or a parenteral route results in the formation of sensitizing antibodies called *reagins*. The primary reagin involved appears to be immunoglobulin E (IgE), produced by plasma cells and lymphoid tissue in response to the antigen. IgE antibodies bind to the surface of tissue mast cells and basophils found in the mucosa of the nasopharynx and airways and sensitize lung tissue.

An antigen-antibody reaction then takes place on the surface of these mast cells and basophils. This causes the release of *primary mediator substances*, including histamine, slow reacting substance of anaphylaxis (SRS-A), and others, as listed in Table 7–4. The release of primary mediators into surrounding tissues causes contraction of smooth muscle (muscle spasm) and tissue edema from increased capillary permeability. When the primary mediator eosinophilic chemotactic factor of anaphylaxis (ECF-A) is released, it attracts circulating eosinophils to the site of the hypersensitivity reaction. (Sputum or blood eosinophilia is common in extrinsic asthma, but it also occurs in intrinsic asthma.)

Simultaneously, the release of primary mediators stimulates local irritant receptors along airways, causing *reflex bronchoconstriction* via the vagus nerve. Nerve impulses travel up afferent pathways of the

Table 7–4. MEDIATOR SUBSTANCES IN HYPERSENSITIVITY REACTIONS*

Primary Mediators	Secondary Mediators
Histamine	Prostaglandins
Slow reacting substance of anaphylaxis (SRS-A) composed of leukotriene C_4, D_4, and E_4	Serotonin
Eosinophil chemotactic factor of anaphylaxis (ECF-A)	Bradykinin
Neutrophil chemotactic factor of anaphylaxis (NCF-A)	Other vasoactive amines
Platelet activating factor (PAF)	
Kallikrein	

*Ziment, 1978

vagus nerves to the brain stem and back down vagal efferent pathways to muscle cells. Muscle contraction by this mechanism potentiates the effects of the already released mediators. (In 1982, however, Leff reported that the role of reflex bronchoconstriction is small in the allergic form of asthma.)

Two other physiological events occur. First, goblet cells and bronchial glands secrete thick mucus into airway lumens, plugging up peripheral airways. Second, the release of primary mediators causes the release of secondary mediators (see Table 7–4), setting off the incompletely understood biochemical reactions of the hypersensitivity reaction and reinforcing the actions of the primary mediators.

Exactly how the release of mediators, vagal stimulation, or both affects bronchoconstriction or bronchospasm is unknown. Somehow, more calcium (Ca^{++}) is made available to smooth muscle for contraction. At present, researchers believe that *intracellular* Ca^{++} *availability* is the main determinant of the magnitude of the contractile response and degree of bronchoconstriction (Leff, 1982).

More recently, *leukotrienes,* a group of compounds originating from leukocytes, have been proposed as major bronchoactive components in eliciting hypersensitivity responses and allergic asthma (Griffin et al, 1983). Perhaps the most potent compound is slow reacting substance of anaphylaxis (SRS-A). Though the exact location of its synthesis is still unknown, SRS-A is now understood to be composed of three different bronchoconstrictors; leukotrienes C_4, D_4, and E_4 (see Chapter 1). This discovery may prompt the development of leukotriene agonists or other pharmacologic interventions for clinical management of asthma (Leitch, 1982).

Other Hypersensitivity Reactions. The allergic reaction described represents only one type of hypersensitivity reaction, i.e., the *type I, immediate hypersensitivity reaction.* Some asthmatics experience *delayed* reactions hours after exposures to antigens via inhalation or skin tests. This type of reaction is called the type III, immune complex–mediated reaction (Table 7–5). Much research is in progress to further understand the physiological mechanisms involved in the type I and type III reactions as well as the type II and type IV immunopathological or hypersensitivity reactions of other types of pulmonary disease.

Intrinsic Asthma

Intrinsic asthma is the nonallergic form of asthma. In essence, all etiologies for asthma except for allergy fall into this category. In past years, it has been called *infective asthma* because of its association with upper and, less frequently, lower respiratory tract infections. Asthmatic episodes are precipitated by viral and, rarely, bacterial infections.

This category may have outlived its usefulness, however, because more recent investigations clearly indicate that other etiologies in addition to infections are responsible for the nonallergic reactions. Moreover, many if not most patients do not fall into either category but represent a mix of the two, with more than one etiological factor responsible for asthmatic episodes. Because of the many etiological factors and their complex pathophysiological interrelationships, asthma is now described as a "syndrome rather than a single disease with bronchoconstriction as the final common pathway" (Leff, 1982). Nevertheless, until this syndrome is further defined, the extrinsic-intrinsic

Table 7–5. HYPERSENSITIVITY REACTIONS IN THE LUNG

Type	Name	Antibodies Involved	Main Mechanism	Reaction Time	Example of Disease
I	Immediate hypersensitivity reaction	IgE IgE in some individuals	Antigen-antibody reaction causes release of chemical mediators from mast cells and basophils	10 to 20 minutes, lasting 1 to 2 hours	Anaphylactic reaction, asthma, hay fever
II	Cytotoxic reaction	IgG IgM	Antibody (primarily IgG) reacts directly with a cell surface antigen to produce cellular damage (autoimmune response)	Variable	Autoimmune diseases, e.g., Goodpasture's syndrome
III	Immune complex–mediated reaction	IgG IgM	Lysosomal enzyme release or production of toxic metabolites by polymorphonuclear lymphocytes causes bronchial wall inflammation. Mast cells release mediator substances	Usually 4 to 8 hours, lasting 24 to 96 hours	Asthma (delayed onset), hypersensitivity pneumonitis, systemic lupus erythematosus
IV	Cell-mediated delayed reaction	No antibody identified; involves sensitized T lymphocytes (type of white blood cell)	Antigen binds with T cells and results in liberation of lymphokines (mediators). Attracted macrophages release hydrolytic enzymes and cause inflammation.	48 hours	Granulomatous diseases, such as tuberculosis; lymphokines may induce inflammatory reaction in any chest disease with a hypersensitivity reaction.

classification conveniently separates allergic and nonallergic components of the disease, a beginning step in the determination of etiology for asthma in any patient.

Exercise-Induced Asthma. Virtually *all* asthmatics as well as others with respiratory diseases have some increase in airway obstruction after exercise. Those that demonstrate *marked* airway obstruction, i.e., decrease in expiratory flow rates (PEFR or FEV_1*) of greater than 10 to 15%, measured by a pulmonary function test, are said to have *exercise-induced asthma.* Bronchoconstriction is triggered by *heat loss* due to cold air, changes in water vapor content of inspired air (dry air), and hyperventilation. The response occurs during the first few minutes of exercise: airways dilate slightly, and airway resistance falls. Thereafter, however, airways begin to constrict, and resistance to airflow increases. On cessation of a 5- to 8-minute period of exercise, airflow to the lungs continues to decrease. Airway resistance is at its highest (and airflow and lung volume measurements at their lowest) about 5 to 7 minutes after exercise in children and 7 to 12 minutes after exercise in adults (Anderson, 1980). This type of response causes a mild decrease in PaO_2. For unknown reasons, the response is greatest after running, less after bicycling, and substantially less after swimming (swimmer's inhaled air is usually warmer and more humidified). Bronchoconstriction may be abolished or inhibited by an aerosol (sympathomimetic or cromolyn drug) given 15 to 30 minutes before exercise.

*PEFR = peak expiratory flow rate; FEV_1 = forced expiratory volume in one second.

Dominance of the Parasympathetic Nervous System. The parasympathetic nervous system appears to play a dominant role in bronchoconstriction in intrinsic asthma, particularly in episodes precipitated by emotional upset, infection, and airway hyperirritability. When the autonomic nervous system is functioning properly, input from sympathetic and parasympathetic nervous systems is in proper balance to produce *normal bronchomotor tone*: bronchial smooth muscle is in slight contraction, producing slight bronchoconstriction. The asthmatic is characterized by an inherent or acquired *increase* in bronchomotor tone. Any further increase in this tone from parasympathetic stimulation may cause asthmatic attack via reflex bronchoconstriction (described previously and illustrated on the left of Figure 7–8). If bronchospasm is already present from

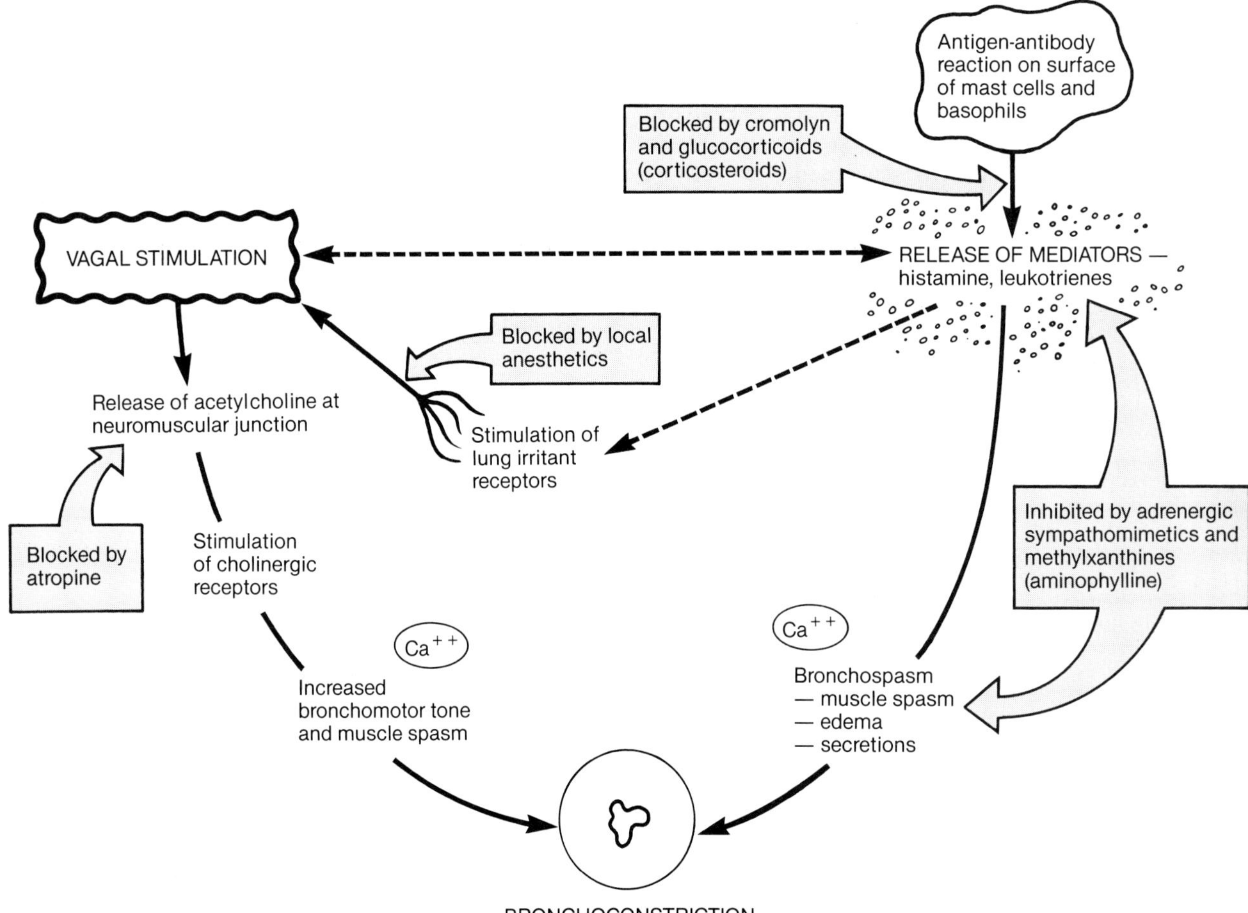

Figure 7–8. Mechanisms of bronchoconstriction in asthma. The broken lines indicate interactions that are not well established.

an antigen-antibody reaction, parasympathetic stimulation greatly enhances it and the severity of clinical signs and symptoms.

Asthma and Airway Hyperreactivity *(Hyperresponsiveness)*

As previously mentioned, asthma is characterized by increased bronchomotor tone and *airway hyperreactivity*, also called airway hyperresponsiveness. The exact mechanism is unknown, but the increased responsiveness is probably due to some abnormality in the autonomic regulation of airway smooth muscle.

Special emphasis must be placed on the fact that *not all persons with airway hyperreactivity have asthma*. An otherwise healthy individual may have hyperreactive or "twitchy" airways after a viral respiratory infection or upon exposure to oxidizing pollutants. The patient's only symptom may be an occasional irritating cough caused by the stimulation of lung irritant receptors along the tracheobronchial tree. Because signs and symptoms are few and nonspecific and the pulmonary function tests show airflow limitation (as in asthma), differentiation between the disease asthma and mere airway hyperreactivity may be difficult if not impossible without historical and other data. Furthermore, in a work or an industrial setting, a relatively asymptomatic person may demonstrate normal pulmonary function test results, but airway hyperresponsiveness on a bronchial provocation test, as defined in the summary box (Wanner, 1986).

AIRWAY HYPERREACTIVITY (HYPERRESPONSIVENESS)

DEFINITION
Exaggerated bronchoconstrictive response to various stimuli

COMMON STIMULI (TRIGGERS)
Viral respiratory infection, cigarette smoke, air pollution, occupational irritant, cold air, exercise, drugs, antigens

CLINICAL MANIFESTATIONS
Unexplained cough (with normal pulmonary function test), asthma symptoms

DIAGNOSIS
A 20% decrease in forced expiratory volume (1 second) on a bronchial provocation test. This test involves administration of a standard dose of a bronchoprovocative agent, such as methacholine (drug), cold air, or irritant; or administration of increasing strengths of a stimulus, with pulmonary function measurements after each one.

Main Pathophysiology

In asthma, the airway obstruction produced by bronchospasm is not uniformly distributed throughout the lungs and involves both large and small airways. Airway resistance rapidly increases in large airways and rapidly returns to normal after acute attacks. In smaller airways, airway resistance tends to gradually increase and remain more intense and persistent even after acute attacks. The net result of these changes is different rates of improvement and deterioration in the functioning of small and large airways.

With mild to moderate obstruction, ventilation of alveoli is normal to reduced due to bronchoconstriction and plugging of peripheral airways with mucus. Perfusion of underventilated alveoli is diverted to better ventilated areas of the lung to maintain a normal overall V/Q ratio for the lungs. During an acute asthmatic attack, airway obstruction becomes widespread. Lung ventilation is grossly reduced. Perfusion increases, assuming that the individual has enough cardiopulmonary reserve to increase cardiac output as a compensatory mechanism. This mismatching of ventilation to perfusion produces a decreased V/Q ratio, as in Figure 7–9A. In some cases, cardiac output increases by as much as 50% as an acute response to bronchodilator drugs given for an asthmatic attack. The increased perfusion to poorly ventilated alveoli decreases the V/Q ratio even more, causing severe arterial blood gas disturbances (Wagner and West, 1980).

During the later stages of an asthmatic attack, pulmonary artery pressure rises, adding a pressure load against which the right ventricle must pump. Also, as airways become obstructed, the trapping of air in terminal respiratory units causes the lungs to hyperinflate.

All of these changes vary in degrees in individuals with moderate to severe chronic asthma. Acute episodes produce such grossly abnormal V/Q ratios that respiratory arrest becomes imminent without immediate treatment with oxygen, pulmonary medications, and appropriate respiratory therapy.

In an otherwise relatively healthy individual, pathological changes and lung functions may completely return to normal between acute episodes (Fig. 7–9B).

Main Signs and Symptoms/Progression of Disease

The dominant symptom during an acute episode is shortness of breath accompanied by coughing and wheezing. Once an attack is well under way, the individual coughs up thick sputum. These signs and symptoms may appear abruptly or more gradually over a few days. They typically disappear between acute episodes. Even the individual with stable but abnormal pulmonary function between acute episodes may give little to no apparent clues regarding the presence of disease except for an occasional cough (Fig. 7–10).

Asthma demonstrates a variable disease course

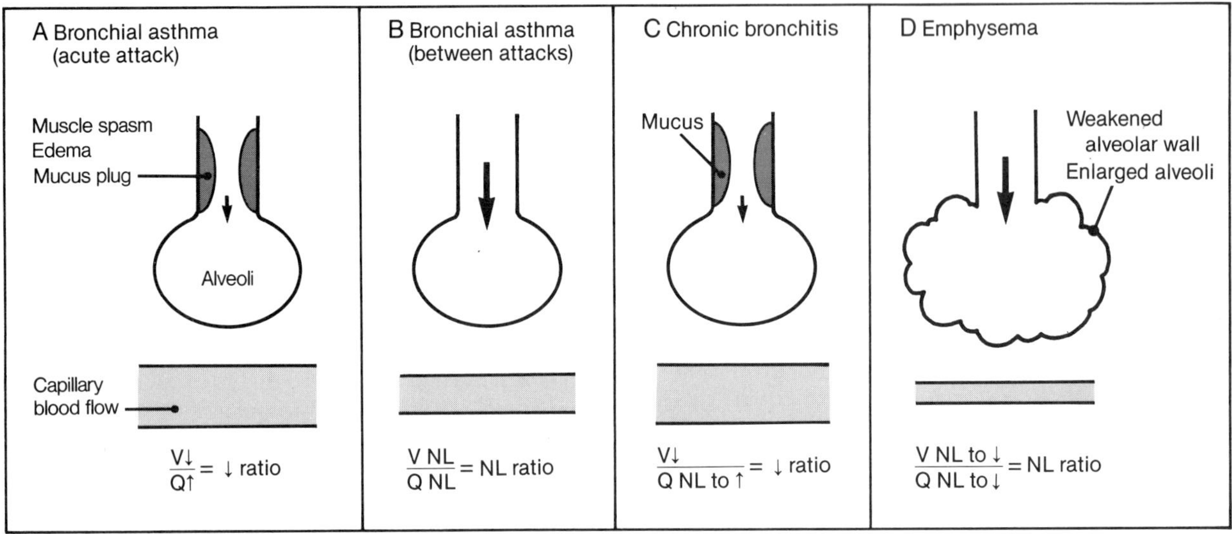

Figure 7–9. Ventilation/perfusion (V/Q) ratios in chronic obstructive pulmonary disease (COPD).

among different patients and within the same patient. Symptoms may disappear by the time a child reaches puberty; they may remain continuous with relatively constant airway obstruction; or they may wax and wane throughout life, with no apparent pattern. Remissions in severe asthmatics may occur unexpectedly. Conversely, the disease may recur at any time upon exposure to a lung irritant, such as air pollution, because even in asymptomatic asthmatics, airways tend to be hyperirritable.

A small percentage of patients develop *status asthmaticus*, defined as unresponsiveness to ordinary bronchodilator medications, such as sympathomimetic drugs and theophylline derivatives. This condition is a medical emergency because death may result even with optimal therapy. In some cases, status asthmaticus lasts for days to weeks.

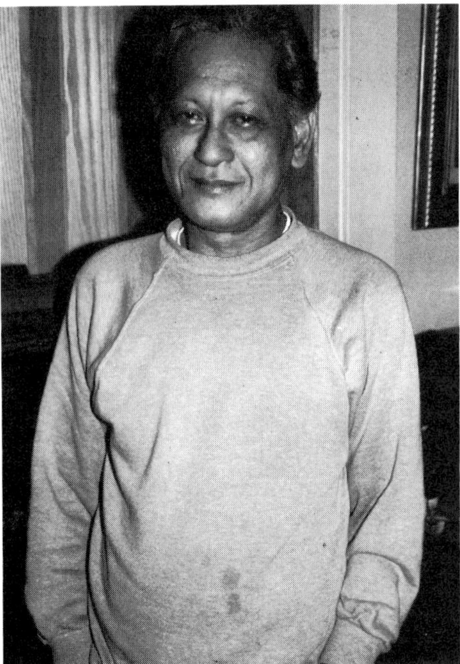

Figure 7–10. Individual with chronic asthma. Signs of disease appear absent except for watery eyes, suggesting allergy or hypersensitivity.

As a general rule, however, intermittent rather than constant symptoms characterize bronchial asthma. Prognoses are much better for individuals with labile symptoms and intermittent attacks than for individuals with continuous symptoms and relatively fixed obstructions.

Groups at increased risk for death due to asthma are, first, *individuals between 40 and 60 years of age*; they frequently have intrinsic asthma with only a short history of attacks. Second, *children under 2 years of age* are at increased risk. They have extremely labile physical conditions during acute illnesses and tend to have narrower airways than adults. Severe bronchospasm and thick mucous plugs are more likely to cause complete airway obstruction. Third, *individuals who overuse aerosol bronchodilator medications* are at increased risk for sudden death. These medications can produce life threatening arrhythmias, causing cardiac arrest.

In conclusion, emphasis must be placed on the fact that asthma is a *reversible* disease. Asthmatic components commonly exist in patients with mixed chest pathology and in others with a completely different disease. Asthma is a chest disease with symptoms that may be completely reversed with appropriate pulmonary medication and respiratory therapy. Improvement in the patient's psychological and physical well being is often dramatic. Patients and their families may have limited understanding regarding the effectiveness of modern medicine to treat different forms of asthma. For their benefit, it is especially important for the nurse to identify the individuals with asthma or asthmatic components and facilitate as much as possible access to medical care.

CHRONIC BRONCHITIS

In its simple form, chronic bronchitis is a common problem affecting about 10 to 25% of the adult population (Hinshaw and Murray, 1980). The majority of patients with moderate to severe bronchitis have some degree of emphysema. Because these two diseases often coexist, little is known about the exact pathogeneses of the two separate diseases. It cannot be established which disease appears first, although certain features of bronchitis seem to predispose the patient to emphysema.

Generally, the etiological factors for emphysema and bronchitis are the same. They include *cigarette smoking, atmospheric pollution,* an occupation involving *exposure to lung irritants, infection,* and *genetic factors.* Cigarette smoking is the prime cause of the disease and is perhaps the most aggravating factor for chronic pulmonary disease in general. Upon rare occasion, etiological factors cannot be determined. For example, a patient may present with severe emphysema despite a lack of history for all of the aforementioned etiological factors, including cigarette smoking. Etiological factors are almost always evident in chronic bronchitis.

Bronchitis, in general, is defined by the American Thoracic Society (1975) as a non-neoplastic disorder of structure or function of the bronchi resulting from infectious or noninfectious irritation. Basically, it is an airway disease with both acute and chronic forms. *Acute bronchitis* represents an acute exacerbation of chronic bronchitis, or it can occur in a relatively healthy individual upon exposure to some infectious or noninfectious lung irritant.

Chronic bronchitis is defined as a chest disease associated with the following:

1. *Prolonged exposure to bronchial irritants*
2. *Mucus hypersecretion*
3. *Structural alterations of the bronchi* (described subsequently)

In the clinical setting, chronic bronchitis is diagnosed when an individual demonstrates *cough or sputum production on most days for at least three months of the year for two successive years.*

Pathologic Features

Pathologically, the most characteristic feature of chronic bronchitis is an increase in the size and number of submucous glands in large bronchi. In most cases, the thickness of the bronchial submucosa may become *twice* as thick as that seen in normal individuals. Although goblet cells in the surface epithelial layer usually increase in number and are responsible for secreting mucus, submucous glands are considered the main source of secretions. The presence of secretions can cause considerable obstruction and narrowing of the airway lumen (Figure 7–11). Large quantities of thick mucus interfere with the functioning of the mucociliary escalator, causing the stasis of mucus in the lungs and predisposing the patient to mucous retention. This problem becomes severe when infection or bronchospasm is superimposed on an uncomplicated case of chronic bronchitis. In severe cases, an intensive program of deep breathing and coughing or even of endotracheal suctioning is necessary to clear airway secretions and improve ventilation of the lungs.

Pathologic changes are thought to occur first in small airways. Small bronchi and bronchioles become narrowed with plugs of thick mucus and inflammatory changes, including cellular infiltration (largely lymphocytes and plasma cells) and airway edema. Granulation tissue is present, and fibrosis around bronchioles may develop. Moreover, the narrowing and plugging of small airways with mucus may be more significant than the mucus hypersecretion in large airways. The small airway obstruction is associated with clinical disability and development of emphysema (Fraser and Paré, 1979).

Patients with chronic bronchitis do not always demonstrate the histologic findings of inflammation. The term chronic *bronchitis,* literally meaning inflammation of the bronchi, is misleading because inflammation may or may not be present. Hinshaw and Murray (1980) further explain "The term chronic bronchitis indicates that the patient has symptoms related to excess secretions and cough; any of these terms—bronchorrhea, chronic hypersecretion of mucus, or chronic production of phlegm—might be substituted to clarify the functional disorder of chronic bronchitis."

Main Pathophysiology

Alveolar ventilation is reduced in chronic bronchitis, mainly because of obstructive secretions in airways. Cardiac output (perfusion) remains normal to increased, depending on the individual's cardiopulmonary reserves. The decrease in ventilation and increase in perfusion produce a grossly decreased V/Q ratio (see Figure 7–9C), particularly when acute bronchitis is superimposed on chronic bronchitis.

Oxygenation remains a major problem for the patient with severe chronic bronchitis because airways are blocked—air cannot reach alveoli where gas exchange takes place. Though the patient tries to compensate for the low Pa_{O_2} by increasing cardiac output, this mechanism has limited effectiveness. The V/Q abnormality remains because many capillaries are in contact with underventilated alveoli. In addition, mucus retention seems to be a persistent problem, predisposing the patient to infection and necessitating an ongoing program of bronchial hygiene to keep airways clear of secretions.

With advanced disease, a grossly abnormal V/Q ratio produces a gradual decrease in Pa_{O_2}, a corresponding increase in Pa_{CO_2} (a measure of alveolar ventilation), and the development of fluid retention problems from right heart failure. The heart failure is usually precipitated by the low Pa_{O_2}, which in turn causes pulmonary vascular narrowing, increased pulmonary artery pres-

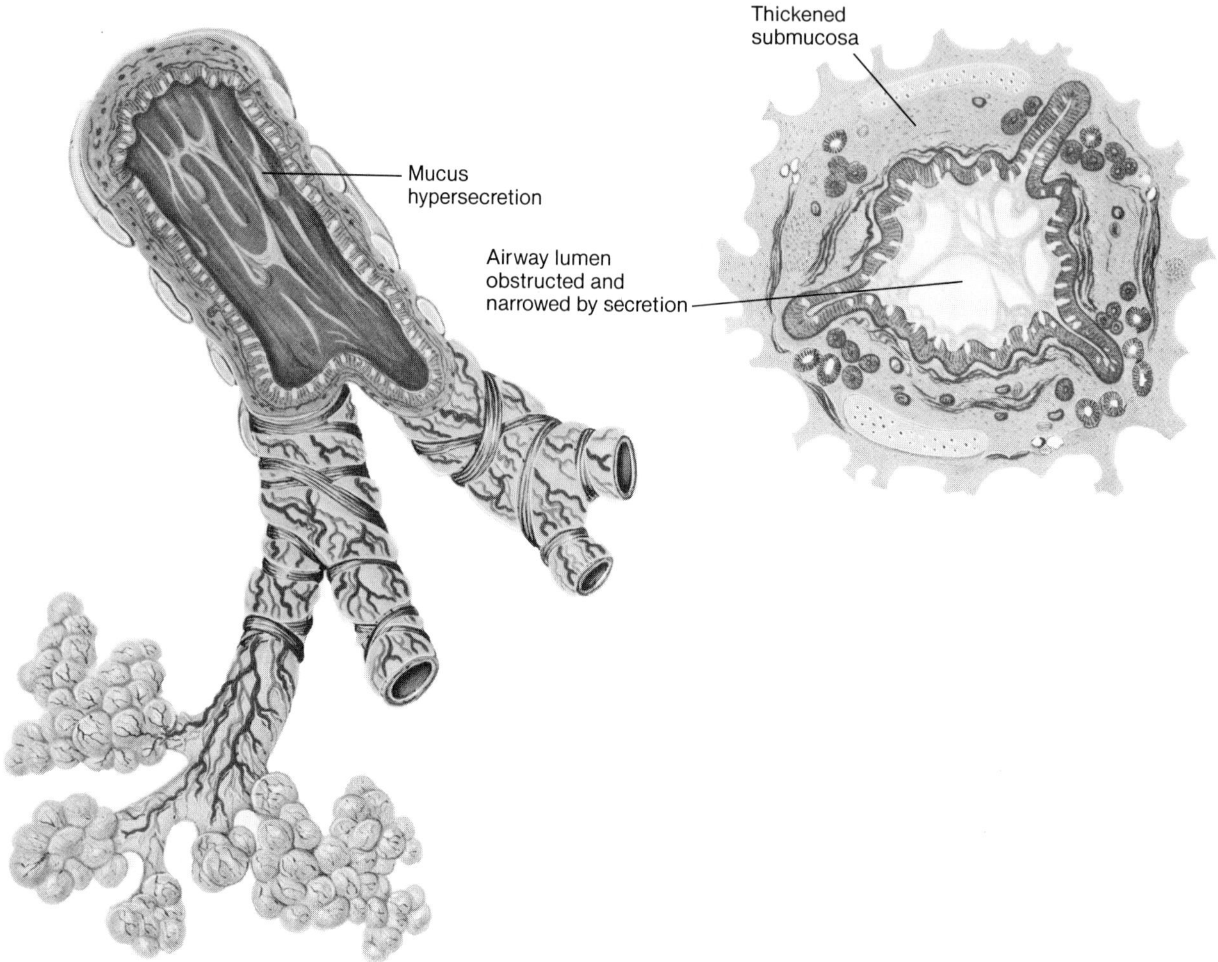

Figure 7–11. A terminal bronchiole (left) and a cross section of a bronchiole (right) in chronic bronchitis. (Reproduced by permission from American College of Chest Physicians, 1974.)

sures, polycythemia, and other events that exacerbate the oxygenation problem (see Chapter 9).

The bronchitic has been labelled a "blue bloater" because oxygenation problems produce a blue-tinged or cyanotic appearance, and a stocky build and a plethoric condition cause a "bloated" appearance. The patient in Figure 7–12 demonstrates the characteristic features of a blue bloater. ["The Pink Puffer" is described in Figure 7–13 and subsequently for comparison.]

Signs and Symptoms/Progression of Disease

The onset of cough and sputum production can appear in individuals between the ages of 25 and 45 years; it more commonly appears in individuals 40 to 55 years of age, with a predilection for men. Shortness of breath develops much later with mucus retention in the lungs and the complication of right-sided heart failure.

Once symptoms appear, the course of disease is *variable*. For example, the condition of the chronic bronchitic may remain relatively stable for a few years. Then, the next year may be marked by frequent episodes of acute bronchitis precipitated by infections or other factors. When pathology impairs oxygenation, right heart failure may be the event that prompts hospitalization.

In conclusion, it is important for the nurse to recognize a bronchitic component in mixed chest pathology because it can be greatly reversed or at least controlled by medications; treatments; and the practice of preventive measures, such as drinking plenty of fluids, avoiding others with chest infections, and implementing an ongoing program of bronchial hygiene. Often the bronchitic patient has an asthmatic component that flares up with chest infections. In this case, the patient is said to have *asthmatic bronchitis*. Both asthmatic and bronchitic components are relatively responsive to appropriate treatment when compared

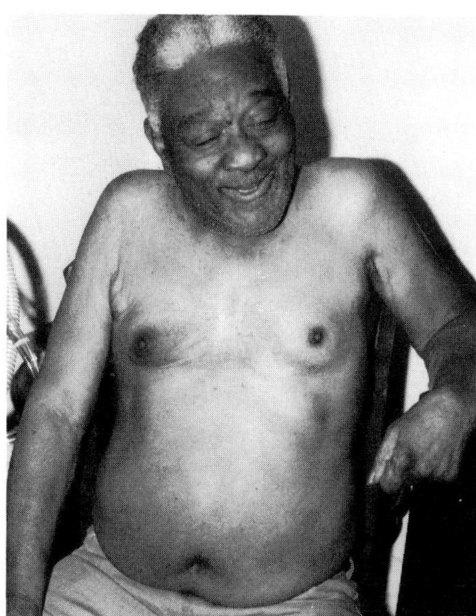

Figure 7–12. Individual with *chronic bronchitis* and all the classic findings listed below of the "blue bloater." In addition, slight gynecomastia and petechiae are present in the midsternal area, both side effects of high-dose oral corticosteroid therapy. The patient's shoulders are raised, and muscles are tensed, from shortness of breath and increased work of breathing.

The Blue Bloater

Stocky body build, no history of marked weight loss.
Age of onset of signs and symptoms: 40 to 50 years.
Main complaint: sputum production.
Clinical course: variable.
Low PaO_2 and high $PaCO_2$, cyanosis present.
Frequent episodes of right ventricular failure, dependent edema.

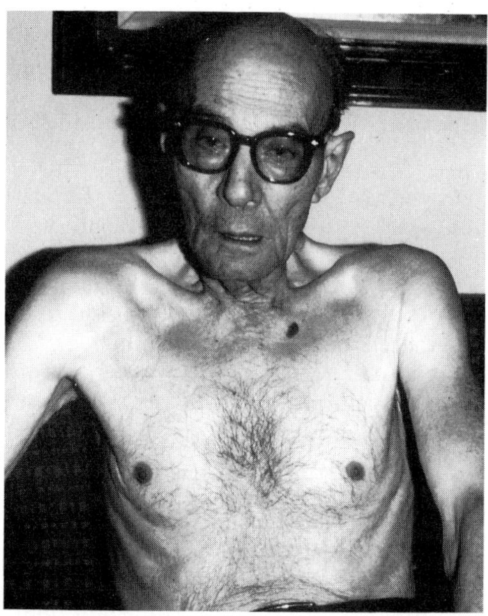

Figure 7–13. Individual with *emphysema* and all the classic findings listed below of the "pink puffer." Use of accessory muscles of respiration (intercostal, neck, and shoulder muscles) and the cachectic appearance reflect two factors: (1) shortness of breath, patient's most disturbing complaint, and (2) the tremendous increased work of breathing necessary to increase minute ventilation and maintain normal arterial blood gases.

The Pink Puffer

Cachectic appearance, history of major weight loss.
Age of onset of signs and symptoms: 50 to 75 years.
Main complaint: shortness of breath and cough.
Persistent downhill clinical course once symptoms appear.
Normal PaO_2 and $PaCO_2$, normal skin coloration.
No history of right ventricular failure, except terminally; no edema.

with the irreversible effects of other chest diseases, such as emphysema.

EMPHYSEMA

Bronchial asthma and chronic bronchitis are *airway* diseases. In contrast, emphysema is a disease that occurs at the *alveolar* level and directly affects the alveolar-capillary bed. It is diagnosed through history and physical examination with supporting evidence from chest x-ray and pulmonary function test results. Diagnosis sometimes is prompted by a specific finding on the chest x-ray (e.g., presence of bulla). Since it is defined in morphologic terms, the *exact* cause typically is discovered during autopsy, when lung tissue is necropsied to determine the precise pulmonary pathology.

The incidence of emphysema in the general population cannot be accurately determined because it commonly coexists with chronic bronchitis. Also, both diseases are known to be underdiagnosed and underreported. Surveys of postmortem data indicate that emphysema, in particular, is a common finding, especially in aged lungs. In many cases, the autopsy findings reveal substantial emphysematous changes in individuals with no documented medical diagnoses of emphysema or COPD.

Pathologically, emphysema in characterized by *destructive changes of the alveolar walls* (septa) and accompanying *enlargement of air spaces.*

The most widely acknowledged explanation for the development of emphysema is the *protease pathogenesis hypothesis* (Hoidal and Niewoehner, 1983). This hypothesis maintains that progressive tissue destruction is due to an alteration in the protease-antiprotease balance in the lower airways, as described subsequently. Upon exposure to lung irritants, such as cigarette smoke, inflammatory cells (e.g., neutrophils and alveolar macrophages) release an excess of proteolytic enzymes. These enzymes digest and destroy the alveolar interstitium, acting unopposed because of the unavailability of proteolytic inhibitors. In addition, exposure to some irritants may cause inactivation of *alpha$_1$-antitrypsin.* In health, this important enzyme protects the lung by inactivating free proteases that digest lung tissue and possibly by reducing inflammatory responses (Cockcroft and Horne, 1982).

Main Types

Emphysema is divided into three main types based on the location of structural changes within the acinus (Fig. 7–14).

In *centrilobular emphysema* (CLE), disease is located in the central part of the acinus, involving the respiratory bronchioles, and sparing the more distal alveolar ducts and alveolar sacs. In its earliest stages, CLE usually begins in the upper lobes, particularly the apical and posterior segments, and progresses downwards. It is associated with cigarette smokers who show evidence of chronic bronchitis.

In *panlobular emphysema* (PLE), the *entire* acinar unit demonstrates disease. Disease is randomly distributed throughout the lungs with some predilection for the lower lobes and anterior zones. PLE is more common in the elderly. It is also associated with cigarette-smoking bronchitics and individuals with family histories of emphysema due to a deficiency of alpha$_1$-antitrypsin. Panlobular emphysema from this enzyme deficiency is an inherited disease. The affected individual becomes symptomatic at a relatively young age (about 40 years) for an emphysema patient. The disease typically occurs with an absent or a small bronchitic component.

In *paraseptal emphysema,* disease is located in the distal part of the acinus, involving alveolar ducts and sacs. Since the disease selectively involves the periphery of the lung deep to the pleura and along interlobar septa, it tends to be well localized and usually does not give rise to pulmonary symptoms. Paraseptal emphysema is associated with the formation of air-filled cavities (bulla) and spontaneous pneumothorax in the diseased region of the lung. In the case of spontaneous pneumothorax, diseased lung tissue develops one or more blebs. A *bleb* is a collection of air within the visceral pleura that is less than 1 to 2 cm. Without any inciting event, communication of a bleb with the adjacent pleural space produces *pneumothorax*—filling of the pleural space with air—and collapse of the underlying lung.

One must be aware that lung pathology may not fall under one of the three types of emphysema just described. A combination of types may be involved. Moreover, the acinus may be irregularly diseased, and tissue destruction may not occur simultaneously with acinar dilatation. Dilatation alone is commonly found in the aging lung, and in many cases is thought to represent an early stage of emphysema.

Pathologic Features

Four pathologic processes account for the shortness of breath and increased work of breathing associated with emphysema.

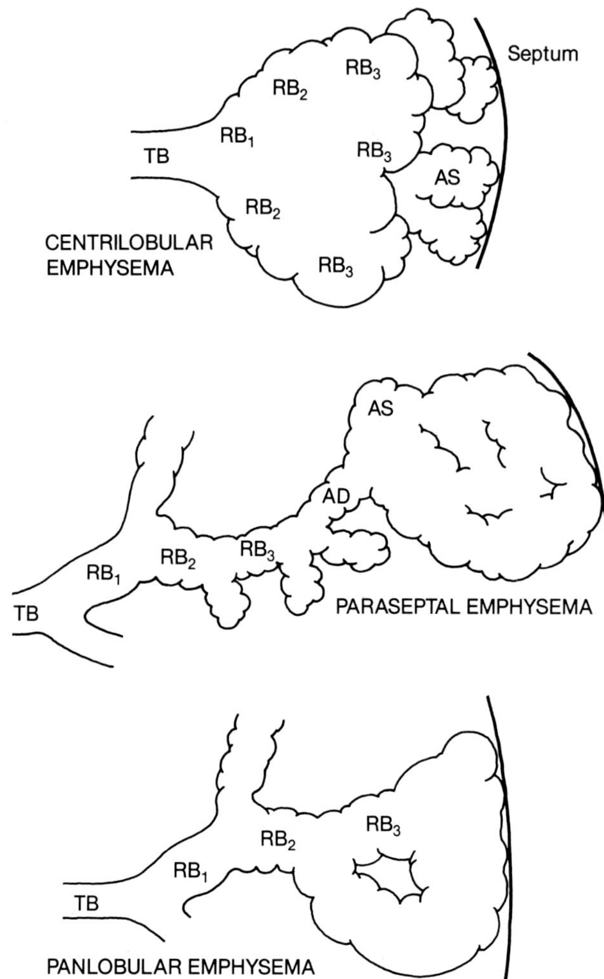

Figure 7–14. Types of emphysema. In centrilobular emphysema, the *respiratory bronchioles* (RB) of the acinus are involved in disease. In paraseptal emphysema, the *alveolar ducts* and *distal alveoli* are mostly affected. In panlobular emphysema, the acinus is more or less uniformly involved. (Reproduced and adapted from Thurlbeck, W.: Chronic bronchitis and emphysema—the pathophysiology of COLD. Basics of Respiratory Disease, 1974, 3:1,3.)

1. *Formation of bullae.* The destruction of alveolar septa coalesces acinar units, producing the formation of bullae (Figure 7–15A). *Bullae* are air-filled, thin-walled spaces or holes in lung tissue that are greater than 1 to 2 cm in diameter and are diagnosed clinically through chest x-ray findings.

2. *Loss of lung elasticity.* A destruction of lung tissue and a postulated connective tissue defect cause the loss of lung elasticity or lung elastic recoil, subsequent enlargement of alveolar air spaces, and the loss of radial traction (see previous section Peribronchial Obstruction).

3. *Lung hyperinflation.* The lung does not recoil to its normal resting position during expiration. It remains inflated above its resting volume, producing *lung hyperinflation* (Fig. 7–15B), and *barrel chest* deformity (see Chapter 12).

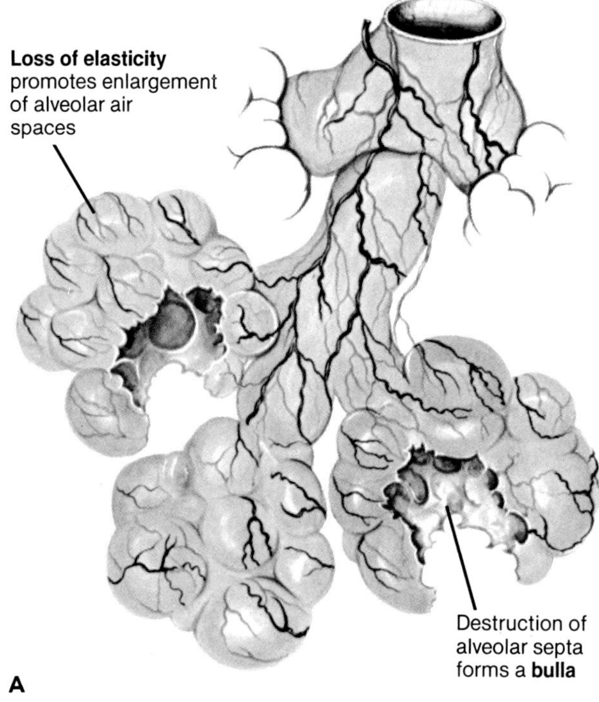

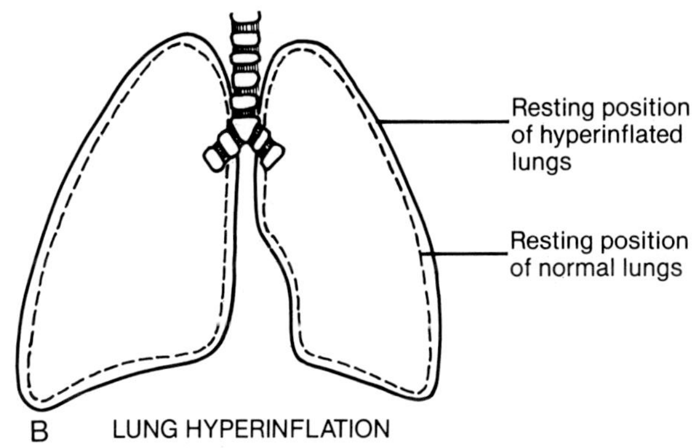

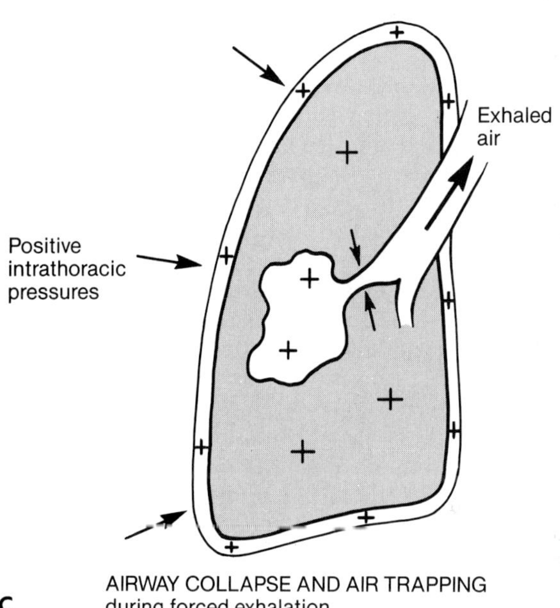

Figure 7–15. Pathologic processes in emphysema. *A*, Formation of bullae and loss of lung elasticity. *B*, Lung hyperinflation. *C*, Airway collapse and air trapping during forced exhalation. (*A*, reproduced by permission from American College of Chest Physicians, 1974.)

4. *Airway collapse and air trapping.* With lung hyperinflation, intrapleural pressures remain more positive, and greater muscular effort is necessary to exhale completely. Airways usually remain open during quiet breathing at rest, but during coughing or forced exhalation the generated positive intrathoracic pressures collapse airways, trapping air more peripherally in acinar units (Fig. 7–15C). In emphysema, airways are especially prone to collapse, since they tend to be narrowed from the loss of elasticity and radial traction around the airway.

Main Pathophysiology

The emphysema patient's main problem lies in altered mechanics of breathing due to dead space ventilation.

Dead Space Ventilation. Emphysema is often described as a classic example of a *dead space producing disease* (see Chapter 5). Because of the destruction of alveolar septa and formation of large bullae, all inspired air does not come into contact with capillary blood flow. The air that does not participate in gas exchange is considered wasted ventilation. In order to keep alveoli adequately ventilated, the patient strives to keep the minute ventilation at high levels by increasing respiratory rate and tidal volume. Increasing respiratory rate is an automatic response and is more or less effective because the airways are patent. Increasing tidal volume is much more difficult because the lungs at their resting volume are already hyperinflated with air, owing to the loss of lung elastic recoil. With severe disease, the patient must exert muscular effort to "squeeze" air out of the lungs, thus expiring air beyond resting lung volume.

Normal V/Q Ratio. Amazingly, a patient with mild to moderate disease maintains a sufficiently high, minute ventilation to maintain normal alveolar ventilation. Most patients with severe disease even manage to maintain a normal V/Q ratio for the lungs as a whole, in spite of abnormal V/Q ratios in many lung regions (see Fig. 7–9D). The exact physiologic mechanism is incompletely understood, but three related mechanisms appear to be involved. *First,* increased ventilation to healthy lung regions compensates for the decreased ventilation to diseased lung regions. *Second,* in diseased regions, alveolar destruction is matched by a corresponding loss of capillary blood flow. Perfusion is redirected to healthy portions of lung and a V/Q mismatch is avoided. *Third,* due to the anatomic loss of pulmonary capillaries, the patient with severe disease is unable to increase blood flow through the lungs. Cardiac *output* remains normal to reduced. The net effect of the reduced alveolar ventilation and reduced perfusion is a normal V/Q ratio (see Chapter 13).

Because a normal V/Q ratio is maintained, the stable emphysema patient maintains *normal* gas exchange. Arterial blood gas tensions remain normal to near normal. This concept is often new to an acute care nurse because he or she typically sees a patient when emphysema is complicated with recent pneumonia or acute bronchitis. It is not until the disease reaches a *very* advanced state that arterial blood gas tensions become abnormal, lung ventilation becomes significantly reduced, and oxygenation becomes problematic. These changes occur only with extensive destruction of lung tissue.

Increased Work of Breathing. The ability to increase minute ventilation to compensate for lung destruction as well as the limited ability to increase cardiac output is not without cost. The work of breathing is tremendous, and some clinicians claim that the work of breathing and associated shortness of breath are increased in emphysema more than in any other chronic obstructive disease of the lower airways.

Nevertheless, emphysema patients *do* adapt physiogically. They have been labelled "pink puffers," and "fighters." Within the pink puffer label, the "pink" refers to the patient's normal pink skin coloration, which is in contrast to the blue-tinged skin of the oxygen-starved blue bloater, already described. The "puffer" part of the label describes the huffing and puffing (shortness of breath) from the increased work of breathing. The "fighter" label refers to the patient's increased effort and relentless drive to breathe for maintenance of normal alveolar ventilation.

The individual with emphysema in Figure 7–13 demonstrates the shortness of breath and body cachexia so characteristic of the pink puffer. The cachexia is due to the dramatic increase in the patient's work of breathing complicated by the tendency towards poor nutrition due to dyspnea.

Comparison of distinguishing features listed in Figure 7–12 and Figure 7–13 will help the reader further understand the basic differences between the blue bloater and the pink puffer.

Main Signs and Symptoms/Progression of Disease

Unquestionably, the emphysema patient's main symptom is *shortness of breath.* It is accompanied by cough and *minimal* sputum production, particularly in the early morning. Besides shortness of breath and cough, perhaps the next most noticeable sign of emphysema is an abnormal chest configuration (barrel chest) caused by lung hyperinflation.

Signs and symptoms appear later in emphysema than in any other chronic obstructive disease so far discussed. This fact may largely account for the reason why emphysema goes unnoticed and remains undiagnosed in many individuals. Shortness of breath appears relatively late at 50 to 75 years of age, marking the beginning of a *persistent* downhill course with gradual increasing shortness of breath and physical disability. There are no remissions and no variability in the progression of disease—only acute exacerbations of a superimposed bronchitic or asthmatic component. Recurrent bronchopulmonary infections mark the onset of advanced pulmonary disease.

When oxygenation problems develop, the patient begins to experience episodes of right-sided heart failure. Yet, emphasis must be placed on the fact that right-sided heart failure occurs only with very advanced pulmonary disease—it is characteristic of the blue bloater rather than the pink puffer because the former develops oxygenation problems much earlier in the progression of the disease than the latter.

It is important for the nurse to recognize a patient with primary emphysema because it is an *irreversible* disease. The destruction of tissue has already taken place, and comprehensive respiratory care may not significantly improve the patient's condition, unless an asthmatic or bronchitic component is present. Health team members must be careful not to set treatment goals that are too high until the patient receives a thorough medical evaluation to determine the exact diagnosis and the potential benefits of the various forms of respiratory intervention.

When the physical condition has stabilized, the COPD patient is a candidate for a formal or informal pulmonary rehabilitation program. Rehabilitative care helps the patient to achieve optimal level of functioning. For the emphysema patient, retraining of breathing to control the disabling shortness of breath is of utmost importance. Exercise reconditioning can also reduce the work of breathing by increasing the efficiency with which skeletal muscles utilize available oxygen.

Though the outlook for the emphysema patient has been bleak in the past, recent advances in respiratory care, including new exercise techniques and more convenient and aesthetic oxygen therapy devices, can dramatically reduce dyspnea, increase exercise tolerance, improve overall quality of life, and in some cases prolong life.

Finally, individuals with restrictive disease may develop emphysematous changes in the lungs. In most cases, cigarette smoking is responsible for the pathology. In some cases, however, emphysematous changes occur when the individual is not a smoker and does not have emphysema. For example, in various advanced restrictive diseases, lung pathology may be so extensive that tissue destruction results in air-filled cysts similar to the bulla characteristic of emphysema.

BRONCHIOLITIS

Whereas bronchitis relates to irritation or inflammation of *major* bronchi, *bronchiolitis* relates to inflammation of bronchioles or *small* airways. Acute bronchiolitis is commonly seen in children less than 3 years of age and in adults with preexisting chronic respiratory disease. Often, bronchiolitis is accompanied by inflammation of the trachea and bronchi. The usual etiological agent is a virus, notably the influenza virus during epidemics, but sometimes it is *Mycoplasma pneumoniae* or a bacterium. Air pollution or exposure to chemical aerosols may cause bronchiolitis, typically in individuals with preexisting chronic airflow limitations. In most mild cases due to smog, pulmonary symptoms abate when the heavily polluted smog clears from the geographic area. However, bronchiolitis with extensive inflammation and destruction of small bronchioles is potentially fatal in children and adults. Without prompt medical treatment, infants and children especially are likely to develop acute respiratory failure requiring mechanical ventilation.

Pathologically, in addition to inflammation and destruction of small bronchioles, inflammation may extend to adjacent alveoli and into peribronchiolar tissues. Goblet cells increase in number, secreting mucus into the lumens of small airways. The presence of mucus plugs and inflammatory edema of bronchial and bronchiolar walls leads to airway obstruction. In severe cases of bronchiolitis, *bronchiolectasis* (abnormal dilatation of bronchioles) develops, and *bronchiolitis obliterans* may develop. The latter refers to permanent occlusion of the airway.

BRONCHIECTASIS

Bronchiectasis is defined in anatomic terms as *abnormal dilatation of the bronchi.* It occurs in two forms as follows: *cylindric* and *saccular* (Kremsdorf, 1980), based on radiologic appearances of *bronchograms* taken during bronchography. Bronchography is a diagnostic test involving inhalation of a radiographic substance to identify irregularities in the structure and function of airways. This test is used because findings for bronchiectasis on ordinary chest x-ray films are absent or nonspecific.

In *cylindric* bronchiectasis, bronchi are tubular shaped with lumens ending abruptly rather than gradually tapering in size towards the periphery, as in the normal lung. This form of disease is the potentially reversible one seen in acute inflammatory diseases, such as pneumonia. Airways return to normal 2 to 4 months after initial treatment for bacterial pneumonia. Only a small percentage of patients with cylindric bronchiectasis develop saccular bronchiectasis.

In *saccular* (or *cystic*) bronchiectasis, airways develop outpouchings ("sacs") or grape-like dilatations. These destroy the normal tapering of bronchi towards the periphery and sometimes actually make distal airways much *larger* than more central airways. This *irreversible* form of bronchiectasis results from many different etiologic factors and is seen in diverse clinical disease states; e.g., cystic fibrosis, an inherited disease; chronic bronchitis, with repeated chest infections; and localized severe chest infections in debilitated individuals, in particular. In children, this form of bronchiectasis may occur from pneumonia developing as a complication of measles, whooping cough (pertussis), or other childhood disease.

The following discussion of bronchiectasis focuses on the irreversible saccular or cystic form of disease, i.e., the form with pathology extending beyond simple bronchial dilatation.

Pathologic Features

The four main pathologic features responsible for signs and symptoms of irreversible bronchiectasis are briefly described next. Of those listed, *bronchial wall destruction* and *abnormal dilatation of bronchi* are most characteristic (Fig. 7–16).

1. *Bronchial wall destruction.* The normal bronchial epithelium is replaced by nonciliated low cuboidal or squamous epithelium. Destruction or fragmentation of elastic, muscular, and sometimes cartilaginous components of bronchial walls results in unsupported "flabby" airways. Inflammation from infection is believed to be responsible for these destructive changes and for distortion of the normal contour of airways. Fibrosis around airways commonly develops as an end result.

2. *Accumulation of respiratory secretions.* Destruction of bronchial walls impairs the mucociliary escalator. Secretions tend to accumulate in the lungs. This pathologic feature is not present in the asymptomatic or "dry" form of bronchiectasis in which the individual is unproductive of respiratory secretions. (Perhaps the most frequent causes of this dry form are the granulomatous diseases, e.g., tuberculosis.)

3. *Abnormal dilatation of bronchi.* The destruction of tissue and the accumulation of large amounts of mucus increase intralumenal pressures and promote airway dilatation. Also, obstructive secretions impair alveolar ventilation. Underventilated alveoli tend to collapse, allowing adjacent bronchi to expand and dilate. Then, the patient's forced expiratory efforts

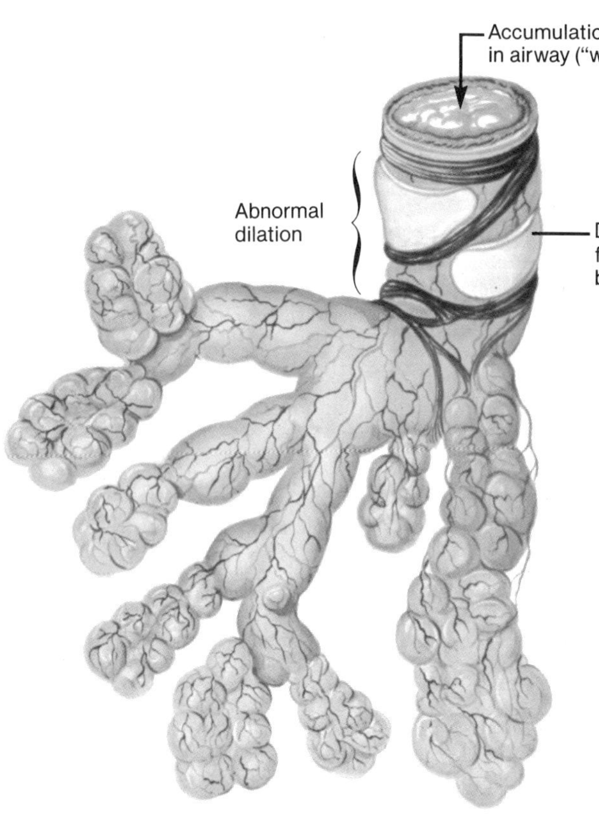

Figure 7–16. Airway pathology in bronchiectasis. (Reproduced by permission from American College of Chest Physicians, 1974.)

against extremely high airway resistance also promote dilatation.

4. *Enlarged bronchial arteries.* In bronchiectasis, bronchial arteries may become enlarged, proliferated, and tortuous. These changes are from high systemic and pulmonary pressures distending the vessels. Systemic pressures may be transmitted to the lung through the bronchial circulation's systemic origin, particularly during coughing episodes (see Chapter 4). High pulmonary pressures from severe pulmonary hypertension are transmitted through the bronchial artery-pulmonary capillary anastamoses.

Coughing may precipitate hemoptysis (coughing up blood) when the destruction of airway walls involves adjacent blood engorged vessels, primarily the bronchial arteries with their higher intralumenal pressures. Hemoptysis occurs in 50% to 70% of individuals with bronchiectasis.

Etiologic Factors

The main etiologic factors responsible for the development of bronchiectasis are summarized in Table 7–6. The listed conditions may be *directly* or *indirectly* responsible for disease. On the one hand, bronchopulmonary infection from pneumonia directly causes disease because infectious microorganisms cause inflammation and destructive changes. On the other

Table 7–6. ETIOLOGICAL FACTORS FOR BRONCHIECTASIS

Conditions	Specific Examples
Bronchopulmonary infection due to specific microorganisms	*Klebsiella*, *Staphylococcus*, pertussis, measles, tuberculosis, influenza, various viruses, and fungi
Other inflammatory and destructive processes	Aspiration pneumonia, inhalation of irritant gases or particles, diffuse interstitial fibrosis
Localized bronchial obstruction	Foreign body, tumor, enlarged lymph nodes, mucoid impaction
Severe chronic obstructive disease	Chronic bronchitis with repeated chest infections
Immune-deficiency states	Deficiency of IgG and IgM in the blood; immunosuppression from drugs
Main hereditary conditions	Cystic fibrosis, Kartagener's syndrome (bronchiectasis, situs inversus, and sinusitis)
Anatomical, congenital, or hereditary disorders	Pulmonary vascular abnormalities; defective development of airways (bronchial hypoplasia, deficiency of bronchial cartilage); lymphatics (lymphatic hypoplasia, yellow nail syndrome); and pulmonary vessels
Unknown etiology	Idiopathic bronchiectasis

hand, bronchial obstruction from a tumor *indirectly* causes disease—the *effects* of obstruction rather than the obstruction per se cause disease. More specifically, airway obstruction decreases alveolar ventilation, promotes alveolar collapse (atelectasis), and impairs the mucociliary escalator. Secretions accumulate that then predispose the patient to bronchopulmonary infection, the actual cause of bronchiectasis. Similarly, immune-deficiency states indirectly cause bronchiectasis by increasing susceptibility to chest infections.

Signs and Symptoms/Progression of Disease

Bronchiectasis is now recognized as relatively common in patients with histories of pulmonary disease. In some cases (e.g., inactive tuberculosis), the patient may be asymptomatic and unaware of any past pulmonary problem. In general, the finding is clinically significant only if infection or hemoptysis is present.

Signs and symptoms vary depending on etiology. The main signs and symptoms are *cough*, purulent *sputum production*, *fever* with the presence of infection, and *hemoptysis*. Also, nasal stuffiness and discharge from sinusitis are commonly seen in association with bronchiectasis. In an adult with a chronic pulmonary process, the presence of *Pseudomonas aeruginosa* in bronchial secretions indicates the presence of underlying bronchiectasis (Rivera and Nicotra, 1982).

Most cases fall in or somewhere between the classic "wet" and "dry" forms of the disease. The wet form is characterized by *cough* and *sputum production* with intermittent fever. Some patients cough up such large quantities of sputum (200 to 300 ml per day) with such foul smelling purulence that family members and health professionals may avoid approaching the bedside. These symptoms may be accompanied by wheeze and shortness of breath. The severity of symptoms seems to depend on the amount of accompanying chronic bronchitis and the amount of lung collapse and destruction resulting from the chest infection. In the majority of cases, bronchiectasis occurs in dependent lobes, where the drainage of secretions is impaired. The most common site is the left lower lobe, followed by the lingular segments, right lower lobe, and right middle lobe in that order (Kremsdorf, 1980).

In the dry form of bronchiectasis, the patient may have absent symptoms or dry cough with intermittent episodes of hemoptysis months or years apart. The hemoptysis may occur without warning or in association with mild respiratory infection. The most common sites of lung involvement are the upper lobe segments, sites that permit continual dependent drainage of pathological areas.

The disease progression of bronchiectasis varies, depending on etiology. Infectious processes may be successfully treated or controlled by antibiotics, other medications, and various respiratory therapy interventions. Fifty years ago, vaccines and potent antimicrobial drugs were not available to control infections and associated signs and symptoms. Affected individuals were likely to die between the ages of 20 and 45 years. Now, with more refined therapy, the incidence of at least the classic wet form of bronchiectasis is decreased, and the life span of the affected individual lengthened.

Severe bronchiectasis may be treated by surgical resection, when pathology is well localized in one lobe or two adjacent lobes and when no contraindications to surgery exist. Bronchiectasis is assumed to be severe if bronchography has been ordered to document its presence and extent. This diagnostic test is usually performed only when surgical intervention is considered a realistic treatment for the patient.

CYSTIC FIBROSIS

Cystic fibrosis (CF), also called *fibrocystic disease of the pancreas* or *mucoviscidosis*, is one of the chief causes of bronchiectasis. It is a more generalized disease involving many organs besides the lungs. The lungs may not be involved at first, but eventually bronchiectasis develops. Death is caused by the effects of repeated pulmonary infections.

Special mention must be made of CF because it is the most frequently occurring lethal genetic disease in whites and is the main cause of chronic lung disease in children. Fifty years ago, CF was considered a rapidly progressive disease whereby patients died before reaching adulthood. Now affected individuals are diagnosed earlier, and control of infections with medications and implementation of modern therapeutic regimens have slowed the progression of CF. At least half of children born today with CF live to be 20 years of age or older. Many reach their thirties; a few reach their forties. About 20% of CF patients in the United States are adults; therefore, CF no longer is considered to be solely a pediatric disease (Davis, 1983). Furthermore, its incidence is increasing in the general population. About 4 to 5% of the general population are carriers of the gene transmitting this disease.

CF is inherited as an *autosomal recessive disease*. The parents are *heterozygotes* or carriers and are not affected by the disease; the patients are *homozygotes* and are affected to varying degrees. Each conception by heterozygote parents is associated with a 25% chance of producing a symptomatic offspring (Fig. 7–17).

At present, no known cost effective and accurate screening method exists to identify carriers of the trait in the general population. Only individuals manifesting disease are diagnosed.

General Features

Basically, pathology is due to an inborn error of metabolism in which a *generalized dysfunction of exocrine glands* exists in the body. The organs and

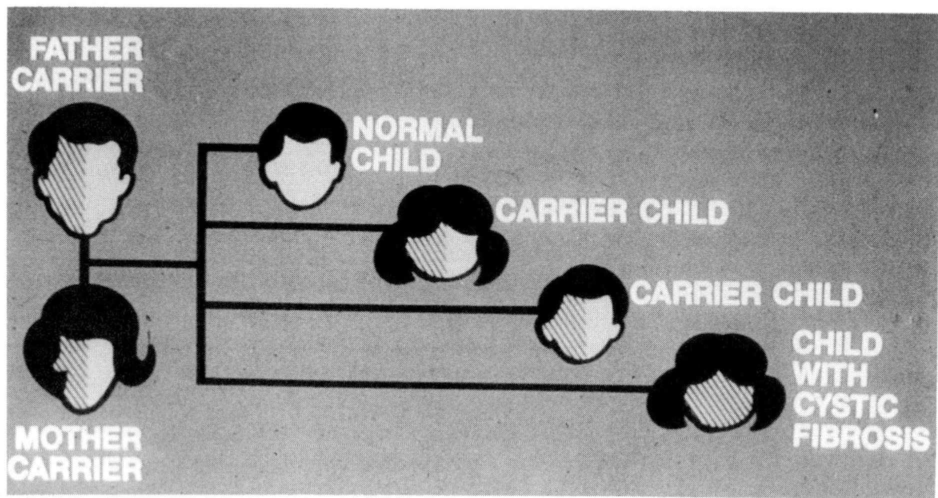

Figure 7–17. Genetics of cystic fibrosis. (Reproduced by permission from Guide to Diagnosis and Treatment of Cystic Fibrosis of the Pancreas, National Cystic Fibrosis Foundation, Professional Education Committee, Rockville, Md., 1987.)

glandular systems involved include the pancreas, respiratory system, salivary glands, gastrointestinal tract, paranasal sinuses, reproductive tract, and sweat glands.

The following two mechanisms are responsible for pathological changes in the different organs and glandular systems. *First,* exocrine gland ducts (e.g., pancreatic ducts) or passageways receiving exocrine gland secretions (e.g., bronchioles, bronchi, small intestine) become obstructed with thick tenacious secretions. *Second,* electrolyte concentrations in certain exocrine secretions make body secretions abnormal. This second mechanism is the basis for diagnosing CF from positive sweat chloride test results. A positive test result is one in which chloride levels are elevated above 60 mEq/L in children and above 80 mEq/L in adults. Negative test results in normal individuals yield unequivocally normal values, ranging from 19 mEq/L in infants to 32 mEq/L in adults.)

A medical diagnosis of CF is rarely made without positive results from a properly collected and accurately measured quantitative sweat test. However, other findings are needed to confirm the diagnosis. Two of the following criteria must be present for a positive medical diagnosis: (1) *positive sweat test results* (at least two separate elevated values are required); (2) *presence of obstructive pulmonary disease* determined by history or recent clinical findings; (3) *exocrine pancreatic insufficiency* determined by history of gastrointestinal signs and symptoms and by specialized laboratory test results; and (4) *family history of CF.*

How the thick abnormal secretions of CF affect different body organs and produce clinical manifestations is beyond the scope of this text. CF is a highly complicated disease because of its multisystem involvement and its variable clinical manifestations. Many theories have been proposed to explain the pathogenesis of CF in the various organs, including the lungs. The discussion presented next focuses on pathologic changes in the lungs.

Pulmonary Pathologic Features

The pathogenesis of pulmonary abnormalities appears to be related to the following features:

1. *Excessive secretion of abnormal mucus.* The secreted mucus is unlike that in chronic bronchitis. Purulence from the products of inflammation is present in both diseases, but the mucus in CF has other unique qualities that predispose the patient to respiratory problems. The mucus in CF is always relatively dehydrated by nature. In addition, it has abnormal organic constituents (highly sulfated and acidic components) and abnormal electrolyte concentrations (elevated calcium and potassium content, reduced sodium and chloride content) that make the mucus especially thick and viscid (sticky).
2. *Impairment of the mucociliary escalator.* This feature is largely due to a defect in the ciliary action, a phenomenon called *ciliary dyskinesis.* In this defect, the abnormal movement of cilia slows the mucociliary escalator. The rate of movement of particles from the lower respiratory tract is five to ten times lower in patients with CF compared with normal subjects of the same age (Wood et al., 1976). Secretions accumulate in airways, predisposing the patient to airway obstruction and infection.
3. *Airway obstruction.* Thick, viscid secretions plug airways and promote the trapping of air in distal airways. The nature and stasis of the mucus in airways provide an excellent environment for the growth of bacteria and the development of chest infection.
4. *Bacterial infection.* Infection initiates a vicious circle of destructive pathologic changes (described subsequently). The infection may be responsible for the initial pulmonary abnormalities in neonates (Taussig and Landau, 1979).

Pathophysiology

Currently, the initial pulmonary insult in the neonate or child is unknown. It is somehow related to infections, excessive secretions, or both. In any case, the earliest pulmonary abnormality involves peripheral airways. Hyperplasia of goblet cells and hypertrophy of mucous secreting glands occur in the bronchioles. These structures hypersecrete mucus, predisposing individuals to the formation of mucus plugs and bronchiolar obstruction. Because peripheral alveoli become underventilated, infection (usually pneumonia) develops, followed by additional mucus production and a vicious cycle. As the disease progresses, the larger airways and the bronchi become involved in the same manner (Fig. 7–18). Recurrent infections cause bronchiolectasis, saccular bronchiectasis, and fibrosis (scarring) around airways.

CF is a self perpetuating type of pulmonary disorder because of the vicious cycle of changes just described. In the stable patient, however, exacerbations occur. They are precipitated by the development of chest infection, acute bronchiolitis, or acute bronchitis. Chest infections from bacteria are responsible for the progression of disease, but viruses play an indirect part by initiating or exacerbating existing bacterial infections. Influenza and the common cold are examples of common viral infections. Also, exacerbations may be related to exposure to air pollution, causing acute bronchiolitis, which in turn predisposes the patient to retained secretions and chest infection.

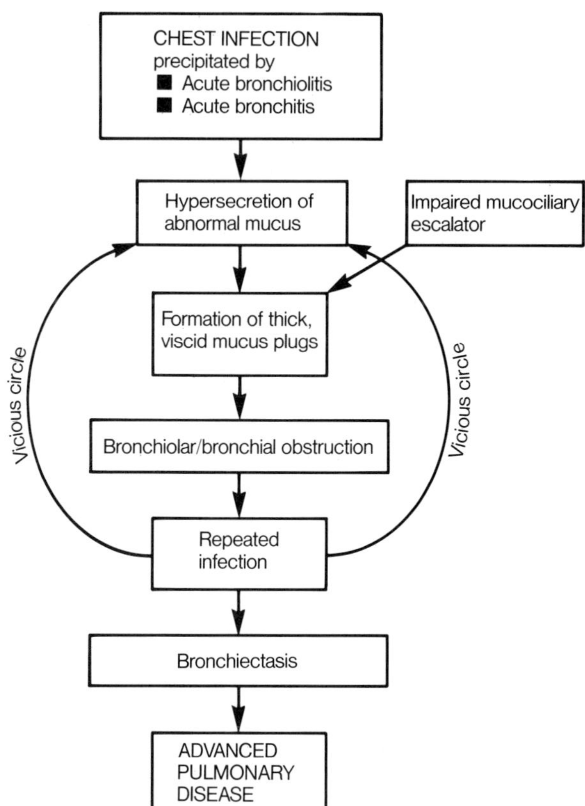

Figure 7–18. Basic pathophysiology of cystic fibrosis.

The bacterial microorganisms *Staphylococcus aureus* and *Pseudomonas aeruginosa* are the most common microorganisms cultured from tracheobronchial secretions. *Pseudomonas* is a common finding in patients with CF. The patient's increased susceptibility to this microorganism appears to be related to the alveolar macrophage's decreased ability to phagocytize and kill it. The presence of *Pseudomonas* should always arouse the suspicion of the presence of CF in undiagnosed patients.

Once recurrent infections develop, the main pathological features of bronchiectasis appear. These features have already been summarized in the preceding section covering bronchiectasis (see page 113). However, changes in CF tend to be more severe than changes in an uncomplicated case of bronchiectasis because of the self perpetuating nature of CF. The patient is never rid of the thick, viscid secretions. These secretions predispose the CF patient to more complications. Airways tend to become impacted with mucus. Abscess formation, cyst formation, and airway collapse (atelectasis) are likely to occur if infection persists or if daily bronchial hygiene measures to keep airways clear of the large amounts of obstructive secretions are not practiced.

Further comparison of CF and uncomplicated bronchiectasis helps clarify differences in clinical manifestations. In bronchiectasis, lung tissue shrinks owing to tissue fibrosis and localized areas of atelectasis, producing a normal to *reduced* lung volume (total lung capacity), depending on the severity of disease. Chest configuration may appear normal.

In contrast, CF produces a normal to an *increased* lung volume (total lung capacity). As mucus plugs trap air peripherally, the increase in intralumenal airway pressures dilates alveoli and bronchioles. The more the mucus plugging and the more the airway dilatation, the greater the lung hyperinflation and the more visible the abnormality in chest configuration (barrel chest).

Because of its pathophysiology, CF tends to produce a greater change in lung volume and a more visible change in chest configuration compared with bronchiectasis.

Thus far, pathologic features unique to CF as well as those attributed to bronchiectasis in general have been mentioned. The patient with advanced CF also ends up with many of the *general* pathological features of emphysema. Emphasis must be placed on the word "general" because specific pathologic findings differ. The two diseases differ greatly in pathogenesis as well as in specific locations of the destructive processes. *Airways* are destroyed in CF; *alveolar septa* are destroyed in emphysema. General pathological features in common include *loss of lung elastic recoil, airway collapse with cough and forced exhalation, lung hyperinflation,* and *formation of bullae.* Both diseases may be complicated by pneumothorax from the rupture of bullae.

The net effect of pathophysiologic events discussed previously is airway obstruction and impaired ventilation. These processes increase airway resistance to a level that reflects the extent and severity of pulmonary disease. Severe airway obstruction greatly increases airway resistance, reduces alveolar ventilation, and yields a grossly abnormal V/Q ratio. Advanced pulmonary disease sets in when repeated chest infections produce persistent oxygenation and ventilatory problems.

Main Signs and Symptoms

Pulmonary signs and symptoms are essentially the same as those for bronchiectasis. Fever is rare, however, despite evidence of pneumonia on the chest x-ray. Hemoptysis may be easily precipitated by minor trauma or increased infection. Cough is the most consistent finding; it is dry and repetitive at first. As disease progresses, it then becomes loose and productive. In an infant, wheezing may be the first presenting pulmonary sign, presumably because of the small size of the airways.

Pulmonary signs and symptoms are late manifestations of disease in most individuals. Other common signs and symptoms alert clinicians to the possible presence of CF. These include the following: salty breath; salty skin from excess sodium and chloride secreted by sweat glands; heat prostration; failure to thrive; voracious appetite; abdominal pain; foul, bulky, and fatty stools; persistent runny nose; and infertility.

Beckerman and Berdan (1980) report that about 98% of young males with CF are infertile, probably because of anatomical abnormalities of the spermatic cord and epididymis and a low sperm count. The female infertility rate is not known, but some clinicians estimate it at 30 to 50%. In a woman, infertility is believed to be due to tenacious cervical and vaginal mucous secretions, blocking the passage of sperm; it is not due to any anatomic defect.

Progression of Disease

The onset and progression of pulmonary disease is variable owing to the heterogeneity of the genetic defect. Some individuals do not manifest pulmonary involvement until late childhood or early adulthood. This finding is especially true if an early diagnosis of CF is made, if the patient receives close medical supervision, and if the patient receives adequate counseling and prophylactic treatment before the onset of irreversible lung damage. Some children remain stable and suddenly deteriorate. Others deteriorate progressively to advanced pulmonary disease. Still others are relatively asymptomatic and may demonstrate mild pulmonary involvement limited to minimal pathologic changes in the upper lobes, commonly the right upper lobe.

The onset and progression of CF involving other body systems are also variable. Individuals with CF are thought to have morphologically normal lungs at birth. The earliest possible problem is intestinal obstruction (from meconium ileus) in neonates between 24 and 48 hours of age; it occurs in 7 to 25% of newborns with CF (Wood et al, 1976). Pancreatic insufficiency is responsible for most signs and symptoms during the first 2 years of life. The lack of pancreatic enzymes results in poor digestion (especially of fat) and is responsible for the frequent, loose, bulky, fatty stools plaguing both children and adults with CF. Gastrointestinal problems are controlled by diet and medication, but stable patients may still have difficulties gaining or maintaining body weight despite voracious appetites. Maldigestion contributes to the development of decreased muscle mass, protuberant abdomen, poor growth, and delayed maturation. Many individuals successfully maintain nutrition by eating two to three times as much as a normal individual the same age. When inevitable pulmonary infections develop, caloric needs increase but appetite and food intake decrease, predisposing the patient to malnutrition. The state of malnutrition correlates with the deterioration in pulmonary status more so than with the appearance of excessive stools from gastrointestinal problems.

As children mature, clinical manifestations of pancreatic insufficiency become less overt. Concern is focused more on the development of pulmonary problems, but the presence of pancreatic insufficiency must not be neglected because it can affect the functioning of all body systems, including the respiratory system.

In conclusion, CF is a complicated disease with multisystem involvement. Reviewing pulmonary pathophysiology helps one to understand the relationship of CF to other main obstructive diseases; it also makes one realize the complexity of the pulmonary abnormalities and the challenge CF presents to all members of the health care team. Early diagnosis is crucial to a more favorable prognosis. Comprehensive and continuing respiratory intervention is essential to help the patient and family cope with the myriad psychosocial and pathophysiologic problems associated with this disease. Although an experienced pulmonary nurse can effectively work with others to assess problems and intervene appropriately, data suggest that patients who receive some or all of their care in a CF center tend to do better than those who receive none of their care in such a center (Taussig and Landau, 1979). Efforts should be made to refer CF patients to these centers for more intensive respiratory care and specialized individual and group counseling sessions.

Goals and Interventions

Basic goals and interventions for treatment of COPD are summarized in the box.

Though this list of interventions gives the nurse a general idea about appropriate therapy for COPD, specific interventions depend on the patient's specific chest pathology and associated respiratory problems. Subsequent chapters clarify indications for each intervention.

GOALS AND INTERVENTIONS FOR OBSTRUCTIVE PULMONARY DISEASE

GOALS

- Decrease or eliminate bronchoconstriction, airway obstruction, or airflow limitation
- Decrease or eliminate mucus production and retention
- Maintain highest possible level of functional activity

INTERVENTIONS

- Smoking cessation
- Pulmonary medications: bronchodilators, corticosteroids (in severe disease), antibiotics
- Bronchial hygiene program
  - Deep breathing and controlled coughing
  - Hydration
  - Balanced diet
  - Environmental control
  - General relaxation
  - Breathing retraining
  - Postural drainage with percussion/vibration
  - Aerosol
- Progressive exercise conditioning
  - Gravity resistance or range of motion exercises
  - Walking, bicycling, swimming, and so forth
  - Arm ergometry (arm bicycle)
- Immunotherapy or hyposensitization treatments (in extrinsic asthma)
- Oxygen therapy
- Mechanical ventilation (in severe disease)
- Self-care education

Conclusion

In summary, the nurse can expect to encounter obstructive pulmonary disease in most clinical settings. Acute disease produces life-threatening cardiopulmonary signs and symptoms. Chronic disease may be mild to severe; the patient presents with either a relentlessly progressive or a variable disease course. Variability is usually attributed to repeated bronchopulmonary infections. In most COPD patients, chest infections occur frequently, typically beginning with a common cold affecting the upper respiratory tract and settling into the chest within a few days. Moreover, it has been said that once significant shortness of breath develops in COPD patients, severe disability follows within 5 to 10 years. Because of recent diagnostic and therapeutic advances, many patients now can live fairly comfortably within the limitations of their diseases. Hence, the onset of disability varies from individual to individual and can rarely be accurately predicted by the physician. Endstage disease is marked by the development of right ventricular hypertrophy (cor pulmonale), severe oxygenation problems, right-sided heart failure, and ventilatory failure. These disorders are explored in subsequent chapters.

REFERENCES

American College of Chest Physicians: *Diseases of the respiratory system.* (Pamphlet.) Lincoln, Nebraska, Dorsey Laboratories, 1974.

Anderson, S.: Exercise and the asthmatic patient. *Respiratory Therapy,* 10:3, 68–75, 1980.

Beckerman, R. and Berdan, M.: Overview of a lethal genetic disease: cystic fibrosis. *Respiratory Therapy,* 10:2, 20–26, 1980.

Chen, W.Y. and Chai, H.: Airway cooling and nocturnal asthma. *Chest,* 81 (6): 675, 1982.

Cherniack, R.: Chronic and acute asthma—keys to successful management. *Postgraduate Medicine,* 75(2): 87–98, 1984.

Cockcroft, D.W. and Horne, S.L.: Localization of emphysema within the lung. *Chest,* 82(4): 483–487, 1982.

Davis, P.: Cystic fibrosis—clinical manifestations in older patients. *Clinical Notes on Respiratory Diseases,* 21(4): 3–12, 1983.

Davis, P. and di Sant' Agnese L.: Diagnosis and treatment of cystic fibrosis. *Chest,* 85(6): 802–809, 1984.

Feist, J., Johnson, T., and Wilson, R.: Acquired tracheomalacia: etiology and differential diagnosis. *Chest,* 68:3, 340, 1975.

Fishman, A.: *Pulmonary Diseases and Disorders.* New York, McGraw-Hill Book Co., 1980.

Fraser, R.G. and Paré, J.A.: *Diagnosis of Diseases of the Chest,* vol. three, 2nd ed. Philadelphia, W.B. Saunders Co., 1979.

Griffin, M., Weiss, J.W., et al: Effects of leukotriene D on the airways in asthma. *New England Journal of Medicine,* 308(8): 436–439, 1983.

Heidorn, A.: Diagnosis and management of croup. *Respiratory Therapy,* 10:6, 43–44, 1980.

Hinshaw, H.C. and Murray, J.F.: *Diseases of the Chest,* 4th ed. Philadelphia, W.B. Saunders Co., 1980.

Hoidal, J.R. and Niewoehner, D.E.: Pathogenesis of emphysema. *Chest,* 83(4): 679–685, 1983.

Homma, H. et al.: Diffuse panbronchiolitis—a disease of the transitional zone of the lung. *Chest,* 83 (1): 63–69, 1983.

Huang, N. and Palmer, J.: Management of patients with cystic fibrosis. *Respiratory Therapy,* 11:1, 49, 1981.

Kremsdorf, R.: Bronchiectasis. In *Manual of Clinical Problems in Pulmonary Medicine* (eds., Bordow, R., Stool, E., and Moser, K.). Boston, Little, Brown & Co., 1980.

Leff, A.: Pathogenesis of asthma—neurophysiology and pharmacology of bronchospasm. *Chest,* 81:2, 224–229, 1982.

Leitch, A.G.: Asthma—mechanisms and management. *Clinical Notes on Respiratory Disease,* 21(1): 3–9, 1982.

Loughlin, G. and Taussig, L.: Upper airway obstruction. *Seminars in Respiratory Medicine,* 1:2, 131–146, 1979.

McCullough, D.: Surgical management of acute upper airway obstruction. *Seminars in Respiratory Medicine,* 2:1, 6–11, 1980.

McFadden, E.R.: Asthma: pathophysiology. *Seminars in Respiratory Medicine,* 1:4, 297–302, 1980.

Morris, L., Mascia, A., and Farnsworth, P.: Cystic fibrosis: making a correct and early diagnosis. *Journal of Family Practice*, 6:4, 749–756, 1978.

Nelson, H.: Review—Gastroesophageal reflux and pulmonary disease. *Journal of Allergy and Clinical Immunology*, 73(5): 547–556, 1984.

Netter, F.: *The CIBA Collection of Medical Illustrations, vol. 7: Respiratory System*. New York, CIBA Pharmaceutical Co., 1979.

Petty, T. and Scoggin, C.: Diseases with chronic airflow limitation. *Seminars in Respiratory Medicine*, 1:1, 18–27, 1979.

Rivera, M. and Nicotra, M.B.: *Pseudomonas aeruginosa* mucoid strain. *American Review of Respiratory Disease*, 126(5): 833, 1982.

Simon, R.: Drug, food, additive asthma syndromes. (Postgraduate Course 1: Recent Advances in Asthma.) Kansas City, Missouri, Annual Meeting of the American Lung Association—American Thoracic Society, 1986.

Soffer, A. (ed.): Supplement to the 22nd Aspen Lung Conference: Chronic obstructive pulmonary disease. *Chest*, 77:2, 1980.

Spector, S.: Psychological factors in asthma. *Practical Cardiology*, 12(2): 150–159, 1986.

Taussig, L., Cota, K., and Kaltenborn, W.: Different mechanical properties of the lungs in boys and girls. *American Review of Respiratory Disease*, 123:6, 640, 1981.

Taussig, L. and Landau, L.: Cystic fibrosis. *Seminars in Respiratory Medicine*, 1:2, 167–182, 1979.

Thurlbeck, W.: Chronic bronchitis and emphysema—the pathophysiology of COLD. *Basics of Respiratory Disease*, 3:1, 3, 1974.

Wagner, P. and West, J.: Ventilation-Perfusion Relationships. In *Pulmonary Gas Exchange, vol. one* (Ed., West, J.). New York, Academic Press Inc., 1980.

Wanner, A.: Bronchial provocation testing in clinical practice. *Respiratory Care*, 31(3): 207–212, 1986.

Welch, M.: Obstructive Diseases. In *Pulmonary Medicine*, 2nd ed. (eds., Guenter, C., and Welch, M.). Philadelphia, J.B. Lippincott Co., 1982.

West, J.: *Pulmonary Pathophysiology: The Essentials*, 2nd ed. Baltimore, Williams & Wilkins, 1982.

Whitcomb, M.: Role of immunologic mechanisms in diffuse alveolar wall diseases. *Clinical Notes on Respiratory Diseases*, 19(1):3–11, 1980.

Wood, R., Boat, T., and Doershuk, C.: State of the art: Cystic fibrosis. *American Review of Respiratory Disease*, 113, 833–862, 1976.

Ziment, I.: *Respiratory Pharmacology and Therapeutics*. Philadelphia, W.B. Saunders Co., 1978.

Restrictive Pulmonary Disease

8

Main Objectives

1. **Define the term restrictive pulmonary disease.**
2. **Define *extrapulmonary* restriction and *pulmonary* restriction, giving at least three unrelated examples of diseases that fall into each of these categories.**
3. **List and describe the three pathologic processes causing restrictive pulmonary disease.**
4. **Explain how decreased tissue distensibility alters lung compliance, lung elastic recoil, and lung volume.**
5. **State and explain the physiologic formula for static lung compliance. Differentiate this measurement from dynamic compliance.**
6. **Define the following terms: parenchymal disease, atelectasis, pneumonia, diffuse interstitial fibrosis, pneumoconiosis, benign tumors, malignant tumors, metastatic tumors, pulmonary edema, pulmonary embolism, pulmonary infarction.**
7. **For diffuse interstitial fibrosis**

a. Identify patients who may already have clinical findings or who are at increased risk.
b. Name the characteristic pathologic defect.
c. List the main signs and symptoms.
d. Describe the general progression of disease.

8. Name and describe the three stages of cardiogenic pulmonary edema.

9. Compare and contrast treatment goals and basic interventions for chronic obstructive pulmonary disease (COPD) and restrictive pulmonary disease.

The first part of this chapter provides an overview of restrictive pulmonary disease. It emphasizes four aspects as follows:

1. The extrapulmonary and pulmonary classifications of restrictive disease
2. The pathologic processes responsible for abnormal lung function
3. The crucial concept of lung/chest wall compliance
4. The main pathophysiology, the main signs and symptoms, and the general disease progression for diffuse interstitial fibrosis, a classic example of a restrictive disease.

The second half of the chapter presents a broad range of specific diseases to familiarize the nurse with certain types of patients who have or are at risk to develop restrictive pulmonary disease.

As with the previous chapter, emphasis is placed on pathophysiology to facilitate a deeper understanding of pulmonary disease in general. Restrictive pathologic processes are not limited to pulmonary diseases classified as *restrictive*—they commonly occur in *obstructive* pulmonary disease as well. For example, the COPD patient may develop the restrictive disease of *pneumonia* or *atelectasis* (collapse) as a complication; the patient with acute upper airway obstruction may develop atelectasis of peripheral lung tissue. Atelectasis itself is such a common pulmonary disorder in the acute setting that a basic knowledge of its pathogenesis is essential for all nurses, regardless of their areas of specialization.

Overview of Restrictive Pulmonary Disease

Restrictive pulmonary disease is not a specific clinical entity. It is produced by a variety of diseases and disorders affecting the chest wall, pleural space, lung parenchyma, and other areas peripheral to the lungs.

DEFINITION

The common denominator in all restrictive diseases, regardless of etiology or pathologic process, is a *decrease in lung volume*. More specifically, a restrictive disorder is *any condition that limits lung expansion and produces a pattern of abnormal function defined by a decrease in lung volume, i.e., total lung capacity (TLC)* on the pulmonary function test.

CLASSIFICATION OF DISEASE

Diseases producing pulmonary restriction may be *acute* or *chronic* and *extrapulmonary* or *pulmonary* in location.

Acute restrictive diseases, such as *pneumothorax* and *pulmonary edema,* are so acute and episodic that they require immediate recognition and treatment by knowledgable and competent clinicians. Nurses are usually more familiar with these diseases than with chronic diseases because signs are overt, treatment is aggressive, and they are directly involved in the care of patients so affected.

Chronic or recurring restrictive pulmonary disease is present within a broad range of clinical disorders, many involving other body systems in addition to the respiratory system, e.g., *sarcoidosis, rheumatoid arthritis,* and *quadriplegia.* The chronic restrictive processes in these diverse disorders tend to remain neglected because pulmonary signs and symptoms are chronic and vague. Many times, clinical manifestations appear unrelated to lung dysfunction. For example, a secondary problem rather than a pulmonary sign prompts hospital admission, e.g., the sarcoidosis patient is hospitalized for ulcerated skin sores. Unless nurses and other health team members recognize that the presenting complaint is related to *pulmonary* disease, respiratory assessment and intervention are overlooked. Similarly, efforts to assess and optimize pulmonary function in a neurologic patient (hemiplegic or quadriplegic) tend to be overshadowed by efforts to deal with the other more obvious problems, such as mobilization of paralyzed limbs, prevention of bed sores, and bladder and bowel control. Particularly in acute settings, where chronic needs are secondary to acute ones, knowledge of the broad range of chronic restrictive pulmonary disease is essential for comprehensive care.

Extrapulmonary and Pulmonary Restriction

Restrictive pulmonary disease is classified according to location of pathology into two categories, as follows: *extrapulmonary restriction* and *pulmonary restriction* (see box).

The *extrapulmonary restriction* category includes disorders in which the etiologies or primary pathologic areas lie *outside* the lungs, peripheral to the visceral pleura. Commonly seen examples of cases of extrapulmonary restriction usually involve the pleural space, chest wall, or both.

The *pulmonary restriction* category includes disorders with etiologies that lie *within* lung tissue itself, involving to varying degrees the alveolar space and the interstitial space, capillary bed, or both. More specifically, this category consists of all *parenchymal* diseases—those disease processes located peripheral to the conducting airways. It comprises a whole host of disorders with varying etiologies and underlying pathologies. Usually, parenchymal disease tends to be *infiltrative* in nature, as in pneumonia from infection—alveoli fill with the products of inflammation; the disease also may be *granulomatous/fibrotic* in nature, as in granulomatous disorders (sarcoidosis and tuberculosis), characterized by the presence of *granulomas* (granular tumors or growths), and in other disorders (diffuse interstitial fibrosis and collagen diseases), characterized by *fibrosis* (scarring or thickening of alveolar interstitium).

This system of classifying restrictive diseases is patterned after Gold's classification system (1968). Division of disorders into extrapulmonary and pulmonary groups is an extremely useful way of classifying disease because it correlates well with the concept of measuring chest wall or lung compliance in the pulmonary function laboratory. Conceptualization of various disease processes and their abnormal patterns of lung function is facilitated.

In spite of its usefulness, from a pulmonary function perspective, this classification system can only serve as a *guide* to understanding. It has its limitations, some of which are mentioned subsequently. Some disorders, such as *sleep apnea syndrome,* may not fall perfectly into any of the listed categories. Many pulmonary restrictive diseases may be classified into more than one category, depending on the nature and extent of the disease entity, e.g., *pneumoconiosis* disease that appears with *diffuse interstitial fibrosis.* Some disease states may be placed into two categories because a restrictive process, such as acute atelectasis, becomes superimposed on an underlying chronic *extrathoracic* disease (e.g., kyphoscoliosis) or on an acute or chronic *pulmonary* restrictive disease (e.g., pneumonia). Many diseases represent combined processes, and some may as yet be unsuitable for classification according to causes because researchers incompletely understand the pathogenesis of the disease.

CLASSIFICATION OF RESTRICTIVE PULMONARY DISEASE

I. EXTRAPULMONARY RESTRICTION

- A. ***Pleural disease***—pleural effusion, hemothorax, chylothorax, empyema, pneumothorax, fibrothorax, pleuritis
- B. ***Chest wall stiffness***—kyphoscoliosis, pectus excavatum, ankylosing spondylitis, obesity
- C. ***Respiratory muscle weakness***—muscular dystrophy, amyotrophic lateral sclerosis, Guillain-Barré syndrome, myasthenia gravis, hemiplegia, quadriplegia
- D. ***Other causes***—abdominal distention, abdominal tumor, pregnancy, chest binders or body braces, disorders affecting CNS control of breathing

II. PULMONARY RESTRICTION

- A. ***Surgical resection***—pneumonectomy and lobectomy postoperatively
- B. ***Atelectasis***—air obstruction, abnormal breathing pattern, compression of lung tissue
- C. ***Pneumonia***—hypersensitivity pneumonitis, infectious pneumonias
- D. ***Diffuse interstitial fibrosis***—heterogeneous group of diseases of *known* etiology (e.g., inhalants, drugs, infectious agents) and of *unknown* etiology (e.g., idiopathic pulmonary fibrosis)
- E. ***Granulomatous disease***—sarcoidosis, pulmonary tuberculosis, eosinophilic granuloma disease, coccidioidomycosis, blastomycosis
- F. ***Collagen disease***—rheumatoid arthritis, systemic lupus erythematosus, scleroderma
- G. ***Pneumoconioses***—occupational lung diseases, e.g., silicosis, asbestosis, coal worker's pneumoconiosis
- H. ***Neoplastic disease***—benign tumors (e.g., hamartomas, papillomas), malignant tumors (e.g., bronchogenic carcinoma), metastatic tumors, granulomatous lesions
- I. ***Vascular disease***—pulmonary edema (cardiogenic and noncardiogenic), adult respiratory distress syndrome, pulmonary embolism, pulmonary infarction, other vascular diseases

MAIN PATHOLOGIC PROCESSES

The main pathologic processes responsible for restrictive disease are *loss of lung tissue, loss of functioning alveoli,* and *decreased lung/chest wall compliance.*

Actual Loss of Lung Tissue

Actual loss of lung tissue by surgical removal, as in pneumonectomy, or by replacement of lung tissue with tumor, results in a decrease in lung volume.

Loss of Functioning Alveoli

Loss of functioning alveoli decreases lung volume because alveoli fill with mucus or fluid, as in pneumonia or pulmonary edema; they become nonfunc-

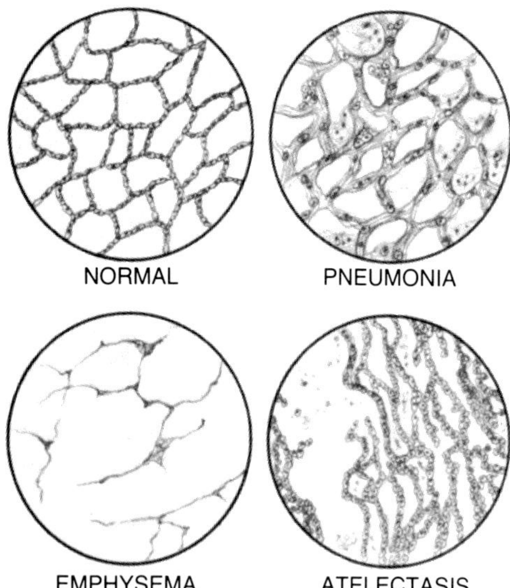

Figure 8–1. Histologic sections of normal and diseased alveoli. (Reproduced by permission from Jacob, S. W., Francone, C. A., Lossow, W. J.: Structure and Function in Man, 5th ed. Philadelphia, W. B. Saunders Co., 1982.)

tional by collapsing, as in atelectasis. Both of these processes alter lung distensibility and lung compliance (described subsequently) because porous, air-filled tissue is replaced with denser matter, which in turn makes the lungs stiffer and more difficult to expand (see both the normal lung and the lung with pneumonia or atelectasis in Figure 8–1).

Decreased Lung/Chest Wall Compliance

Decreased lung/chest wall compliance causes a decrease in lung volume by one or more of the following physiologic mechanisms:

1. A disease process makes the lung stiffer.
2. A disease process occupies the intrathoracic space.
3. Various factors decrease chest wall distensibility.

UNDERSTANDING ELASTIC RECOIL, DISTENSIBILITY, AND COMPLIANCE

To understand how compliance becomes decreased, one must understand what is meant by the terms *elastic recoil*, *distensibility*, and *compliance*. A basic understanding of these terms is crucial to understanding the main pathophysiology of restrictive disease. It also prepares the clinician for interpretation of compliance measurements.

Elastic Recoil

Elastic recoil or elasticity pertains to how well tissue returns to a resting position after stretching. A thick rubber band that immediately returns to its normal length after stretching a considerable distance is said to have *increased elastic recoil*. Similarly, edematous or fibrotic lung tissue will demonstrate increased elastic recoil during expiration, when compared with normal air-filled lung tissue.

Distensibility

Distensibility pertains to *stretchability*—the ease with which tissue can be stretched by an external force. An extremely thick rubber band is not as distensible or stretchable as a thin one. Likewise, edematous or fibrotic lung tissue is more difficult to distend or expand on inspiration than normal lung tissue. A thick chest wall, as in obesity, is more difficult to distend or mobilize outwardly while underlying lungs expand than a thin chest wall.

To better understand the concept of distensibility, consider this example. If one stretches a rubber band using a force of two units, the rubber band stretches two units in distance. If one uses four units of force, the rubber band stretches four units in distance because output (distance stretched) is directly proportional to the input (force applied to the rubber band). This linear relationship is maintained until an *elastic limit* is reached (Fig. 8–2), and a rubber band breaks with further stretching.

Normal lungs act like a bunch of rubber bands. A linear relationship exists between the *force* or *pressure* necessary for lung expansion and the *volume* of air inhaled. This concept is illustrated by the pressure/volume curve for normal lungs in Figure 8–3. As the force or muscular effort to mobilize the chest cage increases X units, volume change during inspiration also increases X units. A 1:1 ratio is maintained until towards the end of inspiration (top flat portion of the curve). Here, high pressures effect little change in volume because the lungs, similar to a bunch of rubber bands, have reached their elastic limit. Unlike rubber bands, however, various mechanical factors, such as changes in *surfactant*, act to reduce surface tension and promote lung deflation rather than alveolar rupture.

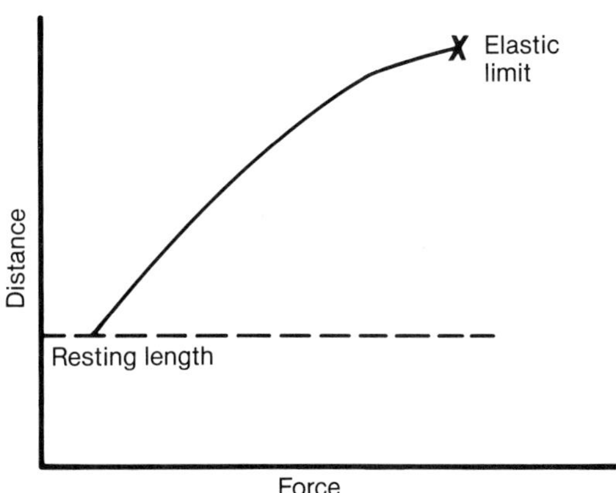

Figure 8–2. Graph illustrating the elastic behavior of a rubber band according to Hooke's law.

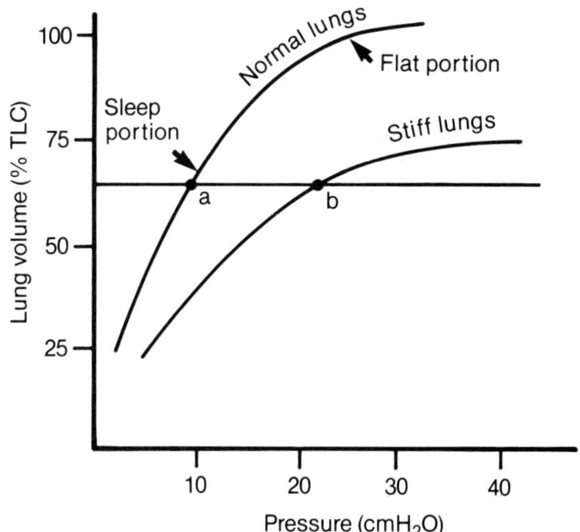

Figure 8–3. Pressure/volume curves for normal lungs and for stiff lungs with restrictive disease. (TLC = total lung capacity.)

In the example of the rubber band, if more than two units of force are required to stretch the rubber band the same distance of two units, then the rubber band is said to be less distensible—it is "stiffer" and more difficult to stretch, just as stiff springs are difficult to stretch. The rubber band is *less* distensible towards its elastic limit because *proportionally more force is required to effect a distance change.* Similarly, normal lungs are stiffer and *less* distensible at high expanding pressures (top flat portion of the curve) because *proportionally greater pressures are required to effect a volume change.* The lungs are *more* distensible at lower pressures, where the curve is steep and lung volume reduced.

The lungs of a patient with restrictive lung disease act like a bunch of stiff rubber bands or a set of stiff springs. The stiff lungs represented in Figure 8–3 are less distensible than normal because more pressure is necessary to distend them to the same volume received by normal lungs. Hence, the slope of the pressure/volume curve is different than that for normal lungs. If, for example, a relatively healthy individual develops pulmonary edema, the lungs fill with fluid and become stiff and less distensible (although lung elastic recoil is increased). *The stiffer the lungs become, the more horizontal the slope of the pressure volume curve.* For any given volume (60% of TLC is the example in Figure 8–3), the patient moves from *point a,* which represents normal compliance, to *point b,* which represents compliance of stiff lungs. When the patient is on a mechanical ventilator, twice as much pressure is necessary to deliver a given volume of air. In the clinical setting, stiff lungs are often equated with "noncompliant" lungs.

Compliance

Compliance is defined in Chapter 6 as the *volume change per unit of pressure change.* The physiologic formula for compliance of the lungs (C_L) is written as follows:

Compliance of the Lungs

$$C_L = \frac{\text{change in volume}}{\text{change in pressure}} \text{ or } \frac{\Delta V}{\Delta P}$$

The meaning of this mathematic formula is difficult to explain simply because of the interrelationship of concepts involved. Although C_L is considered a measure of *distensibility,* it is largely determined by the amount of *elastic recoil,* which must be overcome before lung inflation is possible. Change in pressure (ΔP) is actually stated (measured) in terms of elastic recoil (transpulmonary pressure), as described next and illustrated in Figure 8–4.

What is most important, at this point, to understand is the *inverse relationship between elastic recoil and compliance* (distensibility). On the one hand, fibrotic or edematous tissue with *increased* elastic recoil is less distensible, as explained, and hence demonstrates a *decrease* in lung compliance. On the other hand, the lung tissue of emphysema demonstrates a *decrease* in elastic recoil because of the loss of tissue elasticity from the destruction of tissue and enlargement of air spaces. Tissue density is reduced, as illustrated by the emphysematous lung section in Figure 8–1. The lung is thus easier to distend, and it demonstrates an *increase* in compliance. Note in Figure 8–5 that for any given volume, the emphysematous lung requires less pressure for inflation compared with the normal lung and fibrotic lung. Also, the curve for emphysema is steeper, and it starts at a higher resting volume (over 25% TLC), since the diseased lungs are already somewhat hyperinflated at their resting volume.

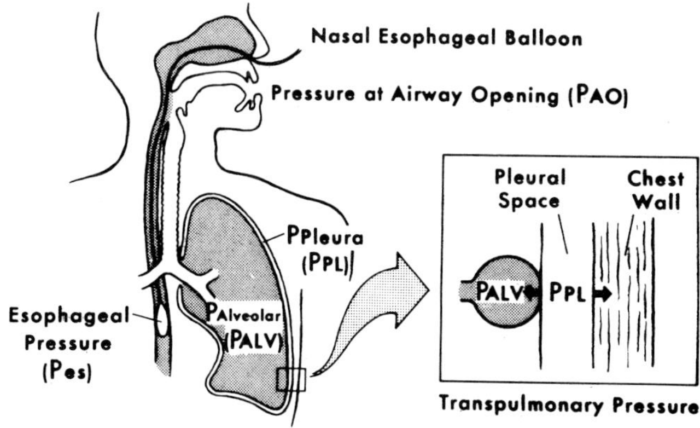

Figure 8–4. Measurement of static compliance of the lung by means of a nasal esophageal balloon. P_{es} or esophageal pressure is used to measure P_{pl} or pleural pressure. P_{ao} is equivalent to the P_m, i.e., pressure at the open mouth with the glottis open and no airflow. (Reproduced by permission from Warren, C. P. W.: Lung Restriction. In Pathophysiology of Respiration (Kryger, M. H., ed.). New York, John Wiley & Sons Inc., 1981.)

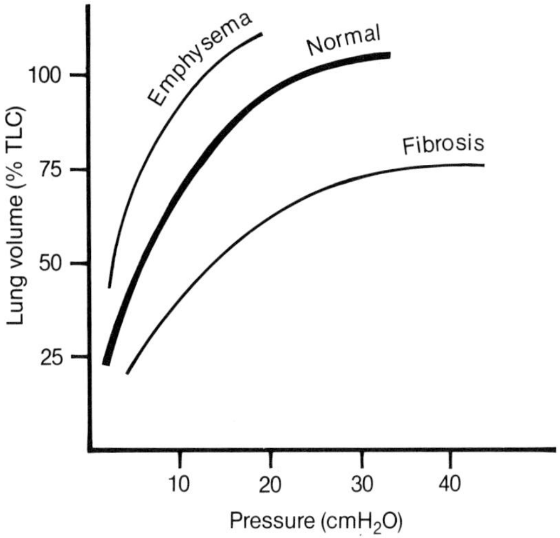

Figure 8–5. Pressure/volume curve for normal lungs compared with curves for stiff fibrotic lungs and emphysematous lungs.

One must remember that the described inverse relationship between elastic recoil and compliance is true under *static* or "no flow" conditions—when the patient is not moving air.

MEASUREMENT OF COMPLIANCE

Compliance of the lungs is measured in L/cmH_2O, as shown next.

Measurement of C_L

$$C_L = \frac{\Delta V\ (L)}{\Delta P\ (cmH_2O)}$$

Static Compliance

Static compliance is most accurately measured in a well-equipped pulmonary function laboratory. *Change in volume* is measured with a spirometer at various "no flow" points when the patient is holding his breath and not moving air. *Change in pressure* is a measurement of *transpulmonary pressure:* P_{ALV} (alveolar) pressure minus P_{pl} (pleural) pressure.

$$C_L = \frac{\Delta V}{\Delta\ (P_{ALV} - P_{pl})}$$

Transpulmonary pressure is assumed to equal pleural pressure because alveolar pressure equals zero under no flow conditions. (At this time, alveolar pressure equilibrates with zero atmospheric pressure at the mouth.) Pleural pressure is assumed to be about equal to pressure in the lower intrathoracic esophagus. Hence, a nasogastric esophageal balloon with a pressure manometer is passed to a midesophageal position to obtain pressure readings at the various no flow points (see Fig. 8–4).

Static compliance of the lung for a normal adult is as follows:

$$C_L = \frac{0.2\ L}{1\ cmH_2O} = 0.2\ L/cmH_2O$$

This formula indicates that during normal breathing, a transpulmonary pressure change of 1 cmH_2O will overcome the lung elastic recoil pressure and cause a change in lung volume of 0.2 L (200 ml). Remember, 0.2 L/cmH_2O (200 ml/cmH_2O) value represents compliance within the tidal volume range—the value is reduced at higher levels of lung inflation, such as at the end of a *full* inspiration. Also, static compliance is lower (about 0.16 L/cmH_2O) in the supine position because of increased pulmonary blood volume, which decreases lung recoil, and small airway closure at lower lung volumes (Behrakis et al, 1983).

In restrictive lung disease, the patient must produce greater transpulmonary pressure to overcome the increased elastic recoil of "stiff" tissues. Compliance measurements of *less than 0.15 L/cmH_2O* are observed. In contrast, emphysema is characterized by decreased elastic recoil and increased lung compliance, often *above 0.35 L/cmH_2O* (Ayers et al, 1974).

Critical Care Setting. Static compliance may be routinely measured in a patient on mechanical ventilation in the critical care setting, but such measurements are used more for monitoring changes in pulmonary status rather than for medical diagnosis (see Chapter 28 for measurement procedure). Values are considered estimations rather than precise measurements because the standard deviation for the normal value is large. Static compliance for a patient with normal lungs who is ventilated mechanically is 70 to 100 ml/cmH_2O (0.07 to 0.10 L/cmH_2O). In addition, there are logistic difficulties in producing a truly no flow situation in the patient who is mechanically ventilated. Measurements are unreliable if the patient makes respiratory efforts (Guenter and Welch, 1982).

Dynamic Compliance

The previous discussion of compliance helps one to understand the pathology of restrictive lung disease, in particular, and its effect on pulmonary function. It must be remembered, however, that static compliance is different than *dynamic compliance,* a measurement taken during breathing. Once air moves in and out of the lungs, compliance becomes affected by *airway resistance* as well as by elastic recoil. As discussed in Chapter 6, the work of breathing involves overcoming these two resistances of the respiratory system, as follows: *airway resistance,* the major component of nonelastic resistance, and *nonelastic resistance,* pertaining to elastic recoil of the lung.

Though typically present in obstructive disease, increased airway resistance occurs in other situations as well. It was pointed out in Chapter 7 that a restrictive disease may introduce an obstructive component. Fibrous tissue, tumors, pleural effusions, and other restrictive processes can constrict, compress, or impinge on airways, thus contributing to airflow limitation and airway resistance. In addition, airway resistance increases further if an endotracheal tube is present, owing to the narrowed airway diameter and the increase in airway turbulence caused by the tube.

During normal breathing, dynamic compliance may be normal in patients with diseases characterized by increased airway resistance or regional abnormalities in compliance, and *normal* results may be observed on the pulmonary function test in patients with diseases affecting small airways, such as mild asthma or early chronic bronchitis. During rapid breathing, however, increased airway resistance occurs, causing a decrease in dynamic compliance.

In the normal adult, values for dynamic compliance and static compliance are about the same. With an increase in airway resistance, the value for dynamic compliance may be far lower than that for static compliance. Emphysema is a classic example. Although static compliance is much higher than normal, the dramatic increase in airway resistance during breathing and especially *rapid* breathing greatly reduces (dynamic) compliance. In this case, a further reduction in dynamic compliance reflects increasing *airway* resistance from a more rapid breathing or some obstructive process; increasing *elastic* resistance from a superimposed restrictive process that decreases tissue distensibility, e.g., interstitial pulmonary edema; or both.

Critical Care Setting. In the critical care setting, dynamic compliance is measured in the ventilator-dependent patient by monitoring peak tidal volume (change in volume) and inspiratory pressure (change in pressure) on the ventilator's pressure dial (see Chapter 28 for *effective (dynamic) compliance* measurement procedure). Normal dynamic compliance is about 50 to 100 ml/cmH_2O (0.05 to 0.10 L/cmH_2O) or usually no more than about 10 ml/cmH_20 more than the value just obtained for static compliance. As in the pulmonary function laboratory, the value for dynamic compliance is dependent upon respiratory rate—an increased respiratory rate decreases dynamic compliance. Hence, since measurement is *not* made under no flow conditions, any decrease in dynamic compliance may represent a considerable increase in airway resistance from rapid breathing through the ventilator system rather than an actual change in lung compliance (lung elastic resistance).

In the respiratory care unit, bedside measurement of both dynamic and static compliance enables the clinician to determine the presence and magnitude of airway resistance. A large difference between the two measurements indicates an increase in airway resistance from some pathologic process, from rapid breathing, from the patient/ventilator circuit, or from all these conditions.

SUMMARY OF DECREASED LUNGS/CHEST WALL COMPLIANCE

Discussion, thus far, has focused mainly on *lung compliance* (C_L) (listed earlier in the chapter as decreasing compliance) and restrictive processes that make lung tissue stiffer. In addition, C_L may become reduced by pathology in the intrathoracic space compressing on underlying lung tissue, e.g., a large mediastinal mass impinging on lung tissue or air or fluid in the pleural space.

Disorders that increase chest wall stiffness produce a decrease in *chest wall* or *thoracic cage compliance,* abbreviated C_{cw} and C_{tc}, respectively. When the stiff chest wall compresses underlying lung tissue, as in marked pectus excavatum or severe kyphoscoliosis, the patient has a decreased C_L as well as a decreased C_{tc}.

Total Compliance. In the pulmonary function laboratory, the sum of C_L and C_{tc} is the *total compliance* (C_T) of the entire lung and thoracic cage system.

In essence, restrictive disease decreases C_T by decreasing C_L, by decreasing C_{tc}, or by decreasing both components simultaneously to varying degrees. Unfortunately, in the average monitoring situation, it may be difficult if not impossible to determine which component is contributing the most to the decreased C_T.

MAIN PATHOPHYSIOLOGY

Of the three pathologic processes previously discussed—actual loss of lung tissue, loss of functioning alveoli, and decreased lung/chest wall compliance, the last is primarily responsible for most restrictive defects. Stiff lungs or a stiff chest wall prevents full lung expansion and produces a *decrease in lung volume.* Not only is total lung capacity (TLC) reduced, as explained in Chapter 14, but other volumes become reduced also.

Figure 8–6 illustrates how a pulmonary restrictive disease, such as diffuse interstitial fibrosis, produces a

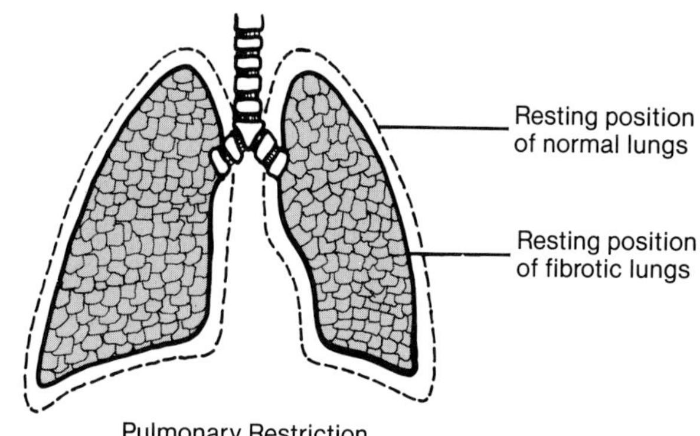

Figure 8–6. Example of pulmonary restriction. Shrunken, fibrotic lung tissue from diffuse interstitial fibrosis results in decreased lung volume (total lung capacity).

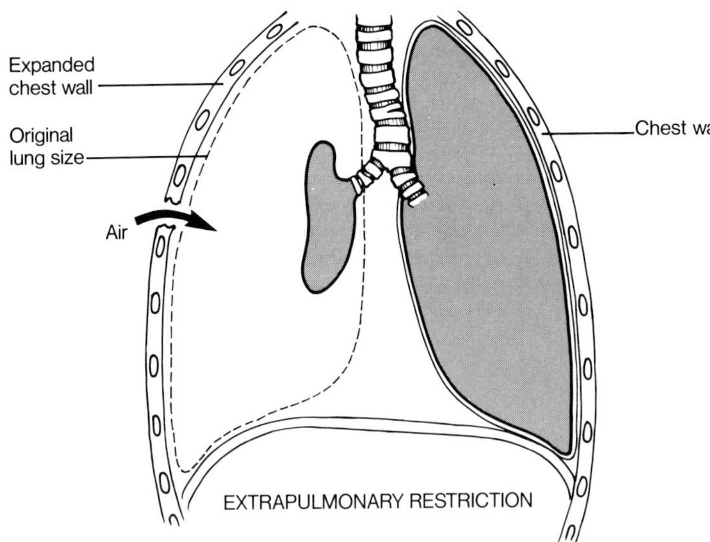

Figure 8–7. Example of extrapulmonary restriction. A chest wall injury permits air to enter the pleural space (open pneumothorax). The lung collapses and cannot reexpand owing to surrounding atmospheric pressure. A drastically reduced lung volume results.

decrease in lung volume. Figure 8–7 demonstrates an extrapulmonary disorder involving the pleural space (open pneumothorax) restricting lung expansion and resulting in a decreased lung volume.

Beyond the mention of decreased compliance and decreased lung volume it is difficult to generalize about the main pathophysiology because so many diverse diseases fall under the restrictive disease category. Discussion here refers primarily to diffuse interstitial fibrosis because (1) it is a classic example of restrictive disease and (2) it is found in other restrictive diseases, such as sarcoidosis, collagen diseases, and the last stage of resolving aspiration pneumonia (see also Diffuse Interstitial Fibrosis).

Uneven Pathology

In brief, the most characteristic defect in restrictive pulmonary disease is *uneven distribution of pathology* in the lungs. Some areas of lung are stiffer than others. In interstitial fibrosis, thickening of the alveolar interstitium is accompanied by obliteration of nearby capillaries and loss of functioning alveolar-capillary units. At any given time, however, the fibrotic process is at different stages in different areas of lung tissue. Where alveolar-capillary units are already lost or extensively damaged, both ventilation and perfusion may be totally absent. Where disease is less extensive, lung tissue is ventilated and perfused to varying degrees, depending on the rate and extent of disease in various groups of alveolar-capillary units. Where healthy lung tissue exists, alveoli are fully ventilated and fully perfused.

Ventilation/Perfusion (V/Q) Ratio

This pathology produces a *normal V/Q ratio* for the lungs as a whole in the case of mild to moderate disease and a *normal to decreased overall V/Q ratio* in the case of advanced interstitial fibrosis (Fig. 8–8).

Two factors account for the normal V/Q ratio found in mild to moderate disease. Although pathology throughout the lung may appear unevenly distributed upon gross examination, fibrotic changes affecting alveolar walls are *equally* matched by the obliteration of nearby capillaries. Also, sufficient numbers of healthy

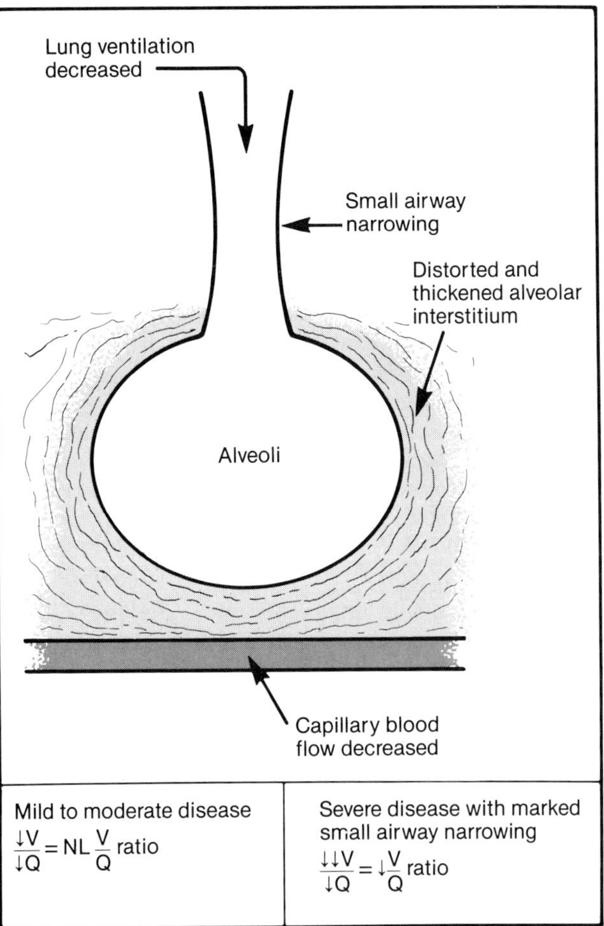

Figure 8–8. Lung pathology and its effect on ventilation/perfusion (V/Q) ratios (see Chapter 1) in diffuse interstitial fibrosis.

alveolar capillary units remain to compensate for diseased regions.

In the case of severe disease *perfusion* is reduced because the obliteration of capillaries significantly decreases the size of the pulmonary capillary bed. However, *ventilation* may be decreased to a *greater* degree owing to extensive fibrosis and accompanying *small airway narrowing*. Perfusion in excess of ventilation decreases the V/Q ratio.

Small airway narrowing associated with fibrosis is now known to occur in many interstitial lung diseases, including *idiopathic pulmonary fibrosis, sarcoidosis, hypersensitivity pneumonitis, asbestosis,* and *coal worker's pneumoconiosis.* The etiology of the obstructive process is not fully understood, but it is believed to be due to the fibrotic process itself, the loss of airway support, or both (Crystal et al, 1981). Small airway obstruction at least partially explains the development of inflammatory airway disease, airway clearance problems, and chest infections that occur late in the disease process.

Normal to Decreased Pa_{O_2}

In interstitial fibrosis, Pa_{O_2} may be normal at rest and decrease only during exercise. As disease progresses, the patient becomes hypoxemic at rest as well as during exercise.

At rest, the decreased Pa_{O_2} may be largely explained by the abnormal V/Q ratio. Lung ventilation is decreased proportionately more than cardiac output, because some alveolar-capillary units in diseased lung regions are perfused but remain completely or nearly unventilated (see Chapter 13 for V/Q abnormality as a cause of hypoxemia).

Particularly *during exercise,* however, this V/Q mismatching is believed to play a minor role in producing a decreased Pa_{O_2}. Two other factors contribute to the drop in Pa_{O_2} during exercise as follows: *diffusion impairment* and *decreased cardiac output* (Wagner and West, 1980).

The diffusion of gases across the alveolar-capillary membrane becomes impaired because the interstitial thickening characteristic of interstitial fibrosis slows gas diffusion. Now researchers believe that a thickened interstitium affects Pa_{O_2} in this way *only* during exercise *not* at rest, as previously thought. Yet, this mechanism's contribution to the drop in Pa_{O_2} is small and was estimated by Wagner and West to be 15% of the total alveolar-arterial P_{O_2} difference.

In advanced disease, perhaps the most limiting factor in the patient's ability to oxygenate body tissues is the *decreased cardiac output.* The heart has a limited ability to increase cardiac output since disease has decreased the size of the pulmonary capillary bed. Although cardiac output may be normal at rest, during exercise or stressful events, the heart is unable to significantly increase cardiac output to permit full oxygenation of blood. Because the body's oxygen-starved tissues extract most of the oxygen from circulating systemic blood, the P_{O_2} of mixed venous blood returning to the right side of the heart drops below the normal level. This drop in the P_{O_2} of mixed venous blood can drastically worsen the patient's oxygenation problem.

Patent Airways and Alveolar Ventilation

The patient with restrictive disease typically has relatively normal airway mechanics and absent ventilatory problems until end-stage disease. Though the patient may be short of breath, major airways remain patent and unobstructed by secretions; air is able to reach acinar units for gas exchange. Pa_{O_2} may drop as previously described, but alveolar ventilation or Pa_{CO_2} remains within normal limits.

If lung compliance or Pa_{O_2} becomes greatly reduced, however, Pa_{CO_2} drops, as lung reflexes stimulate a rapid shallow breathing pattern and alveolar hyperventilation.

MAIN SIGNS AND SYMPTOMS

The aforementioned pathologic changes produce increased work of breathing. The patient breathes rapidly (tachypnea) and shallowly (decreased tidal volumes) to increase minute ventilation and maintain normal alveolar ventilation. *Tachypnea* and *decreased tidal volumes* are the characteristic signs of restrictive pulmonary disease. The main symptom is *shortness of breath,* at first only during exertion and later at rest. Accompanying symptoms depend on the patient's specific chest disease. Generally, they tend to be vague and may include *chest pain, fatigue, irritating nonproductive cough,* and *weight loss.* Sometimes, a decreased Pa_{O_2} is the only objective clinical manifestation of disease (Table 8–1).

PROGRESSION OF DISEASE

The courses of individual diseases and survival rates are variable. With chronic disease, such as diffuse interstitial fibrosis, the disease process has already significantly altered lung pathology by the time shortness of breath appears. Patients with acute forms of disease may die within 1 year of onset. Others may

Table 8–1. MAIN SIGNS AND SYMPTOMS OF RESTRICTIVE PULMONARY DISEASE (DIFFUSE INTERSTITIAL FIBROSIS)

Signs	Symptoms
Increased respiratory rate (tachypnea)	Shortness of breath
Decreased tidal volume	Cough
Normal to decreased Pa_{O_2}	Chest pain or discomfort
	Fatigue
	History of weight loss

live 10 or more years after symptoms appear. The mean survival time for a patient with idiopathic pulmonary fibrosis from the onset of symptoms until death is about 4 years (Keogh and Crystal, 1981). Generally, the more fibrosis present in the lung, the more irreversible the disease and the shorter the survival time.

In many cases of interstitial fibrosis, the progression of disease is a persistent downhill course, as in emphysema. In others, disease activity waxes and wanes. Relapses may occur after months to years of apparent stability. Sometimes, the physician may not know exactly how advanced the patient's disease is because the traditional and readily available physiologic tests help determine disability but cannot be used for accurate staging of the disease. Currently, the best method to initially stage the disease is the *open lung biopsy*, an invasive, uncomfortable, somewhat risky, and costly procedure. It is done in the hospital, usually only once in the patient's disease course for diagnostic purposes.

Often, what prompts the patient to seek medical care is sputum production and other symptoms associated with *acute bronchitis*. Patients with moderate to severe disease commonly experience episodes of acute bronchitis. In addition, *bacterial* or *fungal chest infections* may occur late in the disease course, when the patient is highly susceptible to such infections. Small airway obstruction is commonly present, as previously mentioned, making it more difficult for the patient to keep distal airways and alveoli clear of secretions. Lung volumes are reduced to such a degree that generating adequate air flow for an effective cough becomes difficult. Also, the body's defense mechanisms have been weakened by disease. Any superimposed bacterial infection may be fatal to the patient because of his or her already compromised lung function and overall physical condition. Hence, sputum production and other signs of possible infection or air flow limitation must be promptly reported to the physician so that the patient can receive early and aggressive treatment for the bronchitic component, infection, or other process.

The patient in Figure 8–9 demonstrated all the classic findings of one with restrictive pulmonary disease. Her medical diagnosis was diffuse interstitial fibrosis secondary to radiation treatments for Hodgkin's disease. Signs and symptoms gradually worsened over the last 10 years of her life. Because of ventilatory failure, she spent the last several years at home supported by a volume ventilator and supplementary oxygen. In a stable state, she breathed very shallowly and rapidly at a rate of 25 to 35 respirations/min while on the ventilator most of the day. The ventilator used extremely high pressures (peak pressures of over 30 mmHg) to deliver the preset volume of air to her stiff, noncompliant lungs. This patient complained only of shortness of breath during physical exertion and cough and sputum production early in the morning. Shortness of breath at rest developed after 30 to 120 minutes off the ventilator, often while playing cards with visiting friends. Generally speaking, this patient's pulmonary signs and symptoms deteriorated only when she developed the complications of acute bronchitis and pneumonia from retained secretions and right heart failure associated with advanced pulmonary disease.

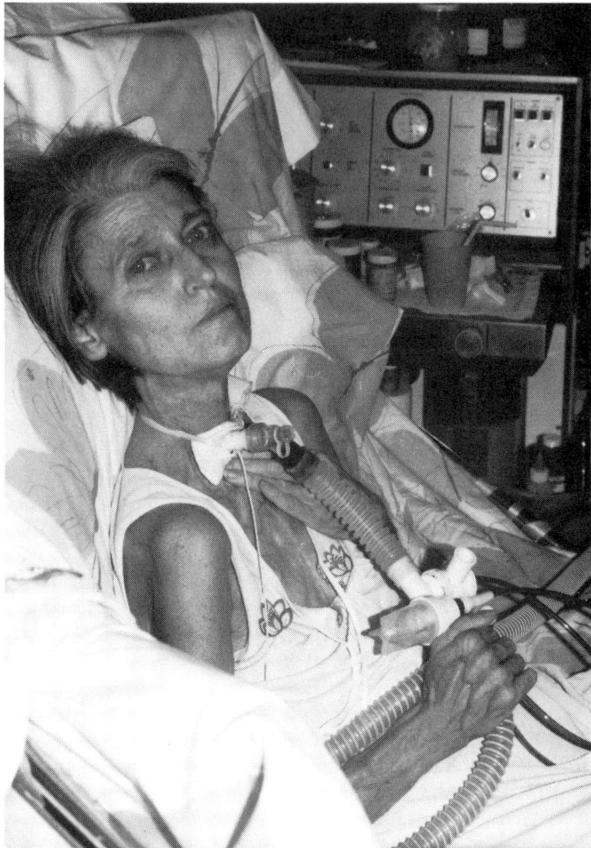

Figure 8–9. Patient with restrictive pulmonary disease on mechanical ventilation at home.

GOALS AND INTERVENTIONS

Basic goals and interventions for restrictive pulmonary disease are summarized in the box and explained in subsequent chapters.

In the summary presented, note that interventions are similar to those already given for chronic obstructive pulmonary disease (COPD) in Chapter 7, with a few exceptions. First, bronchodilator medications are not routinely used in restrictive disease, unless the patient has an accompanying obstructive component. Second, coughing and postural drainage techniques are not used in restrictive disease, unless lobar pneumonia or chronic bronchitis is also present.

Last, as in COPD, breathing retraining is implemented to improve respiratory muscle strength as well as ventilation and oxygenation. However, in restrictive disease, it is currently implemented *without* pursed-lip breathing. Pursed-lip breathing is a technique used

GOALS AND INTERVENTIONS FOR RESTRICTIVE PULMONARY DISEASE

GOALS

- Promote normal oxygenation
- Maintain patent airways and fully inflated alveoli
- Maintain highest possible level of functional activity

INTERVENTIONS

- Pulmonary medications—corticosteroids or none, unless an obstructive disease component is present.
- Bronchial hygiene program
  - Deep breathing
  - Hydration
  - Balanced diet
  - Environmental control
  - General relaxation
  - Breathing retraining
- Progressive exercise conditioning
  - Gravity resistance or range of motion exercises
  - Walking, bicycling, and so forth
  - Arm ergometry (arm bicycle)
- Oxygen therapy
- Mechanical ventilation (severe disease)
- Self-care education

by patients with obstructive disease to improve oxygenation and ventilation, relieve dyspnea, and thus increase activity tolerance. When performed appropriately, the use of pursed lips creates positive pressure in the lungs and prevents airway collapse during expiration, a problem in COPD. Also, it increases tidal volume and decreases respiratory rate, with minute ventilation remaining about the same. Research findings suggest that in many patients, increased tidal volume and decreased respiratory rate alone, without the extra positive airway pressure, may be enough to improve PaO_2 during pursed-lip breathing (Tiep et al, 1986). The implication is that patients with restrictive disease may in fact benefit from use of pursed-lip breathing, as a way to decrease anatomic dead space ventilation from their rapid shallow breathing pattern, thereby increasing PaO_2.

Conclusion

Restrictive pulmonary disease represents a wide variety of acute and chronic clinical entities. Mild to moderate chronic disease may go unrecognized because the patient has minimal to no complaints; pulmonary problems are overshadowed by more visible disease affecting other bodily organs. Shortness of breath develops in moderate to severe forms of disease. End-stage disease is marked by the development of pulmonary hypertension, right ventricular hypertrophy (cor pulmonale), severe oxygenation problems, right-sided heart failure, and ultimately ventilatory failure. These disorders are further explored in subsequent chapters.

The remainder of this chapter reviews extrapulmonary and pulmonary restrictive diseases listed in the box on page 123. By providing an overview of main diseases and related pathology, this section facilitates cue interpretation in decision-making processes discussed in the last part of this book. The content on diffuse interstitial disease clarifies the numerous terms used to describe chronic interstitial lung diseases and stresses features common to all types, regardless of the specific disease entity involved.

Extrapulmonary Restriction

PLEURAL DISEASE

Common pleural disorders are defined next. These disorders and others may be diagnosed as idiopathic findings, as separate disease entities, or more commonly as associated with other pulmonary or extrapulmonary diseases.

Pleural Effusion

Excessive amounts of fluid in the pleural space are known as pleural effusions. The disorder is a frequent manifestation of serious cardiopulmonary disease and occasionally is the first evidence of an important extrathoracic or systemic disease.

Hemothorax

Blood in the pleural space or hemothorax is usually from chest trauma or as a postoperative complication after major chest surgery.

Chylothorax

The accumulation of thoracic duct lymph or chyle, in the pleural space, usually from injury or obstruction of the thoracic duct, is defined as chylothorax. This disorder is associated with trauma, malignancy, or occasionally congenital abnormalities in newborn infants.

Empyema *(Pyothorax)*

Empyema is the accumulation of pus in the pleural cavity. Although the pus usually is infected with microorganisms, uninfected purulent pleural effusions may occur contiguous to an inflammatory process.

Pneumothorax

The presence of gas in the pleural space, occurring from trauma with a pathologic process or without a known inciting event, is termed pneumothorax. Gas usually enters the pleural space by (1) perforation of the visceral pleura and entry of gas *from within* the lung, (2) penetration of the chest wall and parietal pleura and entry of gas *from outside* the body, and (3) formation of gas within the pleural space by gas-forming microorganisms in an empyema (Hinshaw and Murray, 1980). When pneumothorax occurs from an internal cause (e.g., perforation of the visceral pleura and entry of gas from within the lung), the communication between the pleural space and tracheobronchial tree is termed a *bronchopleural fistula. Traumatic pneumothorax* usually occurs as a result of a knife stab, gunshot wound, or other similar wound that penetrates from outside the chest. The pneumothorax is defined as *open* when air moves freely in and out of the pleural space during respiration (Fig. 8–7). It is referred to as *closed* when no air movement takes place (the chest wall remains intact, as in perforation of the visceral pleura and entry of gas from within the lung).

Spontaneous pneumothorax, by far the commonest form of pneumothorax, occurs without an inciting event, in most cases from spontaneous rupture of a small and usually undetectable subpleural alveolar cyst or bleb. The patient is typically a young adult male, and the event occurs most frequently in the lung apex, where mechanical stresses and strains within the lung are greatest. In patients over 40 years of age, spontaneous pneumothorax is most frequently in association with COPD, when tissue destruction and bullae are present. In a small percentage of patients, spontaneous pneumothorax may be a recurrent disorder.

Tension pneumothorax occurs when air in the pleural space is under tension—air enters the pleural space on inspiration but cannot exit on expiration.

Fibrothorax *(Pleural Thickening)*

Fibrothorax is the formation of nonelastic fibrous tissue within the pleural space as a result of an incompletely drained previous hemothorax or empyema or as a result of recurrent pneumothoraces. When an abnormal coat of fibrous tissue covers the lung, resembling the peel of an orange, it is often referred to as *pleural peel.* The presence of pleural peel may require a surgical operation called *decortication* defined as *surgical removal of the fibrous peel from the pleura.*

Pleuritis *(Pleurisy)*

Inflammation of the pleura usually occurs acutely often in association with a serious disease, such as pneumonia, pulmonary embolism, tuberculosis, and malignant disease. Since the term pleurisy also is defined as inflammation of the pleura, some clinicians use the two terms synonymously. Others use the term *pleurisy* loosely to refer to any inconsequential thoracic pain and *pleuritis* to refer to more acute localized pain from a serious disease. Because of the serious implications, the presence of acute pleuritis requires the physician to reach an exact diagnosis without delay.

In a patient with clinical manifestations of pleural disease, air, as in pneumothorax; fluid, as in pleural effusion; or a tumor may occupy the pleural space, limiting expansion of underlying lung tissue. In the case of a large pneumothorax affecting more than 50% of a single lung, air in the pleural space compresses underlying lung tissue, causing lung collapse. With great reductions in lung volume, the patient eventually is unable to move enough air in and out of the lungs to maintain adequate blood oxygenation. The critically ill patient, especially one with limited cardiopulmonary reserve, cannot adequately increase cardiac output to compensate for greatly impaired lung ventilation: a severe ventilation/perfusion abnormality occurs. Without immediate treatment, such gross pleural pathology produces respiratory distress and respiratory failure in minutes to hours.

With minor pleural pathology (e.g., a small pleural effusion of less then 200 ml of fluid and a small benign tumor), lung function may remain normal or near normal, and the patient may be completely asymptomatic. In the critical-care setting, the patient with minor pleural problems is not critically ill from the small pleural effusion, for example, but from the underlying disease process. Pleural effusion is a common manifestation of many serious illnesses, including congestive heart failure, constrictive pericarditis, lupus erythematosus, cirrhosis, and malignant disease. Furthermore, it is a common postoperative complication of thoraco-abdominal surgery.

In contrast, other pleural diseases may develop over a period of weeks, months, or years, some eventually producing life-threatening disease. Small localized areas of nonelastic fibrotic tissue may have no effect on lung function. But, if this type of tissue eventually lines a large part of the lung's surface, lung expansion becomes markedly restricted, and ventilatory function becomes impaired.

CHEST WALL STIFFNESS

Musculoskeletal abnormalities affecting the trunk of the body, as in kyphoscoliosis, can produce a very stiff, noncompliant chest wall. Respiratory muscles become ineffective because they are unable to fully mobilize the thoracic cage during respiration. Underlying lung tissue cannot fully expand. With the resulting impaired ventilation and gradually diminishing lung volumes, the patient's respiratory rate and work of breathing increases. Impairment of lung function may be accompanied by impairment of cardiac function.

Chapter 12 reviews various musculoskeletal abnormalities that affect chest configuration. Of those listed, abnormalities most likely to produce significant restrictive lung disease are mentioned next. (The first two, kyphoscoliosis and pectus excavatum, are discussed in further detail in Chapter 12 in relation to abnormal chest configurations.)

Kyphoscoliosis

Kyphoscoliosis is a progressive musculoskeletal deformity characterized by lateral and posterior angulations of the spine. Gradual disability results from impairment of pulmonary and eventually cardiac function.

Pectus Excavatum *(Funnel Chest)*

Pectus excavatum (funnel chest) is depression of the lower end of the sternum, creating a hollow pit in that area, displacement of intrathoracic structures, and abnormal development of the anterior portion of the diaphragm. The condition usually is a congenital malformation. Respiratory failure can result from pronounced deformity.

Ankylosing Spondylitis *(Marie-Strümpell Disease)*

Ankylosing spondylitis is a progressive inflammatory disease similar to rheumatoid arthritis, involving the spine, particularly the joints between articular processes; the costovertebral joints; the sacroiliac joints; the adjacent soft tissues; and other structures. The exact etiology of this disease is unknown, but it is thought to be related to the presence of a particular antigen in the body (HLA-B27 antigen). It is most commonly found in young males, manifesting itself clinically in the second or third decade of life. Progression of the disease up the spinal column to the thoracic spine results in fixation of the chest cage in the inspiratory position and lung hyperinflation. Kyphosis develops and becomes more marked, as the spinal column fuses in position. Occasionally associated with pulmonary fibrosis in the upper lobes and cavitary infiltrations, ankylosing spondylitis can cause significant impairment of pulmonary function—vital capacity on the pulmonary function test may be reduced to 70% or less of predicted values (Fraser and Paré, 1979).

Obesity

Obesity is defined as an increase in body weight 20 to 30% over the individual's average weight for age, sex, and height, due to excessive food intake or some endocrine or metabolic abnormality within the body. In gross obesity, the noncompliant thick chest wall is largely responsible for restricted lung expansion, reduced lung volume, and increased work of breathing. Other abnormalities that contribute to impaired ventilation include the following:

1. Less efficient functioning of respiratory muscles.
2. Airway closure in dependent areas of the lungs, particularly in the lower lobes, where a protuberant abdomen pushes upward to compress lung tissue and restrict lung expansion.
3. Increased oxygen consumption, increased carbon dioxide retention (alveolar hypoventilation), and increased minute ventilation necessary to provide adequate tissue oxygenation to the greater body mass.

These physiologic changes predispose the patient to pulmonary complications, such as atelectasis and retained secretions, especially when lung function becomes compromised by complete bed rest, anesthesia, surgical procedures, or respiratory depressant medications.

Gross obesity with alveolar hypoventilation and daytime somnolence is now known to represent the *obstructive type* of the *sleep apnea syndrome* (discussed subsequently). In the past, it has been commonly referred to as the *pickwickian syndrome*, a name stemming from Charles Dickens's portrayal of Joe, the fat, somnolent, red-faced boy in *Pickwick Papers*. Patients with this disorder are especially prone to cardiopulmonary problems, including increased work of breathing, increased cardiac workload, muscle deconditioning, atelectasis, and mucus retention.

RESPIRATORY MUSCLE WEAKNESS

Extrapulmonary restrictive disease may be due to respiratory muscle weakness from a variety of causes. Related to neuromuscular dysfunction, most disorders in this category are characterized by a decrease in lung volume due to malfunctioning of the respiratory muscles themselves or of their neural pathways. Some may involve brain stem respiratory centers, as in bulbar poliomyelitis. The nature and extent of the muscle weakness and paralysis determine the severity of the respiratory dysfunction. Respiratory impairment may be *partial*, with selective muscle involvement; *complete*, with complete muscle involvement and complete paralysis; *transitory*, as in Guillain-Barré; or *permanent*.

The neuromuscular diseases that affect lung function produce ineffective breathing patterns, limited ability to sigh or cough effectively, decreased Pa_{O_2}, increased Pa_{CO_2}, and eventually ventilatory failure when the body's compensatory mechanisms cannot restore arterial blood gases to relatively normal levels. In the chronic condition and especially in the case of the persistent cigarette smoker, ineffective coughing and impaired lung ventilation predispose the patient to the accumulation of respiratory secretions, repeated chest infections, and eventual development of obstructive pulmonary disease.

Some neuromuscular disorders that commonly produce respiratory problems are summarized in the subsequent sections.

Muscular Dystrophy

A genetically determined degenerative disease characterized by atrophy and wasting of muscles. The various types of muscular dystrophy are differentiated on the basis of the predominant muscle groups involved, the age of onset of symptoms, and the rate at which the disease progresses. Selective weakness of trunk muscles leads to postural problems, skeletal distortion, and in severe cases all of the problems associated with kyphoscoliosis. If expiratory muscles are weakened, cough becomes impaired. Progressive muscular weakness not only involves respiratory muscles but often involves heart muscle as well.

Amyotrophic Lateral Sclerosis *(Charcot's disease or Lou Gehrig's disease)*

A severe disease characterized by muscular weakness and muscle atrophy with spasticity and hyperreflexia due to degeneration of motor neurons of the spinal cord, medulla, and cortex. This disease is a chronic progressive one of unknown etiology, occurring in middle-aged individuals. Once the initial symptoms of weakness and wasting of the extremities (usually the upper extremities) occurs, the disease course is progressively downhill and without remission. When the respiratory muscles become affected, mechanical ventilation becomes necessary. Survival time from the onset of symptoms is about 3 years.

Guillain-Barré Syndrome *(Infectious Polyneuritis)*

This syndrome is a disorder of unknown etiology characterized by ascending muscular weakness, impairment of reflexes, and sensory disorders. It usually begins with fever, usually from an upper respiratory tract infection, which precedes the onset of paralytic symptoms by 1 to 3 weeks. The extent of muscle weakness varies depending on the severity of individual cases. When paralysis of respiratory muscles, dysphagia, and speech difficulties develop, mechanical ventilation becomes necessary. Most patients with this disease recover in weeks to months with minimal to no residual impairment of lung function.

Myasthenia Gravis

This is a chronic disease characterized by progressive fatigability and muscle weakness (without atrophy), especially involving the facial, ocular, laryngeal, pharyngeal, and respiratory muscles. The disease occurs with periodic relapses and remissions and most commonly affects females in their twenties. Acute exacerbations may be precipitated by upper respiratory tract infections, emotional upset, fatigue, or alcohol intake. In this disease, nerve impulses fail to induce normal muscle contractions, owing to a lack of acetylcholine or an excess of cholinesterase at the myoneural junction. The specific etiology is unknown.

Hemiplegia

Hemiplegia is defined as paralysis of half the body, commonly as a result of a stroke or brain lesion. Patients with hemiplegia have less pulmonary vasculature in addition to limited diaphragmatic and intercostal mobility on the affected side (Haas et al, 1979). They also tend to have low PaO_2 levels, especially during exercise, and abnormal pulmonary function values, as determined by a pulmonary function test. Respiratory dysfunction has gone relatively unrecognized in these patients until recently.

Quadriplegia

This type of paralysis involves all four extremities, occurring most frequently from trauma—automobile accidents, diving accidents, other sports-related mishaps, and gunshot wounds. Other causes are congenital deformities, infections involving the spinal cord, neoplasms, and vascular anomalies.

If the area of damage lies below the third cervical vertebrae (C3), the complete quadriplegic has a partially or completely intact diaphragm but totally paralyzed intercostal and abdominal muscles; pulmonary function remains relatively normal during rest, but forced expiratory maneuvers, such as coughing, are impaired.

The quadriplegic patient with injury above the C3-C5 level demonstrates partial or complete diaphragmatic paralysis because the diaphragm is enervated by C3-C5 motor neurons.

Respiratory failure is common in the immediate postinjury period in a patient with high cervical cord involvement due to direct injury to the area or due to tissue edema spreading upward from a lower cervical injury. Flaccid paralysis of respiratory muscles may cause paradoxical retraction of the chest cage, which limits lung expansion and further impairs ventilation. These processes stabilize within the first year after the causative traumatic event. With little to no ability to cough, the patient may begin to accumulate respiratory secretions in the lungs, especially during the postinjury period of immobility. Without proper bronchial hygiene, the presence of secretions predisposes the patient to chest infections and atelectasis.

OTHER CAUSES

Other extrapulmonary conditions can also restrict lung expansion and impair ventilation. Lung volumes are reduced in patients with abdominal distension from ascites, abdominal tumors, large ovarian cysts, and the later stages of normal pregnancy. In the medical-surgical patient, abdominal distention hinders diaphragmatic movement and, in severe cases, compresses lung tissue to produce airway collapse and pooling of respiratory secretions in dependent areas of the lungs. Chest binders and body braces can have the same effects on underlying lung tissue.

Hypoventilation due to dysfunction of automatic control of breathing may be considered an extrapulmonary disorder. Because of primary alveolar hypoventilation (Ondine's curse) or neurologic disease affecting the brain and central nervous system (CNS), hypoventilation is characterized by a slow respiratory rate and shallow breathing, at times interrupted by apnea (cessation of breathing), especially during sleep.

Sleep Apnea Syndrome

This syndrome actually belongs in a category of its own because it is neither a pure restrictive nor a pure obstructive disorder. The syndrome is placed in this section since one underlying physiologic mechanism involves a CNS control of breathing dysfunction that results in hypoventilation and apnea during the night.

The *sleep apnea syndrome* must be differentiated from *sleep apnea.* On the one hand, brief periods of *sleep apnea* at night are not uncommon in normal individuals (see Chapter 12 for the normal breathing pattern during sleep). Apneic episodes may vary greatly in duration and frequency among individuals; they are considered normal and do not require treatment.

The *sleep apnea syndrome,* on the other hand, is considered a disorder manifested by apneic episodes that are so numerous and prolonged that the patient usually requires medical treatment. More specifically, the syndrome is defined as *30 or more apneic episodes, lasting at least 10 seconds, observed during 7 hours of nocturnal sleep* (Guilleminault et al, 1976). Patients have 200 to 500 episodes of prolonged apnea each night, and commonly more than 50% of the time slept is without effective alveolar ventilation (Sanders, 1980). This syndrome was once associated with obese patients (pickwickian syndrome); it is now known to occur in nonobese individuals also. Sleep apnea syndrome is associated with a broad range of disorders, including *sudden infant death syndrome (SIDS),* a cause of "crib death."

Although the etiology is currently under investigation, the syndrome in adults appears to be an exaggeration of normal phenomena during sleep. Sleep apnea that lasts longer than 15 to 120 seconds is a concern because the drop in Pa_{O_2} and alveolar hypoventilation contributes to the development of pulmonary hypertension and chronic cor pulmonale. Sinus bradycardia or other cardiac arrhythmias may precipitate cardiopulmonary arrest.

Types of Sleep Apnea. Three main types of sleep apnea are summarized in Table 8–2. Because a CNS disorder is involved in *all* types of sleep apnea, patients are categorized depending on which of the following type predominates: *obstructive, central,* or *mixed.*

In *obstructive apnea,* respiratory drive is present, but the tongue is sucked back into the upper airway, possibly because of malfunctions of the genioglossus muscle, which normally contracts during inspiration to prevent airway obstruction. In addition, the lateral pharyngeal walls collapse inward. Although air flow ceases, respiratory muscular efforts persist, and the patient generates large intrathoracic pressures—up to 100 cmH_2O—in an attempt to move air past the obstruction. Apneic episodes severe enough to precipitate a drop in Pa_{O_2} occur primarily in obstructive apnea rather than in central apnea.

Central apnea is less common than the obstructive type. The patient stops breathing due to an incompletely understood CNS abnormality affecting respiratory centers in the brain. Unlike the obstructive type, no thoracic or abdominal respiratory effort to breathe is exerted.

In *mixed apnea,* central apnea is followed by obstructive apnea. No disorders are listed in the mixed category in Table 8–2 because usually either the central or obstructive type is found to predominate in most patients; there are no clear criteria for the mixed apnea category.

In all three types, each apneic episode is followed by incomplete awakening, with resumption of respiratory efforts in the central type. In the obstructive type, relief of the upper airway obstruction permits resumption of air movement with each respiratory effort.

A definitive medical diagnosis is made by studying

Table 8–2. TYPES OF SLEEP APNEA

Type	Characteristic Feature	Associated Disorders
Obstructive	Cessation of air flow in spite of respiratory (muscular) effort (upper airway obstruction)	Obesity Enlarged tonsils and adenoids Enlarged tongue, as in myxedema Deviated nasal septum Vocal cord paralysis Laryngeal stenosis Mandibular malformations Sudden infant death syndrome (in older infants)
Central	Cessation of air flow without respiratory effort (primary CNS abnormality)	Idiopathic alveolar hypoventilation (Ondine's curse) Brain stem diseases: poliomyelitis, encephalitis, brain stem infarction, and neoplasm Spinal cord disorders: cervical chordotomy and anterior spinal cord surgery Sudden infant death syndrome
Mixed	Central apnea followed by obstructive type	Any disorder with both obstructive and central apneas

the individual during sleep by polysomnography in the hospital, out-patient clinic, or sometimes the physician's office. *Polysomnography* involves monitoring a number of measurements noninvasively, as the individual passes through the various stages of sleep during a single night. Monitoring parameters may include the electroencephalogram (EEG), right and left electro-oculograms, genioglossal electromyogram, airflow at the mouth or in the upper airway as well as diaphragmatic or chest wall movement, and oxygen saturation (using oximetry). The essential measurements are EEG, airflow at the mouth or in the upper airway, and diaphragmatic or chest wall movement.

Pulmonary Restriction

SURGICAL RESECTION

Surgical resection of lung tissue causes significant long-term pulmonary restrictive disease only when large amounts of lung tissue are removed. *Pneumonectomy*, defined as total removal of a lung, results in a drastic reduction in lung volume. Over a period of 6 to 8 months, the remaining lung maximally hyperinflates to accommodate for the loss of alveolar capillary surface area. Lung volumes and flow rates on the routine pulmonary function test drastically improve over this period of time but never become completely normal. Following a *lobectomy* (removal of a lobe of a lung), lung volumes are only temporarily reduced. In 6 weeks to a few months, the remainder of the lung hyperinflates until it is normal or near normal in size. Lung function returns to normal or near normal provided that the rest of the lung is healthy. For both pneumonectomy and lobectomy, accompanying atelectasis in the postoperative period will further decrease lung volume, worsening the restrictive defect.

ATELECTASIS

Atelectasis is incomplete expansion of the lung resulting in collapse of lung tissue. Primary atelectasis may occur as a result of failure of the lung to expand at birth, but most cases occur later in life after the lung has been fully inflated.

A patient may develop atelectasis from one or more of the following processes: *airway obstruction*, *abnormal breathing pattern*, and *compression of lung tissue*. Pathology for these processes is discussed subsequently, and adventitious lung sounds on physical examination are reviewed in Table 12–15.

Airway Obstruction

Obstruction of a main stem or lobar bronchus from a large tumor, foreign object, mucus plug, or other process may cause *partial* or *complete* occlusion of the airway. In complete bronchial obstruction, gas may be totally absorbed into the pulmonary circulation from alveoli distal to the obstruction, producing what is known as *absorption atelectasis* (Fig. 8–10). With partial bronchial obstruction, atelectasis is likely, and its extent is related to the degree to which alveolar ventilation becomes impaired. When obstruction of a segmental or smaller bronchi occurs, the extent of atelectasis depends on the extent of collateral ventilation keeping alveoli open.

One must remember that bronchial obstruction does not always cause atelectasis. Sometimes, in partial obstruction, the airway remains patent during inspiration but totally occludes during expiration owing to the normal airway narrowing during this phase of respiration. When air gets in but cannot get out, the affected lung overdistends distally to the site of the obstructive lesion.

Lung overdistention or *hyperinflation* also is observed in the *check-valve* type of partial bronchial obstruction. In Figure 8–11, pathology, such as an endobronchial tumor, is attached to the bronchial wall by a peduncle that acts as a one-way valve or trap door. With normal air way widening during inspiration, air easily passes over the peduncle (see Fig. 8–11). During expiration, however, normal air way narrowing as well as the shape of the peduncle contributes to complete occlusion, blocked expiratory air flow, and eventual lung overdistention (hyperinflation), as represented in Figure 8–11.

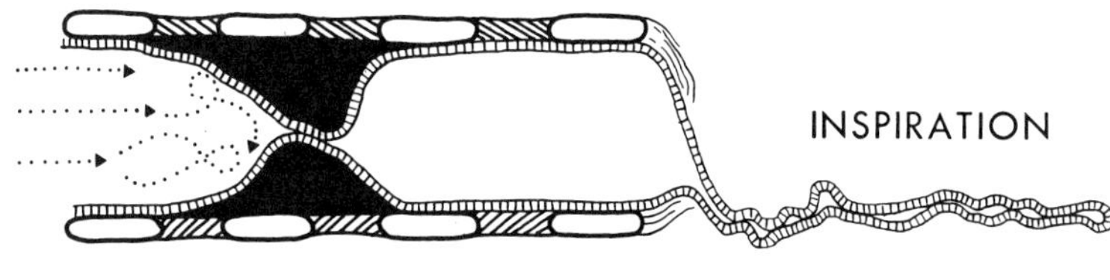

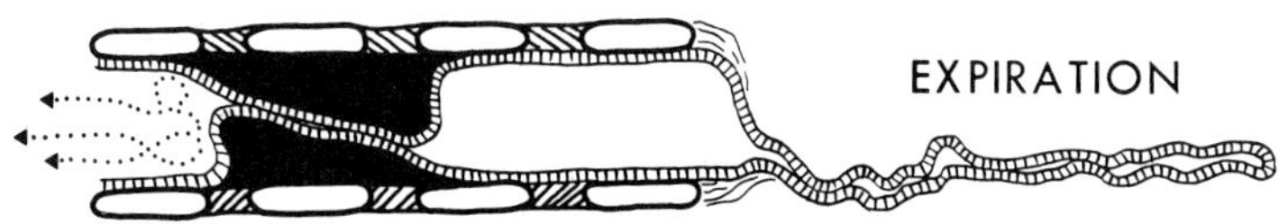

Figure 8–10. Total bronchial obstruction resulting in absorption atelectasis distal to the site of obstruction. (Reproduced by permission from Cherniack, R. and Cherniack, L.: Respiration in Health and Disease, 2nd ed. Philadelphia, W. B. Saunders Co., 1983.)

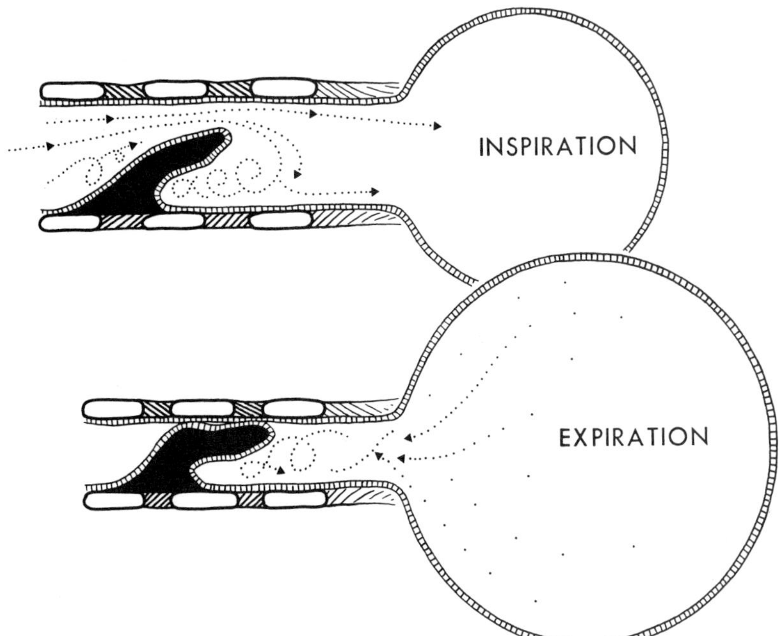

Figure 8–11. Check-valve, partial bronchial obstruction resulting in lung over distention (hyperinflation). (Reproduced by permission from Cherniack, R. and Cherniack, L.: Respiration in Health and Disease, 2nd ed. Philadelphia, W. B. Saunders Co., 1983.)

Abnormal Breathing Pattern

Different patterns of abnormal breathing described in Chapter 12, including hypoventilation and bradypnea (i.e., decreased respiratory rate), may result in incomplete expansion of the lungs and atelectasis. Atelectasis results from very shallow and monotonous breathing patterns, as seen during immobility: use of sedative, hypnotic, or tranquilizer medications: and abdominal or chest pain. Thoraco-abdominal surgical patients splint from pain postoperatively, producing the monotonous breathing pattern shown in Figure 8–12A. Note this pattern is characterized by reduced tidal volumes and the absence of normal periodic signs characteristic of a normal breathing pattern (Fig. 8–12B). Since postoperative atelectasis is a major concern of hospital nurses, it is briefly discussed further in the section so identified.

Compression of Lung Tissue

Another cause of atelectasis is *compression of lung tissue*. Gross pathologic processes that lie just peripheral to lung tissue, such as a large pneumothorax, an abdominal distention, or a large pleural effusion, compress adjacent lung tissue and prevent full lung expansion. Gross obesity can cause atelectasis due to a restrictive thick chest wall and compression of tissue in the lung bases from a large abdomen. Furthermore, space-occupying lesions in the lung parenchyma, such as large tumors or large air cavities (pneumatoceles), fall under this category. A *pneumatocele* is an air cavity larger than a bulla, occupying a volume of about one third of a lung. It is a rare finding but can occur in destructive processes, such as advanced emphysema and severe lung infections with tissue necrosis. Atelectasis develops when the walls of the large lesion or cavity compress surrounding lung tissue and prevent full lung expansion.

Postoperative Atelectasis

Of the four main types of postoperative pulmonary complications—atelectasis, pneumonia, pulmonary embolism, and pulmonary edema—*atelectasis* is by far the most frequent. Basic information about the pathogenesis of this disorder is summarized, as follows:

1. Atelectasis and associated pulmonary sequelae (e.g., low Pa_{O_2}, mucus retention, pneumonia) are most

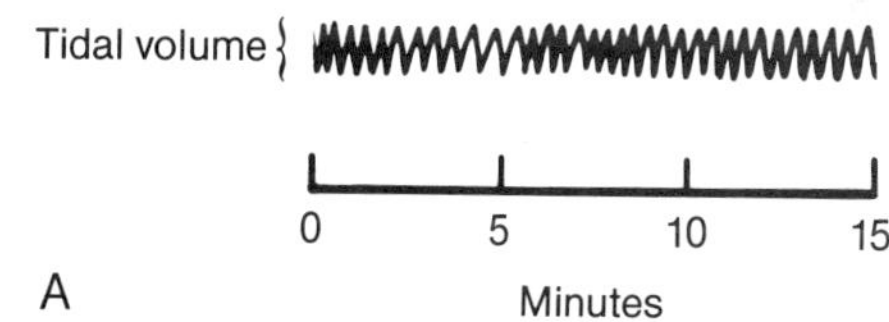

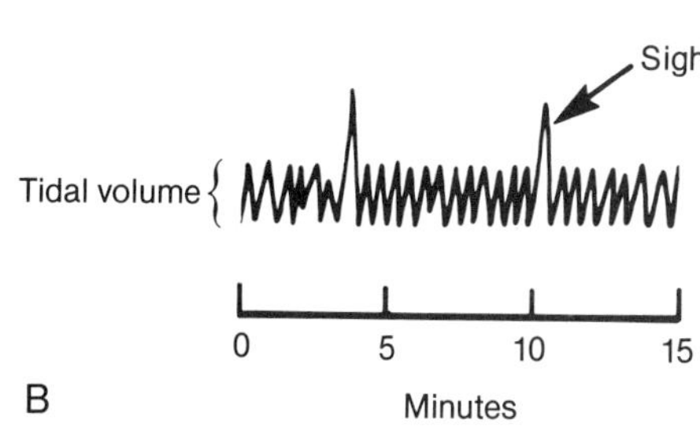

Figure 8–12. Monotonous breathing pattern *(A)*, with reduced tidal volumes and absence of sighs, compared with normal breathing pattern *(B)*, with larger tidal volumes and sighs or yawns every 5 to 10 minutes.

likely in individuals with any of the risk factors listed in Table 8–3.

2. Abnormal breathing pattern, usually the previously mentioned monotonous one typically seen in a postsurgical patient, appears to be the main source of postoperative pulmonary complications (Risser, 1980).

3. Ventilation at low tidal volumes *without* periodic signs can lead to atelectasis within *1 hour* (Bartlett, 1973).

4. In the postoperative lung, atelectasis occurs *first*. Mucus retention is secondary to collapsed alveoli. Hence, signs of mucus retention suggest the presence of atelectasis in addition to the presence of mucus in the lungs.

5. Atelectasis can appear abruptly, but it usually appears gradually and progressively.

6. Figure 8–13 summarizes the pathogenesis of early postoperative atelectasis; Figure 8–14 summarizes the postoperative pulmonary changes and signs of atelectasis in individuals with normal lungs compared with those expected in high risk individuals.

PNEUMONIA *(Pneumonitis)*

Pneumonia is the inflammation of the lung parenchyma, usually associated with alveolar filling with fluid. It may result from inhalation of viral, bacterial, or mycoplasmal pathogenic organisms, but it has several other etiologies, e.g., radiation therapy; parasitic infections; fungal or protozoan infections, such as *Pneumocystis carinii;* chemical irritation from inhalation of

Table 8–3. RISK FACTORS FOR ATELECTASIS AND OTHER POSTOPERATIVE PULMONARY COMPLICATIONS*

Risk Factor	Explanation
Fixed Risk Factor	
Increased age	The lungs become less compliant, airways close earlier during expiration (closing volume increases), and resting Pa_{O_2} progressively drops.
Thoracic or upper abdominal operative site	The patient so affected overrides the normal sigh reflex because thoracic expansion or depression of the diaphragm on the upper abdomen during inspiration causes pain. Postoperative pulmonary complications are reported in 20 to 80% of all patients who have undergone abdominal or thoracic operations.
Long duration of operation†	Schlenker and Hubay (1973) report a 50% incidence of severe atelectasis when anesthesia duration exceeds 4 hours compared with a 19% incidence in association with a 2 hour duration.
Operation performed on an emergency basis	Probably related to the acuteness of the patient's preoperative condition and to the lack of preoperative pulmonary and bowel preparation.
Alterable Risk Factor	
Obesity	Enlarged abdomen and thick chest wall interfere with lung expansion, resulting in lower lung volumes and V/Q abnormality.
Pre-existing respiratory problems (e.g., chronic bronchitis, COPD, respiratory infection, chronic restrictive disease)	Pulmonary complications are associated with a large amount of preoperative secretions (the reason for preoperative bronchial hygiene programs), bacterial colonization of the lower respiratory tract (Schlenker and Hubay, 1973), and abnormal preoperative PFTs (decreased FVC, FEV_1, and MVV) or ABGs. Chronic respiratory disease is the most important risk factor, but acute problems including the common cold may predispose the patient to complications.
Smoking	Cigarette smoking damages the ciliated epithelium of the tracheobronchial tree, increases the rate of mucus secretion, impairs the mucociliary escalator, and decreases the amount of alveolar surfactant. Also, it increases blood coagulability and hence risk of pulmonary embolism. Smoking cessation for weeks to months is preferable to reverse smoking-induced changes and to significantly decrease risk for postoperative pulmonary complications (Wheatley et al, 1977).
Perioperative and Postoperative Risk Factor	
Use of narcotic analgesics	
Decreased consciousness	
Muscular weakness	
Hypotension	
Sepsis	
Blood transfusions	
Postoperative use of nasogastric tube	

*Adapted from Risser, N.: Preoperative and postoperative care to prevent pulmonary complication. *Heart and Lung*, 9:57–67, 1980.
†Note: Choice of anesthesia does not appear to alter risk for postoperative pulmonary complications.

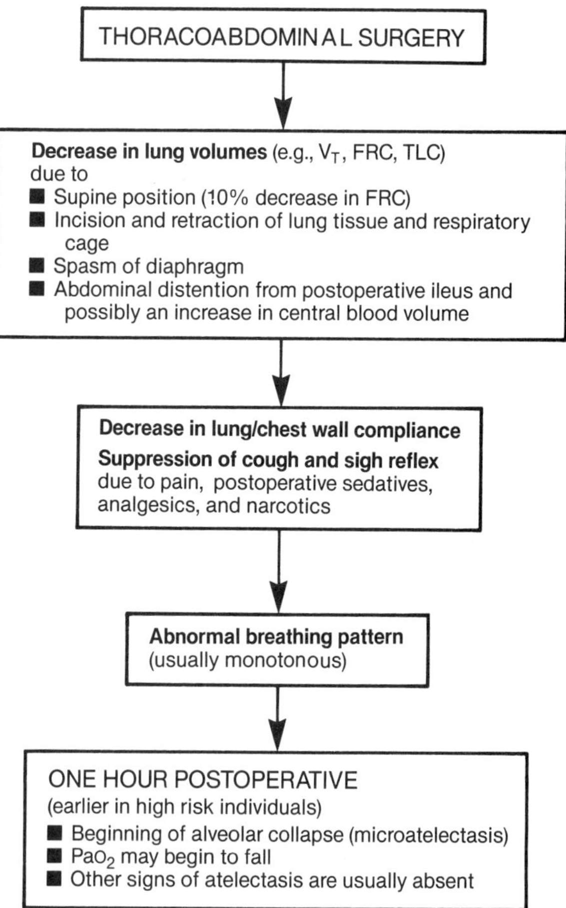

THORACOABDOMINAL SURGERY
Decrease in lung volumes (e.g., V_T, FRC, TLC) due to
■ Supine position (10% decrease in FRC)
■ Incision and retraction of lung tissue and respiratory cage
■ Spasm of diaphragm
■ Abdominal distention from postoperative ileus and possibly an increase in central blood volume
Decrease in lung/chest wall compliance
Suppression of cough and sigh reflex due to pain, postoperative sedatives, analgesics, and narcotics
Abnormal breathing pattern (usually monotonous)
ONE HOUR POSTOPERATIVE
(earlier in high risk individuals)
■ Beginning of alveolar collapse (microatelectasis)
■ PaO_2 may begin to fall
■ Other signs of atelectasis are usually absent

Figure 8–13. Basic pathogenesis of early postoperative atelectasis. All the pathophysiologic developments leading to alveolar collapse are incompletely understood.

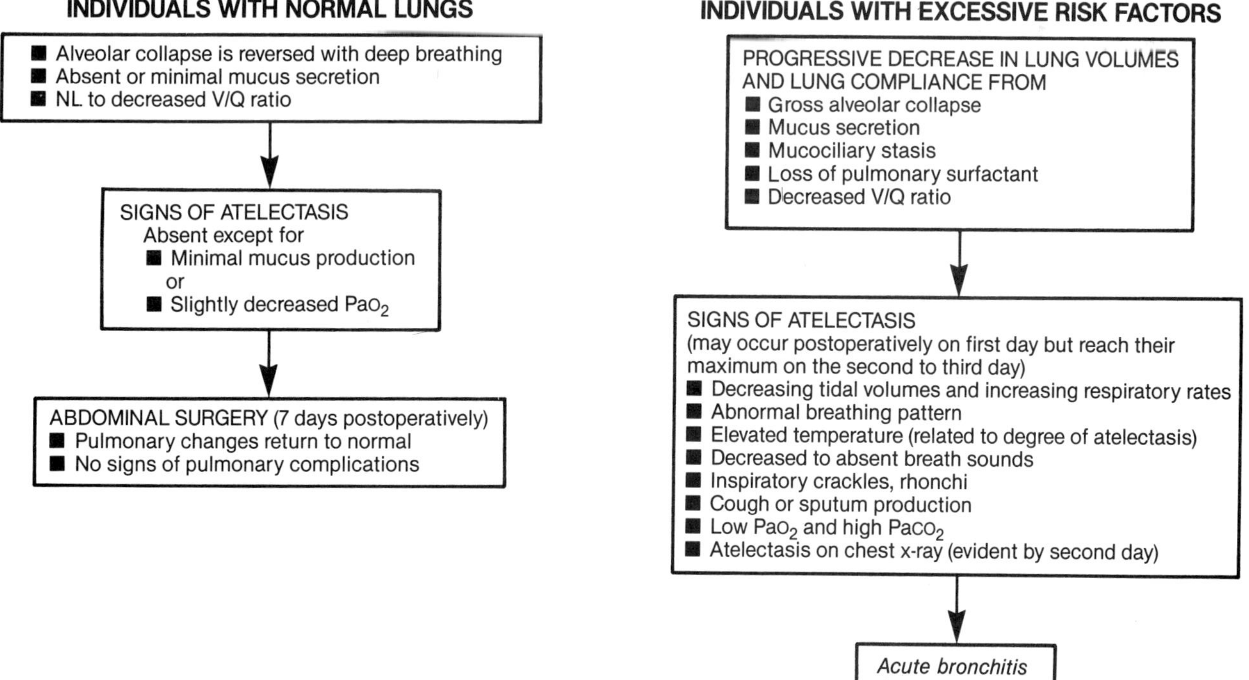

INDIVIDUALS WITH NORMAL LUNGS
■ Alveolar collapse is reversed with deep breathing
■ Absent or minimal mucus secretion
■ NL to decreased V/Q ratio
SIGNS OF ATELECTASIS
Absent except for
■ Minimal mucus production
or
■ Slightly decreased PaO_2
ABDOMINAL SURGERY (7 days postoperatively)
■ Pulmonary changes return to normal
■ No signs of pulmonary complications
INDIVIDUALS WITH EXCESSIVE RISK FACTORS
PROGRESSIVE DECREASE IN LUNG VOLUMES AND LUNG COMPLIANCE FROM
■ Gross alveolar collapse
■ Mucus secretion
■ Mucociliary stasis
■ Loss of pulmonary surfactant
■ Decreased V/Q ratio
SIGNS OF ATELECTASIS
(may occur postoperatively on first day but reach their maximum on the second to third day)
■ Decreasing tidal volumes and increasing respiratory rates
■ Abnormal breathing pattern
■ Elevated temperature (related to degree of atelectasis)
■ Decreased to absent breath sounds
■ Inspiratory crackles, rhonchi
■ Cough or sputum production
■ Low PaO_2 and high $PaCO_2$
■ Atelectasis on chest x-ray (evident by second day)
Acute bronchitis
Acute pneumonia

Figure 8–14. Postoperative pulmonary changes and signs of atelectasis in normal versus high-risk individuals.

noxious fumes, and aspiration of gastric contents. In addition to the inhalational route of entry into the body, infectious pneumonias may develop from infectious organisms that are transported via the blood stream to the lungs from a peripheral infectious site.

Hypersensitivity Pneumonitis

Pulmonary disease due to inhalation of organic dusts results in *hypersensitivity pneumonitis*, also known as *allergic alveolitis* or *extrinsic fibrosing alveolitis*. Ex-

Table 8–4. MAIN TYPES OF INFECTIOUS PNEUMONIAS

Bacterial
Classic or typical pneumonia
Streptococcus pneumonia (pneumococcus)—gram-positive bacteria
Accounts for 70% to 80% or more of primary bacterial pneumonias. The microorganism is found in the oropharynx of 10% to 70% of normal adults (Frame, 1982).
Klebsiella pneumoniae (Friedländer's bacillus)—gram-negative bacteria
The most common gram-negative pneumonia acquired outside a hospital setting. Common in alcoholics—they have impaired ciliary function, changes in pharyngeal florae, and impaired body defenses.
Staphylococcus aureus—gram-positive bacteria
Accounts for 1% of primary bacterial pneumonias in unhospitalized patients and about 10% in hospitalized patients. Often occurs after a viral infection. A principal cause of pneumonia in children. Between 20% and 40% of the population carry *S. aureus* in the anterior nares.
Haemophilus influenzae—gram-negative bacteria
Most often seen in children younger than 10 years of age and individuals with COPD or immune defects.
Atypical pneumonia
Legionella pneumophila (legionnaires' disease)—gram-negative bacteria
A relatively rare disease with a mortality rate of 15%. Associated with contaminated air-conditioning systems. Most often seen in older adults, smokers, or others with impaired lung defenses.
Aspiration pneumonia—usually polymicrobial
From aspiration of pharyngeal/oral secretions in patients with altered consciousness, alcoholism, laryngeal dysfunction, or respiratory muscle paralysis. *In the unhospitalized patient*, anaerobic bacteria (e.g., *Bacteroides spp.*) normally dominate oral flora. *In the hospitalized patient*, aerobic bacteria (*staphylococci* or various aerobic gram-negative species) commonly dominate because the flora of their oropharyngeal secretions becomes altered.
Other bacterial pneumonias common in hospitalized, debilitated, or antibiotic-treated individuals
Pseudomonas aeruginosa—the microorganism thrives in moist environments, e.g., hospitals, respiratory therapy equipment, and even food.
Serratia marcescens
Acinetobacter sp.
Escherichia coli, Enterobacter, Proteus, enteric gram-negative aerobes

Fungal
Histoplasma capsulatum, Coccidioides immitis, Cryptococcus neoformans and *Aspergillus spp.* are soil organisms. Spores are produced in the soil, carried by the wind, and inhaled, producing *histoplasmosis, coccidioidomycosis,* and *aspergillosis.* Bronchopulmonary aspergillosis is a common fungal pneumonia seen in debilitated patients and as a complication in patients with bronchial asthma and cystic fibrosis.
Blastomyces dermatitidis—the airborne microorganism causes *blastomycosis* (see Chapter 10).
Candida albicans—pulmonary candidiasis is rare.

Mycoplasma
Mycoplasma pneumoniae (primary atypical pneumonia)
Most *M. pneumoniae* are restricted to pharyngitis and bronchitis, but 5% to 10% of infected patients develop pneumonia (Frame, 1982), which accounts for 20% to 40% of pneumonias in adults outside the hospital. Rare in children.

Protozoan
Pneumocystis carinii—causes *Pneumocystis* pneumonia
Associated with renal transplantation, advanced autoimmune disease, and immunologic deficiencies. Occurs in 42% of children with severe combined immune deficiency disorder, 4.1% of children with cancer, 11% of bone marrow transplant recipients, and 15% of patients with Kaposi's sarcoma (Hughes, 1984). Seen in at least 50% of patients with acquired immune deficiency syndrome (AIDS) (Witek et al, 1984).

Viral
Influenza—types A, B, and C
Uncommon in normal adults, usually occurring during epidemics. Viral infection is more likely to lower the patient's resistance and facilitate bacterial invasion, causing a bacterial rather than a viral pneumonia.
Adenovirus pneumoniae
Known to occur in association with the crowded conditions of military camps.

posure to organic antigens from moldy tree bark, as in maple stripper's lung, or moldy hay, as in farmer's lung, produces an immunologic response in the body and probably a type of nonimmunologic inflammation of tissues mostly at the alveolar and small bronchiolar level. Exposure to forced-air heating, air conditioning, or room humidification is another source of organic antigens (e.g., thermophilic actinomycetes and thermotolerant bacteria), causing hypersensitivity pneumonitis. The chronic form of this disease may be clinically indistinguishable from idiopathic diffuse interstitial fibrosis defined subsequently in this chapter.

Infectious Pneumonias

Main infectious pneumonias are classified according to causative microorganism (Table 8–4). Nurses need to be familiar with infectious pneumonia since it is still the most common infectious cause of death in the United States, even though modern medical practices, including the use of antibiotics, have reduced the mortality rate for the most common type (pneumococcal) from about 40% to between 5% and 10% (Frame, 1982). Furthermore, pneumonias are becoming more difficult to treat medically because of their increased incidence due to unusual pathogens, particularly those acquired in the hospital. Unusual or mixed pathogens require the use of broad-spectrum antibiotics. As the administration of broad-spectrum antibiotics is increasing, more hospital-acquired pneumonias are caused by antibiotic-resistant organisms. Mortality tends to be high because of difficulties in medical treatment. Hospitalized patients tend to have weakened lung and body defenses. They are prime candidates for infection, perhaps more so now than in the past; modern medicine and life-support technology have lengthened the survival time of today's patients, producing more patients with impaired defenses.

The basic pathology of acute *bacterial pneumonia* is inflammation of alveoli and increased capillary permeability, with marked increased interstitial and alveolar fluid. Alveoli fill with an exudate comprised of fibrin-containing fluid, bacteria, polymorphonuclear leukocytes, and red blood cells.

Once the appropriate antibiotic eradicates the infection and stops the alveolitis, the disease stabilizes, and the parenchyma is either restored to its original structure or remains with residual scarring (fibrosis). This type of fibrosis is *nonprogressive* in nature, unlike the fibrosis of diffuse interstitial fibrosis (described subsequently). Virtually all infectious agents can result in localized fibrosis at the site of infection, depending on the severity of disease.

Most *pneumococcal* pneumonias resolve completely. Other types, such as *Staphylococcus* and *Klebsiella*, are more destructive and can produce a fatal illness in the compromised host. When *suppuration*—the process of pus formation—occurs, tissue necrosis may cause a lung *abscess*. Residual fibrosis is more likely in the more destructive types.

Generally, in bacterial pneumonias, the pneumonia is severe if the patient has an acutely elevated temperature; a low or very high white blood cell count; a positive blood culture for bacteria; a case of jaundice (from hemolysis); or a large area of consolidation, as observed on the chest x-ray film.

The disease is likely to be more severe and more dangerous in the elderly; younger infants; debilitated or immunosuppressed individuals; and individuals with pre-existing disease, notably COPD.

Acquired Immune Deficiency Syndrome (AIDS). Though an immunologic disorder, AIDS is mentioned briefly since opportunistic pneumonia is a key clinical finding and the usual cause of death. The causative microorganism is most commonly *Pneumocystis carinii;* this infection is the primary diagnosis in 64% of patients with AIDS and occurs at least once in up to 80% of patients (Murray et al, 1987). In addition to *Pneumocystis* pneumonia, other infections may develop in AIDS patients and in carriers of the AIDS virus, as shown in the box, Pulmonary Complications of HIV Infection. The mortality rate for AIDS patients ranges

*PULMONARY COMPLICATIONS OF HIV INFECTION**

OPPORTUNISTIC INFECTIONS DIAGNOSTIC OF AIDS

Pneumocystis carinii pneumonia
Pulmonary toxoplasmosis
Extraintestinal strongyloidiasis (e.g., pulmonary)
Bronchopulmonary candidiasis
Pulmonary cryptococcosis
Disseminated histoplasmosis
Disseminated *Mycobacterium avium* complex or *M. kansasii*
Cytomegalovirus pneumonia
Herpes simplex pneumonia

HIV-RELATED PULMONARY INFECTIONS

Tuberculosis
Nocardiosis

PRESUMED HIV-RELATED PULMONARY DISORDERS

Pyogenic bacterial pneumonia
Lymphoid interstitial pneumonitis†

AIDS-RELATED PULMONARY NEOPLASIA

Kaposi's sarcoma
Non-Hodgkin's lymphoma

*Reproduced by permission from Murray, J., Garay, S., et al: Pulmonary complications of the acquired immunodeficiency syndrome: an update. *American Review of Respiratory Disease*, 135:2, 105, 1987.

†Diagnostic of AIDS when occurring in a child 13 years of age or less with positive HIV antibody test results.

from 40% to over 90%, depending on the medical source and on how long the patient has been diagnosed. A mortality rate in excess of 90% is typical for patients with one or more opportunistic infections (Gottlieb, 1984).

Though the pathophysiology of the syndrome is incompletely understood, the AIDS virus has been identified as the human immunodeficiency virus (HIV), previously known as the human T-lymphotropic virus-III/lymphadenopathy-associated virus (HTLV-III/LAV). Other information is given in the box for quick reference, i.e., Summary of Acquired Immune Deficiency Syndrome (AIDS).

Since the recent AIDS epidemic has raised numerous health concerns and misconceptions about risk factors, this information will help the nurse answer questions posed by patients, family, and others about the nature and transmission of this publicly dreaded syndrome. The onset of opportunistic infections typically marks the beginning of clinical deterioration, eventually requiring mechanical ventilation.

Roentgenologic Classification of Pneumonia

Infectious and noninfectious pneumonias are classified into the following three types based on morphologic and roentgenologic characteristics:

1. *Alveolar* or *airspace pneumonia* (lobar pneumonia) affects peripheral alveoli, where inflammatory edema spreads through intra-alveolar collateral channels, producing fluffy white infiltrates on the chest x-ray (see Fig. 15–47 for pattern). Though common, the term lobar pneumonia is not recommended as a synonym of alveolar pneumonia; alveolar pneumonia is seldom lobar in extent. Examples of causative microorganisms are pneumococcus *(Streptococcus)* and *Klebsiella*.
2. *Bronchopneumonia* (lobular pneumonia) incites an inflammatory response in the conducting airways of the lung and surrounding parenchyma. *Staphylococcus* commonly causes bronchopneumonia. The characteristic features on the x-ray film are patchy areas of consolidation from alveolar filling *without* a lobar or segmental pattern.
3. *Interstitial pneumonia* incites an inflammatory response in the interstitial space of the lungs. It mainly involves viral organisms or *Mycoplasma*. Interstitial pneumonia has acute as well as chronic forms. In many diseases, the chronic form represents the noninfectious chronic alveolitis associated with diffuse interstitial fibrosis (see Fig. 15–50 for the interstitial pattern).

DIFFUSE INTERSTITIAL FIBROSIS

Diffuse interstitial fibrosis is a general term commonly employed to describe a heterogeneous group of diseases characterized by thickening or fibrosis of the alveolar interstitium.

Some diseases are associated with rapid development of fibrosis once acute illness has stabilized, e.g.,

*SUMMARY OF ACQUIRED IMMUNODEFICIENCY SYNDROME (AIDS)**

DEFINITION

A viral infection that destroys the body's immune system, leaving the body vulnerable to opportunistic infections. The syndrome is characterized by a deficiency of helper T–lymphocytes and a decrease in the helper to suppressor T–cell ratio.

MEDICAL DIAGNOSIS

Usually depends on presence of the two following criteria: (1) opportunistic infection (or Kaposi's sarcoma, a rare type of skin cancer) in a person with no known reason for immune suppression and (2) antibodies to the AIDS virus.

HIGH RISK CATEGORIES

Gay and bisexual males; heroin and other intravenous drug users because of unsterile techniques; hemophiliacs receiving frequent blood products; heterosexual contacts; transfusion recipients; infants or fetuses with virus-infected mothers; and others for unknown reasons.

AGE GROUP AFFECTED

Most prevalent age groups 30 to 39 years; 90% of adult patients are 20 to 49 years of age.

MODE OF TRANSMISSION

Exposure of abraded mucous membrane to the virus or direct inoculation into the blood stream. Common modes of transmission include receptive anal intercourse, use of contaminated needles during intravenous drug abuse, and sexual intercourse with an HIV-infected heterosexual partner.

SIGNIFICANCE OF A POSITIVE HIV BLOOD TEST

A positive test means that the individual has been exposed to the AIDS virus and has produced antibodies to it; it does not mean that the person has AIDS.

About 25% of persons with a positive test develop symptoms of *AIDS-related complex* (ARC) over months to years. ARC symptoms include unexplained fever, malaise, weight loss, night sweats, diarrhea, lymphadenopathy, idiopathic thrombocytopenic purpura, autoimmune hemolytic anemia, and oral thrush.

About 10 to 15% of ARC patients develop AIDS.

*Data from the National Jewish Hospital and Research Center/National Asthma Center: Immunology: its rapid evolution holds clinical promise for AIDS. Medical/Scientific Update, 4(4):2–8, 1985 and Murray, J., Garay, S., et al: Pulmonary complications of the acquired immunodeficiency syndrome: an update. *American Review of Respiratory Disease*, 135:2, 105, 1987.

adult respiratory distress syndrome. However, the majority of diseases develop fibrosis over months to years. Hence, the terms diffuse interstitial fibrosis and chronic interstitial lung disease may be used interchangeably in the clinical setting.

To put diffuse interstitial fibrosis in proper perspective, the reader must be aware that experts are only beginning to understand the entity's pathogenesis. Hence, in past years when little was known about these many diseases, little agreement existed as to how to describe, classify, and label them. Numerous terms were and in many cases still are, used to describe what we now know as the same overall syndrome. For example, although the topic is still controversial, many experts now believe that the *Hamman-Rich syndrome* (originally described by Hamman and Rich), *cryptogenic fibrosing alveolitis, desquamative interstitial pneumonitis*, and *usual interstitial pneumonitis* are not separate disease entities but may represent different aspects or different stages of the same disease, i.e., *idiopathic pulmonary fibrosis* (Fulmer and Crystal, 1979).

Furthermore, the term *pulmonary fibrosis* rather than diffuse interstitial fibrosis may be a more appropriate one for the interstitial diseases. First, fibrosis may be localized in one or more lung regions rather than throughout all lung regions, depending on the disease process. Also, we now know that the fibrosis may involve other areas besides the alveolar interstitium, e.g., alveolar epithelial cells, pulmonary capillary endothelial cells, small airways (as described previously in this chapter), and sometimes arteries and veins.

Important facts to remember about interstitial lung disease are summarized as follows:

1. Interstitial lung disease is more common than previously thought. It represents about 15% of diseases in all patients seen by pulmonary physicians in the United States (Crystal et al, 1981).

2. Some medical sources use these two terms interchangeably as follows: *pneumonia* or *pneumonitis* represents any infectious type of alveolitis, and *alveolitis* represents the noninfectious type of alveolitis associated with interstitial fibrosis. This approach is confusing, even though an alveolitis is involved in both cases, pathology and treatment are different. After reflecting on the difference between these two types of alveolitis, one sees that interstitial lung disease commonly refers to diseases that are diffuse, chronic, and *not* associated with active infection. The trend is to use *alveolitis* rather than pneumonia or pneumonitis to emphasize the noninfectious nature of chronic interstitial diseases.

3. There are more than 130 defined interstitial lung diseases. Now, the trend is to classify them according to etiology; etiology can be identified in about 35% of cases of interstitial lung disease (see Table 8–5). For the majority of patients (65%), however, the specific etiologic agent responsible for disease cannot be identified, and the disease falls into the "unknown etiology" category.

Table 8–5. INTERSTITIAL LUNG DISEASES ACCORDING TO KNOWN AND UNKNOWN ETIOLOGIES*

Known Etiologies	Unknown Etiologies†
Occupational and Environmental Inhalants	Idiopathic pulmonary fibrosis
Inorganic dusts, e.g., silica, asbestos, talc, kaolin (China clay)	Chronic interstitial disease associated with collagen-vascular disorders, e.g., rheumatoid arthritis, systemic lupus erythematosus
Organic dusts‡, e.g., organic antigens from living sources, e.g., moldy hay, duck and chicken feathers, wood dust or wood pulp.	Sarcoidosis
Gases (e.g., oxygen), fumes (e.g., oxides of zinc and iron), vapors (e.g., mercury), aerosols (e.g., fats and oils)	Histiocytosis-X
Drugs Producing Chronic Disease	Goodpasture's syndrome
Cytotoxic and immunosuppressive agents, e.g., busulfan, bleomycin, methotrexate, cyclophosphamide	Inherited disorders, e.g., familial pulmonary fibrosis, neurofibromatosis
Antimicrobial agents, e.g., nitrofurantoin, sulfonamides, penicillin, aminosalicylic acid	Liver disease associated with interstitial lung disease, e.g., chronic active hepatitis
Neuroactive and vasoactive agents, e.g., diphenylhydantoin, ganglionic blocking agents (e.g., hexamethonium), beta-blocking agents (e.g., practolol, propranolol)	Lymphocytic infiltrative disorders
Others, e.g., chlorpropamide, gold salts, hydrochlorothiazide	Pulmonary vascular disorders associated with interstitial lung disease, e.g., pulmonary veno-occlusive disease, some diseases with vasculitis
Poisons	Bronchopulmonary aspergillosis§
Paraquat	Wegener's granulomatosis
Radiation	Chronic eosinophilic pneumonia
Therapeutic and inhaled (e.g., nuclear accident)	Other less common or unclassified disorders
Infectious Agents	
Bacteria, mycobacteria, fungi, viruses, *Mycoplasma*, and parasites	
Other Causes	
Chronic pulmonary edema, chronic uremia	

*Adapted from Keogh, B. and Crystal, R.: Chronic interstitial lung disease. In Current Pulmonology, vol. 3. (Simmons, D., ed.). New York, John Wiley & Sons Inc., 1981; and Fulmer, J. D. and Crystal, R.: Interstitial lung disease. In Current Pulmonology, vol. 1, (Simmons, D., ed.) Boston, Houghton Mifflin Professional Publishers, 1979.

†Limited list.

‡The resulting interstitial disease is known as *hypersensitivity pneumonitis* or *extrinsic allergic alveolitis*.

§Interstitial changes develop secondary to the primary airway disease.

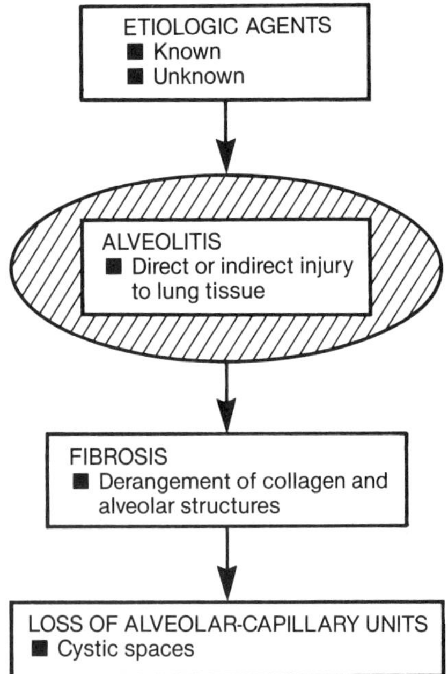

Figure 8–15. Basic pathogenesis of interstitial lung disease. (Adapted from Keogh, B. and Crystal, R. Chronic Interstitial Lung Disease. In Current Pulmonology, vol. 3. (Simmons, D., ed.) New York, John Wiley & Sons Inc., 1981.)

4. In the unknown etiology category, most patients have *sarcoidosis*, interstitial lung disease associated with *collagen-vascular disease*, or *idiopathic pulmonary fibrosis (IPF)*. Each of these entities, including each different type of collagen disorder, is now known as a specific disease entity with characteristic clinical features (Keogh and Crystal, 1981). Of these, IPF is considered the classic example of a fibrotic lung disease. It is localized in the lungs, whereas the other two, and many others mentioned elsewhere in this chapter, represent systemic diseases.

5. The main pathologic feature of interstitial fibrosis is thickening of the alveolar interstitium, which eventually destroys the alveolar architecture and obliterates nearby capillaries. However, most interstitial diseases pass through a series of pathologic changes that represent different stages of a disease (Fig. 8–15). These pathologic features are important to remember as medical prognosis and treatment depend on which pathologic feature is dominant (e.g., alveolitis, fibrosis, and loss of alveolar-capillary units) and the specific nature and intensity of disease activity in each of these stages.

Alveolitis

The etiologic agent first causes *alveolitis*. Acute alveolitis may produce direct toxicity to lung tissue, indirect injury mediated through various inflammatory and immune systems, or both. Within days to years, chronic alveolitis develops. The initial proliferation and activation of inflammatory and immune-effector cells from acute alveolitis dramatically alters constituent cells in the interstitium and within alveolar air spaces. In IPF, early disease is marked by alveolar filling with macrophages and other mononuclear cells, a process called *desquamation*. As the disease progresses, the aggregates of cells in alveoli decrease and seem to disappear with severe fibrosis.

In this alveolitis stage, recovery of different numbers and types of inflammatory and immune-effector cells by *bronchoalveolar lavage* helps to diagnose the type and intensity of the alveolitis and the specific disease entity. Bronchoalveolar lavage is a diagnostic procedure involving the instillation of saline solution into the lungs and aspirating it back out of the lungs to examine lower respiratory tract cellular constituents mixed in the solution. *Neutrophilic alveolitis*, characterized by increased numbers of neutrophils in the saline solution, is found in diseases such as IPF, several collagen disorders, and asbestosis. *T-lymphocytic alveolitis* is associated with granulomatous lung diseases, e.g., sarcoidosis.

As long as alveolitis is present, cellular alterations and injury continue. If the epithelial and endothelial basement membranes remain intact, however, the lungs are likely to return to normal with appropriate and aggressive treatment of the disease. Corticosteroid drugs are used to modulate the inflammatory and immune effector processes. Sometimes, cytotoxic drugs may be used, but this therapy is controversial particularly when the alveolitis is of low intensity (e.g., progressive systemic sclerosis). In such a case, even steroids may not slow the progressive nature of the disease.

Fibrosis

Alveolitis eventually causes *fibrosis*, characterized by irreversible derangement of interstitial collagen. In IPF, the lungs produce increased quantities of a certain type of collagen (type I) that happens to be the less compliant of the collagen types in the lungs. The total amount of interstitial collagen, however, remains unchanged. This feature and the changes in the types and locations of various interstitial, alveolar, and muscle cells produce a twisted and frayed interstitium, fragmented islands of smooth muscle cells, and a distorted alveolar structure. Furthermore, specific diseases may have distinguishing histologic features, e.g., granulomata in the granulomatous diseases.

Most important, in any given patient, the more fibrosis present in the lung, the more irreversible the disease.

Loss of Alveolar-Capillary Units

Eventually, groups of alveolar-capillary units reach this last stage of the disease. Alveolitis and fibrosis result in the obliteration of alveolar-capillary units and formation of nonfunctional *cystic spaces*, the hallmarks of end-stage disease (see Fig. 9–4A). Once many regions of lung reach this last stage (disease activity varies among alveolar-capillary units), it may be impossible to discern the underlying type of interstitial disease. Characteristic histologic features of specific diseases (e.g., granulomata) may be absent. The cystic spaces and adjacent thickened interstitium may give the diseased tissue a "honeycomb" appearance, resembling a honeycomb built by honeybees. Evidence of a honeycomb appearance may be seen on a routine chest x-ray film and is a manifestation of late rather than early interstitial disease (see Fig. 15–49B). It is usually localized in specific areas of the lungs—often the lung bases—or it may be scattered throughout the lung fields.

Patients whose lungs manifest primarily fibrosis and cystic spaces rather than alveolitis and healthy lung tissue have end-stage lung disease. Grossly, their lungs are shrunken, very stiff, and noncompliant, which in turn accounts for the greatly reduced lung volumes on the pulmonary function test.

Importance of Early Medical Diagnosis

Because of the progressive and fatally destructive nature of diffuse interstitial fibrosis, early medical diagnosis is crucial. In many cases, the individual can be removed from exposure to the causative agent once it is identified. The alveolitis may be successfully treated and the disease process arrested or at least slowed. Supplementary oxygen can treat any oxygenation problem.

Complicating chest infections that commonly develop later in the disease course can be treated before they cause further deterioration in lung function and further deterioration in the overall physical condition of the patient. Such prompt treatment may at least partially determine whether the disease progresses rapidly or slowly, remains the same, or reverts toward normal. For IPF, early treatment is likely to slow the progression of the disease or at least ease the signs and symptoms and thereby improve the overall quality of life for the patient. In a few select cases, it may reverse the disease process.

GRANULOMATOUS DISEASE

Granulomatous disease is a disorder characterized by the presence of *granulomas,* defined as granular tumors or growths, usually composed of lymphoid or epithelioid cells. The disease often involves the lung parenchyma; two such diseases are described further. Other diseases characterized by the presence of granulomas include *eosinophilic granuloma disease,* a form of what is known as *histiocytosis X,* and various fungal diseases, such as *coccidioidomycosis* and *blastomycosis,* found most commonly in farmers, construction workers, and others who live in dusty environments where infective spores from various sources become airborne and easily inhaled.

Sarcoidosis

A multisystem granulomatous disorder of unknown etiology, usually affecting young adults 20 to 40 years of age, especially black females. The patients present most frequently with mediastinal or hilar lymph adenopathy, pulmonary infiltration that is usually interstitial, and cutaneous or ocular lesions (Israel and Atkinson, 1978). The disease is a chronic *noncaseating* one. A caseating disease is one in which necrotic tissue develops and is converted into a granular amorphous mass resembling cheese. Roentgenographic evidence of pulmonary involvement in sarcoidosis is observed in about one third of cases.

Medical diagnosis of sarcoidosis is made through chest x-ray findings, biopsies of affected organs, or both. A scale for staging sarcoidosis using these two assessment parameters is shown in Table 8–6. Most young individuals who initially present with sarcoidosis are at Stage 1. Treatment with corticosteroids is recommended for patients who are in Stage II or Stage III for 6 to 12 months. However, Hillerdal and coworkers (1984) report in their 15-year study of patients with sarcoidosis that the value of this treatment is questionable. Restoration to normal can be expected in most cases even without corticosteroid treatment. Only 6% of patients in Stage III progress to Stage IV, the one associated with end-stage disease and disability. Hence, most patients recover from sarcoidosis, though resolution of pathology seen on x-ray (e.g., lymphadenopathy) may take from 15 months up to several years.

Pulmonary Tuberculosis

An infectious disease of the lung parenchyma is caused by the organism *Mycobacterium tuberculosis.* The disease is transmitted by the airborne spread of droplet nuclei containing *tubercle bacilli* surrounded by respiratory tract secretions. Coughing or speaking by infected persons makes these droplets airborne and available for inhalation by friends, relatives, and others living or working in close proximity. Recent findings

Table 8–6. STAGING FOR SARCOIDOSIS*

Stage 0	Normal chest x-ray film Positive tissue biopsy findings
Stage I	Chest x-ray film shows bilateral hilar adenopathy alone
Stage II	Chest x-ray film shows bilateral hilar adenopathy and pulmonary infiltrates
Stage III	Chest x-ray film shows pulmonary infiltrates with normal hilar lymph nodes Positive tissue biopsy findings
Stage IV	Chest x-ray film shows overt parenchymal destruction, such as shrinkage, emphysematous blebs, or both

*Adapted from Hillerdal, G., Nou, E., et al: Sarcoidosis: epidemiology and prognosis. *American Review of Respiratory Disease,* 130:29–32, 1984.

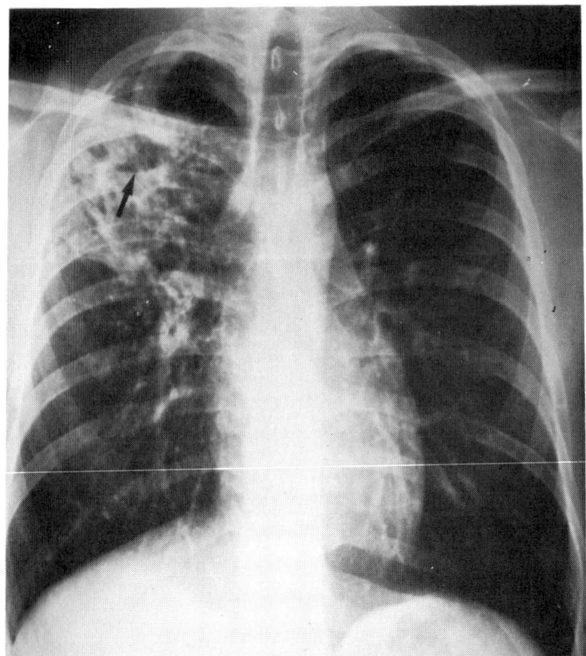

Figure 8–16. Cavitary pulmonary tuberculosis in a 23-year-old man. The lung fields and cardiac silhouette are unremarkable except for the patchy area of consolidation in the right upper lobe. There is an internal air-fluid level (arrow) in the middle of the consolidation.

indicate, however, that uninfected persons must be exposed to an infectious case of tuberculosis for many weeks before the chance of infection becomes appreciable. As Glassroth (1981) points out, even then only about 30% of close contacts are found to be infected. Furthermore, the likelihood of transmission is related to the concentration of droplet nuclei in the air. Hence, patients with large numbers of tubercle bacilli are highly infectious, and those who do not cough or who have no bacilli in their sputum (negative sputum smear results) are significantly less infectious.

If tubercle bacilli in the inhaled droplet are not cleared from the lungs by macrophage ingestion and the mucociliary escalator, they reach a susceptible site, such as the respiratory bronchiole or alveoli, and begin to multiply. The small area of bronchopneumonia that develops at the site of deposition is called the *primary focus.* Tubercle bacilli from the primary focus drain into regional lymph nodes, producing inflammation and enlargement (lymphadenopathy).

Most primary foci develop in the lung apices or sometimes in the superior segments of the lower lobes. The predilection for the apices is thought to be due to the high oxygen content normally present in that location, which in turn favors the growth of bacilli; it may be due to the decreased pulmonary blood flow to the apices (see Chapter 5). In the last case, the accompanying lymph stasis impairs the clearance of antigenic substances (Goodwin and Des Prez, 1983).

After initial exposure to the tubercle bacilli, the patient is typically asymptomatic and the primary focus largely or completely resolves without the patient even knowing of the infection. In about 5% of infected persons, the disease process becomes radiographically or clinically apparent (Glassroth, 1981). The granulomatous form of response occurs 2 to 10 weeks after initial infection. The primary focus may undergo necrosis (caseation), producing large fluid-filled *cavities* in the lung. Yet even with this *cavitary tuberculosis* evident on the chest x-ray findings (Fig. 8–16), the patient may be relatively asymptomatic, except for chest pain associated with inflammation of the pleura.

In some cases, the bacilli enter the pulmonary lymphatics and pulmonary capillaries and are carried to other parts of the lungs and body, producing a disseminated form of tuberculosis called *miliary tuberculosis.* This form produces a potentially fatal illness. The term miliary comes from the miliary pattern—diffuse, uniform, discrete nodular shadows about the size of a millet seed (2 mm)—characteristically seen on the chest x-ray (Fig. 8–17). If the infection spreads systemically, other parts of the body may also become involved.

After medical treatment of tuberculosis by appropriate drugs or after the individual acquires immunity on his own (in unrecognized cases), infected areas resolve. The healing process occurs over a period of

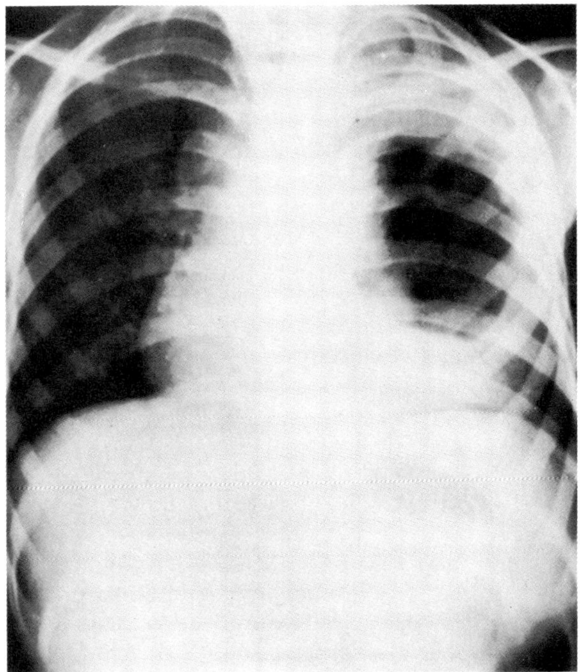

Figure 8–17. Cavitary pulmonary tuberculosis with miliary dissemination throughout the lung fields in a South African infant. Many of the discrete nodules are not visible, but the large consolidation containing a central cavity is quite evident in the lower half of the left lung. The patient has enlarged mediastinal lymph nodes, resulting on the film in a widened mediastinum. *Mycobacterium tuberculosis* was recovered from gastric washings. (Reproduced by permission from Fraser, R. G. and Paré, J. A.: Diagnosis of Diseases of the Chest, vol. 3. Philadelphia, W. B. Saunders Co., 1979.)

months with the formation of *fibrous scars* and ultimately *calcifications*. Such calcifications are readily identified on the chest x-ray findings and may be the only evidence of a past granulomatous disease. In a minority of cases (4 to 15%), one of these inactive residual areas (granulomata) breaks down and reactivates the disease. A precipitating factor might be malnutrition, immunosuppression, silicosis, diabetes mellitus, or other unknown factors.

COLLAGEN DISEASE

Collagen or *collagen-vascular* disorders are connective tissue disorders that frequently affect the lung interstitium, pleura, or both. Interstitial changes are similar to those found in idiopathic diffuse interstitial fibrosis. Other lung changes may include nodular lung lesions, patchy infiltrations, and pleural inflammation with or without pleural effusion or fibrosis.

About 20% of patients with *rheumatoid arthritis* have evidence of interstitial disease on the chest x-ray (Keogh and Crystal, 1981). An affected individual tends to have a much milder form of disease compared with an individual with IPF; many are unaware of its presence. Clinical manifestations of pleuropulmonary involvement may precede the onset of arthritis or appear years later.

Pleuropulmonary involvement occurs in 50% to 90% of cases of *systemic lupus erythematosus* (SLE), a chronic and usually fatal disease characterized by skin rash and pathologic collagen alterations in the vascular system. The untreatable collagen disease, *progressive systemic sclerosis* (scleroderma), involves the lung in about 70% to 90% of those examined at autopsy (Guenter and Welch, 1982). Diffuse interstitial fibrosis with honeycombing in severe cases is prominent pathologically, and it is sometimes accompanied by pleural changes.

PNEUMOCONIOSIS

Pneumoconiosis is a lung disease caused by retention of inhaled dust in the lungs accompanied by tissue reaction. Since pneumoconiosis commonly is seen in an individual with dust exposure at the place of employment, it is also known as a type of *occupational lung disease*.

The pathologic mechanism responsible for tissue injury begins with inhalation and retention of particles. Small dust particles (1 to 5 μm) are most likely to be retained in the lungs and are produced by disruptive processes in work settings, such as in those where crushing, grinding, drilling, cutting, or smoothing of natural minerals takes place. Prolonged exposure (months to years) to high concentrations of particles is most likely to cause detectable disease. Depending on the chemical and physical properties of a particular substance, deposition and retention of particles may or may not produce lung damage. When lung damage occurs, it is usually from an inflammatory and sometimes immunologic reaction leading to tissue fibrosis. Permanent retention of particles potentially exerts a continuing biologic effect for the lifetime of the individual. If the retained substance is *carcinogenic* (cancer causing), prolonged exposure may result in malignancy as much as 20 to 30 years after the last date of occupational exposure. The three main types of pneumoconioses are defined and described in the next sections.

One must remember, however, that other pneumoconioses exist. Substances other than coal and silica may cause active pneumoconiosis—some examples are nonasbestos silicates, tungsten carbide, graphite, aluminum, beryllium, and nickel carbonyl. Furthermore, substances such as tin, iron, fiberglass, barium, and cement cause and are placed under the category *inert pneumoconioses*. Inhalation of tin, iron, or barium dust, for example, may produce significant chest x-ray changes with little to no pathologic changes, unless fibrogenic (fibrosis causing) substances are simultaneously inhaled (Mitchell, 1979).

Silicosis

Silicosis is a pulmonary disease caused by exposure to silica, a specific compound of the element silicon. Next to oxygen, silica is the most common and widely distributed element in the earth's crust. Inhalation of silica dust occurs in miners, sandblasters, stonemasons, and anyone else who handles silica-containing materials, such as quartz, sandstone, coal, and others.

Acute silicosis is seen in an individual with a brief (weeks to months) but intense exposure to silica dust. Rock drillers, sandblasters, and tunnelers may develop this acute, rapidly progressive form of silicosis, which leads to severe disability and death within 5 years of diagnosis.

Silicosis most commonly develops as a chronic disease in miners, foundry workers, and others who have inhaled relatively low concentrations of silica dust for 1 to 20 years. In this *simple* form, the patient is usually completely asymptomatic except for some breathlessness during exercise. When silica particles are deposited in the lungs, alveolar macrophages ingest them. But the macrophages are then killed by intracellular liberation of enzymes, which in turn produces materials that attract more macrophages: this process repeats itself as macrophages continue to engulf silica particles. Eventually, fibrous nodules 2 to 5 mm in size develop in the lungs, located primarily near the respiratory bronchioles with a predilection for the upper lobes.

In *complicated silicosis*, these nodules form large conglomerate masses of fibrotic tissue sometimes exceeding the volume of an upper lobe (Fig. 8–18). When this occurs, the patient is said to have developed *progressive massive fibrosis* (PMF), the most severe form of interstitial fibrosis in a pulmonary patient.

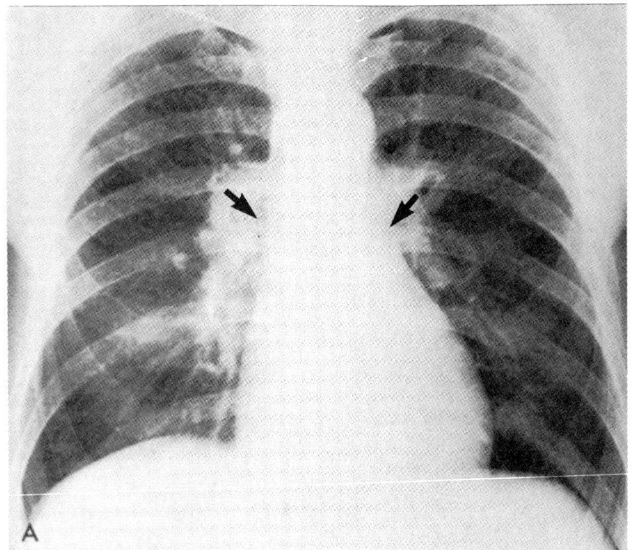

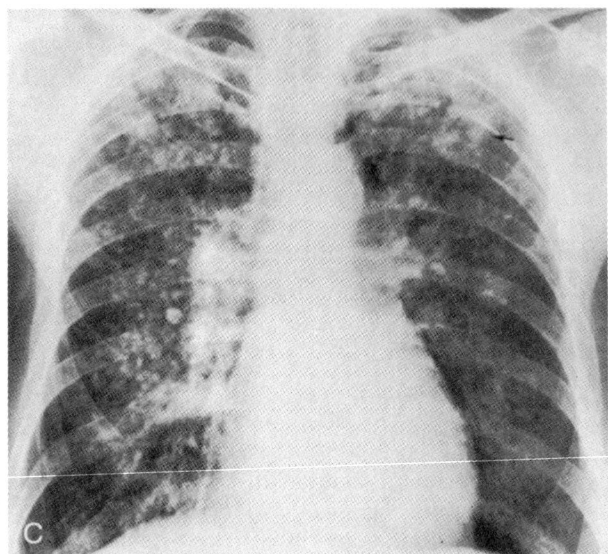

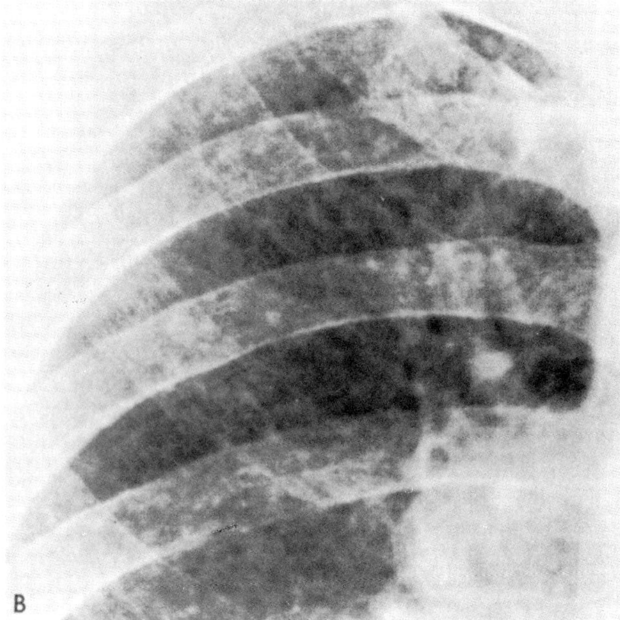

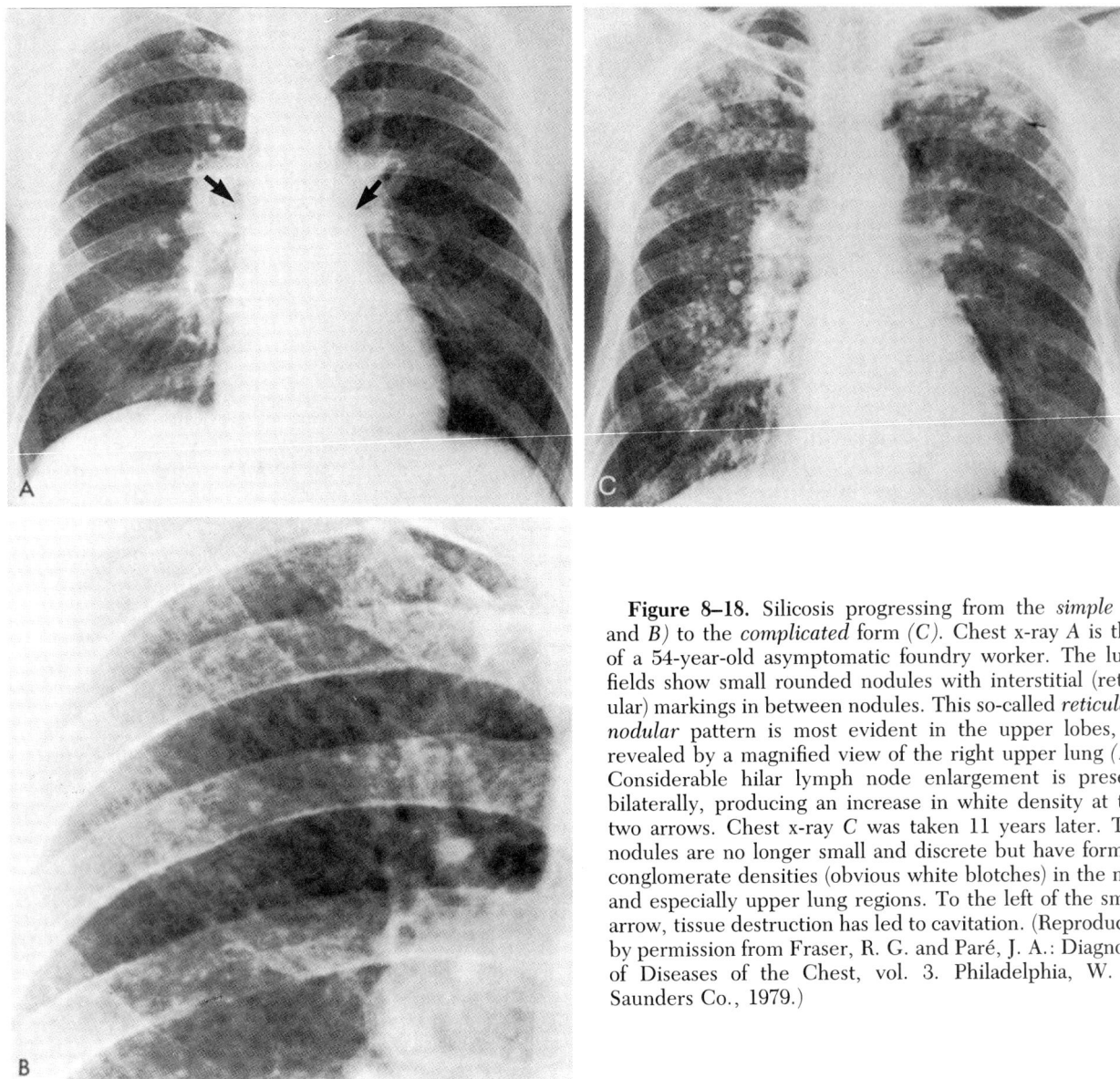

Figure 8–18. Silicosis progressing from the *simple* (*A* and *B*) to the *complicated* form (*C*). Chest x-ray *A* is that of a 54-year-old asymptomatic foundry worker. The lung fields show small rounded nodules with interstitial (reticular) markings in between nodules. This so-called *reticular-nodular* pattern is most evident in the upper lobes, as revealed by a magnified view of the right upper lung (*B*). Considerable hilar lymph node enlargement is present bilaterally, producing an increase in white density at the two arrows. Chest x-ray *C* was taken 11 years later. The nodules are no longer small and discrete but have formed conglomerate densities (obvious white blotches) in the mid and especially upper lung regions. To the left of the small arrow, tissue destruction has led to cavitation. (Reproduced by permission from Fraser, R. G. and Paré, J. A.: Diagnosis of Diseases of the Chest, vol. 3. Philadelphia, W. B. Saunders Co., 1979.)

Emphysematous bullae from tissue destruction are frequently seen on the chest x-ray in the upper lobes, especially if the individual has a history of heavy cigarette smoking. Lymph nodes may become calcified and the pulmonary arteries enlarged from pulmonary hypertension. Also, patients with silicosis, especially those with the disabling complicated form, have increased predispositions to tuberculosis and autoimmune collagen disorders.

Asbestosis

Asbestosis is a restrictive disease characterized by diffuse interstitial fibrosis induced by inhalation of asbestos fibers. Asbestos is a general term that refers to a number of different fibrous silicates that are extremely resistant to chemical and physical influences. It can be woven into fireproof, heat resistant sheets that are used in automobile clutch facings, brake linings, and fire resistant textiles. Until recently and before its toxic properties were recognized, asbestos was employed freely as an insulation material for buildings and for ships, and in the home for cookware items, such as hot pads and "simmering" pads to keep food warm on the stove. The process of "rip-out," i.e., removal of asbestos-containing insulation materials around piping systems on board ships, has been responsible for numerous cases of asbestosis among employees in naval shipyards. Building demolition produces clouds of dust high in asbestos content, which are inhaled by workers. Fibrous glass is now used in place of asbestos, and precautionary measures are used to protect against dust inhalation during rip-out or demolition of old asbestos materials. However, the risk of developing asbestosis is still of prime public concern. Since extensive mining and use of the mineral has occurred only in the last 100 years, the disease asbestosis and other asbestos-related diseases have only recently been recognized. Effective surveillance programs have only recently been implemented to identify hazardous environmental conditions as well as individuals who manifest disease or are at risk to develop disease. Currently, increasing numbers of newly diagnosed cases are found in shipyard workers, military personnel, and others who were exposed to asbestos 20 to 30 years ago. Hence, it is important for the nurse to become familiar with this chest disease and its implications.

In asbestosis, long narrow asbestos fibers are deposited in alveoli arising directly from the respiratory bronchioles. About 25% of these fibers become coated with iron-rich proteinaceous materials, forming yellow-to-brown "asbestos bodies." They are often found in sputum of persons recently exposed to asbestos and exert little to no fibrogenic reaction, presumably because the coating inactivates the asbestos fibers inside. The 75% of fibers that remain uncoated cause alveolitis and fibrosis by several proposed mechanisms, including mechanical irritation by the long pointed fibers and activation of various inflammatory and immune systems. The exact physiologic mechanism is unknown. In addition to causing interstitial fibrosis, primarily in the lower lobes, uncoated asbestos fibers "needle" their way to the lung periphery to produce *pleural fibrosis*, commonly observed as *bilateral pleural thickening* on the chest x-ray.

Although asbestos bodies may occur in the sputum as early as 2 months after first exposure, the disease may not appear for 20 to 30 years. The long latent period applies to individuals with years of exposure as well as to those with limited but intense exposure (e.g., 2 months). Affected individuals and possibly exposed individuals without disease are at increased risk to develop lung cancer, especially cigarette smokers. The most serious form of asbestosis is *mesothelioma*, a malignant tumor of the pleura, peritoneum, or both that leads to death usually within 1 year of diagnosis. Also, exposure to asbestos is related to cancer of the gastrointestinal tract, larynx, and possibly other organs.

Asbestos-Related Disease. Exposure to asbestos may produce *asbestos-related disease* rather than asbestosis. This entity is defined as disease due to inhalation of asbestos fibers, producing pathology *other than* classic diffuse interstitial fibrosis. The classic example is the asymptomatic patient who demonstrates *no* lung pathology at all except for a *pleural plaque*, a small, irregular area of mostly collagenous connective tissue that usually contains granular deposits of calcium along the collagen fibers (calcifications). On the chest x-ray, the presence of bilateral widespread pleural plaques, and especially calcified diaphragmatic pleural plaques, is almost always diagnostic of exposure to asbestos. Sometimes, a pleural effusion is present in asbestos-related disease.

COAL WORKER'S PNEUMOCONIOSIS
(Black Lung)

This chest disease is due to inhalation of coal dust and is further defined by its specific radiographic presentation. It is very similar to silicosis in that it progresses from a simple form to a complicated one. In fact, the two diseases often coexist; coal is composed of many substances including silica. About 10% of coal miners develop *simple coal worker's pneumoconiosis* (CWP) without symptoms. Inhaled coal dust settles within aleveoli, later accumulates in the vicinity of the respiratory bronchioles and forms coal macules, aggregates of coal dust, dead and dying macrophages, fibroblasts, and connective tissue. Coal macules are characteristic of all forms of CWP. The macules form a diffuse nodular pattern on the chest x-ray, especially in the upper lobes of the lung. When the nodules become 1 cm or more in diameter, a diagnosis of *complicated CWP* is made. The nodules become large masses of black fibrous tissue. As in complicated silicosis, emphysematous changes occur along with the progressive massive fibrosis. With the fibrosis and shrinking of heavily involved portions of lung, the great decrease in lung volume produces a very disabling restrictive pulmonary disease. To complicate matters, the peribronchial fibrosis in this interstitial disease introduces an obstructive component to the underlying restrictive process. Luckily, a very small percentage of coal miners develop the complicated form. Complications of CWP are chronic bronchitis (commonly present), rheumatoid arthritis, tuberculosis, and secondary chest infections.

NEOPLASTIC DISEASE

Disorders characterized by *new abnormal tissue formation*, such as a tumor or growth, fall under the category of *neoplastic disease*. In general, tumors of the chest may arise within any intrathoracic structure including the lungs, mediastinum, pleura, and chest wall. Large tumors involving the pleura and chest wall may restrict expansion of underlying lung tissue and hence serve as examples of extrapulmonary restrictive disease. Multiple or large solitary infiltrative tumors located within the lung parenchyma cause a pulmonary rather than an extrapulmonary restrictive defect. In this case, healthy air-filled lung tissue is replaced with solid, more noncompliant mass of tissue, making the lungs stiffer and preventing full lung expansion during inspiration. While tumors generally cause a restrictive defect, the nurse must remember that small tumors may have little to no effect on lung function. The patient with a small benign *fibroma*, for example, is typically asymptomatic and demonstrates a normal pulmonary function test. Occasionally, an obstructive rather than a restrictive process may result from a tumor, depending on the nature, location, and extent of the neoplastic disease. For example, a malignant tumor called *epidermoid carcinoma*, often causes lumenal obstruction of a large bronchus. Then, as seg-

Table 8–7. SOME BENIGN LUNG TUMORS*

Name	Description	Main Location
Hamartoma (most common benign tumor)	Disorganized collection of normal lung tissues, mostly cartilage	Peripheral lung parenchyma
Fibroma	Tumor of fibrous connective tissue	Lung parenchyma Bronchial lumen Pleura
Hemangioma	Vascular lesion receiving blood supply from pulmonary arteries	Lung parenchyma
Lipoma	Fatty tumor, sometimes quite vascular	Lung parenchyma Bronchial lumen Pleura
Papilloma	Epithelial tumor	Larynx Sometimes trachea and main bronchi
Bronchogenic (bronchial) cysts	Fluid-filled or air-filled or both type cysts lined with bronchial epithelium; from congenital or acquired cystic disease	Lung parenchyma may communicate with bronchial tree

*Except for hamartoma, all of these tumors may become malignant in rare instances.

mental or lobar pneumonia develops distal to the site of the obstruction (as is often the case), a restrictive process is added to an obstructive one. Accompanying atelectasis will worsen the restrictive defect.

Benign Tumors

These are tumors or growths that are not malignant and have a relatively harmless effect on the body. Some benign tumors of the lungs and chest wall are listed and described in Table 8–7. Except for *hamartomas*, benign thoracic tumors are not commonly found. Histologic identification is always important because some of these tumors may mimic the clinical presentations of cancer or later become malignant. The patient may be asymptomatic or present with progressive disease with alarming symptoms including hemoptysis. The patient with *papillomas* may present with signs of bronchial obstruction, since this type of benign tumor is most likely to obstruct major airways.

Malignant Tumors

These are cancerous growths with a harmful effect on the body, eventually producing death in the later stages of disease. Although the following may accompany benign tumors, a malignant tumor is always suspected in the following situations:

1. When a new lesion (less than 2 years old) appears on chest x-ray, particularly in an individual over 35 years old.
2. When a chest lesion of indeterminant age shows no signs of calcification.
3. When a patient coughs up blood—small amounts are as ominous as large amounts.
4. When pneumonia is recurrent or responds in an unusually slow manner to appropriate treatment.

Malignant tumors that first arise in the lungs are *primary malignant tumors*. Different types of primary malignancies are classified in the box, according to laboratory-determined histologic types. Note that *bronchogenic carcinomas* make up the first five classifications, and as a group account for more than 90% of all primary malignancies of the lung. They have dramatically increased in incidence over the past 50 years and are the leading cause of death from cancer in men. By the late 1980s, they may surpass breast cancer as the leading killer in women. At least 80% of cases are attributed to the effects of cigarette smoking. In general, the more one smokes, the greater the injury to the bronchial epithelium and the greater the risk of lung cancer. Persons who stop smoking remain at high risk of developing bronchogenic carcinoma for a few years, but the risk becomes near normal in about 10 years.

In addition to histologic types, tumors are classified

*CLASSIFICATION OF PRIMARY MALIGNANT TUMORS**

BRONCHOGENIC CARCINOMAS

I. Epidermoid carcinomas
II. Small cell undifferentiated carcinomas (includes oat cell carcinomas)
III. Adenocarcinomas (includes alveolar cell carcinoma)
IV. Large cell undifferentiated carcinomas
V. Combined epidermoid and adenocarcinoma

OTHERS

VI. Bronchial adenomas (includes carcinoid and bronchial gland tumors)
VII. Papillary tumors of the surface epithelium
VIII. "Mixed" tumors and carcinosarcomas
IX. Sarcomas
X. Unclassified
XI. Mesotheliomas
XII. Melanomas

*Adapted from the World Health Organization Classification System.

Table 8–8. TUMOR-NODE-METASTASIS (TNM) STAGING OF LUNG CANCER*

Stage	Code
Occult cancer	$T_XN_0M_0$
Stage 1	$T_{IS}N_0M_0$ $T_1N_0M_0$ $T_1N_1M_0$ $T_2N_0M_0$
Stage 2	$T_2N_1M_0$
Stage 3	T_3 with any N or M N_2 with any T or M M_1 with any T or N

*Adapted from the World Health Organization.

by stages of development. The American Joint Committee for Cancer Staging has developed a simplified system of classification based on the presence and extent of primary tumor in the lung, the extent of hilar or mediastinal lymph node involvement, and the evidence of metastases (spread) to other parts of the body. The classification system is called the *tumor-node-metastasis* (TNM) system for staging of lung (bronchogenic) cancer (Table 8–8). The glossary in the box helps to interpret TNM codes utilized to describe a patient's disease state (Hinshaw and Murray, 1980; Bone and Balk, 1982).

Clinical findings in patients with primary malignancies vary considerably owing to different pulmonary and extrapulmonary pathologic features. Symptoms related to the local effects of malignant lung tumors include *cough, dyspnea, chest pain,* and *hemoptysis* accompanied by *weight loss* and *general weakness.* Five to ten years may elapse from the time a tumor begins development from a single cell until it becomes detectable in the lungs; when the patient develops any of the aforementioned symptoms, there has been ample time for metastases.

Other types of primary malignancies in addition to bronchogenic carcinomas are listed in the box. Many of these are extremely malignant, such as *mesotheliomas* and *small cell undifferentiated carcinomas.* Others, such as *carcinoid tumors* and certain types of bronchial gland tumors *(cylindromas),* are considered to be far less malignant but are locally invasive and, upon occasion, may metastasize. These tumors have an endobronchial location and are often called *bronchial adenomas.*

Lung tumors that develop by spread from malignancies involving other parts of the body are called *metastatic tumors.* Metastases commonly spread from the breast, kidney, prostate gland, testicle, gastrointestinal tract, and other sites. This spread of malignant cells to the lungs and surrounding thoracic structures is via four major routes, as follows: (1) the arterial and venous circulatory system; (2) the lymphatic system; (3) the direct local invasion of nearby structures; and (4) the tracheobronchial system, as in metastases from the larynx, oral cavity, and paranasal sinuses.

Likewise, primary lung tumors may spread to other organ systems as well as to other parts of the lungs by the same routes. The presence of lymph node metastases outside the thoracic cavity, as determined by scalene lymph node biopsy, indicates incurable and unresectable disease.

Granulomatous Lesions

Tuberculoma, coccidioidoma, and *histoplasmoma* are residual masses of necrotic debris or old granulomatous tissue in the lung parenchyma. This type of lesion commonly presents as a single peripheral lesion on the chest x-ray in a patient with a history of *tuberculosis, coccidioidomycosis,* or *histoplasmosis.*

*GLOSSARY FOR THE TMS CLASSIFICATION OF LUNG CANCER**

T Refers to local tumor characteristics.
N Refers to regional hilar and mediastinal lymph node involvement.
M Refers to distant metastasis.

CODES

T_X Occult cancer. Malignant cells are present on sputum cytology but are not detected by x-ray or bronchoscopy.
T_{IS} Carcinoma *in situ.*
T_1 Solitary nodule less than 3 cm in greatest diameter. No bronchoscopic evidence of invasion proximal to a lobar bronchus.
T_2 Nodule greater than 3 cm diameter or any size lesion that invades visceral pleura or has obstructive pneumonitis or atelectasis associated with it but not involving an entire lung. Bronchial lesion must be 2 cm distal to carina. No pleural effusion.
T_3 Any size tumor with direct extension to parietal pleura, chest wall, diaphragm, or mediastinum. A lesion involving the main stem bronchus less than 2 cm from the carina. Associated atelectasis or obstructive pneumonitis involving an entire lung. Malignant pleural effusion.
N_0 No extension of tumor to hilar or mediastinal nodes.
N_1 Metastasis to peribronchial or ipsilateral hilar lymph nodes.
N_2 Mediastinal lymph node involvement.
M_0 Absence of distant metastasis.
M_1 Metastasis outside the thorax, for example, to scalene, cervical, or contralateral hilar lymph nodes, brain, bone, and liver or to the contralateral hilar lymph nodes or lung.

*Tumor-node-metastasis classification system adopted by the World Health Organization to stage lung cancer.

Old lesions are usually calcified and may be responsible for reactivated granulomatous disease in debilitated or immunosuppressed patients. Although this lesion is typically benign, *scar carcinoma* can arise in its vicinity.

VASCULAR DISEASE

Pulmonary Edema

Pulmonary edema is defined as an *abnormal increase in the amount of extravascular fluid in the lungs.* This disease is a major complication of many cardiopulmonary diseases. In its acute form, pulmonary edema is a life-threatening medical emergency that frequently requires endotracheal intubation and mechanical ventilation: it may be *cardiogenic* or *noncardiogenic* in origin.

Cardiogenic Pulmonary Edema. Cardiogenic pulmonary edema is due to hemodynamic alterations. The characteristic feature is a rise in pulmonary capillary pressure, as a result of one or more of the following: (1) *elevated left ventricular end-diastolic filling pressure,* as in aortic valve disease, hypertension, coronary artery disease, and cardiomyopathies; (2) *elevated left atrial pressure,* as in mitral valve disease; and (3) *elevated pulmonary venous pressures,* as in *pulmonary veno-occlusive disease.* The last term refers to a rare condition, affecting mainly children and young adults, in which numerous pulmonary veins and venules are narrowed or completely obliterated by dense connective tissue.

The most common causes of cardiogenic pulmonary edema are left ventricular failure and mitral valve disease. *Left ventricular failure (congestive heart failure)* results from the inability of the left ventricle to pump out sufficient blood for metabolic demands of the body. It is usually due to some acute precipitating event, such as *acute myocardial infarction,* in which the patient passes through all the stages of cardiogenic pulmonary edema in minutes to hours.

In contrast, *mitral stenosis* is a chronic form of pulmonary edema that gradually becomes worse over a period of years. The stenotic mitral valve impedes the forward flow of blood into the left ventricle. Blood begins to accumulate in the left atrium, gradually increasing left atrial pressure and then pulmonary venous pressures until interstitial edema occurs in the lungs. The slow progression of the disease and the associated clinical signs and symptoms usually allow time for the patient to seek medical help before the alveoli fill with fluid and produce *acute pulmonary edema.*

In any case, the pulmonary patient does *not* typically present with left ventricular failure unless he has accompanying cardiac disease. Yet, in the acute situation, whenever left ventricular function is compromised, and this stress is in addition to already compromised lung function, pulmonary edema is likely, as a complication.

The three stages of cardiogenic pulmonary edema from left ventricular failure are pulmonary vascular congestion, interstitial pulmonary edema, and alveolar flooding or alveolar pulmonary edema (Fig. 8–19). The following sections explain these stages in relation to the movement of fluid into different locations in the lung and in relation to corresponding changes in selected clinical signs. The movement of fluid from pulmonary capillaries into interstitial and alveolar spaces occurs due to a change in net filtration pressure as explained by the Starling equation; this equation is

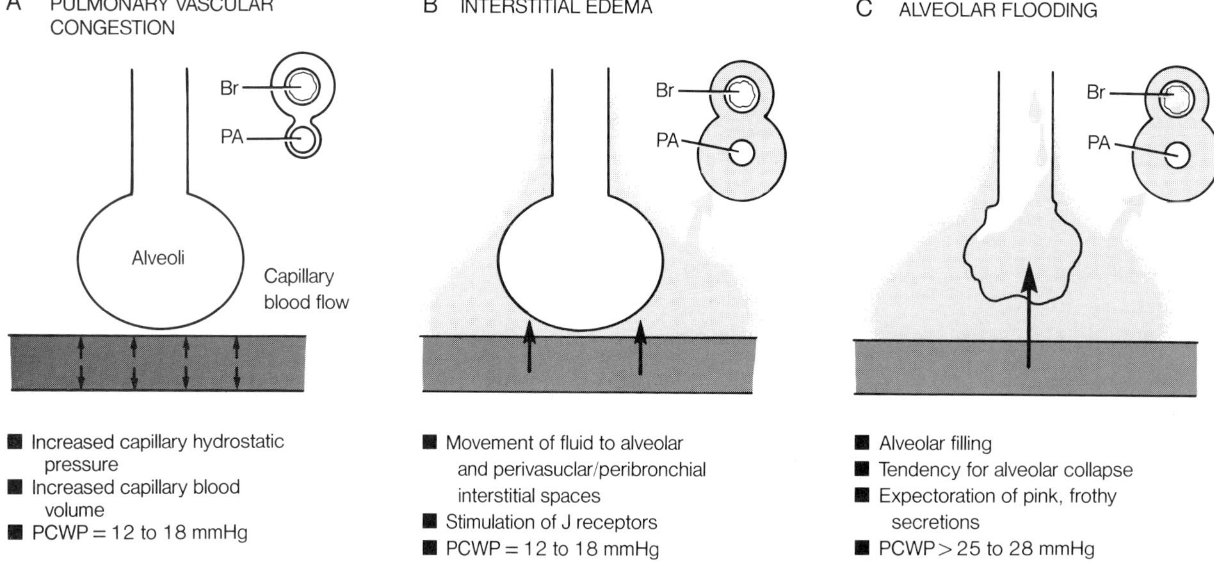

Figure 8–19. Three stages of cardiogenic pulmonary edema. (If necessary, review Figure 2–23 for identification of alveolar and perivascular/peribronchial interstitial spaces.) PCWP = pulmonary capillary wedge pressure; Br = bronchus; PA = pulmonary artery.

introduced in Chapter 4 and describes the lung-fluid balance in the lung. In essence, pulmonary edema appears when pulmonary capillary hydrostatic pressure exceeds plasma oncotic pressure.

Pulmonary Vascular Congestion. In the first and relatively asymptomatic stage of disease, hydrostatic pressure increases and exerts an outward pressure on the walls of pulmonary capillaries. This increase in pressure is accompanied by an increase in capillary blood volume due to the back-up of blood from the left ventricle. *Pulmonary vascular congestion* begins to develop (see Fig. 8–19A).

Interstitial Pulmonary Edema. With further increases in hydrostatic pressure, fluid moves into the alveolar interstitial space (see Fig. 8–19B). This interstitial edema becomes worse as lymphatics draining interstitial spaces dilate, become incompetent, and fail to remove the excess fluid filtered across the capillary membrane. Much of the extra fluid is shunted to the peribronchial and perivascular interstitial spaces, producing peribronchial "cuffs" that show up on the x-ray film around terminal bronchioles, especially around those located centrally near the hila. The swelling in the alveolar interstitial space or the decreased compliance stimulates juxtacapillary or J receptors. This stimulation is responsible for the sensation of dyspnea, which prompts the patient to increase his respiratory rate.

In this stage of interstitial edema, the patient may be able to maintain adequate alveolar ventilation and oxygenation by increasing respiratory rate and minute ventilation. Also, the normal anatomic structure of the alveolar septum is particularly conducive to excellent gas exchange. While fluid collects on the "thick side" of the alveolar-capillary membrane where the alveolar interstitium is located, the "thin side" can continue its main function of gas exchange. With this optimal arrangement, the lung may have up to three times the normal extravascular fluid content without clinical signs, such as breathlessness, increased respiratory rate, and hyperventilation (Lind et al, 1981).

Yet, interstitial edema can cause significant *shunting* (perfusion in excess of ventilation), as the interstitium continues to fill up with fluid, especially if the patient has been critically ill with other problems in the intensive care unit. Abnormal blood gases may be evident in this stage, particularly a decrease in Pa_{O_2}. In some cases, however, the patient passes so quickly through the three stages of pulmonary edema that chest x-ray signs of interstitial fluid are not evident either because a chest x-ray is unavailable or because they are seen in combination with signs of alveolar flooding.

Alveolar Pulmonary Edema. Alveolar flooding occurs when the interstitial spaces become completely filled with fluid, and filtration exceeds removal by the lymphatics. Edema develops when the pulmonary capillary "wedge" pressure, a pressure reflecting left atrial pressure, increases to *25 to 28 mmHg* (normal, 5 to 15 mmHg), as measured by a pulmonary artery catheter that has been wedged in a small pulmonary artery (see Chapter 29). Researchers still do not know exactly how and where fluid leaks into the alveoli. But pathologic specimens show that alveoli either fill completely with fluid or remain completely air filled; partial filling of alveoli with fluid is not characteristic.

As alveoli fill with fluid, disruption of surfactant that lines alveoli predisposes them to collapse (see Fig. 8–19C). "Foam" is created, as fluid and air intermix. The tiny bubbles of the classic pink- or red-tinged foamy sputum of pulmonary edema are from the presence of surfactant with its low surface tension. Although the permeability of the capillary membrane remains relatively intact, blood from a few ruptured vessels is thought to account for the pink or reddish tinge of the sputum.

The aforementioned physiologic changes produce very stiff, edematous lungs that are unable to fully expand. Lung volumes, especially the vital capacity measured at the bedside, are greatly reduced. When excess fluid obstructs the passage of air through airways, an obstructive process is present in addition to the severe restrictive defect. Shunting and alveolar hypoventilation are responsible for an abnormal V/Q ratio, a marked reduction in Pa_{O_2}, and an increased Pa_{CO_2}.

Basic Changes in the Chest X-ray Film. Figure 8–20 displays chest x-ray films of a cardiac patient passing through the three stages of cardiogenic pulmonary edema. One can easily see that in early heart failure (Fig. 8–20A), the lung fields are essentially clear and the heart in the middle of the film appears enlarged. In Figure 8–20B, the lung fields show white interstitial markings from interstitial fluid, and the heart has become larger. The last chest x-ray film (Fig. 8–20C) was taken as fluid was moving from the interstitial space into the alveoli, producing an *alveolar-interstitial* chest x-ray pattern. (See Chapter 15 for chest roentgenology.)

Adult Respiratory Distress Syndrome. Pulmonary edema is also due to a variety of noncardiogenic causes. Perhaps the most common cause is *adult respiratory distress syndrome* (ARDS), also known as *shock lung* and *wet lung.* This disorder is not a separate disease but a syndrome associated with a heterogeneous group of disorders, including shock of any cause, gram-negative sepsis, pneumonia, trauma, near drowning, drug overdose, inhalation of chemicals or high concentrations of oxygen, massive blood transfusion, air or fat emboli, and many others (Table 8–9). The common denominator in these disorders is *injury to alveolar-capillary units* with subsequent increased pulmonary capillary and epithelial permeability. Capillary membrane damage creates a "capillary leak," alveolar flooding, and acute pulmonary edema. (See Said [1985] for details of acute lung injury.)

The clinical course of ARDS is similar to that of cardiogenic pulmonary edema, except ARDS is characterized by a *normal* pulmonary capillary wedge pressure and the cardiogenic type, an *elevated* wedge pressure. Mortality rate is extremely high for this critical illness—about 50%, even in treatment centers

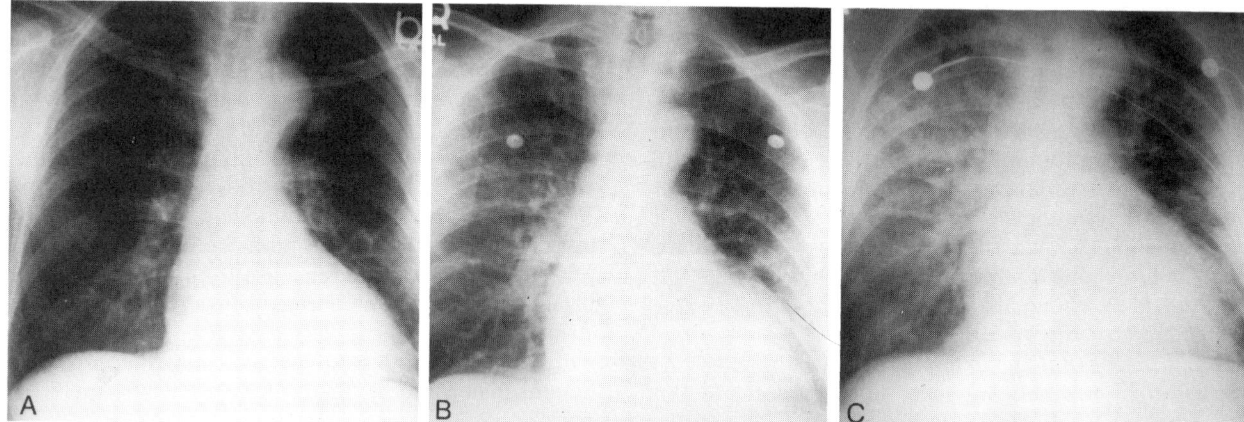

Figure 8–20. Basic changes in the chest x-ray from the pulmonary vascular congestion stage with an enlarged heart *(A)* to interstitial pulmonary edema *(B)*, to the beginning of alveolar flooding, *(C)* and then alveolar pulmonary edema. *C* demonstrates a combined alveolar-interstitial pattern in the lung field.

providing experienced care. The rate is higher for debilitated patients with multiple problems (Lind et al, 1981).

ARDS patients usually require mechanical ventilation; oxygenation; fluid replacement; corticosteroids, although no controlled studies prove the drug's efficacy; and possibly other drugs. Numerous problems may arise in the treatment of ARDS, including anxiety, fluid and electrolyte imbalance, renal failure, congestive heart failure, myocardial infarction, gastrointestinal bleeding, bacterial colonization, superinfection, malnutrition, and other complications of mechanical ventilation.

Knowledge of the basic pathophysiology of ARDS and oxygen toxicity (see Chapter 13) helps the nurse to understand treatment of hypoxemia and other res-

Table 8–9. DISORDERS ASSOCIATED WITH ADULT RESPIRATORY DISTRESS SYNDROME

Disorders	Clinical Findings
Shock (any cause)	Hypotension, blood loss
Infectious causes Pneumonia Gram-negative sepsis	Fever, chills, purulent body secretions, positive cultures of body fluids, antibodies to viral antigens
Aspiration of gastric contents	History of difficulty swallowing, leaking tracheal cuff, stomach distention, loss of consciousness, seizures, vomiting
Oxygen toxicity	Prolonged exposure to high concentrations of oxygen
Drug overdose Heroin Methadone Barbiturates Colchicine Tricyclic antidepressants	History of drug abuse, mental depression, suicidal thoughts
Transfusion reaction	Recent blood transfusion, agglutinins in cross-matched specimen, multiple blood transfusions
Trauma Lung contusion Fat emboli Nonthoracic	History of recent trauma, history of long-bone trauma with petechiae and lipuria (fat emboli)
Pancreatitis	Abdominal pain, ascites, elevated serum amylase level
Uremia	Oliguria, rising blood urea nitrogen (BUN) and creatinine levels
Increased intracranial pressure (ICP)	Seizures, increased ICP readings, head trauma
Other Disorders and Conditions	
Abscess (intra-abdominal)	Heat stroke
Amniotic fluid embolism	High altitude
Aspirin intoxication	Lymphangiography
Burns	Lymphangitic carcinomatosis
Cardiopulmonary arrest	Paraquat ingestion
Cardiopulmonary by-pass	Postcardioversion
Chemical fume inhalation	Radiation pneumonitis
Disseminated intravascular coagulation	Smoke inhalation
Drug reactions, e.g., to thiazides, ampicillin	Surgery (prolonged)
Eclampsia	Transplantation

piratory problems associated with the syndrome. In 48 to 72 hours after the initial tissue injury, *hyaline membranes* form from alveolar epithelial cell debris. In survivors, edema fluid may persist in the interstitium, and leakage of blood proteins into the interstitium increases protein osmotic pressures there, which in turn draws in more fluid. The presence of large protein molecules in the interstitial space predisposes the patient to interstitial fibrosis during the recovery period.

Although many ARDS survivors appear to recover completely, one third have permanent reductions in pulmonary function, e.g., obstruction to airflow and reduced vital capacity. All survivors may have at least some residual interstitial or vascular abnormalities, manifested by abnormal gas exchange during exercise, i.e., a widened alveolar arterial oxygen difference (Rinaldo and Rogers, 1982).

Some patients with ARDS may develop clinical manifestations similar to those of bronchopulmonary dysplasia (BPD), a disorder seen in the newborn, characterized by obliteration or marked epithelial metaplasia of bronchioles and the formation of large cystic air spaces with thick fibrous walls. BPD is actually a later stage of *infant respiratory distress syndrome* (IRDS). The early stages of IRDS and ARDS are morphologically, radiographically, and physiologically similar. The cause of BPD in the neonate is unknown, but high inspired oxygen content (see Chapter 13), use of high ventilator pressures, and lung immaturity appear to be contributing factors (Churg et al, 1983).

Re-expansion Pulmonary Edema. This unpredictable, uncommon disorder may result as a complication following evacuation of large amounts of air (pneumothorax) or fluid (pleural effusion) from the pleural space. Prolonged collapse of lung or application of excessive negative pressure during the evacuation is thought to precipitate its development. The pathophysiology of the disorder is unknown, but abnormal pulmonary capillary permeability seems to be involved (Mahajan, 1983).

Neurogenic Pulmonary Edema. *Neurogenic pulmonary edema* is due to a central nervous system (CNS) problem rather than a problem related to heart or lung pathology. The exact physiologic mechanism involved is not completely understood. One theory is that the increased intracranial pressure associated with head trauma or CNS injury initiates a centrally mediated, via the hypothalamus, massive sympathetic nervous system discharge (Milley et al, 1979). The sympathetic discharge briefly increases systemic and pulmonary vascular pressures, resulting in the shift of blood from the systemic to the low resistance pulmonary circulation. The increase in pressures may last only 5 to 15 minutes. However, it is so dramatic that it damages pulmonary capillary walls, producing the persistent leak of fluid out of capillaries into alveoli and airways, even though vascular pressures return to normal. Left ventricular failure does *not* occur—it is averted as vascular pressures return to normal. Therefore, the left ventricle does not dilate as in cardiogenic pulmonary edema, and it remains normal in size on the chest x-ray. This feature helps to identify neurogenic pulmonary edema in the clinical setting.

Pulmonary Embolism

Pulmonary embolism is the plugging of pulmonary vessels with an embolus, defined as a mass of undissolved matter transferred to the lungs by blood or lymphatic vessels. Emboli may arise within the body or gain entrance from without. Occasionally, an embolus or thrombus arises within the lung itself in the pulmonary arterial system, as occurs in *pulmonary vasculitis* caused by infections, foreign bodies, and immunologic responses. Emboli appear in solid, liquid, and gaseous forms and can be categorized into one of the following different types:

1. *Thrombotic* emboli from thrombi (blood clots) arising in the venous system, notably the deep veins of the lower extremities, the pelvic area, and the right side of the heart.
2. *Fat* emboli from droplets of fat, as in single or multiple fractures of the lower extremities or pelvis.
3. *Amniotic fluid* emboli, a collection of fluid, hair, and other debris, as may occur in a difficult or complicated labor in an older and multiparous woman.
4. *Air* emboli entering the venous system through an intravenous catheter or needle.
5. *Tumor* emboli from fragmented pieces of malignant tissue.
6. *Foreign material* emboli from substances accidentally entering the venous system from diagnostic studies. Also, foreign bodies (e.g., bullets, sutures, and tips of indwelling catheters that break off or fragment) enter the venous system and lodge in the lungs. Drug abusers may inject medications intended for oral use. Foreign particles, commonly common fibers through which dissolved heroin is filtered, may be injected along with the injectate.
7. *Septic* emboli from infected or contaminated tissues, substances, or foreign bodies.
8. *Parasitic* emboli from parasites that migrate through the lungs during their life cycle in the human host.

Under normal circumstances, the lungs efficiently filter blood clots and other particles that are larger in diameter than the formed elements in the blood. Small clots are easily dissolved because of the lung's fibrinolytic mechanism, but a single large clot or multiple small ones cause respiratory distress with symptoms of *dyspnea*, *chest pain*, *acute anxiety*, *cough*, and *hemoptysis*. The extent of symptoms depends on the size of the embolus obstructing pulmonary blood flow and the underlying condition of the patient. Symptoms range from none at all in the case of occasional small emboli to tachypnea; deep substernal chest pain, with occcasional radiation to the arms and shoulders; sudden drop in blood pressure; and respiratory arrest, with acute massive emboli. Because of the variability in extent of pathology and accompanying symptoms. pulmonary embolism is considered to be frequently misdiagnosed or undiagnosed by physicians.

Predisposing Factors. Actually pulmonary embolism is not a primary disease but a consequence of some other pathologic event in the body, usually venous thrombosis with or without associated inflammatory reaction. The physiologic factors that predispose patients to thromboses were delineated over 100 years ago by the pathologist Virchow. The three factors are as follows:

1. Venous stasis or sluggish blood flow
2. Increased blood coagulability
3. Damage to the vessel wall, especially the endothelial surface

These factors are listed in the box along with specific situations and disorders predisposing the patient to pulmonary embolism. Several of the situations and disorders are commonly found in pulmonary patients as well as in other types of patients with unrelated diseases. In any situation, *bed rest* promotes venous stasis and thrombosis by delaying the removal of activated clotting factors from the veins in which they are formed. Activated coagulation factors are likely to become even more increased if *immobilization* of all or part of the body is necessary for recovery from an acute illness.

Congestive heart failure in patients with advanced pulmonary disease also promotes peripheral venous stasis as well as formation of clots in the right ventricle. If *atrial fibrillation* (cardiac arrhythmia) is present, *mural* thrombi may form on the endothelial surfaces of the right atrium owing to blood stasis and incomplete emptying of the atrium with each contraction. However, since most thrombotic emboli arise from the lower extremities rather than from the heart or the upper extremities, perhaps of greater concern is venous problems of the lower extremities, specifically *thrombophlebitis* manifested by swelling of the affected limb with local tenderness and sometimes inflammation. Thrombosis may extend proximally to the thigh and pelvis. Although venous problems are often detectable because of calf tenderness, about 85% to 95% of pulmonary emboli arise from the ileofemoral veins. Moreover, pulmonary patients with chronic arterial blood gas disturbances (high carbon dioxide and low oxygen levels) typically demonstrate *polycythemia*, an increase in red blood cell count. Flow of thick blood is sluggish, predisposing the patient to clot formation. Finally, *trauma* including chest trauma from accidents and various other mishaps, as well as major surgical operations, may cause damage to vessel walls and initiate clot formation. About 50% of clots in surgical patients form during, rather than after, the operation.

Sequelae. When a large clot becomes dislodged from its peripheral site, it travels through the venous circulatory system, the right side of the heart, and lodges in the lungs in a branch of one of the pulmonary arteries. Such a clot often rests in the lower lobes, more commonly the right lower lobe, because of their normally increased blood flow. The clot may break up and lodge in several of the smaller vessels. Pulmonary artery pressure rises owing to this mechanical obstruction of vessels and possibly to the active vasoconstriction due to neurohumoral stimuli. In a *normal* individual, at least half of the cross-sectional areas of the pulmonary circulation must be obliterated before pulmonary artery pressure begins to rise. Pulmonary artery pressure is likely to rise sooner in many pulmonary patients because of their already elevated pulmonary artery pressures from underlying chronic lung diseases. The resulting increase in pulmonary vascular resistance decreases cardiac output and causes hypotension. The rapid shallow breathing that is often transient and episodic is thought to be reflexive in origin, possibly related to stimulation of the previously mentioned J receptors in the lung interstitium.

MAIN PREDISPOSING FACTORS FOR PULMONARY EMBOLISM

VENOUS STASIS

Prolonged bed rest
Immobilization
Prolonged sitting with knees flexed
Vascular disorders
  Thrombophlebitis of lower extremities, pelvic area
Congestive heart failure
Cardiac arrhythmias; atrial fibrillation

INCREASED BLOOD COAGULABILITY

Oral contraceptives
Pregnancy
Polycythemia
Malignant diseases

DAMAGE TO VESSEL WALL

Blunt trauma
Penetrating wounds
Bone fractures with soft tissue (vessel) injury
Surgical procedures, especially hip surgery, extensive pelvic or abdominal surgery, and cardiovascular surgery
Obstetric manipulations during labor and delivery

Pulmonary Infarction

Pulmonary infarction results when pulmonary embolism is extensive enough to produce the necrosis (death) of lung parenchyma. Infarction occurs in only about 10 to 15% of cases of pulmonary embolism. Pulmonary infarction is most likely in patients (1) of advanced age; (2) with septic embolism and the associated inflammatory process in the lungs; (3) with preexisting diseased pulmonary arteries, as in COPD and pulmonary vasculitis; and (4) with reduced blood flow to the bronchial arteries, supplying the lungs, as in congestive heart failure and prolonged shock. The infarction is accompanied by the appearance of hemoptysis (hemorrhage) and pleurisy (inflammation of the pleura). A pleural effusion may develop; low grade fever is common. The course of the disease is such that *hemorrhage* develops within 12 hours after embolization, *areas of hemorrhagic consolidation* and *atelectasis* within 24 hours, and *necrosis* and *swelling* later. In some cases, necrotic tissue may liquefy and form a cavity, which is observed on the chest x-ray film. Repair of tissue begins in 2 weeks, and necrotic tissue is replaced gradually with scar tissue. The term *incomplete infarction* describes the situation in which tissue is ischemic and hemorrhagic but healthy enough to heal without formation of scar tissue.

Other Vascular Diseases

Other vascular diseases include *primary pulmonary hypertension,* a rare disorder of unknown etiology that is seen mostly in females in the age range of 20 to 40 years (see Chapter 9); *pulmonary vasculitis,* inflammation of pulmonary blood vessels (arteries) often seen in scleroderma and other collagen diseases; and *pulmonary veno-occlusive disease,* a rare disease of unknown origin characterized by widespread narrowing of small- and medium-sized veins by fibrous occlusions. The characteristic pathologic features of the aforementioned vascular diseases are *occlusion of blood vessels* and *local tissue reactions.* This pathology can result in a decrease in lung distensibility, especially if the adjacent interstitial space becomes involved in the disease process.

REFERENCES

American Lung Association. (Anderson, J. M.): Occuptional Lung Diseases—An Introduction. New York, American Lung Association, 1979.

Ayers, L., Whipp, B., and Ziment, I.: Pulmonary compliance. A Guide to the Interpretation of Pulmonary Function Tests. New York, Projects in Health, Inc., 1974.

Bartlett, R. H., Gazzaniga, A., and Geraghty, T.: Respiratory maneuvers to prevent postoperative pulmonary complications: a critical review. *Journal of the American Medical Association,* 224:7, 1017–1021, 1973.

Bates, D., Macklem, P., and Christie, R.: Respiratory Function in Disease, 2nd ed. Philadelphia, W. B. Saunders Co., 1971.

Behrakis, P., Baydur, A., et al: Lung mechanics in sitting and horizontal body positions. *Chest,* 83 (4): 643–646, 1983.

Biomedical Information Corporation: Postoperative pulmonary complications—atelectasis. Kansas City, Marion Laboratories, Inc., 1978.

Bone, R. and Balk, R.: Staging of bronchogenic carcinoma. *Chest,* 82 (4): 473–480, 1982.

Breslin, E. H.: Prevention and treatment of pulmonary complications in patients after surgery of the upper abdomen. *Heart and Lung,* 10:3, 511–519, 1981.

Briggs, D.: Pulmonary infections. *Medical Clinics of North America,* 61:6, 1163–1181, 1977.

Burton, G. and Hodgkin, J. (eds): Respiratory Care—A Guide to Clinical Practice, 2nd ed. Philadelphia, J. B. Lippincott Co., 1984.

Cherniack, R. and Cherniack, L.: Respiration in Health and Disease, 2nd ed. Philadelphia, W. B. Saunders Co., 1983.

Churg, A., Golden, J., et al: Case reports—bronchopulmonary dysplasia in the adult. *American Review of Respiratory Diseases, 127*(1): 117–120, 1983.

Crofton, J. and Douglas, A. (eds.): Respiratory Diseases. Oxford, Blackwell Scientific Publications, 1981.

Crystal, R., Gadek, J.: Interstitial lung disease: current concepts of pathogenesis, staging and therapy. *The Americn Journal of Medicine,* 70:542–568, 1981.

Drage, C.: Respiratory Medicine for Primary Care. New York, Academic Press, 1982.

Findley, L., Kreis, P., Ancoli-Israel, S., and Kripke, D.: Sleep apnea in hospitalized medical patients. American review of respiratory disease, 125:4, 101, 1982.

Fishman, A.: Pulmonary Edema. Pulmonary Diseases and Disorders, vol. I. New York, McGraw-Hill Book Co., 733–753, 1980.

Forester, R., II, Dubois, A., Briscoe, W., and Fisher, A.: The Lung—Physiologic Basis of Pulmonary Function Tests, 3rd ed. Chicago, Year Book Medical Publishers, Inc., 1986.

Frame, P.: Acute infectious pneumonia in the adult. *Basics of Respiratory Disease,* 10:3, 1982.

Fraser, R. G. and Paré, J. A.: Diagnosis of Diseases of the Chest, vols. 3 and 4, Philadelphia, W. B. Saunders Co., 1979.

Fulmer, J.: The interstitial lung diseases. *Chest,* 82 (2): 172–178, 1982.

Fulmer, J. D. and Crystal, R.: Interstitial Lung Disease. In Current Pulmonology, vol. 1 (Simmons, D., ed.). Boston, Houghton Mifflin Professional Publishers, 1979.

Garay, S., Rapaport, D., et al: Regulation of ventilation in the obstructive sleep apnea syndrome. *American Review of Respiratory Disease,* 124:4, 451–457, 1981.

Glassroth, J.: Tuberculosis: a review for clinicians. *Clinical Notes on Respiratory Diseases* 20:2, 5–13, 1981.

Gold, W.: Restrictive lung disease. *Physical Therapy,* 48:5, 455–466, 1968.

Goodwin, R. and Des Prez, R. M.: Apical localization of pulmonary tuberculosis, chronic pulmonary histoplasmosis, and progressive massive fibrosis of the lung. *Chest,* 83(5):801–806, 1983.

Gottlieb, M.: Pulmonary disease in the acquired immune deficiency syndrome. *Chest,* 86(3): 29S–35S, 1984.

Guenter, C. and Welch, M.: Pulmonary Medicine, 2nd ed. Philadelphia, J. B. Lippincott Co., 1982.

Guilleminault, C., Tilkian, A., and Dement, W. C.: The sleep apnea syndromes. *Annual Review of Medicine,* 27:465, 1976.

Haas, A., Pineda, H., et al: Restrictive Pulmonary Diseases. In Pulmonary Therapy and Rehabilitation: Principles and Practice. Baltimore, Williams & Wilkins, 1979.

Hillerdal, G., Nöu, E., et al: Sarcoidosis: epidemiology and prognosis. *American Review of Respiratory Disease,* 130(1): 29–32, 1984.

Hinshaw, J. C. and Murray, J. F.: Diseases of the Chest, 4th ed. Philadelphia, W. B. Saunders Co., 1980.

Hughes, W.: *Pneumocystis carinii* pneumonitis. *Chest,* 85(6): 810–813, 1984.

Israel, H. and Atkinson, G. W.: Sarcoidosis. *Basics of Respiratory Disease,* 7(1):1–6, 1978.

Katz, J. A., Zinn, S., Ozanne, G., and Fairley, H., et al: Pulmonary, chest wall, and lung-thorax elastances in acute respiratory failure. *Chest,* 80:3, 304–311, 1981.

Keogh, B. and Crystal, R.: Chronic interstitial lung disease. In Current Pulmonology, vol 3. (Simmons, D., ed.). New York, John Wiley & Sons, Inc., 1981.

Lind, T., McDonald, J., and Avioli, L.: Adult respiratory distress syndrome. *Archives of Internal Medicine,* 141:13, 1749–1753, 1981.

Mahajan, V.: Re-expansion pulmonary edema. *Chest,* 83(1):4–5, 1983.

Milley, J. R., Nugent, S., and Rogers, M.C.: Neurogenic pulmonary edema in childhood. *Journal of Pediatrics,* 94:5; 706–709, 1979.

Mitchell, R.: The pneumoconioses. *Seminars in Respiratory Medicine,* 1:1; 55–58, 1979.

Morton, A., Hansen, P., and Baker, A. B.: Postoperative pulmonary compliance. *Anaesthesia and Intensive Care,* 5:2; 149–152, 1977.

Moser, K. (ed.): Pulmonary Vascular Diseases. New York, Marcel Dekker Inc., 1979.

Murray, J., Garay, S., et al: Pulmonary complications of the acquired immunodeficiency syndrome: an update. *American Review of Respiratory Disease,* 135:2; 504–509, 1987.

National Jewish Hospital and Research Center/National Asthma Center: Immunology: its rapid evolution holds clinical promise for AIDS. *Medical/Scientific Update,* 4(4): 2–8, 1985.

Netter, F.: The CIBA collection of medical illustration, vol. 7, respiratory system. New York, CIBA Pharmaceutical Co., 1979.

Rinaldo, J. and Rogers, R.: Adult respiratory distress syndrome—changing concepts of lung injury and repair. *New England Journal of Medicine,* 306 (15): 900–909, 1982.

Risser, N.: Preoperative and postoperative care to prevent pulmonary complication. *Heart and Lung,* 9:1, 57–67, 1980.

Said, S. (ed.): The Pulmonary Circulation and Acute Lung Injury. Mount Kisco, N.Y., Future Publishing Co. Inc., 1985.

Sanders, M.: Apnea associated with sleep. *Clinical Notes on Respiratory Diseases,* 19:3; 3–9, 1980.

Schlenker, J. D. and Hubay, C. A.: Colonization of the respiratory tract and postoperative pulmonary infections. *Achives of Surgery,* 107:2; 313–318, 1973.

Schlenker, J. D. and Hubay, C. A.: The pathogenesis of postoperative atelectasis. *Archives of Surgery,* 107:6, 846–850, 1973.

Tiep, B., Burns, M., et al: Pursed lips breathing training using ear oximetry. *Chest,* 90(2): 218–221, 1986.

Wagner, P. and West, J.: Ventilation-perfusion relationships. In Pulmonary Gas Exchange, vol. 1, (West, J., ed.). New York, Academic Press, Inc., 1980.

Warren, C. P. W.: Lung restriction. In Pathophysiology of Respiration, (Kryger, M. H., ed.). New York, John Wiley & Sons, 1981.

West, J.: Pulmonary Pathophysiology—The Essentials, 2nd ed. Baltimore, Williams & Wilkins, 1982.

Westerman, D. and Fanburg, B.: Sleep related respiratory disorders. *Respiratory Therapy,* 10:6: 57–63, 1980.

Wheatley, I. C., Hardy, K. J., and Barter, C. E.: An evaluation of preoperative methods of preventing postoperative pulmonary complications. *Anaesthesia and Intensive Care,* 5:1: 56–59, 1977.

Witek, T., Young, K., et al: The acquired immune deficiency syndrome (AIDS): current status and implications for respiratory care practitioners. *Respiratory Care,* 29(1): 35–45, 1984.

Pulmonary Heart Disease

9

Main Objectives

1. **Define the following terms: pulmonary hypertension, cor pulmonale, hypoxic vasoconstriction, pulmonary capillary wedge pressure, and right ventricular ejection fraction.**
2. **Name the five physiologic events in the pathogenesis of cor pulmonale.**
3. **State and explain three principal mechanisms responsible for increased pulmonary vascular resistance. For each mechanism, name two diseases that exemplify physiologic events.**
4. **Describe the hemodynamic effects of the lack of oxygen.**
5. **Name two situations in which the pulmonary patient develops left ventricular dysfunction.**
6. **Define and differentiate between acute and chronic cor pulmonale, giving an example of one restrictive and one obstructive disease for each of these categories.**
7. **State the signs and symptoms for pulmonary hypertension, cor pulmonale, and right ventricular failure.**
8. **Describe basic medical treatment and prognosis for cor pulmonale *with* and *without* right ventricular failure.**

Previous chapters explain how lumenal obstruction, intrinsic airway narrowing, and peribronchial obstruction cause obstructive pulmonary disease and how loss of lung tissue, loss of functioning alveoli, and decreased compliance cause restrictive pulmonary disease.

The purpose of this chapter is to describe how obstructive and restrictive diseases progress to *pulmonary heart disease*, more commonly referred to as *cor pulmonale* in medical literature. Knowledge of the pathogenesis of cor pulmonale helps one understand the progression of pulmonary disease from mild to severe. Emphasis is placed on the physiologic chain of events and their basic recognition in the clinical setting.

Definition

Researchers and clinicians have defined the term cor pulmonale differently in the past, applying different criteria for cardiac enlargement. The most popular definition seems to be as follows: "Alteration in structure or function of the right ventricle resulting from disease affecting the structure or function of the lung or its vasculature, except when this alteration results from disease of the left side of the heart or congenital heart disease" (Behnke et al, 1970). Pulmonologists define cor pulmonale as the *enlargement of the right ventricle from hypertrophy, dilatation, or both secondary to disorders that affect the structure or function of the lungs.*

Several important points are implied in this definition. First, the etiology of the right ventricular enlargement varies. Enlargement may be due to some intrinsic pulmonary disease involving the lung parenchyma or airways, or it may be due to an extrapulmonary disorder affecting lung function, more specifically control of breathing (central nervous system disorders) or dysfunction of the chest bellows (diaphragm, chest wall, and neuromuscular structures).

Second, although etiology varies, the common denominator in the initial sequelae of events is dysfunction of the breathing apparatus, which results in pulmonary hypertension. Regardless of the underlying disease, it is the respiratory dysfunction that causes cor pulmonale.

Third, the resulting right ventricular *enlargement* may be from *dilatation* (acute enlargement of the chamber), from *hypertrophy* (chronic increase in muscle mass), or from *both* processes. Right ventricular dilatation may exist alone, depending on the degree and duration of the pulmonary hypertension.

Fourth, cor pulmonale is due to *respiratory* rather than cardiac disease. Cardiac disease can cause pulmonary hypertension also, but it derives from two mechanisms not discussed in this chapter, i.e., *increased left atrial pressure* (e.g., mitral stenosis and left ventricular failure) and *increased blood flow through the lungs* (e.g., congenital heart defects, such as ventricular and atrial septal defects). The last category includes cases of left-to-right cardiac shunts with developing pulmonary vascular changes, pulmonary hypertension, and in some the reversal of the shunt to right-to-left, when pulmonary pressures become excessively high over a period of many years (so-called Eisenmenger's syndrome).

Incidence

The incidence of cor pulmonale in general cannot be accurately estimated because it often goes unrecognized both clinically and at autopsy. Cor pulmonale makes up a very small percentage (about 6% to 7%) of all types of adult heart disease (Fishman, 1980). Incidence is higher in countries and regions where cigarette smoking is prevalent, air pollution is severe, and chronic obstructive pulmonary disease (COPD) is common. Brashear (1981) estimated that 40% of patients with bronchitis, emphysema, or both have right ventricular hypertrophy. The value is probably higher for cor pulmonale, since the 40% excluded cases of right ventricular dilatation.

Table 9–1. MAIN DISEASES LEADING TO COR PULMONALE*

Physiologic Mechanism	Obstructive Diseases	Restrictive Diseases
Lack of oxygen with normal lungs	Upper airway obstruction	Gross obesity (in some patients) Neuromuscular diseases affecting the respiratory center or respiratory muscles Chronic mountain sickness Severe kyphoscoliosis
Lack of oxygen with abnormal lungs	COPD Bronchial asthma Cystic fibrosis Bronchiolitis	Chest trauma
Removal of lung tissue	—	Pneumonectomy (when remaining lung is diseased)
Obliteration of vessels from destruction of capillaries	Emphysema	Diffuse interstitial fibrosis: idiopathic form, granulomatous diseases (sarcoidosis), pneumoconioses, other disorders causing massive fibrosis Metastatic carcinoma of the lung
Mechanical obstruction of vessels causing partial or complete occlusion	—	Multiple pulmonary emboli Pulmonary vasculitis (arteritis) collagen disease, especially scleroderma Primary pulmonary hypertension Pulmonary veno-occlusive diseases

*Classified by physiologic mechanism.

Diseases Leading to Cor Pulmonale

Main obstructive and restrictive diseases that are apt to lead to cor pulmonale are listed in Table 9–1. One can see that the spectrum of disease is broad and diverse.

Physiologic Chain of Events

The physiologic chain of events in the pathogenesis of cor pulmonale is still under investigation. The basic chain of events is summarized in Figure 9–1. Many aspects of each event are incompletely understood, and some aspects are vigorously debated, such as whether COPD impairs left in addition to right ventricular function.

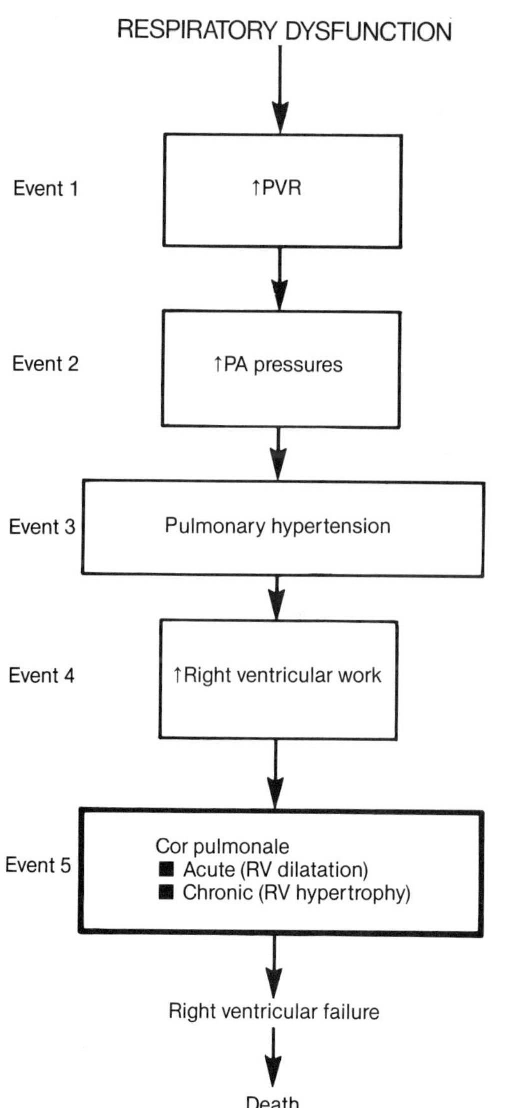

Figure 9–1. Physiologic events in the pathogenesis of cor pulmonale. (PVR = pulmonary vascular resistance; PA = pulmonary artery; and RV = right ventricular.)

The rate of progression from event 1 through event 5 (see Fig. 9–1) depends mostly on the nature and severity of the causative disorder. On the one hand, in acute severe bronchitis or upper airway obstruction, as the heart enlarges from dilatation, the patient may move through all five events within a relatively short period of time (days or weeks). On the other hand, in long-standing obstructive and restrictive disease, such as emphysema and coal worker's pneumoconiosis, the heart gradually enlarges (hypertrophy) over several decades. In contrast, relentlessly progressive chronic diseases with diffuse interstitial fibrosis can cause massive right ventricular hypertrophy within 1 to 4 years.

In addition, the progression of disease depends on the patient's general state of health. Debilitated multiproblem patients tend to progress quickly through each event to cor pulmonale and are more likely to ultimately develop right ventricular failure. Young healthy individuals who sustain substantial lung damage may rapidly adapt to the increase in right ventricular work without the development of right heart failure.

Each of the events in Figure 9–1 leading to cor pulmonale, and the main physiologic mechanisms responsible for disease progression, are discussed in this chapter. Some readers may wish to review the content of Chapter 4 on the pulmonary circulation to facilitate the understanding of more detailed concepts explained here.

INCREASED PULMONARY VASCULAR RESISTANCE

Increased pulmonary vascular resistance (PVR) is the first event in the pathogenesis of cor pulmonale. PVR is measured using a pulmonary artery catheter and the following formula (presented in Chapter 4):

$$\text{PVR} = \frac{\text{mean PAP} - \text{LAP (PCWP)*}}{\text{Q}}$$

The primary defect involved is narrowing of pulmonary vessels, primarily *pulmonary arterioles*, sometimes capillaries, and rarely veins. Extensive narrowing of vessels from various pulmonary abnormalities decreases the cross-sectional area of the pulmonary vascular bed. Blood ejected from the right ventricle encounters resistance to flow because it cannot easily pass through the narrowed vessels in the lungs.

The three main mechanisms responsible for increased PVR are *lack of oxygen, destruction or surgical resection of lung tissue,* and *mechanical obstruction of vessels* from vascular changes. Of these, lack of oxygen is perhaps most central, as shown in Figure 9–2.

*Pulmonary vascular resistance equals mean pulmonary artery pressure minus left atrial pressure (measured clinically as pulmonary capillary wedge pressure) divided by cardiac output.

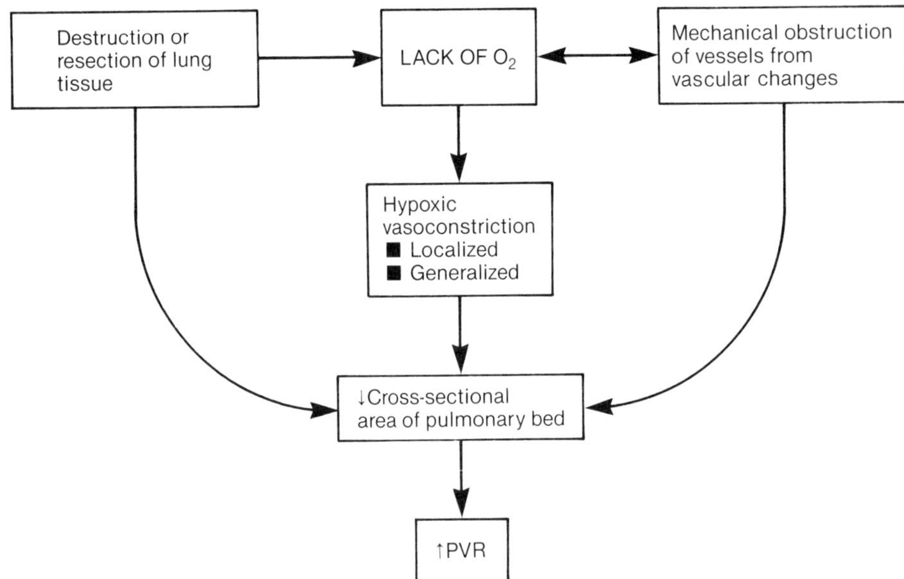

Figure 9–2. Main mechanisms causing increased (↑) pulmonary vascular resistance (PVR).

Lack of Oxygen

The lack of oxygen and associated abnormal blood gas values appear to be the main determinants of pulmonary hypertension in pulmonary disease (Brashear, 1981).

It is the low *alveolar* PO_2 (rather than low arterial PO_2) that initiates the incompletely understood active response in tissue surrounding affected alveoli. Smooth muscle in the walls of small arterioles contracts. This process is called *vasoconstriction.* Vasoconstriction narrows vessels and further impairs the local transfer of O_2 and CO_2 across the alveolar-capillary membrane because blood flow becomes reduced in affected areas of the lung. Local tissue hypoxia (lack of O_2) occurs. This local tissue reaction is called *hypoxic vasoconstriction.* Acidosis (low blood pH) in the capillary vessels often accompanies tissue hypoxia and augments vasoconstriction. Also, the local release of chemical mediators from perivascular tissue may contribute to vasoconstriction, as in asthma and pulmonary embolism. In pulmonary embolism, mediator release is believed to be responsible for producing both bronchoconstriction and pulmonary vascular spasm in nonembolized segments of the lung (Robin, 1982).

Localized Hypoxic Vasoconstriction. In many diseases, particularly restrictive parenchymal diseases, hypoxic vasoconstriction appears to be localized because disease is localized in certain regions of the lungs, and the body readily adapts to the abnormality. Both ventilation (V) and perfusion (Q) are reduced proportionally in diseased regions, producing a relatively normal V/Q ratio. (see Chapter 5 for explanation of V/Q ratio.) Also, pulmonary blood flow is redirected *away* from diseased regions and *toward* normal or near normal alveolar capillary units, where blood can become fully oxygenated. The overall V/Q ratio for the lungs as a whole as well as total PVR remains normal or near normal.

Generalized Hypoxic Vasoconstriction. Adaptation is more difficult when hypoxic vasoconstriction is generalized to most or all regions of the lungs owing to more extensive lung disease or pathology that limits the exposure of otherwise healthy alveolar-capillary units to O_2, e.g., upper airway obstruction, mountain sickness. In the case of extensive lung disease, PVR increases because few healthy areas of lung remain to compensate for diseased areas. Some diseases characteristically produce generalized hypoxic vasoconstriction and more dramatic increases in PVR. In *upper airway obstruction,* the lesion obstructs air flow to both lungs, and all alveoli are uniformly underventilated and underoxygenated. PVR continues to rise until medical treatment relieves the obstruction. In *mountain sickness from high altitude,* all alveoli are exposed to ambient air low in O_2 concentration. With acclimatization, the low PaO_2 causes mountain residents to chronically hyperventilate, driving $PaCO_2$ to low levels. For unknown reasons, some of these individuals lose their ventilatory drive to breathe. An abnormality in CNS regulation of the control of breathing is implicated. $PaCO_2$ rises, and PaO_2 drops to lower levels, making hypoxic vasoconstriction worse and greatly increasing PVR.

Destruction or Resection of Lung Tissue

In emphysema, the destruction of alveoli is matched over time by the loss of nearby capillaries as well. Similarly, in diffuse interstitial fibrosis, the thickening of the interstitium and alteration in alveolar structure are matched by the obliteration of nearby capillaries and sometimes small arteries. Such *destructive processes* eventually and completely obliterate capillaries in diseased areas of the lungs, leaving cystic spaces or bullae, as explained previously.

Although this organic basis is one mechanism for increased pulmonary vascular resistance, more than one mechanism is commonly involved. There may be no correlation between the extent of certain destructive diseases, such as emphysema, and the extent of right ventricular hypertrophy or dilatation. For example, cor pulmonale may occur when only 14% of the lung is destroyed by centrilobular emphysema and when 40% to 70% of the lung is destroyed in panlobular emphysema (Hicken et al, 1966). The higher incidence for the centrilobular group is probably related to the higher incidence of accompanying bronchitis in patients with this type of emphysema. Secretions from bronchitis block air flow and drastically reduce alveolar ventilation. Whenever an accompanying obstructive process, such as bronchitis, is involved, localized vasoconstriction becomes more widespread, increases in PVR become more marked, and the overall V/Q ratio becomes more abnormal.

Surgical resection of lung tissue (pneumonectomy) also decreases the cross-sectional area of the pulmonary vascular bed and may increase resistance to blood flow through the remaining lung. However, if the remaining lung is healthy, the rise in PVR may not be large enough to increase pulmonary arterial pressure. Previously underperfused vessels in the remaining lung are recruited to accommodate the entire cardiac output.

Mechanical Obstruction of Vessels

This mechanism refers to the complete or partial occlusion of pulmonary vessels by vascular changes (described subsequently). Although occlusion by vascular changes may occur in response to the first mechanism—the lack of O_2—it is the causative mechanism characteristic of various vascular diseases, such as *pulmonary emboli, pulmonary vasculitis, pulmonary veno-occlusive diseases,* and *primary pulmonary hypertension.*

Primary pulmonary hypertension is discussed to help explain the pathogenesis of mechanical obstruction. This disease is a relentlessly progressive one of unknown etiology characterized by a persistent rise in pulmonary vascular pressures. Symptoms include exertional dyspnea, excessive fatigue, and sometimes syncope during physical effort. Death usually is within 2 to 8 years after onset of symptoms. Primary pulmonary hypertension is considered a distinct disease entity because of its tendency for familial occurrence, its predilection for young to middle-aged women, and evidence that it can be induced by some drugs.

Vicious Circle of Vascular Changes. In primary pulmonary hypertension, once pulmonary pressures begin to steadily increase, the upward trend is difficult if not impossible to stop because of progressive secondary changes in arteries. The primary vascular change is an increase in smooth muscle that lines the walls of small arteries. Muscular thickening narrows vessels, promoting the stasis of blood and hypoxic vasoconstriction. These effects become much worse as the intima (innermost lining) of vessels proliferates, becomes fibrous, and sometimes obliterates the lumens of vessels. Blood stasis predisposes the patient to the formation of thrombi and further narrowing of vessels due to the presence of obstructive intralumenal thrombi and the release of various vasoconstricting substances, such as histamine and serotonin. Hence, a *vicious circle* develops in which each pathologic event promotes further narrowing of vessels. Once started, this circle accelerates disease and accounts for the relatively poor prognosis for patients with progressive vascular diseases.

Most important, this vicious circle of vascular changes seems to be operating to some degree in *any* patient with progressive or severe pulmonary hypertension. Pulmonary hypertension always begets more pulmonary hypertension. Hence, the reduction of PVR and pulmonary arterial pressures becomes all the more crucial to prolonging the patient's life.

Unfortunately, event 1—increased pulmonary vascular resistance—is the clinically silent event in the pathogenesis of cor pulmonale. Patient and physician may be totally unaware of the presence of disease because of the absence of signs and symptoms.

INCREASED PULMONARY ARTERY PRESSURE

Severe and extensive pathology must be present before pulmonary vascular resistance rises sufficiently to cause the sustained increase in pulmonary artery (PA) pressures and the appearance of signs and symptoms. In fact, *up to 60% to 70% of the vascular bed must become obstructed or obliterated before PA pressures rise substantially* (Hinshaw and Murray, 1980).

The slow development of increasing PA pressures is attributed to the unique design of the pulmonary circulation. As pointed out in Chapter 4, the pulmonary circulation is a low pressure system that can easily adjust to the narrowing of vessels, obliteration of vessels, and corresponding decrease in the cross-sectional areas of the pulmonary vascular bed. In fact, when pulmonary abnormalities cause an increase in pulmonary artery pressure, pulmonary vascular resistance tends to *decrease* rather than increase.

The decrease in resistance is due to two main mechanisms. *First,* pulmonary arteries and their branches are extremely distensible because they are thin walled and contain relatively little of the smooth muscle found in systemic arterioles. Pulmonary arteries can easily distend or expand in response to greater pressures. Distension increases the lumen of vessels and decreases the resistance to blood flow. *Second, the opening up or recruitment* of previously closed vessels expands the surface area of the pulmonary vascular bed. The normal lung contains about 2000 capillaries/alveolus, and only about 25% of these capillaries are perfused at rest (Tisi, 1980); the rest remain underperfused or closed and unavailable to conduct blood. As pressures rise, these vessels are recruited—

they begin to conduct blood and cause a decrease in PVR. Hence, compensatory mechanisms decrease PVR and tend to lower any recent elevations in PA pressure.

Key Role of the Lack of Oxygen

Both physiologic mechanisms—destruction or resection of lung tissue and mechanical obstruction of vessels from vascular changes—decrease the cross-sectional area of the pulmonary vascular bed by organic means. However, when the underlying disease is advanced, the abnormal V/Q ratio results in an oxygenation problem. Hence, these two mechanisms eventually contribute to the main mechanism in Figure 9–2—the lack of O_2. Furthermore, the lack of O_2 contributes to other *hemodynamic alterations* that further increase PA pressures and become more marked as PaO_2 continues to decrease, and heart failure becomes imminent or clinically evident. Hemodynamic alterations related to the lack of O_2 are summarized in Figure 9–3.

CNS Response. The pathway labelled *A* in Figure 9–3 represents the CNS response to poorly oxygenated blood in the systemic and coronary circulations. When peripheral chemoreceptors sense a low PaO_2, they cause the hypothalamus of the brain to stimulate adrenergic nerves to the lung vasculature. Sympathetic nervous stimulation of alpha-adrenergic receptors, in particular, causes vasoconstriction primarily of large pulmonary arteries. Simultaneous stimulation of beta-adrenergic receptors in the heart causes an increase in heart rate. Together, these changes represent an increase in *sympathetic vasomotor tone*; they serve to increase blood flow through the lungs, increase cardiac output, and increase pulmonary artery pressures.

Changes in Body Fluids. The pathway labelled *B* represents anticipated changes in body fluids, when blood remains poorly oxygenated for a long period of time. The lack of O_2 in the blood stimulates bone marrow to produce more red blood cells, thus increasing the patient's red blood cell mass or *hematocrit* (Hct) and producing *polycythemia*.

Polycythemia may be accompanied by a proportionate rise in plasma volume, causing marked *hypervolemia*, a rise in total circulating blood volume. The presence and extent of hypervolemia is modulated by the disease processes involved. In right heart failure, as PaO_2 drops and the heart fails, blood flow is redistributed *away* from the periphery and *towards* vital organs. Renal blood flow becomes reduced. A subsequent decrease in glomerular filtration leads to an increase in aldosterone secretion by the adrenal cortex and, eventually, a retention of sodium and water by the renin/angiotensin mechanism. The extra water adds to total blood volume.

Together with the greater sympathetic vasomotor tone (pathway *A* in Fig. 9–3), hypervolemia increases mean vascular pressures, thereby causing greater venous return to the heart, ventricular diastolic filling, and ultimately cardiac output. The increase in flow through the pulmonary circulation elevates the PA pressures.

Keep in mind that the hemodynamic alterations discussed thus far may vary among patients. For example, total blood volume may remain relatively normal rather than increased if fluid moves out of vessels and into interstitial spaces. The movement of fluid within and between fluid spaces is governed by numerous factors, including hydrostatic and osmotic pressures, position of the patient, degree of liver dysfunction, and degree of polycythemia.

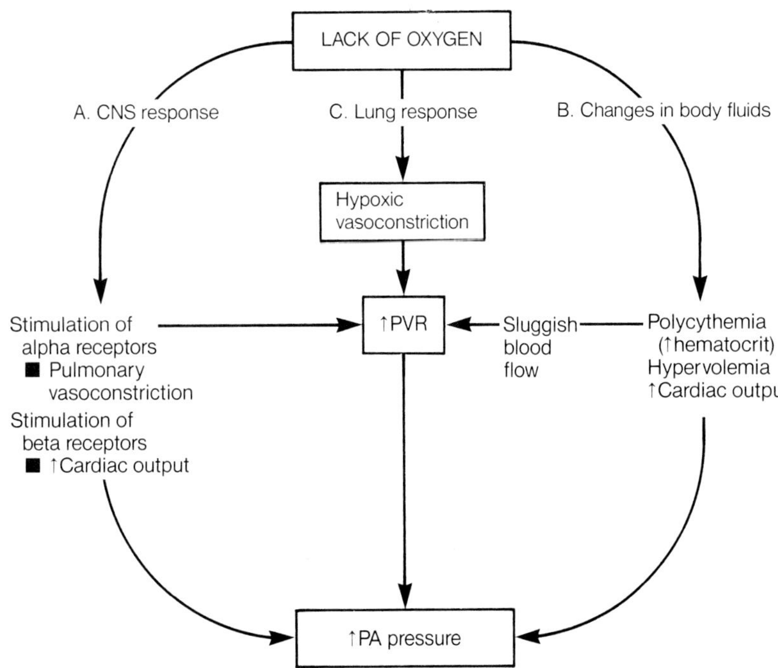

Figure 9–3. Hemodynamic alterations related to the lack of oxygen in pulmonary disease.

The Lung's Response. The pathway labelled C represents the lung's response to the lack of O_2. Hypoxic vasoconstriction leads to mechanical obstruction of vessels from vascular changes, as previously described. The vessel narrowing, obstruction, or both grossly decreases the cross-sectional area of the pulmonary vascular bed, thus increasing PVR. This effect is more dramatic when the cross-sectional area has already been reduced by preexisting pulmonary disease or major surgical procedure (e.g., lung resection).

In addition, polycythemia contributes to increased PVR. The higher number of red blood cells causes the blood to become extremely thick and to move sluggishly, particularly through small vessels; it also impedes the forward flow of blood through the pulmonary capillary bed. When the blood hematocrit level rises to greater than 55% to 60%, PVR rises to the point of decreasing cardiac output. In the clinical setting, one strives to promptly identify marked polycythemia because it is predictive of heart failure in pulmonary patients. When polycythemia is severe, the physician may perform small phlebotomies (withdrawal of about 250 ml of venous blood) to reduce the red blood cell mass and avoid possible thromboembolism. Sometimes, however, the pressure of polycythemia is not identified because the hematocrit level remains near normal as a result of the dilutional effect of accompanying increases in plasma volume.

PULMONARY HYPERTENSION

Pulmonary hypertension is defined as a prolonged increase in PA pressures above normal at rest or during exercise. Pulmonary artery systolic pressure must be above 30 mmHg, and mean pressure above 18 mmHg, as measured by a catheter in the main pulmonary artery (Fraser and Paré, 1979).

Mild Pulmonary Hypertension

The mild form of pulmonary hypertension is mostly due to vasoconstriction from the *lack of* O_2, *acidosis*, or both. The hypertension may be respiratory or metabolic in origin. Except in the case of relentlessly progressive diseases, it is generally considered to be reversible because the administration of O_2, vasodilator drugs in select cases, and the normalization of arterial blood gases either partially or completely return PA pressures to normal. This effect is the physiologic basis for the administration of continuous O_2 to relieve pulmonary hypertension and prevent the development of cor pulmonale.

The identification of mild hypertension is no easy task because the patient typically remains asymptomatic, sometimes even with mean pressures as high as 24 mmHg. The results of other assessment parameters, specifically the chest x-ray, electrocardiogram, and physical examination, are normal. Even if a catheter were placed in a pulmonary artery to measure mean pressure, the reading may not be helpful because with mild disease, pressure at rest remains normal—the distension and recruitment of pulmonary vessels easily compensates for disease. Pressure rises only when the patient exercises. Patients in critical condition cannot exercise because they are too ill. Ambulatory patients can exercise, but insertion of a pulmonary artery catheter is an invasive diagnostic procedure that is inappropriate as a general screening measure. Hence, many patients with early disease remain undiagnosed.

It is important to understand more specifically why exercise testing is required to diagnose early pulmonary vascular disease. In the normal lung, exercise greatly increases the cross-sectional area of the pulmonary vascular bed because closed capillaries are recruited and become fully dilated to accommodate increased blood flow through the lungs. PVR decreases while PA pressure increases only slightly. In mild pulmonary hypertension, exercise does not cause such a large increase in cross-sectional area since many of the vessels are narrowed by vascular changes and cannot be fully recruited—compensation mechanisms at rest have already recruited many of these vessels. The lung's ability to decrease vascular resistance during exercise becomes impaired. Therefore, PA pressure rises significantly.

Moderate to Severe Pulmonary Hypertension

In moderate to severe pulmonary hypertension, mean pressures are from 27 to 60 mmHg or higher. This more serious form of hypertension is reversible when associated with an acute pulmonary disorder or an acute episode of heart failure. Moderate to severe pulmonary hypertension is irreversible or only partially reversible if the patient has long-standing pulmonary disease with progressive hemodynamic worsening. Little can be done to arrest progressive vascular changes that partially obstruct and obliterate the pulmonary capillary bed. Mean PA pressures may stabilize or improve somewhat if the use of long-term O_2 relieves much of the hypoxic vasoconstriction.

In the critical care setting, elevated *systolic*, *diastolic*, and *mean* pulmonary artery pressures all confirm the presence of moderate to severe pulmonary hypertension. However, the *pulmonary capillary wedge pressure*, a measure of left atrial pressure, remains normal because left ventricular function is typically normal in pulmonary hypertension and cor pulmonale. All these measurements are taken utilizing a catheter positioned in a branch of the pulmonary artery (see Chapter 29).

In spite of the pulmonary artery catheter's diagnostic value, most patients will *not* have pulmonary artery catheters in place. It is an invasive form of monitoring, and even in the critical care setting, it is reserved for use in specific situations, possible early left ventricular failure, to assess hemodynamic function and to achieve maximum efficacy with current therapies, such as intravenous fluid administration. Hence, the clinician must rely on other clinical findings to diagnose pulmonary hypertension.

Signs and Symptoms

The main signs and symptoms of pulmonary hypertension are present to varying degrees (Table 9–2), depending on the severity and duration of the pulmonary hypertension. Signs and symptoms of the underlying obstructive or restrictive disease may also be present, many times appearing more marked than the clinical manifestations of pulmonary hypertension (e.g., sputum production in chronic bronchitis).

When physical examination findings and other diagnostic evidence are normal or inconclusive, it is often the chest x-ray film that arouses the suspicion of the presence of moderate to severe hypertension. The pulmonary arteries and right ventricle appear enlarged, and the contour of the vessels may appear abnormal, particularly when serial chest films are compared.

The patient demonstrates O_2 desaturation on the exercise stress test, but the exercise stress test is not a routine monitoring parameter in many settings.

INCREASED RIGHT VENTRICULAR WORK

High PVR and high PA pressures increase the work of the right ventricle. As pressures rise, the right ventricle successfully accommodates the extra workload by increasing heart rate and force of contraction. If any right ventricular dysfunction occurs, it occurs during exercise, when the workload is greater and pressures higher. With the development of severe pulmonary hypertension, the heart has much more difficulty pumping adequate volumes of blood through the high resistance pulmonary vascular system. The increased cardiac workload impairs the efficient pumping or *ejection* of blood from the right ventricle out through the main pulmonary artery.

Table 9–2. MAIN SIGNS AND SYMPTOMS OF PULMONARY HYPERTENSION

Signs	Symptoms
Systolic lift of lower parasternal area	Dyspnea on exertion
Pulsation in second intercostal space (from pulmonary valve closure)	Substernal chest pain
Loud pulmonary closure sound (P_2)	Syncope during exercise
Abnormal splitting of second heart sound (S_2)	
Prominent jugular venous A-wave (from increased pressure during atrial contraction)	
Prominent pulmonary arteries on the chest x-ray	
Other abnormal heart sounds may be present, e.g., right-sided S_4, pulmonary diastolic murmur	

Signs and Symptoms

Presence of the signs and symptoms of pulmonary hypertension are indications of greater right ventricular work. Other clinical manifestations may be present, such as tachycardia, high systemic blood pressure, increased respiratory rate, and general fatigue, but these and others are all indirect and nonspecific manifestations that might be found in any patient adapting to another systemic disease or a stressful event. Furthermore, when signs and symptoms of pulmonary hypertension are present, they are not accurate measures of the extent of right or left ventricular dysfunction. Currently, with available bedside monitoring techniques, clinicians cannot determine at what point increased pulmonary hypertension begins to affect right ventricular function. Increased right ventricular work remains a relatively unmonitored step in the pathogenesis of cor pulmonale. Without specific measurements, the nurse can only assume the presence of increased right ventricular work and possible right ventricular dysfunction when clinical manifestations of pulmonary hypertension and cor pulmonale appear.

Radionuclide Imaging

Various radionuclide imaging techniques have recently been developed to help assess the right and left ventricular function and the effect of pulmonary hypertension on the right ventricular myocardium. The relatively new noninvasive technique called *first-pass radionuclide angiography* measures right and left ventricular function. Although some studies suggest it may be sensitive enough for early detection of right ventricular dysfunction in COPD, its use has been limited mostly to research studies. First-pass radionuclide angiography is not routinely done in the clinical setting because of its recent development, its expense, and its requirements of sophisticated equipment and continuous monitoring in a special procedures room.

In this type of angiography, a bolus of radioisotope is injected into a peripheral vein. Images of the right and left ventricles at end-diastolic and end-systolic volumes are obtained, as the bolus traverses the central circulation. *Right* and *left ventricular ejection fractions* are calculated from the data collected.

An *ejection fraction* is the ratio of ventricular stroke volume to end-diastolic volume. In normal adults, the right ventricular ejection fraction averages about 55% (range of 45% to 65%), while the left ventricular ejection fraction is greater than 55% and averages about 69% (range of 58% to 70%) (Berger et al, 1978).

Right and left ventricles have different stroke volumes and ejection fractions per heart beat, since their respective chambers have different geometries and pump mechanics. However, the pump mechanics are such that both chambers eject the same amount of blood *per minute*, thus ensuring the forward flow of blood through these chambers.

In general, an *increased* ejection fraction reflects improved cardiac performance and the heart's ability to adapt to a greater workload by increasing contractility and stroke volume. A *depressed* ejection fraction indicates a trend towards ventricular failure.

Right Ventricular (RV) Ejection Fractions

Currently, the RV ejection fraction is the most accurate measurement of RV function. A *depressed RV ejection fraction* indicates the RV's limited ability to sustain an increased workload and to maintain adequate blood flow through the lungs. The patient with a depressed fraction is likely to already have cor pulmonale, but this is not always the case, as Berger and associates have shown.

These workers used radionuclide angiography to study right and left ventricular performance in 50 normal adults and 36 patients with COPD. Their study showed that all ten COPD patients with the diagnoses of cor pulmonale had depressed RV ejection fractions. Also, nine additional COPD patients with severe ventilatory impairments but *without* evidence of cor pulmonale had depressed fractions. All COPD patients with greatly depressed fractions had lower PaO_2 values and usually, but not always, lower pulmonary function values (forced expiratory volume) than COPD patients with normal right ventricular function. This finding supports the key role of the lack of O_2 in the pathogenesis of cor pulmonale. No relationship was found between abnormalities in right and left ventricular ejection fractions.

The results of this study and others reflect four important concepts. First, mild pulmonary disease yields normal left and RV ejection fractions at rest (Slutsky et al, 1980). Second, right ventricular dysfunction occurs before clinical manifestations of cor pulmonale. This order is logical since PVR and mean PA pressures rise significantly before signs and symptoms of pulmonary hypertension. Third, the severity of pulmonary hypertension with accompanying hemodynamic alterations varies with the severity of disease and the degree of arterial blood gas disturbances. Patients with severe disease and especially those with severe arterial blood gas disturbances (e.g., low PaO_2 and high $PaCO_2$) demonstrate the most severe hemodynamic alterations and greatly depressed RV ejection fractions (between 20% and 40%). Fourth, patients with cor pulmonale have normal left ventricular functions and normal left ventricular ejection fractions, as long as hemodynamic relationships in the body remain normal, e.g., blood pressure and circulating blood volume remain normal, and no heart failure exists. If the left ventricular ejection fraction is reduced, it is because the chamber is receiving less output from the dysfunctional right ventricle. In select cases (e.g., advanced cystic fibrosis), bulging of a massive right ventricle into the left ventricular cavity is responsible for reduced left ventricular ejection fractions (Jacobstein et al, 1981).

Left Ventricular Involvement in Pulmonary Disease

As mentioned at the beginning of this chapter, the presence and extent of left-sided heart involvement in pulmonary patients are controversial. Researchers are in the process of experimenting with the use of more sensitive indices than ejection fractions to more thoroughly evaluate left ventricular dysfunction in particular. Until the facts are sorted out and conflicting evidence is explained, the following basic points are most useful for clinical practice:

1. Cardiac dysfunction in most pulmonary patients is limited to the *right* side of the heart. Hence, monitoring focuses mostly on *right* ventricular function rather than left ventricular function.
2. The left side of the heart is involved in the *presence of coexisting cardiovascular disease*; e.g., the older pulmonary patient with coexisting arteriosclerosis and systemic hypertension. Also, a granulomatous disease, such as sarcoidosis, may invade the myocardium, and thereby affect left ventricular function.
3. The left as well as the right side of the heart is involved in the presence of a *severe* oxygenation problem, cardiac arrhythmia, and acute and extensive chest disease, e.g., acute almost complete upper airway obstruction and massive pulmonary embolism. In these situations, the heart and lung compensatory mechanisms may be insufficient to maintain adequate cardiac output. PaO_2 continues to drop, and the myocardium becomes more and more ischemic. Cardiopulmonary arrest or congestive heart failure ensues.

COR PULMONALE

Sustained increased right ventricular work eventually results in cor pulmonale.

Acute Cor Pulmonale

Acute form of cor pulmonale is present when hemodynamic alterations occur intensely over a period of hours, days, and sometimes weeks. The right ventricle *dilates*—it expands and increases the size of its chamber. This adaptive response allows the right ventricle to increase force of contraction to maintain cardiac output to the diseased lungs. It is only a temporary response because dilatation is *not* accompanied by more muscle mass to sustain the greater workload over a long period of time. After the acute illness resolves, the right ventricle returns to its normal size. Examples of pulmonary diseases leading to acute cor pulmonale include upper airway obstruction, pulmonary embolism, severe chronic pneumonia, and bronchitis.

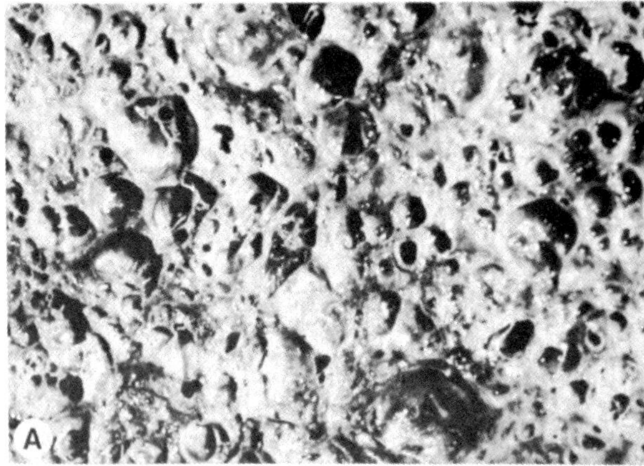

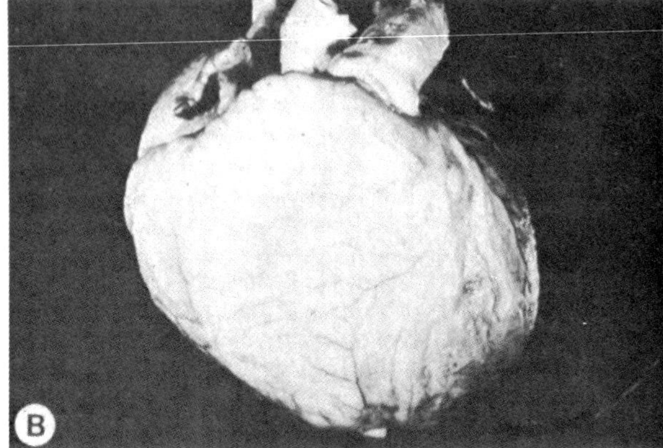

Figure 9–4. Advanced idiopathic pulmonary fibrosis. *A*, The lung's surface showing multiple cystic spaces and diffuse fibrosis. *B*, An enlarged heart with right ventricular hypertrophy. (Reproduced by permission from Crystal, R., Gader, J., et al: Interstitial lung disease: current concepts of pathogenesis, staging and therapy. *The American Journal of Medicine*, 70:543, 1981.)

Chronic Cor Pulmonale

The chronic form of cor pulmonale occurs with the gradual and persistent rise in pulmonary artery pressure over months to years, or it occurs when acute illness becomes prolonged over weeks to months. The long time period allows the right ventricle to *hypertrophy*—increase the size of its muscle mass—to better withstand the high pressure workload without cardiac decompensation (Fig. 9–4B). Examples of conditions leading to chronic cor pulmonale include upper airway obstruction, COPD, cystic fibrosis, diffuse interstitial fibrosis, neuromuscular diseases involving the CNS control of breathing (e.g., idiopathic alveolar hypoventilation) or the nerves and muscles of breathing (e.g., poliomyelitis and myasthenia gravis), hypoventilation from gross obesity, chronic mountain sickness, and others.

Acute Cor Pulmonale Superimposed on Chronic Disease

Hospitalized pulmonary patients commonly have acute disorders, such as right ventricular failure and acute asthma, superimposed on a chronic disease, such as COPD. In these cases, acute cor pulmonale (RV dilatation from failure or asthma) is superimposed on chronic cor pulmonale (RV hypertrophy from the underlying chronic disease). After medical treatment, RV enlargement from dilatation disappears, leaving RV enlargement from hypertrophied muscle. Note that right ventricular failure is an example of cor pulmonale, but cor pulmonale is *not* synonymous with right heart failure.

Main Involved Chest Diseases

Of the diseases listed in Table 9–1, COPD is the most common cause of cor pulmonale. It is most characteristic of the *chronic bronchitic patient* because this patient typically has the most abnormal V/Q ratio, the most acidotic and hypoxic capillary bed, and the most abnormal arterial blood gases. Hence, it is the bronchitic, rather than the asthmatic or emphysematous patient, who experiences frequent episodes of *acute* right ventricular failure (acute cor pulmonale) because of his persistent oxygenation problem.

Cor pulmonale is not common in *asthmatics* unless they have accompanying bronchitis or emphysema.

Cor pulmonale is not found in the *emphysematous patient* until *very* advanced disease, since he develops an abnormal V/Q ratio with abnormal arterial blood gases much later than the bronchitic patient. The pink puffer may have considerable destruction of lung tissue and may be breathless for years before pulmonary hypertension and cor pulmonale develop; sometimes, cor pulmonale does not develop. As with other chest diseases, pulmonary hypertension seems to correlate with development of the lack of sufficient O_2 in the blood, a situation that is largely reversible with the administration of O_2, even in emphysema (Fishman, 1976).

Cor pulmonale is likely to develop in *vascular diseases* that obliterate pulmonary vessels (e.g., multiple pulmonary emboli, primary pulmonary hypertension, and pulmonary arteritis), since they tend to produce gross elevations in PA pressures. PA pressures may reach or surpass systemic blood pressures, while left atrial pressures and cardiac output remain normal to decreased. The obliteration of vessels is central to the pathogenesis of cor pulmonale in these diseases because the extent of pathology is widespread.

In other chronic restrictive diseases, particularly *diffuse interstitial fibrosis*, cor pulmonale develops late in the progression of disease along with V/Q abnormalities and arterial blood gas disturbances.

Cardiac Output

In cor pulmonale, cardiac output in general is normal to lowered. However, if the lack of O_2 is a chracteristic feature of a particular disease, as it is in chronic bronchitis, then cardiac output tends to be greater, owing to polycythemia, hypervolemia, and other hemodynamic effects previously described in this chapter (Ferrer, 1975).

A recent study suggests that peripheral O_2 delivery in chronic lung disease is a function of cardiac output, and cardiac output is primarily a function of right ventricular systolic function (Morrison et al, 1986). Based on this assumption, measurement of the RV ejection by fraction radionuclide methods has been proposed as a noninvasive way to assess continuous low flow O_2 therapy. A cor pulmonale patient on O_2 therapy may demonstrate substantial improvement in O_2 delivery to tissues (assessed by cardiac output) and a small improvement in PaO_2.

Clinical Manifestations

The medical diagnosis of cor pulmonale depends on two criteria, as follows: (1) *the presence of a respiratory disease with associated pulmonary hypertension* and (2) *the evidence of an enlarged right ventricle*. The isolated finding of right ventricular enlargement is significant because it indicates the presence of pulmonary hypertension from primary pulmonary hypertension; from some other undiagnosed respiratory disorder; or possibly from a pulmonary artery disorder, valvular disorder, or cardiac shunt disorder.

Determination of right ventricular enlargement is not always straightforward since pulmonary symptoms are associated with the underlying disease process and are not specific for right ventricular enlargement. Specific signs are few and may be absent (Table 9–3).

In right ventricular hypertrophy, cardiac enlargement is usually so gradual that it may escape clinical detection. Often what suggests the presence of cor pulmonale is the appearance of signs and symptoms of abnormal arterial blood gases, e.g., paleness, cyanosis, drowsiness, and inappropriate behavior, which are confirmed by abnormal blood gas values. The chest x-ray film may show right ventricular enlargement, as shown in the case study below. However, in COPD, notably severe emphysema, cardiac enlargement may not be evident—lung hyperinflation compresses and distorts the shape of the heart and pulmonary arteries, thus making them smaller. Heavy reliance is placed on the electrocardiogram, but this diagnostic tool has its limitations, especially in COPD patients. Fishman (1980) reports that "the standard criteria for right ventricular enlargement have been found in only one third of patients with chronic bronchitis and emphysema who have been shown to have right ventricular hypertrophy at autopsy." In essence, cor pulmonale may not be evident until the right ventricle actually fails, yielding overt signs of right ventricular failure.

Table 9–3. CLINICAL MANIFESTATIONS OF RIGHT VENTRICULAR ENLARGEMENT

Physical examination
Systolic lift of lower parasternal area
Chest x-ray
Enlargement of right ventricle, pulmonary arteries, or both
Electrocardiogram
Enlarged or peaked P-waves (P-pulmonale) in leads II, III, AVF
*Right QRS axis deviation of 110 degrees or greater**
Incomplete right bundle branch block
Large R-wave in V_1 or poor R-wave progression across the precordium
S_1Q_3 *pattern**
$S_1 - S_2 - S_3$ *pattern**
*R/S ratio in V_6 of 1.0 or less**
T-wave inversion in V_{1-3}
Arrhythmias may be present from underlying pulmonary disease, e.g., wandering atrial pacemaker, multifocal atrial tachycardia
Echocardiogram: Two-dimensional images, including a view through subxiphoid region
Increased size of right ventricular and right atrial chambers and pulmonary artery
Increased dimensions for right ventricular wall, sometimes evident
Radionuclide angiography, supporting evidence
Depressed right ventricular ejection fraction

*Reliable ECG criterion in the presence of COPD (Murphy and Hutcheson, 1974).

CASE STUDY

This case study shows changes in the chest x-ray findings from a case of clinically stable COPD (A and B) to the development of acute cor pulmonale from right ventricular failure (C and D).

EXPLANATION

The posterior-anterior view (*A*) and left lateral view (*B*) are chest x-ray films of a 49-year-old female outpatient with severe, but clinically stable, COPD (emphysema and chronic bronchitis).

The cardiac silhouette and mediastinum are normal. The lung fields demonstrate no infiltrates or pleural effusions. The most impressive finding is *lung hyperinflation*, readily apparent on the lateral view (*B*) from the *increased anterior-posterior diameter, increased size of the retrosternal air space* (RAS), and the completely right (R) and left (L) *hemiflattened diaphragms* (arrows). In the posterior-anterior view (*A*), the hyperinflated lungs have depressed the hemidiaphragms so much that portions appear inverted, and numerous diaphragmatic *muscle slips* (attachments) have become visible (arrows).

The patient remained relatively stable for several years, except for occasional episodes of acute bronchitis.

Five Years Later (at age 54 years). The patient is admitted to the respiratory care unit; she is experiencing ventilatory failure with hypoxemia (low PaO_2) and cor pulmonale from right ventricular failure. The hematocrit is 76, and pitting edema is observed from toes to pelvic brim.

The entire heart appears enlarged due to *expansion of the right heart border* towards the arrows in the frontal view. This expansion to the right is a sign of *right ventricular enlargement.*

STABLE COPD

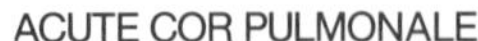

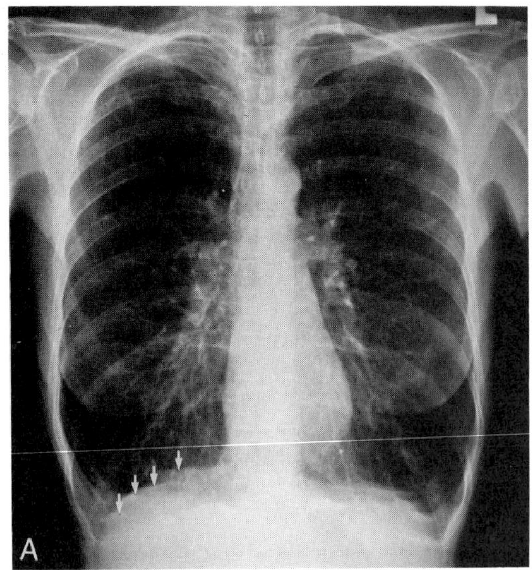

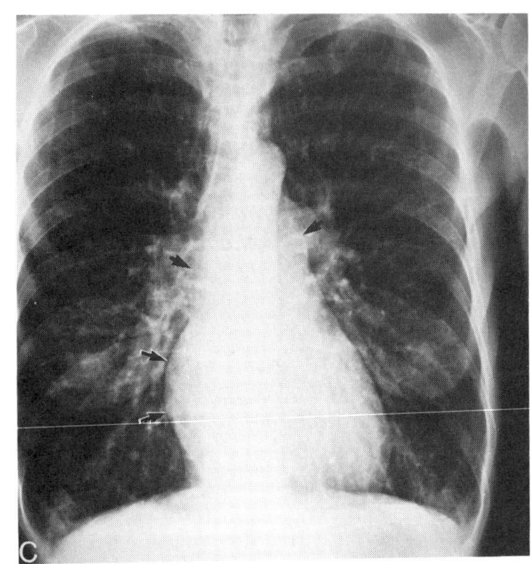

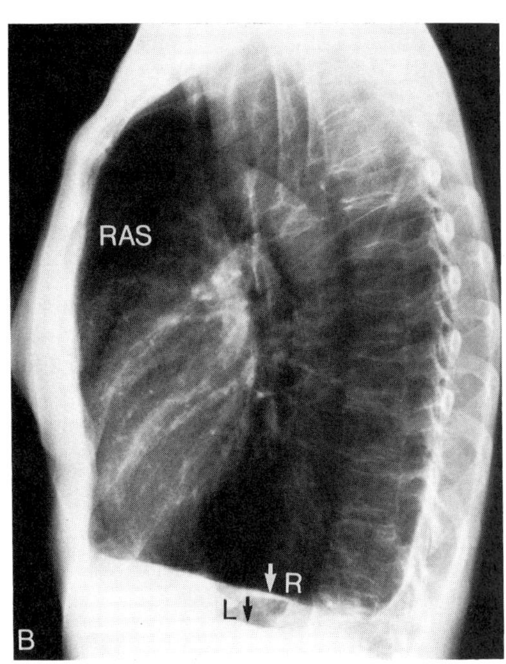

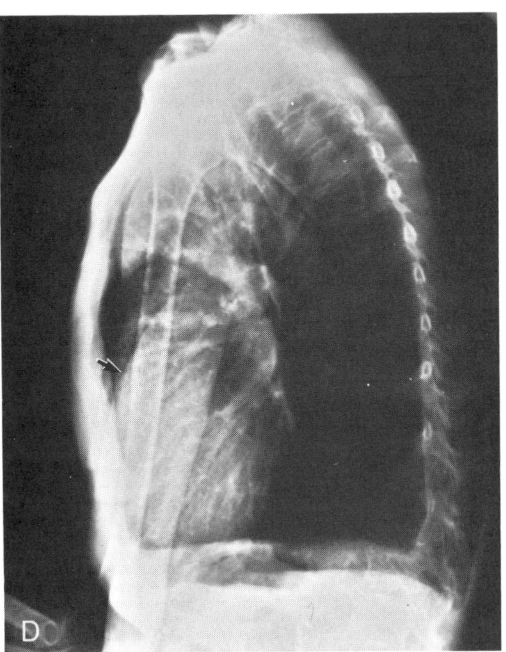

As the right ventricle expands, it begins to *"climb the sternum,"* encroaching on the retrosternal air space in the lateral view (*D*). The superior border of the right ventricle is at the tip of the white arrow. A little more posteriorly, note the arm crossing the chest—the patient was unable to lift her arms for the chest x-ray.

Five years ago in *C* and *D*, the lungs do not appear as hyperinflated as in *A* and *B*. In these more recent films, the patient was unable to take a deep inspiration, owing to severe dyspnea and decreased lung compliance from mucus retention in the lungs. In *C*, the hemidiaphragms are not as depressed and have regained some normal curvature. In *D*, lung volume and anterior-posterior diameter are reduced, compared with these findings in *B*.

In *C*, other signs indicate a worsening pulmonary status, e.g., *enlarged hilar vessels* (thick arrows) from worsening pulmonary hypertension and more *prominent bronchovascular markings* in the lung fields.

RIGHT VENTRICULAR FAILURE

When the right ventricle can no longer sustain the increased right ventricular work, it fails. Failure is usually associated with worsening arterial blood gases and an O_2-starved myocardium no longer capable of pumping an adequate blood volume into the right resistance pulmonary vascular network. In the COPD patient, mean pulmonary artery pressure increases from about 27 mmHg to a value between 40 and 50 mmHg (Israel, 1978). Hypoxic vasoconstriction is much worse with minimal exercise, causing further dramatic elevations in pressure.

Right ventricular diastolic (filling) pressure rises, as the heart fails. Blood backs up from the right ventricle into the right atrium, superior and inferior vena cava, and peripheral venous system, producing venous engorgement or congestion in many of the body's organs (Fig. 9–5). As the heart fails, cardiac output decreases.

When the liver becomes congested with the back-up of fluid, particularly if the patient has accompanying liver disease, liver dysfunction may result in *hypopro-*

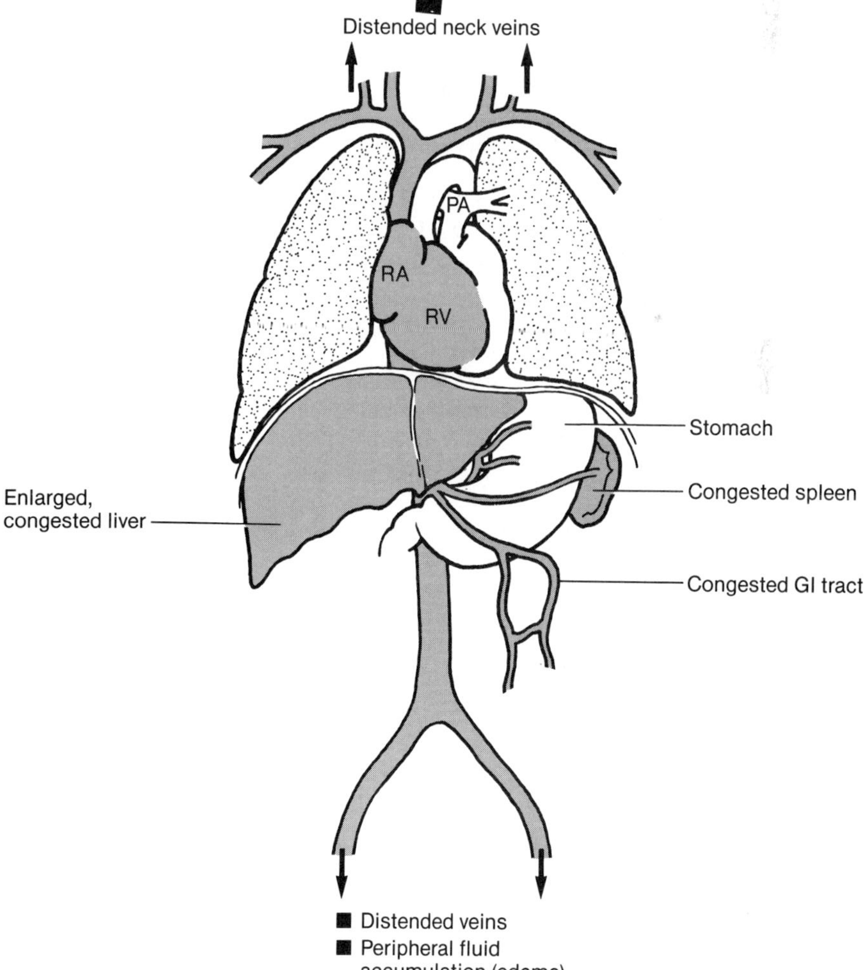

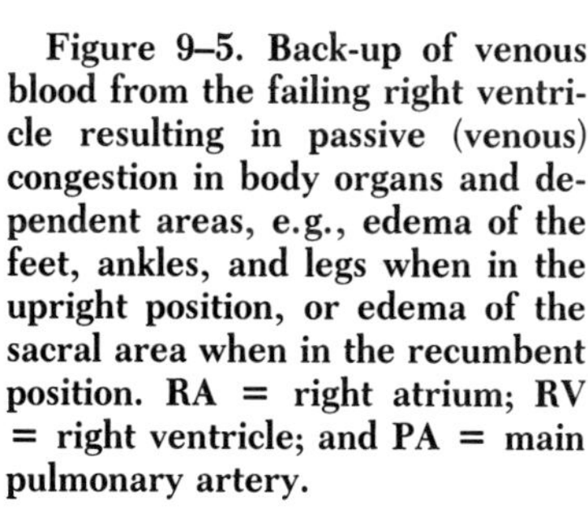

Figure 9–5. Back-up of venous blood from the failing right ventricle resulting in passive (venous) congestion in body organs and dependent areas, e.g., edema of the feet, ankles, and legs when in the upright position, or edema of the sacral area when in the recumbent position. RA = right atrium; RV = right ventricle; and PA = main pulmonary artery.

Table 9–4. SUMMARY OF RIGHT VENTRICULAR FAILURE

Signs and Symptoms	Goals and Interventions
Main signs and symptoms Fatigue Weight gain Edema in dependent areas of the body Dyspnea or dizziness on exertion **Other signs and symptoms** Chest x-ray Right ventricular and right atrial enlargement Distended azygos vein and superior vena cava Cardiovascular Systolic lift of lower parasternal area Neck vein distention Hepatojugular reflux Right-sided S_3 gallop heart sound and murmur of tricuspid insufficiency Peripheral edema Cyanosis from increased O_2 extraction by tissues Increased central venous pressure (greater than 10 cmH_2O) Hepatic Enlarged, tender liver from venous congestion Jaundice and hyperbilirubinemia from liver dysfunction Ascites Gastrointestinal (GI) Anorexia, nausea, vomiting, "fullness" after meals from venous congestion of GI tract or digitalis toxicity Constipation from inactivity Other Urine output and frequency Decreased during the day due to salt and water retention—urine specific gravity is high Increased at night due to diuresis—urine specific gravity is low Somnolence or mental confusion from increased venous pressure, decreased cerebral blood flow, or abnormal blood gases	**Goals** Correct blood gas abnormalities Reduce the workload of the heart and increase cardiac output Eliminate excess peripheral fluid accumulation Identify and treat the underlying disease process as well as precipitating factors, e.g., excessive salt intake, failure to take medications **Interventions** O_2 therapy to increase $Pa{O_2}$ Respiratory therapy (e.g., aerosol treatment) as needed to stabilize the underlying pulmonary disease Fluid restriction as needed Drugs Diuretics to prevent fluid retention associated with decreased cardiac output Electrolyte replacement for potassium and chloride loss from diuresis Digitalis use is controversial. It is administered as an adjunct rather than a main treatment. Theophylline preparation to bronchodilate and increase right and left ventricular ejection fractions in COPD patients Small phlebotomies (250 ml) for excessive polycythemia due to chronically low $Pa{O_2}$ Dietary support Sodium restriction Adequate intake of nutritious food Bedrest and then early ambulation to prevent mucus retention in the lungs and peripheral venous stasis Monitoring for signs of fluid retention, e.g., weight gain, edema Self-care education regarding causes or precipitating factors and treatment of disease process Psychologic support

teinemia. The decrease in colloid osmotic pressure promotes the leakage of fluid or "third spacing" of fluid *out* of vessels and *into* peripheral body tissues. This mechanism worsens any peripheral edema already present and decreases plasma volume as well as total blood volume.

Clinical Manifestations

The main signs and symptoms for right ventricular failure are listed in Table 9–4. (Physical findings are discussed in detail in relation to content on the physical examination of the chest in Chapter 12.) Also, since right ventricular failure is actually an example of cor pulmonale, clinical manifestations of right ventricular enlargement may become evident or more marked.

Right Ventricular Failure in Perspective

Emphasis must be placed on the vacillating position of right ventricular failure in the pathophysiologic chain of events in cor pulmonale. From one perspective, it is only one example of cor pulmonale. Like many other chest diseases, its acute form may cause cardiac dilatation when no underlying hypertrophy is present from an underlying chronic disease (event 5 in Fig. 9–1). Appropriate medical treatment (see Table 9–4) usually reverses the failure, and PA pressures return to previous levels. In critically ill pulmonary patients, especially those with accompanying cardiac diseases, worsening arterial blood gases and increased blood volumes in the periphery may cause oxygen-starved left ventricles to fail as well.

From another perspective, right ventricular failure can be seen as the *final common pathway* for all patients with end-stage chronic pulmonary disease. Right ventricular failure is the last event before death (see Fig. 9–1). The chronically ill patient is afflicted with occasional to frequent episodes of acute right ventricular failure that usually respond well to treatment. Eventually, some patients, e.g., those with chronic bronchitis, may gradually develop chronic right ventricular failure. Right ventricular failure is controlled by medications, but it sometimes becomes acute when the blood gases and the underlying chest disease become worse.

Treatment and Prognosis for Cor Pulmonale

GOALS

The goals of medical treatment of cor pulmonale include correction of the blood gas abnormalities, identification and treatment of the underlying disease process, reduction of the workload of the heart, and a reduction of the pulmonary vascular resistance.

INTERVENTIONS

Interventions focus on (1) *O_2 therapy* to increase PaO_2 and (2) other interventions that eliminate or control problems associated with the disease that causes the cor pulmonale.

It is unknown whether O_2 administration prevents cor pulmonale, but it is certain that long-term O_2 therapy (continuous or 15 hours a day scheduled to coincide with normal sleeping hours) rather than short-term O_2 therapy is needed to deal with the organic remodeling of the pulmonary capillary bed associated with severe pulmonary hypertension and chronic cor pulmonale.

In COPD, O_2 decreases blood hematocrit, prevents further rise in PVR, and improves other parameters, such as the patient's sense of well being, appetite, and alertness (Medical Research Council Working Party, 1981). When O_2 is given *continuously* in patients with severe respiratory failure, it may improve the survival rate to a level about twice that in patients receiving O_2 15 hours daily (Nocturnal Oxygen Therapy Trial Group, 1980). (See Chapter 23 for discussion of O_2 therapy.) In some cases, long-term oxygen therapy may completely reverse the right ventricular hypertrophy (Reid, 1986).

Anticoagulant drugs are used if recurrent pulmonary emboli are present or likely from a thrombosed pulmonary vascular bed.

Vasodilators may be helpful in reducing pulmonary vasoconstriction, PVR, and mean PA pressures, and in reducing cardiac output in primary pulmonary hypertension and cor pulmonale. Examples of such vasodilators include *hydralazine*, *phentolamine*, *isoproterenol*, select *prostaglandins*, *nitrates* (e.g., nitroglycerin), and *calcium channel blockers* (e.g., nifedipine). Though these drugs may improve hemodynamics, they have an uncertain and investigative role in the treatment of cor pulmonale. Therapeutic failures and unwanted side effects have occurred, and long-term effects of vasodilator therapy have not yet been established (Hyman and Kadowitz, 1984). Currently, vasodilators are reserved for select patients who have persisting signs of pulmonary hypertension or right ventricular failure, despite aggressive medical treatment (Murphy and Bone, 1984).

PROGNOSIS

Prognosis for cor pulmonale without heart failure has not been determined because evidence for this condition is often not appreciated until autopsy and even then the right ventricular hypertrophy is easily overlooked. It appears, however, that prognoses for restrictive diseases that obliterate pulmonary vessels are worse than those for COPD. In vascular diseases, treatment may alleviate signs and symptoms and at times slow the destructive process somewhat, but these diseases still are relentlessly progressive. Also, an individual residing at high altitude has a shorter survival time for the same degree of COPD than an individual residing at sea level.

The following points are generally agreed upon:

1. Survival time is worse for patients with cor pulmonale compared with those without cor pulmonale. This finding holds true irrespective of the amount of airway disease present.
2. The higher the PVR, the higher the mortality rate.
3. The presence of right ventricular failure significantly worsens prognosis, although exactly by how much is debatable.

Stevens and coworkers (1963) estimate that mean survival time of patients with cor pulmonale is 45.6 months after the initial appearance of peripheral edema. Vandenbergh and associates (1965) observed that patients with chronic bronchitis die about 16 months after the first episode of heart failure. Most medical authorities agree, however, that prognosis for COPD is generally improved owing to modern medical treatment and recent use of long-term continuous O_2 therapy. Rather than a stepwise worsening of pulmonary hypertension after episodes of heart failure, clinicians now more typically observe an improved clinical condition with appropriate medical treatment. Some clinicians have estimated prognosis for COPD patients with right ventricular failure at 5 to 17 years (Ferrer, 1975). More recently, because of variable survival rates reported in the literature and numerous factors, such as amount of CO_2 retention, that might affect survival, physicians avoid providing patients and families with specific life expectancy estimates (Hodgkin and Petty, 1987).

Cor Pulmonale in Perspective

This overview of the pathogenesis of cor pulmonale helps the nurse understand how pulmonary disease progresses to advanced or end-stage disease. When confronted with a breathless patient, one may tend to conjure up visions of physical debilitation, terminal illness, and death. Many of these patients do become respiratory "cripples" as they develop chronic cor pulmonale with repeated episodes of acute cor pulmonale from right-sided heart failure and acute ventilatory failure (see Chapter 13).

Yet, this review of physiologic events indicates that the pulmonary patient need not be a respiratory cripple. The early identification and treatment of abnormal arterial blood gases alone may prevent the onset of cor pulmonale. If the patient is already debilitated, appropriate treatment with medications, O_2, and other forms of respiratory therapy can ameliorate blood gas abnormalities, relieve distressing signs and symptoms, and help provide a more enriching life. Once the goal of reducing right ventricular work has been attained, the patient is less likely to experience as much breathlessness, mental depression, and loss of control over a seemingly relentlessly progressive disease.

Cor pulmonale is clearly a preventable form of heart disease. Nurses are becoming more involved in the identification of individuals at risk to develop cor pulmonale from various respiratory complications, such as pulmonary emboli, upper airway obstruction, and right ventricular failure. More emphasis is placed on monitoring PVR, PA pressures, and arterial blood gases. Monitoring pulmonary artery catheter readings has remained an important nursing function; monitoring PVR is receiving increasing attention. Clinicians sometimes monitor this parameter in patients during exercise preoperatively to determine their risk for complications postoperatively. Fee and colleagues (1978) documented that COPD patients whose PVR increases markedly during exercise have a higher mortality rate during elective thoracotomy for lung resection compared with those whose PVR does not increase during exercise. Most important, monitoring of blood gas measurements has become a basic and absolute necessity in caring for respiratory patients because, as previously discussed, hypoxia and hypoxemia remain central in the pathogenesis of pulmonary hypertension and cor pulmonale. Herein lies an important rationale for increasing proficiency at blood gas interpretation to aid in the prompt identification of respiratory problems.

Conclusion

Although obstructive and restrictive diseases have diverse pathophysiologies, they both progress through the same basic physiologic chain of events described in this chapter. Goals for nursing and medical interventions relate to slowing and if possible reversing progression through the five steps leading to cor pulmonale. It is my intention to impress the nurse with the reversible aspects of pulmonary hypertension and cor pulmonale. Even the dyspneic respiratory cripple must be approached with a hopeful attitude until medical evaluation determines the exact nature of disease. Conversely, one must be equally aware of the relentlessly progressive nature of pulmonary vascular disease once pathologic changes occur in pulmonary vessels. Whatever the case, the nurse plays an important role in detecting and evaluating clinical manifestations of pulmonary hypertension and cor pulmonale and in participating in comprehensive and continuing care of the patient.

REFERENCES

Alpert, J.: Pulmonary hypertension and cardiac function in chronic obstructive pulmonary disease. (Editorial.) *Chest*, 75:6, 651–652, 1979.

Behnke, R. H., et al: Primary prevention of pulmonary heart disease. Report of pulmonary heart disease study group. *Circulation*, 41:June, A17–A23, 1970.

Berger, H., Matthay, R., et al: Assessment of cardiac performance with quantitative radionuclide angiocardiography: right ventricular ejection fraction with reference to findings in COPD. *American Journal of Cardiology*, 41:5, 897–905, 1978.

Brashear, R. E.: Chronic obstructive pulmonary disease: cor pulmonale and left ventricular function. In Current Pulmonology, vol. 3, (Simmons, D., ed.), New York, John Wiley & Sons, Inc., 1981.

Crystal, R., Gadec, J., et al: Interstitial lung disease: current concepts of pathogenesis, staging and therapy. *The American Journal of Medicine*, 70:3, 543, 1981.

Fee, H. J., Holmes, E., et al: Role of pulmonary vascular resistance measurements in preoperative evaluation of candidates for pulmonary resection. *Journal of Thoracic and Cardiovascular Surgery*, 75:4, 519–523, 1978.

Ferrer, M. I.: Cor pulmonale (pulmonary heart disease): present-day status. *American Heart Journal*, 89:5, 657–664, 1975.

Fishman, A.: Cor Pulmonale: General Aspects. In Pulmonary Diseases and Disorders, vol. 1. New York, McGraw-Hill Book Co., 1980.

Fishman, A.: State of the art—chronic cor pulmonale. *American Review of Respiratory Disease*, 114:4, 775–794, 1976.

Fraser, R. G. and Paré, J. A.: *Diagnosis of Diseases of the Chest*, vol. 2, 2nd ed. Philadelphia, W. B. Saunders Co., 1979.

Hartman, R.: Pulmonary heart disease—pathophysiology, diagnostic signs and therapy. *Postgraduate Medicine*, 66:3, 58–71, 1979.

Hicken, P., Heath, D., and Brewer, D.: The relation between the weight of the right ventricle and the percentage of abnormal air space in the lung in emphysema. *Journal of Pathology and Bacteriology*, 92:524, 1966.

Hinshaw, H. C. and Murray, J. F.: Pulmonary hypertension and cor pulmonale. *Diseases of the Chest*, 4th ed. Philadelphia, W. B. Saunders Co., 1980.

Hodgkin, J. and Petty, T.: Chronic Obstructive Pulmonary Disease—Current Concepts. Philadelphia, W. B. Saunders Co., 1987.

Hyman, A. and Kadowitz, P.: Vasodilator therapy for pulmonary hypertensive disorders. *Chest*, 85(2):145–147, 1984.

Israel, E. J. (ed.): Clinical conferences at the Johns Hopkins Hospital—cor pulmonale. *The Johns Hopkins Medical Journal*, 143:5, 171–177, 1978.

Jacobstein, M. D., Hirschfeld, S. S., et al: Ventricular interdependence in severe cystic fibrosis. *Chest*, 80:4, 399, 1981.

Medical Research Council Working Party: Long-term domiciliary oxygen therapy in chronic hypoxic cor pulmonale complicating chronic bronchitis and emphysema. *Lancet*, 1:8222, 681–686, 1981.

Morrison, D., Henry, R., and Goldman, S.: Preliminary study of the effects of low flow oxygen on oxygen delivery and right ventricular function in chronic lung disease. *American Review of Respiratory Disease*, 133(3):390–395, 1986.

Murphy, M. and Bone, R.: Cor Pulmonale in Chronic Bronchitis and Emphysema. Mount Kisco, New York, Futura Publishing Co., 1984.

Murphy, M. and Hutcheson, R.: The electrocardiographic diagnosis of right ventricular hypertrophy in COPD. *Chest*, 65:6, 622, 1974.

Nocturnal Oxygen Therapy Trial Group: Continuous or nocturnal oxygen therapy in hypoxemic chronic obstructive lung disease. *Annals of Internal Medicine*, 93:3, 391–398, 1980.

Olivey, S., Reduto, L., et al: First pass radionuclide assessment of right and left ejection fraction in chronic pulmonary disease. *Chest*, 78:1, 4–9, 1980.

Reid, L.: Structure and function in pulmonary hypertension—new perceptions. *Chest*, 89(2): 279–288, 1986.

Robin, E. D.: Special report—some basic and clinical challenges in the pulmonary circulation. *Chest*, 81:3, 357–363, 1982.

Rounds, S. and Hill, N.: Pulmonary hypertensive diseases. *Chest*, 85(3):397–405, 1984.

Slutsky, R. A., Ackerman, W., et al: Right and left ventricular dysfunction in patients with chronic obstructive lung disease. *American Journal of Medicine*, 68:2, 197–205, 1980.

Stevens, P., Terplan, M., Knowles, J.: Prognosis of cor pulmonale. *New England Journal of Medicine*, 269:1289–1291, 1963.

Tisi, G. M.: Pulmonary Physiology in Clinical Medicine. Baltimore, Williams & Wilkins, 1980.

Vandenbergh, E., Van De Woestijne K. P., and Billiet, L.: Evolution et pronostic de la bronchite chronique au stade de la rétention de CO_2. *Bulletin de Physiopathologie Respiratoire*, 1:260–272, 1965.

Weitzenblum, E., Hirth, C., and Rasaholinjanahary, J.: Course of pulmonary hemodynamics in patients with chronic obstructive pulmonary disease. *Chest*, 75:6, 656–662, 1979.

West, J. B.: Pulmonary Pathophysiology—The Essentials, 2nd ed. Baltimore, Williams & Wilkins, 1982.

West, J. B.: Respiratory Physiology—The Essentials, 2nd ed. Baltimore, Williams & Wilkins, 1979.

Wynn, J. W.: Cor Pulmonale. In The Respiratory System—A Core Curriculum (Gong, H. and Drage, C., eds.). Norwalk, Connecticut, Appleton-Century-Crofts, 1982.

BASIC ASSESSMENT PARAMETERS

Part Three

Parts one and two of this book provide a foundation for an understanding of the basic respiratory assessment parameters discussed in Part Three. Chapters 10 through 17 explain *what* data to observe for decision-making throughout the nursing process and, specifically, *how* to implement individual assessment parameters in the clinical setting.

Basic assessment parameters include the *pulmonary history, pulmonary pharmacology, complete chest examination, blood gases, pulmonary function tests, chest roentgenology, patient motivation,* and *self-care education.* These are the basic parameters the nurse utilizes most often for respiratory nursing diagnosis and intervention. Information related to laboratory and diagnostic studies, other important parameters, is integrated throughout other sections of this book. Since the role of the nurse is to evaluate the appropriateness and effectiveness of medications prescribed by the physician, the topic of pulmonary pharmacology is included as an assessment parameter rather than in relation to basic intervention.

This section of the book is the most crucial, because of the key role of assessment in the nursing process and in comprehensive respiratory care. Careful study of each chapter in several short study sessions will facilitate comprehension of this large and important body of knowledge. When these chapters are considered with the clinical application chapters at the end of the book, they will help the nursc (1) to collect a comprehensive data base, (2) to identify respiratory problems and their etiologies, and (3) to provide rationales for interventions that pertain to reassessment and evaluation.

Numerous clinical examples and case studies are integrated throughout these chapters to enhance the comprehension of individual assessment parameters. For the parameters that are more difficult to learn (pulmonary pharmacology, blood gases, and pulmonary function tests), study questions are provided at the end of the chapter, with answers listed in Appendix II at the end of the book. These study questions are designed to help refine practical decision-making skills relating to the individual assessment parameter.

Glossary of Commonly Used Terms in Basic Assessment Parameters

Commonly used assessment terms are listed in the following glossary.

A-aO_2 gradient (A-aDO_2)—alveolar to arterial pressure gradient (difference); a measurement of intrapulmonary shunting, normally 5 to 20 mmHg.

ABGs—set of arterial blood gas results.

alpha receptor—adrenergic receptor; stimulation produces a vasopressor effect, decongestant effect, mild bronchoconstriction, and increase in rate and force of heart contraction.

anticholinergic—bronchodilator agent, such as atropine, that acts by blocking bronchoconstriction in the cholinergic response.

antihistamine—agent that counteracts histamine.

antitussive—anticough agent, such as codeine (narcotic) or dextromethorphan (non-narcotic).

AP chest x-ray—portable frontal chest x-ray taken with the film cassette against the back (anterior-posterior view).

AP diameter—anterior-posterior diameter of the chest. An increased diameter results in a barrel chest, a sign of COPD.

atelectasis (absorption)—alveolar collapse from the rapid absorption of high concentrations of oxygen into the pulmonary circulation.

base excess—blood gas measurement that reflects bicarbonate concentration (base) in the body; normally between -2 and $+2$. Negative values reflect base deficiency (i.e., excess of fixed acid). Positive values reflect base excess.

beta 1 receptor—an adrenergic receptor. Stimulation is responsible for cardiac side effects, such as tachycardia, to pulmonary medications.

beta 2 receptor—an adrenergic receptor. Stimulation produces bronchodilatation, the main goal of pulmonary pharmacology.

bronchial breath sound—hollow tubular sound heard on chest auscultation indicates pulmonary consolidation (e.g., pneumonia) or compression of tissue (e.g., pleural effusion).

bronchodilator—agents used for relief of bronchoconstriction and airflow limitation. Main types include autonomic active agents, methylxanthines, corticosteroids, and cromolyn agents.

chest examination (complete)—physical examination of the thorax and lungs supplemented with extrathoracic and precordial examinations.

chest tightness—chest discomfort associated with wheezing and bronchospasm.

clubbing—enlargement of the last phalanges of the fingers. A sign of chronic cardiopulmonary disease, e.g., pulmonary fibrosis, cystic fibrosis, and congenital heart disease.

CO_2 narcosis—respiratory and CNS depression due to alveolar hypoventilation.

corticosteroid—anti-inflammatory agent with a bronchodilating effect.

crackles (rales)—discrete "popping" sounds auscultated during inspiration indicate atelectasis, inflammation, fluid, or mucus in small airways and alveoli.

cyanosis—blue-tinged coloration of the skin or mucous membranes.

decongestant—usually an alpha-adrenergic sympathomimetic used to treat nasal congestion or upper respiratory tract mucosal edema.

diffusion capacity of the lung (DL)—pulmonary function test that measures gas transfer across the alveolar-capillary membrane.

diffusion defect—impairment of gas exchange across the alveolar-capillary membrane manifested by a reduced DL.

dyspnea—complaint of shortness of breath.

emotional state of action—anxiety, anger, or other emotional state associated with increased energy expenditure and increased demand for lung ventilation.

emotional state of nonaction—apathy, depression, or other emotional state associated with decreased energy expenditure and hypoventilation.

emotional straight jacket—term used to describe the COPD patient's emotional state and avoidance of extreme states of action and nonaction.

$FEF_{25\text{-}75\%}$ (forced midexpiratory flow)—airflow rate over the middle half of the forced vital capacity; a reflection of airflow in small airways.

FEV_1 (forced expiratory volume in 1 second)—volume of air exhaled during the first second of the forced vital capacity; a reflection of airflow in large airways.

flow-volume loop—graphic display of airflow rate versus volume during a forced expiration followed by a forced inspiration.

FVC (forced vital capacity)—volume of air exhaled forcefully after a maximal inspiration.

HCO_3^- (bicarbonate ion)—a base substance and important buffer regulated primarily by the kidneys.

Health Belief Model of Health Behavior—a motivational model that stresses the role of patient perceptions in shaping health-seeking behavior.

hypocapnea (hypocarbia)—low levels of carbon dioxide in the blood.

lateral chest x-ray (left)—chest x-ray of the upright patient, with the left side of the chest against the film cassette.

learning objective—statement of what the patient is to learn in behavioral objective form.

MDD (metered dose device)—cartridge inhaler.

metabolic acidosis—acid-base abnormality associated with a low blood HCO_3^- level and low blood pH.

metabolic alkalosis—acid-base abnormality associated with a high blood HCO_3^- level and high blood pH.

methylxanthine—theophylline agent, such as Theo-Dur and aminophylline, used to promote bronchodilatation, to relieve dyspnea, and to improve diaphragmatic contractility.

motivation—internal force within a person that prompts goal attainment.

mucokinetic—an agent that promotes mobilization and removal of secretions from the respiratory tract.

normal (vesicular) breath sound—breezy sounding breath sound normally heard throughout the chest except over central airways.

orthopnea—dyspnea when reclining from upright to supine position.

PA chest x-ray—frontal chest x-ray taken with the film cassette against the anterior chest (posterior-anterior view).

pack years of cigarette smoking—years of cigarette smoking multiplied by packs smoked per day.

paroxysmal nocturnal dyspnea—sudden onset of shortness of breath after going to sleep in the recumbent position; a sign of left ventricular failure.

patient education—health education that stresses professional guidance, dependent role of the learner (patient), and compliance with prescribed treatment.

pleural friction rub—grating or scratching adventitious lung sound produced by inflamed visceral and parietal pleurae rubbing against each other during respiration.

pleuritic chest pain—chest pain during inspiration, often associated with a pleural friction rub.

pH—symbol used to express hydrogen ion concentration in solution. Normal blood pH is 7.40. Blood pH decreases as hydrogen ion concentration increases and vice versa.

psychologic coping mechanism in COPD—response patterns, such as social isolation, denial, and repression, used by COPD patients to cope with their disease.

pulmonary function test (PFT)—series of breathing maneuvers and measurements to assess lung volumes, mechanics of breathing, gas diffusion, arterial blood gases, and overall lung function.

pulmonary history—gathering of subjective data to diagnose or rule out respiratory problems.

purulent—containing pus from infection.

question categories—categories to guide the gathering of signs and symptoms during the pulmonary history, including chronology, bodily location, quality, quantity, setting, associated phenomena, and alleviating and aggravating factors.

quick chest examination—selective inspection and auscultation of the chest for quick overall nursing assessment.

respiratory acidosis—acid-base abnormality associated with a high blood CO_2 and low blood pH.

respiratory alkalosis—acid-base abnormality associated with a low blood CO_2 and high blood pH.

respiratory failure—failure of the pulmonary system to provide adequate gas exchange; a clinical diagnosis based on deteriorating signs and symptoms.

rhonchus—low-pitched coarse sound auscultated during expiration indicates fluid or mucus in large airways.

self-care education—health education that stresses patient involvement in care and patient rather than staff responsibility for learning.

spirogram—graphic tracing of a lung volume measurement.

spirometer—breathing device for measuring lung volumes and capacities.

spirometry—pulmonary function test that measures selected lung volumes and mechanics of breathing, e.g., slow VC, forced VC, FEV_1, and $FEF_{25\text{-}75\%}$.

stridor—loud musical sound of constant pitch heard without a stethoscope or auscultated over the upper airway; a sign of upper airway obstruction.

teaching-learning process—six steps that guide staff teaching and patient learning as follows: (1) identify need to learn, (2) identify readiness to learn, (3) set learning goals, (4) implement interventions, (5) evaluate outcome, and (6) reteach and relearn.

theophylline level—measure of theophylline in the blood; normal therapeutic range is about 10 to 20 mcg/ml.

total lung capacity (TLC)—total volume of air in the lungs after maximal inspiration; a reduced TLC indicates restrictive disease.

venous admixture—perfusion in excess of ventilation; alveolar ventilation is reduced but not totally absent.

ventilatory failure—$PaCO_2$ greater than 50 mmHg.

vital capacity (VC)—total volume of air exhaled after a maximal inspiration.

wheeze—high-pitched musical sound auscultated usually during expiration; a sign of bronchoconstriction.

work of breathing—percentage of total body oxygen consumption used for breathing; normally less than 5% in the resting adult.

Pulmonary History

10

Main Objectives

1. **Name three purposes of the pulmonary history.**
2. **Describe an appropriate setting for interviewing a pulmonary patient.**
3. **Discuss the nurse's approach to questioning, listening, and observing the pulmonary patient during history taking.**
4. **Name and define seven question categories for pulmonary signs and symptoms.**
5. **Describe how the nurse takes a detailed account of signs and symptoms from their earliest onset to the present.**
6. **Name six pulmonary signs and symptoms and explain their significance.**
7. **Explain how investigation of *other components* of the pulmonary history helps to identify actual or potential respiratory problems. These other components are family history, residence or recent travel, smoking history, immunizations, allergies, occupation, environmental factors, and pulmonary medications and treatments.**
8. **Name four main areas of focus that serve as guides to history taking.**

This chapter reviews the interviewing process adapted to respiratory patients; it also reviews the components of the pulmonary history, emphasizing the collection of subjective data necessary to identify and assess a broad range of respiratory problems.

Nurses in advanced practice and many others in practices involving ambulatory settings take detailed pulmonary histories to assess patients comprehensively. In contrast, the acute care nurse may shorten the pulmonary history to a few questions, because the patient lacks the physical stamina for participation in prolonged conversation. Whenever full exploration of all aspects of a pulmonary history is impossible, the nurse gathers crucial information related to present complaints and postpones further discussion until the patient's condition or situation permits a more detailed interview that is more apt to shed light on long-standing pulmonary problems. In any case, whether gathered over several minutes or days, a detailed pulmonary history is essential to insure comprehensive assessment. Furthermore, in some cases, the pulmonary patient may be neither psychologically ready to acknowledge the severity of disease nor to discuss certain aspects of associated problems. When such a patient finally sends verbal cues indicating readiness to talk about respiratory problems, or when the nurse unexpectedly discovers a patient at risk to develop pulmonary problems, the nurse must know beforehand how to implement appropriate sections of the pulmonary history to gather information.

Definition and Purpose

A pulmonary history pertains to those aspects of a complete nursing history that help diagnose or rule out respiratory problems. The pulmonary history focuses on *subjective* information related to a respiratory patient's present complaints as well as the description and interpretation of events leading up to the present condition.

As part of a more complete nursing history, the pulmonary history serves several purposes. First, it *initiates data collection*, helping the nurse begin to understand the nature and extent of the patient's respiratory problems. Second, in providing clues as to which elements in a comprehensive assessment need particular attention, it helps the nurse decide *how to approach the physical examination of the chest* and *how to review a complete set of laboratory data and diagnostic tests*. For example, if a patient complains of sharp chest pain on deep inspiration located in the right lateral chest area, the nurse remembers to thoroughly assess that area during the physical examination. Similarly, subjective complaints of lethargy, headache, and shortness of breath indicate the need to interpret arterial blood gas results to more thoroughly assess the patient's condition. Third, the taking of a pulmonary history helps *establish rapport with the patient*. Not only does the interview situation establish communication between patient and pulmonary nurse, but it also gives the pulmonary nurse a chance to express special understanding of the patient's respiratory problems as well as genuine concern for his personal welfare. Fostering a relationship of mutual trust is essential—the patient is more likely to give a more detailed and accurate history, to become actively involved in his own care from the very beginning, and to cooperate with health professionals throughout the process of diagnosis and intervention.

Interviewing Pulmonary Patients

APPROPRIATE SETTING

The nurse interviews the patient in a quiet, comfortable, and private environment where the patient can freely discuss personal information. Although this ideal environment is not always available, one strives to provide as much privacy as possible and to guard against distractions that might interrupt the interview and might hinder active nurse-patient interaction.

Optimally, the nurse sits in a chair 3 to 4 feet from the patient—closer distances usually are socially uncomfortable, whereas a chair on the other side of the room does not facilitate the exchange of information and may alienate the patient. The optimal distance is modified depending upon individual situations. To effectively communicate with acutely ill patients, the nurse may have to stand 1 to 2 feet away to maintain the patient's attention. To interview a chronically ill, depressed patient, the nurse may sit 1 foot away and touch the patient to give psychologic reassurance while asking crucial questions. If the patient is angry and upset, the nurse sits farther away (4 to 6 feet) until the patient openly verbalizes negative feelings and is ready to actively listen.

The interview setting often includes the presence of family or significant others. The nurse elicits much of the history from family members if the patient is too ill to talk. This practice conserves the patient's energy and, in some cases, leads to more accurate descriptions of respiratory problems. Because chronically ill respiratory patients often tend to relinquish responsibility for their personal well being to nearby supportive family members, the nurse should address early questions *directly* to the patient whenever possible. The dyspneic patient must be given adequate time to collect his thoughts and to fully express his ideas without being interrupted by an impatient interviewer or an overly attentive family member in the same room. Early attention to the patient is essential to develop rapport and a feeling of mutual trust between patient and nurse. It also prompts the patient to become involved in his own care. Family members should be asked to leave the room if their presence prevents the nurse from establishing rapport with the patient and eliciting appropriate subjective data.

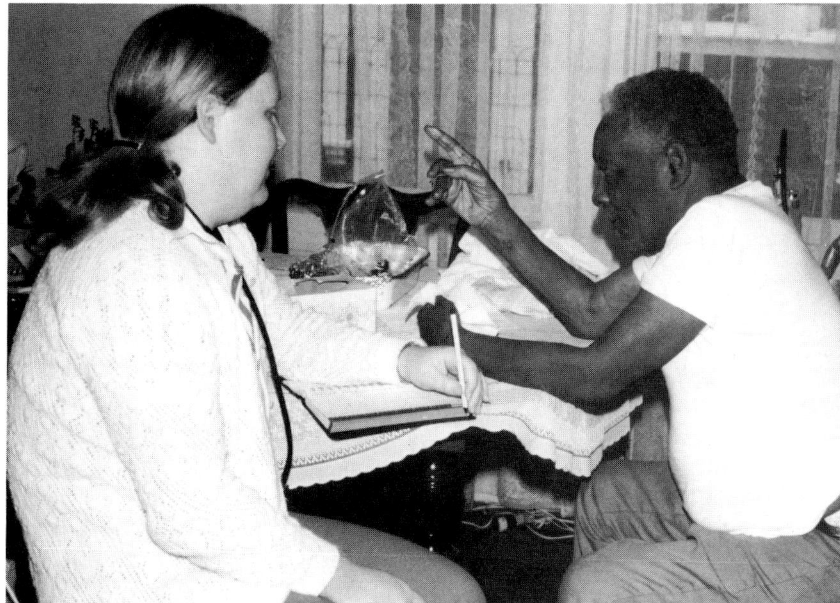

Figure 10–1. Visiting nurse taking a health history in the home setting. Attentive listening encourages the dyspneic patient to communicate problems and concerns as he views them.

The time of day makes a difference. Mornings are less than ideal for the typical respiratory patient who coughs, expectorates sputum, and feels more shortness of breath upon rising until he is able to clear his chest of secretions accumulated during the night. Such patients usually have more energy and longer attention spans in the afternoon when they feel better.

QUESTIONING AND LISTENING WITHOUT BIAS

The nurse questions and listens to the respiratory patient without prejudging behavior. This approach puts the patient at ease, helps develop a relationship of trust, and prevents the nurse from missing important information because of unwillingness to accept or explore an unpleasant aspect of the patient's life.

Interviewing without negative bias is difficult for many health professionals because our society fosters discriminatory attitudes towards disabled persons, in general, by stressing such values as cleanliness, physical ability, and health, and, therefore, many respiratory patients appear undesirable to work with because they are disabled and are aesthetically unpleasing. They may continuously spit up unpleasant looking secretions, gasp for air, and experience accompanying emotional problems; they appear physically weak. They make poor conversationalists because they are too short of breath to effectively communicate ideas. Chronically ill patients may not reward the staff with words of appreciation for the excellent care delivered—some overtly reject care because, although they experience some physical improvement, they have not been cured of their disease as they expected; they have not returned to a socially acceptable level of physical and psychologic functioning. When patients reject treatment or continue to smoke in spite of warnings about the ill effects this has on the body, some health professionals harbor feelings of anger and resentment against such patients.

To interview without negative bias, the nurse first recognizes any personal negative feelings related to respiratory patients. Negative feelings are acceptable as long as the nurse deals with them in a healthy way and does not project them onto the patient. Rather than reacting to unpleasant situations or undesirable comments, the nurse holds negative feelings in check. A conscious effort is made to determine the meaning behind the patient's undesirable statements or behaviors. For example, instead of verbally or nonverbally disapproving of a patient's smoking habits, the nurse focuses on gathering information to identify the patient's reasons for smoking.

To collect unbiased information, the nurse allows the patient to communicate problems and concerns in his own words. Use of good eye contact, nods, gestures, and occasional comments encourages the dyspneic patient to elaborate on important aspects of the history (Fig. 10–1).

Questions are asked without prompting the patient to respond in a certain manner. For example, instead of asking "You take four pills a day, don't; you," the nurse asks "How many pills a day do you take?" This unbiased approach helps the patient freely admit that he has not been taking his medications as prescribed. An accurate assessment of the situation cannot be made unless the patient gives accurate information.

ATTENTION TO SPECIFICS

The nurse asks for specific information. Global or open-ended questions are used to begin to explore a topic and to give the patient the opportunity to focus on areas of concern. Because many COPD patients use denial as a psychologic coping mechanism, continued use of general questions may yield falsely negative findings. To the question "How do you feel?" the patient may answer "Fine." When the nurse merely comments "I see you are slightly short of breath," the patient may respond "Oh, it's nothing—this smoggy weather makes me a little short winded." Crucial information is collected only when the nurse pursues general topics by asking specific questions to more thoroughly describe signs and symptoms and to identify or to rule out common respiratory problems.

The following case illustrates the importance of rephrasing questions to obtain more specific information. A nurse asked Mrs. B., a 65-year-old woman with COPD, whether she slept soundly all night and whether she had difficulties doing housework.

Nurse: Mrs. B., do you ever have difficulty sleeping at night?

Mrs. B: No.

Nurse: How many pillows do you sleep on during the night?

Mrs. B: I don't use any at all.

Nurse: Are you able to do housework regularly without breathing difficulties?

Mrs. B: Yes. I get a little tired, but I manage just fine.

At this point, it appears that the patient's pulmonary status has not affected her sleeping patterns nor her ability to perform household duties. More specific questions yielded crucial information necessary to more thoroughly assess the situation.

Nurse: Mrs. B., how do you normally sleep?

Mrs. B: Well, since this breathing problem has gotten worse, I sit in my rocking chair in the living room and cover myself up with a few blankets, and I am quite comfortable sleeping there all night. I'm just too short of breath when I lie down to sleep in my bed. Besides, now I can't even climb the stairs to get to my bedroom upstairs—I get too short of breath.

Nurse: Tell me when, and exactly how, you do your housecleaning.

Mrs. B: I clean my house about once every 2 weeks. Usually it takes a couple of hours to vacuum and dust the downstairs area. (Pause.) It used to take me a lot longer than that, but now I've learned to take frequent rest periods to better conserve my energy. (Pause.) Also, I wear a kerchief as a mask so I don't breathe dust into my lungs. Dust makes me short of breath. Now I think I do okay.

Nurse: Do you ever wheeze or cough up sputum while performing housework?

Mrs. B: Not usually—only when I do not take frequent rest periods.

With this patient, specific questioning and cross examination uncovered problems that might have been missed if the nurse had maintained the previous general line of questioning.

Upon occasion, even with skillful cross examination, the patient may not be able to give specific information. The nurse with beginning-level interviewing skills who is confronted with the task of gathering a complete data base is often frustrated when persistent questioning yields very vague or questionable information. In this case, further cross examination may send out cues to the patient that only certain information is desirable and acceptable to health professionals. Such persistent questioning leads the patient to think that maybe the nurse did not believe his first response. To avoid creating an atmosphere of labelling responses as right or wrong or an atmosphere of mistrust, the nurse accepts the patient's response and mentally notes to ask the same question again but from a different perspective later in the interview when a related topic is discussed.

Obtaining specific information for a complete data base is difficult when the nurse interviews a pulmonary patient who rambles about his life experiences. In such a case, the interview may resemble psychologic treatment whereby the patient expresses his innermost feelings and relates daily happenings in detail. The patient may identify the nurse as the only person who truly understands his pulmonary problems and who offers to listen. The nurse has difficulty structuring an interview with such a patient and gathering crucial data within the time allotted and leaving the patient's bedside or home, in the case of the visiting nurse, without appearing impolite or disrespectful.

Certainly in many interview situations, helping the patient to verbalize his feelings is appropriate and most therapeutic. But to maintain a primary focus on data collection upon one's first encounter with the patient, the nurse introduces herself and states the purpose of the desired interview in addition to the amount of allotted time. *Setting a time limit is essential!* If the patient begins to concentrate on tangential matters, the nurse verbally recognizes his feelings and thoughts and indicates the desire to pursue the matter after the interview, if time permits. The nurse then refocuses the interview back to the essentials of the pulmonary history. To maintain a relationship of trust, the nurse must remember to pursue the identified areas of concern and to ask the patient to bring up the topic at an agreed upon time at a later date.

NONVERBAL CUES

During the interview, the nurse notes the patient's physical appearance to help evaluate the chief complaints and the impact of the illness on his life at the present time.

Facial expressions may reflect the patient's emotional state and comfort level. Dyspneic patients may grimace with the increased work of breathing and the worsening pulmonary condition. Chronically ill patients may rarely smile. A blank stare often accompanies a total body fatigue, grossly elevated $Pa{CO_2}$ (CO_2 narcosis), and hopelessness associated with terminal illness.

Clothes and style of dress may reflect such personal attributes as age, socioeconomic status, occupation, and prevailing mood. Depressed patients, who appear tired and somewhat disheveled, may pay little attention to such details as matching the color of their clothing and completely tucking in a shirt. Patients with early morning cough, sputum production, and breathing discomfort may remain in pajamas and robe until late morning or noon.

Body posture may indicate breathing problems. Dyspneic patients appear tense. Some feel unable to breathe comfortably without sitting up and leaning forward with elbows resting on the knees or on a nearby table.

Distracting eye movements, persistent head nods, and frequent shifts in position may mean that the patient does not wish to continue the interview or subject matter under discussion. Patients with unstable chest conditions may retreat to their beds in the middle of the interview because they are unable to physically and emotionally cope with the interviewer or potentially threatening information; such nonverbal cues must be respected. Potentially threatening information is better investigated when the patient's condition has improved, and he is willing and better able to express himself.

CHECKING IMPORTANT INFORMATION

The nurse checks the patient's history for consistency. If information given early in the history conflicts with information given later, the patient may be confused owing to an arterial blood gas disturbance; he may be trying to portray a negative history so that he will be discharged from the hospital earlier. Respiratory patients with poor psychosocial assets or an inadequate support system of family and friends may make up histories of pulmonary symptoms to ensure continued contact with sympathetic health professionals. Occasionally, an individual with alleged exposure to lung irritants in an occupational setting will complain of respiratory symptoms in an attempt to strengthen his case for claiming disability insurance. When the patient's history is inconsistent with the usual progression of signs and symptoms of suspected respiratory problems, the nurse questions its reliability. Inconsistent histories are checked for reliability by interviewing family, friends, and health professionals who know the patient. Also, other assessment findings, such as physical findings and laboratory data, usually help to identify malingerers.

Yet, even in the case of a seemingly reliable pulmonary history, the nurse uses other sources whenever convenient, to check on its crucial aspects. Because many patients do not recognize or tend to minimize the extent of their physical ailments, their spouses or significant others can be very helpful in providing details relating to pulmonary symptoms. Often these supportive persons provide more objective information describing the degree to which symptoms interfere with activities of daily living. For example, different types of sleep apneas (periods of no breathing) are evaluated by collecting information from the spouse as well as the patient in regard to the patient's breathing patterns during the night.

In some cases, history taking of itself is inadequate unless it is accompanied simultaneously by direct observation. For example, some information pertaining to assessment of various forms of respiratory therapy must be verified by direct observation. Since proper care of respiratory equipment in the home is a continual problem and is crucial to the prevention of chest infections, the nurse asks the patient to bring the equipment to the hospital or clinic, if possible. Direct observation of breathing circuits for the presence of medication stains and residual droplets of water quickly confirms the inadequacy of cleaning procedures. Even when the patient denies problems, the nurse asks to inspect equipment. Because of inadequate education regarding maintenance and use of respiratory equipment, many patients are not able to identify potentially hazardous situations. Furthermore, inspection of equipment is best done during questioning so that the patient observes how you identified potential or actual problems related to the care of equipment.

In summary, checking important information is done tactfully by specific cross examination; by use of other sources of information; and by inspection during the interview, without suggesting incompetence or unreliability. Minor inconsistencies in the pulmonary history are best discussed after the nurse has established good rapport with the patient.

Main Components

CHIEF COMPLAINT

The chief complaint (cc) indicates which pulmonary signs and symptoms the individual is currently most distressed about—cough, sputum production, shortness of breath, hemoptysis, wheezing, pleuritic pain, or change in voice. It is most important to realize that the cc represents the *patient's*, not the nurse's, point of view. On the one hand, the cc is a more general symptom, such as fever, chills, and weight loss, or it involves another body system, such as muscle weakness, cardiac palpitations, and stomach upset. On the other hand, some individuals who are evaluated for evidence of cardiopulmonary disease may have no complaints at all.

In a *chronic ambulatory setting* the nurse determines the patient's cc by using an open-ended, neutral question or statement, e.g., "What is bothering you?" or "Tell me how things have been with you." If the patient identifies several complaints, the nurse prompts him to select the *most* bothersome symptom—this symptom usually gives a better indication of what the primary pulmonary problem might be.

The nurse is brief and specific when recording the cc. Complaints are preferably written in quotation form to preserve the patient's subjective impressions. Some examples of chief complaints common to chronically ill respiratory patients are as follows:

1. Wheezing with exertional exercise.
2. "I felt so short of breath I had to open the window to get some air."
3. "My chest feels tight when I get up each morning."

Alternatively, in an *acute care setting*, the nurse who is not responsible for collecting a complete data base in a limited period of time uses a different approach. To ask a general, open-ended question at the beginning of a shift in an intensive care unit often leads the acutely ill patient to think that the nurse is either unfamiliar with his problems or does not realize that he is too sick to fully respond to the question. Acutely ill patients as well as those with limited attention spans must be questioned more directly and specifically with use of short, easy-to-understand sentences. The nurse might ask a newly admitted patient who has not yet seen a physician "What is your main problem?" or "What is the matter?" or "What is bothering you the most?" If the nurse knows the patient's chief complaint, more specific questioning is used, such as "How is your chest pain?" or "Is your pain better, the same, or worse?" This type of question allows the dyspneic, acutely ill patient to respond in one or two words. If the patient is unable to talk because of placement of an endotracheal tube for mechanical ventilation, the nurse reads the patient's lips and encourages him to use nonverbal communications as well as pencil and paper, if necessary. Common chief complaints of acute ill respiratory patients are as follows:

1. Continuous sputum production when lying supine.
2. "I'm suffocating."
3. "The ventilator is not giving me enough air."

HISTORY OF PULMONARY SIGNS AND SYMPTOMS

The patient's chief complaint and related information are fully explored by taking detailed account of the progression of symptoms and associated phenomena from their earliest onset to the present. If the nurse is using a system's approach to history taking, the gathered data is usually recorded under the heading *History of Present Illness* or *Present Health Status*, if the individual is well. Otherwise, the history of pulmonary signs and symptoms may be gathered and recorded in another fashion, depending on the model or conceptual framework chosen to gather and record the complete nursing history. Whatever form of nursing history is used, during the interview, the nurse asks questions about each pulmonary sign and symptom using all the question categories summarized in the box.

QUESTION CATEGORIES

Chronology

Chronology refers to the sequence of signs, symptoms, and related events; it includes the patient's present and past pulmonary history.

The patient who is seen in a clinic for mild or questionable pulmonary problems may not have an extensive pulmonary history. In this case, the nurse may choose to begin the chronologic story at the time of the very earliest complaint of any symptoms. The patient can complete his entire chronology without fatigue and shortness of breath interrupting his speech pattern.

Present History. The chronically ill respiratory patient with moderate to severe lung disease has a long medical history and may not be able to relate it completely owing to physical fatigue, shortness of breath, or disinterest. To conserve the patient's energy and to allow enough time to explore crucial details, the nurse *first* explores events related to the patient's *present* condition or the period immediately prior to hospital admission; this time period is called the *present history*.

To facilitate history taking, the clinician divides the present history into two time periods—*recent onset* and *course since onset*.

Recent Onset. Recent onset is thoroughly investigated as outlined in the box (see I.B.). To document the recent onset of symptoms, the nurse follows a broad question, such as "How did it start?" with a specific one, such as "Exactly what day and at what time did you first notice the chest pain?" The nurse also notes whether the manner of the symptom's appearance was *gradual* or *sudden*. An attack of wheezing is relatively abrupt. The onset of cough and sputum production may appear gradually over a period of a few days if an asthmatic or emphysematous patient catches a cold and develops acute bronchitis. *Duration* of symptoms is determined by simply asking "How long did it last?" Finally, *precipitating factors* are best investigated by asking the patient what *he* thinks caused the problem. An asthma attack may be precipitated by a variety of stimuli, such as different allergens, emotional upsets, physical exertion, and certain drugs. An attack of shortness of breath may be precipitated by an aerosol, if the patient reacts adversely to

QUESTION CATEGORIES FOR PULMONARY SIGNS AND SYMPTOMS

I. Chronology
  A. Time periods
    1. Present history; recent onset; course since onset.
    2. Past history; time of earliest pulmonary sign or symptom to recent onset.
  B. Thorough investigation of recent onset
    1. Specific date and time
    2. Manner of appearance—gradual or sudden
    3. Duration
    4. Precipitating factors
  C. Course since onset
    1. Incidence (frequency)
    2. Manner of appearance
    3. Duration
    4. Patterns of remissions and exacerbations
II. Bodily location; localized areas, radiation
III. Quality; unique properties, color, texture, composition, appearance, and odor
IV. Quantity; size, extent, number, or amount
V. Setting; home, work, hospital, other particular situation
VI. Associated phenomena; symptoms or events
VII. Alleviating and aggravating factors
  A. Health habits
  B. Body position
  C. Activity
  D. Medications and treatments

the aerosol drug or if thick secretions move more centrally and temporarily plug airways. When the patient does not identify a precipitating factor, the nurse continues to search for one, while chronologically reviewing activities during the week or day the symptoms first appeared. When possible, family or significant others should be consulted to identify or rule out suspected precipitating factors.

This detailed line of questioning applies to all cardiopulmonary signs and symptoms the patient complains of at the time of recent onset. It permits both the clinician and patient to fully understand the situation under investigation and serves as a reference point to determine whether individual symptoms during the course of the problem since onset became better, worse, or remained the same.

Course Since Onset. This part of the present medical history is investigated in the same manner, with emphases on the items outlined in the box (see I.C.). *Incidence* or frequency is specified in times a day, week, month, or year. *Duration* of symptoms may be short, average, long, or "all of the time." Patients who vaguely state that they have symptoms "all the time" may mean all during the day and not during the night, ten times a day, once a month, and so forth. To obtain more specific information on duration, the nurse asks the patient to provide the time meant as specifically as possible, in minutes, hours, days, or weeks. One avoids suggesting answers, but sometimes leading questions are necessary, such as "Does your cough and sputum production last *all* morning?" If course since onset is weeks to months, the nurse notes any periods of *remission* (abatement of symptoms) and *exacerbation* (aggravation of symptoms). Acute exacerbations are investigated in a manner similar to recent onset of symptoms, noting dates and times, manner of appearance, duration, and precipitating factors.

Past History. After investigation of the present history, the nurse reverts to *past history*, beginning with the earliest pulmonary signs or symptoms noticed by the patient and ending with the time of recent onset of symptoms. This time period is explored in exactly the same manner as the present history. Since the earliest symptoms might have occurred 20 to 30 years ago in the elderly patient, the nurse is encouraged to make use of past medical records to avoid overexerting or possibly annoying patients unnecessarily. If the old hospital chart contains a detailed history of past medical problems, the nurse uses it for background information and then questions the patient to verify crucial details (e.g., causes of acute exacerbations) and to explore any nebulous areas (e.g., care of respiratory equipment and activity level). Although the hospital chart helps one to understand the patient's past medical history, it may not give a history of preventive health habits between hospitalizations. This information is crucial for a comprehensive nursing assessment.

Emphasis on Present History. Certainly, investigation of past history helps one to understand how the patient physiologically and psychosocially copes with disease. But present history is of prime importance. In most cases, more interviewing time should be devoted to its thorough investigation for two reasons. First, accurate and detailed information is necessary to promptly diagnose and treat *present* problems. These problems tend to be acute, physiologically based, and often life threatening, since patients tend to wait until physical ailments become severe before seeking medical help. Second, in many cases, patients are more ready and able to relate information, identify problems, and seek long-term solutions. By seeking help, the patient is admitting to a problem. He is more likely to admit that he might have to change his health habits and life style to more effectively and realistically cope with lung disease. Furthermore, a health-seeking individual is more likely to give a thorough history that assists the nurse evaluate how well he understands and follows preventive measures and how well he lives within the limitations of the disease. Teaching-learning needs can be identified.

Because the present illness is so crucial, it is advisable to fully explore it first to avoid becoming overinvolved in the less relevant details of past history.

Chronology is complete once the nurse obtains a clear picture of the progression of signs and symptoms. Using the aforementioned time periods as frameworks for interviewing, one simultaneously explores the other question categories in the summary box to identify the exact nature and extent of the pulmonary problems.

Bodily Location

The nurse asks the patient to describe the *exact location* of a sign or symptom. Often this is not possible for the patient because many of the pulmonary symptoms, such as cough and shortness of breath, cannot be localized. Yet, the patient with chest pain can usually point to an exact area of pain and trace its radiation, if present, with the finger. The wheezing patient may localize substernal chest discomfort. The patient with lobar pneumonia may feel chest discomfort over the area of pathology.

Quality

Quality refers to *unique properties* of a sign or symptom. Signs, such as sputum production and hemoptysis, are characterized in terms of *color, texture, composition, appearance,* and *odor.* Symptoms are more difficult to describe because they cannot be seen or touched. Chest pain may be characterized as *dull, aching, sharp, throbbing, stabbing,* and *squeezing.* Respiratory patients with significant airway obstruction may deny chest pain but admit to chest discomfort. Although certain qualities tend to characterize certain cardiopulmonary symptoms, descriptions vary owing to different perceptions and abilities to verbalize subjective feelings. Whenever appropriate, the nurse records descriptions as direct quotations.

Quantity

Quantity refers to the *size, extent, number,* or *amount* of a sign or symptom. Descriptions such as "a little," "a lot," and "a couple" have different meanings to different people and must be restated in more specific terms.

Signs, such as mucus production and hemoptysis, are quantified as specifically as possible using measurements, such as ounces, milliliters, teaspoons, tablespoons, and cups; cups each day are specified in fractions—1/4, 1/2, or 3/4.

Symptoms, such as pain and shortness of breath (dyspnea), are best evaluated in two ways. First, the nurse uses a rating scale, such as the Borg Scale in Table 10–1, to estimate the perceived intensity of a symptom at a specific moment. Though this scale was developed for estimation of perceived exertion during exercise, it is sometimes used for estimation of dyspnea at rest, for chest pain of cardiac or pulmonary origin,

Table 10–1. THE BORG SCALE FOR ESTIMATION OF SUBJECTIVE SYMPTOMS*

Number Rating	Description of Associated Intensity	Interpretation
0	Nothing at all	
0.5	Very, very weak	Just noticeable
1	Very weak	
2	Weak	Light
3	Moderate	
4	Somewhat strong	
5	Strong	Heavy
6		
7	Very strong	
8		
9		
10	Very, very strong	Almost maximal
•	*Maximal*	

*Reproduced by permission from Borg, G.: Psychophysical bases of perceived exertion. *Medicine and science in sports and exercise,* 14(5):377–381, 1982.

and for leg muscle fatigue during exercise. To use the scale, the nurse might ask "On a scale of zero to ten, how do you rate your shortness of breath? Zero means no shortness of breath, and ten means maximal shortness of breath."

In addition, the nurse evaluates symptoms, such as dyspnea and pain, in relation to rest and activity. What does the patient do when he experiences the symptom? Does he stop all activity? Sit down? Lie down? Or continue what he is doing? How has the symptom altered his normal activities during the day? The nurse notes what activities of daily living the patient performs *without* experiencing symptoms and what activities he avoids because of the onset of symptoms. Does the symptom keep the patient awake all night?

Setting

Setting refers to a certain time and place or particular situation that has a physical or psychologic effect on the patient such that his condition worsens. For example, most respiratory patients do extremely well when they are given comprehensive and individualized care in the hospital. Sometimes, when the severely disabled patient returns home without the support of family or friends, the patient's condition worsens. The setting of his being home alone with sole responsibility for following a rigorous treatment regimen automatically triggers symptoms to facilitate readmission to the hospital where psychologic and physical support are readily available. Also, the setting becomes important in the case of an employee who complains of symptoms every Monday morning when he begins to work at his job site. In this case, the symptoms may pertain to an occupational health hazard in the work environment.

Associated Phenomena

Associated phenomena are symptoms or events that occur with the chief complaint. There may be other cardiopulmonary symptoms, general symptoms, or symptoms that are totally unrelated to lung disease. Usually, more cardiopulmonary symptoms develop as the patient's respiratory status worsens. Other associated phenomena occurring with pulmonary symptoms might include stomach fullness, weight loss, emotional tension, muscle incoordination, inability to concentrate, and excessive fatigue.

Alleviating and Aggravating Factors

In a nonjudgmental manner, the nurse asks specifically, *"What makes symptoms better?"* and *"What makes symptoms worse?"* Questions focus on the following four areas: health habits, body position, activity, and medications plus treatments.

Health Habits. Certain health habits tend to aggravate or alleviate symptoms. Alcohol ingestion can depress the respiratory center and cause the patient to breathe shallowly and slowly (hypoventilation). The lungs become underventilated, which in turn impairs the optimal functioning of the mucociliary escalator, fostering the accumulation of respiratory secretions in the lungs. Over a period of days to weeks, the patient may develop a chest infection from retained secretions. The habit of eating large meals tends to cause stomach discomfort and increase shortness of breath. Poor eating habits result in severe weight loss in a cystic fibrosis patient and may precipitate respiratory problems. While most patients admit that cigarette smoking aggravates respiratory symptoms, some claim that whenever they light up a cigarette, they feel much more relaxed. Identification of poor health habits is essential to determine what preventive measures the patient might take to improve his condition.

Good health habits are areas that need positive reinforcement. For example, the cystic fibrosis patient with significant sputum production and little bronchospasm may report that running alleviates chest discomfort—he runs, becomes short of breath, coughs, expectorates sputum, and feels 100% better.

Body Position. In the acute setting, position changes—turning the patient to the far right or left or adjusting the head of the bed—may aggravate or alleviate symptoms. Acutely ill respiratory patients may become short of breath when the head of the bed is lowered. This response is most likely with inadequate oxygenation or mucus retention problems, especially if the patient coughs ineffectively or if the lungs and upper airway have not recently been suctioned. Many respiratory and cardiac patients have difficulties lying completely flat even with supplemental oxygen. Patients with localized lung pathology (e.g., postoperative thoracotomy and bronchiectasis) may complain of increasing shortness of breath while lying on one particular side.

Activity. The nurse determines what level of activity alleviates or aggravates symptoms. How much walking distance (in feet or in city blocks) or what normal activities of daily living increase or decrease symptoms? By how much or to what extent? Is rest necessary before symptoms improve? How much rest is necessary before symptoms abate and completely disappear? The time period for rest is estimated in minutes, hours, or days.

Medications and Treatments. While taking the history of the present illness, the nurse carefully notes the prescribed medications and treatments the patient was taking when symptoms increased or decreased. Sometimes a cause and effect relationship can be established—the patient undergoes an aerosol treatment and claims that during and immediately afterwards he feels better. Other times, gradually worsening symptoms indicate that the patient's entire medication and treatment program needs to be reevaluated and adjusted to changing needs.

Even when a direct cause and effect relationship seems evident, the nurse must be careful to reserve judgment regarding any medication or treatment the patient claims worsens symptoms, until other assessment parameters are evaluated. For example, the patient may attribute problems to use of the nebulizer device when in fact other factors, such as low PaO_2 and retained secretions, precipitated shortness of breath during the aerosol treatment. Rather than immediate discontinuation of the aerosol, the patient may require supplemental oxygen during treatments for the oxygenation problem and hydration for liquefaction of thick mucus plugs obstructing airflow through airways.

In a nonjudgmental manner, the nurse asks the patient what medications or treatments, other than those prescribed, alleviate or aggravate symptoms. Many patients resort to home remedies when medical care is unavailable or seems to be ineffective. Over-the-counter drugs and vitamin supplements are popular. Such remedies as hot showers, the next door neighbor's "breathing pills," home vaporizers, air purifiers, and commercial hand vibrators may help some patients with postural drainage. Severely disabled respiratory patients may have tried a variety of home remedies before agreeing to try prescribed medications and treatments. The type of home remedy also helps to identify respiratory problems. For example, the patient who uses a hot shower in the morning to cough up mucus probably has a mucus retention problem. The heat, humidity, and resultant mist from the shower helps to loosen these retained secretions in the chest and facilitate expectoration. The patient may not experience cough and sputum production except during or shortly after this effective and inexpensive form of mist therapy.

PULMONARY SIGNS AND SYMPTOMS

The nurse verifies with the patient the presence or absence of *shortness of breath* (SOB), *wheeze, pleuritic chest pain, cough, sputum production, hemoptysis,* and *voice change.* These are the main pulmonary signs and symptoms discussed in the following sections. Presence of one or more of these indicates that the patient either has respiratory problems or is at risk to develop problems.

Shortness of Breath

SOB, also called *dyspnea*, is perhaps the most common complaint of all pulmonary patients. This discussion focuses on *pathologic* dyspnea, defined as the "unpleasant, distressing sensation of labored breathing which is usually associated with cardiac or pulmonary disease" (Burki, 1980). It must be distinguished from *physiologic* dyspnea or breathlessness, defined by Burki as the "pleasant, not distressful, sensation felt by healthy subjects on exercise or excitement."

Subjective Descriptions. Pathologic dyspnea is difficult to evaluate because it is so subjective. It is most important for the nurse to remember that the patient's perception of dyspnea or shortness of breath may have no relation to the patient's appearance. On the one hand, the patient who complains of dyspnea—most commonly described as *shortness of breath, breathlessness, "short-winded,"* or *vague chest discomfort*—may not appear dyspneic at all. On the other hand, a patient with chronic lung disease may completely deny dyspnea when they obviously appear affected, since the accessory muscles of breathing are used. Patients with long-standing chest disease have become so accustomed to the feeling of dyspnea that, over a period of time, it becomes more and more difficult for them to recognize its presence. In these cases, although dyspnea is denied, patients usually admit to an *increased respiratory rate* or *"breathing faster"* than normal with activity. Others describe dyspnea as a distressing *feeling of suffocation.* Its presence elicits anxiety because the lungs and their vital function of breathing are associated with life and survival. Recognizing the possibility of complete breathlessness and perhaps even death, the dyspneic patient may panic at the slightest feeling of dyspnea and subsequently lose control of breathing. Other pulmonary patients complain of suffocation only when in acute respiratory distress due to increasing obstruction from airway secretions or bronchospasm. Because the meaning of dyspnea has different nuances to different people, the nurse may have to use other terms, as described, to identify subjective complaints.

Causes or Associations. Causes of dyspnea are nonspecific in nature. The patient may have one or more of a number of cardiopulmonary physiologic abnormalities. Conversely, the symptom may be due entirely to psychosomatic illness or severe anxiety and fear associated with acute emotional or long-standing psychologic problems. In some cases dyspnea is unexplainable.

Several theories have been proposed to elucidate the genesis of the sensation of dyspnea. Those related to increased work of breathing, intercostal muscle fatigue, increased oxygen cost of breathing, abnormal drive to breathe, and asynchrony of intercostal muscles and diaphragm, are only some. Generally speaking, however, two basic physiologic mechanisms have been associated with dyspnea as follows: (1) hypoxemia—the lack of oxygen in arterial blood (low PaO_2) and (2) increased work of breathing.

Hypoxemia is found in almost any pulmonary, cardiac, or noncardiopulmonary disease when inadequate pulmonary gas exchange develops in acute or end-stage disease (see Chapter 13). Emphasis must be placed on the *association* of hypoxemia with dyspnea rather than on the cause and effect relationship. Hypoxemia may cause dyspnea but not always. In fact, the degree of hypoxemia correlates poorly with the degree of dyspnea. Severely hypoxemic individuals may complain of only slight dyspnea. In some illnesses hypoxemia may not be evident (e.g., thyrotoxicosis), but excessive demand for oxygen to the tissues exists, and the patient does complain of dyspnea.

Increased work of breathing produces dyspnea when demand for lung ventilation brought about by changes in blood gases is out of proportion to the patient's ability to respond to the demand. With acute or progressively worsening restrictive or obstructive disease, abnormal lung mechanics brings about more uncomfortable or labored breathing to achieve adequate pulmonary gas exchange.

Whether or not dyspnea has a physiologic basis, the nurse labels dyspnea as a problem until it is proved otherwise. An emotional problem as a cause of dyspnea is a diagnosis made by exclusion. Similar to the concept of pain, dyspnea is a reality to the patient experiencing it and must be treated whether the cause is deemed physiologic or psychologic. Untreated, an anxious individual may develop *hyperventilation syndrome* manifested by prolonged periods of hyperventilation; symptoms of dyspnea; numbness of the arms, hands, and lips; and tetany in severe cases. Even if emotional problems appear to be responsible for hyperventilation, other cardiopulmonary problems may contribute to the severity of symptoms.

In conclusion, during the investigation of causes of dyspnea, the nurse considers the possibility that respiratory therapy prescribed for the treatment of disease may be causing or aggravating shortness of breath. Table 10–2 reviews the main respiratory treatments that may cause dyspnea and other associated symptoms. The onset of symptoms indicates patient intolerance to the treatment, inappropriate administration, or side effects that must be either treated medically or eliminated by discontinuation of the treatment.

Orthopnea and Paroxysmal Nocturnal Dyspnea. During the investigation of complaints of dyspnea, the nurse directs questions to the patient to determine the presence or absence of orthopnea and paroxysmal nocturnal dyspnea (PND).

Orthopnea. This symptom is defined as dyspnea when reclining from the upright position to the supine position. Orthopnea is suspected whenever a patient

Table 10–2. RESPIRATORY TREATMENTS CAUSING SHORTNESS OF BREATH

Causes	Associated Complaints	Interventions
IPPB TREATMENT (Pressure limited ventilator)		
Hyperventilation*	Rapid respiratory rate Dizziness Tingling of extremities	Instruct patient to relax, inspire air slowly, and pause between breaths.
Adverse circulatory effects (more common with low Pao_2, hypovolemia, pharmacologic depression, and intravenous infusion of vasopressor medications).	SOB only when cardiac output severely reduced	
Decreased blood pressure from positive pressure to airways during deep, prolonged inspirations. Positive pressure decreases blood return to the right ventricle.	Rapid pulse Faintness	Coach patient to inspire with minimal effort or decrease volume of inspired air by reducing present peak pressure by 2 to 6 cmH_2O. Check blood pressure.
Arrhythmias from decreased blood pressure, decreased cardiac output, and inadequate blood oxygenation.	Faintness Weakness Rapid or irregular pulse Heart palpitations Dusky appearance	Hold treatment and consult physician; for continued circulatory effects, provide supplementary O_2.
Arrhythmia as a side effect to pulmonary medication aerosolized in nebulizer.*	Rapid or irregular pulse Heart palpitations	Hold treatment if there are more than 4 irregular beats per minute or if heart rate increases by over 20 beats per minute. Consult physician.
Increased airway obstruction from the following:		
Mobilization of mucus centrally to larger airways; mostly in patients with thick, tenacious respiratory secretions.*	Rapid respiratory rate and pulse Chest discomfort Cough Beginning sputum production	Encourage coughing and deep breathing during and after treatment to expectorate mucus and clear airways.
Bronchospasm as a side effect to aerosolized medication.*	Feeling of suffocation Chest tightness Wheezing Rapid respiratory rate and pulse	Hold treatment and consult physician.
Increased work of breathing in critically ill or weak patients and in those with difficulties taking treatments.*	Fatigue Distressed appearance Rapid respiratory rate or pulse Diaphoresis Chest pains in cardiac patient IPPB—difficulty maintaining mouth seal and inspiring to present peak pressure Manual aerosol treatments—inability to deep breathe and coordinate delivery of aerosol with inspiration.	Hold treatment and consult physician. For manual aerosol treatments, consider change to IPPB to more efficiently deliver aerosol.
Overinflation of lungs—increases risk for pneumothorax.	Fatigue Chest discomfort on inspiration High ventilator peak pressures on inspiration (greater than 30 cmH_2O) Difficulty maintaining mouth seal during treatment due to excessive pressure in lungs	Coach patient to inspire with minimal effort. Decrease volume of inspired air by reducing peak pressure by 2 to 6 cmH_2O.
OXYGEN THERAPY		
Inadequate oxygenation (hypoxemia).	Rapid respiratory rate Rapid or irregular pulse Orthopnea Dusky appearance or cyanosis Depressed mental function Disorientation Behavior changes	Call physician and check blood gas results. Within prescribed orders, increase O_2 percentage of inspired air by 30 to 50% or double liter flow of O_2.
Over oxygenation in COPD patients receiving supplementary O_2.	Slow or shallow respirations Periods of no breathing Flushed skin (from CO_2 retention) Depressed mental function	Call physician and check blood gas results. Provide low flow O_2 (1 to 3 L/min via nasal prongs or Venturi mask at 24 to 28% O_2 concentration).

Table continued on following page

Table 10–2. RESPIRATORY TREATMENTS CAUSING SHORTNESS OF BREATH *Continued*

Causes	Associated Complaints	Interventions
BLAND AEROSOL (MIST THERAPY)		
Increased airway obstruction from airway irritation or bronchospasm from irritant effect of small aerosolized particles, heat, inadequate nebulization, or type of aerosolized liquid.	Feeling of suffocation Chest tightness Coughing Wheezing Rapid respiratory rate and pulse	Check setup for proper functioning. Hold treatment and consult physician.
Increased airway obstruction from liquefication and mobilization of secretions to larger airways.	Rapid respiratory rate and pulse Chest discomfort Cough Beginning sputum production	Encourage coughing and deep breathing during and after treatment to clear airways. SOB disappears after effective therapy. Encourage oral fluids for hydration so that bland aerosol may be discontinued.
POSTURAL DRAINAGE		
In reclining positions, **increased airway obstruction** from the drainage of secretions to larger airways; inadequate oxygenation.	Rapid respiratory rate Rapid or irregular pulse Orthopnea Chest discomfort Dusky appearance	Provide supplementary O_2 during treatment. Encourage coughing and deep breathing to clear airways. Modify postural drainage positions to relieve SOB and maintain bronchial relaxation.

*Items also apply to aerosol treatments administered by hand bulb nebulizer or compressed air devices. (See Part Four of this book for further descriptions of treatments.)

states he must use more than one pillow to sleep comfortably at night. In the cardiac patient with congestive heart failure, orthopnea is due to increased venous return to the heart, increased hydrostatic pressures in the upper lung regions, and decreased lung volumes in the recumbent position. In COPD, orthopnea is due to displacement of abdominal organs toward the chest cavity and reduced lung volumes; both cause increased work of breathing in the recumbent position.

Paroxysmal Nocturnal Dyspnea. This symptom is defined as the sudden onset of shortness of breath (SOB) after going to sleep in the recumbent position. PND is considered a classic symptom of left ventricular heart failure. The cardiac patient has no difficulty going to sleep, but 1 to 2 hours later, acute SOB causes him to sit upright in bed and sometimes to run to an open window to catch a breath of fresh air. He may then sleep undisturbed for the rest of the night.

In this case, the sudden acute dyspnea represents the development of alveolar pulmonary edema. Several hours after the episode, although the patient may be resting confortably, the chest x-ray may show evidence of pulmonary congestion, sometimes with evidence of interstitial edema.

Pulmonary patients do not typically experience PND as described unless the pulmonary disease is complicated by cardiac problems affecting left ventricular function. An acute asthmatic episode may similarly occur, but it often occurs sporadically at night or in the early morning; such an episode requires a longer period of time to subside, with administration of bronchodilators for relief of airway obstruction. The COPD patient with emphysema and bronchitis may wake up during the night, but the associated dyspnea is rarely so sudden in onset and is usually in the early morning hours after mucus has had time to accumulate in the lungs and cause enough airway obstruction to disturb sleep. In this case, dyspnea is accompanied by cough and mucus production.

Onset and Patterns of Dyspnea. The nurse notes whether onset of dyspnea is *sudden* or *gradual.* The sudden appearance of SOB might indicate PND associated with congestive heart failure as described, or it may be due to other acute events, such as pulmonary embolism, pneumothorax, and myocardial infarction with acute ventricular failure. All these conditions require immediate medical attention. Whenever acute dyspnea occurs in a patient during the post-surgical or post-partum period or in a patient undergoing treatment for heart failure, acute pulmonary edema is automatically suspected. The gradual onset of dyspnea over a period of months or years suggests chronic lung disease. If the pulmonary patient recently notices an increase in dyspnea, one suspects heart disease, notably heart failure, or pulmonary complications, notably pneumothorax, atelectasis, and possible chest infection.

The individual's age at the time of onset of dyspnea, as well as patterns of remissions and exacerbations, are also important. Various obstructive and restrictive diseases appear in certain age groups and demonstrate certain patterns of disease progression.

Quantification. To quantify dyspnea, the nurse determines if it occurs only during physical activity (i.e., *dyspnea on exertion* or DOE) and if it also occurs at rest. Deterioration from DOE to dyspnea at rest indicates progressive disease. The patient with significant COPD may not complain of dyspnea at rest. However, physical activity increases the body's demand for oxygen in general. As activity stimulates hyperirritable airways and secretions in the chest, dyspnea develops. In contrast, the patient with advanced diffuse interstitial fibrosis without an obstructive component usually has dyspnea at rest that is exaggerated by exercise.

Further quantification is achieved by asking how many feet or city blocks the patient can walk on level ground *without* becoming SOB. Similarly, the nurse asks whether the patient climbs stairs, and if he does, how many stairs or flights of stairs can he climb *without* becoming SOB. It is also helpful to note whether the patient must rest periodically during activity. Many patients stop exercising when experiencing significant dyspnea. Others rarely stop to rest, and continue to exercise far beyond the point at which chest discomfort and dyspnea appears.

To determine the degree to which dyspnea limits daily activities, the nurse asks the following questions:

1. What activities cause dyspnea?
2. How much dyspnea? (Use the Borgs scale to estimate intensity.)
3. What activities does the patient avoid to prevent the sensation of dyspnea?

This information is collected by direct interview with or without the use of a patient questionnaire.

The questionnaire in Table 10–3 is used by health team members at the University of California, San Diego, Medical Center to assess SOB as well as the general medical and educational needs of pulmonary patients recently enrolled in a Pulmonary Rehabilitation Program. The first four sections of the questionnaire help identify patients who cannot perform certain activities, such as cooking, climbing stairs, and shaving, because of their inability to control SOB. These patients may benefit from breathing retraining and energy conservation techniques to control SOB related to the performance of basic household chores and personal hygiene measures (see Part Four).

Information gained from the answers to the questionnaire may be used to rate the patient on a dyspnea-disability scale, such as the one in Table 10–4. Classification provides an overall assessment of the patient. A goal of medical and nursing interventions is to reduce the patient's classification towards Class I.

Normal or Abnormal? Eventually, the nurse must make a judgment as to whether the symptom of dyspnea is normal or abnormal for a particular patient. Any change in amount or nature of dyspnea indicates abnormality. Is it increased or decreased? Are alleviating and aggravating factors different? Changes in behavior patterns are significant—they may be designed to avoid dyspnea. For example, a patient may take an elevator to a third-floor laundry room to eliminate the experience of dyspnea associated with stair climbing. A woman may decide to see a hairdresser every week rather than cope with the dyspnea associated with caring for her own hair. Comparison of the patient with peers the same age is also a key in identifying abnormality. Poor physical fitness and advancing age may explain exercise intolerance. However, they do not explain the inability to run as far as a peer, especially if the same distance caused no breathing difficulties the previous year. Furthermore, mild dyspnea as a solitary finding may not indicate an abnormality unless it is accompanied by other cardiopulmonary signs and symptoms. Presence of other signs and symptoms is much more helpful in diagnosing specific respiratory problems.

WHEEZE

Subjective complaints of wheezing are not as common as objective findings of wheezing detected by auscultation of the chest. Frequently, the patient denies wheezing when it is auscultated by stethoscope, or the patient denies wheezing but admits to chest tightness or chest discomfort.

Complaints of wheezing almost always indicate disease of the lower airways from bronchoconstriction. Bronchoconstriction may be from a number of obstructive processes, but it most typically is associated with bronchospasm or airway narrowing from excess mucus or fluid. If bronchoconstriction is found in an adult, especially in one over 40 years of age, congestive heart failure is suspected. Wheezing due to heart disease is called *cardiac asthma*.

In pulmonary patients, wheezing is most commonly found in those with bronchial asthma or those with an asthmatic component to the mixed chest pathology. Although the onset of wheezing and associated dyspnea may be relatively abrupt, it usually occurs more gradually over hours to days. Individuals are essentially asymptomatic during periods of remission until provocative factors, such as allergens, foods (commonly shellfish), emotional upsets, and physical overexertion, stimulate already hyperirritable airways.

While wheezing is a classic finding of lower airway obstruction, it also may be encountered in cases of intrathoracic upper airway obstruction due to dynamic compression of the airway during respiration. If wheezing is present with extrathoracic lesions, it is usually overshadowed by stridor. The presence of wheezing in these so affected patients may mislead clinicians to think that respiratory problems are due to asthma rather than to upper airway obstruction.

Finally, the point must be made that even though wheezing is a classic finding in asthma, its absence does not exclude the diagnosis. Cough and dyspnea may be the only manifestations of asthma. Nonwheezing asthmatics have less airway reactivity than wheezing asthmatics (Pratter et al, 1981). The topic of wheezing is more fully discussed as an adventitious chest sound in Chapter 12.

Pleuritic Chest Pain

Pleuritic chest pain ranges from intense pain or discomfort during slight inspiratory effort to sharp pain at the end of maximum inspiratory effort. The pain is aggravated by deep breathing and coughing. Pleuritic chest pain indicates the presence of pleural inflam-

Table 10–3. PULMONARY REHABILITATION PROGRAM PRE-PROGRAM QUESTIONNAIRE*

Name________________________________

Date________________________________

Rehab. No.___________________________

Instructions: Check the category that most closely describes the patient's response to the situations given, according to the following scale:
0 = none, 1 = small, 2 = moderate, 3 = large, 4 = severe.

A. Shortness of Breath

	0	1	2	3	4
1. Rest					
To what degree do you get short of breath at rest?					
2. Walking					
To what degree do you get short of breath					
a. walking on level at your own pace?					
b. walking on level with others your age?					
c. walking up a hill?					
d. walking up stairs?					

	0	1	2	3	4
3. Activities of Daily Living					
To what degree do you get short of breath					
a. eating?					
b. standing up from a chair?					
c. picking up and straightening?					
d. brushing teeth?					
e. shaving or brushing hair?					
f. showering or bathing?					
g. dressing					
h. doing dishes					
i. sweeping or vacuuming?					
j. making bed?					
k. shopping?					
l. doing laundry?					

B. Overall Limitations

To what degree do these limit you in your daily life?	0	1	2	3	4
1. shortness of breath					
2. attacks of coughing or wheezing					
3. fatigue					
4. "bone or joint" problems					
5. "heart" problems					
6. fear of "hurting myself"					
7. fear of shortness of breath					
8. suggestions (or demands) of family and friends					

C. Hobbies

List, e.g., golfing, sewing, bowling, and gardening

Hobby	**How often?**	**Limitations**

Table continued on opposite page

Table 10–3. PULMONARY REHABILITATION PROGRAM PRE-PROGRAM QUESTIONNAIRE* *Continued*

D. Walking

1. How *many times* do you walk daily?__________
2. How *long* (time) do you walk each time?__________
3. How *far* (distance) do you walk each time?__________

E. Sputum

Amount/day__________ Most in am, pm, or both?__________Usual color__________

Consistency:

0	1	2	3	4
(Saliva-like)				(Too thick to get up)

F. Appetite (check one)

0	1	2	3	4
(Poor)				(Excellent)

G. Weight__________

H. Employment

1. Are you employed now?__________
2. If not, did you retire because of lung disease?__________
3. Limitations on job:__________
4. Have you recently changed jobs because of lung disease?__________

I. Smoking

1. Do you smoke now?__________
2. If not, when stopped?__________
3. How many packs a day?__________
4. How many years?__________

*Reproduced by permission from University Hospital and the Pulmonary Medicine Department of the University of California, San Diego Medical Center. Courtesy of Carol Archibald, R.N., Pat Hansen, R.N., and Kenneth Unger, M.D.

mation, malignant disease, or pneumothorax and is often accompanied by a pleural friction rub that is discovered during physical examination of the chest.

The source of pleuritic pain is the parietal pleura, which is richly supplied with sensory nerves from intercostal nerves and nerves to the diaphragm. Lung tissue and the visceral pleura lack sensory nerves to detect pain.

Table 10–4. DYSPNEA-DISABILITY SCALE*

Classification	Criteria
Class I	No significant restriction of normal activities but dyspnea on strenuous exertion.
Class II	Not dyspneic with essential activities of daily living; dyspneic with climbing stairs and inclines but not level walking.
Class III	Dyspnea with some activities of daily living (e.g., showering, dressing) but can perform all such activities without assistance. Able to walk at his own pace for a city block but cannot keep up while walking with others of his own age.
Class IV	Dependent on others in some activity of daily living; not dyspneic at rest but dyspneic with minimal exertion.
Class V	Dyspneic at rest; dependent on assistance from others for most activities of daily living.

*Adapted from Moser, K.: Rehabilitation of the COPD patient. Weekly update: pulmonary medicine, Lesson 40, New Jersey, Biomedia, Inc., 1979.

In pleurisy, pneumonia, and pulmonary infarct affecting the pleura, the irritated pleura lies directly under the general area where the pain is perceived. However, if the diaphragm is involved, pain may be referred to other areas of the body. Irritation of the *central portion* of the diaphragmatic pleura refers pain to the neck and upper parts of the shoulder, whereas irritation of the *outer portion* refers pain to the lower thorax, lumbar region, and upper abdominal region.

Because pleuritic chest pain may be mistaken for other types of chest pain, basic knowledge of these other types of chest pain is essential.

Chest Wall Pain. This type of chest pain may occur from rib fractures and from damaged intercostal muscle fibers (myositis or fibrositis) due either to chest trauma or to no known, obvious precipitating cause. Generally, when patients complain of this type of pain, the affected area can be localized to a very small area of damaged muscle or bone. In contrast, pleuritic pain may not be accompanied by tenderness to palpation over the identified painful area. When tenderness is present, it usually cannot be localized to a very small area of muscle or bone within the chest wall. From this perspective, pleuritic pain is a more subjective sensation than chest wall pain.

In addition, localized muscle tenderness or pain may be associated with infection of the upper respiratory tract and a dry, often paroxysmal, cough. This pain is frequently localized in the anterolateral chest area; localized muscle tenderness or pain can be differentiated from true pleuritic pain because it increases little or not at all during deep inspiration—it may be aggravated by coughing or trunk movement and usually does not disappear between coughing episodes.

Cardiac Chest Pain. The nurse must also differentiate pleuritic pain from chest pain of cardiac origin. Cardiac pain has many different clinical presentations and may be due to a variety of causes, such as angina pectoris from ischemic heart disease, myocardial infarction, dissection of the aorta, and acute pericarditis. The nurse commonly encounters the patient situation in which chest pain of myocardial ischemia must be distinguished from chest pain of pleuritic or chest wall origin. Pain from myocardial ischemia is classically characterized as an *aching*, *heavy*, or *squeezing* sensation, with *pressure* or *tightness* in the substernal region or across the anterior portion of the upper part of the chest. Induced by exertion and relieved by rest, it generally radiates into the neck and down one or both arms. Although a patient with chest pain from myocardial ischemia presents differently than one with chest pain from pulmonary causes, when found in mild forms without radiation, it may closely resemble the chest discomfort typically found in pulmonary patients.

Psychologic Origin. Chest pain in the cardiac or pulmonary patient may be of psychologic origin—*anxiety* is the most common cause of chest pain, in general. Information from a complete history, physical examination, and laboratory test results helps to further assess possible pulmonary, cardiac, and psychologic origins.

Cough

Chronic cough is difficult to evaluate because an occasional cough may be a normal finding in healthy persons. In addition, patients may not report its presence unless asked specifically. To quantify the complaint, the nurse focuses on quality—a *"loose" sounding* cough indicates the presence of secretions; a *dry, hacking* cough indicates airway irritation from airway obstruction; and a *harsh, barky* cough similar to a seal's suggests upper airway obstruction from limited vocal cord movement secondary to subglottic edema. Although some patients may not relate a characteristic quality, they usually can relate whether the cough is *weak* or *strong* and *productive* or *unproductive* of secretions. Many will openly associate coughing with cigarette smoking, the most common cause of coughing in addition to bronchitis.

Temporal relationships are important. Cough and sputum production of chronic bronchitis occurs on most days, 3 months of the year, for 2 consecutive years. It is worst on awakening in the morning and may be associated with SOB and sometimes with wheezing, if airway narrowing (bronchoconstriction) occurs from bronchospasm or excessive mucus in airways. Cough and sputum production shortly after the patient goes to bed indicate a significant mucus retention problem and usually a need to intensify bronchial hygiene measures before bedtime to promote uninterrupted sleep during the night.

Paroxysmal coughing, usually during early morning hours, is typical of many asthmatics. The reclining position in general tends to cause coughing and the onset of wheezing, possibly due to two mechanisms as follows: (1) the decreased neural discharge from the sympathetic nervous system in the reclining position—the parasympathetic discharge takes over, stimulates receptors along the tracheobronchial tree, and causes bronchospasm—and (2) the accumulation of mucus plugs during the night—the patient awakens abruptly with cough and wheeze. He sits on the edge of the bed and begins to develop the sensation of suffocation and chest tightness. After coughing up mucus plugs, symptoms may abruptly abate.

Paroxysmal coughing also occurs in other conditions. An episode of paroxysmal coughing and SOB may herald the onset of left ventricular failure. COPD patients with hyperirritable airways may cough violently when taking a walk in extremely cold weather; inclement weather aggravates symptoms. Exposure to various paint fumes, dusts, animal hairs, and other allergens can also precipitate attacks of coughing and wheezing.

Nasal discharge that drips down the back of the throat from head trauma, hay fever, or the common cold often causes a "scratchy" throat and may stimulate coughing, especially during sleep. When the patient is unconscious or asleep, uncontrolled postnasal drip may result in aspiration and development of chest infection.

Special emphasis must be placed on the relatively high incidence of postnasal drip as the cause of chronic persistent cough in adults. Irwin and associates (1981) report the incidence of causes of chronic cough in 49 patients as follows: chronic postnasal drip from a variety of conditions in 29%, asthma in 25%, postnasal drip plus asthma in 18%, chronic bronchitis in 12%, gastroesophageal reflux in 10%, and miscellaneous disorders in 6%.

Sputum Production

Information pertaining to sputum is crucial to the diagnosis of respiratory problems associated with mucus production and retention. Although a positive history indicates a mucus *production* problem, it only suggests the possibility of a mucus *retention* problem—physical examination of the chest (e.g., presence of rhonchi and decreased breath sounds) and the chest x-ray film (e.g., presence of signs of lung consolidation) confirm one's suspicion of retained secretions in the chest.

The nurse evaluates sputum production by investigating the following question categories.

Amount. Sputum production is quantified in teaspoons, tablespoons, or cups per day. If the patient has a sputum cup at the bedside, quantification is usually in cubic centimeters (cc) or in ounces (oz) per day or per nursing shift. Usually, only patients with severe bronchitis with bronchiectasis keep sputum cups at home to collect and monitor sputum—up to 8 oz per day in severe cases, which is considered a large quantity.

Unless a sputum cup is used, estimations of sputum production are very subjective. For the ambulatory patient, the nurse might begin the questioning by asking whether he coughs up minimal, small, moderate, or copious amounts of sputum with each episode. Then, the patient is asked to quantify these terms in teaspoons, tablespoons, or cups. Although patients can usually quantify sputum per episode of coughing in the morning, afternoon, or at night, they frequently need help to quantify amounts per 24 hours. The nurse suggests a likely amount, starting with a higher one and working down to a lower, less likely amount in view of the patient's complaints—Two cups per day? One cup? One-half cup? The opposite approach can be taken for patients who may tend to exaggerate signs and symptoms.

To assess the amount of sputum produced, the nurse must first decide whether sputum production is normal or abnormal for the patient in question. Well individuals do not normally cough up sputum. For them, sputum production suggests the onset of pulmonary or cardiac disease.

For patients with pulmonary disease, sputum production is normal or abnormal depending on the lung disease or mixture of lung pathology. The patient with pure anatomic emphysema does not normally cough up sputum; if he does, it usually is of minimal amount when he awakens in the morning. The patient with asthma does not normally cough up sputum between attacks when he is feeling good; however, during attacks he may cough up minimal to moderate amounts of very thick mucus. Also, patients with restrictive diseases, such as myasthenia gravis and sarcoidosis, do not characteristically produce mucus.

Bronchitic Component. In pulmonary disease, a *bronchitic component* is present when a patient begins to produce mucus or show other signs of bronchitis. As discussed in previous chapters, lung disease often appears in a mixed rather than pure form. For example, the emphysematous patient may enter the hospital with acute bronchitis. Other pulmonary patients develop respiratory problems when their normally absent or mild bronchitic component worsens owing to an advancing disease or inadequate program of medications and treatments at home or in the hospital.

For a patient with a bronchitic component to the disease process, the nurse questions carefully to determine how much sputum is normally produced on "good days" as well as "bad days," when he is feeling poorly. These parameters provide baseline values to help assess worsening or improving conditions.

Chest Infection. Sputum production is also a common sign of a chest infection, typically pneumonia. Patients with bacterial pneumonia classically present with the abrupt onset of cough, sputum production, chills, fever, and pleuritic pain. This type of pneumonia is a major cause of death but represents only a very small percentage of respiratory infections. Most respiratory infections result from viral infections, characterized by more gradual onset of symptoms without high fever, chills, and pleuritic chest pain. Otherwise healthy individuals suffer mild to severe discomfort from viral pneumonias. Mortality remains extremely low.

Signs and symptoms as well as manner of appearance vary in patients with pneumonia, depending on the type of pneumonia, causative agent, and individual susceptibility to disease. *Alveolar (lobar) pneumonia* from *Diplococcus* (pneumococcus) microbes shows a predilection for older, debilitated, and alcoholic patients. Symptoms start abruptly with fever as high as 106°F, shaking chills, and cough, which is nonproductive at first and then productive of bloody, rusty, or greenish sputum. The majority of patients report upper respiratory infections prior to the abrupt onset of these symptoms. In *bronchopneumonia* from *Staphylococcus aureus*, the classic symptoms of pneumonia vary depending on the patient's age, degree of debilitation, and whether the pneumonia is superimposed on an influenzal infection. Symptoms may appear abruptly in the ambulatory patient. In contrast, they appear more gradually when the patient develops pneumonia in the hospital and when the patient with chronic lung disease on corticosteroids or multiple antibiotics develops pneumonia as a complication. In the latter case, cough, fever, and blood-streaked sputum are rarely accompanied by chest pain and chills. Finally, in *interstitial pneumonias*, sputum production is more typically absent or minimal unless the patient has a chest infection or superimposed lower airway problem that stimulates mucus hypersecretion along the tracheobronchial tree.

Thus far, one can see that sputum production is of great concern to the nurse—the respiratory patient may have severe chronic bronchitis that requires comprehensive and continuing respiratory care; he may have acute bronchitis that may develop into pneumonia if microorganisms grow in retained secretions in the lungs; or he may have an acute chest infection from pneumonia or some other infectious process, such as lung abscess.

Changes in Amount Produced. Once sputum production is noted, the nurse notes any *increase or decrease in amount produced.* An increase in sputum production might indicate the new appearance of a chest infection or ineffectiveness of antibiotic medications used to treat an already existing infection. Accompanied by improving chest assessment findings on physical examination, it indicates a resolving mucus retention problem. Then sputum production gradually decreases as the patient's condition continues to improve. However, it is most important for the nurse to realize that *minimal sputum production may not indicate an improving or less severe chest condition.* First, sputum production in dehydrated patients may remain minimal until increased fluid intake causes rehydration and liquefaction of lung secretions, thus facilitating expectoration. Second, *minimal* amounts of expectorated sputum may be *grossly* infected with microorganisms, as evidenced by laboratory test results. Third, a patient may produce minimal amounts of thick sputum because it remains consolidated in the lung. All of these situations illustrate the importance of evaluating sputum production in light of other physical findings and laboratory data.

Finally, in assessing the amount of sputum produced, the nurse notes any *sudden increases or decreases.* A sudden decrease in sputum production might be due to obstruction of a draining bronchus by thick mucus plugs or an episode of bronchospasm, causing severe airway narrowing. The patients so affected are usually in critical condition. A sudden increase in sputum volume might be due to dramatic relief of airway obstruction by aspiration of mucus plugs or administration of bronchodilators by intravenous infusion. A sudden increase in sputum might also be due to rupture of a pulmonary abscess or an empyema into the bronchial tree.

Color. The most important point to remember is that *any change in the color of sputum is significant.* The change may be from the normal anticipated sputum color (clear or slightly whitish) or from the patient's particular baseline color. The tenacious mucoid sputum of a cigarette smoker is usually clear to gray in color, sometimes spotted with specks of brown tobacco. The postoperative patient without underlying lung disease demonstrates clear to whitish sputum. The COPD patient may normally demonstrate clear, whitish, or slightly yellow sputum, especially in the morning upon rising. If the patient reports any change from clear or gray to slightly yellow or from slightly yellow to obviously yellow, the patient may develop a chest infection. It does not mean he *has* a chest infection—he may *develop* one unless he receives appropriate medical and nursing respiratory care. Furthermore, if the sputum changes to any other color—pink, red, brown, or green—cardiopulmonary complications must be suspected.

Purulent Sputum. This type of sputum is generally yellow or green. It is found in lung abscess, acute bronchitis, and pneumonia when the inflammatory process produces pus from infection.

Mucopurulent Sputum. This sputum contains mucus from airway disease (e.g., bronchitis, bronchiectasis, and cystic fibrosis) and green or yellow pus from infection. It is commonly seen in patients with cystic fibrosis because the sputum typically grows *Pseudomonas aeruginosa,* a gram-negative bacillus. Since *Pseudomonas* organisms tend to grow rapidly in liquid media, patients using any respiratory therapy equipment are prone to such infections, if moisture-laden equipment is not regularly disinfected and dried. If an ambulatory patient reports the new appearance of green or yellow mucus, the nurse thoroughly investigates the cleaning procedure used for respiratory equipment at home. Usually, respiratory therapy personnel regularly monitor the adequacy of respiratory sterilization procedures in the hospital.

Pink, Watery, Frothy Sputum. This type of sputum is typical of an acute episode of pulmonary edema (left ventricle failure). If, however, acute pulmonary edema is not fully developed, pulmonary congestion yields blood-streaked sputum owing to the ruptured pulmonary capillaries from high intravascular pressures.

Pink to Red-Tinged Saliva or Sputum. This type of saliva or sputum is occasionally noticed in patients who are using the bronchodilator medication, Bronkosol (isoetharine), for an inhaled medication via intermittent positive pressure breathing (IPPB), or hand held nebulizer.

Consistency. The nurse determines whether the expectorated sputum is thick, thin, or frothy. *Thick, tenacious sputum* sticks to the sides of alveoli and airways, making expectoration more difficult and predisposing the patient to a mucus retention problem. Such a patient must be encouraged to increase fluid intake (providing he is not on restricted fluids) to liquefy respiratory secretions and facilitate expectoration.

Thin, watery secretions indicate adequate hydration of respiratory secretions, sometimes inappropriate use of expectorant medications, or possibly improper coughing technique that yields mostly saliva and upper respiratory tract secretions, such as postnasal drip and sinus drainage. If the patient reports *frothy secretions,* the nurse questions further regarding an associated pink-tinged color and other signs and symptoms of pulmonary edema.

Evaluation of Purulence. Evaluation of sputum consistency is important in evaluating purulence. One cannot *always* assume that a chest infection is present if secretions appear or are reported to be purulent. Certainly one suspects a chest infection, but this is not always the cause. There are two types of pus as follows: (1) *infectious pus,* seen in pneumonias, and (2) *noninfectious pus,* commonly seen in allergies with reversible airway obstruction or asthma. On microscopic examination, sputum with noninfectious pus demonstrates mostly eosinophils (i.e., leukocytes that stain readily with acid stain) and Charcot-Leyden crystals, important noncellular components of sputum formed by the coalescence of granules from disintegrating eosinophils. In contrast, infectious pus demonstrates neutrophils (i.e., leukocytes that stain readily with neutral dyes). Two purulent plugs of mucus—one of each type of pus—may appear exactly the same. But sputum with noninfectious pus is different in that it is extremely tenacious and adhesive. In a sputum cup, small plugs may remain stuck together in a worm-like appearance. If a small amount is placed on a microscope slide, resistance to compression occurs when a coverslip is placed on top of the sample, and pressure is applied. Hence, thick purulent plugs may represent the noninfectious, eosinophilic sputum of an asthmatic patient rather than the sputum of a respiratory patient with a chest infection.

Odor. Most sputum specimens are odorless. Cherniack (1983) claims that ". . . purulent sputum may occasionally have a sweet odor. A rotten, decomposed stench indicates an anaerobic putrefactive process, although infections by certain coliform organisms are also occasionally associated with a foul odor." Generally, a foul odor suggests an infectious process as in lung abscess. However, assessing odor is not crucial because color, consistency, and amount signal a respiratory problem that needs further assessment by a physician. Yet, some odors are so strong that they are difficult to ignore. Since *Pseudomonas* is common in chronically ill cystic fibrosis patients and hospitalized patients who develop pneumonia, many nurses and physicians claim they can identify its characteristic odor when working with such patients. The presence of a strong odor may indicate a need to evaluate disposal procedures for freshly expectorated or endotracheally suctioned respiratory secretions. Inadequate secretion disposal procedures are of concern because they may unnecessarily expose staff and the patient's family to infectious microorganisms, thus increasing the risk for others to develop pneumonia. Also, unless secretions are properly disposed, their odors can permeate a room, creating an aesthetically unpleasant and uncomfortable environment for everyone.

Hemoptysis

Hemoptysis is the coughing up of blood in the form of gross blood, of frankly bloody sputum, or of blood-tinged sputum. Hemoptysis is a main complaint in 10% of patients who visit chest disease clinics (Podnos and Chappell, 1985). Because it indicates cardiopulmonary disease and in some cases a potentially life-threatening bleeding problem, the nurse promptly notifies the physician of its presence or of any increase in amount of expectorated blood.

Blood coughed up from the lungs is usually bright red in color because its presence in the lung usually stimulates a cough reflex, facilitating immediate expectoration. Sometimes, however, it may appear dark red or rusty brown when a longer interval exists between the actual bleeding and expectoration of sputum, as in severe pneumonia with lung consolidation. Moreover, true hemoptysis usually contains at least some frothy portions of bright red blood and is followed by blood-streaked sputum for several days while the pathologic site in the lungs heals.

The type and amount of bloody sputum expectorated helps to identify possible cardiopulmonary problems. *Blood-streaked* sputum is common in bronchitis and pneumonia caused by *Staphylococcus* or *Klebsiella* organisms. *Frankly bloody* sputum with little if any mucoid content is seen in tuberculosis, bronchogenic carcinoma, and pulmonary infarction. Hemoptysis accompanied by *purulent* sputum suggests an infectious disease, such as pneumonia, lung abscess, and severe bronchitis with bronchiectasis, when the patient is chronically infected with microorganisms.

Hemoptysis may occur in large amounts (over 5 to 10 ml per coughing episode) in bronchial adenoma, bronchiectasis, tuberculous cavities, mitral stenosis, and lung cancer because the pathologic sites tend to have a very accessible or a richly vascular blood supply or both. Massive hemoptysis is present when more than 600 ml of blood is coughed up within a 48-hour period of time. It is most likely to occur in certain vascular conditions, such as aortic aneurysm and vascular congenital abnormalities, when the vessels gain access to a major airway.

In addition to bacterial infections, vascular conditions, and lung cancer, excluding most metastatic carcinomas except for choriocarcinoma and osteogenic sarcoma, hemoptysis is observed in other conditions. These include various parasitic diseases and fungal infections of the lungs (e.g., aspergillosis, coccidioidomycosis, and candidiasis), cystic fibrosis, and Goodpasture's syndrome, an immunologic condition involving the lungs and kidneys. In the presence of disease, patients on anticoagulant therapy may cough up blood as blood anticoagulation levels approach the desired therapeutic level.

Identification of the Bleeding Source. When taking a history from a patient with hemoptysis, the nurse attempts to determine the source of bleeding. Blood usually originates from one of three places as follows: (1) the *lungs and adjacent structures,* (2) the *upper respiratory tract,* and (3) the *stomach.* Discussion thus far has focused on the lungs, where pathology exists at the alveolar level, in the pulmonary circulation, and along the tracheobronchial tree. However, blood in the upper respiratory tract from the nose, gums or periodontal disease, tumor of the tongue or pharynx, or traumatized pharyngeal tissue, may appear to come from the lungs. In the critically ill patient, physical examination is especially necessary to identify these other sources of bleeding. Furthermore, *hematemesis,* the vomiting of blood from the stomach, may simulate hemoptysis; Table 10–5 helps to differentiate these two entities.

Precipitating Events. The nurse questions the patient to learn if any event triggered hemoptysis. Along with vigorous coughing in a suceptible individual or recent chest trauma to lung tissue, hemoptysis occasionally is due to respiratory treatments, such as IPPB and postural drainage with percussion and vibration. In IPPB, increased pressures in the lungs from me-

Table 10–5. DIFFERENTIATION OF HEMOPTYSIS FROM HEMATEMESIS*

Hemoptysis	Hematemesis
History of cough and respiratory problems may be present.	History of gastric problems, liver disease, or both, especially alcoholism, may be present.
May be preceded by chest discomfort.	Preceded by nausea and vomiting.
Blood is coughed up. Nausea and retching may be stimulated.	Blood is vomited. Coughing may be stimulated.
Blood is bright red to rusty brown in color and at least somewhat frothy.	Blood is dark red in color and never frothy.
Mucus or pus may be seen in specimen.	Food particles may be seen in specimen.
Continued blood-streaked sputum lasts for several days.	Blood-streaked sputum is usually not present.
Blood is alkaline in reaction.	Blood is acid in reaction.

*Adapted from Lyons, H.: Differential diagnosis of hemoptysis and its treatment. *Basics of respiratory disease*, 5:2, 1976.

chanical ventilation and subsequent coughing episodes may further irritate and inflame airways of the COPD patient and cause hemoptysis. Being placed in the Trendelenburg position for postural drainage, with vigorous percussion and vibration applied to the chest, may have a similar effect. As secretions drain into more proximal airways, more coughing is stimulated. This maneuver is usually well tolerated by an otherwise normal individual with acute bronchitis. But a COPD patient with already inflamed and dilated airways from bronchitis and bronchiectasis may bleed along the airways as a result of overly exertional activities and uncontrolled coughing. In these cases, the respiratory treatment is automatically discontinued at any sign of hemoptysis, and the physician is notified.

Medical Treatment. Because severe pulmonary hemorrhage has a reported mortality of 50 to 100% (Lyons, 1976), a patient with hemoptysis must be thoroughly evaluated by a physician to determine underlying cause.

Initial medical management includes diagnostic *bronchoscopy*, i.e., the visualization of bronchi through a bronchoscope to determine the location and nature of the bleeding. Bed rest is instituted when hemoptysis approaches 20 ml per coughing episode. Endotracheal intubation and mechanical ventilation are required when massive bleeding increases the risk of respiratory distress and asphyxiation. Other interventions may include vasopressin injection (*Pitressin*) and *bronchial artery embolization*, a relatively new procedure involving injection of an absorbable gelatin sponge into areas of angiographically localized bleeding.

Surgical elimination of the source is reserved for life-threatening bleeding, as in lung abscess with massive hemoptysis. The reason for current emphasis on more conservative therapy rather than surgery relates to the 37% death rate in patients who bleed heavily from their operation. Also, medical and surgical interventions for massive bleeding have comparable mortality rates (Podnos and Chappell, 1985).

During medical evaluation, ambulatory patients are cautioned to avoid situations that might worsen hemoptysis. For example, the nurse might advise the patient with cystic fibrosis or bronchiectasis on ways to avoid violent coughing episodes. Alternatives for mucus expectoration include slow-controlled deep breathing, hot showers, mist therapy, and increasing fluid intake, which also helps loosen secretions in the lungs. These interventions may also be appropriate for immunosuppressed patients and others with mucus retention and bleeding tendencies.

Voice Change

During the interview, the nurse notes any change in the patient's voice. Subtle change in voice is usually indicated by hoarseness. Hoarseness is a classic sign of upper airway obstruction in both children and adults. In its mild form and without associated signs and symptoms, it may be of little consequence. Extremely conversational individuals may complain of hoarseness that is alleviated with resting the voice. But medical evaluation is needed when voice change occurs acutely, in association with vocal cord dysfunction or in association with other signs and symptoms, especially stridor. *Stridor* is a harsh whistling sound during inspiration usually caused by upper airway obstruction from edema or inflammation or from a mass in the pharynx, larynx, or trachea.

Several acute disorders of the upper airway cause hoarseness. Hoarseness indicates *viral laryngitis* when it occurs acutely and in association with symptoms of infection of the upper respiratory tract. In cases of *epiglottitis*, hoarseness is often seen with accompanying signs and symptoms including high fever, sore throat, dyspnea, drooling, dysphagia, subdued cough, and sometimes stridor. These signs and symptoms may become severe in less than 8 hours, causing complete upper airway obstruction.

Subglottic edema from inflammation of the airway below the larynx also causes voice change, but the voice tends to be more muffled rather than hoarse, as long as the vocal cords are not affected. Accompanied by a barky cough and stridor, this type of hoarseness is more typically observed in children with laryngotracheobronchitis (childhood croup). It also follows short-term or long-term intubation after removal of an endotracheal or tracheostomy tube. During the intubation period, the tube causes irritation and inflammation of the subglottic area; its removal allows the mucosa to swell even more, potentially causing complete upper airway obstruction in severe cases.

Chronic or milder forms of hoarseness may result from the effects of a mediastinal lesion (e.g., tumor from bronchogenic carcinoma and enlarged lymph nodes), involving the recurrent laryngeal nerve. This nerve innervates the larynx (glottic and subglottic areas) as well as the mucous membranes of the upper part of the trachea. The left laryngeal nerve has a

particularly long intrathoracic course, traversing downward into the mediastinum and looping below the aortic arch before ascending upward to innervate the left vocal cord. Metastatic disease in the mediastinum is more likely to produce hoarseness by affecting this left branch.

An infrequently seen pulmonary cause of hoarseness is from secondary laryngeal lesions that develop in some cases of pulmonary tuberculosis with cavitation.

For persistent change in voice, the physician performs a technical procedure (*laryngoscopy*) to inspect the vocal cords and surrounding area for evidence of a neoplastic or granular tumor as well as a neurologic dysfunction of the vocal cords (e.g., unilateral abductor palsy).

GENERAL SIGNS AND SYMPTOMS

The following signs and symptoms are nonspecific in nature but may indicate pulmonary disease.

Fever, Chills, Night Sweats

A high temperature in a pulmonary patient suggests a chest infection. A high fever in the evening or at night, with nearly normal temperature in the morning, chills, and drenching night sweats, is found in pulmonary tuberculosis and eosinophilic pneumonia, a chest disease with an allergic or immunologic response.

Weakness, Fatigue

A patient will sometimes deny the presence of cardiopulmonary symptoms but admits to feeling more fatigued in general over the past few weeks or months. He may admit to increasing weakness or fatigue while performing specific activities of daily living.

Change in Body Weight

Weight loss is seen in many chest diseases, such as tuberculosis, eosinophilic pneumonia, granulomatosis from the metal beryllium, and carcinoma of the lung. A steady and sometimes dramatic reduction in weight over a few months to 1 or 2 years is found in end-stage chronic lung diseases. In the end-stage patient, even well-balanced meals with supplementary snacks fail to prevent cachexia.

Weight gain indicates a possible fluid retention problem (right ventricular failure). In the case of obesity, obstructive sleep apnea must be suspected, particularly if severe snoring during the night is reported, and even if the individual is otherwise asymptomatic (Block, 1981).

Anxiety, Depression, Anorexia

These problems are commonly accompanied by weight loss. They may have a physiologic basis (e.g., medications such as aminophylline and steroids), or they may represent psychologic difficulties in coping with acute or chronic illness.

Thus far, pulmonary signs and symptoms that form the main components of the pulmonary history have been discussed in detail. Before the discussion of other components of the history, the next brief section reviews main cardiac symptoms. Because of the close interrelationships between pulmonary and cardiac systems, cardiac signs and symptoms are considered with pulmonary ones in the overall pulmonary assessment.

REVIEW OF MAIN CARDIAC SYMPTOMS

Throughout an interview, the nurse notes the presence or absence of each of the following symptoms that suggest cardiac problems:

1. Shortness of breath
2. Fatigue
3. Chest pain
4. Syncope
5. Palpitations
6. Nocturia
7. Peripheral edema
8. Anorexia and vomiting

Since shortness of breath, fatigue, and chest pain are common in pulmonary disease as well as cardiac disease, the nurse may not be able to determine whether a problem is of pulmonary or cardiac origin based on the history alone. Many times, the presence of other pulmonary signs and symptoms supports a pulmonary nursing diagnosis, whereas the presence of other cardiac signs and symptoms supports a cardiac nursing diagnosis. If no other cardiopulmonary signs or symptoms exist, the nurse suspects pulmonary or cardiac problems based on associated complaints and unique characteristics of the cardiopulmonary symptoms being assessed.

Other Components

The other components of the pulmonary history discussed subsequently help to identify etiologies of problems, aggravating and alleviating factors, and general circumstances under which problems developed.

FAMILY HISTORY

The nurse inquires about the health of the patient's family members, including maternal and paternal grandparents, parents, siblings, aunts, uncles, spouse, and children. This information helps to identify pulmonary diseases of environmental, genetic, and familial nature that might have implications for the patient's current and future pulmonary problems.

Some pulmonary diseases have a familial incidence due to genetic transmission. A family history of COPD appears to place an individual at increased risk for

COPD. Some studies suggest that first-degree relatives of patients with known COPD are at excess risk. A study by Madison and colleagues (1980) reports equal deterioration in lung function in first- through third-degree relatives of patients with COPD.

Some obstructive diseases are more consistently inherited by successive generations. *Cystic fibrosis* (mucoviscidosis), a hereditary disease transmitted as an autosomal recessive trait, is the most common, lethal, genetically transmitted syndrome among white children; it is now seen in the adult population as well. About 1 in 20 individuals in the white population are genetic carriers (see Fig. 7–17).

Panlobular emphysema caused by an alpha-antitrypsin deficiency is clearly hereditary.

Kartagener's syndrome, a pulmonary disease consisting of situs inversus (complete reversal of chest structures), paranasal sinusitis, and bronchiectasis, has a high familial incidence, but transmission does not appear to occur in successive generations.

Other hereditary pulmonary diseases include alveolar microlithiasis, pulmonary myomatosis, and some forms of diffuse interstitial fibrosis.

Acute, highly contagious pulmonary diseases have a high familial incidence when they occur in home environments that foster the spread of disease, e.g., crowded conditions, poor room ventilation, and poor sanitary conditions. Tuberculosis and many acute viral chest infections may be disseminated throughout households unless proper preventive measures are taken and other family members or significant others are identified and adequately protected.

RESIDENCE AND RECENT TRAVEL

The nurse questions the patient regarding present and past geographic areas of residence as well as any recent intrastate, interstate, and foreign travel in regions with endemic pulmonary diseases. *Pulmonary tuberculosis* is worldwide in distribution, but it is more common in poverty-stricken individuals living in crowded regions that lack modern sanitary conveniences. *Coccidioidomycosis,* a highly infectious fungal disease of the lung, is found in the Western Hemisphere, mostly in California (notably the San Joaquin Valley), Arizona, northern Mexico, and western Texas. This granulomatous disease is caused by inhalation of the fungal organism from contaminated soil that is typically alkaline, free from severe frost, and exposed to a dry season following a wet one. Epidemics can occur after disturbance of such soil in preparation for construction projects.

Histoplasmosis, a fungal pulmonary disease caused by inhalation of saprophytic organisms in soil, is endemic to the central and eastern portions of North America, notably the Ohio, Mississippi, and St. Lawrence River valleys. It is also found in other regions of the world, such as South America and Central America, India, and Cyprus. The saprophytic organisms live in moist soil of appropriate chemical composition, frequently in areas of bird roosts.

Blastomycosis, a systemic fungal pulmonary disease with extrapulmonary spread to the skin, is primarily found in southeastern and midwestern regions of the United States but also is found in Canada, Central America, and Africa. Farmers and agricultural workers often develop this disease by inhaling air-borne infective spores from the soil.

Parasitic pulmonary diseases should be suspected in individuals who have emigrated from foreign countries noted to have pulmonary parasitic diseases less frequently seen in individuals who live in the United States.

SMOKING HISTORY

The nurse asks the patient to report any history of smoking cigarettes, pipes, cigars, or any other type of inhalant besides tobacco. Toxic substances in tobacco smoke include carbon monoxide, nicotine, and ammonia.

Cigarette smoking is the largest avoidable cause of death and disability in the United States (American Thoracic Society, 1985). Smokers are at increased risk of developing carcinoma of the lung, larynx, oral cavity, and esophagus. Several studies have shown that the risk of a smoker's dying from lung cancer is as high as 14 times that of a nonsmoker (Ayres, 1975). In addition, smokers compared with nonsmokers are at increased risk for COPD, notably chronic bronchitis and emphysema; heart disease; and postoperative pulmonary complications. They experience a 70% greater death rate due to coronary artery disease compared with nonsmokers. Maternal smoking is associated with a low infant birth weight, complications during pregnancy, and increased perinatal mortality (American Thoracic Society, 1985).

Cigarette smoking generally has worse effects on the body than pipe or cigar smoking. However, since risk for disease depends on numerous factors, particularly the dose-response relationship with duration and amount of smoking, comparisons are difficult to make.

Marijuana is now the third most frequently used psychoactive substance in the United States, after alcohol and tobacco. The contribution of marijuana smoking to pulmonary disease is still not entirely clear. Marijuana smoking dilates airways for minutes to hours, but long-term effects on the lung (e.g., chronic bronchitis) may be as harmful or more harmful than the effects of cigarette smoking. It may be a cancer-causing substance, since it contains more carcinogenic materials than tobacco smoke.

Quantification

To quantify cigarette smoking history, the nurse asks at what age the patient began smoking, whether he still smokes, and at what age he stopped smoking. The

number of packs smoked each day is estimated. Then the patient's *pack year history of smoking* is calculated as follows:

Formula:
Years of smoking × packs smoked per day = pack years

Example:
30 years × ½ pack per day = 15 pack years

As a general rule, an individual with a pack year history of over 20 years may already have COPD. The patient with an 8-pack-year history is likely to have obstructive changes in the lungs, even with an asymptomatic history.

Variable Effects of Smoking

To keep the positive finding of smoking in perspective, the nurse must remember that the effects of smoking on the body are highly variable. On the one hand, a heavy cigarette smoker (e.g., 20 pack years or more) with a history of cough and sputum production may show little to no impairment of lung function on a routine pulmonary function test. On the other hand, an occasional smoker may demonstrate significant lung impairment on a pulmonary function test.

Variable findings may be explained by several factors, some of which are summarized as follows:

1. Smoking habits, including *depth of inhalation, number of puffs taken per cigarette, use of a filter,* and *brand* or *type* of cigarette, largely determine the amount of inhaled carbon monoxide and tar deposited in the lungs. The chain smoker who deeply inhales smoke from an unfiltered cigarette is more at risk to develop pulmonary problems than the smoker who rarely inhales and smokes a filtered, low-tar brand of cigarette.
2. The presence of other major risk factors (e.g., history of allergy and presence of air pollution) in addition to cigarette smoking greatly enhances the risk for cardiopulmonary disease.
3. A symptomatic individual with no abnormality evident on a *routine* pulmonary function test may actually have lung impairment—specialized tests must be ordered to detect more subtle changes in lung function.
4. Variable findings and incongruities among smoking history, severity of pulmonary symptoms, and degree of impaired lung function may be unexplainable.

In light of the variable and still unknown effects of smoking as well as the limited and sometimes conflicting research findings on the topic, the claim that there is no safe cigarette may have some validity. Shaman (1981) reports that there is no clear evidence that low-tar, low-nicotine cigarettes reduce the risk of disease other than lung cancer. Such cigarettes may be more dangerous because of the increased amount of smoking and the inclusion of unknown chemical additives intended to enhance tobacco flavor. The additives are not identified on the cigarette package, and some have been implicated as possible lung irritants or carcinogenic substances.

More attention is now given to clinical screening for the presence of *passive* smoking. Although the patient may not smoke, contact with a cigarette smoker in an enclosed environment may predispose the patient to upper and lower respiratory problems, including the symptoms of eye irritation, rhinitis, headache, cough, wheezing, sore throat, and hoarseness. Very young children who live with smokers in the home have an increased incidence of lower respiratory tract infections. Moreover, nonsmokers who live with smokers may have a higher risk for lung cancer compared with nonsmokers who do not live with smokers (Lefcoe et al, 1983).

IMMUNIZATIONS

The nurse takes a history of immunizations, including booster inoculations and dates. The nurse notes immunizations against the usual childhood communicable diseases, such as measles, mumps, pertussis, and chickenpox, as well as influenzal and pneumococcal pneumonia. An individual with a usual childhood disease may develop pulmonary complications.

Influenza, a viral infection of the upper airway and sometimes the lungs, places the heavy smoker or individual with preexisting lung disease at increased risk to develop serious respiratory complications, including pneumonia, respiratory failure, and death, in severe cases. For protection against influenza, annual vaccination immediately preceding the winter months is recommended for elderly persons over 65 years of age and for persons with chronic disorders involving compromised lung function. Others who may benefit from this vaccine include (1) residents of nursing homes and long-term care facilities; (2) persons who have been hospitalized in the previous year for diseases that affect metabolism (e.g., diabetes, anemia, immunosuppressive diseases); and (3) physicians, nurses, and others who have extensive contact with those at risk for contracting influenza.

The pneumococcal pneumonia vaccine is recommended for sickle cell disease patients and older individuals with pulmonary disease. Though it protects against a major cause of bacterial pneumonia, it does not protect against other types of pneumonias more commonly seen in ambulatory patients. Unlike the influenzal vaccine, the pneumococcal pneumonia vaccine provides life-long immunity and is given only once.

ALLERGIES

The nurse questions the patient in regard to any known allergies to foods, various environmental factors

(discussed in Occupation and Environmental Factors), and drugs. Once the patient reports an allergy, more specific information is gathered about the causative factor, nature of the reaction, therapy, and sequela. Drug reactions are carefully assessed to determine whether an allergic reaction truly occurred or whether symptoms can be attributed to an inappropriate dose, a side effect, or a drug interaction with another concurrently administered drug.

Allergic reactions vary in different individuals. A reaction can range from allergic rhinitis or localized skin rash to systemic, life-threatening anaphylactic reaction with dyspnea, cyanosis, sometimes convulsions, unconsciousness, and death without immediate medical treatment.

Food reactions are assessed by asking questions about foods involved, methods of preparation, frequency and reproducibility of reactions, severity and nature of symptoms, and timing between food ingestion and onset of symptoms. Reactions may occur within 2 to 4 hours or for 4 hours to weeks after ingestion (National Jewish Center for Immunology and Respiratory Medicine, 1986). The sequence of signs and symptoms is as follows: (1) pruritus and edema of the lips; (2) nausea, vomiting, and abdominal cramps; (3) cutaneous reactions; (4) respiratory problems; and (5) anaphylaxis.

Asthmatics may be allergic to food or drug additives and preservatives, such as monosodium glutamate, often added to Chinese food, and the metabisulfites (see Chapter 7). Metabisulfites are sulfiting agents that serve as preservatives in various drugs, including bronchodilator solutions (e.g., isoetharine and metaproterenol), local anesthetics (e.g., lidocaine), and epinephrine (e.g., Adrenalin) in multidose vials. Metabisulfites are found, as preservatives, in many beverages (e.g., beer, wine, citrus drinks); convenience foods (e.g., prepared vegetables, dried fruits); and restaurant foods, especially shrimp and other seafoods; peeled and processed potatoes; and salads. Though the recent governmental ban on metabisulfites in fruits and vegetables potentially eliminates the risk of related breathing problems, complete success in this regard depends on the food industry's compliance with federal regulations. Moreover, metabisulfites have not been eliminated from beverages and other foods.

When allergy is suspected, the nurse asks whether the patient has ever had skin tests to document the presence and magnitude of an allergic reaction. In addition, the nurse asks whether *immunotherapy* or *hyposensitization therapy* was used to minimize allergic signs and symptoms. Immunotherapy is a series of injections of antigen extracts (e.g., pollens, molds, and dusts) given over an extended period of time to alter the patient's IgE response to specific allergens. It is one of the main treatments for hay fever and asthma; however, only 50% or 60% of patients respond.

OCCUPATION

The nurse notes the patient's past and present occupations because certain ones are associated with increased incidence of *occupational lung disease* (OLD). An OLD is a disease caused by inhalation of lung irritants or allergens in the work place. Table 10–6 lists a variety of causes of OLD, yet this list is by no means complete. There are thousands of pollutants in work places throughout the United States that are occupational lung hazards. The list for causes of occupational asthma alone is quite extensive; however, it must be used only as a guide. Because of individual susceptibility to disease, what causes a hypersensitivity reaction in one person may have no observable effect in another.

Table 10–6. CAUSES OF OCCUPATIONAL LUNG DISEASE

Substance	Occupation	Disease
Animal hair, dander, urine of animals, including insects and birds	Animal handlers, e.g., farmer, veterinarian, laboratory worker	Asthma
Asbestos fiber	Asbestos miner Shipyard worker Construction worker Demolition worker Insulation worker Electrician Brake mechanic	Asbestosis Lung cancer (mesothelioma)
Coal dust	Coal miner	Coal worker's pneumoconiosis (black lung)
Cotton dust	Textile worker	Asthma (byssinosis or brown lung)
Diisocyanates		
Toluene diisocyanate (TDI), diphenylmethane diisocyanate, hexamethylene diisocyanate	Automobile worker TDI manufacturer Foundry core worker Polyurethane foam worker Painter	Asthma
Drugs		
Ampicillin, penicillin, glycyl-containing compounds, piperazine	Pharmacist Pharmaceutic industrial worker	Asthma
Enzymes		
Subtilisin Trypsin, pancreatin	Detergent manufacturer Pharmacist Pharmaceutic industrial worker	Asthma
Formaldehyde	Laboratory worker Fur, tanning, and clothing industrial workers Home insulation worker	Asthma
Grain dust and flour	Baker Miller Farmer	Asthma

Table continued on opposite page

Table 10–6. CAUSES OF OCCUPATIONAL LUNG DISEASE *Continued*

Substance	Occupation	Disease
Henna extract	Hairdresser	Asthma
Insoluble gases		
Phosgene, nitrogen oxides, and so forth	Industrial worker Participants in chemical warfare (phosgene)	Chemical pneumonia Pulmonary edema
Irritant gases		
Chlorine, sulfur dioxide, ammonia, and so forth	Industrial worker Housekeeper, maid	Upper respiratory tract symptoms; bronchitis
Metal oxides		
Copper, zinc, magnesium, cadmium, iron, manganese, and mercury	Welder Industrial worker	Metal fume fever
Metallic salts		
Nickel	Metal plating worker	Asthma
Chromium	Cement, tanning, and metal plating workers	
Aluminum	Aluminum fluoride and sulfate workers	
Nitrogen dioxide in filled silos, closed welding spaces, and chemical laboratories	Farmer Welder Laboratory technician	Silo filler's disease Nitrogen dioxide exposure
Polyvinyl chloride	Meat wrappers	Asthma
Rosin (colophony)	Electronics worker	Asthma
Silica	Sandblaster Foundry worker Jeweler Stonemason Pottery maker Ceramist Construction worker Miner	Silicosis
Spores from moldy hay	Farmer	Farmer's lung
Wood dusts	Carpenter Wood carver Construction worker Mill worker	Asthma

Since occupational asthma is much more common than many realize, the nurse is on the alert for complaints of the characteristic symptoms of dyspnea, wheezing, chest tightness, and cough occurring during or after work. Because wheezing is worst on Mondays (or the first work day of the week) and may be accompanied by a low grade fever, this type of asthma is often referred to as "Monday fever." Symptoms gradually improve as the week progresses and may completely abate on weekends and during vacations when exposure to the inhalant is avoided. Upper respiratory tract symptoms—runny nose, sore throat, eye irritation, and headache—may antedate the onset of asthma by several weeks to months.

Occupational lung diseases may cause acute illness—hypersensitivity reaction, chemical pneumonia, or pulmonary edema—or it may cause a chronic diffuse interstitial fibrosis—silicosis, coal worker's pneumoconiosis, or asbestosis. Exposure to some industrial substances increases risk for lung cancer, especially if the individual is a cigarette smoker.

ENVIRONMENTAL FACTORS

Occupation is perhaps the most overt clue that suggests the presence of OLD, but it is not the most reliable one. Many times it is the worker in a totally unrelated occupation who develops disease. For example, a maintenance man may be sweeping the floor in a poorly ventilated room in the vicinity of a welder who is fully protected against metal fumes. In this case, if the maintenance man has no protective mask to guard against inhalation of metal fumes, he is more likely to develop respiratory problems than the welder. Hence, questions to assess *environmental conditions* are needed to further explore occupations related to OLD and to discover hazardous environmental conditions that might not be considered for a particular occupation.

The Work Place

Evaluation of the patient in relation to the work place and its environment begins by asking the following: "Have you been exposed to chemicals or particles in the form of dusts, fumes, vapors, or exhausts?" If the patient responds positively, ask for the name of the chemical or dust; a worker usually knows the name of the substance with which he works. The nurse proceeds to explore all the question categories for symptoms to obtain a detailed account of the progression of symptoms and associated phenomena, noting alleviating and aggravating factors as well as periods of remission and exacerbation. A detailed account of job duties is taken to determine the amount and extent of exposure in hours per day, week, month, and year. Questioning is terminated once the nurse has a clear history of the patient's past and present daily job activities and associated symptoms.

In most cases, the interview situation yields sufficient information to screen the patient for OLD. Yet, consultation with appropriate personnel in the work place may be necessary to identify possible environmental hazards, such as poorly ventilated rooms and inadequate protective masks and clothing that might serve as causative or aggravating factors in the development of pulmonary symptoms.

The Home Environment

Exposure to lung irritants or allergens in the home environment is just as important as exposure on the

Table 10–7. INTERVIEW FORM FOR HOME ASSESSMENT OF POTENTIAL ALLERGENS OR LUNG IRRITANTS

Instructions: To complete this form, please provide the appropriate information by filling in the spaces and checking the appropriate boxes.

1. General description of home:

   Years of occupancy__________ Number of occupants__________

2. Occupants who smoke in home__________

3. Pets__________

4. House plants or cut flowers__________

5. Air indoors

   Heating system: Electric ☐ Radiant ☐ Forced air ☐

   Cooling system: Air conditioning ☐ Electric fans ☐

   Filters present?__________

   Frequency of cleaning air vents__________ Filters__________

   Humidifier__________

6. Floors: Wood or linoleum ☐ Carpet: High pile ☐ Medium pile ☐ low pile ☐

   Throw rugs ☐ Type of fabric__________

7. Windows: Venetian blinds ☐ Shades ☐ Curtains or drapes ☐

   Mold on window frames?__________

8. Walls: Leaking pipes or ceilings__________

   Dust catchers__________

9. Furniture: Dust catchers__________

   Stuffed furniture__________

   Any new furniture or items left by previous occupants that may be source of allergens?__________

10. Bathroom: Presence of mold__________

    Irritating aerosol air fresheners__________

11. Kitchen: Cleanliness of refrigerator__________

    Mold growth?__________

    Vent for escape of cooking fumes?

12. Bedding: Type of pillows__________ Type of blankets__________

    Type of mattress and box spring__________

13. Storage areas: Locations__________

    Condition of closets__________

    Doors kept open ☐ closed ☐

14. House cleaning habits:

    By whom:

    Frequency:

    Means: Vacuuming ☐ Dry dusting (mopping) ☐ Wet dusting ☐

15. Outdoor sources of allergy: (i.e., plants, trees, grasses, weeds)

16. Other:

17. Overall assessment with recommendations:

job site. This fact is especially true when assessing small children, housewives, or retired individuals who spend most of their time at home. Some of the OLDs listed in Table 10–6 may be related to hobbies in the home (e.g., pottery, ceramics, and wood carving) rather than to duties in the work setting. Without proper protective clothing, workers may transport lung irritants home via contaminated clothing. There have been cases of asbestosis in family members who presumably inhaled air-borne asbestos fibers while handling or laundering contaminated work clothes. Moreover, environmental conditions at home—paint fumes from a freshly painted room or dusts from nearby construction work—may precipitate an acute asthmatic attack in hypersensitive individuals.

Allergens or irritants in the home environment that precipitate pulmonary symptoms are relatively easy to assess when the patient readily identifies the source of allergy. But when sources of allergy cannot be readily identified by interviewing in the hospital or clinic setting, the visiting nurse may be asked to interview the patient at home, inspecting the home environment for potential allergens or lung irritants. Table 10–7 is an interview form for home assessment of commonly found potential allergens and irritants. Explanations that correspond to the same numbered items on the form are as follows:

1. Untidy, cramped living quarters tend to cause accumulation of more potential allergens than well-kept, spacious quarters. Long-term occupancy by several persons might also create the same situation if they are not good housekeepers.
2. Nonsmokers are at increased risk to develop pulmonary symptoms when in contact with smokers in a poorly ventilated room. Young children are clearly more sensitive to smoke; a positive correlation exists between smoking parents and increased incidence of pulmonary problems in children. Recent related literature stresses the point that respiratory symptoms and pulmonary function abnormalities from exposure to sidestream cigarette smoke seem to be more marked in individuals with preexisting airway hyperreactivity or asthma. Normal individuals may show no change in pulmonary function when exposed to cigarette smoke (Dahms et al, 1981).
3. Pet hair and dander are common sources of allergy.
4. Pollen from blooming house plants or cut flowers may cause allergy. Also, mold grows easily on the surface of potting dirt and on the sides of pots.
5. Forced air heating systems may aggravate breathing problems, especially if no filter exists to filter out air-borne dust particles—in such cases, patients may have to switch to portable electric heaters. Radiant heating is ideal, but more expensive. Filtered air conditioning systems are also ideal to help alleviate respiratory symptoms during hot, smoggy weather; the filters must be cleaned regularly to avoid the growth of molds and to insure effective filtering. Electric fans are less than ideal because they stir up and recirculate dust. For optimum effectiveness in reducing dust circulation, filters on air systems should be changed as often as every 2 weeks, depending on the frequency of use and manufacturer recommendation. Dirty air vents provide a continual source of dust. Humidifiers may be sources of infection if they are not cleaned regularly, with the water changed daily.
6. High pile carpets or throw rugs are notorious collectors of dust, animal hairs, and other allergens. For highly allergic individuals, wood or linoleum floors are recommended because they can be more easily and thoroughly cleaned. Throw rugs should be of low pile material or of machine washable fabric. Carpet padding should not be made of animal hair.
7. Other notorious dust catchers are draperies and Venetian blinds. Asthmatics who also have allergies may be advised to use washable cotton or synthetic roll-up window shades or washable cotton or fiberglass curtains. Mold may grow on window frames in areas with a warm, humid climate; bathrooms are common sources of mold.
8. Inspect wallpaper for swelling, indicating the presence of underlying mold. Pictures on the walls, especially those with broad frames, may collect dust.
9. Fabric upholstered furniture collects dust and may have to be replaced by rubberized canvas or plastic upholstered furniture. Foam rubber pillows may grow moldy in damp areas. Kapok and feathers in pillows are common allergens and may be replaced with Dacron or other synthetics in pillows.
10. Mold may be found near leaky faucets, bathtubs, and shower areas.
11. Mold may grow on food stored for long periods, in drip pans under the refrigerator, and on surfaces exposed to steam from cooking. Patients who complain of dyspnea from cooking fumes are advised to use overhead fans to vent fumes to the outside or open windows. Higher concentrations of nitrogen dioxide are reported in homes where gas is used for cooking than in homes where electricity is used. More men, especially nonsmokers, than women appear to develop respiratory symptoms from the gas used for cooking (Comstock et al, 1981).
12. Bedding for allergic individuals may include synthetic filling for pillows rather than kapok or feathers; washable cotton or synthetic blankets rather than wool or fuzzy surface blankets, and, for severe asthmatics, specially made allergen-proof encasings for pillows, mattresses, and box springs.
13. Untidy, crowded closets with open doors, storage areas under beds, and large pieces of furniture tend to collect dust and other allergens.
14. If vacuuming or dusting aggravates the patient's

pulmonary symptoms, someone else should house clean when the patient is not in the immediate area. Since dusting with a dry mop or cloth stirs up and redistributes allergens, wet dusting is preferred. Depending on the degree of airway hypersensitivity, cleaning may have to be done once or twice a day to once or twice a week to effectively control the level of dust and other allergens in the home. If no one else is available to house clean, the patient should wear a protective mask or kerchief to guard against allergen inhalation. If the whole house looks untidy, advise the patient to concentrate the cleaning on the bedroom or other rooms where the most time is spent.

15. Blooming flowers, shrubs, trees, grasses, and weeds are common sources of allergy. Determine whether contact with allergens and associated pulmonary symptoms are seasonal. Allergies that exacerbate in *spring* are usually due to flower, shrub, or tree pollens. *Late spring-early summer* allergies are usually due to grasses, while *late summer* allergies are usually due to weeds.
16. Other potential allergens might be stuffed toys, perfumes, insect sprays, tar paper, or camphor. Allergens or lung irritants from hobbies, e.g., wood carving, jewelry making, and ceramics, may cause or aggravate pulmonary symptoms.
17. The following questions help assess the overall situation in the home:
    a. Which of the aforementioned potential allergens or irritants do you think is causing or aggravating pulmonary symptoms?
    b. Do symptoms indicate a lung problem, such as asthma (e.g., wheezing, chest tightness, dyspnea), or a more local response such as hay fever?
    c. Can the allergen or irritant be eliminated from the home? Should house cleaning habits be modified?

If inspection of the premises is not possible, the nurse can still use the form as a guide to interview the patient in more detail and identify pulmonary symptoms that might be associated with any of the potential sources listed. Furthermore, if review of allergy skin test results reveals the allergen responsible for pulmonary symptoms, the form can be used to help identify specific sources of the known allergen in the home. The allergen then can be either eliminated completely (e.g., replacement of down pillows with synthetic) or controlled to tolerable levels (e.g., appropriate house cleaning acivities to control dust accumulation). Hence, this form helps to more thoroughly assess an allergic component of a patient's pulmonary disease. If allergy test results and home assessment results are negative, emotional factors may be responsible for some episodes of increased airway obstruction.

The interview form is also appropriate for assessment of patients with severe chronic lung disease who are not diagnosed asthmatics but who still complain of pulmonary symptoms upon exposure to dusts or fumes associated with daily chores in the home. The nurse interviews to determine the source of the lung irritation (dust or cooking fumes in most cases) and how successful the patient has been at eliminating or controlling the source in the home.

Animals

Animals, especially pets, are common sources of respiratory problems. More specifically, animal hairs and dander are common precipitating factors in asthma as well as hay fever, an upper respiratory tract disorder. Contact with excreta from pigeons may lead to *cryptoccosis*, especially in breeders. Contact with birds, especially parrots, may lead to *psittacosis*, a viral disease also called *ornithosis* or *parrot fever*. Contact with dusts contaminated by sheep or cattle may cause *Q fever* in ranchers or others living in nearby rural areas.

Air Pollution

In more populated cities, *air pollution* due to reliance on private vehicles for transportation and growth of industry, has become increasingly recognized by the general public and scientific community as a significant factor in aggravation of pulmonary symptoms. It does not seem to have much influence on nonsmokers, but it has a significant additive or synergistic influence on cigarette smokers. Air pollution can aggravate mucus hypersecretion along the tracheobronchial tree and, in susceptible individuals, cause impairment of respiratory function. Hot, smoggy weather in an industrial region or urban city is a common precipitating factor of acute respiratory failure in ambulatory COPD patients. Major industries that tend to contribute the most to air pollution, in the form of sulfur oxide, nitrogen dioxide, and particulate matter, are electric utilities, iron and steel producers, copper smelters, pulp and paper producers, petroleum refiners, and chemical producers. Other sources of air pollution include motor vehicle exhaust and exposure to combustion products, e.g., smoke from wood-burning stoves.

PULMONARY MEDICATIONS AND TREATMENTS

The nurse questions the patient regarding past and present prescribed and nonprescribed over-the-counter pulmonary medications and treatments, noting dates and reasons for starting and discontinuing each. Simultaneously, the nurse tries to determine the patient's level of compliance with prescribed therapy. Does the patient's past history indicate that all therapies are strictly adhered to? Are some therapies sporadically or rarely followed? To make an accurate assessment of the patient's situation, a history of actual medications and treatments taken must be gathered. Since pharmalogic assessment is of crucial importance, it is covered separately in Chapter 11.

Areas of Focus

Taking a pulmonary history may be quite time consuming, especially when it is integrated into the broader nursing history covering other body systems and psychosocial aspects. A comprehensive interview including the pulmonary history of a multiproblem patient often takes 30 to 60 minutes. In the acute care setting, interview time may be broken up into periodic short conversations with the patient when he is feeling well enough to converse about the course of his illness and his past health habits. Because of the various constraints that inevitably arise in the clinical setting, the nurse must be prepared to conduct short productive interviews, keeping in mind the main historical findings of respiratory disease (Table 10–8) and focusing on the main areas of concern. The pointers enumerated subsequently serve as guides to the process of history taking. They will help the nurse mentally process information, as it is gathered from the patient, family, and medical chart.

1. *Focus on chief complaints and try to determine cause and effect relationships.* Primary problems are usually centered on chief complaints. The crucial question then becomes "What *really* caused the disorder in the first place?" or "What *really* precipitated the exacerbation of signs and symptoms?" Pulmonary signs and symptoms may be due to the natural progression of disease, but in many cases extrinsic factors trigger acute problems. Examples of extrinsic factors are discontinuation of a pulmonary medication, mental depression, lack of transportation to the physician's office, and lack of education.

2. *Differentiate between upper airway disease and lower airway disease.* In most cases, specific signs and symptoms of *upper airway disease* include rhinitis (runny nose); sore throat; sneezing spells; nasal obstruction; stridor, for extrathoracic obstructive lesions; and voice change. Specific signs and symptoms of *lower airway disease* usually are as follows: wheeze, pleuritic chest pain, cough and sputum production, and hemoptysis. Shortness of breath is a vague symptom and must be evaluated in light of other findings.

3. *Identify individuals who may have infections.* Individuals who have infections may be afebrile, or they may report chills, night sweats, or high temperatures. Other signs of infection may include a change in amount, color (to yellow, green, or brown), or quality of sputum. Infected individuals need immediate medical treatment. Isolation precautions may need to be taken to protect nearby susceptible individuals from exposure to infectious airborne microorganisms.

4. *Identify individuals with chronic or recurrent disease.* Take note of patients with repeated hospital admissions for respiratory problems. Once acute problems are effectively treated and controlled, the nurse focuses subsequent conversation on full exploration of the circumstances surrounding exacerbations.

Table 10–8. MAIN HISTORICAL FINDINGS IN RESPIRATORY DISEASE

Disease	Dominant Symptoms	Other Symptoms
Atelectasis	Acute: sudden onset of SOB, cyanosis, fever if infection is present Chronic: usually no symptoms	Nonspecific
Bacterial pneumonia	Sudden onset of high fever and shaking chills Cough, nonproductive at first Pleuritic chest pain	Bloody, rusty, or greenish sputum SOB at times
Bronchial asthma	Episodic SOB	Cough and wheezing (before SOB) Thick mucus plugs Chest tightness Sense of suffocation
Bronchogenic carcinoma	Depend on the size, extent, and type of tumor as well as presence or absence of systemic complications Patient may be asymptomatic for 5 to 10 years	Weight loss and fatigue One or more of the following: cough, SOB, chest pain, and hemoptysis
Chronic bronchitis	Cough and sputum production	Hemoptysis from bronchiectasis Wheezing at times SOB in early morning
Cystic fibrosis	Cough and purulent sputum production	Hemoptysis Wheezing (most common in infants) Loose, bulky, fatty stools, voracious appetite, abdominal pain, salty breath and skin, runny nose, poor physical growth
Diffuse interstitial fibrosis	SOB first on exertion; then at rest also	Other symptoms depend on specific chest disease May complain of vague symptoms of chest pain, fatigue, nonproductive cough

Table continued on following page

Table 10–8. MAIN HISTORICAL FINDINGS IN RESPIRATORY DISEASE *Continued*

Disease	Dominant Symptoms	Other Symptoms
Emphysema	SOB	Cough Minimal sputum production, if any
Lung abscess	Cough Sputum production Fever	Sudden severe illness, e.g., *Staphylococcus* and *Klebsiella* infections, pulmonary infarction Progressive illness with cough, weight loss, weakness, and low-grade fever, e.g., tuberculosis, fungal infections, most bronchogenic carcinomas History of aspiration, pneumonia, or recent unconsciousness (from alcoholism, drug overdose, surgical procedure)
Mycoplasmal pneumonia	Gradual development (3–4 days) of fever, headache, malaise, sore throat, nasal ingestion, and cough	May have skin rash or complain of ear problems (erythema or tympanic membrane or bullous myringitis) Scanty sputum production—may be purulent
Pleural effusion	Patient may be asymptomatic Pleuritic chest pain or shoulder pain often precedes effusion	SOB if effusion is large Other symptoms depend on underlying cause
Pneumothorax (spontaneous)	Sudden onset of pleuritic chest pain referred to shoulder or arm on involved side	Associated SOB Sometimes only vague chest discomfort and dry cough
Pulmonary edema	Acute SOB Orthopnea Frothy, blood-tinged sputum	Objective data are crucial, e.g., cyanosis, diaphoresis, anxiety, tachycardia, chest x-ray findings
Pulmonary embolism	Variable Usually SOB	Pleuritic or substernal chest pain Nonproductive cough Hemoptysis with incomplete infarction Anxiety Fever Syncope
Pulmonary hypertension	SOB with strenuous effort; then with slight effort or at rest	Dull substernal aching chest pain, commonly effort induced (with increased pulmonary arterial pressure) Syncope with exercise Cough or other symptoms associated with underlying disease Signs of right ventricular failure with prolonged or severe pulmonary hypertension
Pulmonary tuberculosis	Patient is commonly asymptomatic but has a history of exposure to tuberculosis Cough, nonproductive at first	May have only nonspecific complaints of fatigue, weight loss, anorexia, and irritability Purulent and sometimes bloody sputum production Pleuritic chest pain when pleurisy is present Symptoms of chronic infection; low-grade fever, night sweats, headache, vague digestive disturbances
Right ventricular failure	Dependent edema Weight gain	Nocturia—oliguria in daytime Anorexia, bloating, exertional right upper abdominal pain, and jaundice Weakness, headache, and mental aberration (see Table 9–5)
Sarcoidosis	SOB first on exertion; then at rest also Patient may be asymptomatic	Skin lesions (i.e., erythema nodosum) Dry cough Joint pains Fever
Sleep apnea syndrome	Loud sonorous snoring in obstructive apnea Daytime hypersomnolence Morning headache	Difficulty arising in morning Poor concentration ability or disorientation, improving during the day Abnormal motor behavior during sleep; peculiar postures, flailing limbs Personality changes; irritable or aggressive behavior
Viral pneumonia (influenza)	Sudden onset of chills, followed by *fever* (essential feature) prostration, myalgias, backache, and headache *Cough*, nonproductive at first (essential feature)	Purulent sputum production May have anorexia and nausea; rhinitis, epistaxis, slight conjunctivitis, and photophobia May develop signs of bacterial superinfection (tracheobronchitis or pneumonia)

Conclusion

A pulmonary history typically yields a large body of subjective data. Yet, it is only the initial step towards the collection of a complete data base from which respiratory problems or nursing diagnoses are made. Sometimes, the pulmonary history indicates the exact nature of respiratory problems, e.g., mucous production is fairly easy to document on the basis of history. In most cases, however, the clinician waits to gather objective data before interpreting this subjective data.

REFERENCES

American Thoracic Society: Cigarette smoking and health. 132(5):1133–1138, 1985.

Ayres, S. M.: Cigarette smoking and lung diseases: an update. Basics of respiratory disease, 3(5), 1975.

Barbee, R.: The medical history in pulmonary disease. *Basics of respiratory disease,* 11(3), 1983.

Billingsley, J., et al.: Screening asymptomatic patients at risk. *Patient care,* 13:6, 40–59, 1979.

Block, A. J.: Is snoring a risk factor? *Chest,* 80:5, 525, 1981.

Borg, G.: Psychophysical bases of perceived exertion. *Medicine and science in sports and exercise,* 14(5): 377–381, 1982.

Buist, A. S.: The relative contributions of nature and nurture in chronic obstructive pulmonary disease. *Western journal of medicine,* 131:2, 114–120, 1979.

Burki, N.: Dyspnea. In Williams, M. H. (ed.), *Clinics in chest medicine,* 1:1, 47–55, 1980.

Cherniack, R., and Cherniack, L.: Respiration in Health and Disease. Philadelphia, W. B. Saunders Co., 1983.

Comstock, G. W., et al.: Respiratory effects of household exposures to tobacco smoke and gas cooking. *American review of respiratory disease,* 124:2, 143, 1981.

Dahms, T., Bolin, J. F., and Slavin, R. G.: Passive smoking—effects on bronchial asthma. *Chest,* 80:5, 530, 1981.

doPico, G. A.: Occupational asthma. *Advances in asthma, allergy and pulmonary diseases,* 5:4, 2–9, 1978.

Doyle, N. C.: Marijuana and the lungs. *American lung association bulletin,* November, 1979.

Dudley, D., and Sitzman, J.: Psychosocial and psychophysiologic approach to the patient. *Seminars in respiratory medicine,* 1:1, 59–83, 1979.

Fraser, R. G., and Paré, J. A.: Diagnosis of Diseases of the Chest, vol. 1, (2nd ed.). Philadelphia, W.B. Saunders Co., 1979.

Glauser, F.: Signs and Symptoms in Pulmonary Medicine. Philadelphia, J.B. Lippincott Co., 1983.

Herman, S.: Can we afford to clean up our air? *American lung association bulletin,* December, 1979.

Irwin, R., Corrao, W., and Pratter, M.: Chronic persistent cough in the adult: the spectrum and frequency of causes and successful outcome of specific therapy. *American review of respiratory disease,* 123:4, 413, 1981.

Lefcoe, N., et al: The health risks of passive smoking—the growing case for control measures in enclosed environments. *Chest,* 84(1): 90–95, 1983.

Loudon, R. G.: Cough: a symptom and a sign. *Basics of respiratory disease,* 9:4, 1981.

Loughlin, G., and Taussig, L.: Upper airway obstruction. *Seminars in respiratory medicine,* 1:2, 131–146, 1979.

Lyons, H.: Differential diagnosis of hemoptysis and its treatment. *Basics of respiratory disease,* 5:2, 1976.

Madison, R., Zelman, R., and Mittman, C.: Inherited risk factors for chronic lung disease. *Chest,* 77:2, 255–257, 1980.

Malasanos, L., et al.: Health Assessment, 2nd ed. St. Louis, C. V. Mosby Co., 1981.

Moller, D., et al.: New directions in occupational asthma caused by small molecular weight compounds. *Seminars in respiratory medicine,* 7(3): 225–239, 1986.

Moser, K.: Evaluation of Patients with Acute or Chronic Dyspnea. Respiratory Emergencies, 2nd ed. (Moser, K. and Spragg, R. eds.). St. Louis, C. V. Mosby Co., 1982.

Moser, K.: Rehabilitation of the COPD patient. *Weekly update: pulmonary medicine,* Lesson 40, New Jersey, Biomedia, Inc., 1979.

National Jewish Center For Immunology and Respiratory Medicine: Adverse reactions to food not always "food allergy." *Medical/scientific update,* 5(1): 1–5, 1986.

Podnos, S. and Chappell, T.: Hemoptysis: a clinical update. *Respiratory care,* 30(11): 977–985, 1985.

Pratter, M., et al: Less airway reactivity in nonwheezing asthmatics compared to wheezing asthmatics. *Respiratory care,* 26:8, 739, 1981.

Shaman, D.: Getting out the antismoking message. *American lung association bulletin* 67:7, 11, 1981.

Splitter, S.: Nonsmokers (involuntary smokers): the silent majority. *Heart briefs,* American Heart Association, Winter, 1976.

Vachon, L.: The smoke in marijuana smoking. *New England journal of medicine,* 294:3, 160–161, 1976.

Ziskind, M.: *Clinical symposia-occupational pulmonary disease.* New Jersey, Ciba Pharmaceutical Co., 1978.

Pulmonary Pharmacology

11

Main Objectives

1. **Identify the seven question categories that serve as guides for pharmacologic assessment.**
2. **State four goals of pulmonary drug intervention.**
3. **Describe the pharmacology of bronchodilators and how different agents act at different sites to increase cellular levels of cyclic adenosine monophosphate (cAMP).**
4. **Describe clinical uses for the following drug groups: adrenergic sympathomimetics, anticholingergics, methylxanthines, corticosteroids, cromolyn sodium, decongestants, antihistamines, antitussive agents, respiratory stimulants, mucokinetic agents, and antibiotics.**
5. **Explain why bronchodilators are crucial to the management of obstructive disease.**
6. **For adrenergic sympathomimetics, explain how to anticipate drug action, bronchodilator effectiveness, and possible side effects by noting the degree of alpha-, beta 1–, and beta 2–receptor activities.**
7. **For methylxanthines, anticipate drug effectiveness by calculating the daily anhydrous theophylline dosage and interpreting the blood theophylline level.**
8. **Describe the physiology of the hypothalamic-pituitary-adrenal axis. Explain the rationale for**

daily corticosteroids at 8:00 am, alternate day steroids, and use of inhaled steroids.

9. **Given a pulmonary patient's medication list, do the following:**
   a. **Classify by drug group.**
   b. **Identify common over-the-counter pulmonary drugs.**
   c. **State the possible rationale for the use of each drug.**
   d. **Anticipate drug effectiveness, side effects, and possible adverse reactions.**

This chapter discusses pulmonary medications in relation to pharmacologic assessment. Emphasis is placed on bronchodilators, though decongestants, antihistamines, mucokinetic agents, and other drugs are reviewed. The case study at the end of the chapter is designed to help implement pharmacologic assessment, before the nurse even approaches the patient for the history and physical examination. Once pharmacologic assessment is refined, intervention naturally follows in a more efficient and effective way.

Pharmacologic Assessment in The Clinical Setting

Drug regimens for pulmonary patients range from long lists of different types of pulmonary medications to an occasional over-the-counter "cold remedy." Whatever the case may be, pharmacologic assessment involves reviewing the medical chart, interviewing the patient, and consulting the physician, if necessary, to answer the pharmacologic assessment questions provided in Table 11–1.

The clinical setting determines how these questions are asked by the nurse and answered by the patient. For example, in ambulatory and home settings, pharmacologic assessment is part of history taking (see Chapter 10). Questions may be asked and answered in a straightforward fashion. Information obtained is usually sufficient for problem identification. However, other information, such as chest assessment findings, pulmonary function tests, financial status, family support systems, and health beliefs, may be necessary to refine assessment and plan pharmacologic intervention.

In an acute case, the patient may be too short of breath to answer questions. A few crucial ones about preadmission medications must suffice, until the patient's condition improves and he can supply more details about medications used at home and possible compliance problems.

In the critical care setting, the nurse may interview family or friends, when the patient is comatose, intubated, and unable to communicate. In life-threatening situations, pharmacologic assessment focuses *first* on monitoring for drug effectiveness. Objective parameters, such as the chest examination and chest x-ray findings are relied upon to answer basic pharmacology-related questions and identify problems. Once the patient's condition stabilizes, the nurse returns to history taking to determine exactly what events precipitated the acute exacerbation and what interventions are needed to prevent reoccurrence.

The remainder of the chapter presents basic principles of pulmonary pharmacology so that the nurse can ask more specific questions in each of the categories listed in Table 11–1. Issues related to patient compliance are reviewed in Chapter 16 in relation to patient motivation.

Table 11–1. PHARMACOLOGIC ASSESSMENT QUESTIONS

Question Category	Questions
Type of drug	What is the rationale for use of the drug? Which problem is it intended to treat, e.g., infection, bronchoconstriction, mucus retention, or alveolar hypoventilation? Is the drug for prophylaxis or treatment of chest disease? Has the individual self prescribed any over-the-counter drugs?
Dosage	Is the dosage appropriate? Too much? Too little?
Administration	Is the mode of administration appropriate, e.g., intravenous, oral, rectal, aerosol via inhaler, handheld nebulizer, or IPPB? Are dosages and administration times arranged for maximum therapeutic response with little to no side effects?
Side effects	Are side effects present? If so, have they been minimized to a tolerable level?
Proper use of PRN drugs	Does the patient use PRN drugs appropriately to successfully prevent or control disease exacerbations?
Patient knowledge of drugs	Does the patient have a basic and accurate knowledge base regarding his drugs, e.g., drug name, purpose, dosage, and side effects?
Patient compliance	Are there any discrepancies between drugs and dosages prescribed in the medical chart and those actually taken by the patient?

Goals of Drug Intervention

The four goals of pulmonary drug intervention are presented in the box.

> *PHARMACOLOGIC GOALS*
>
> 1. Relief of bronchoconstriction and promotion of bronchodilatation
> 2. Improvement of mucociliary transport and removal of secretions from the lungs
> 3. Improvement in alveolar ventilation and oxygenation
> 4. Promotion of a normal breathing pattern

These goals are of varying importance, depending upon the chest disease and specific respiratory problems involved. In asthma and COPD, the overall goal is to keep chronic airflow limitation (airway obstruction) to a minimum, using the lowest possible drug dosage.

Drug Groups—Clues to Patient Problems

In any clinical situation, involving a list of pulmonary medications, the first step in pharmacologic assessment is categorization by drug group (Table 11–2). Drug group is the clue to the existence of a respiratory problem. For example, the patient on a bronchodilator probably has a bronchoconstrictive problem and possibly a mucus retention problem and chest infection. The patient taking an antitussive agent may have an uncontrollable cough from postnasal drip or from a chest condition, such as asthma. The patient on a respiratory stimulant may be hypoventilating, if the drug is ineffective, or hyperventilating, if the drug produces excessive respiratory stimulation.

Bronchodilators

Bronchodilators are the most frequently prescribed medications in pulmonary disease. They are used for relief of bronchospasm (bronchoconstriction) and chronic airflow limitation.

IMPORTANCE

Knowledge of bronchodilators is important because bronchoconstriction or bronchospasm is a problem of top priority in respiratory care. Unless bronchodilators open constricted airways, alveolar hypoventilation in peripheral lung regions will lead to mucus accumulation and retention. In this situation, intensive bronchial hygiene measures, including coughing, deep breathing, and postural drainage, will never completely drain peripheral lung regions, unless bronchodilators are given to keep airways open, thus allowing mucus to be expectorated or drained out of the lungs.

Furthermore, knowledge of bronchodilators must be extensive because of the numerous types of available drugs, the confusion among health professionals over which drugs to use, and the complexities of monitoring patients. Because the clinical use of bronchodilators is largely dictated by the physician's experience, the nurse may encounter patients who have the same diagnosis and the same extent of disease, but who are on different bronchodilator medications. Some of these various drug regimens may be appropriate, since there is more than one way to effect bronchodilatation. However, others may be inappropriate and may lead to inadequate bronchodilatation and disease exacerbation.

The confusion over the appropriate use of bronchodilators has been compounded by the proliferation of a variety of drug preparations (e.g., sustained release and sprinkles), the inconsistent manufacturer's guidelines, and the absence of meaningful regulation by the appropriate governmental agencies (Hendeles and Weinberger, 1983). Many effective adrenergic sympathomimetic and anticholinergic bronchodilators (defined subsequently) have been used for years outside the United States, and many of these drugs are still not available here. If available, they have not been formally approved by the Food and Drug Administration (FDA).

The clinical use of bronchodilators is an important, complex, and changing topic. Keeping up-to-date information on the main agents is essential to the rapid assimilation of new therapies into clinical practice. The use of new agents, such as the anticholinergics, may spare the patient unresponsive to standard bronchodilators the feeling of hopelessness and the suffering associated with chronic pulmonary disease.

MAIN TYPES

The main types of medications promoting bronchodilatation are listed in the box.

> *MEDICATIONS PROMOTING BRONCHODILATATION*
>
> Autonomic active
> - Adrenergic sympathomimetics (e.g., epinephrine and isoetharine)
> - Anticholinergics (e.g., atropine)
>
> Methylxanthines (e.g., theophylline)
> Corticosteroids
> Cromolyn sodium

Table 11–2. PULMONARY DRUG GROUPS AND ASSOCIATED PATIENT PROBLEMS

Drug Groups	Possible Problems	Key Questions
Bronchodilators	Bronchoconstriction Bronchospasm Mucus retention Chest infection	Is bronchoconstriction accompanied by mucus retention and a chest infection?
Antitussive agents	Airway irritation Postnasal drip Mucus retention Bronchospasm	What is stimulating the coughing—a minor upper respiratory tract problem or major pulmonary problem?
Respiratory stimulants	Alveolar hyperventilation Alveolar hypoventilation Ventilatory failure Hypoxemia Acidosis Mucus retention	Have samples for arterial blood gas analysis been drawn to help assess ventilation and oxygenation?
Respiratory depressants	Ventilatory failure Hypoxemia Acidosis Mucus retention	Are signs of ventilatory failure, hypoxemia and acidosis, present?
Mucokinetic agents	Mucus retention Excessive mucus production Airway irritation Bronchospasm	Is the agent facilitating secretion hydration and removal—or is it causing airway irritation, excessive mucus production, and other problems?
Antibiotics	Chest infection	Are signs of a chest infection present, e.g., fever, yellow mucus, and change in sputum?
Over-the-counter drugs	Nasal congestion Rhinitis, sinusitis, watery and itchy eyes Cough Headache Fever and muscular aches Bronchoconstriction Mucus retention Inability to control dyspnea	Why is the patient taking the drug—for hay fever, a minor cold ailment, or major uncontrolled pulmonary problem?
Paralyzing agents	Increased work of breathing Excessive tissue oxygen demands Breathing asynchrony (with ventilator) Uncontrollable combativeness Upper airway obstruction (pre-endotracheal intubation) Increased intracranial pressure (neuromuscular disorder) Respiratory muscle weakness or atrophy Situational anxiety and helplessness	Is the need for paralysis still present—or can it be discontinued and more conservative measures be taken to control the patient?

The three main bronchodilator groups include the (1) *adrenergic sympathomimetics* (e.g., epinephrine), (2) *anticholinergics* (e.g., atropine), and (3) *methylxanthines* (e.g., aminophylline). The first two groups—adrenergic sympathomimetics and anticholinergics—are classified as autonomic active drugs (see box), because they act on the autonomic nervous system.

Corticosteroids are anti-inflammatory drugs with bronchodilating effects. They are used in treatment of severe chronic disease and life-threatening acute disease.

Cromolyn sodium is a prophylactic anti-asthma drug, with a possible slight bronchodilating effect.

PHARMACOLOGY

The pharmacologic actions of bronchodilators are best understood by first reviewing the mechanisms of bronchoconstriction (see Chapter 7, especially Fig. 7–8 on page 104).

Bronchoconstriction and Sites of Drug Intervention

In Figure 7–8, the shaded boxes represent the main sites of drug intervention. Some of these drugs act directly to inhibit bronchoconstriction and promote bronchodilatation. For example, the anticholinergic drug, atropine, directly blocks the action of acetylcholine, a substance that indirectly (reflexly) causes bronchospasm. Other drugs also act indirectly, e.g., the adrenergic sympathomimetics counteract the effects of mediator release on bronchial muscle. Action appears directed more towards muscle cells rather than the mast cells and basophils that released the mediators in the first place. The exact mechanism is incompletely understood, but the antimediator action is thought to hinder the further release of histamine and other mediators, thereby preventing chemical events leading to bronchospasm.

Biochemical Reactions Controlling Bronchomotor Tone

The main bronchodilators—adrenergic sympathomimetics, methylxanthines, and anticholinergics—act by influencing the biochemical reactions that control bronchomotor tone.

Normal bronchomotor tone is largely determined by the balance of two chemical substances in the body, namely, cyclic 3′, 5′ adenosine monophosphate (cAMP) and cyclic 3′, 3′ guanosine monophosphate (cGMP). These two substances are structurally similar, but they act through different enzyme systems and produce opposite effects, as diagrammed in Figure 11–1. Currently, the cAMP system is considered more powerful and more important in drug intervention, partly because there appears to be more cAMP than cGMP in normal muscle cells.

Pharmacologic Goal. The goals of bronchodilator therapy are as follows:

1. To increase cellular levels of cAMP.
2. To decrease cellular levels of cGMP.

Increasing cAMP may be considered the main goal, since cAMP dominance means that less cGMP is available to constrict airways. Bronchodilators act at different sites within the two cyclic systems to reverse bronchospasm.

Bronchodilatation by the Adrenergic Sympathomimetics

The adrenergic sympathomimetics (beta 2–adrenergics) increase cAMP by stimulating beta 2–adrenergic receptors.

The beta 2–receptors are located on the cell surfaces of mast cells next to muscle fibers. These are the sites of the enzyme *adenylate cyclase* (formerly, *adenyl cyclase*). In the presence of magnesium, receptor stimulation activates this enzyme. Activation prompts two reactions:

1. Sequestration of calcium either intracellularly or extracellularly, which in turn decreases calcium availability to muscle cells. Low levels of calcium are associated with increased bronchomotor tone (Leff, 1982).
2. Catalysis of the conversion of intracellular *adenosine triphosphate* (ATP) into cyclic AMP.

The increase in cyclic AMP promotes bronchodilatation, as shown in Figure 11–1. In this chain of events, the enzyme adenylate cyclase plays a central role, but electrolytes and other incompletely understood factors are also important because they modify the contractile response (Shenfield, 1982).

Bronchospasm by Beta Blockers. Beta blockers, such as the cardiac drugs *propranolol* and *atenolol*, block both beta 1– and beta 2–receptor activities. The blocking of beta 2 stimulation decreases cAMP and induces bronchospasm in persons with preexisting chronic lung disease (see Fig. 11–1). This action does not occur in those with normal lungs. Beta blockers are contraindicated in pulmonary patients, but they may be used inadvertently in cardiac patients with undiagnosed chronic lung disease.

Bronchodilatation by Methylxanthines

The methylxanthines bronchodilators (e.g., aminophylline) increase cAMP by inhibiting its metabolic breakdown.

Normal levels of cAMP in the body are maintained by a balance between metabolic production and breakdown. An intracellular enzyme *phosphodiesterase* breaks down cAMP to produce the inactive nucleotide, 5′ adenosine monophosphate (5′AMP). Inhibition of this enzyme's action by *phosphodiesterase inhibitors*, such as the methylxanthines, will slow the breakdown of cAMP, allow it to accumulate intracellularly, and thereby promote bronchodilatation.

Bronchodilatation by the Anticholinergics (Antimuscarinics)

The anticholinergics block bronchoconstriction caused by increased levels of cGMP, as shown in Figure 11–1. The sympathetic nervous system (the cAMP enzyme system) is allowed to dominate the parasympathetic nervous system (cGMP enzyme system). In the illustration, note that when the parasympathetic system dominates, strong cholinergic stimulation results in increased levels of the neurotransmitter *acetylcholine*. Acetylcholine in turn stimulates the cell wall enzyme *guanyl cyclase*, and the increase in cGMP causes bronchoconstriction.

Implications for Clinical Practice

In the clinical setting, most patients who have asthma or an asthmatic component to mixed chest pathology receive bronchodilators. Mild or acute intermittent asthma may be reversed with adrenergic

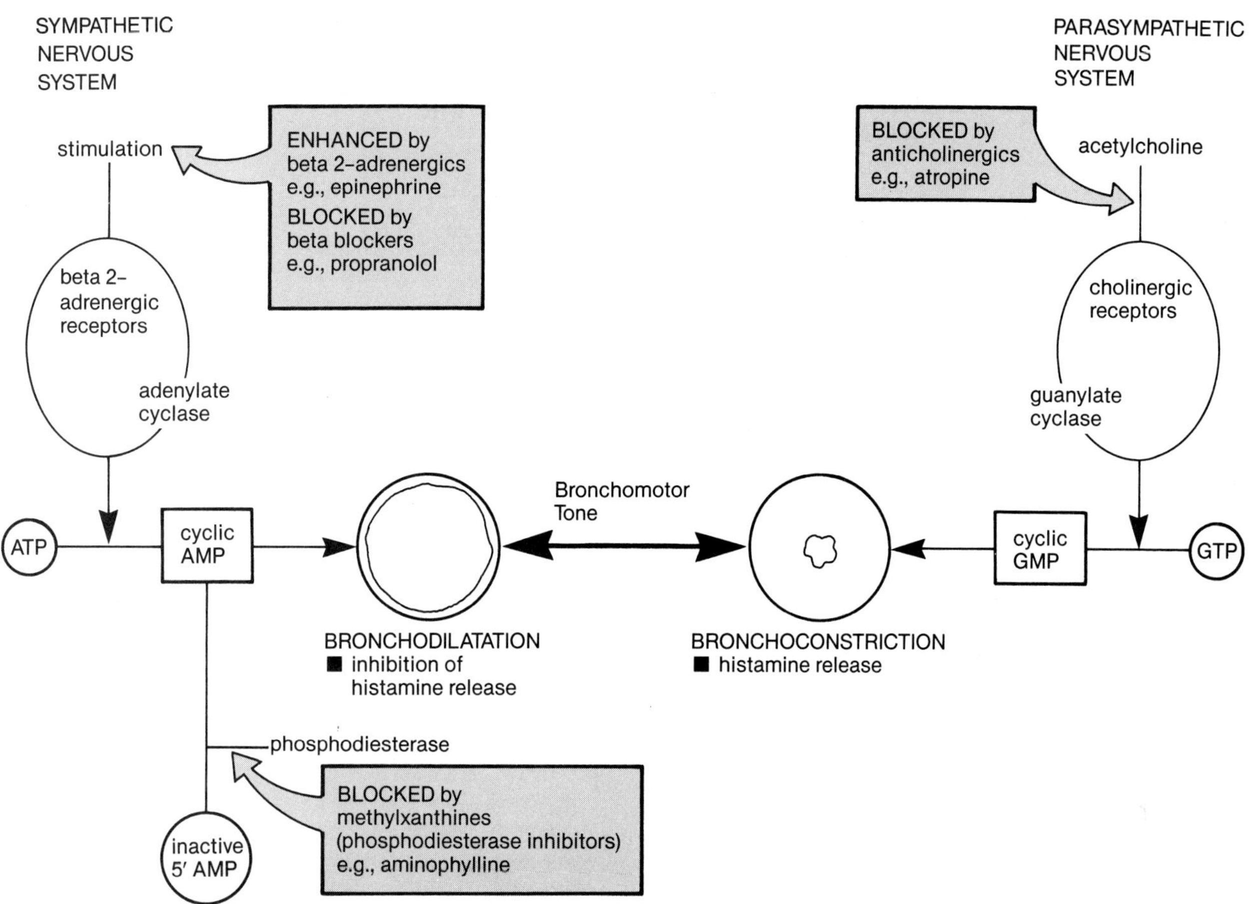

Figure 11–1. Pharmacological control of bronchial muscle tone—the classic view. The balance between the sympathetic nervous system (cyclic AMP system) and parasympathetic nervous system (cyclic GMP system) largely determines bronchomotor tone. Also, it influences the release of histamine and other mediators. ATP = adenosine triphosphate; AMP = adenosine monophosphate; GMP = guanosine monophosphate; GTP = guanosine triphosphate. (Adapted from Shenfield, G.: Combination bronchodilator therapy. *Drugs*, 24(5):414–439, 1982.)

sympathomimetics alone (Fig. 11–2). When bronchospasm persists, a methylxanthine (e.g., theophylline) or an oral beta 2–drug is added to further increase cAMP (see Fig. 11–2). In severe COPD, corticosteroids and drugs from all bronchodilator groups are used to act at different sites within the cAMP and cGMP systems. In a very few select cases, other drugs (not elaborated here) may be used, e.g., anti-mediator drugs and alpha-adrenergic blockers.

Clearly, the rationale for combination bronchodilator therapy pertains to the many pharmacologic routes by which bronchodilatation can be achieved. Moreover, the bronchodilating effect of different drug combinations is usually additive and sometimes synergistic (i.e., combined effect exceeds the sum of individual effects). In this manner, maximal bronchodilatation may be achieved without the toxic side effects that accompany high dose, single drug therapy.

ADRENERGIC SYMPATHOMIMETICS

The adrenergic sympathomimetics are referred to as sympathomimetics because their effects mimic the effects of the sympathetic nervous system.

The sympathetic nervous system produces bronchodilatation by stimulation of adrenergic nerves and release of norepinephrine or epinephrine at various receptor sites. The adrenergic or so-called flight-or-fight sympathetic response includes relaxation of the bronchi, the desired response from sympathomimetic drugs. It also includes other responses (listed in the box Sympathetic Response).

SYMPATHETIC RESPONSE

Relaxation of bronchi
Pupil dilatation
Increased heart rate
Increased blood pressure
Decreased gastric motility
Skin pallor

The sympathetic response is mediated via three types of receptors in the body (see the box Adrenergic Receptors).

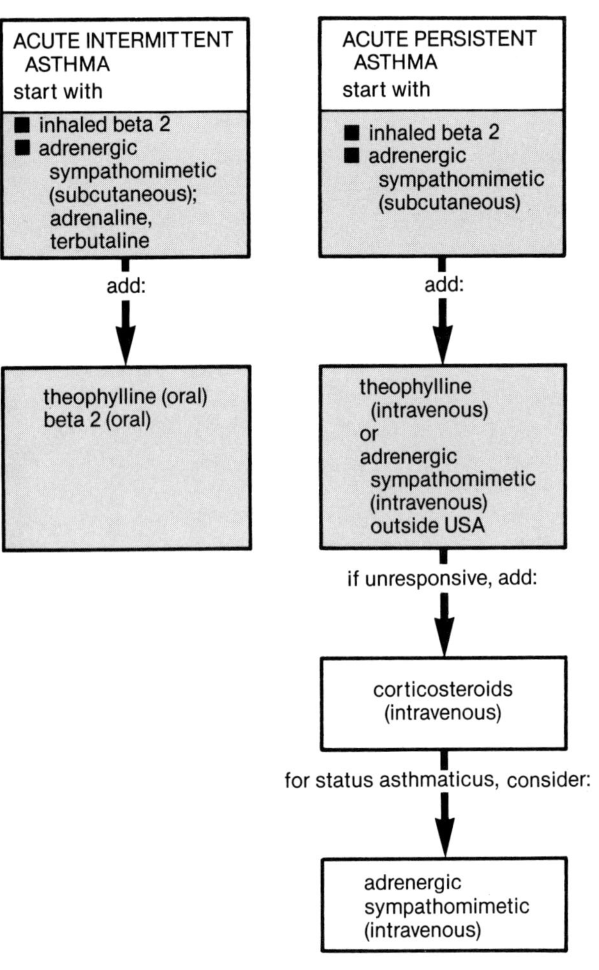

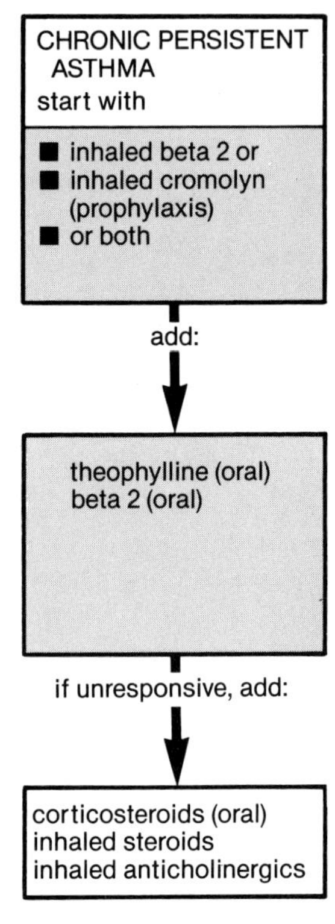

Figure 11–2. Combination bronchodilator therapy in asthma. If primary drugs (gray boxes) do not reverse bronchospasm, the clinician resorts to secondary drugs (white boxes).

ADRENERGIC RECEPTORS

1. Alpha receptors
2. Beta 1–receptors
3. Beta 2–receptors

Each type of receptor is selective in activity and produces specific effects as summarized in Table 11–3.

Adrenergic drugs stimulate the three types of adrenergic receptors to varying degrees, as noted by the relative potencies given in Table 11–4. The potency of receptor site stimulation determines the favorable and unintended effects of the numerous adrenergic drugs on the market.

The actions and clinical uses of adrenergic bronchodilators administered for acute bronchospasm are presented in Table 11–5, for quick reference. Because this list is long and changes with the addition of new agents, the best introduction to adrenergic agents must be based on knowledge of receptor site activity. When a new or unfamiliar drug is encountered, the nurse can knowledgeably verify it in an appropriate information resource, note the receptors stimulated (e.g., alpha, beta 1, and beta 2), and anticipate bronchodilator effectiveness, possible side effects, and implications for monitoring the patient.

In the following discussion of adrenergic drugs and their adrenergic receptor stimulation, keep in mind that *the "best" adrenergic bronchodilators selectively stimulate beta 2–receptors along the tracheobronchial tree.*

Drugs with Alpha Receptor Activity

Adrenergic drugs that stimulate primarily alpha receptors are called *alpha-adrenergic sympathomimetics.*

Alpha receptors are located mainly in peripheral smooth muscle (Table 11–3). However, stimulation of other receptors in mucosal blood vessels causes respiratory *decongestion*, the relief of mucosal edema along upper and lower respiratory tracts. More specifically, muscular contraction of arterioles and small arteries

Table 11–3. EFFECTS OF ADRENERGIC RECEPTOR STIMULATION*

Receptor	Receptor Sites (limited list)†	Effects of Receptor Stimulation	Related Clinical Side Effects
Alpha	Peripheral smooth muscle†	Vasoconstriction (vasopressor effect)	Hypertension
	Bronchial smooth muscle	Mild bronchoconstriction	Signs of increased airway obstruction
	Cardiac muscle	Small increase in rate and force of contraction	Tachycardia
	Mucosal blood vessels	Contraction of bronchial blood vessels (decongestant effect)	Rebound congestion with repeated dosages
Beta 1	Cardiac muscle†	Increase in rate and force of contraction	Tachycardia and other arrhythmias
	Mucosal blood vessels	Dilation of bronchial blood vessels	Increased airway obstruction Decreased Pa_{O_2}
Beta 2	Bronchial smooth muscle†	Bronchodilatation Improved mucociliary transport	—
	Peripheral smooth muscle	Vasodilatation	Slight hypotension, reflex tachycardia, decreased Pa_{O_2}
	Skeletal muscle	Decreased duration of skeletal muscle fiber contraction	Muscle tremor
	Central nervous system (indirect)	Stimulation	Nervousness, anxiety, insomnia
	Uterus	Relaxation	Inhibition of uterine contractions
	Other: glycogenolysis and glycolysis biochemical processes	Stimulation	Aggravation of diabetes mellitus and ketoacidosis

*Date from Ahrens, R. and Smith, G.: Albeterol: an adrenergic agent for use in the treatment of asthma pharmacology, pharmacokinetics and clinical use. *Pharmacotherapy*, 4(3):105–120, 1984.
†Main site.

Table 11–4. ADRENERGIC SYMPATHOMIMETICS: ACTIONS AND ADMINISTRATION ROUTES*

	Relative Potencies of Receptor Site Stimulation†				Administration Routes			
Agent	alpha	beta 1	beta 2	Duration of Action‡	SQ/IV	Oral	Metered Inhaler	Nebulizer
Epinephrine (Adrenalin, Suprarenin)	+ + +	+ + + +	+ + +	Short	×		×	×
Racemic epinephrine (Micronefrin, Vaponefrin)	+ +(+)	+ + +(+)	+ +(+)	Short			×	×
Ephedrine	+ +	+ + +	+ + +	Long		×		
Isoproterenol (Isuprel)	(+)	+ + + +	+ + + +	Short	(×)	(×)	×	×
Isoetharine (Bronkosol, Bronkometer)	—	+(+)	+ + +	Medium	0	0	×	×
Metaproterenol (Alupent, Metaprel)	—	+ +(+)	+ +(+)	Medium-long		×	×	×
Terbutaline (Brethine, Bricanyl)	—	+(+)	+ + +(+)	Long	×	×	×	0
Albuterol (Salbutamol, Proventil, Ventolin)	—	+(+)	+ + + +	Long	0	×	×	×
Fenoterol (pending FDA approval, Berotec)	—	+(+)	+ + + +	Long		0	0	0
Bitolterol (Tornalate)	—	+(+)	+ + + +	Long			×	

*Adapted from Ziment, I.: Respiratory Pharmacology and Therapeutics. Philadelphia, W. B. Saunders Co., 1978.
†+ = one unit of relative potency
(+) = one unit of possible relative potency
— = no clinical effect
‡Varies in different subjects or in same subject at different times in the illness; therefore, comparisons are only approximate.
§× = FDA approved; (×) = rarely used or unreliable; 0 = available in other countries.

Table 11–5. ADRENERGIC SYMPATHOMIMETIC BRONCHODILATORS FOR ACUTE BRONCHOSPASM

Drug*	Dosage‡	Onset of Action	Peak Action	Duration of Action	Special Uses	Monitoring Considerations
Epinephrine (Adrenalin)						
Subcutaneous epinephrine HCl, 1:1000 solution	0.1 to 0.5 ml. Repeat in 30 minutes to maximum of 1.0 ml q4 to 6 h. (Sus-Phrine 0.1 to 0.3 ml q6h.)	5 min	30 min or more	1 to 2 h	Asthmatic attack Anaphylactic reaction	Other bronchodilators are needed if unresponsive after two or three injections. Less effective in the presence of acidosis. May increase the viscosity of mucus plugs (Webb-Johnson and Andrews, 1977). *Side effects*: tachycardia, arrhythmias, palpitations, hypertension, tremors, nausea, headache, sweating, pallor, hypokalemia. *Caution* with coronary artery disease, hypertension, arrhythmias, cerebrovascular disease, hyperthyroidism, diabetes, glaucoma, prostatic hypertrophy, and patients susceptible to hypokalemia. *Contraindicated* in patients on antihypertensive or antidepressant drugs with monoamine oxidase inhibitors.
Nebulized racemic epinephrine HCl 2.25% solution†:	0.3 to 1.0 ml in normal saline q2 to 4h.	1 to 5 min	5 to 15 min	1 to 3 h	Laryngotracheo-bronchitis (for alpha effects) Postendotracheal tube extubation	*Side effects*: same as above.
Vaponefrin, Micronefrin, Solution A, Asthmanefrin 0.25 and 0.5% solution†: **Adrenalin, Asthmolin**						
Inhaler epinephrine bitartrate suspension	1 to 2 puffs q4 to 6 h. Maximum of 12 puffs per day.	1 to 5 min	5 to 15 min	1 to 3 h	Quick relief from asthmatic attack: however, use of a more selective beta 2–adrenergic is preferable, e.g., isoetharine.	In emergency, no more than 6 puffs over 1 h. *Side effects*: same as above. Watch for arrhythmias in particular.
Medihaler-Epi (Riker), 0.16 mg/puff† Other preparations†: **Primatene Mist, Bronitin Mist, Asthmahaler**						
Terbutaline						
Subcutaneous terbutaline sulfate, 1.0 mg/ml solution **Brethine** (Geigy), **Bricanyl** (Merrell Dow)	0.25 ml. Repeat in 15 to 30 min to maximum of 0.5 ml q4h.	5 to 15 min	30 to 60 min	2 to 4 h	Asthmatic attack—more powerful than subcutaneous epinephrine, but more side effects may be experienced.	*Side effects*: same as for subcutaneous epinephrine.

Table continued on opposite page

Table 11–5. ADRENERGIC SYMPATHOMIMETIC BRONCHODILATORS FOR ACUTE BRONCHOSPASM *Continued*

Drug*	Dosage‡	Onset of Action	Peak Action	Duration of Action	Special Uses	Monitoring Considerations
Nebulized unavailable—injection solution substituted	1.0 to 2.0 ml in normal saline q2 to 4 h.	5 to 30 min	2 h	4 to 6 h		Side effects are few and usually mild. Tachycardia, hypertension, arrhythmias, tremor, insomnia, and CNS stimulation may occur.
Inhaler **Brethaire** (Geigy), 0.20 mg/puff	1 to 2 puffs q4 to 6h.	5 to 30 min	2 h	4 to 6 h		Same as above.
Isoproterenol						
Nebulized						
Isuprel 1:200 solution and 1:100 solution	0.25 to 0.50 (up to 1.0) ml in 2 ml normal saline: q4 to 6 h. If refractory, use 1:100 solution: 0.10 to 0.50 in 2 ml normal saline.	2 to 5 min	5 to 30 min	2 h	Asthmatic attack in persons without cardiovascular problems	*Side effects*: palpitations, nervousness, and tachycardia are common; nausea, vomiting, arrhythmias, chest pain, dizziness, flushing of skin. Watch for tachyphylaxis and excessive cardiac stimulation in particular.
Inhaler **Isuprel Mistometer** (Winthrop-Breon), 0.131 mg/puff **Medihaler-Iso** (Riker), 0.08 mg/puff	1 to 3 puffs q4 to 6 h.	2 to 5 min	5 to 30 min	2 h		One puff is equivalent in effectiveness to 5 to 7 nebulized breaths of 1:100 solution. Throat irritation may occur from alcohol content in inhaler. In emergency, no more than 6 puffs over 1 hour.
Intravenous **Isuprel** 1:5000 solution and 0.2 mg/ml	0.03 to 0.2 mcg/kg/min. Mix 1 to 2 mg in 250 ml 5% dextrose.	Immediate	—	Lasts as long as infusion continues.	Status asthmaticus refractory to other measures. Bronchospasm during anesthesia (initial dose 0.01 to 0.02 mg; may be repeated.)	*Side effects*: same (as above). Initial side effects of flushing of face, mild tremor, tachycardia, palpitations, headache may disappear. Titrate dosage to relieve airway obstruction, without increasing heart rate over 110–120 beats/minute, causing arrhythmias, decreasing blood pressure, or adversely affecting other hemodynamic parameters.
Isoetharine						
Nebulized						
Isoetharine HCl **Bronkosol** (Winthrop Breon), 1% solution	0.25 to 1.0 ml in 2 to 3 ml normal saline q3 to 6h.	Within 5 min	15 to 60 min	2 to 3 h	Less potent and has fewer cardiac side effects than isoproterenol. Shorter acting compared with metaproterenol. Watch for tachyphylaxis and excessive cardiac stimulation with ql to 2h treatments.	*Side effects*: tachycardia, arrhythmias, palpitations, tremor, nausea, headache, dizziness, and changes in blood pressure.
Inhaler Isoetharine mesylate, 0.61 %	1 to 2 puffs q3 to 6h.	Within 5 min	15 to 60 min	2 to 3 h		Same as above.

Table continued on following page

Table 11–5. ADRENERGIC SYMPATHOMIMETIC BRONCHODILATORS FOR ACUTE BRONCHOSPASM *Continued*

Drug*	Dosage‡	Onset of Action	Peak Action	Duration of Action	Special Uses	Monitoring Considerations
Bronkometer (Breon), 0.34 mg/puff	Maximum of 12 puffs per day.					
Metaproterenol *Nebulized* **Alupent** (Boehringer Ingelheim), 5% solution	0.2 to 0.3 ml in 2 ml normal saline q3 to 6 h. Unit dose vial equivalent to 0.3 ml Alupent in 2.2 ml normal saline.	Within 5 to 10 min	30 to 90 min	4 h	The unit dose vials are without metabisulfites. Though they are more expensive than nebulizer solution in a bottle, they may eliminate problems related to measuring medication.	*Side effects*: same as for isoetharine.
Inhaler **Alupent** (Boehringer Ingelheim) 0.65 mg/puff	2 to 3 puffs q3 to 6h.	Within 5 to 10 min	30 to 90 min	4 h		Same as for isoetharine.
Albuterol (Salbutamol) *Inhaler* **Ventolin** (Glaxo),§ **Proventil** (Schering), 0.90 mg/puff‖	2 puffs q4 to 6 h.	Within 15 min	60 to 90 min	4 to 6 h	A preferred beta 2–adrenergic for ambulatory use; may be more efficacious, produce fewer side effects than theophylline or alternative drugs, or both (Ahrens and Smith, 1984).	*Side effects*: same as for isoetharine; usually limited to mild tachycardia and transient tremor.
Bitolterol *Inhaler* **Tornalate** (Winthrop-Breon), 0.37 mg/puff	2 puffs q4 to 6h or 3 puffs q6h.	Within 15 min	60 to 90 min	5 to 8 h	May have a longer duration of action compared to albuterol. May permit q 8 hour dosing for asthma prophylaxis.	*Side-effects*: transient tremor, mild tachycardia, palpitations, nausea, throat irritation, and cough.

*Brand name (**bold faced**): manufacturer in parentheses.

†Nonprescription drug.

‡Dosages represent typical clinical ranges. Inhaler dosages may be gradually increased to 16 to 24 puffs per day in patients who are not on oral beta adrenergic agents (American Thoracic Society, 1987).

§A sulfite-free, 0.5% Ventolin solution is now available for nebulization. Manufacturer-recommended dosage is 2.5 mg albuterol (0.5 ml in 2.5 ml NS) TID or QID.

‖0.5% Proventil solution in both multidose and unit-dose vials is now available for nebulization. Dosage is 2.5 mg albuterol (0.5 ml in 3 ml NS or one 3 ml unit-dose vial) TID or QID.

decreases blood flow to affected areas. The reduced capillary hydrostatic pressure prevents fluid from moving into tissues and thereby causing nasal passage or airway edema.

Because of their selective alpha receptor stimulation, decongestants are not classified as bronchodilators, though they produce a bronchodilating effect. They are most commonly administered for upper respiratory tract decongestion (see Decongestants and Antihistamines).

In pulmonary disease, decongestants are used for lung decongestion only in combination with a beta 2–drug. For example, the alpha stimulator *phenylephrine* is added to isoproterenol in an inhaler called *Duo-Medihaler*. Here, phenylephrine prolongs isoproterenol's beta 2 bronchodilating effect and counteracts its beta 1 bronchial vasodilating effect.

However, in past years, the value of adding an alpha stimulator to beta 2–drugs has been questioned. Alpha stimulation may worsen airway edema. Some alpha receptors are located on the venous side of the pulmonary circulation. Stimulation can cause excessive venoconstriction, increased capillary pressure, leakage of fluid into tissues, and airway edema (Paterson et al, 1979).

Stimulation of alpha receptors is associated with side effects shown in Table 11–3, including hypertension, tachycardia, and a phenomenon called *rebound congestion*. Rebound congestion is the return and worsening of mucosal edema, after repeated drug administrations. One postulate is that this type of congestion is caused by the dominance of the beta-receptor vasodilating effect, after short-lived, alpha-receptor stimulation. Overuse of prescription and over-the-counter topical decongestants, especially nasal sprays, is likely to cause this phenomenon. Drug discontinuation may be necessary to reverse the worsening of upper respiratory tract symptoms.

Drugs with Beta 1–Receptor Activity

Beta 1–receptors are located mainly in the heart. Adrenergic bronchodilators stimulating these receptors are likely to produce the unwanted cardiac side effects of tachycardia and other arrhythmias. Hence, clinicians either avoid or prescribe judiciously drugs such as epinephrine and isoproterenol (Isuprel) because repeated administrations stimulate intense beta 1 activity, particularly in the patient with a history of cardiac problems.

Drugs with beta 1 activity have the potential of increasing airway obstruction. Stimulation of beta 1–receptors in mucosal blood vessels may cause bronchial vasodilatation. The vasodilatation in turn increases capillary hydrostatic pressures in the lungs, promotes leakage of fluid into tissues, and worsens airway edema. This process is more likely when cardiac stimulation greatly increases the cardiac output to the lungs and the capillary hydrostatic pressure, pushing fluid into tissues. As in other types of bronchodilators, such as atropine and aminophylline, PaO_2 may drop significantly, as excessive perfusion to underventilated alveoli causes a reduced V/Q ratio.

Drugs with Beta 2–Receptor Activity

Beta 2–receptors are located mainly in bronchial smooth muscle. Their stimulation produces the desired effects of *bronchodilatation* and possibly *increased mucokinesis.*

The best adrenergic sympathomimetic bronchodilator is one with the *most* beta 2 activity and the *least* alpha and beta 1 activity. Note in Table 11–4 that most of the short-acting and medium-acting adrenergics have significant beta 1 activity, symbolizing beta 1 side effects. The longer-acting drugs, such as metaproterenol, terbutaline, albuterol, and fenoteral, have stronger beta 2 effects with weak beta 1 side effects.

Currently, isoetharine hydrochloride (Bronkosol) and metaproterenol (Alupent) are commonly used nebulized drugs for control of acute bronchospasm (Fig. 11–3). Though both have some effect within 3 to 8 minutes, metaproterenol is often favored because of its longer duration of action. Isoetharine may be more appropriate for acutely ill patients who require frequent (every 1 to 3 hours) aerosol treatments.

Inhaled metered preparations, such as isoetharine mesylate (Bronkometer), metaproterenol (Alupent), albuterol (Ventolin and Proventil), and bitolterol (Tornalate), are all used for the ambulatory patient with bronchoconstriction. They may be given with an aminophylline drug, an oral adrenergic preparation, such as metaproterenol or terbutaline, or with both (Table 11–6). These oral bronchodilators may act on peripheral airways not reached by topical aerosol. In the United States, however, ephedrine and ephedrine combinations are not recommended because central nervous system (CNS) side effects limit the dosage given, resulting in suboptimal dosages and inadequate bronchodilatation.

In addition to bronchodilatation, stimulation of beta 2–receptors may cause adverse side effects (see Table 11–3). For example, stimulation of beta 2–receptors in skeletal muscle is responsible for the tremor seen in patients on oral bronchodilators, particularly terbutaline. The tremor usually decreases after 2 weeks of therapy.

Stimulation of beta 2–receptors in peripheral smooth muscle may cause peripheral vasodilatation, venous pooling, and decreased cardiac output. A subsequent drop in blood pressure may cause reflex tachycardia, particularly when oral doses are given. The reflex

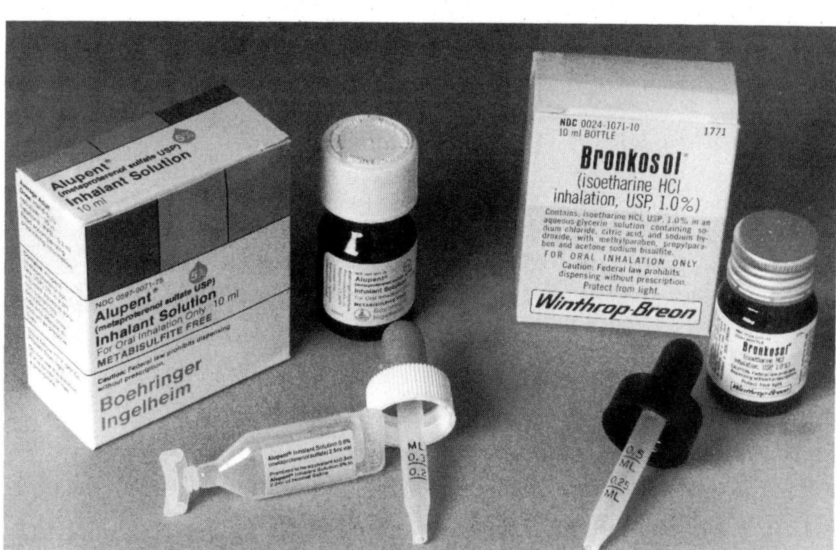

Figure 11–3. Examples of nebulized adrenergic sympathomimetic bronchodilators. **Left:** metaproterenol (Alupent) multidose vial with dropper and unit dose vial. **Right:** isoetharine (Bronkosol) multidose vial with dropper.

Table 11–6. ORAL ADRENERGIC SYMPATHOMIMETICS

Drug	Adult Dosage	Action*	Specific Uses	Monitoring Considerations
Ephedrine (sulfate) TABS, 25 mg, 50 mg	12.5 to 50 mg TID or QID	O, over 1 h P, varies D, 4 h	Used alone or in combination drugs containing theophylline, a tranquilizer, and other agents. Nasal decongestion	Recommended only for bronchodilatation in mild asthma When used for decongestion, watch for excessive CNS stimulation, tachycardia, hypertension, and tachyphylaxis.
Albuteral (Ventolin, Proventil) TABS, 2 mg, 4 mg Syrup, 2 mg/5 ml	2 to 4 mg TID or QID Maximum of 8 mg QID	O, 30 min P, 2 to 3 h D, 4 to 6 h	Added to oral theophylline and inhaled beta 2–agent for additive effect.	Side effects: nervousness, tremor (common), headache, tachycardia, palpitations, muscle cramps, insomnia, nausea, hypertension, anginal pain, and hypokalemia. May inhibit uterine contractions in pregnant women.
Metaproterenol (Alupent) TABS, 10 mg, 20 mg Syrup, 10 mg/5 ml	10 to 20 mg TID or QID	O, 30 min P, 1 to 2 h D, 3 to 5 h	Same as albuterol Preferred oral adrenergic in pediatric patients Dose, 1 teaspoon (under 60 lbs) to 2 teaspoons TID to QID	Watch for nervousness, tachycardia, tremor (common), nausea, hypertension, palpitations, and muscle cramps.
Terbutaline (Brethine, Bricanyl) TABS, 2.5 mg, 5 mg	2.5 to 5.0 mg TID	O, 30 min P, 2 to 3 h D, 4 to 8 h	Same as albuterol	Watch for nervousness, tremor (common), tachycardia, headache, palpitations, nausea, sweating, muscle cramps. Side effects usually improve or disappear after 1 to 2 weeks of therapy.

*Onset (O); Peak (P); Duration (D)

tachycardia in turn may increase pulmonary blood flow, decrease V/Q ratio, and decrease PaO_2, particularly if the drug has accompanying beta 1 activity.

Other adverse effects of beta 1–drugs include the following:

1. *Drug resistance.* The loss of bronchodilating effect with continued drug administration or with worsening disease. In status asthmaticus, resistance necessitates the addition of theophylline and corticosteroid medications.
2. *Drug tolerance* or *tachyphylaxis.* Increasing dosage is necessary to achieve the same degree of bronchodilatation. Some drugs are more likely to cause tachyphylaxis than others, e.g., ephedrine and isoproterenol.
3. *Paradoxical effect.* Isoproterenol and other adrenergics may increase rather than decrease bronchospasm and airflow limitation. However, if this effect does occur, it is extremely rare.

Administration Routes and Delivery Systems

Adrenergic drugs may be given via one or more of the following administration routes: intravenous, subcutaneous, oral, and inhaled. Oral and injected routes produce more adverse side effects than inhaled (aerosol) routes. For example, 20 to 80 times the dose of the same drug must be administered in the oral form to achieve a comparable effect to the aerosolized form (Tobin et al, 1982). The systemic distribution of large doses accounts for the increase in side effects. Side effects are minimized by delivery of a smaller dose of aerosol drug directly into the airway and onto the target organs, the lungs.

Aerosol drugs may be delivered in several different ways (see the box). (These and other delivery systems are discussed in detail in Chapter 18 and Chapter 22.)

COMMON DELIVERY SYSTEMS

Inhaler—a metered dose device (MDD) or metered dose inhaler (MDI).

Hand-held nebulizer—attached to compressed gas source.

Intermittent positive pressure breathing—IPPB device

The efficacy of these delivery systems has been vigorously debated over the past 20 years. Research is in progress to determine the best delivery system and the specific factors responsible for aerosol deposition in the lung periphery rather than in the mouth. Main factors affecting aerosol delivery are mentioned in Table 11–7.

In spite of the large quantity of available research, findings suggest that no one aerosol delivery system is best. Each system has advantages and disadvantages that vary, depending on the clinical situation (Newman, 1983; Stiell and Rivington, 1983; Cherniack and Svanhill, 1976). For example, use of a MDD may be optimal for a young asthmatic patient with a busy work schedule, but highly ineffective for an older asthmatic patient who cannot coordinate the required breathing pattern.

Monitoring Patients on Adrenergic Sympathomimetics

Monitoring patients on adrenergic sympathomimetics involves the assessment of lung sounds, pulmonary function tests (spirometry), arterial blood gases, and other parameters for signs of improvement. Also, it involves observation for adverse side effects. The presence of adverse side effects indicates the need to adjust the patient's medication regimen. Adjustments may include the following: (1) drug discontinuation, (2) change in administration route, (3) decrease in dose, and (4) possibly the addition of another type of bronchodilator.

Side effects may include any of those mentioned in Table 11–5 and Table 11–6.

The interventions in Table 11–8 serve as guides to maximize bronchodilatation by the inhaled route. Keep in mind that although aerosol deposits mostly on large central airways, a number of studies suggest that inhaled bronchodilators can effectively treat obstructions in small airways at all grades of severity (Clark, 1982).

Continuous monitoring of the patient is of utmost importance, considering past experiences with use of adrenergic bronchodilators. In the mid 1960s, a 50% to 300% increase in deaths from asthma occurred in England, Wales, and Australia (Inman and Adelstein, 1969; Campbell, 1966). Several theories were proposed to explain the increase in mortality. Some clinicians postulated that asthmatic patients developed a false sense of security with use of the then nonprescription inhalers, such as isoproterenol, and failed to seek medical care during disease exacerbations. Excessive beta 1 side effects were likely because the nonprescription isoproterenol preparation in the 1960s was about ten times as strong as present day Isuprel, which is now a prescription drug.

Other workers argued that the *Freon propellants* in the inhalers caused cardiac arrhythmia and sudden death in aerosol overusers. Freons are fluorinated hydrocarbons closely related to chloroform and halothane. Subsequently, simulated studies demonstrated

Table 11–7. FACTORS AFFECTING AEROSOL DEPOSITION

Factors	Relative Importance
Particle Size Optimal size is probably between 1 and 5 microns (Newman, 1983). Smaller particles are exhaled before deposition. Larger ones tend to impact in large proximal airways. Particle size is largely determined by the delivery system.	Important
Aerosol qualities Tonicity, density, temperature, and electrostatic charge	Less important
Patient factors Breathing technique, correct use of delivery device, airway patency, variations in airway anatomy, and airway susceptibility of bronchospasm	Most important
Equipment factors Aerosol formulation, complexity of operating and cleaning instructions	Of variable importance

Table 11–8. MAXIMIZING BRONCHODILATATION BY THE INHALED ROUTE

Interventions	Rationale
Work with the patient to optimize administration technique. (See Chapters 18 and 22 for proper breathing technique and evaluation criteria for patient teaching.)	Breathing technique is crucial because only about 10% of each aerosol dose is deposited in the lungs. More specifically, 80% is deposited in the mouth, 10% in the aerosol actuator, 9% in the lungs, and 1% is expired. Moreover, up to 70% of adults use incorrect inhaler techniques (Newman et al, 1981; Sackner and Kim, 1985).
If the patient cannot handle a metered dose device (MDD), try a hand held nebulizer device.	Wet nebulization delivers a much larger dose of drug per treatment (up to 6 to 8 times the MDD dose). Hence, a greater portion of drug may reach the lungs (Paterson et al, 1979).
For nebulization, eliminate extra mechanical dead space from breathing circuits.	Extra tubing between the nebulizer and patient promotes aerosol deposition before the drug reaches the patient.
Be on the alert for patients on over-the-counter (OTC) aerosols, such as *Bronitin Mist*, *Primatene Mist*, and *Medihaler-Epi*. Also, note use of oral OTC adrenergic agents, such as *Bronkaid* tablets.	Ambulatory or patients at home with OTC drugs tend to overuse them and develop cardiac side effects and tachyphylaxis. OTC bronchodilators are more dangerous than prescribed bronchodilators, not only because of their more potent beta 1 side effects but also because patients using them usually lack proper medical and nursing supervision.

Table continued on following page

Table 11–8. MAXIMIZING BRONCHODILATATION BY THE INHALED ROUTE *Continued*

Interventions	Rationale
Respect the patient's need to keep an inhaler at the bedside or in his pocket for PRN use.	Use of the inhaler as a PRN "security blanket" promotes general relaxation and confidence that relief of shortness of breath is readily available. Also, though inhalers have the potential for abuse, proper use promotes patient involvement in activities outside the home.
Notify the physician of any factors that appear to limit aerosol deposition in the lungs. Watch for faulty administration technique, ineffective breathing pattern, excessive fatigue, obstructive secretions, and bronchospasm.	The patient may need more aggressive bronchodilator therapy or a temporary change to nebulization by IPPB instead of MDD or hand held nebulizer.
Notify the physician of patients at home on IPPB or hand held nebulizaton, who lack the knowledge, skill, or resources to properly clean the nebulizer and tubing every 24 hours. (See Chapter 21 for cleaning instructions.)	The device must be discontinued. When equipment is not properly cleaned, the patient is at risk to develop a chest infection from microorganisms growing in water droplets. Instead, a metered inhaler or an oral bronchodilator may be indicated.
Continue to monitor the patient! During monitoring (1) always suspect suboptimal breathing technique until proved otherwise and (2) always suspect tachyphylaxis or drug toxicity in patients using a metered inhaler, who have an elevated or irregular pulse and show little improvement in lung sounds.	Dyspneic patients tend to unknowingly administer either too much or too little drug owing to insufficient patient education, inadequate supervision, and sometimes altered mental status from an acid-base disorder and low PaO_2.

that there is actually little if any hazard from fluorocarbons, if inhalers are used as recommended. A patient would have to take a puff of aerosol on every breath for a sequence of 12 to 24 breaths for Freon to adversely affect the heart (Paterson et al, 1979).

Though controversy still exists about the exact cause of past fatalities with metered inhalers, experts agree on one following point: *inhalers should not be prescribed without patient education and ongoing supervision* (Ahrens and Smith, 1984). A key role of the nurse is to assess inhaler technique, offer suggestions for improvement, and encourage the patient to seek medical attention when pulmonary symptoms become worse or when side effects develop.

ANTICHOLINERGICS

Anticholinergics dilate the bronchi by blocking bronchoconstriction in the cholinergic response (Table 11–9). More specifically, they block the action of the neurotransmitter acetylcholine at the neuromuscular junctions of effector cells. Main effector organs include exocrine glands, cardiac muscle, and smooth muscle.

Though the intended anticholinergic response is relaxation of the bronchi, thereby producing bronchodilatation, other responses may be present (see Table 11–9). In the pulmonary patient on an inhaled anticholinergic, the intensity and extent of the anticholinergic response depends on the drug given, the dosage, and the degree of systemic absorption.

Atropine

Atropine is a plant alkaloid found in belladonna (an extract from the deadly *Atropa belladona* plant), in stramonium (from the Jamestown weed or Jimson weed, *Datura stramonium*), and in the formerly marketed Asthmador antiasthma cigarettes made from both of these plant sources.

Atropine-related drugs have been used for many centuries for the treatment of asthma. Until 1900, atropine was commonly used orally, subcutaneously, and by smoke inhalation of the aforementioned plant extracts. Currently, atropine is mostly used for ophthalmic problems, for bradycardias, and for preanesthesia to prevent bradycardia, bronchospasm, and increased respiratory secretions.

A resurgence of interest in atropine's respiratory uses has led to the further development of inhaled anticholinergic drugs to control bronchospasm. Though not approved by the FDA for inhalation, atropine has been a valuable secondary drug in the treatment and prophylaxis of bronchospasm. Also, it has other special uses listed in Table 11–10. Unfortunately, however, the optimal dose of 2.5 mg is likely to result in side effects, such as dryness of mouth, tachycardia, palpitations, and blurred vision due to miosis. Similar to many oral adrenergic agents, administration of therapeutic doses of atropine may not be possible because

Table 11–9. CHOLINERGIC AND ANTICHOLINERGIC RESPONSES

Cholinergic Response (from parasympathetic stimulation)	Anticholinergic Response (from parasympathetic block)
Pupillary constriction	Pupillary dilatation
Decreased heart rate	Increased heart rate
Bronchoconstriction	*Bronchodilatation*
May increase respiratory secretions or induce rhinorrhea	Decrease in respiratory secretions and rhinorrhea; thickens mucus and saliva.
Urinary bladder spasm (intense stimulation)	Relief of bladder spasm
Gastrointestinal spasm (intense stimulation)	Decrease in gastrointestinal spasm
Increase in sweating	Decrease in sweating
Cholinergic drugs (*methacholine, carbachol*) are used to induce bronchospasm during bronchial provocation challenge in the pulmonary function laboratory.	*Anticholinergic drugs*: atropine, ipratropium.

Table 11–10. ANTICHOLINERGIC BRONCHODILATORS

Drug	Dosage	Action	Specific Uses	Monitoring Considerations
Atropine sulfate				
Nebulized Not FDA approved, but injection solution is commonly substituted for nebulization, 1.0 mg/1 ml.	1 to 2 mg in 2 ml normal saline or 0.025 mg/kg	Onset, within 15 min Peak, 15 to 60 min Duration, 4 h	Perennial childhood asthma Bronchospasm caused by cholinergic agents, beta blockade, and psychogenic factors Chronic bronchitis and emphysema Cystic fibrosis Poor or adverse response to theophylline or adrenergic agents	Side effects are dose related: dryness of mouth is common. Use of high doses causes rapid systemic absorption manifested by tachycardia and blurred vision, followed by speech and swallowing problems, difficulty voiding (men), and mental changes (confusion or excitement). Use with caution in patients with glaucoma, prostatic hypertrophy, bladder-neck obstruction, and arrhythmias.
Ipratropium bromide*				
Inhaler Atrovent FDA approved 18 mcg/puff	2 puffs QID (usual dose)	Onset, within 15 min Peak, 1 to 2 h Duration, 3 to 6 h	Same as for atropine	Side effects; dryness of mouth and cough are the most common. Others may include headache, dizziness, nausea, gastrointestinal distress, paradoxical bronchospasm, and nervousness. Use with caution in patients with glaucoma, prostatic hypertrophy, and bladder-neck obstruction.

*Data from Boehringer Ingelheim Atrovent inhalation aerosol—prescribing information and instructions for use. St. Paul, Minnesota, Riker Laboratories, Inc/3M, 1986.

of significant blood levels and associated systemic side effects.

Ipratropium Bromide (Atrovent)

This drug was recently approved for use in the United States, after numerous findings suggested that anticholinergic agents appear more effective in stable chronic obstructive pulmonary disease (COPD) than the most potent adrenergic agent (Gross, 1987). While adrenergic agents alone achieve the most available bronchodilatation in asthmatic patients, anticholinergics alone, given in sufficient dosage, achieve all available bronchodilatation in COPD (e.g., emphysema and bronchitis) patients.

At present, ipratropium is expected to supplant atropine because of the convenient metered dose device (MDD) form and because of its relative freedom from side effects. Though dryness of mouth occurs as with atropine, ipratropium does not affect mucus secretion or mocociliary transport in the tracheobronchial tree. It does not affect intraocular tension, unless sprayed into the eye by mistake, nor is the drug associated with significant hemodynamic changes, arrhythmias, tremor, or tachyphylaxis, as are adrenergic agents.

Gross concludes that anticholinergic agents are now the most potent bronchodilators for maintenance therapy in COPD patients and possibly for acute exacerbations. They are best utilized as secondary therapy in asthma, except possibly in the cases of beta blockade and psychogenic asthma.

METHYLXANTHINES

Chemically, the methylxanthines are methylated *xanthines* made of *caffeine, theophylline,* and *theobromine*; the same substances found in the popular beverages, such as coffee, tea, cola, and cocoa. Although the methylxanthines are a naturally occurring class of plant alkaloids, most are produced synthetically and are related to the prototype *theophylline*. Theophylline constitutes most oral preparations on the market; its main salt *aminophylline* constitutes the common intravenous preparation given in emergency situations.

Indications

Theophylline is primarily used as a bronchodilator in the prophylaxis and treatment of asthma. Because theophylline also acts as a respiratory and myocardial stimulant, it may be used in a number of different situations, as shown in the box.

The use of theophylline in patients with irreversible airway obstructions (e.g., cystic fibrosis, bronchitis and emphysema) is controversial. Though no improvement may be observed in pulmonary function tests, administration over a 2- to 4-week trial period may relieve dyspnea, decrease the work of breathing, or improve biventricular performance (Hendeles and Weinberger, 1983).

Theophylline is contraindicated in the following situations: tachyarrhythmias, unstable blood pressure, history of seizure, extreme tremulousness, hepatic failure, peptic ulcer or gastrointestinal bleeding, nau-

INDICATIONS FOR THEOPHYLLINE ADMINISTRATION

Acute and chronic asthma
 to dilate airways and increase alveolar ventilation
Cheyne-Stokes respiration to increase the rate and regularity of respirations
Apnea and bradycardia episodes in newborns to prevent recurrent apnea and excessive periodic breathing in sudden infant death syndrome (SIDS)
Acute pulmonary edema
 to dilate airways, relieve paroxysmal dyspnea, stimulate myocardium, and promote diuresis
Acute respiratory failure
 to improve diaphragmatic contractility and prevent respiratory muscle fatigue, particularly during weaning from mechanical ventilation (Viires et al, 1984)

sea and vomiting, glaucoma, hyperthyroidism, and hypersensitivity to ethylenediamine (drug additive). In addition, the drug is not prescribed, unless the patient can be monitored for drug effectiveness, side effects, and dosage adjustments.

Absorption

The methylxanthines are readily absorbed after oral, rectal, and intravenous administration. Specific absorption rates depend on the theophylline derivative, specific preparation, and route of administration.

Theophylline Derivatives. Theophylline derivatives have anhydrous theophylline contents ranging from 48% to 100% (Table 11–11). Derivatives with low theophylline content are likely to produce less bronchodilatation than those with high theophylline content. Hence, 100 mg of *aminophylline* will be less effective than 100 mg of a pure theophylline drug, such as *Slo-Phyllin* and *Theo-Dur*. Similarly, a 100 mg tablet of Choledyl will be less effective than 100 mg of Slo-Phyllin, because the former contains less anhydrous theophylline. Many clinicians prescribe only aminophylline and anhydrous theophylline derivatives because of the higher theophylline content and the greater potential for maximal bronchodilatation.

Some theophylline derivatives are better absorbed than others. For example, aminophylline is better absorbed than *dyphylline* (*Lufyllin* and *Dilor*), a derivative that is actually a chemical variation of theophylline rather than a simple salt. Dyphylline is a poor bronchodilator, with less than half the potency of theophylline. Nevertheless, it is sometimes prescribed in patients prone to arrhythmias from theophylline and in patients with liver dysfunction, since the drug is excreted unchanged in the urine. Unlike theophylline, dyphylline's pharmacokinetics and plasma levels are not affected by factors that affect liver function and hepatic enzyme activity, such as smoking, age, and congestive heart failure.

Administration Routes and Dosage Forms. In the acute care setting, theophylline has several acceptable forms as follows: plain, uncoated tablets; alcohol-free oral liquids; rectal solutions; and intravenous solutions (Table 11–12). The *slow-release* preparations, also called *sustained action* (SA) or *sustained release* (SR) preparations, are most appropriate for ambulatory and home settings. Intermediate action SR preparations, such as Theo-Dur, are often initiated in the hospital, after bronchospasm has been successfully controlled by quick-acting intravenous aminophylline and an inhaled beta 2–adrenergic bronchodilator.

Dosage forms not listed in Table 11–12 either are not recommended or are contraindicated in most clinical situations. Enteric coated tablets and rectal suppositories, of a cocoa-butter base, are not recommended because of delayed, erratic, or incomplete absorption patterns.

Oral elixirs (e.g., elixophyllin elixir) are available but are not recommended or are used with caution because of their 5% to 20% alcohol content. They may

Table 11–11. MAJOR THEOPHYLLINE DERIVATIVES

Generic Name Chemical Name	Brand Name Examples	Anhydrous Theophylline Content (%)
Aminophylline (anhydrous) Theophylline ethylenediamine	Aminophylline Somophyllin	80 (range 78 to 86)
Dyphylline (chemically related) Dihydroxypropyl theophylline	Lufyllin Dilor	None (manufacturers claim 70)
Oxtriphylline Choline theophyllinate	Choledyl Brondecon	65
Theophylline (anhydrous)	Slo-Phyllin Theo-Dur	100
Theophylline calcium salicylate	Quadrinal Verequad	48

THEOPHYLLINE PEAK PLASMA CONCENTRATIONS

DOSAGE FORM	*PEAK PLASMA CONCENTRATION*
Intravenous solution	Within 30 minutes
Oral liquid	30 minutes to 2 hours
Plain, uncoated tablets	1 to 3 hours
Slow-release capsules or tablets	
Intermediate action	3 to 7 hours
Once-a-day	4 to 13 hours (highly variable)

Table 11–12. THEOPHYLLINE PREPARATIONS

Dosage form (brand name, manufacturer, theophylline strength)	Specific Uses	Dosing Interval (Hours) Children and adults with rapid metabolism	Infants and nonsmoking adults	Administration Tips
Plain uncoated tablets				
Slo-Phyllin (Rorer) 100 mg, 200 mg Theolair (Riker) 125 mg, 250 mg Theophyl Chewable (McNeil) 100 mg Aminophylline (Searle) 79 mg, 158 mg	Used with an inhaled beta adrenergic for immediate relief of dyspnea or wheezing.	q4 to 6	q6 to 8	These and other rapid release preparations may be used interchangeably. Chewable tablets may be divided into 25 mg portions, chewed, and swallowed rapidly with water to avoid bitter aftertaste.
Alcohol-free oral liquids				
Elixicon Suspension (Berlex) 20 mg/ml Slo-Phyllin GG syrup (Rorer) 10 mg/ml Slo-Phyllin 80 Syrup (Rorer) 5.3 mg/ml Theolair Liquid (Riker) 5.3 mg/ml	Acute care use for infants, children, and elderly; nasogastric tube administration.	q4 to 6	q6 to 8	Shake well before use to insure uniform concentration.
Rectal solutions				
Somophyllin (Fisons) (aminophylline enema)	Acute care use for vomiting children, preoperative patients.	PRN	PRN	Supplied with calibrated syringe and disposable rectal tips.
Slow-release (SR) preparations				
Intermediate action preparations Constant-T (Geigy) 200, 300 mg Theo-Dur (Key) 100, 200, 300 mg Theolair-SR (Riker) 200, 250, 300, 500 mg Theo-Dur Sprinkle (Key) 50, 75, 125, 200 mg Respbid (Boehringer Ingelheim) 250, 500 mg Slo-Phyllin gyrocaps (Rorer) 60, 125, 250 mg	Long-term use, preferred over rapid release preparations because of longer dosing intervals, less variation in serum theophylline levels, and better symptom control.	q8 to 12	q8 to 12	SR products acting for 12 rather than 8 hours are preferred, e.g., Slo-Bid, Sustaire, and Theo-Dur. No timed-release preparations should ever be chewed or crushed; crushing increases rate of absorption. Bead-filled capsules (sprinkles) may be swallowed whole or opened and the tiny beads sprinkled on soft food, such as applesauce.
Once-a-day preparations Theo-24 (Searle) 100, 200, 300 mg Uniphyl (Purdue-Frederick) 200, 400 mg	Long-term use, may be preferred for normal or slow theophylline metabolizers with noncompliance problems. Not recommended for rapid metabolizers requiring 900 mg or more (Spector et al, 1986).	q24	q24	Schedule dose in the morning not at night. (Theophylline clearance is more rapid during the day than at night.) Patients with subtherapeutic or variable theophylline levels should be changed to a standard BID SR preparation.
Intravenous solution				
Aminophylline (Searle) 20 mg/ml Theophylline (Travenol) 0.4–4 mg/ml	Acute care use	Constant infusion	Constant infusion	Administer by metriset or infusion pump for increased safety.

produce a therapeutic serum theophylline level within a relatively short period of time. However, the sugar content or associated sedative effect may be contraindicated in the alcoholic, diabetic, obese person, child, or person on sedatives or antihistamines.

The intramuscular route is not used for theophylline because of drug precipitation at the injection site, local irritation, and slow systemic absorption.

When theophylline is given, peak plasma concentrations are achieved; the fastest are obtained with use of an intravenous solution and the slowest with use of an oral slow release preparation, as shown in the box (see page 228).

Rate of absorption and peak plasma concentration are most unpredictable with once-a-day SR preparations, such as Theo-24 or Uniphyl. Hendeles and coworkers (1985) state that absorption is incomplete, erratic, or too rapid to achieve relatively constant plasma concentrations over a 24-hour dosing interval. In spite of this problem, however, once-a-day preparations may be preferred for patients who are normal or slow theophylline metabolizers (e.g., young smokers), particularly those with noncompliance problems.

Metabolism and Excretion

About 90% of each theophylline dose is metabolized in the liver and excreted in the urine in an inactive form. About 10% is excreted unchanged in the urine. The status of renal function does not appreciably alter theophylline elimination from the body (Smith, 1983).

Theophylline is eliminated from the body at different rates. This variability explains why dosage adjustment in the clinical setting is difficult, if not impossible, to achieve safely without continuous monitoring and periodic measurement of blood theophylline levels. Factors that alter theophylline metabolism and excretion include age, smoking history, disease, diet, and other medications (Table 11–13). On the one hand, note that cigarette smokers and children metabolize and eliminate theophylline rapidly. They are prone to low theophylline levels, unless dosage is appropriately increased to sustain bronchodilatation to the next administration time. On the other hand, persons with severe COPD or liver disease eliminate theophylline more slowly than normal nonsmoking adults. Drug toxicity may occur, unless the normal dosage is reduced.

Side Effects

A patient on theophylline may experience two types of side effects; (1) less serious caffeine-like induced side effects and (2) more serious adverse side effects that prompt either a decrease in dosage or discontinuation of the drug.

Caffeine-like induced side effects may occur after an initial loading dose of theophylline. Clinical manifestations may include minor CNS stimulation, slight nausea, and stomach queasiness. Signs and symptoms are not directly related to the blood theophylline level. They disappear spontaneously or are well tolerated by treating minor complaints, e.g., acetaminophen (Tylenol) for a headache, food or antacids for a queasy stomach, and a quiete environment for nervousness and agitation.

More serious side effects are related to drug toxicity or to hypersensitivity reactions. The easiest way for the nurse to recall important adverse effects is to first recall the effects of theophylline on key body systems. Then, the nurse notes related adverse effects that help determine how to monitor the patient (Table 11–14).

Table 11–13. PATIENT SITUATIONS ASSOCIATED WITH HIGH AND LOW SERUM THEOPHYLLINE LEVELS

High Theophylline Levels (Decreased Dosage Required)	Low Theophylline Levels (Increased Dosage Required)
Elderly	Babies, children, women, adolescents with cystic fibrosis
Diets high in chocolate, cola, tea, coffee	Cigarette and marijuana smokers (may require 50 to 100% increase in dosage)
Low protein, high carbohydrate diet	High protein, low carbohydrate diet
Liver disease; cirrhosis, acute hepatitis, cholestasis	Hyperthyroidism
Congestive heart failure, severe airway obstruction, cor pulmonale, pneumonia	Charcoal-broiled beef
Fever, shock, hypoxia	Drugs: isoproterenol, phenobarbital, phenytoin, carbamazepine, rifampin
Antibiotics: erythromycin, troleandomycin, lincomycin, clindamycin	
Other drugs: allopurinol, cimetidine, oral contraceptives (with moderate amounts of estrogen)	

Standard Theophylline Dosages

Standard theophylline dosages are based on its serum *half-life*, abbreviated $T_{1/2}$. Half-life is the duration of a drug's pharmacologic activity, which in this case is bronchodilatation. More specifically, it is the *time required for the drug serum level to fall to 50% of peak activity level.* Drug dosages are given at time intervals approximating twice a drug's half-life. Theophylline has a mean half-life of 3 to 4 hours in children and 7 to 8 hours in nonsmoking adults (Smith, 1983).

The steps that follow may be taken to start a patient on a theophylline drug.

History. Take a history to determine theophylline and other drugs taken in the last 24 to 48 hours. Note medical conditions, such as congestive heart failure, that alter theophylline clearance.

Loading Dose. If the patient's history is negative for the aforementioned, give a full loading dose of theophylline orally, via nasogastric tube or, in the case of severe bronchospasm, intravenously (American Thoracic Society, 1987).

LOADING DOSE

4 to 6 mg/kg theophylline
5 to 7 mg/kg aminophylline

TARGET BLOOD THEOPHYLLINE LEVEL

10 to 20 mcg/ml (normal range)

A typical loading dose is usually between 200 and 500 mg of aminophylline. An intravenous dose is mixed with 50 ml of fluid and infused over 20 to 30 minutes.

In emergency situations and when theophylline in-

Table 11–14. MAIN EFFECTS OF THEOPHYLLINE ON BODY SYSTEMS

Main Effects	Monitoring Considerations
Respiratory	
Relaxes bronchial smooth muscle Stimulates respirations and mucociliary transport Inhibits mediator release of histamine Vasodilates pulmonary vessels and decreases pulmonary hypertension Decreases diaphragmatic muscle fatigue	Goal for intervention: improved oxygenation and alveolar ventilation, as evidenced by normal or increased PaO_2, increased breath sounds, decreased wheezing, normal skin coloration, normal baseline pulmonary artery pressures, and normal breathing pattern.
Cardiovascular	
Increases heart rate, force of contraction, and cardiac output Vasodilates coronary vessels	Monitor for related adverse effects: palpitation, tachycardia, other arrhythmias; hypertension and headache; hypotension, vasomotor collapse, and shock.
Vasoconstricts cerebral vessels Variable effect on blood pressure Rapid intravenous administration may cause hypotension, headache, flushing, palpitations, dizziness, hyperventilation, precordial pain, or sudden cardiac arrest. The release of catecholamines may contribute to tachycardia, increased blood pressure, and diaphoresis.	Give loading dose slowly over 30 minutes to avoid hypotension, mild caffeine-like side effects as well as life-threatening reactions.
Renal	
Promotes diuresis	Monitor for dehydration, proteinuria, and hypokalemia. Replace fluids and potassium, as indicated by the situation.
Nervous and Musculoskeletal	
Stimulates the central nervous system and skeletal muscle	Monitor for restlessness, irritability, anxiety, headache, insomnia, tremulousness, maniacal behavior, muscle twitching, convulsions.
Gastrointestinal	
Increases gastric acid secretion	Monitor for nausea, vomiting, abdominal pain, hematemesis, and melena when history of ulcer disease is present. If anorexia and stomach discomfort occur, advise antacids between meals or oral theophylline administration with a few crackers.
Other	
Hypersensitivity reaction Usually from ethylenediamine in aminophylline preparations	Discontinue drug when rash, dermatitis, or other signs of allergy appear.

take is a possibility in the last 24 hours, give half the normal loading dose or 2.5 mg/kg theophylline.

Maintenance Dose. Immediately follow the intravenous loading dose with a continuous infusion of theophylline, e.g., 500 mg aminophylline in 500 ml 5% dextrose in water (D5W) via infusion pump. Continuous infusion is better than intermittent boluses because it maximizes bronchodilatation without great fluctuations in blood theophylline levels. Appropriate infusion rates are listed in Table 11–15 under calculated mg/kg/day.

For patients on theophylline, draw a blood sample to determine theophylline level *before* administering additional theophylline. The loading dose is calculated using a separate formula, the patient's current theophylline level, and the target level, estimated conservatively at 10 to 15 mcg/ml (Smith, 1983). Normally, each mg/kg of ideal body weight of theophylline administered results in a 2 mcg/ml increase in the blood theophylline level.

The patient is given an oral preparation in 1 to 5 days after bronchospasm is under control. SR preparations are stated immediately after the intravenous infusion is discontinued or within 1 to 2 hours, depending on theophylline level and dose prescribed. They are continued on an 8- to 12-h schedule. Fast acting oral preparations are started 2 to 3 hours after infusion discontinuation; they are administered every 4 to 6 hours. Individual doses are determined by dividing the total daily theophylline requirement by the number of desired daily administrations.

Blood Theophylline Levels

The decision to alter a patient's theophylline dosage depends on the desired therapeutic response, the presence of side effects, and the blood theophylline level.

Most clinicians monitor peak rather than trough theophylline levels. A *peak level* is observed during peak pharmacologic activity as follows: (1) 30 minutes after completion of an intravenous loading dose, (2)

Table 11–15. MAINTENANCE INTRAVENOUS THEOPHYLLINE AND AMINOPHYLLINE DOSAGES*

	Theophylline		Aminophylline	
	Calculated (mg/kg/h)	Typical Dose (mg/day)	Calculated (mg/kg/h)	Typical Dose (mg/day)
Nonsmokers	0.4 to 0.6	800	0.5 to 0.7	900
Smokers	0.75	1100	0.9	1300
Cimetidine use	0.25 to 0.3	500	0.3 to 0.4	600
Cor pulmonale	0.2 to 0.25	400	0.25 to 0.3	500
Hepatic insufficiency	0.18 to 0.2	350	.2 to 0.25	450

*Adapted by permission from the American College of Chest Physicians— American Thoracic Society: Standards for the diagnosis and care of patients with chronic obstructive pulmonary disease (COPD) and asthma. *American review of respiratory disease,* 136(1):233, 1987.

Table 11–16. INTERPRETATION OF BLOOD THEOPHYLLINE LEVELS

Blood Theophylline Level	Clinical Effect	Theophylline Dose Adjustment
Subtherapeutic range		
Less than 5 mcg/ml	No effect	Discontinue theophylline *or* Give a loading dose and reschedule maintenance doses
5 to 10 mcg/ml	Mild bronchodilatation	Increase theophylline to therapeutic range IV: increase dose by 25% (± 50 mg) Oral: Increase doses by 50 to 100 mg, every 2 or 3 days or decrease dosing interval, e.g., TID (q8h) instead of BID (q12h). *or* Continue low dose theophylline and add a beta adrenergic for an additive effect.
Therapeutic range		
10 to 20 mcg/ml or 8 to 20 mcg/m recommended by the American Thoracic Society (1987)	Maximal bronchodilatation	Continue present dose, as tolerated.
Mild toxicity		
20 to 30 mcg/ml	Nausea, vomiting, abdominal pain, diarrhea, anorexia, nervousness, headache, tachycardia	Decrease doses by 50 to 100 mg or skip one to two doses and decrease subsequent doses by 25% (± 50 mg), as tolerated.
Severe toxicity		
30 to 50 mcg/ml	Tachycardia, occasional premature ventricular beats	*A medical emergency*: HOLD THEOPHYLLINE! Skip next two or three doses and check theophylline level for guidance in further dosage requirement. Give activated charcoal.
Greater than 40 mcg/ml	Ventricular tachycardia, premature ventricular beats, grand mal seizures	

about 2 hours after an oral dose, (3) 4 hours after a SR dose (i.e., intermediate action), and (4) 12 hours after a once-a-day SR dose. In the acute care setting, blood is drawn every 24 to 48 hours for this purpose or 8 hours after a change in the infusion rate. In an ambulatory setting, blood is drawn after a change in theophylline dosage, when a steady state has been reached. The criteria for *steady state* include the following:

1. No missed doses in the previous 36 to 48 hours (72 hours for once-a-day preparations).
2. Equal dosing intervals.
3. Absence of other mediations or new problems that might alter theophylline elimination from the body.

Thereafter, the theophylline level is checked every 6 to 12 months or as indicated by the patient's situation.

A *trough level* occurs just before a maintenance dose. In routine cases, this determination is not needed because clinical symptoms, such as increased wheezing and dyspnea, usually appear to indicate subtherapeutic theophylline levels. However, in severe bronchospasm, a trough blood level of theophylline permits more precise titration of large doses of theophylline, with less risk of drug toxicity.

Interpreting Theophylline Levels. Various ranges for blood theophylline levels are summarized in Table 11–16 with implications for adjustment of subsequent theophylline doses.

As previously mentioned, the normal therapeutic range for theophylline is 10 to 20 mcg/ml. Many clinicians aim for a level close to 10 mcg/ml and then gradually increase the dose until the patient complains of a minor symptom, such as headache or slight stomach discomfort, or until the theophylline level approaches 20 mcg/ml. At levels close to 20 mcg/ml, a patient demonstrates more improvement in pulmonary function and requires intravenous theophylline for a shorter period than a patient maintained at levels close to 10 mcg/ml (Vozeh, 1982).

Presence of a theophylline level of less than 5 mcg/ml usually indicates a need to either discontinue the drug or give a loading dose to achieve a therapeutic blood concentration. Similarly, a level between 5 and

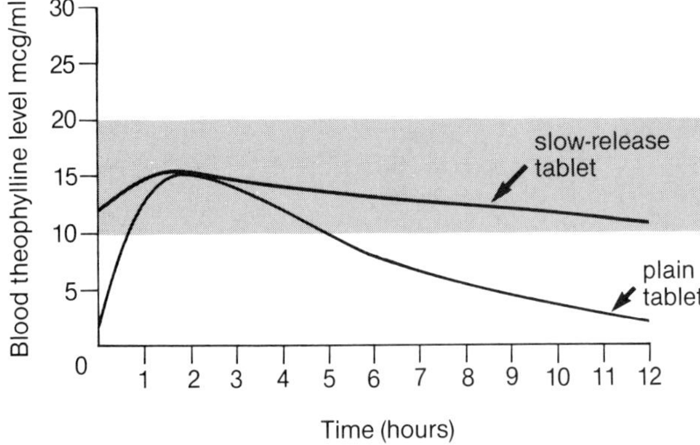

Figure 11–4. Theophylline levels for a patient receiving a plain uncoated tablet versus a slow-release product (Theo-Dur) every 12 hours. The gray area marks the normal therapeutic range.

10 mcg/ml is still below the therapeutic range and usually requires an increase in the daily theophylline dose. However, if side effects prevent an increase in theophylline, *low dose theophylline* is an acceptable alternative. This approach involves subtherapeutic doses of theophylline (e.g., 200 mg Theo-Dur BID) in combination with a beta-adrenergic drug, such as albuterol. Research indicates that half a dose of these two drugs given together will at least equal the effectiveness of a full dose of one of them (Shenfield, 1982; Wolfe et al, 1978). (The American Thoracic Society (1987) recommended 8 to 20 mcg/ml rather than 10 to 20 mcg/ml as the therapeutic theophylline range, in recognition of the mild bronchodilatation possible at the lower end of the therapeutic range.)

A theophylline level over 20 mcg/ml is in the toxic range: theophylline doses are then held or skipped. However, some patients may tolerate and need higher levels for clinical improvement. Subsequent doses are decreased until a therapeutic serum concentration is reached, without significant side effects. Most important, *a blood level of theophylline over 30 mcg/ml is a medical emergency*, requiring not only the withholding of theophylline but the careful monitoring of toxic reactions. Convulsions and ventricular arrhythmias may suddenly appear, *without* previous signs of mild toxicity. The patient with a toxic level is given activated charcoal orally to decrease rapidly the level to therapeutic range. In addition, toxic levels are rechecked by venipuncture in an extremity different from the extremity of the intravenous infusion site to assure a reliable laboratory result and to guide the clinician in further dosage requirements.

Monitoring Patients on Methylxanthines

The nurse collaborates with the physician and respiratory therapist to monitor the patient on methylxanthine. Monitoring involves the interventions presented in Table 11–17.

Fixed Combination Drugs

The nurse may encounter a variety of different fixed combination theophylline preparations in the clinical setting. A few common preparations are listed in Table 11–18 along with their constituents. Theophylline is the primary bronchodilator. It is accompanied by at least one other drug (e.g., ephedrine), a tranquilizer or sedative (e.g., phenobarbital), an expectorant (e.g., guaifenesin or potassium iodide), and alcohol. Ephedrine, a beta adrenergic, is included to potentiate bronchodilatation and promote decongestion. However, ephedrine may simultaneously potentiate the CNS stimulant effects of theophylline and significantly increase side effects. A sedative, such as phenobarbital, is included to counteract the CNS effects of ephedrine. Yet, phenobarbital may decrease the effectiveness of some drugs, such as steroids, by inducing their metabolism; along with the alcohol constituent, it may pro-

Table 11–17. MONITORING PATIENTS ON METHYLXANTHINES

Interventions	Rationales
Be on the alert for excessively low and excessively high blood theophylline levels.	Low levels indicate a possible noncompliance problem. High levels indicate drug toxicity.
Assess each patient separately.	Though the normal 10 to 20 mcg/ml level serves as a good guide, specific therapeutic and toxic levels are different for each patient.
Report all possible side effects and adverse reactions.	Remember, *toxicity can occur at any theophylline level.* Also, a small change in theophylline dosage or clearance may cause toxicity, because toxicity appears only slightly above each patient's therapeutic level.
Calculate each patient's daily anyhydrous theophylline dosage. Multiply the derivative dose by percentage anhydrous theophylline content in Table 11–11. *Example*: Aminophylline 200 mg = 200 × 0.80 = 160 mg theophylline	The effectiveness of a methylxanthine depends on its theophylline content.
Assess the patient's daily theophylline requirement. As a rule of thumb, the normal requirement is 900 mg/day or 13 mg/kg/day 400 mg/day in patients with cardiac decompensation, cor pulmonale, liver dysfunction* Watch for toxicity when theophylline level exceeds 900 mg/day (about 1 gm aminophylline). Suspect inadequate bronchodilatation when it falls below this limit.	Consideration of the normal daily theophylline requirement helps the nurse confirm optimal and safe bronchodilator doses, when theophylline levels are unavailable.
Seek ways to promote 24-hour bronchodilatation.	Around-the-clock bronchodilatation keeps the serum theophylline concentration within the therapeutic range at all times.
Schedule doses at equal intervals.	Equal intervals prevent peaks and valleys in theophylline levels and the appearance of pulmonary symptoms between maintenance doses.
Monitor the patient for increased wheezing and dyspnea prior to giving maintenance doses.	An increase in pulmonary symptoms suggests a low trough level. Increased dosage or shorter dosing intervals is needed. For the patient on a once-a-day preparation, a change to an intermediate action preparation with BID dosing usually eliminates wide theophylline peak-trough

Table continued on following page

Table 11–17. MONITORING PATIENTS ON METHYLXANTHINES *Continued*

Interventions	Rationales
	differences and associated wheezing.
Promote use of SR preparations that act for 12 hours, e.g., Slo-bid, Sustaire, Theo-Dur.	Long-acting preparations result in fewer fluctuations in blood theophylline levels (Fig. 11–4), fewer side effects, and greater improvement in clinical signs and symptoms, when compared with short-acting preparations.† Also, they promote uninterrupted sleep at night and patient compliance, since dosing intervals are longer.
Monitor the patient for signs of heart failure, worsening airway obstruction, liver failure, and other conditions that alter theophylline clearance from the body.	When signs appear, a theophylline level is needed to help assess changing daily theophylline requirements. A therapeutic theophylline dose may quickly become a toxic one, unless dose adjustments are made.
Encourage the chronic patient to see his physician regularly, even though he says he feels fine, and especially during periods of emotional stress or disease exacerbation.	COPD patients tend to deny increasing pulmonary symptoms and gradually become undermedicated, as disease progresses over days, weeks, months, or years. Stress and disease exacerbations both contribute to increased bronchodilator requirements.
Call the physician, if breath sounds, wheezing, and other pulmonary signs and symptoms do not improve.	The patient probably requires corticosteroids and more aggressive bronchodilator therapy.
Discourage use of fixed combination theophylline preparations, e.g., Bronkotabs, Tedrol, and Marax.	Such preparations promote submaximal bronchodilatation and increased side effects, as described in the text.

*From Matthay, R. and Depew, C.: Rational therapy for asthma with theophylline agents. *Respiratory therapy*, 10(5):53–59, 1980.

†From Andrasch, R. and Schmitz-Schumann, M. Short-acting versus a long-acting preparation of theophylline ('Xantivent') in the treatment of reversible bronchospasms. *Pharmatherapeutica*, 3(10):668–677, 1984.

mote respiratory depression or drug addiction. The value of expectorant constituents is largely undocumented. The medical literature indicates that expectorants induce no marked or consistent change in bronchial toilet (Yeates, 1980). When included in fixed combination drugs, expectorants exist in doses too small to effectively hydrate mucus and facilitate expectoration (Ziment, 1978).

Most important, the problem with fixed combination preparations is that theophylline cannot be increased without also increasing other constituents and thereby risking more side effects. The side effects limit dosage. Hence, patients on these combination preparations tend to be submaximally bronchodilated. Physicians revert to pure theophylline derivatives for safer and easier titration of dosage. For these reasons, the disadvantages of fixed combination drugs usually outweigh the advantages.

CORTICOSTEROIDS

Corticosteroids are anti-inflammatory drugs with antibronchoconstrictor effects. Pharmacologic actions in pulmonary patients are reviewed in Table 11–19.

Steroids have profound effects on the body, as evidenced by the many therapeutic effects listed in Table 11–19 and the side effects discussed in this section. Proper use may save a patient's life and permit his return to a normal or near normal life style. Since misuse can result in more adverse effects than beneficial effects, careful monitoring by knowledgeable health professionals is required for initiation and ongoing evaluation of steroid therapy.

Indications

Corticosteroids are widely used to treat the critical stages of acute chest disease and to control the symptoms of disabling chronic disorders. They are most useful in relieving bronchoconstriction associated with type III (delayed hypersensitivity) reaction. They may not inhibit the type I anaphylactic (immediate hypersensitivity) reaction. Though commonly prescribed for asthma, steroids may be used in a variety of other disorders (see box).

Most pulmonary patients on steroids fall under one or more of the following categories:

1. Poor response to conservative bronchodilator therapy
2. Previous treatment with steroids, particularly within the past 12 months. These so treated patients may have impaired adrenocortical function.
3. Poor tolerance to adrenergic sympathomimetic or methylxanthine side effects

INDICATIONS FOR STEROIDS

Acute or severe asthma, status asthmaticus, hypersensitivity pneumonitis, allergic bronchopulmonary aspergillosis (fungal disease with asthmatic component)

Severe COPD (variable effect)

Active interstitial lung disease (sarcoidosis, collagen-vascular diseases, pneumoconioses, idiopathic interstitial fibrosis)

Overwhelming illness or potentially fatal infection (a controversial indication)

Adult respiratory distress syndrome (a controversial indication), tracheitis, and some malignant lung diseases

Table 11–18. COMMON COMBINATION BRONCHODILATORS

Drug	Content	mg per tablet	mg per 5 ml or tsp
			Elixir
Bronkotabs	Theophylline	100	15
Bronkolixir (Wintrop-Breon) over-the-counter drug	Ephedrine	24	12
	Phenobarbital	8	4
	Guaifenesin (glyceryl guaiacolate)	100	50
	Alcohol		(19%)
			Syrup
Marax (Roerig)	Theophylline	130	32.50
	Ephedrine	25	6.25
	Atarax (hydroxyzine HCl)	10	2.50
	Alcohol		(5%)
			Suspension
Quadrinal (Knoll)	Theophylline (theophylline calcium salicylate, 130 mg)	65	32.50
	Ephedrine	24	12
	Phenobarbital	24	12
	Potassium iodide	320	160
			Suspension
Tedral (Parke-Davis)	Theophylline	130	65
	Ephedrine	24	12
	Phenobarbital	8	4

4. Critical illness
5. History of hay fever, allergic rhinitis, conjunctivitis, and atopic eczema

The decision to initiate steroid therapy involves weighing the risks against the potential benefits. Some patients (e.g., those with history of atopy, inflammatory wheal on skin testing, asthma with wheezing, sputum or blood eosinophilia, and improvement after bronchodilator inhalation) do remarkably well on steroids. In these patients, whose symptoms cannot be controlled by "simpler" drugs, benefits usually far outweigh risks. The patient is routinely treated with steroids when adrenergic sympathomimetics and methylxanthines prove ineffective or when severe and persistent bronchospasm (e.g., status asthmaticus) warrants the immediate and simultaneous use of steroids with other bronchodilators (see Fig. 11–2).

Steroids are often resorted to in COPD, though the

Table 11–19. PHARMACOLOGIC ACTIONS OF STEROIDS

Pharmacologic Actions	Therapeutic Effects and Significance
Prevent the release of lysosomal enzymes in the type III delayed hypersensitivity reaction; may inhibit type I reaction.	Recommended for prophylaxis of type III reactions, status asthmaticus, and some forms of intrinsic asthma.
Inhibit vasodilatation Decrease circulatory lymphocytes, eosinophils, and tissue mast cells	Given to decrease inflammation, bronchoconstriction, and airway hyperirritability.
Decrease the migration of phagocytes and macrophages Inhibit formation, storage, and release of histamine and other mediators. Affect Ca^{++} transport.*	Total eosinophil counts guide management of steroid-dependent asthmatics. Normal blood counts average 122/mm^3; counts from active asthmatics *off* steroids are greater than 350/mm^3; and counts from asthmatics *on* steroids are greater than 85/mm^3.†
Increase 3′5′ cAMP. May interfere with cholinergic and alpha-adrenergic receptor stimulation.	Promote relaxation of bronchial smooth muscle.
Decrease mucus volume, alter mucus composition, and increase mucociliary transport.	Help alleviate mucus retention problems.
Lower the stimulation threshold of beta 2–receptors. Inhibit	Enhance sympathomimetic responsiveness.
the enzyme COMT (catechol-*O*-methyl transferase), which breaks down catecholamines in the body.	Improve the effectiveness of adrenergic and methylxanthine medications.
Increase the heart's force of contraction. Improve circulatory function.	Improve cardiovascular function in acute conditions, such as shock.
Improve general sense of well being.	Relieve stress, anxiety, and depression associated with pulmonary disease.
Reduce serum angiotensin converting enzyme (ACE), a measure of disease activity in sarcoidosis.	ACE levels are used to monitor steroid effectiveness in sarcoidosis patients.‡

*Morris, H. Mechanisms of glucocorticoid action in pulmonary disease. *Chest*, 1335–1415, 1985.

†Horn, B. et al: Total eosinophil counts in the management of bronchial asthma. *New England journal of medicine*, 292(22):1152–1155, 1975.

‡Estepan, H. and Libby, D.: Glucocoticoid therapy of pulmonary disease. *Drug therapy*, 12(10):109–118, 1982.

benefits may barely outweigh the risks of side effects and steroid dependency. In many cases, steroids improve general sense of well being without other objective signs of clinical improvement.

Whenever possible, corticosteroid therapy is avoided in children and in adults with uncontrolled peptic ulcer, generalized osteoporosis, psychoses, severe brittle diabetes, increased susceptibility to infection, glaucoma, and cataracts.

Physiology of Corticosteroids

Naturally occurring corticosteroid hormones are secreted by the adrenal cortex. The hormones are classified into three groups as follows:

1. *Glucocorticoids* (e.g., cortisol or hydrocortisone and cortisone) affect glucose metabolism and have an extraordinary range of anti-inflammatory properties.
2. *Mineralocorticoids* (e.g., aldosterone) affect fluid and electrolyte balance.
3. Certain *sex hormones* (e.g., androgens and estrogens).

It is the *glucocorticoids*, simply called *steroids*, that are used in respiratory care. More specifically, the synthetic derivative of *hydrocortisone* is the prototype drug, because of its powerful anti-inflammatory property and few mineralocortocoid properties.

The natural secretion of hydrocortisone in the body (described in the following section) is important because it guides the administration of synthetic steroids further discussed.

Hydrocortisone's Diurnal (Daily) Rhythm. Hydrocortisone has a diurnal (daily) rhythm with blood levels ranging from a low of 5 mcg/100 ml in late evening hours (up to 2:00 am) to a high of about 30 mcg/100 ml (about 8:00 am). During stressful situations, levels can increase fivefold to tenfold, but usually they do not exceed 60 mcg/100 ml.

The *hypothalamic-pituitary-adrenal* (HPA) *axis* is responsible for these variations in blood hydrocortisone levels. During a person's normal cycle of sleep and wakefulness, the hypothalamus in the brain begins to produce more *corticotropin-releasing hormone* (CRH) in the hours after midnight (Fig. 11–5). This hormone causes the anterior pituitary to release increasing amounts of *adrenocorticotropic hormone* (ACTH) also called *corticotropin*. ACTH reaches a peak in blood plasma by 6:00 am.

ACTH secretion in turn causes the two adrenal cortices to secrete large amounts of glucocorticoids between the hours of 4:00 am and 8:00 am. Note in Figure 11–3 that hydrocortisone peaks at about 8:00 am, the time when daily synthetic steroids are given in the clinical setting.

Glucocorticoids circulate to peripheral tissues and reach the brain, suppressing further production of CRH by the hypothalamus, ACTH by the anterior pituitary, and glucocorticoids by the adrenal cortex.

This whole cycle repeats itself, when the hypothalamus senses that hormone levels have fallen below normal. Low hormone levels prompt it to begin production of more CRH. Peak and trough cortisol levels

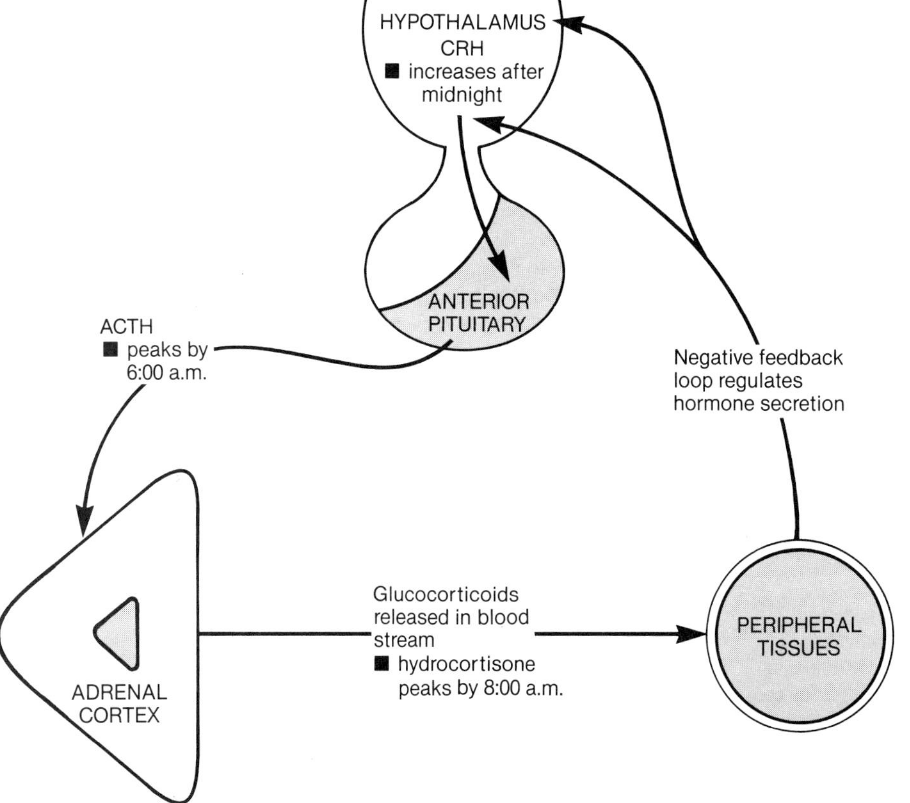

Figure 11–5. Conceptual drawing of the hypothalamic-pituitary-adrenal axis.

correspond with changes inherent in this negative feedback system. A total of 10 to 25 mg of cortisone (hydrocortisone) is produced each day via this mechanism.

Absorption, Metabolism, Excretion

The plasma half-life of ACTH is about 15 minutes. Intravenously administered ACTH is inactivated in body tissues, rapidly disappearing from the circulatory system without a trace excreted in the urine. This hormone is not given orally, because gastrointestinal enzymes destroy it before absorption can take place.

The plasma half-lives of various glucocorticoid preparations vary, ranging from ½ hour (*cortisone*) and 1½ hours (hydrocortisone) to over 5 hours (*dexamethasone*). Cortisol (hydrocortisone) is transported in plasma by albumin and *corticosteroid binding globulin* (CBG). Metabolic degradation occurs mostly in the liver, and the metabolites are excreted in the urine.

Various drugs and disorders alter glucocorticoid metabolism and require a change in steroid dosage or steroid preparation (Table 11–20). Liver disease may require increased dosages because it decreases the rate of steroid metabolic breakdown in the liver and impairs the conversion of *prednisone* to *prednisolone.* (Prednisone is biologically inactive until it is converted to prednisolone.) However, hypoalbuminemia may counterbalance this effect. It requires decreased steroid dosages because less cortisol binds to serum albumin, making more steroids available to body tissues.

Side Effects

Side effects usually appear after days or weeks of steroid therapy. The side effects discussed subsequently may be minimized by the use of the lowest possible steroid dose. However, some side effects are unavoidable and may develop into severe adverse reactions.

Impaired Immunologic Status. *Immunosuppression* increases the patient's susceptibility to infection, particularly to nosocomial, viral, or fungal infectious diseases. Beginning infection may become systemic and fulminant with little warning, because immunosuppression tends to mask early signs and symptoms of infection.

Table 11–20. DISORDERS AND DRUGS REQUIRING MODIFIED STEROID DOSAGES

Increased Dosage Required	Decreased Dosage Required
Liver disease—specific effect on prednisone. A change to prednisolone may be indicated.	Low serum albumin
Barbiturates	Cromolyn (slight decrease)
Ephedrine—specific effect on dexamethasone	Estrogens
Dilantin (phenytoin)	Macrolide antibiotics, e.g., erythromycin and troleanolomycin, which has a specific effect on methylprednisolone.
Rifampin	Preparations with the preservative parabens
Tranquilizers, e.g., diazepam, nitrazepam, hydroxyzine	High dose salicylates

Other related problems that accompany steroid therapy include severe reactions to immunizations, conversion of a positive tubercular skin test result to a negative one, and reactivation of inactive granulomatous disease (e.g., tuberculosis). When an aggressive course of steroids is anticipated for a patient with positive tubercular skin test results, prophylactic antituberculosis drugs are usually prescribed to decrease the risk of reactivation of tuberculosis.

Cushingoid Effects (Hypercortisonism). Long-term moderate to high dose steroids result in *Cushing's syndrome*, a condition that simulates adrenal cortex hypersecretion and the effects listed in the box.

CUSHINGOID EFFECTS

Weight gain
Swelling or moon-like appearance of the face
Central obesity with buffalo hump over back and neck
Widened cardiac borders from mediastinal fat pads on the chest x-ray
Skin changes, e.g., stretch marks over limbs and trunk; acne and hirsutism; thin fragile skin susceptible to bruising, ecchymosis, and poor wound healing.

Cushingoid effects may cause body image problems for patients. Women may become concerned with weight gain and hirsutism and other unfeminine qualities that prompt them to discontinue the steroid or reduce the dosage without consulting their physicians.

Emotional Responses. Emotional responses occur with the high dose steroids or the tapering or discontinuation of dosages, particularly if the patient has a preexisting personality disorder. High doses can cause euphoria, nervousness, insomnia, personality changes, and psychoses. Low doses can cause severe mental depression, apathy, and emotional lability, with periods of crying for no apparent reason. If the patient realizes the connection between depression and decreasing doses, he may take larger doses than prescribed to improve his physical and psychologic sense of well being. This behavior may result in psychologic dependence on steroids to maintain an emotional "high."

Gastrointestinal Effects. Ten to 50% of patients on steroids experience minor gastrointestinal disturbances, such as stomach discomfort, nausea, and vomiting (Richards et al, 1979). The patient is at increased risk for ulcerative disease, particularly if he is on long-term high dose therapy and has COPD, a disease associated with ulcerative disease. Antacids or an H_2 blocker (e.g., cimetidine) may be prescribed, though the benefits of this practice are controversial (Spiro, 1983).

Osteoporosis. Loss of calcium from bones promotes osteoporosis and increases the likelihood of bone fractures and aseptic bone necrosis. Compression fractures of weakened thoracic and lumbar vertebrae occur in 10 to 15% of patients, especially in elderly inactive females on steroids longer than 1 year (Gilston, 1980). Back problems are of special concern because associated back pain restricts breathing, promotes atelectasis, and can precipitate ventilatory failure.

Growth Retardation. Children on systemic steroid therapy may experience marked slowing of skeletal maturation and linear growth unless alternate-day steroids are used. The exact mechanism responsible is incompletely understood, but cessation of therapy may permit a compensatory growth spurt.

Myopathy. Muscle weakness and atrophy may rarely occur, but are noticeably in the proximal muscle groups in the shoulder and pelvic girdle. These adverse effects usually reverse within 3 to 4 weeks after steroid discontinuation. In severe COPD, steroids may limit the degree of muscle retraining possible in pulmonary rehabilitation, especially if the individual is already cachectic from end-stage lung disease.

Hyperglycemia. Steroids readily initiate or aggravate hyperglycemia. Occasional blood and urine glucose determinations are performed on patients who have accompanying diabetes mellitus or a family history of diabetes.

Fluid-Electrolyte Disorders. Sodium and water retention may cause edema, nocturia, and hypertension. However, salt restriction and potassium supplementation are usually not necessary, unless large steroid doses are used or unless the patient is taking diuretics.

Steroid Dependency. Psychologic dependence may be accompanied by physical dependence on steroids. Normally, the diurnal rhythm of the HPA axis allows blood cortisol levels to fall below normal. This triggers adrenal gland stimulation and cortisol production via the mechanism described previously in this chapter. Administration of large steroid dosages or daily steroid administration prevents cortisol levels from falling below normal. The adrenal gland becomes suppressed and no longer is stimulated to secrete natural hormones on its own. The body's reliance on regularly administered synthetic derivatives fosters drug dependency. Subsequently, the tapering and discontinuation of dosages causes adrenal insufficiency and withdrawal symptoms until the adrenal cortex once again begins to secrete glucocorticoids on its own. Patients on daily steroids for many years become permanently dependent on them for hormone replacement. Drug discontinuation always results in adrenal insufficiency, though the degree of insufficiency varies among patients. Some patients experience little to no signs of steroid withdrawal. Others may experience many of the signs and symptoms in the box above, including disease exacerbation.

Typical signs and symptoms, such as *general malaise*, *anorexia*, *joint tenderness*, and *mental depression*, are most likely when the steroid dose is completely discontinued or when it is tapered too rapidly to low doses. Yet, signs of withdrawal can also appear after a single moderately large steroid dose or when the dosage is not increased during surgery or some other physical or emotional stress.

SIGNS AND SYMPTOMS OF STEROID WITHDRAWAL

Mental depression, emotional "letdown"
Lethargy, muscle weakness, fatigue
General malaise, headache, fever
Backache and joint problems; tenderness, stiffness, pain
Anorexia, nausea, vomiting
Orthostatic hypotension, dizziness, fainting
Hypoglycemia
Weight loss
Exacerbation of primary or secondary disease

Table 11–21. PHARMACOLOGIC ACTIVITY OF INTRAVENOUS AND ORAL GLUCOCORTICOIDS*

Drug	Relative Glucocorticoid Potency	Relative Mineralocorticoid Potency	Equivalent Oral Dose (mg)	Serum Half-Life (min)	Biologic Half-Life† (h)
Short-acting					
Hydrocortisone	1	1	20	80 to 120	<12
Cortisone	0.8	0.8	25	30	<12
Intermediate acting					
Prednisone	3.5	0.8	5	60	12 to 36
Prednisolone	4	0.8	5	120 to 250	12 to 36
Methylprednisolone	5	0.5	4	80 to 180	12 to 36
Triamcinolone	5	0	4	>200	12 to 48
Long-acting					
Dexamethasone	25 to 40	0	0.75	110 to >300	36 to >48
Betamethasone	25 to 30	0	0.60	>300	36 to >48

*After Ziment, I.: Respiratory Pharmacology and Therapeutics. Philadelphia, W. B. Saunders Co., 1978.
†Measures biologic activity in body tissues.

Table 11–22. COMMONLY USED INTRAVENOUS AND ORAL GLUCOCORTICOIDS

Glucocorticoid	Daily Dosage (Average)	Loading Dose	Maintenance Dosage
Hydrocortisone Intravenous (Solu-Cortef)	1.5 to 2.0 gm Up to 4 to 6 gm	Severe asthma: 4 mg/kg or 300 mg	0.5 mg/kg/h by continuous infusion* or 100 to 200 mg q3 to 6 h. Dosage may be increased until blood cortisol level rises to 100 to 150 mcg/ 100 ml.
Methylprednisolone Intravenous (Solu-Medrol) Tablets (Medrol)	300 mg Up to 0.9 to 1.2 gm	Severe asthma: 0.8 mg/kg	0.1 mg/kg/h* or 300 mg/24 h
Prednisone Tablets	5 to 80 mg	Mild asthma attack: 40 to 60 mg	20 mg q4 to 6h Tapered to QD or QOD Doses given at 8:00 am

*American Thoracic Society, 1987.

Other Adverse Effects. Steroids can cause numerous other adverse effects, including menstrual irregularities, cataracts, papilledema, and heart failure.

Main Glucocorticoids

The pharmacologic activities of numerous glucocorticoids on the market are reviewed in Table 11–21. Preparations most commonly used in respiratory disease are listed in Tables 11–22 and 11–23.

Intravenous Steroids. Intravenous *hydrocortisone* is preferred in the treatment of status asthmaticus and other acute chest diseases because of its rapid onset of action. Symptomatic relief begins to occur within 1 hour, but peak action occurs in 5 hours (± 2 to 4 hours). Because of this delayed peak action, effectiveness largely depends upon prompt administration in the emergency room, after inadequate response to routine bronchodilators.

Methylprednisolone may be preferred over hydrocortisone for hypersensitivity reactions, collagen diseases, status asthmaticus, aspiration pneumonia, and ARDS. It has less mineralocorticoid activity, resulting in less sodium retention and potassium loss. Also, it is believed to stabilize cellular membranes, though clinical advantages of this effect have not been convincingly shown.

Intravenous *ACTH* is sometimes used in chronic asthma (particularly in children), allergic disorders, and other conditions, but its main use is in diagnostic tests that evaluate adrenal function.

High dose intravenous steroids can be given for 48 hours without serious side effects or dependency. After the acute disease is stabilized, dosages are rapidly tapered and discontinued within 5 days, provided other agents are continued to keep the patient bronchodilated.

Oral Steroids. *Prednisone* is the drug of choice because it is relatively inexpensive and intermediate acting. In liver disease, however, oral *prednisolone* is preferred because of the diseased liver's impaired ability to convert prednisone to prednisolone, the biologically active form.

The critical care patient is given prednisone when oral intake is initiated. In other clinical settings, acute disease exacerbations are controlled by doubling or tripling the patient's daily prednisone to about 40 to 60 mg/day. Though a single 40-mg dose may be

Table 11–23. INHALED GLUCOCORTICOIDS

Preparation	Mcg per Puff (Actuation)	Minimum Puffs per Inhaler	Average Daily Dosage	Typical Schedule
Beclomethasone				
Oral inhaler (Vanceril, Beclovent)	42	200	4 to 16 puffs, up to 1000 to 2000 mcg	2 to 4 puffs BID, TID, or QID
Intranasal inhaler (Beconase, Vancenase)	42	200	168 to 336 mcg	1 puff in each nostril BID, TID, or QID
Flunisolide*				
Oral inhaler (AeroBid)	250	100	4 puffs	2 puffs BID, not to exceed 4 puffs BID (2000 mcg daily)
Intranasal inhaler (Nasalide)	25	200	200 to 300 mcg	2 puffs in each nostril BID or TID
Triamcinolone*				
Oral inhaler (Azmacort)	200 (100 actually delivered)	240	4 to 8 puffs	2 puffs BID, TID, or QID up to 16 puffs daily (1600 mcg)

*Recently approved for clinical use by the FDA. Doses are based on manufacturer's guidelines.

sufficient to treat an asthmatic episode, usually 1 to 3 days of high dose therapy is required.

After acute disease stabilization, prednisone is tapered to about 5 to 10 mg every 1 to 2 days. When ⅛ the initial loading dose is reached, tapering progresses cautiously at a much slower rate—0.5 to 1.0 mg/day—or by as little as 1 to 5 mg/month in a steroid-dependent individual.

Daily steroid doses are gradually reduced to once a day, given at 8:00 am to mimic normal functioning of the HPA axis and to avoid adrenal suppression.

Reasonable attempts are made to initiate *alternate-day steroids* to minimize adrenal suppression and serious side effects as much as possible. On the "low-dose day," dosage is gradually reduced to zero (or at least below 7.5 mg), even if the amount given on the "high dose day" must be increased.

Some patients with severe chronic disease need long-term steroids indefinitely to prevent disease exacerbations. In these patients and others with histories of steroid therapy within the past 12 months, changes in physical or emotional status may trigger a need for more steroids. Acute adrenal insufficiency causes signs of steroid withdrawal, requiring temporary return to high dose therapy. In rare cases, adrenal insufficiency is due to impaired adrenal cortical functioning without a known triggering event.

Inhaled Steroids. Several inhaled glucocorticoid preparations are available in the United States, as shown in Table 11–23.

Beclomethasone dipropionate (Vanceril and *Beclovent)* is a commonly used drug in chronic asthma and steroid dependency. It has been available for a much longer period of time than flunisolide and triamcinolone. One to 4 puffs of this inhaled steroid QID from a metered dose device permits most patients to discontinue or at least reduce daily oral steroid doses. Sometimes the drug is used as an alternative to cromolyn sodium, a prophylactic asthma drug, or as a substitute for oral steroid therapy in the patient with responsive disease. Other uses for beclomethasone dipropionate include intranasal application to control perennial and seasonal rhinitis and to decrease the size of nasal polyps.

Inhaled steroid preparations have two related advantages over oral steroid preparations as follows: (1) minimal to absent systemic absorption and (2) few side effects. Because it is poorly absorbed from the pharyngeal and bronchial mucosae, little if any of the drug is absorbed into the blood stream. Hence, adrenal suppression does not occur, except at doses over 1000 mcg daily (Brogden et al, 1984).

Side Effects. The side effects of inhaled steroids are usually minor. Intranasal application may cause nasal irritation, sneezing, slight epistaxis, and headache. Moreover, the patient may need an antihistamine or decongestant for the first 1 to 2 weeks of therapy or until the steroid is effective.

When steroids are inhaled through the mouth, side effects are limited to oropharyngeal fungal infection with *Candida* or *Aspergillus*, hoarseness, and sore throat. Mouth infections may be avoided by rinsing the mouth and gargling with a mouthwash high in alcohol content (e.g., Listerine and Cepacol). When infection develops, the steroid is discontinued, or the infection is treated, or both. Treatment includes administration of topical nystatin, clotrimazole (Mycelex troches), or amphotericin B in extreme cases. In addition, an extension device or spacer may be prescribed for attachment to the patient's inhaler to reduce aerosol deposition in the mouth.

Use During the Tapering of Oral Steroids. An inhaled steroid is started during the slow tapering of oral prednisone, e.g., 2.5 mg each week. Gradual tapering may continue, but complete discontinuation of prednisone is never implemented until after 2 to 4 weeks. This overlapping period is necessary to prevent adrenal failure and to allow time for patient education. The patient must learn and perfect a breathing technique that will reduce aerosol deposition in the mouth and increase deposition in the lungs. Also, as previously mentioned, slow tapering of prednisone helps minimize signs and symptoms of steroid withdrawal and decreases the likelihood of disease exacerbation.

During the change from oral to inhaled steroids, a patient with a previous history of sinusitis or rhinitis may complain of nasal stuffiness. This sign of withdrawal is due to the loss of systemic steroid effect on the nasal mucosa. The patient may need an antihistamine, a decongestant, or a intranasal steroid preparation to clear nasal passages and sinuses and to prevent postnasal drip.

If increased wheezing and decreased breath sounds prevent the further tapering of prednisone, the physician may discontinue the inhaled steroid and increase the oral steroid, until the patient's condition stabilizes.

When the patient is wheezing, but his overall condition is unchanged, the physician may increase a steroid, such as beclomethasone, up to 2000 mcg daily (Brogden, 1984). A 1- to 2-month trial period is usually necessary to determine beclomethasone effectiveness. When more than 15 mg/day of prednisone is required, beclomethasone is less likely to result in complete withdrawal of prednisone. Nevertheless, the clinical goal is always to reduce oral maintenance dose as much as possible and eventually to change from QID to QOD dosing to reduce HPA axis suppression. These interventions may substantially decrease side effects and improve the patient's condition.

Monitoring Patients on Steroids

Special monitoring considerations for the pulmonary patient on steroids are summarized as follows:

1. For the critical care patient, monitor fluid and electrolytes and blood glucose levels every day.
   a. Replace potassium loss.
   b. Control hyperglycemia with insulin administration.
   c. When fluid balance is positive, determine

whether sodium and fluid retentions are contributing to heart failure.

2. Closely monitor breath sounds, wheezing, and pulmonary symptoms in these critical situations as follows:
   a. Steroid tapering, especially at low steroid doses.
   b. Steroid discontinuation on the "low dose day" (alternate-day steroids) and during physical stress, surgery, major medical illness, e.g., colds and other minor ailments.
   c. Emotional stress.
3. Remember, no steroid dosage should be considered as fixed!
   a. Call the physician when one of the aforementioned conditions appears responsible for a worsening clinical condition.
   b. Home patients should have an ample supply of oral prednisone to allow for dosage adjustments and to avoid such situations as running out of pills on the weekend.
4. Encourage steroid-dependent individuals to obtain Medic Alert bracelets. In emergencies, these individuals typically need immediate steroid administration.
5. Monitor for signs of gastrointestinal disturbances.
   a. When stomach discomfort first appears, encourage the patient to eat some crackers with oral steroid administration and to take antacids between meals.
6. During steroid tapering, monitor for signs of steroid withdrawal.
   a. Encourage the patient to avoid stressful activity and utilize family and friends for psychologic support during this difficult period.
   b. Remind the depressed patient that mental depression and emotional lability are normal responses that will pass after the body has adapted to medication changes.
   c. Advise acetaminophen (Tylenol) and hot tub soaks and other forms of relaxation to help ease minor aches and pains.
   d. Call the physician when signs and symptoms of withdrawal become severe or persist days after steroid adjustment.
7. Work with the patient on inhaled steroids to enhance breathing technique (see Chapter 18). To enlist full patient cooperation, stress the special advantages of inhaled steroids, including weight reduction and other positive body changes in the steroid-dependent patient (Fig. 11–6).
8. Schedule inhaled steroids at optimal times.
   a. Encourage use of equal dosing intervals (adapt typical schedules in Table 11–23). In stable cases of asthma, a 400 mcg daily dose may be divided into two doses (200 mcg BID) without loss of effectiveness (Brogden et al, 1984).
   b. Schedule inhalations a few minutes after the beta 2 or anticholinergic bronchodilator inhalations and after the patient has cleared obstructive secretions from the lungs. This regimen promotes deeper aerosol deposition in the lungs and increased effectiveness.
   c. Warn the patient that inhaled steroids are not used for acute bronchospastic episodes. Since a steroid inhaler looks very much like inhalers with other drug groups (Fig. 11–7), patients tend to use it inappropriately.
9. Be on the alert for the noncompliant patient.
   a. Encourage BID dosing schedules for noncompliant patients on inhaled steroids.
   b. Remember that cost may be a factor in noncompliance. Prednisone is far cheaper than inhaled steroid preparations. When cost or suboptimal inhaler technique is a factor, the patient on inhaled steroids may be best managed on QOD prednisone.
   c. Make sure the patient has an adequate supply of medication at home. Warn the patient when his inhaler will empty. *To determine how many days a new inhaler will last* divide puffs per inhaler (see Table 12–23) by prescribed puffs per day. As a reminder, some patients find it helpful to date new inhaler cartridges when they first begin to use them.

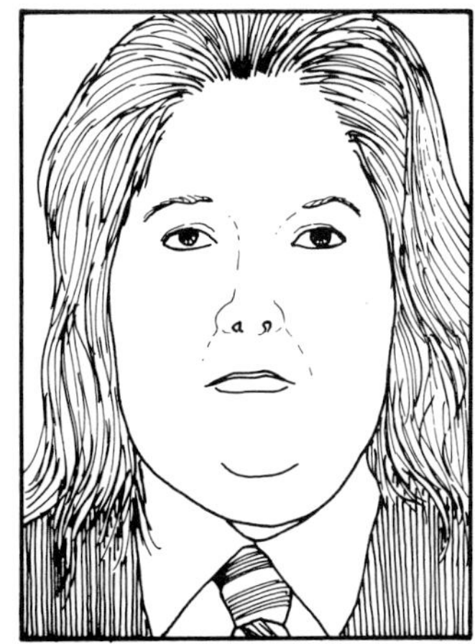
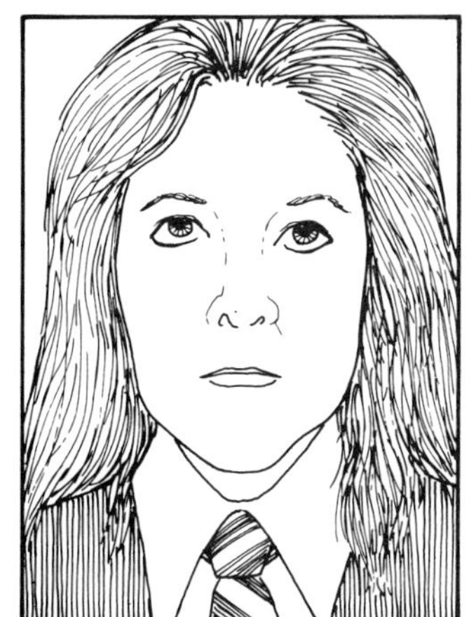

Figure 11–6. Physical appearance during long-term oral corticosteroids (left) and 6 months after changing to inhaled steroids (beclomethasone dipropionate or Vanceril). The patient reported a 28-lb weight loss and an increase in psychological well-being after the change in therapy. (Redrawn. The Schering Corporation.)

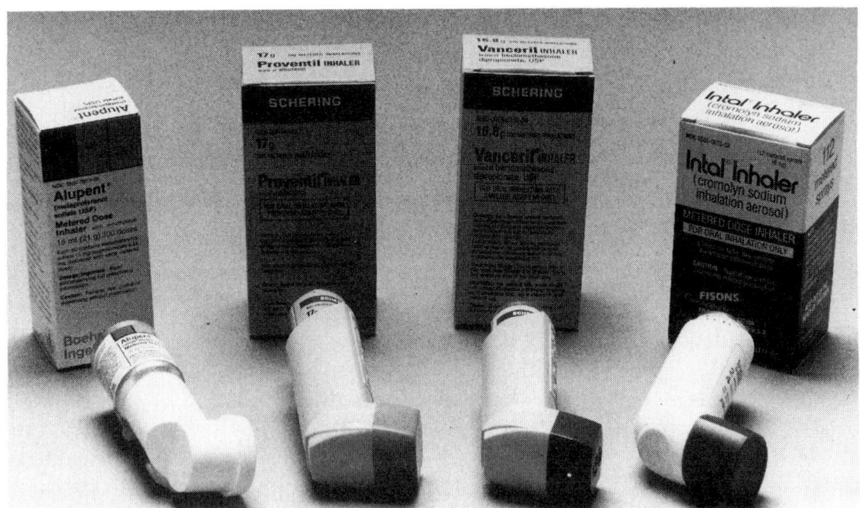

Figure 11–7. The patient may easily mistake a steroid inhaler (third from left), such as beclomethasone dipropionate or Vanceril), for an adrenergic sympathomimetic inhaler (first and second from left) or for a cromolyn inhaler (fourth from left).

CROMOLYN

The inhaled drug *cromolyn sodium* (disodium cromoglycate), known under the brand name as *Intal*, is a prophylactic agent in chronic asthma.

Pharmacologically, cromolyn prevents the type I immediate hypersensitivity reaction, while prophylactic doses of glucocorticoids prevent mainly the delayed Type III reaction. More specifically, cromolyn blocks mast cell release of the mediators of bronchoconstriction by preventing the influx of calcium ions into these cells. As alluded to, calcium influx is necessary for the degranulation of cells and release of mediators. Cromolyn is not indicated in acute asthma because the drug exerts no clinical effect once mediators have already been released in the antigen-antibody reaction.

Cromolyn is primarily administered in extrinsic, steroid-dependent, occupational, and exercise-induced asthma. It is particularly effective in children and others with labile asthma, which is difficult to control with routine bronchodilators and steroids. Success rates range from 33% to over 80% in persons with chronic perennial asthma and histories of allergy (Nicholson, 1976).

Cromolyn Preparations

Inhaled cromolyn is available in three different forms as follows: (1) 20 mg gelatin capsules (filled with a white powder), (2) nebulizer solution, and (3) metered dose device (Table 11–24).

In addition, the asthmatic may be on an intranasal or ophthalmic cromolyn preparation for treatment of a secondary disorder, e.g., *Nasalcrom* for allergic rhinitis or *Opticrom* for allergic conjunctivitis associated with hay fever, atopic dermatitis, or eczema.

Administration

Guidelines for the administration of inhaled cromolyn are largely based on clinical experience with the powdered form of the drug. Each 20 mg gelatin capsule is administered by a special *turbo-inhaler*, also called a *Spinhaler* (see Fig. 11–8 and Chapter 18 for discussion of inhaler technique). The inhaled powder is deposited in the lungs, absorbed into the blood stream, and completely excreted in the bile and urine within 4 hours.

After acute asthma stabilizes, cromolyn is given on

Table 11–24. CROMOLYN PREPARATIONS

Preparation (Brand Name)	How Supplied	Dosage
Powder capsules (Intal)	20 mg capsules delivered by turboinhaler.	20 mg BID, TID, or QID
Nebulizer solution (Intal)	Individual ampules; each ampule contains 20 mg cromolyn in 2 ml purified water.	20 mg BID, TID, or QID
Metered dose device (MDD) or (oral) inhaler (Intal)	Small MDD delivers 112 puffs. Large MDD delivers 200 puffs. Each puff (actuation) delivers 800 mcg cromolyn.	2 puffs BID, TID, or QID
Intranasal inhaler (Nasalcrom)	MDD delivers 100 puffs. Each puff delivers 520 mcg cromolyn.	1 puff in each nostril TID or QID, up to 6 times a day.
Ophthalmic solution (Opticrom)	10 ml bottle of 4% solution, with dropper.	1 to 2 drops (gtt) in each eye, 4 to 6 times per day.

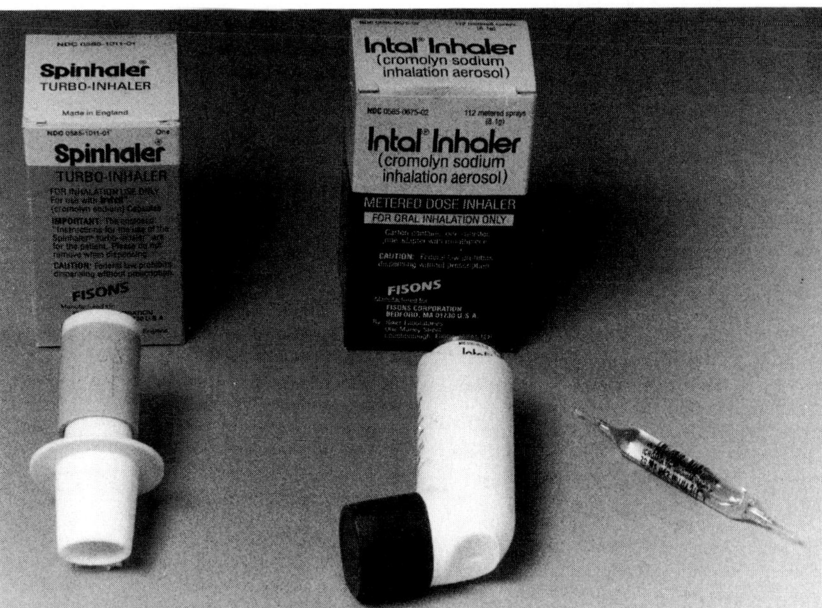

Figure 11–8. Cromolyn sodium is administered by turbo-inhaler (left), by metered dose device (center), or by nebulization of solution from a unit dose vial (right).

a trial basis for 4 to 6 weeks. The initial dosage is 20 mg QID, but five to six administrations per day may be necessary in rare cases. Patients with liver or renal disease may require reduced dosages.

The clinician keeps a record of frequency of asthmatic attacks, degree of disability, chest assessment findings, and pulmonary function test results. Clinical improvement may be as early as a few days or as late as 8 weeks. However, most patients require 4 weeks of therapy before responses can be determined. If the patient does not improve after 4 weeks, the cromolyn dose is increased.

Maintenance doses depend on the patient's situation. For example, some patients tolerate reductions in cromolyn administrations to twice a day and remain at this level indefinitely. Others need only periodic courses of cromolyn during certain seasons of the year. Those who develop bronchospasm after exercise may require only one dose 15 minutes before exercise for effective protection. Similarly, cromolyn may be taken just before exposure to environmental agents, such as cold air or known allergens.

As with steroids, cromolyn dosage is tapered gradually rather than suddenly discontinued, to prevent acute bronchospasm and reinstitution of corticosteroids.

Side Effects and Clinical Problems

Side effects are infrequent and few in number. They include dry throat and mouth; throat and airway irritation; hoarseness; cough; and, rarely, allergic skin rashes. Bronchospastic reactions occasionally occur but tend to be minor, short in duration, and avoidable with bronchodilator inhalation before cromolyn inhalation. In addition, a change to a different cromolyn preparation (e.g., inhaler and nebulizer preparations shown in Figure 11–8) may eliminate bronchospastic reactions associated with cromolyn powder.

Clinical problems with this drug stem from its relative expense, the long-term trials necessary to evaluate its effectiveness, and its inadequate protection in asthmatics with more than one asthmogenic stimulus. In addition, compliance is sometimes a problem for patients on QID therapy or those with difficulty manipulating the administration device.

Other Drug Groups

Other drug groups in addition to bronchodilators may be utilized in respiratory care. The main groups include decongestants, antihistamines, antitussive agents, mucokinetic agents, respiratory stimulants, respiratory depressants, paralyzing agents, and antimicrobial agents.

DECONGESTANTS AND ANTIHISTAMINES

Decongestants are used to treat upper respiratory tract mucosal edema and symptoms of nasal congestion, "stuffy" nose, and "plugged ears." Most decongestants fall under the *alpha-adrenergic sympathomimetic* category, e.g., ephedrine derivatives and phenylephrine (described previously).

Antihistamines are used to treat the hay fever and common cold symptoms of sneezing, runny nose, and watery and itchy eyes.

Decongestants and antihistamines are major constituents of the numerous brands of nonprescription cough and cold medicines available in supermarkets and drug stores. When used according to package directions, common brands, such as *Sudafed* (*pseudoephedrine*) and *Contac* (*phenylpropanolamine, chlorpheniramine*) can safely and effectively relieve bothersome symptoms. Yet, because of the vast number of available products, the question always arises as to which brands are best. Different brands have different constituents. Moreover, each cold or hay fever sufferer may have different drug requirements, depending on the nature and extent of specific signs and symptoms.

In these situations, the nurse should advise the average consumer to carefully read medicine labels and to buy only those brands with constituents indicated for their particular problems (Table 11–25). Single or double constituent brands are preferable because dose can be more easily titrated with changing signs and symptoms. Multiple constituent brands are acceptable as long as the person has a continued need for all the constituents.

Patients with cardiopulmonary disease should consult a physician before taking decongestants and other remedies. Some brands may be contraindicated because specific constituents may exacerbate a medical condition.

For example, the aspirin in *Coricidin* (chlorpheniramine maleate) may irritate the COPD patient's stomach, alter the cardiac patient's blood clotting times, or cause an allergic reaction in the hypersensitive asthmatic. To avoid the sedative-like side effect of most nonprescription antihistamines plus decongestants, the physician may prefer to prescribe *terfenadine* (Seldane). This drug will not cause drowsiness and associated respiratory depression. Moreover, referral to a physician is encouraged because it prompts medical re-evaluation and regulation of the nonprescription drug (if indicated) with the patient's other medications.

ANTITUSSIVE AGENTS

Antitussive agents are used to suppress an ineffective, dry hacking cough. They are not indicated for coughing due to retained secretions. *Topical anes-*

Table 11–25. DRUGS FOR COMMON COLD AND COUGH SYMPTOMS*

Chief Complaint	Appropriate Drug Group	Common Constituents
Nasal congestion, "stuffy nose," "plugged ears"	Decongestant	Ephedrine Phenylephrine Phenylpropranolamine Pseudoephedrine
Sneezing, runny nose, watery and itchy eyes	Antihistamine	Brompheniramine Carbinoxamine Chlorcyclizine Clorpheniramine Dexchlorpheniramine Diphenhydramine (Benadryl) Phenindamine Pheniramine Phenyltoloxamine Promethazine (Phenergan) Pyrilamine Thonzylamine Triprolidine
	Anticholinergic	Atropine Belladonna alkaloids Hyoscyamine
Dry, hacking cough	Antitussive	Codeine (narcotic) Benzonatate Dextromethorphan Hydrocodone bitartrate (narcotic)
Difficulty expectorating thick mucus	Expectorant	Ammonium chloride Guaifenesin (glyceryl guaiacolate) Ipecac Potassium citrate Potassium iodide Terpin hydrate
Muscle aches	Anti-inflammatory agent	Aspirin Salicylamide Nonsteroidal anti-inflammatory drugs
Headache	Analgesic	Acetaminophen Aspirin Salicylamide
Fever	Antipyretic agent	Acetaminophen Aspirin Salicylamide

*After Barreuter, A.: A drug therapy patient guide: how to treat a cold. *Drug therapy*, 10(10):74–77, 1980.

thetics, such as lidocaine (Xylocaine) given via endotracheal tube, act peripherally on lung irritant receptors. Various narcotic and non-narcotic drugs act centrally on the brain's cough center to depress sensitivity to afferent stimuli.

Narcotic antitussives (e.g., morphine) relieve cough and bronchospasm from cardiac asthma but are generally avoided in respiratory patients because of associated respiratory center depression, anticholinergic-like effects (dry mouth and ciliary depression), impaired mucokinesis, and bronchospasm from histamine release.

Codeine, perhaps the most commonly prescribed antitussive agent, has antitussive, sedative, and analgesic actions. Compared with morphine, it is less toxic and less likely to cause drug dependence. Codeine has only one fourth the depressant effect on respirations as morphine.

Dextromethorphan and *benzonatate* are common non-narcotic antitussive constituents in nonprescription cough and cold medicines.

MUCOKINETIC AGENTS

Mucokinetic agents are drugs that promote mobilization and removal of secretions from the respiratory tract. Main types include wetting agents, surface active agents, expectorants, and chemical mucolytics.

Wetting Agents

Wetting agents humidify and lubricate secretions, making expectoration much easier for the patient. *Sterile water* and 5% *hypertonic saline* are airway irritants sometimes administered via ultrasonic nebulizer to induce coughing and facilitate sputum collection for cytology and microbiology. Administration of 3 to 5 ml of *normal saline* (0.9% NaCl) may be done in a small volume nebulizer or IPPB device to promote deep breathing and coughing. *Half normal saline* (0.45% NaCl) is the diluent of choice for continuous aerosol or intermittent ultrasonic nebulization (Shrake and Oltmann, 1980). During nebulization, water evaporation occurs, leaving a more hypertonic solution in the nebulizer. However, this process of *drug concentration*, is not a problem with 0.45% NaCl because the remaining solution approaches a true physiologic saline solution value (0.9% NaCl).

Surface Active Agents (Detergents)

Solutions of *propylene glycol*, *glycerin*, and *sodium bicarbonate* are supposed to stabilize aerosol droplets and facilitate hydration and emulsification of adhesive-like secretions. Although they are effective carrier vehicles for nebulized drugs, "they have little, if any, effect on mucoid or purulent secretions and exert no mucolytic activity per se" (Lehnert and Schachter, 1980).

Expectorants

Expertorants, such as saturated solution of *potassium iodide* (SSKI), *guaifenesin* (glycerol guiaiacolate), and *ammonium chloride*, increase the volume output of respiratory tract secretions and, in doing so, may decrease the viscosity of mucus. They are used alone or as constituents of cough and cold medications.

Currently, the clinical efficacy of expectorants is in question. From one perspective, patients may derive little if any benefit from expectorants. Such agents tend to be used in suboptimal dosages. Long-term use may result in airway irritation, excessive mucus production (bronchorrhea), and toxic side effects. Moreover, simple humidification measures may more effectively and simply treat mucus retention problems.

From another perspective, expectorants may be beneficial, as long as they are reserved for acute care use, as an adjunct rather than a substitute for aggressive bronchial hygiene measures. When given in therapeutic doses (200 to 400 mg q 4 to 6 hours), an expectorant such as guaifenesen may liquefy secretions, facilitate mucus expectoration, and ultimately reduce coughing associated with acute respiratory illnesses (Cohen, 1983).

Mucolytics

The *chemical mucolytic*, *N-acetylcysteine* (Mucomyst, 10% and 20% solutions), produces *mucolysis*. More specifically, it disrupts chemical bonds in mucoid or purulent airway secretions, and in doing so it decreases mucus viscosity and promotes airway clearance. This drug is indicated for mucus retention only when hydration and routine bronchial hygiene measures prove ineffective. Side effects include airway irritation, coughing, bronchospasm (particularly in asthmatics), nausea from the sulfurous taste and odor, and eye irritation. Airway irritation is reduced by use of the less concentrated preparation (10%) or by the simultaneous administration of a bronchodilator (e.g., Mucomyst with isoproterenol). Eye irritation is reduced by keeping exhalation ports and wasted aerosol away from the patient's face.

RESPIRATORY STIMULANTS

Respiratory stimulants stimulate respirations by direct or indirect effects on the medullary respiratory center. Simultaneously, they may cause excessive CNS stimulation, manifested by hypertension, tachycardia, and agitation. Carbon dioxide, adrenergic sympathomimetics, and methylxanthines have this effect, but the largest class of respiratory stimulants is the *analeptics*, which act as restoratives.

Doxapram is one of the most acceptable analeptics. It is given intravenously (1 to 3 mg/min) in acute ventilatory failure to prevent a rise in Pa_{CO_2} with oxygen therapy. Also, it is used to prevent respiratory depression in high risk postoperative patients and to stimulate respirations in the newborn or persons with hypoventilation syndromes.

Oral *medroxyprogesterone* (20 mg TID) may be given to COPD patients (blue bloaters) to prevent nocturnal alveolar hypoventilation (Skatrud et al, 1981) or to others with periodic breathing or oxygen desaturation during wakefulness or sleep. However, its effects are unreliable.

RESPIRATORY DEPRESSANTS

Oxygen, sedatives, and tranquilizers depress respirations to varying degrees, depending on the amount given, drug type, and clinical circumstances (see Chapter 13 for discussion of hazards of oxygen). *Sedatives* are avoided in respiratory care and absolutely contraindicated in respiratory failure because they suppress ventilatory drive and cause respiratory acidosis. In extreme cases, however, intravenous morphine or diazepam (Valium) is used in ventilator patients, when agitation and anxiety increase the work of breathing and interfere with mechanical ventilation. In spontaneously breathing patients, a *tranquilizer*, such as *haloperidol (Haldol)*, can control agitation and combativeness with less risk of respiratory depression compared with sedatives and other tranquilizers. Whenever possible, calm and continual reassurance is provided at the first sign of agitation to avoid need for sedatives, tranquilizers, and paralyzing agents.

PARALYZING AGENTS

Neuromuscular blocking agents, such as succinylcholine (*Anectine*) or pancuronium bromide (*Pavulon*), are used for skeletal muscle relaxation during anesthesia or endotracheal intubation. In the agitated patient on a ventilator, intravenous Pavulon is used to minimize energy expenditure during the critical illness period and to facilitate the mechanical ventilation. The initial dose is 0.04 to 0.1 mg/body weight. Subsequent doses are usually 1 to 2 mg (or start at 0.01 mg/km) given intravenously every 30 to 60 minutes or immediately before the patient shows signs of inspiratory effort. (The assist light on the ventilator goes on.) Side effects are few and are usually limited to mild tachycardia and hypertension. Nevertheless, Pavulon is always used as a last resort, when more conservative measures fail to control the patient. Associated respiratory muscle atrophy during controlled mechanical ventilation may prolong weaning, once the patient recovers from critical illness. Also, being paralyzed and totally dependent on others for basic needs while mentally alert can be a terrifying experience.

ANTIMICROBIAL AGENTS

Antimicrobial drugs used to treat infections involving the lungs are listed in Table 11–26 by causative microorganism. Most of the drugs in this table are *antibiotics*. Antibiotics act by selectively binding to certain vital cell constituents and inhibiting the growth of microorganisms (bacteriostatic agents) or by killing them (bactericidal agents).

The COPD patient is instructed to start antibiotics at the first sign of a chest infection. A typical order is tetracycline or ampicillin, 250 to 500 mg 4 times a day, or one tablet of trimethoprim and sulfamethoxazole (Bactrim) twice a day. Antibiotics are continued for 7 to 10 days, until sputum returns to normal. They may be prescribed cyclically, e.g., the first 10 days of each month or the first 4 days of each week, for prophylactic treatment of persons with chronic lung disease and repeated chest infections.

Aerosol Antibiotics

Aerosol antibiotics are sometimes used as adjuncts to bronchodilators and mucolytics to eliminate colonization of microorganisms along the respiratory mucosa. Specific indications are listed in the box below.

INDICATIONS FOR AEROSOL ANTIBIOTICS

- Microbial colonization without local inflammatory changes or signs of systemic infection
- Chronic respiratory tract infection, e.g., cystic fibrosis
- Limited use of systemic antibiotics due to impaired renal function or sclerosed peripheral veins

Infections with *Pseudomonas* and other gram-negative organisms are usually treated with *polymixin*, *gentamycin*, *amikacin*, or *tobramycin*. *Staphylococcus* species is treated with *bacitracin* or *neomycin*.

Aerosol antibiotics are not always prescribed because routine use favors the development of resistant organisms in the patient and lung sensitization of all persons breathing air in the immediate environment. Also, aerosol does not reach all peripheral lung regions. Though distal deposition is limited, generalized toxic or allergic reactions can occur, causing severe bronchospasm in some individuals.

Antituberculosis Drugs

Drugs for pulmonary tuberculosis are listed in Table 11–27 with associated side effects. They are divided into three categories as follows: primary, secondary, and tertiary. The *primary drugs*, *isoniazid* (INH) and *rifampin*, are basic drugs. They rate high in effectiveness and relatively low in toxicity. *Secondary drugs* are less effective and usually more toxic than primary drugs. They are used in combination with a primary

Table 11–26. ANTIMICROBIAL DRUGS FOR SPECIFIC INFECTIOUS AGENTS*

Microorganisms	Antimicrobial Agents	Alternative Agents
BACTERIA		
Gram-positive cocci (aerobic)		
Staphylococcus aureus		
Nonpenicillinase producing	Penicillin	Vancomycin, cephalosporin (e.g., Cefoxitin, Cefazolin)
Penicillinase producing	Methicillin, nafcillin, oxacillin	Vancomycin, cephalosporin
α-Streptococci (*Streptococcus viridans*)	Penicillin	Erythromycin, clindamycin, cephalosporin
β-*Streptococcus* (Group A, B, C, and G)	Penicillin	Cephalosporin, erythromycin
Enterococcus	Penicillin or ampicillin + aminoglycoside	Vancomycin + aminoglycoside
Streptococcus pneumoniae (pneumococcus)	Penicillin	Erythromycin, vancomycin, cephalosporin, trimethoprim-sulfamethoxazole (Bactrim)
Gram-negative bacilli (aerobic)		
Acinetobacter sp.	Aminoglycoside (e.g., Gentamicin or Amikacin) + carbenicillin	Trimethoprim-sulfamethoxazole
Enterobacter sp.	Aminoglycoside	Third-generation cephalosporin
Escherichia coli	Ampicillin	Cephalosporin, aminoglycoside
Haemophilus influenzae	Chloramphenicol	Ampicillin, trimethoprim-sulfamethoxazole
Klebsiella pneumoniae	Aminoglycoside	Cephalosporin
Legionella sp.	Erythromycin + rifampin	
Proteus mirabilis	Ampicillin	Aminoglycoside, cephalosporin
Other *Proteus* species	Aminoglycoside	Cephalosporin
Pseudomonas aeruginosa	Aminoglycoside + carbenicillin	Third-generation cephalosporin
Salmonella sp.	Chloramphenicol	Trimethoprim-sulfamethoxazole
Serratia marcescens	Aminoglycoside	Third-generation cephalosporin
Anaerobes		
Anerobic streptococci	Penicillin	Clindamycin, chloramphenicol
Bacteroides sp. (oropharyngeal)	Penicillin	Chloramphenicol
Gastrointestinal strains	Clindamycin	Chloramphenicol, metronidazole
Other bacteria		
Actinomyces	Penicillin G	Tetracycline
Nocardia sp.	Trimethoprim-sulfamethoxazole	Minocycline
Mycobacterium tuberculosis	Isoniazid (INH) + rifampin	Ethambutal, streptomycin
FUNGI		
Aspergillus sp.	Amphotericin B	
Blastomyces dermatitidis	Amphotericin B	Ketoconazole
Candida sp.	Amphotericin B	Ketoconazole
Coccidioides immitis	Amphotericin B	
Cryptococcus neoformans	Amphotericin B + flucytosine	
Histoplasma capsulatum	Amphotericin B	Ketoconazole
PROTOZOA		
Pneumocystis carinii	Trimethoprim-sulfamethoxazole	Pentamidine
VIRUSES		
Herpes simplex or zoster	Adenosine arabinoside	Acyclovir
Influenza A	Amantadine	
OTHER MICROORGANISMS		
Mycoplasm pneumoniae	Erythromycin	Tetracycline

*Modified after Chernow, B. and Lake, C.: The Pharmacologic Approach to the Critically Ill Patient. Baltimore, Williams & Wilkins, 1983.

drug to help prevent the development of drug resistance during therapy. *Tertiary drugs* are least effective and most toxic but may be used when other drugs are contraindicated because of toxicity or resistance (Glassroth, 1981).

In recognition of new drug combinations of varying duration, other sources use slightly different labels for the classification of antituberculosis drugs. The American Thoracic Society (1986) employs the label "primary" for both primary and secondary drugs in the initial treatment of tuberculosis (i.e., first-line drugs). The term second-line drugs refers to the tertiary drugs listed in Table 11–27.

Specific antituberculosis drug regimens vary among patients, depending on the extent of disease, the likelihood of drug-resistant microorganisms, the history of compliance, the cost, and other factors. At one time, duration of drug therapy lasted 18 months to 2 years; new drug regimens now permit much shorter courses, lasting only 6 to 9 months in uncomplicated cases, as shown in the current national guidelines (see the box).

Prophylactic INH therapy is indicated for a variety of situations listed in Table 11–28. Dosage is usually 300 mg PO daily or 5 mg/kg (10 mg/kg for children). Duration of therapy is 6 to 12 months for maximal benefit.

NATIONAL CONSENSUS: CHEMOTHERAPY FOR TUBERCULOSIS*

1. A 9-month regimen of isoniazid and rifampin, usually supplemented during the initial phase by ethambutol, streptomycin, or pyrazinamide, should be standard therapy for tuberculosis in the United States and Canada.
2. Infants, children, and adolescents with tuberculosis should be treated with a 9-month regimen of isoniazid and rifampin, which should be supplemented by an initial phase of ethambutol, streptomycin, or pyrazinamide when drug resistance is suspected.
3. When drug resistance is suspected, the initial use of at least three drugs is mandatory.
4. A 6-month regimen of therapy is acceptable if four drugs (isonizid, rifampin, pyrazinamide, and streptomycin or ethambutol) are given for 2 months and followed by an additional 4 months of isoniazid and rifampin, with all drugs given under close supervision.
5. Regimens less than 6 months in duration are not acceptable owing to high rates of failure of treatment and relapse.
6. Studies of drug susceptibility on the initial isolate are always desirable but must be obtained when drug resistance is suspected.
7. Tuberculosis occurring during pregnancy should be treated with a 9-month regimen of isoniazid and rifampin supplemented during the initial phase by ethambutol (streptomycin and pyrazinamide should not be used).
8. Immunosuppressed patients with tuberculosis should be treated with 9 to 12 months of isoniazid and rifampin, supplemented during the initial phase by ethambutol, streptomycin, or pyrazinamide.
9. Extrapulmonary tuberculosis should be treated with the previously stated standard regimens.

*Reproduced by permission from the American College of Chest Physicians—Committee on Chemotherapy of Tuberculosis. *Chest* 87(2):1235, 1985.

Areas of Focus for Pharmacologic Assessment

This chapter has covered respiratory pharmacology with emphasis on bronchodilators, specifically autonomic active agents, methylxanthines, corticosteroids, and cromolyn sodium. This information will sufficiently guide the nurse in all aspects of pharmacologic assessment and intervention.

The following points serve as areas of focus during pharmacologic assessment.

1. *Note whether individuals with signs of chest infections are on antibiotics.* Check for prophylactic use of antibiotics in patients with severe COPD.
2. *Look for signs of drug toxicity as well as undermedication.*
   a. Are several drug groups utilized for maximal bronchodilatation, starting with an aerosol beta 2-drug for mild disease and ending with steroids for severe disease?
   b. Suspect subtherapeutic dosages or unwanted side effects, when combination theophylline drugs are used.
   c. Always interpret historical and physical findings in light of the recent blood theophylline levels.
3. *Identify individuals who omit dosages or discontinue drugs on their own.*
   a. Determine whether discontinuation is due to lack of knowledge, fear of drug dependence, hopelessness, forgetfulness, excess cost of prescribed medications, or other factors.
   b. Remember that pulmonary patients tend to discontinue drugs after recovery from acute exacerbations, without realizing that it is the bronchodilators that are keeping them asymptomatic.
4. *Identify individuals who use over-the-counter drugs.* These individuals may need complete med-

Table 11–27. ANTI-TUBERCULOSIS DRUGS*

Drug	Adult Daily Dosage	Twice Weekly Dosage	Common Side Effects
Primary (First-line)			
Isoniazid (INH)	5 to 10 mg/kg up to 300 mg PO or IM	15 mg/kg PO or IM	Peripheral neuritis (prevented by vitamin B_6); hepatitis, increased transaminases (SGOT, SGPT); anorexia; nausea; malaise; jaundice; hypersensitivity.
Rifampin	10 to 20 mg/kg up to 600 mg PO	NR†	Stains secretions orange. Accelerates catabolism of birth control pills, oral anticoagulants, methadone, and other drugs. Hepatitis, febrile reaction.
Secondary (First-line)			
Ethambutol	15 to 25 mg/kg PO	50 mg/kg PO	Optic neuritis, reversible with drug discontinuation, rare at doses around 15 mg/kg; skin rash.
Streptomycin	15 to 20 mg/kg up to 1 gm IM‡	25 to 30 mg/kg IM	Eight nerve damage (hearing loss, impaired sense of equilibrium), hypersensitivity reaction, nephrotoxicity, discomfort on injection.
Pyrazinamide	15 to 30 mg/kg up to 2 gm PO	NR	Hepatotoxicity, hyperuricemia.
Tertiary (Second-line)			
Capreomycin	15 to 30 mg/kg up to 1 gm IM‡	NR	Similar to streptomycin.
Cycloserine	10 to 20 mg/kg up to 1 gm PO	NR	Psychosis, personality changes, seizures, rash.
Ethionamide	15 to 30 mg/kg up to 1 gm PO	NR	Gastrointestinal upset, hepatotoxicity, hypersensitivity.
Kanamycin	15 to 30 mg/kg up to 1 gm IM‡	NR	Similar to streptomycin.
Para-amino salicylic acid (aminosalicylic acid)	150 mg/kg up to 12 gm PO	NR	Gastrointestinal upset, hepatotoxicity, hypersensitivity, sodium overload.
Viomycin	15 to 30 mg/kg up to 1 gm IM‡	NR	Similar to streptomycin.

*Modified from Glassroth, J.: Tuberculosis: a review for clinicians. *Clinical notes on respiratory diseases*, 20 (2):5–13, 1981 and from Committee on Chemotherapy of Tuberculosis: Standard therapy for tuberculosis 1985. *Chest*, 87(2):117S–124S, 1985.

†NR = Not recommended for twice weekly therapy.

‡Given 2 to 3 times weekly after initial response to therapy.

ical evaluations, adjustments in prescribed medications and treatments, or education about the appropriate use of pulmonary drugs.

5. *Note whether bronchodilator dosages are optimally spaced for around-the-clock bronchodilatation.*
   a. In acute care, check for equal dosing intervals around the clock.
   b. In other settings, the early dose should be scheduled as soon as possible after awakening and the late dose at bedtime. Slow release rather than plain theophylline tablets are best. When needed, PRN bronchodilators should be scheduled in the early morning, when pulmonary signs and symptoms are worse.
6. *Note whether CNS stimulants (e.g., terbutaline and ephedrine) are keeping the patient awake at night.*
   a. Administration of such drugs should be avoided at bedtime.
   b. Some oral beta 2–agents may be changed to aerosol administration to reduce side effects.
7. *Determine whether the patient knowledgeably and skillfully regulated PRN "shortness of breath" drugs.*
   a. Check for indiscriminate use of metered inhalers.
   b. Does the patient know *not* to use inhaled steroids or cromolyn for acute dyspnea?
8. *Identify individuals who may be steroid dependent.*
   a. Maintenance glucocorticoid therapy should be tapered to one 8:00 am dose every day or preferably every other day.
   b. Has the steroid-dependent patient been given a trial of inhaled steroids?
   c. Is the inhaled steroid or cromolyn taken after and not before the inhaled bronchodilator?

Conclusion

This chapter helps the nurse establish and refine skills used in pharmacologic assessment and intervention. It is hoped that this information will facilitate pharmacologic assessment, even before the nurse approaches the patient to interview and examine him. Given a list of pulmonary medications and basic patient information, the nurse should now be able to scan the list of medications, group drugs appropriately, anticipate patient problems, and formulate key questions for more thorough clinical assessment.

The pharmacologic case study presented next will help one apply the information in this chapter and integrate pharmacologic assessment into the pulmonary history. Findings from other respiratory assess-

Table 11–28. ISONIAZID PREVENTIVE THERAPY*

Indications	Contraindications
Conversion of tuberculin skin test results from negative to positive within the past 2 years.	Prior completion of adequate preventive therapy.
Household or other close contact with infected person.	History of adverse reaction to isoniazid.
Less than 35 years of age with positive TB skin test results.	Possible tuberculous disease; multiple drugs required.
Positive TB skin test and x-ray film evidence of previous untreated tuberculosis.	Acute liver disease.
History of inadequately treated tuberculosis.	Pregnancy; preventive therapy is delayed until delivery.
Special situations; e.g., diabetes mellitus; silicosis; postgastrectomy; steroid therapy; immunosuppression; some, hematologic and reticuloendothelial diseases; AIDS and persons with AIDS virus antibodies (i.e., prior positive skin test, unless previously treated); end-stage renal disease; conditions associated with substantial, rapid weight loss or chronic undernutrition.	

*Adapted from Glassroth, J.: Tuberculosis: a review for clinicians. *Clinical notes on respiratory diseases*, 20 (2):5–13, 1981. American Thoracic Society: Treatment of tuberculosis and tuberculosis infection in adults and children. *American review of respiratory disease*, 134(2):355–363, 1986.

ment parameters, particularly the chest examinations (discussed in the next chapter), will facilitate more detailed data collection and confirmation of diagnoses suspected from the pulmonary history.

PHARMACOLOGY CASE STUDY

A 76-year-old COPD patient is admitted to the hospital in acute respiratory distress.

ADMITTING ORDERS

Aminophylline 500 mg in 500 D5W at 40 mg/hr (40 ml/hr)
Tetracycline, 500 mg PO q6h
Solumedrol, 60 mg by intravenous piggyback (IVPB) q6h
Bronkosol, 0.3 ml/2 ml normal saline via IPPB q1h
Oxygen, nasal cannula at 2 L/min
IV, D5W, half normal saline at 100 ml/h

The nursing admission notes included the following data:

VITAL SIGNS

Temperature, 37^5 °C
Monitor, sinus tachycardia 120 beats/min
Respirations, 28/min
Blood pressure, 140/80
Weight, 72 kg

CHEST ASSESSMENT FINDINGS

Labored breathing
Normal breath sounds but with diffuse wheezing over all lung lobes
Coughing up moderate amounts of yellow mucus
Blood theophylline level, 14 mcg/ml
Sputum culture and sensitivity, Gram's stain, results pending

QUESTION

Study the above data base and assess the appropriateness of the patient's pulmonary medications. In your assessment, do the following:

Classify the pulmonary medications by their respective drug groups.

State the probable rationale for use of these drugs. Which problem does each drug treat?

List the most likely patient problems related to drug intervention. How can these problems be avoided?

The most appropriate response to this question is found in Appendix II.

REFERENCES

Ahrens, R. and Smith, G.: Albuterol: an adrenergic agent for use in the treatment of asthma pharmacology, pharmacokinetics and clinical use. *Pharmacotherapy*, 4(3):105–120, 1984.

Al-Bazzar, F.: Practical management of asthma in adults. *Drug therapy*, 10(4):61–72, 1980.

American Thoracic Society: Standards for the diagnosis and care of patients with chronic obstructive pulmonary disease (COPD) and asthma. *American review of respiratory disease*, 136(1):225–244, 1987.

American Thoracic Society: Treatment of tuberculosis and tuberculosis infection in adults and children. *American review of respiratory disease*, 134(2):355–363, 1986.

Andrasch, R. and Schmitz-Schumann, M.: Short-acting versus a long-acting preparation of theophylline ('Xantivent') in the treatment of reversible bronchospasm. *Pharmatherapeutica*, 3(10):668–677, 1984.

Angel, J. (publisher): Physicians' Desk Reference, 38th ed. Oradell, NJ, Medical Economics Co., Inc., 1984.

Barreuter, A.: A drug therapy patient guide: how to treat a cold. *Drug therapy*, 10(10):74–77, 1980.

Bitolterol—a new bronchodilator. *The medical letter on drugs and therapeutics*, 27(088):46–47, May 24, 1985.

Boehringer Ingelheim: Atrovent Inhalation Aerosol—Prescribing Information and Instructions for Use. St. Paul, MN, Riker Laboratories, Inc./3M, 1986.

Brogden, R., Heel, R., Speight, T., and Avery, G.: Beclomethasone dipropionate—a reappraisal of its pharmacodynamic properties and therapeutic efficacy after a decade of use in asthma and rhinitis. *Drugs*, 28 (2):99–126, 1984.

Campbell, A. H.: Mortality from asthma and bronchodilator aerosols. *Medical Journal of Australia*, 2(14):667–669, 1966.

Cherniack, R. and Svanhill, E.: Long-term use of intermittent positive pressure breathing (IPPB) in COPD. *American review of respiratory disease*, 113(6):721–728, 1976.

Chernow, B. and Lake, C.: The Pharmacologic Approach to the Critically Ill Patient. Baltimore, Williams & Wilkins, 1983.

Clark, T. J.: Choice of drug treatment in asthma. *Pharmacology and therapeutics*, 17(2):221–227, 1982.

Cohen, B.: Antitussive effect of guaifenesin. *Chest*, 84(1):119–120, 1983.

Committee on Chemotherapy of Tuberculosis: Standard therapy for tuberculosis 1985. *Chest*, 87(2):117S–124S, 1985.

Cooper, E. and Grant, I.: Beclomethasone dipropionate aerosol in treatment of chronic asthma. *Quarterly journal of medicine*, 46(183):295–308, 1977.

Corticosteroid aerosols for asthma. *The medical letter on drugs and therapeutics*, 27(679):5–6, 1985.

Dasta, J., Mirtallo, J., and Altman, M.: Comparison of standard- and sustained-release theophylline tablets in patients with COPD. *American journal of hospital pharmacy*, 36(5):613–617, 1979.

Estepan, H. and Libby, D.: Glucocorticoid therapy of pulmonary disease. *Drug therapy*, 12(10):109–118, 1982.

Gilston, M.: Clinical Applictions of Respiratory Drugs. Syllabus from Department of Pharmaceutical Services, Hospitals and Clinics of the University of California, Los Angeles, 1980.

Glassroth, J.: Tuberculosis: a review for clinicians. *Clinical notes on respiratory diseases*, 20(2):5–13, 1981.

Goodman, L. and Gilman, A. (eds.): The Pharmacological Basis of Therapeutics, 7th ed. New York, MacMillan Co., Inc., 1985.

Grainger, J. R.: Correct use of aerosol inhalers. *Canadian medical association journal*, 116(6):584–586, 1977.

Gross, N.: Anticholinergic agents in COPD. *Chest*, 91(5):52S–57S, 1987.

Gross, N. and Skorodin, M.: State of the art—anticholinergic, antimuscarinic bronchodilators. *American review of respiratory disease*, 129(5):856–870, 1984.

Hendeles, L., Massanari, M., and Weinberger, M.: Update on the pharmacodynamics and pharmacokinetics of theophylline. *Chest*, 88(2):103S–111S, 1985.

Hendeles, L. and Weinberger, M.: Theophylline—a "state of the art" review. *Pharmacotherapy*, 3(1):2–44, 1983.

Horn, B., et al: Total eosinophil counts in the management of bronchial asthma. *New England journal of medicine*, 292(22):1152–1155, 1975.

Hudson, L.: Management of COPD—state of the art. *Chest*, 84(6):76S–81S, 1984.

Inman, W. and Adelstein, A.: Rise and fall of asthma mortality in England and Wales in relation to use of pressurized aerosols. *Lancet*, 1(7615):279–285, 1969.

Kass, I., Nair, S. V., and Patil, K.: Beclomethasone dipropionate aerosol in the treatment of steroid-dependent asthmatic patients. *Chest*, 71(6):703–707, 1977.

Kirilloff, L. and Tibbals, S.: Drugs for asthma—a complete guide. *American journal of nursing*, 83(1):55–61, 1983.

Küng, M., White, J., and Burki, N.: The effect of subcutaneously administered terbutaline on serum potassium in asymptomatic adult asthmatics. *American review of respiratory disease*, 129(2):329–332, 1984.

Leff, A.: Pathogenesis of asthma—neurophysiology and pharmacology of bronchospasm, *Chest*, 81(2):224–229, 1982.

Lehnert, B. and Schachter, E.: The Pharmacology of Respiratory Care. St. Louis, C. V. Mosby Co., 1980.

Mathewson, H.: Anticholinergic aerosols. *Respiratory care*, 28(4):467–469, 1983.

Mathewson, H.: Risks and benefits of aerosolized steroids. *Respiratory care*, 28(3):325–326, 1983.

Matthay, R. and Depew, C.: Rational therapy for asthma with theophylline agents. *Respiratory therapy*, 10(5):53–59, 1980.

Morris, H.: Mechanisms of glucocorticoid action in pulmonary disease. *Chest*, 133S–141S, 1985.

Nelson, H.: Getting the most out of beta-adrenergics today. *The journal of respiratory diseases*, 3(3):11–19, 1982.

Newman, S.: Factors influencing the efficacy of inhaled bronchodilators. *Respiratory therapy*, 13(4):37–45, 1983.

Newman, S., Pravia, D., and Clarke, S. W.: How should a pressurized beta-adrenergic bronchodilator be inhaled? *European journal of respiratory diseases*, 62(1):3–21, 1981.

Nicholson, D.: A problem in clinical research: asthma and cromolyn sodium. *Heart and lung*, 5(1):71–75, 1976.

Paterson, J., Woolcock, A., and Shenfield, G.: State of the art—bronchodilator drugs. *American review of respiratory disease*, 120 (5):1149–1181, 1979.

Richards, W., Church, J., and Lawrence, R.: Uses and limitations of corticosteroids in asthma. *Drug therapy*, 4(5):52–59, 1979.

Rodman, M., et al: Pharmacology and Drug Therapy, 3rd ed. Philadelphia, J. B. Lippincott Co., 1985.

Sackner, M. and Kim, C.: Auxiliary MDI aerosol delivery systems. *Chest*, 88(2):161S–169S, 1985.

Sahn, S.: Critical review—corticosteroids in chronic bronchitis and pulmonary emphysema. *Chest*, 73(3):389–395, 1978.

Scoggin, C. and Petty, T.: Clinical Strategies in Adult Asthma. Philadelphia, Lea & Febiger, 1982.

Shrake, K. and Oltmann, T.: Effective use of wetting agents, Mucolytics, and bronchodilators. *Respiratory therapy*, 10(6):73–77, 1980.

Shenfield, G.: Combination bronchodilator therapy. *Drugs*, 24(5):414–439, 1982.

Skatrud, J. J., Dempsey, J., Iber, C., and Berssenbrugge, A.: Correction of CO_2 retention during sleep in patients with COPD. *American review of respiratory disease*, 124(3):260–268, 1981.

Smith, G.: How to use theophylline for maximal benefit in pulmonary disease. *Respiratory therapy*, 13(4):31–33, 1983.

Spector, S., Siegel, S., Katz, R., et al: Theophylline dose-dumping. *Chest*, 86(2):317, 1986.

Spiro, H.: Is the steroid ulcer a myth? *New England journal of medicine*, 309(1):45–47, 1983.

Stiel, I. and Rivington, R.: Adrenergic agents in acute asthma: valuable new alternatives. *Annals of emergency medicine*, 12(8):493–500, 1983.

Tobin, M., Jenouri, G., et al: Response to bronchodilator drug administration by a new reservoir aerosol delivery system and a review of other auxiliary delivery systems. *American review of respiratory disease*, 126(4):670–675, 1982.

Viires, N., Aubier, M., et al: Effects of aminophylline on diaphragmatic fatigue during acute respiratory failure. *American review of respiratory disease*, 129(3):396–402, 1984.

Vozeh, S., Kewitz, G. et al: Theophylline serum concentration and therapeutic effect in severe acute bronchial obstruction: the optimal use of intravenously administered aminophylline. *American review of respiratory disease*, 125(2):181–184, 1982.

Webb-Johnson, D. and Andrews, J.: Bronchodilator therapy. *New England journal of medicine*, 297(8):476–482, 1977.

Weiss, E., Segal, M., and Stein, M.: Bronchial asthma—mechanisms and therapeutics, 2nd ed. Boston, Little, Brown & Co., 1985.

Wolfe, J., Tashkin, D., Calvarese, B., and Simmons, M.: Bronchodilator effects of terbutaline and aminophylline alone and in combination in asthmatic patients. *New England journal of medicine*, 298(7):363–367, 1978.

Yeates, D.: Clearance of secretions from the lungs. *Drug therapy*, 10(4):107–111, 1980.

Ziment, I.: Respiratory Pharmacology and Therapeutics. Philadelphia, W. B. Saunders Co., 1978.

The Complete Chest Examination

12

Main Objectives

PRELIMINARY INFORMATION

1. **Name four purposes for physical examination of the chest.**
2. **Describe the use of the chest examination as a vital sign in at least three different clinical settings.**
3. **Draw vertical imaginary lines and lobes of the lungs on pictures of anterior, lateral, and posterior views of the chest. Identify by marking with an X the crucial reference points that help locate boundaries between lobes.**
4. **Describe background patient information and general observations most helpful in providing clues as to how to approach the patient; describe which components of the examination should be emphasized.**
5. **Describe how to collect and examine sputum.**
6. **Name the four basic steps for preparing the patient for the examination.**

EXTRATHORACIC EXAMINATION

7. **Describe how to examine the head and neck, trachea, and extremities for signs of cardiopulmonary disease.**
8. **List at least six extrathoracic signs of respiratory distress.**

9. State the significance of the following abnormal findings: blue-tinged lips, neck lymphadenopathy, subcutaneous emphysema, elevated mean venous pressure, lateral displacement of the trachea, digital clubbing, dependent edema, and asterixis.
10. Describe the physiologic mechanism and presentation of jugular venous distention in right ventricular failure versus chronic obstructive pulmonary disease (COPD).

EXAMINATION OF THORAX AND LUNGS

11. Name the four components of the examination of the thorax and lungs.
12. Describe how to inspect and palpate the chest, including the precordium.
13. List the normal respiratory rate ranges for infants, children, and adults. Describe normal breathing patterns for adults and infants during wakefulness and sleep.
14. Define and state the significance of the following abnormal findings: increased anteroposterior (AP) diameter; kyphoscoliosis; I:E ratios of 1:1, 3:1, and 1:4; labored breathing; minimal and maximal chest excursions; paradoxical chest movements; flail chest; and en bloc chest movement.
15. Define and state the significance of decreased lateral chest expansion, rhonchal fremitus, pleural rub fremitus, and increased and decreased vocal (tactile) fremitus.
16. Identify and describe the precordial pulsations that are characteristically present or absent on the chest's surface in respiratory patients.
17. Differentiate between right-sided and left-sided cardiac auscultatory findings.
18. Identify the anticipated percussion note for each of the following: normal lung tissue, severe emphysema, atelectasis, fibrosis, lobar pneumonia, pleural effusion, pneumothorax, and distended stomach.
19. Describe the ideal stethoscope and its correct usage in the clinical setting.
20. Define and state the significance of bronchophony, egophony, and whispered pectoriloquy.
21. Describe the basic methodology for auscultation of the lungs.
22. Describe the characteristic features, physiologic mechanisms (for sound production and transmission), and clinical significance of basic breath sounds (normal, bronchial, and bronchovesicular) and adventitious sounds (crackles, rhonchi, wheeze, and pleural friction rub).
23. Compare and contrast chest assessment findings for lobar pneumonia and pleural effusion.

CHARTING AND INTERPRETATION OF FINDINGS

24. Using a recording example of a complete chest examination, identify respiratory problems and definitive chest assessment findings that support each problem.

LEARNING CHEST ASSESSMENT

25. Describe the learning prerequisites for successful implementation of chest assessment skills in the clinical setting.
26. Describe how to perform a quick chest examination.

This chapter provides an extensive knowledge base for physical examination of the chest, including examination of the extrathoracic structures most important in respiratory disease as well as the thorax and lungs. It is my hope that it will serve as a guideline for nurses and other health professionals interested in learning or sharpening their chest assessment skills. These skills tend to be underutilized by bedside personnel because, as this chapter points out, they take time, patience, and supervision to learn well enough to use efficiently and appropriately in clinical practice. Yet, of all the respiratory parameters, chest assessment is perhaps the most important because it is noninvasive, cost effective, and otherwise practical. Individual skills can be utilized by all bedside personnel who care for patients as they pass through the health care continuum.

SECTION I—PRELIMINARY INFORMATION

Purpose

Physical examination of the chest has many uses that are directly related to one another.

VERIFICATION OF PATIENT'S HISTORY

Physical examination provides objective data to support subjective complaints, such as chest tightness, wheezing, and shortness of breath. If objective findings are absent, the patient's problems may be restricted to other settings (workplace or home), or they may be psychosocial in nature. When complaints are absent and physical findings are prominent, the patient may be providing an unreliable history, or he may be denying their existence, a common psychologic coping mechanism of patients with chronic obstructive pulmonary disease (COPD). Such uncomplaining patients require closer monitoring than complaining patients.

DOCUMENTATION OF PATIENT'S PROBLEMS

The chest examination may be the nurse's *only* reliable tool for documenting respiratory problems. Unlike the physician, who is aware of the patient's baseline chest assessment findings in addition to other objective findings, the nurse is often without immediate access to the history and physical examination report, blood gas results, and other diagnostic test results. This is a continual problem for emergency room nurses, nurses on evening or night shifts, and visiting nurses in the home; they have limited access to both the physician and the medical chart. Particularly when the patient is asymptomatic or not fully conscious or when symptoms are vague, a conscientious physical examination by the nurse is required to document possible or actual bronchoconstriction, impaired ventilation, hypoxemia, mucus retention, or fluid overload.

DIAGNOSIS OF PULMONARY DISEASES AND DISORDERS

Although the physician has primary responsibility for medical diagnosis, the nurse identifies and reports signs and symptoms that frequently are crucial to diagnosis. The nurse's role in diagnosis is vital in the case of patients who are reluctant to "bother" the physician with seemingly minor complaints. It is also crucial in asymptomatic patients, patients with labile cardiopulmonary conditions, and chronic disease patients who have lived so long with a particular sign or symptom that they think it is normal and nothing to complain about. Moreover, owing to the rising costs of medical care and limited patient access to medical care, some nurses are actively involved in medical diagnosis, as they screen patients for lung disorders under a physician's supervision.

MONITORING RESPIRATORY PROBLEMS

The chest examination is the most inexpensive and practical parameter for monitoring problems associated with respiratory disease. It requires only a skilled individual and a stethoscope, and it is one parameter that does *not* require a physician's order. When combined with vital signs and the patient's complaints, chest assessment findings can indicate the patient's status: better, worse, or unchanged. In some situations, one physical finding is enough to justify alterations in nursing interventions. For example, wheezing on auscultation is typically the sign that prompts the nurse to give a PRN aerosol treatment with a bronchodilator.

Indications

Because physical examination of the chest provides crucial objective data, it is considered a vital sign for *all* cardiopulmonary patients. Indications specific to different settings are described hereafter.

ACUTE CARE UNIT

Nurses on each shift perform a quick chest examination on *all* acute patients during their initial nursing assessment. (See the end of this chapter for the quick chest examination, a short form of the complete examination discussed here.) Further examination is done whenever signs of a changing cardiopulmonary status appear.

GENERAL MEDICAL-SURGICAL WARD

Nurses incorporate the quick chest examination into the standard nursing assessment for all newly admitted patients. An admitting examination establishes baseline chest assessment findings for later comparison should the patient's status change. Otherwise, the nurse routinely examines respiratory patients once a shift and PRN. A second but very important priority is any patient at risk for pulmonary complications, e.g., cardiac, postsurgical, debilitated, and immobile patients, and patients receiving fluid challenges by intravenous infusion.

DIALYSIS UNIT

Nurses perform a quick chest examination on every patient before and after renal dialysis. Pulmonary problems may develop in chronic renal failure patients, in whom lung tissue loses its integrity with advanced renal disease and severe acidosis. The more acidotic and fluid overloaded the patient is before dialysis, the more likely the possibility that excess fluid has leaked into interstitial spaces, alveoli, and the pleural space (i.e., pleural effusion), producing crackles and decreased breath sounds. The chest examination is necessary to assess the presence and extent of this fluid leakage as well as the common complications of heart failure.

Dialysis usually removes excess fluid from the body or at least keeps it to acceptable levels. With the removal of fluid from the lungs and pleural space, chest assessment findings should improve after dialysis and may become normal. If they do not improve markedly, the physician should be notified. The patient's dry weight is reevaluated, and it may be reduced for subsequent dialysis to facilitate fluid removal from the lungs.

The quick chest examination is needed to screen renal patients for underlying chronic lung disease. The presence of COPD complicates the management of acid-base disturbances and exacerbates any existing oxygenation problems. Also, unless problems associated with COPD are routinely monitored, they tend to be overshadowed by concerns related to dialysis and chronic renal disease, and they may remain neglected.

PSYCHIATRIC WARD

The quick chest examination is used once a shift and PRN for all patients with a history of respiratory problems, particularly those on sedatives and tranquilizers. The respiratory depressant effect of these medications can cause alveolar hypoventilation and ventilatory failure in a relatively short period of time in asymptomatic patients with underlying lung disease.

HOME SETTING

The visiting nurse performs at least a quick examination on all new patients whenever a case is officially opened. Patients seen for other than respiratory problems may also have some undiagnosed or uncharted chronic pulmonary disorder, e.g., the orthopedic patient with chronic cough and the renal or cardiac patient with poor exercise tolerance. Furthermore, in the absence of other objective data, a meticulous examination is needed to identify subtle changes in findings, thereby providing sufficient documentation of the need for further monitoring and health care teaching in the home for insurance carriers.

AMBULATORY SETTINGS

Many nurses in ambulatory settings incorporate the physical examination of the chest into a more thorough evaluation of the patient. They utilize most of the components of the complete examination to delineate baseline findings. Subsequently, different components are used as indicated by the situation and as time permits.

Basic Tools—Anatomic Landmarks and Terminology for Charting

Examination of the chest requires a basic knowledge of the anatomy of the bony thorax and anatomic landmarks that serve as reference points for the description of findings. Turn to Chapter 1 and study the anatomy of the lungs within the bony thorax. In particular, note the location of the clavicles, ribs, manubrium, body of the sternum, seventh cervical vertebra, thoracic vertebrae, and the scapulae (see Fig. 1–10). Anatomic landmarks and other reference points used in the identification and description of chest examination findings are discussed here.

VERTICAL IMAGINARY LINES

Vertical imaginary lines are used as reference points to accurately describe and chart the location of normal and abnormal findings, particularly the apical impulse and abnormalities on the surface of the chest.

Anterior Area of the Chest

Anteriorly, three different imaginary lines vertically traverse the chest: the *midsternal line* (MSL), the *midclavicular lines* (MCL), and the *anterior axillary lines* (AAL) (Fig. 12–1). The MSL runs down the center of the sternum. The right and left midclavicular lines (RMCL and LMCL) run down the anterior chest starting from the midpoints of the clavicles. The right and left anterior axillary lines (RAAL and LAAL) run vertically down from the anterior axillary folds.

Lateral Area of the Chest

The *anterior axillary line* (AAL), *midaxillary line* (MAL), and *posterior axillary line* (PAL) are viewed from the side and are used to help describe the location of abnormalities in lateral areas of the chest (Fig. 12–2). The right and left midaxillary lines (RMAL and LMAL) run vertically downward from the centerpoints

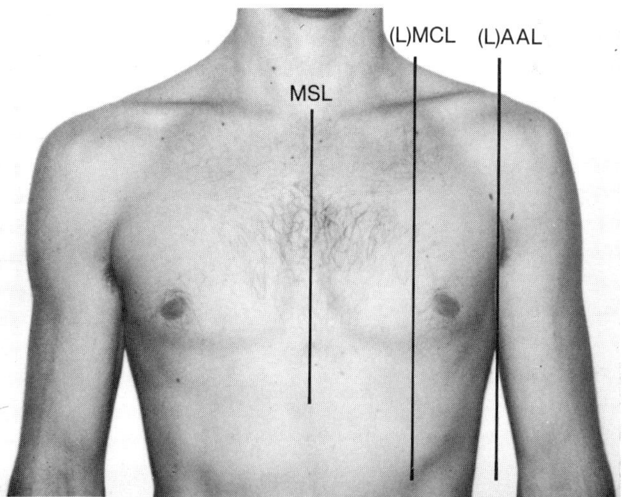

Figure 12–1. Vertical imaginary lines shown on the anterior chest region. MSL = midsternal line; (L)MCL = (left) midclavicular line; (L)AAL = (left) anterior axillary line.

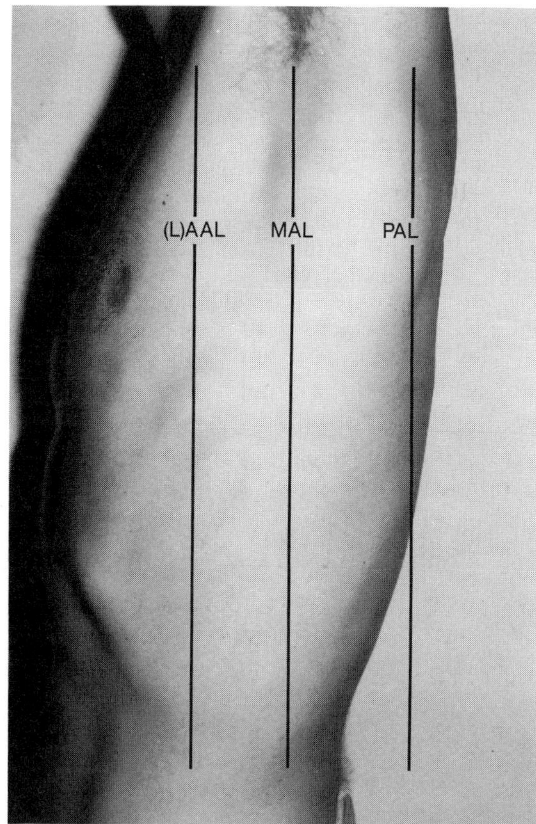

Figure 12–2. Vertical imaginary lines shown on the left lateral side of the chest. (L)AAL = anterior axillary line; MAL = midaxillary line; and PAL = posterior axillary line.

of the axillae. The right and left posterior axillary lines (RPAL and LPAL) run down the posterior axillary folds.

Posterior Area of the Chest

The *vertebral line* (VL) runs along the spinous processes of the vertebrae (Fig. 12–3). The *right scapular line* (RScL) and *left scapular line* (LScL) run through the middle of the inferior angles of the scapulae.

COUNTING RIBS AND INTERCOSTAL SPACES

Ribs and intercostal spaces (ICS) are also used as reference points to describe the location of normal and abnormal physical findings as well as to appropriately place ECG electrodes on the surface of the chest.

To count the ribs of the anterior chest, first find the sternal angle (angle of Louis). This is a bony protuberance where the manubrium joins the body of the sternum. In many thin, elderly people this protuberance is noticeable merely on inspection. In other normal adults, it might be barely identifiable on palpation. *To locate the sternal angle,* firmly place the fingertips of your three middle fingers along the patient's MSL, 2 to 6 cm below the sternal notch. Pressing firmly, move your fingertips up and down until you locate a bump. This bump is sometimes more prominent on the left side of the junction of the manubrium with the body of the sternum. Place a fingertip on the top of the sternal angle. Slowly move it downwards and laterally towards the 4-o'clock position until you feel an ICS. This ICS is the second ICS (Fig. 12–4). The second rib is *above* the second ICS. From the second ICS, count down to the level of other ribs or ICSs adjacent to the finding being described.

CHARTING CHEST SURFACE FINDINGS

When charting findings located on the surface of the chest, use abbreviations whenever possible as well as simple analogies to save time and to make charting more succinct and comprehensible. Some examples are as follows:

1. *Apical impulse visible 5th ICS, MCL.*
2. *Area the size of a quarter tender to palpation 5th rib, RAAL.*
3. *Linear keloid scar runs from MSL to LAAL at the level of the 4th rib.*

LOCATING THE LOBES OF THE LUNGS

To describe the location of auscultatory findings and large areas on the surface of the chest, use the underlying lobes of the lungs as main reference points.

Anterior Area of the Chest

Two basic landmarks—the *right fourth rib* and the *right and left sixth ribs, MCL*—help to identify the

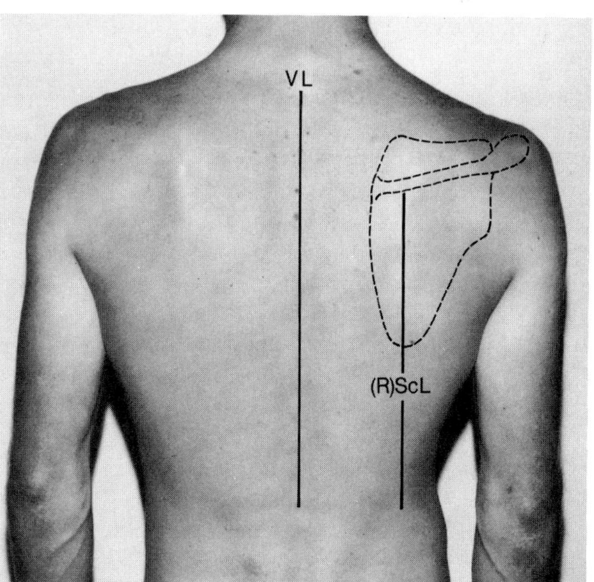

Figure 12–3. Vertical imaginary lines shown on the posterior chest region. VL = vertebral line and (R)ScL = right scapular line.

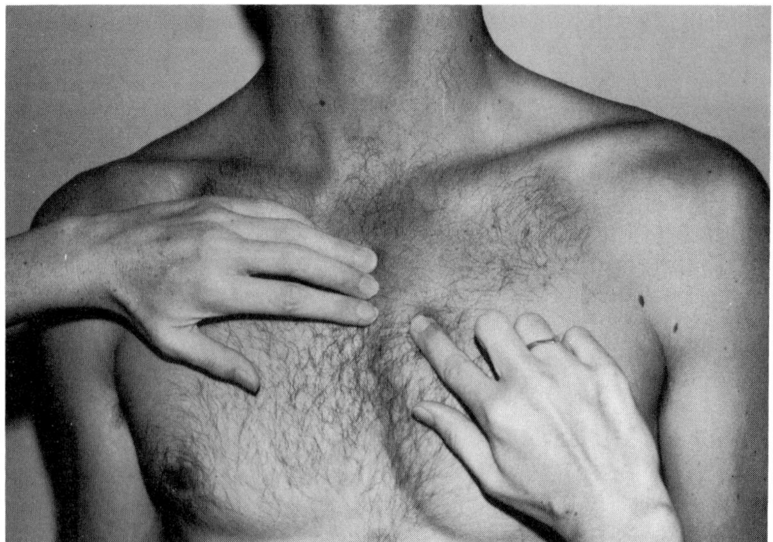

Figure 12–4. Locating the sternal angle and second intercostal space (ICS). Adjust the fingertips of the left hand until the prominence or "bump" marking the sternal angle lies directly under the middle finger. The right index finger marks the 4-o'clock position of the second ICS.

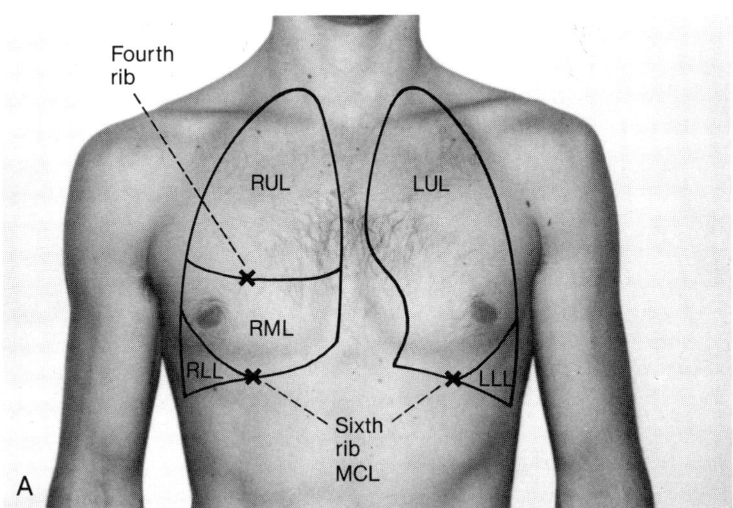

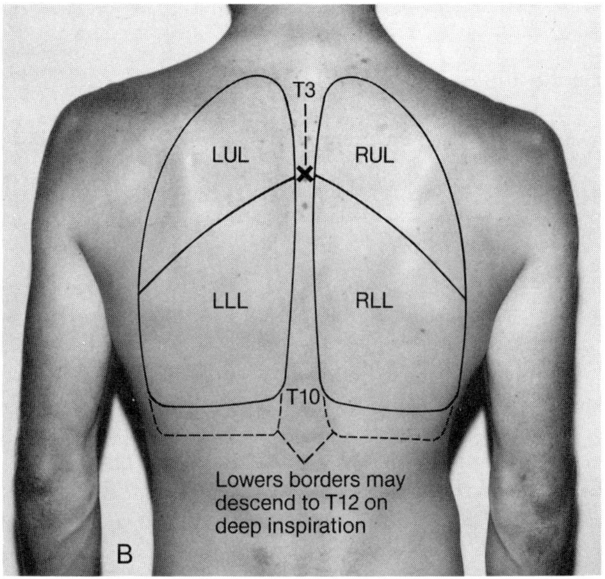

Figure 12–5. Locating the lobes of the lungs in anterior (A) and posterior (B) chest regions and in right and left lateral chest regions (C and D). (RUL = right upper lobe; RML = right middle lobe; RLL = right lower lobe; LUL = left upper lobe; LLL = left lower lobe; MCL = midclavicular line; MAL = midaxillary line; and T = thoracic vertebrae.)

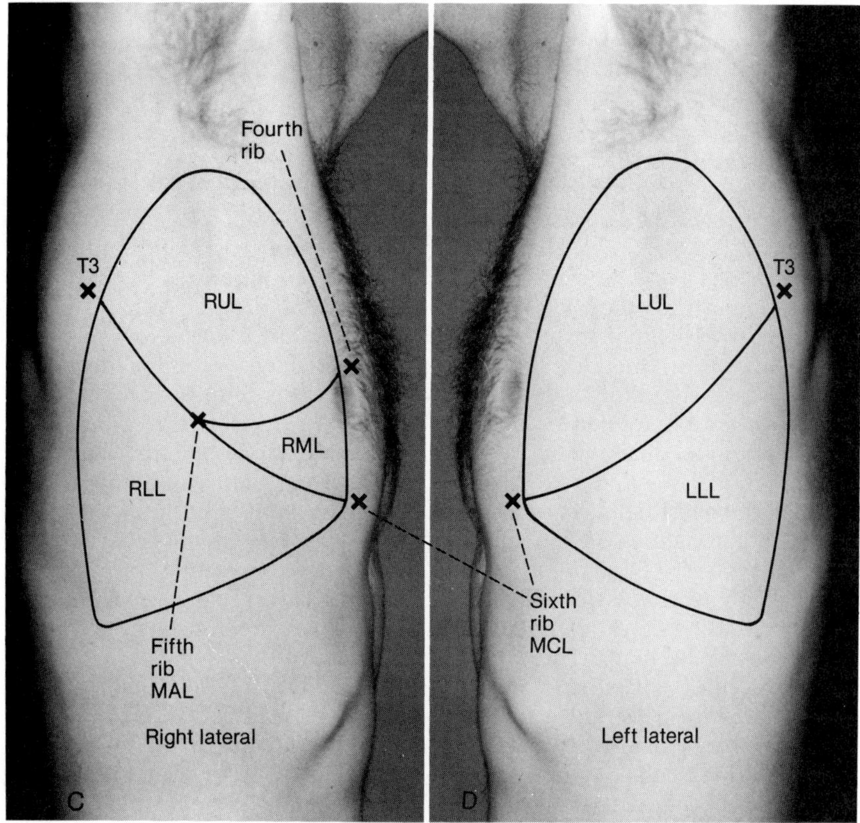

Figure 12–5 *Continued*

underlying lobes of the anterior chest. The right fourth rib is important because it marks the location of the *minor fissure*, which divides the right upper lobe (RUL) from the right middle lobe (RML) below. The right and left sixth ribs are important landmarks because they mark just how far the lower lobes extend anteriorly (Fig. 12–5A). Utilizing these landmarks to identify findings, the nurse might then chart the following: *decreased breath sounds RML* or *mild chest pain on inspiration LLL laterally*.

Lateral Area of the Chest

Study the lateral view of the chest to identify the underlying lobes of the lungs (Fig. 12–5B). Note that the right lower lobe (RLL) and left lower lobe (LLL) occupy the lower lateral chest areas. Also note that only a small wedge of RML extends to the MAL. This lobe lies only in the anterior area of the chest; it does not extend beyond the MAL to the posterior area of the chest. Remember from Chapter 1 that the left lung has no middle lobe; the lingular segments of the left upper lobe correspond to the RML.

Posterior Area of the Chest

To localize findings posteriorly, use these essential landmarks: the *scapulae*, the *spinous process of the seventh cervical vertebra*, and the *spinous processes of the 12 thoracic vertebrae*. The scapulae are familiar landmarks and are easy to palpate.

To count the spinous processes of the vertebrae, ask the patient to flex his neck forward, as in Figure 12–6. The first protuberance palpated in the lower neck

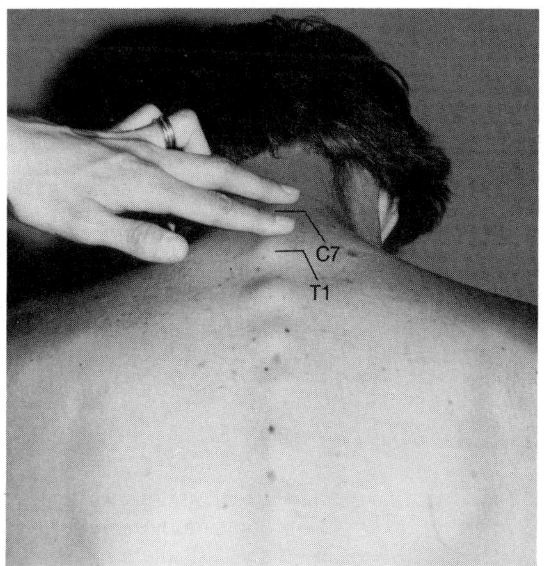

Figure 12–6. A method for counting the spinous processes of the vertebrae.

area is the seventh cervical vertebra (C7). Below a slight depression (intervertebral space), the second protuberance is the spinous process of the first thoracic vertebra (T1). The spinous process of T1 may be more prominent than that of C7. Once C7 and T1 are identified, the other 11 processes follow in order. If they are difficult to palpate, ask the patient to bend over; flexion of the spine makes the processes more protuberant.

For obese patients or elderly patients whose intervertebral cartilages have almost completely calcified, the nurse may not be able to reliably palpate spinous processes or intervertebral spaces. One must estimate the location of the processes using other landmarks as guides. One optional landmark is the inferior angle or tip of the scapula. In most individuals, it lies at the level of the seventh rib.

In the posterior area of the chest, spinous processes may be used to localize abnormalities on the surface of the chest, e.g., *faint red rash 6 cm in diameter noted at the level of the spinous process of T6*. However, they are most frequently used to estimate the location of underlying lobes of the lungs. The *spinous process of T3 or T4* is the most crucial landmark. It lies at the level of the tracheal carina and marks the inferior borders of the upper lobes as well as the superior borders of the lower lobes. Note in the posterior view of the chest (see Fig. 12–5B) that the lower lobes (i.e., superior segments) lie immediately below the *midposterior* chest area, forming the top portion of a symmetric cone or "teepee" with the tip at T3.

Once the nurse is familiar with vertical imaginary lines and other anatomic landmarks previously described, preparation for the physical examination can begin.

Background Patient Information—Clues for Approach to Patient

Background patient information provides clues as to what signs to look for, which components of the complete examination to use, and what areas of the lungs to thoroughly examine. This information is obtained from the nursing history completed beforehand, the medical chart, and a brief, informal interview just before the examination to update the patient's chief complaints. The following points are most important.

MEDICAL DIAGNOSIS

Diagnosis is a prime factor in determining which aspects to emphasize. For lobar pneumonia, the nurse may thoroughly examine pathologic lobes and only inspect and auscultate uninvolved lobes. For myocardial infarction, checking for signs of atelectasis and fluid retention (e.g., in congestive heart failure) in the dependent lower lobes becomes most important. For COPD, the nurse looks for signs of airway obstruction or air flow limitation.

SIGNS AND SYMPTOMS

Presenting complaints or findings reported by others suggest an approach to the patient, as the following examples indicate.

1. *Patient reported coughing up sputum*—check for signs of mucus retention (decreased breath sounds and adventitious sounds).
2. *C/O (complains of) chest tightness*—check for wheezing on auscultation.
3. *Renal patient with 30 pack-year history of cigarette smoking*—check for signs of airway obstruction.
4. *C/O chest pain*—check for signs of impaired lung ventilation (splinting respirations, decreased breath sounds, or crackles over painful area).

PULMONARY MEDICATIONS AND RESPIRATORY TREATMENTS

Since these suggest the existence of a pulmonary disorder, the patient usually requires more than just a quick chest examination. During the examination of the patient, note the time of the last bronchodilator medication, e.g., oral or inhaled via handheld nebulizer or metered dose device (MDD). Chest assessment findings are usually better immediately after respiratory treatments and much worse immediately preceding scheduled treatments with bronchodilator medications.

DIAGNOSTIC TESTS

When available, diagnostic tests indicate pathologic areas requiring thorough evaluation. *Ventilation or perfusion defects* on the lung scan or an *infiltrate* on the chest x-ray indicates areas that must be incorporated into the quick chest examination. *Bullae* on the chest x-ray are also important because the associated regional decrease in alveolar ventilation is conducive to mucus retention if the COPD patient has a significant bronchitic component. In some cases, the chest x-ray may be the *only* indicator of pathology. For example, an infiltrate in the medial segment of the lung is often missed on physical examination because the overlying axillary area is not routinely auscultated.

General Observations

General observations while greeting the patient will help determine how to examine the patient and interpret the data collected.

FIRST IMPRESSIONS

By viewing the patient from the door, the nurse can often determine whether the patient is in any emotional or respiratory distress and whether he will tolerate a complete or quick chest examination. The patient's resting position may suggest the presence of dyspnea, e.g., hunched over the bedside stand or sleeping upright in bed. A positive overall demeanor suggests a stable pulmonary status, whereas a negative demeanor with signs of fatigue and dyspnea suggests worsening chest symptoms.

NEW COMPLAINTS

First impressions might be based solely on the patient's ready complaint of a new symptom, such as a feeling of suffocation, chest tightness, or wheezing. The new complaint may be totally unrelated to signs and symptoms reported upon admission.

PRESENTING SIGNS

At the bedside, the nurse notes *sounds of breathing, cough*, and *sputum production.*

Sounds of Breathing

Normal breathing is quiet except for occasional audible signs. Audible wheezing indicates severe bronchospasm. Gurgling from secretions indicates mucus retention and a need for coughing, repositioning, and possibly other bronchial hygiene measures. The presence of stridor (i.e., high-pitched crowing on inspiration) indicates upper airway obstruction, requiring immediate medical attention.

Cough

Cough is an abnormal finding indicating airway irritation or obstruction with or without the presence of secretions. Note whether the cough is *strong* or *weak, dry* or *hacking*, and *productive* or *nonproductive.*

A *weak cough* may be due to muscle weakness or paralysis of respiratory muscles, both seen in neuromuscular disease. Other causes are anesthesia, use of sedatives or narcotics, fatigue, splinting from abdominal or chest pain, inflammation of the epiglottis, and the presence of an endotracheal tube. The patient with a weak cough is a prime candidate for a chest infection owing to the inability to cough up retained secretions.

The patient with both a *weak cough* and a *poor cough reflex* from neuromuscular disease or drugs is at risk to aspirate saliva, mucus, or gastric contents and develop aspiration pneumonia. The intubated patient with a poor cough reflex may also aspirate secretions, if the endotracheal tube cuff is not adjusted to proper inflating pressures with changes in body position.

A *dry, hacking cough* suggests airway irritation from secretions, atelectasis, or other forms of airway obstruction.

Sputum Production

To evaluate sputum production, ask the patient to cough up sputum into a white tissue (Fig. 12–7A) or down the side of a bedside sputum cup (Fig. 12–7B) for your *direct* observation (never rely on historical data). A sputum cup is a better receptacle than a tissue because it permits closer inspection of sputum color and odor and mucus plugs. Consistency can be evaluated by tipping the cup in two directions; thick mucus tends to stick to the sides of the cup. If the patient is unable to cough up sputum, instruct him to save early morning sputum in a covered cup for later examination. If the patient is suctioned endotracheally, inspect secretions left in the suction catheter and adjoining connecting tubing.

As Chapter 10 points out, estimation of sputum quantity is also important. If a sputum cup is already at the bedside, the nurse notes the *amount produced over the last 24 hours.* Increased amounts might indicate a new chest infection, unresponsiveness to

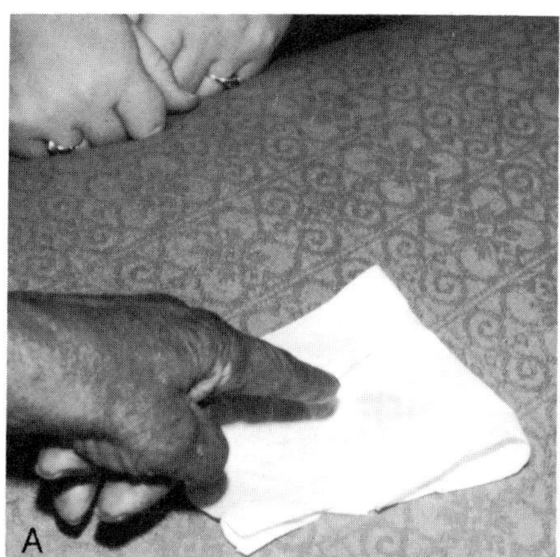

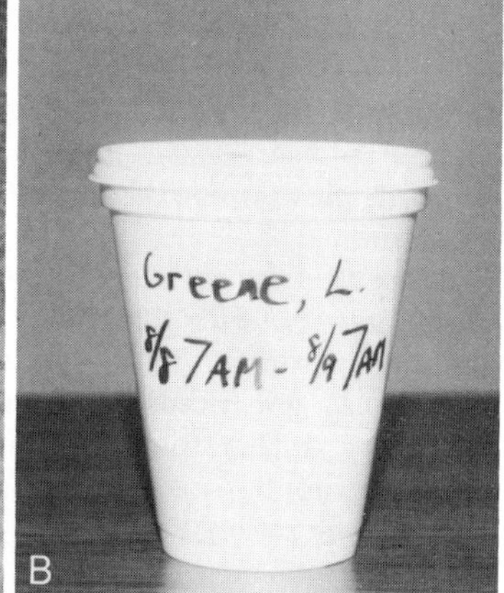

Figure 12–7. A method for monitoring of sputum. *A*, Patient and nurse observe sputum together to agree on its actual appearance—clear versus yellow. *B*, For a patient who regularly coughs up sputum, a daily sputum cup is used to monitor *amount, color, odor*, and *consistency.*

present antibiotic therapy, an increase in airway obstruction, or a worsening bronchitic component.

If direct observation of sputum is not possible, ask staff to start monitoring sputum. A fresh sputum cup is placed at the patient's bedside early each morning before the patient awakens. An early starting time is important because most patients cough up more sputum in the morning—after lying in bed all night more mucus accumulates. Also, an early time insures the collection of *fresh* sputum for morning rounds, a better indicator of recent progress. A clear plastic graduated specimen container may be used to better visualize the contents, but a plain cardboard cup with a lid and white interior can serve the same purpose and is more aesthetic to keep at the bedside. The cup does not have to be sterile, and it should be labelled with the patient's name, the date, and designated period of time for collection as shown in Figure 12–7B.

Preparing the Patient

After general observations, the nurse prepares the patient for the examination.

1. *First, briefly explain the procedure to the patient in simple terms.* Patients may become uncooperative if the purpose and simple logistics are not explained, particularly when patients do not know what the procedure will involve on their part. Some nurses may surprise the elderly patient because, in the past, only the physician ever listened to the lungs or tapped on the chest.

Some nurses have difficulty with this first step because of reluctance to "bother" the patient unnecessarily and lack of self confidence in their ability to perform the procedure efficiently. However, clinical skills cannot be perfected without going through the normal period of "fumbling around" and feeling inefficient. Eventually, practice yields efficiency. To ensure full patient cooperation, the nurse must approach the patient with a positive attitude and explain that the chest examination is a crucial vital sign as well as a therapeutic treatment (deep breathing helps keep the lungs clear).

2. *Provide a warm, comfortable environment.* Close the door of the room for privacy and to eliminate distracting sounds. Pull the bedside curtain around the bed when other patients are in the room. Patients in the home setting may want to move to the bedroom for the physical examination. When cold drafts are present, close open windows to promote comfort and relaxation.

3. *Expose the chest area to adequate light.* Ask male ambulatory patients to undress to the waist. Ask female patients to remove underclothing above the waist and to put on a gown that the examiner can remove when necessary during the procedure. Full exposure with adequate light is necessary to pick up subtle changes in skin coloration, pulsations, and other findings on the surface of the chest.

4. *Position the patient correctly.* To promote patient comfort and careful examination, the nurse examines the anterior area of the chest with the patient resting comfortably at a 30- to 60-degree angle. Then, to examine the posterior thorax and lungs, the nurse asks the patient to sit up, move his arms forward, and place his hands in his lap. This maneuver moves the scapulae laterally and exposes more of the lung fields in the midback area (see Fig. 12–41). The anxious or dyspneic patient may be unable to recline and may prefer to sit on the edge of the bed, leaning on the bedside stand with his arms extended across the stand. Use a position that is most comfortable for both you and the patient. A relaxed patient is easier to examine, less anxious, and more likely to exhibit true baseline chest assessment findings. If the patient prefers to lean over the bedside stand, be sure he does not lean heavily on his elbows or arms when you listen to the upper lobes. Tense, shrugged shoulders can create compression of underlying lung tissue and bronchial breath sounds, not a true baseline finding. Furthermore, if the patient is sitting up or leaning forward at any time during the examination, make sure the two sides of the thorax are on the same horizontal plane; the patient should not lean more to one side than the other. Leaning to one side might create the false positive finding of decreased breath sounds where the movement of the chest is restricted by poor posture. The nurse in the acute care unit usually must get help to lift the patient up and *directly* forward a few inches to listen to the bases of the lower lobes posteriorly.

SECTION II—THE EXTRATHORACIC EXAMINATION

The complete physical examination of the chest begins with the extrathoracic examination. Components of the extrathoracic examination are reviewed in the box on the opposite page.

Head and Neck

The examiner starts with the head and neck and moves outward to the peripheral extremities, using a combination of inspection and palpation to check for the presence or absence of extrathoracic signs of cardiopulmonary disease.

SKIN COLOR

When approaching the bedside, the nurse immediately looks for pallor and cyanosis. *Cyanosis* is bluish or grayish discoloration of the skin caused by a decreased PaO_2. A general cyanotic appearance indicates

THE EXTRATHORACIC EXAMINATION

HEAD AND NECK
Skin color
Cyanosis, pallor, reddish-blue or ruddy complexion, pale or cyanotic mucous membranes
General symmetry
Regular or irregular
Swollen areas
Traumatized or inflamed tissue, tumor, lymphadenopathy, subcutaneous emphysema
Neck veins
Jugular venous distention, mean venous pressure, estimated CVP, venous filling

TRACHEA
Anterior or posterior displacement
Displacement to the right or left

EXTRATHORACIC SIGNS OF RESPIRATORY DISTRESS
Cyanosis or pallor
Neck vein distention
Facial tension
Nasal flaring
Movement of thyroid cartilage (Adam's apple) with respiration
Disconnected speech pattern
Grunting (infant)
Use of neck muscles with suprasternal notch and supraclavicular space retractions
Altered level of consciousness

EXTREMITIES
Skin coloration
Pallor, cyanosis, reddish-blue or ruddy coloration
Nail bed capillary refill
Poor, sluggish
Fingernails and toenails
Tobacco stains, prominent vertical ridges
Clubbing
Early, advanced, hypertrophic pulmonary osteoarthropathy
Peripheral edema
Dependent, pitting, nonpitting
Asterixis, drug-induced tremor from bronchodilators

a *central* oxygenation problem; PaO_2 is decreased throughout the entire pool of blood in the body. It is a sign of respiratory distress and imminent cardiopulmonary arrest. *Pallor* may or may not indicate an oxygenation problem, depending upon the patient's normal skin coloration. Anemic or chronically ill patients may normally appear pale.

Patients with advanced pulmonary disease and polycythemia may demonstrate a *reddish-blue* complexion of the face, mucous membranes, hands, and feet. The color change is due to the combination of an increase in total hemoglobin, an increase in reduced hemoglobin, and a capillary stasis.

A *red* or *ruddy* complexion may occur because of increased blood flow or superficial vasodilatation of blood vessels from fever, blushing, alcohol intake, local inflammation, or excess CO_2 in the tissues (e.g., from high $PaCO_2$). In the last case, the patient with a high $PaCO_2$ may not exhibit a ruddy complexion when a central oxygenation problem is also present, as is typically the case when $PaCO_2$ is high.

In addition to noting general skin color, the nurse specifically looks for subtle changes in the color of the lips, a readily visible structure. Without available blood gas results to identify a low PaO_2, *pale or cyanotic mucous membranes* of the lips, eyes, or under the tongue are the most reliable and sensitive sign of a possible oxygenation problem.

GENERAL SYMMETRY

Note any irregularity in the general symmetry of the head and neck with the patient seated or standing directly in front of you. Then briefly examine the right and left sides of the neck with the neck slightly extended and turned away from the side being examined (Fig. 12–8).

After this general examination, specifically observe for *swollen areas, neck vein abnormalities, tracheal deviation*, and *signs of respiratory distress*.

SWOLLEN AREAS

Swollen areas might indicate traumatized or inflamed tissue or the presence of a tumor or lymphadenopathy. Lymphadenopathy may be due to primary lymph gland tumors, such as Hodgkin's lymphoma, viral or bacterial respiratory tract infections, or metastatic carcinoma.

Asymmetric swollen areas might indicate *subcutaneous emphysema*, also called *crepitation* (i.e., air under the skin), a complication seen in patients with chest trauma, chest tubes, or a new tracheostomy or in patients in critical condition on mechanical ventilation. In severe cases, air moves under the layers of the skin from the thorax or mediastinum to the neck area.

NECK VEINS

Neck veins are best examined by adding contrast lighting to emphasize subtle findings. With the neck slightly extended and turned away from the side being examined, shine the light from a bedside lamp or a flashlight obliquely across the neck area. Oblique

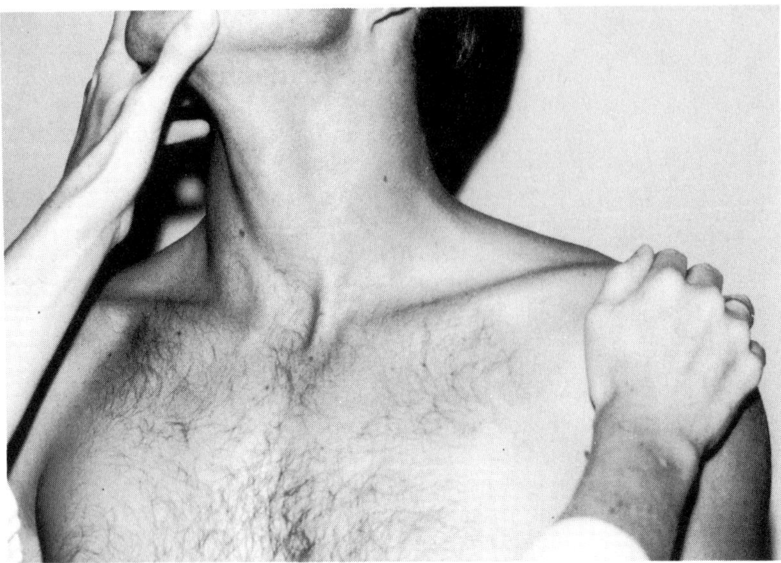

Figure 12–8. An inspection of the left side of the neck is demonstrated.

lighting casts shadows that make neck veins and venous levels more obvious.

Jugular Venous Distention

In Right Ventricular Failure. Neck vein distention is a sign of increased venous pressure and is associated with right ventricular (RV) failure. Venous blood backs up from the failing right ventricle to the jugular veins in the neck, causing *jugular venous distention* (JVD). The nurse suspects cardiac decompensation in a patient exhibiting neck vein distention, sitting at a 45- to 90-degree angle (Fig. 12–9).

In COPD. Neck vein distention also occurs in COPD, only the physiologic mechanism and characteristic finding are different from those in RV failure. The neck veins of a severely dyspneic COPD patient distend on expiration because the increased work of breathing during the prolonged expiratory phase of respiration generates large positive pressures in the chest. And they collapse on inspiration as negative intrathoracic pressures promote the return of venous blood to the heart. If neck veins do *not* collapse on inspiration, the patient may be developing severe airway obstruction, RV failure, or possibly a physical obstruction of a vein.

In Normal Lungs. As in COPD, a normal person in respiratory distress may demonstrate neck vein distention as he tries to generate greater negative and positive intrathoracic pressures to move more air in and out of the lungs.

Evaluation of Venous Pressure

In the patient with heart failure, once neck vein distention has been identified, the nurse proceeds to

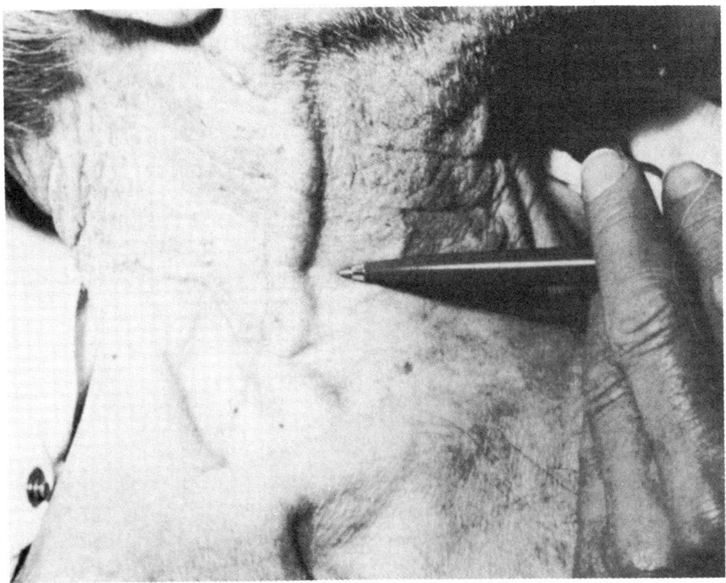

Figure 12–9. Jugular venous distention and marked elevation of venous pressure in a patient with severe right ventricular failure. (Reproduced by permission from Prior, J., Silberstein, J., and Stang, J.: Physical Diagnosis—The History and Examination of the Patient, 6th ed. St. Louis, C. V. Mosby Co., 1981.)

determine the level of *venous pressure* in one of the veins. For a starting point, place the head of the bed at 15 to 30 degrees. Turn the head slightly to the left and observe the right side of the neck with tangential light as previously instructed. The right side of the neck is used because, in normal subjects, compression of the innominate vein by the arch of the aorta (aortic knob) damps and elevates the venous pulse in the left jugular vein. The elevated venous pulse results in a falsely high venous pressure reading on the left side of the neck.

Controversy exists regarding which vein should be used—the external or the internal jugular vein? Since the external jugular vein is much easier to identify in the clinical setting, many nurses automatically use it to estimate venous pressure. Yet many cardiopulmonary experts stress the fact that one should never rely on venous pressure estimations from this vein, especially since in respiratory patients the veins may be distended from the increased work of breathing rather than from heart failure. Whichever vein is used in the clinical setting, the nurse must remember that readings from the external jugular vein represent only *gross* estimations of central venous pressure that are most likely to be accurate when hypovolemia is involved. The internal vein gives more reliable estimations of venous pressure.

Locating the External Jugular Vein. With the head comfortably supported to prevent tense back muscles, the external jugular vein is best seen just above the clavicle between or slightly posterior to the two heads of the sternocleidomastoid muscle (Fig. 12–10A). The venous pressure level corresponds to the apparent blood level in the vein, the point above which the vein appears collapsed. With the head of the bed at 30 degrees, this level is normally, slightly above the level of the clavicle. The pulsation in the vein is gentle and wavelike, unlike the sharp outward thrust of the carotid pulse located more medially and higher in the neck (see arrow Fig. 12–10A). Because of its superficial

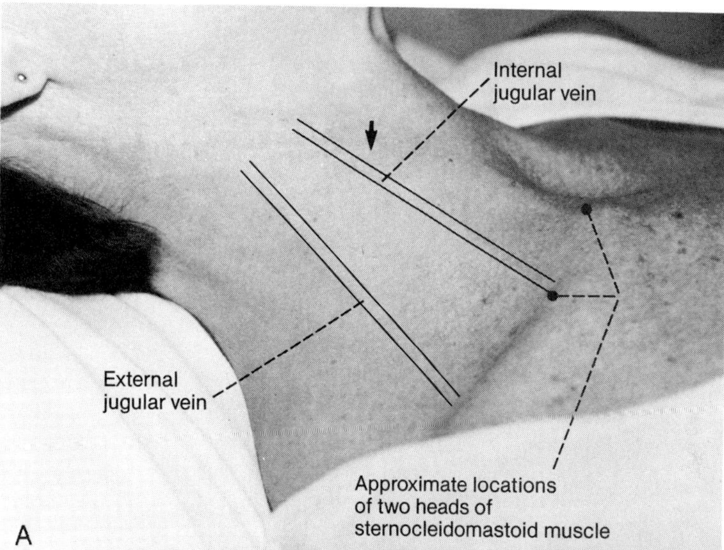

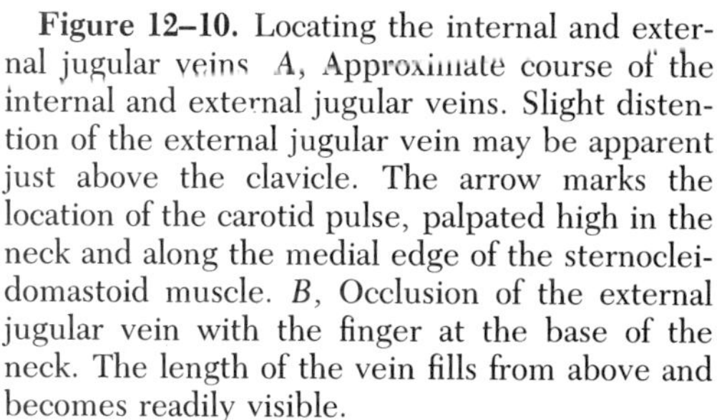
Figure 12–10. Locating the internal and external jugular veins. *A*, Approximate course of the internal and external jugular veins. Slight distention of the external jugular vein may be apparent just above the clavicle. The arrow marks the location of the carotid pulse, palpated high in the neck and along the medial edge of the sternocleidomastoid muscle. *B*, Occlusion of the external jugular vein with the finger at the base of the neck. The length of the vein fills from above and becomes readily visible.

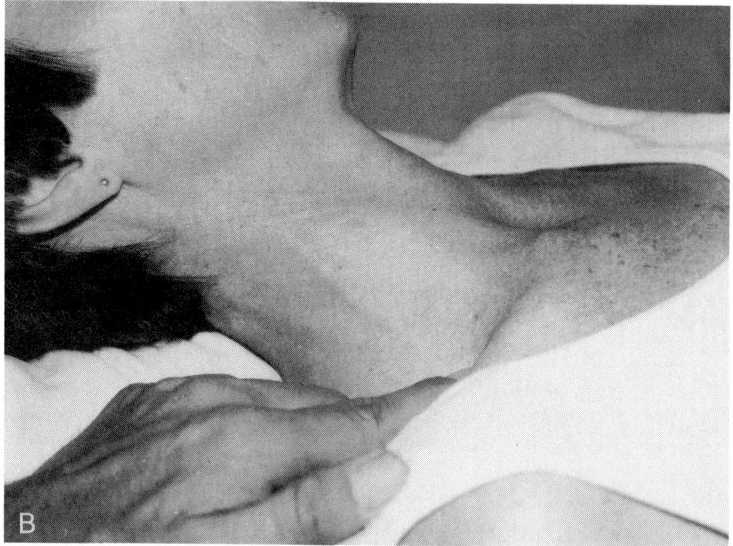

location and distention in dyspneic patients, the external jugular vein is usually easy to locate. Yet, because of its unreliability as explained previously, it is best used *only* if pulsations cannot be identified in the internal jugular vein.

Locating the Internal Jugular Vein. The internal jugular vein is difficult to examine because the length of the vein cannot be observed; it lies deep in the muscle of the neck, anterior to the external jugular vein (see Fig. 12–10A). Instead of looking for the vein itself, the nurse looks for fine oscillations or pulsations in soft tissues near the imagined path of the vein. The level of venous pressure corresponds to the highest point of these fine oscillations. Often the oscillations are barely visible, even in tangential light, and they may not be observable at all in patients with muscular or short, stocky necks.

Adjusting the Head of the Bed. A 15- to 30-degree angle of the bed is a good starting level to examine a patient's neck veins. However, the nurse may have to adjust the head of the bed to find a level that maximizes venous pulsations and makes the level of venous pressure visible above the clavicles but well below the angle of the jaw. If the patient's external jugular veins are not visible, lower the head of the bed until a distinct venous level can be seen. Note that veins become fully distended when the patient lies completely flat. If the patient's veins are fully distended with the head of the bed at 30 degrees, elevate the head of the bed to find the venous level.

Measuring Mean Venous Pressure. Once the venous pressure level is located, the nurse can easily measure *mean venous pressure.* Imagine two horizontal lines—one passing through the sternal angle and the other passing through the identified venous level of a neck vein (Fig. 12–11). Mean venous pressure is the vertical distance in centimeters between these two lines. Although an experienced practitioner can make a good estimation of venous pressure, nurses are encouraged to use a centimeter ruler and, if necessary, a yardstick or other available straight edge to help identify a horizontal line that is truly parallel with the ground. Normal venous pressure is no more than 3 cm above the sternal angle and usually no more than 1 to 3 cm below this angle. The patient in heart failure with obvious neck distention has a venous pressure well over 3 cm. A low pressure reading is due to hypovolemia, a reduction in blood volume.

Charting. The following examples indicate how to chart mean venous pressure:

1. *Internal jugular venous pressure (JVP) = 5 cm above the sternal angle, with the head of the bed (HOB) at 45 degrees.* This pressure is slightly elevated.
2. *External JVP = 2 cm below the sternal angle, with the HOB at 10 degrees.* This pressure is on the low side of normal. The external vein was probably used because the venous level of the internal vein was not visible.
3. *Neck veins flat in supine position.* This finding suggests an extremely low reading and hypovolemia, since normal veins distend in the supine position. A venous pressure level could not be found.

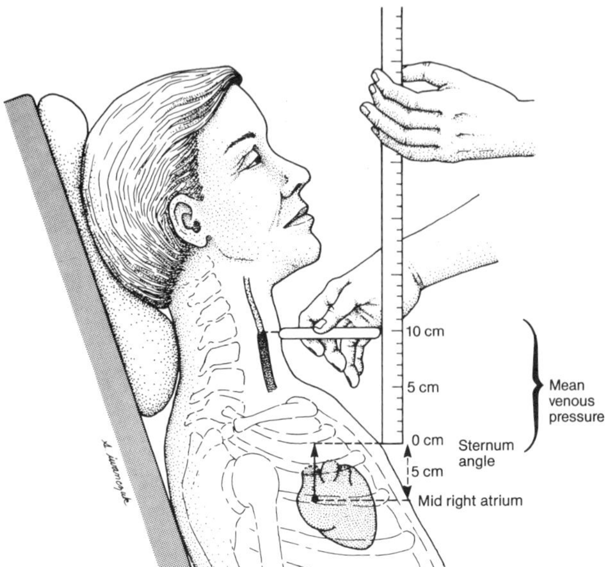

Figure 12–11. Estimation of central (mean) venous pressure using the vertical distance from the sternal angle to the pulsating crest of the internal jugular vein. (Reproduced by permission from Darovic, G. O.: Hemodynamic Monitoring: Invasive and Non-Invasive Clinical Application. Philadelphia, W. B. Saunders Co., 1987.)

Estimated Central Venous Pressure

Some clinicians prefer to estimate a venous pressure by using the right atrium instead of the sternal angle as a reference point for zero. The vertical distance between the estimated level of the right atrium and the identified venous level is called the *estimated central venous pressure* (CVP) (Fig. 12–12). Depending upon the patient's body build, the sternal angle is about 5 to 7 cm above the right atrium. A normal estimated CVP is no greater than 10 cm.

Use of the right atrium rather than the sternal angle as a reference point has its limitations. It may not be reliable because the level of the right atrium must be estimated by viewing the supine patient from the side and assuming that the right atrial level is located at or slightly superior to the middle of the lateral chest. The arm may need to be abducted to expose the area. Also, with use of the right atrial level, the increased vertical distance between reference points leaves more room for error.

Neither a mean venous pressure reading from the sternal angle nor an estimated CVP from the level of the right atrium is as reliable as a direct CVP reading from a catheter placed in the superior vena cava. The reading from a CVP catheter truly reflects pressure in the right atrium and diastolic filling pressure in the right ventricle. If a catheter is in place, no need exists to take readings from the neck veins.

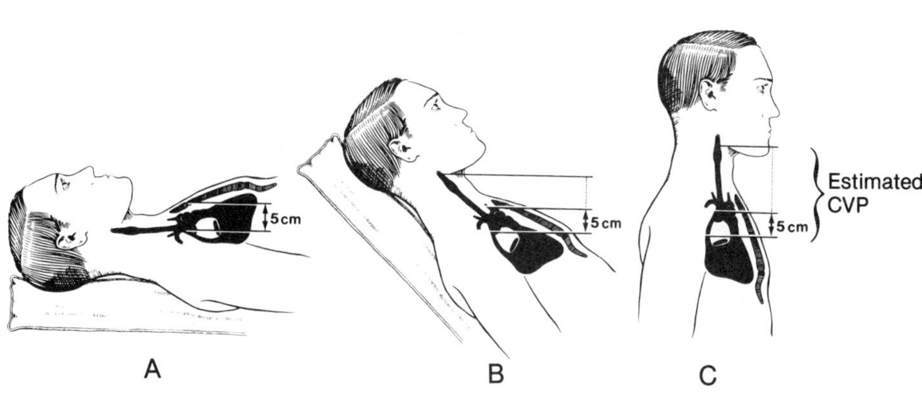

Figure 12–12. Constant distance (5 cm) of sternal angle to right atrium in supine *(A)*, semi-Fowler's *(B)*, and upright *(C)* positions. Note that although the venous level is at the angle of the jaw in both *A* and *B*, mean venous pressure and estimated central venous pressure (CVP) are much greater in the upright position. (Reproduced by permission from Vanden Belt, R., Ronan, J., and Bedynek, J.: Cardiology—A Clinical Approach. Chicago, Yearbook Medical Publishers, Inc. 1979.)

Evaluation of Venous Filling

Occasionally, the nurse will not be able to identify a venous pressure level. Perhaps the head of the bed cannot be moved, or the neck veins appear distended throughout the respiratory cycle. Still, the nurse would like to examine the neck veins to help identify or rule out the possibility of right heart failure in the pulmonary patient. The following vein stripping technique allows the nurse to evaluate the pattern of venous filling and collect additional data.

With your index finger, occlude one external jugular vein at the base of the neck, just above the clavicle, as in Figure 12–10B. Momentarily watch the vein distend as it fills up with blood returning to the heart. Place your second index finger superiorly next to your first one, and strip the vein up to the angle of the jaw. Then release both fingers simultaneously and watch the vein fill with blood. Neck veins fill from above. If the vein fills from below when the fingers are released, suspect RV failure, hypervolemia, or, less commonly, constrictive pericarditis, cardiac tamponade, or superior vena cava obstruction.

Trachea

The nurse examines the *extrathoracic section of the trachea* for signs of tracheal deviation (displacement). This section lies midline in the neck above the sternum and below the thyroid and cricoid cartilages.

With the patient's neck flexed and his chin in the midline position, first inspect this general area and then palpate the trachea at the *base of the neck where it is most mobile, in the suprasternal notch* just above the manubrium. Check for *anterior* displacement of the trachea or a *shallow* suprasternal notch by inserting your fingertip directly in the middle of the suprasternal notch, as shown in Figure 12–13A. Normally the fingertip bumps into the trachea's cartilaginous rings several centimeters posterior to the manubrium. Inability to place a fingertip into this notch indicates anterior displacement. *Posterior* displacement or a *deep* suprasternal notch is present when the entire fingertip fits into the suprasternal notch.

Check for lateral displacement of the trachea by firmly inserting your index finger in the suprasternal notch, *first* on the patient's right side of the trachea and *then* on the left side (Fig. 12–13B). If the trachea is displaced, your fingertip will encounter the tracheal wall on one side, as the trachea is deviated to this side, and only soft tissue on the other side. Some clinicians prefer to check for tracheal deviation by palpating with the thumb and forefinger.

INTERPRETATION OF FINDINGS

Tracheal deviation usually indicates gross pathology of the neck, thorax, lungs, or mediastinum.

Anterior displacement, i.e., shallow suprasternal notch, occurs with mediastinitis; a neoplasm behind the trachea; cervicomediastinal goiter, at times; and a dilated esophagus from achalasia.

A deep suprasternal notch normally occurs in a thin individual with a long chest and neck. However, the trachea may be displaced posteriorly with emphysema, if the patient has a short, thick neck, and with a tumor of the anterior mediastinum in rare cases.

Lateral displacement might indicate an aortic aneurysm, a mediastinal tumor, a tumor in the neck, an enlarged paratracheal lymph node, or a unilateral thyroid enlargement. In respiratory disease, lateral displacement is usually a sign of mediastinal shift due to one or both of the following physiologic processes:

1. *Loss of Lung Volume*—The trachea deviates to the affected side, as in atelectasis, pneumonectomy, unilateral pulmonary fibrosis, severe pleural adhesions, and unilateral elevation of the diaphragm. In Figure 12–14A, right lung atelectasis causes a shift to the right, where pleural pressures are most negative.
2. *Increase in Lung or Thoracic Volume*—The trachea deviates to the side *opposite* the affected lung or thorax, as in tension pneumothorax (lung collapses but

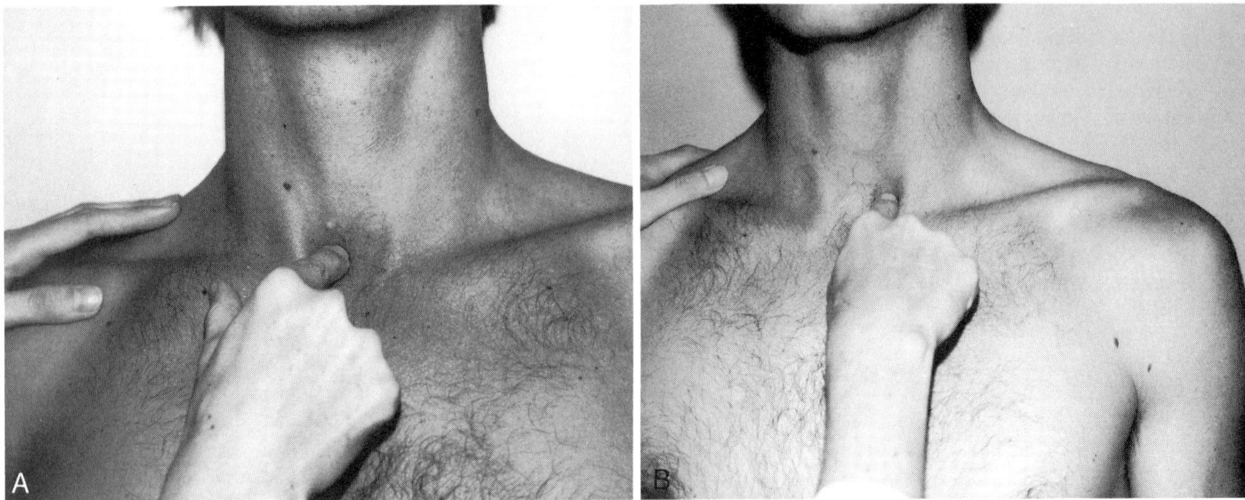

Figure 12–13. Palpation of the trachea. *A*, Checking the trachea for anterior and posterior displacement. *B*, Checking the trachea for lateral displacement.

air fills the pleural space), pulmonary or extrapulmonary tumor, large hemothorax, and large pleural effusion. In Figure 12–14B, the pleural effusion causes end-expiratory pleural pressures on the affected side to rise. The mediastinum and trachea shift to the unaffected left side, where pleural pressures are more negative.

Respiratory pathology that does not cause an increase or decrease in lung or thoracic volume will not cause tracheal and mediastinal shift. For example, in Figure 12–14C, the lung consolidation is large but does not cause tracheal and mediastinal shift because it remains localized within lung tissue without increasing lung size and impinging on mediastinal structures.

To better understand the interpretation of findings, consider a patient who presents with tracheal deviation to the *right*. One or more of the following processes may be involved:

1. The loss of volume and more negative intrathoracic pressures in the right lung pull the trachea to the right.
2. Some space-occupying lesion in the left lung (large LUL tumor) or left pleural space (pleural effusion) pushes the trachea to the right.
3. Deviation is caused by both 1 and 2. For example, the trachea is pulled to the right by atelectasis and simultaneously pushed to the right by pneumothorax or pleural effusion of the left lung.

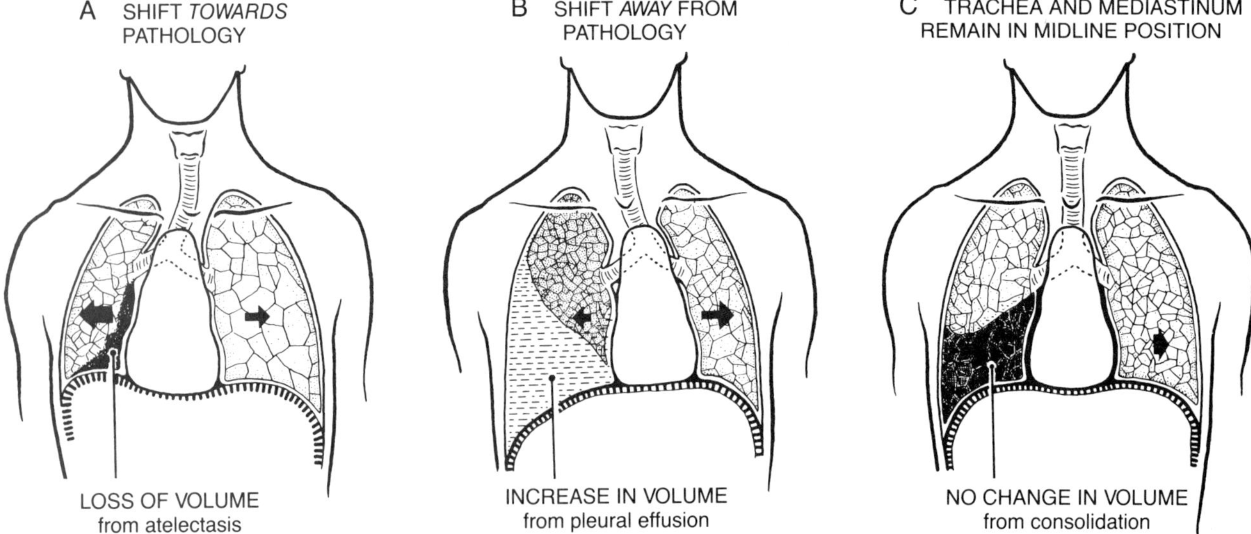

Figure 12–14. Tracheal and mediastinal shift in respiratory disease. In *A* and *B*, the large arrow represents the direction of the shift and the more negative end-expiratory pleural pressures on that side. In *C*, pleural pressures remain about equal for right and left lungs. (Reproduced and adapted by permission from Cherniack, R. and Cherniak, L.: Respiration in Health and Disease, 3rd ed. Philadelphia, W. B. Saunders Co., 1983.)

4. Slight deviation of the trachea to the right is normal for individuals over 65 years of age due to impinging pressure from an unfolding, aging ascending aorta.

Extrathoracic Signs of Respiratory Distress

Before completion of the observation of head and neck area, the nurse observes and mentally notes any extrathoracic signs of respiratory distress. These extrathoracic signs are verified by changing vital signs and other signs found while examining the thorax and lungs. These signs are crucial because unlike auscultation, which involves a technical maneuver, they can be monitored continuously by bedside observation; in many cases respiratory distress is discovered on the basis of positive extrathoracic findings alone. At other times, the clinical nurse suspects respiratory problems in the fully clothed outpatient whose head and neck alone are visible during an initial interview.

Although experienced nurses are expert at utilizing their "sixth" sense to pick up signs of respiratory distress, all nurses are encouraged to refine their technique by looking for specific abnormalities that suggest respiratory distress. As previously discussed, *neck vein distention, increased skin pallor*, and *cyanosis* are important extrathoracic signs. The cooperative, congenial patient without complaints and signs of distress may only exhibit *facial tenseness* or *grimace*. Overt shortness of breath may be accompanied by *nasal flaring* and the *upward and downward movement of the Adam's apple* (thyroid cartilage) with inspiration and expiration. This movement is especially noticeable in the reclined patient who breathes with his mouth open. The COPD patient may unconsciously use *pursed lip breathing* to help keep the airway open during expiration, thus relieving some airway obstruction. The dyspneic patient may interrupt his sentences with 1- to 2-second pauses to catch his breath, creating a *disconnected speech pattern*. Specifically note the *use of neck accessory muscles* and any *retractions of the suprasternal notch and supraclavicular spaces*, both signs of increased work of breathing. Suprasternal notch retraction of the airway and soft tissue is referred to as *tracheal tug*. Also, in the presence or absence of these signs of respiratory distress, the patient may demonstrate an *altered level of consciousness*. Signs may include decreased ability to concentrate, drowsiness, disorientation, lethargy, impaired judgment, restlessness, headache, and nausea.

Extremities

For the lower extremities, the nurse asks the ambulatory patient to remove his shoes and socks and place his feet next to each other in full view. For the upper extremities, examine each hand individually and then hold the two hands side by side for comparison to notice any subtle differences. Visual observations are confirmed immediately by palpating and casually asking the patient pertinent questions.

During the examination, the nurse checks for asymmetric areas, deformities, skin lesions, and general skin coloration.

SKIN COLORATION

Mild pallor is normal. *Ruddy* hands may be seen with the ruddy complexion of the COPD patient with a high $Paco_2$. The fingers may feel slightly warm to the touch from local dilatation of vessels.

Increased pallor or cyanosis indicates a *central* oxygenation problem (low Pao_2) when accompanied by overt signs of respiratory distress or sometimes milder pulmonary signs and symptoms, such as increased respiratory rate and mild dyspnea. In this case, Pao_2 decreases to such a degree that peripheral tissues also suffer from the lack of oxygen, resulting in a decreased tissue Po_2 and peripheral pallor or cyanosis.

As a solitary finding, however, increased pallor or cyanosis of the extremities, including the ears, indicates a *peripheral* oxygenation problem, e.g., low tissue Po_2 with a normal Pao_2. It is usually found in patients with nonpulmonary or vascular diseases that cause circulatory changes in the extremities, e.g., Raynaud's disease, Buerger's disease, arteriosclerosis, thrombophlebitis, and others.

In the evaluation of peripheral pallor or cyanosis, the nurse searches for signs of peripheral vascular problems to help rule out a low Pao_2 from respiratory disease. The absence of other assessment parameters (especially since clinical signs of a low Pao_2 may be absent) may help determine whether the patient really has a serious oxygenation problem at the moment. Patients with chronic arterial insufficiency may exhibit *shiny, atrophic, hairless skin* with a *dusky red coloration* when the extremities (usually the feet) are in the dependent position. Patients with chronic venous insufficiency may exhibit *edematous feet with a brown skin pigmentation* around the ankles. Other distinguishing features of patients with peripheral vascular disorders are *skin ulcerations, varicose veins, prominent, superficial venous patterns*, and *signs of phlebitis*.

NAIL BED CAPILLARY REFILL

Poor capillary refill under the nail beds accompanies increased pallor or cyanosis of the fingers and toes. To check for capillary refill, press on the patient's nail beds and watch for the blanching underneath to return to the patient's baseline skin coloration. If this blanching takes more than 1 second to return to normal, the patient has poor, i.e., sluggish, capillary refill. This finding is present in those with central or peripheral cyanosis as well as in normal individuals walking outdoors in cold weather.

FINGERNAILS AND TOENAILS

The following findings almost always suggest chronic cardiopulmonary problems.

Tobacco-stained fingernails indicate that the individual has been smoking in the recent past. If the patient's history is negative for cigarette smoking, ask for an explanation of the stains in a nonjudgmental manner.

Prominent, vertical ridges along the lengths of the toenails and fingernails are found in some normal individuals. In the absence of other signs, this finding is not significant. In the presence of other signs, such as smoking history, clubbing of the fingers, and cool, pale extremities, it suggests chronic cardiopulmonary disease.

CLUBBING

Clubbing is an abnormality involving the nails and last phalanges of the fingers that produces bulbous formations at the tips of the fingers in severe cases (Fig. 12–15). Although it can be a normal familial trait, manifesting itself shortly after birth, it is usually seen in patients with *congenital heart disease, subacute bacterial endocarditis, bronchiectasis, cystic fibrosis, lung abscess, pulmonary fibrosis, lung cancer,* and other chronic diseases. It is uncommon in patients with COPD unless a suppurative process such as bronchiectasis develops. Yet, even for bronchiectasis, the incidence of clubbing is low, only about 10%. Similarly, other diseases occur with clubbing only when a suppurative process or extensive fibrosis is present (e.g., tuberculosis). Sometimes clubbing is found in other disorders, such as *hepatic cirrhosis, chronic ulcerative colitis, Crohn's disease,* and *hemiplegia.* Although clubbing may suggest chronic hypoxemia, many patients with clubbing have normal resting PaO_2s.

To check for clubbing, the nurse looks at the profile of the fingers, noting the *angle between the nail bed and finger.* This angle is normally no greater than 160 degrees, as illustrated in Figure 12–16. In early clubbing, this angle is lost, and the base of the nail bed may feel soft and spongy. In some cases, the patient does not exhibit overt clubbing because, owing to extremely soft, spongy nail beds, the base of the nail descends to maintain the angle.

Figure 12–17 demonstrates one way to check for a *spongy nail bed* and the *floating of the nail* in a bed of soft vascular tissue; both findings are signs of clubbing. First, the clinician holds the sides of the nail with one hand to check for the floating nail, a sign of advanced clubbing. Movement of the nail may not be evident until direct pressure is applied to the root of the nail with the other index finger. Resiliency at the nail's root indicates a spongy nail bed. Sometimes the nail bed does not feel particularly spongy, but the proximal edge of the nail's root can be felt. The ability to feel this proximal edge is considered a relatively

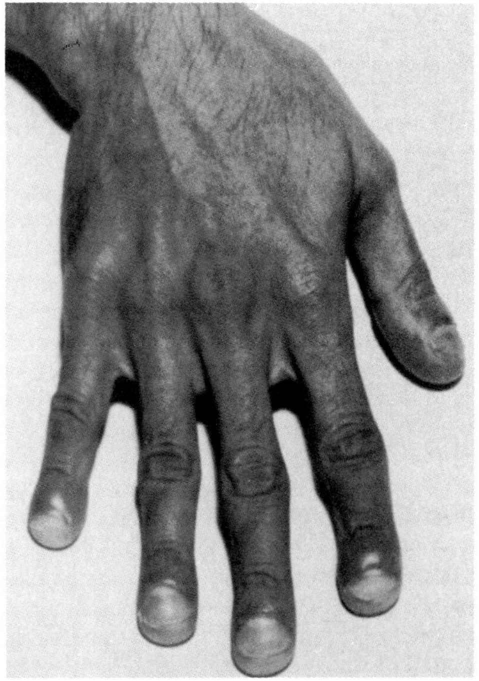

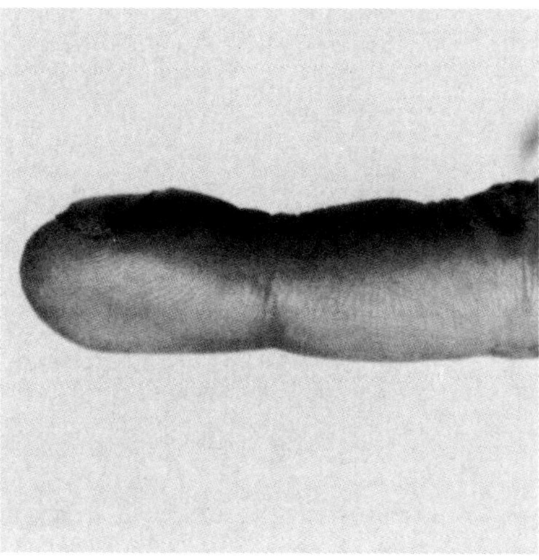

Figure 12–15. Advanced clubbing of the fingers from diffuse interstitial lung disease. (Reproduced by permission from Hinshaw, H. and Murray, J.: Diseases of the Chest, 4th ed. Philadelphia, W. B. Saunders Co., 1980.)

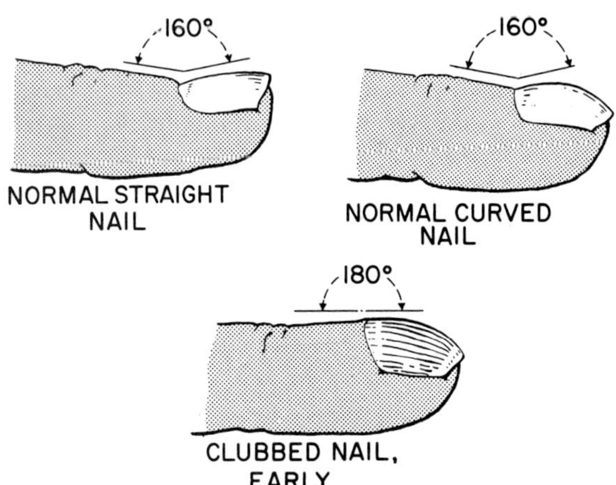

Figure 12–16. Normal and abnormal angles between the base of the nail and the finger. (Reproduced by permission from Cherniack, R. and Cherniak, L.: Respiration in Health and Disease, 3rd ed. Philadelphia, W. B. Saunders Co., 1983.)

early sign of clubbing. Most important, these findings may not be detectable unless the clinician palpates the nail with the index finger pointing *away* from the patient, as demonstrated in Figure 12–17.

Although clubbing is usually bilateral, it can be unilateral or even unidigital in rare cases. It usually affects the thumb and index finger first. In the foot, the great toe is easiest to examine for clubbing because the terminal phalanges of the other toes tend to be misshapen normally.

In advanced clubbing, the angle of the nail bed decreases as the fingertips enlarge. The nail curves longitudinally and transversely (i.e., watch-glass deformity) as the fingertips become wider and rounder, as illustrated in Figure 12–18. The skin overlying the nail bed stretches, loses its normal wrinkles, and may glisten, giving a polished appearance, as in Figure 12–16. Eventually the fingertips become larger than the last interphalangeal joint of the fingers, creating the bulbous appearance of advanced clubbing.

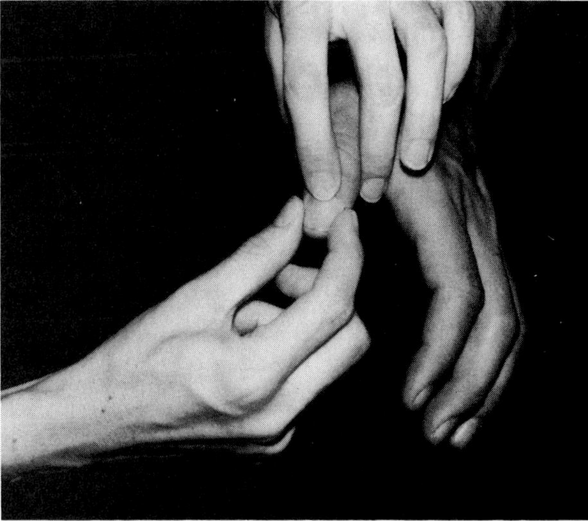

Figure 12–17. Technique for detection of the *floating nail* and the *spongy nailbed*, both signs of clubbing.

HYPERTROPHIC PULMONARY OSTEOARTHROPATHY

In some cases, clubbing progresses to *hypertrophic pulmonary osteoarthropathy*. This is a disorder involving extremities and joints, not just fingertips and toes. Gross digital clubbing is accompanied by enlargement of the ankles, wrists, interphalangeal joints of the fingers and toes, and the distal ends of long bones in the arms and legs. Because the main pathologic finding is bilateral subperiosteal bone formation along long and tubular bones, some clinicians call the disorder *pulmonary periostopathy* rather than hypertrophic pulmonary osteoarthropathy. Joint effusions may appear, but, unlike those seen in rheumatoid arthritis, these effusions are noninflammatory in nature (low leukocyte and neutrophil counts). Clubbed digits are reddened and painful, but pain and swelling are characteristically localized along the long bones of the extremities, particularly the distal third of the legs. Sometimes digital clubbing is absent or delayed in the disease process. Diseases usually associated with clubbing and hypertrophic osteoarthropathy include *primary lung cancer, mesothelioma*, and *neurogenic diaphragmatic tumors*.

PERIPHERAL EDEMA

Edema is defined as excessive fluid in the interstitial spaces of body tissues. *Peripheral edema* involves the extremities and is seen as a complication of end-stage

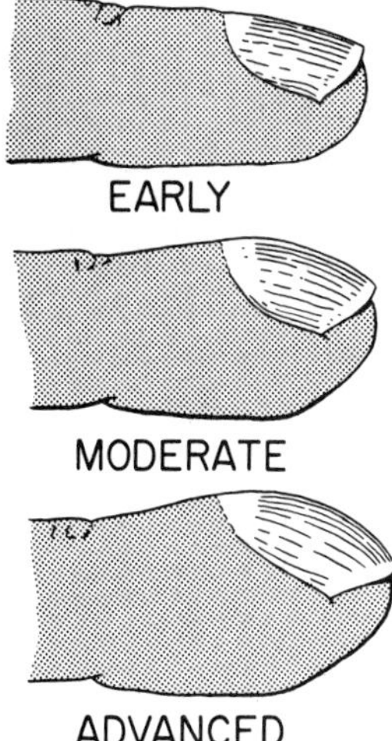

Figure 12–18. Progressive changes in early, moderate, and advanced finger clubbing. (Reproduced by permission from Cherniack, R. and Cherniak, L.: Respiration in Health and Disease, 3rd ed. Philadelphia, W. B. Saunders Co., 1983.)

pulmonary disease and in RV failure as well as other disorders affecting the distribution of body fluids, e.g., vascular disease, lymphatic insufficiency, cirrhosis, nephritis, and pressure on the inferior vena cava caused by ascites or an intra-abdominal mass.

Peripheral edema appears first in dependent areas of the body—the sacral area for the patient on bed rest, and the feet and legs for the ambulatory patient. It is always worse in immobile extremities and physically inactive individuals, particularly in the presence of preexisting venous stasis.

To identify peripheral edema, the nurse first inspects the extremities and then palpates the bony prominences of the feet and lower legs, where edema is easier to identify. Press firmly on the surface of the skin with a thumb for 5 seconds in three specific areas: (1) medial aspect of the foot behind the ankle bone (i.e., medial malleolus), (2) dorsum of the foot where one feels for the pedal pulse, and (3) shin of the leg. When dependent edema is present, the tissues will *pit* (indent) with pressure from the thumb (Fig. 12–19). The edema will also improve significantly if the extremity is elevated for a few minutes. A longer period of time is necessary in severe cases.

To help evaluate the progression of heart failure or fluid overload, the nurse quantifies the severity of edema by describing its *location* and *extent*, e.g., left ankle edema up to the patient's knee. A general scale of 1+ (i.e., minimal pitting edema) to 4+ (i.e., severe pitting edema—the large indent takes longer than 30 seconds to return to normal) is used to estimate and chart the severity of the problem. Use of a standardized scale becomes especially important when different nurses periodically assess the same patient and must decide if the patient is better, worse, or unchanged based on previously charted findings. In some cases, edema in the extremities is accompanied by total body edema, a condition called *anasarca*.

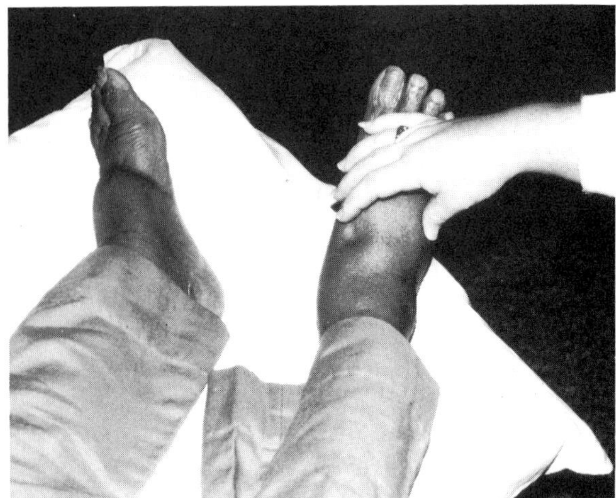

Figure 12–19. Severe pitting edema of the feet caused by right ventricular failure. The thumb imprint (by nurse's index finger) is still visible 40 seconds after palpation. Note the linear mark on the left foot made by the top edge of the patient's bedroom slipper.

When edema is a persistent problem, and particularly when it is accompanied by swelling from inflammation, a type of nonpitting edema, ankle and calf girth are measured and recorded in centimeters to follow the progression of disease.

ASTERIXIS

The nurse examines the upper extremities of the pulmonary patient for *asterixis*, an irregular flapping or shaking tremor caused by the sporadic loss of tone in contracting muscle. Asterixis is a sign of CO_2 retention, but it is also found in patients with liver failure, uremia, and other metabolic encephalopathies.

With the patient sitting or standing, ask him to raise the arms to shoulder level (90 degrees in 0 degree abduction), with the hands pronated and the fingers spread. In asterixis, *flapping* or jerky alternations of extension and flexion occur within 5 seconds at the wrists and interphalangeal joints. The flapping occurs in cycles: a few seconds of quick jerks followed by 1- to 2-second rest periods. The fingers may deviate laterally and exhibit fine tremor. For patients unable to outstretch their arms to 90 degrees, the nurse can ask them to squeeze two of her fingers. With asterixis, the patient will alternately clench and unclench the fingers.

The irregular, gross movements of asterixis must not be mistaken for the more regular and fine hand and arm tremors seen as a side effect of bronchodilator medications, notably terbutaline (Brethine, Bricanyl) or theophylline (aminophylline) derivatives. In asterixis from a high Pa_{CO_2}, the tremor usually disappears when the extended arms return to the patient's sides. In contrast, the drug-induced fine tremor may be continuously present to some degree, becoming accentuated with arm extension or other movements that require coordination. It is typically accompanied by the subjective feeling of jitteriness.

SECTION III—INSPECTION, PALPATION, AND PERCUSSION OF THE THORAX AND LUNGS

After the extrathoracic examination, the nurse proceeds to the following four components of the examination of the thorax and lungs: *inspection*, *palpation*, *percussion*, and *auscultation*. The first three components are discussed here; the most important component, auscultation, is discussed in the following section of this chapter. The following box provides an overview of all four components.

EXAMINATION OF THE THORAX AND LUNGS

INSPECTION
General observations
- Posture
- Chest symmetry
- Chest configuration
- Spinal deformities

Skin surfaces
Respiratory rate and breathing pattern
I:E ratio
Muscles of breathing
Chest movements

PALPATION
General palpation
Fine palpation
Costal angle
Lateral chest expansion
Fremitus
- Rhonchal
- Pleural rub
- Vocal or tactile

PERCUSSION
Lung fields
Diaphragm
- Resting diaphragmatic levels
- Diaphragmatic excursions

AUSCULTATION
Voice sounds
- Egophony
- Bronchophony
- Whispered pectoriloquy

Breath sounds
- Normal
- Bronchial
- Bronchovesicular

Adventitious sounds
- Crackles or rales
- Rhonchi
- Wheeze
- Pleural friction rub

Inspection

Inspection provides important information pertaining to the skin, chest wall, and mechanics of breathing. Often it yields information suggestive of pulmonary signs detectable by one or more of the other components of the examination. It is accomplished by investigating each of the items listed under Inspection in the box.

GENERAL OBSERVATIONS

Posture

The nurse checks for the presence of *normal posture.* The head should be erect, trunk upright, and shoulders level, with the arms hanging loosely at the patient's sides. Any deviation from this norm may indicate a chest wall abnormality, spinal deformity, or pulmonary disease; it may arise from general fatigue, inattention to correct posture, or mental depression without a physiologic basis.

In respiratory disease, postural problems are common in post-thoracotomy patients, who lean to the operative side to splint painful respirations. Dyspneic patients may always reach for a chair, table, or railing to lean on. Patients on bed rest may insist on lying on one side because they cough less, feel less shortness of breath, and claim they sleep better curled up on their favored side. The result may be pneumonia in the dependent lung. COPD patients commonly have tense, slightly shrugged shoulders with the increased work of breathing. Muscle tension and the anxiety associated with shortness of breath interfere with normal relaxed breathing and achievement of normal alveolar ventilation.

Although some postures may allow chronic respiratory patients to better ventilate certain regions of lung, poor posture is generally a concern because some regions are not being fully expanded and alveolar hypoventilation may develop, particularly in hospitalized patients.

Chest Symmetry

The nurse inspects the anterior and posterior chest for general symmetry, standing first *directly* in front of the patient and then *directly* behind him. Although the two sides of the thorax are normally symmetric, no chest is perfect, and some asymmetry may be evident. Right-handed individuals may have more muscle mass on the right side of the chest. The nipples or shoulders may not be exactly at the same level.

Specifically, look for unilateral chest cage *depression* or *overexpansion.* Obvious depression may be caused by pneumonectomy or severe atelectasis (i.e., loss of lung volume). Overexpansion might be from a large pulmonary consolidation, which is rare; tension pneumothorax; and displacement of an endotracheal tube down a main stem bronchus. In the last case, the tube is usually displaced down the more vertical right main stem bronchus. The right hemithorax appears overexpanded, especially when the patient is receiving large tidal volumes from a ventilator; the left hemithorax appears depressed, since the left lung is receiving little inspired air.

Chest Configurations

Normal Infant. The normal infant's thorax is circular in shape with nearly equal diameters from the top to the bottom of the chest. The thorax gradually becomes more elliptic as the infant grows.

The ratio of the anteroposterior (AP) diameter, viewed from the side, to the transverse diameter, viewed from the front, is 1:1 because the chest is circular.

Normal Adult. The normal adult's thorax is elliptic in shape, with a wider diameter at the base than at the top. The AP-transverse chest ratio ranges from 1:2 to 5:7. As a general rule, the transverse diameter is about twice as wide as the AP diameter, as shown in Figure 12–20. Although some clinicians may actually estimate and record chest ratios for respiratory patients, and chest calipers are often used to monitor the chest diameters of children with cystic fibrosis, in adults, visual estimations are highly subjective and chest calipers unnecessary. The purpose of the chest ratio is to identify patients who have *increased AP diameters*, a characteristic finding of COPD patients with lung hyperinflation from air trapping. Patients with chest deformities, such as severe kyphosis, may have this finding but lack the auscultatory findings of COPD.

Barrel Chest (Increased AP Diameter). In COPD, the AP diameter increases until the AP-transverse chest ratio approaches 2:2, and the cross-sectional view of the thorax is circular, looking like a barrel, hence the term *barrel chest*. Since some lung hyperinflation and redistribution of air in the lungs occur in older people as part of the aging process, individuals over 65 years of age may have slightly increased AP diameters and noticeable barrel chests. Most important, this deformity is detected by viewing the chest from the side (Fig. 12–21). It may be more obvious on a lateral chest x-ray than on physical examination.

Pigeon Breast (Pectus Carinatum: Keel Breast). This deformity is abnormal protrusion of the sternum; the sternum juts forward similar to the keel of a ship (Fig. 12–22). Diseases that may cause this deformity include rickets, congenital heart disease, Marfan's syndrome, and severe primary kyphoscoliosis. It may be a congenital or acquired deformity, and it appears in slightly different forms, depending on etiology. In childhood rickets or vitamin D deficiency, the softened upper ribs bend inward, narrowing the width of the thorax and forcing the sternum forward. Most congenital forms of pigeon breast simply cause gradual protrusion of the sternum and costal cartilages with growth. Patients with this simple form are usually asymptomatic, except that some children tend to be more susceptible to respiratory infections. The most common cause of acquired pigeon breast, however, is congenital atrial or ventricular septal defect; about 50% of these patients have this chest cage deformity (Fraser and Paré, 1979). In atrial septal defect, the protrusion occurs unilaterally, directly over the right ventricle. In ventricular septal defect, the deformity symmetrically affects the chest, mainly over the upper part of the sternum; patients usually develop pulmonary hypertension.

Funnel Chest (Pectus Excavatum: Cobbler's Chest). This deformity is the reverse of pigeon breast; the sternum is depressed, owing to its attachment to the spine by a number of fibromuscular bands. In severe cases, the sternum may lie only a few inches away from the spinal column. The depression creates a hollow pit over the bottom half of the sternum, with the ribs on each side protruding slightly above the surface of the chest (Fig. 12–23). Known as a genetically determined abnormality of the sternum and re-

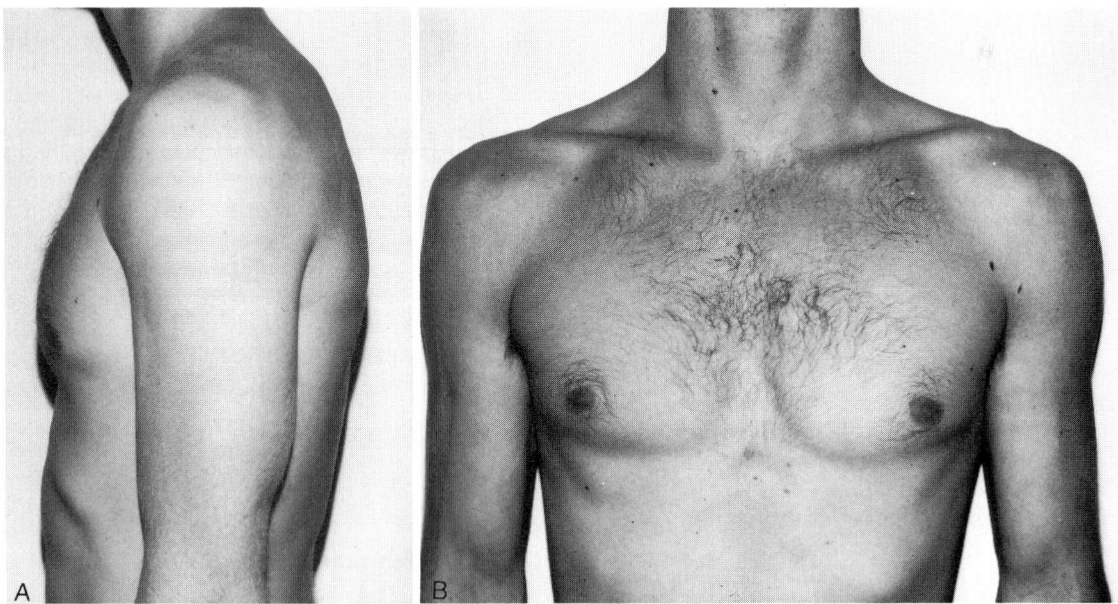

Figure 12–20. A normal adult's chest configuration. The anterior-posterior (AP) diameter in *A* and transverse (T) diameter in *B* compose the normal AP:T ratio of 1:2.

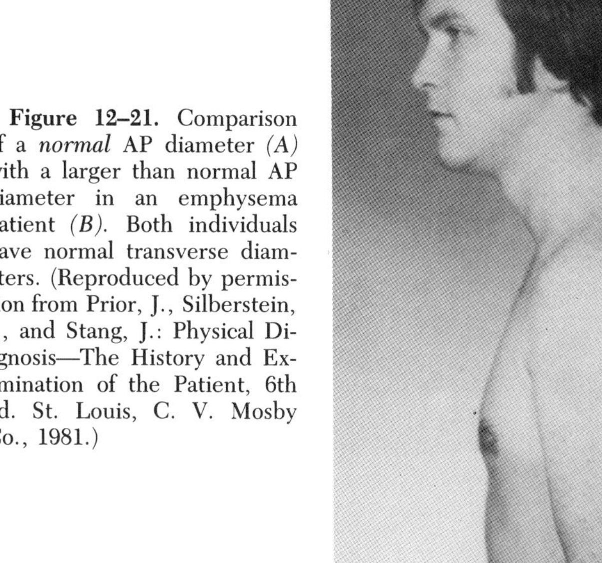

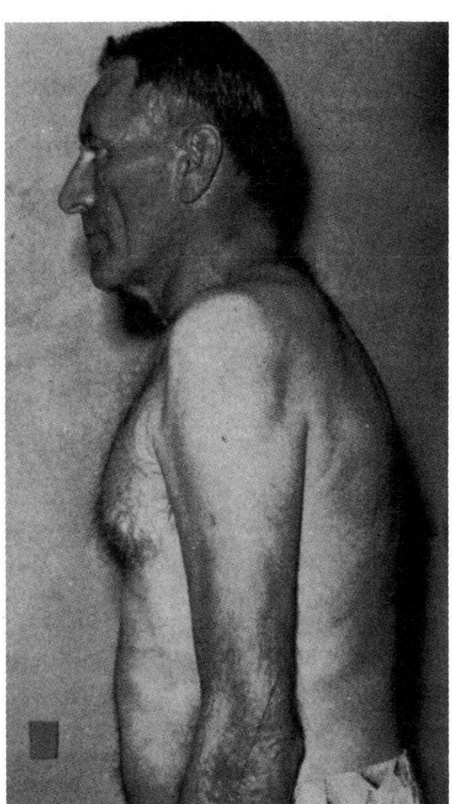

Figure 12–21. Comparison of a *normal* AP diameter *(A)* with a larger than normal AP diameter in an emphysema patient *(B)*. Both individuals have normal transverse diameters. (Reproduced by permission from Prior, J., Silberstein, J., and Stang, J.: Physical Diagnosis—The History and Examination of the Patient, 6th ed. St. Louis, C. V. Mosby Co., 1981.)

lated parts of the diaphragm, funnel chest is found in individuals with and without a positive family history. It is associated with Marfan's syndrome and other congenital connective tissue disorders. Occasionally, it may develop from childhood rickets or from continuous pressure against the sternum; a cobbler may repair shoes in this manner, hence the term *cobbler's chest*. When seen with displacement of the heart to the left,

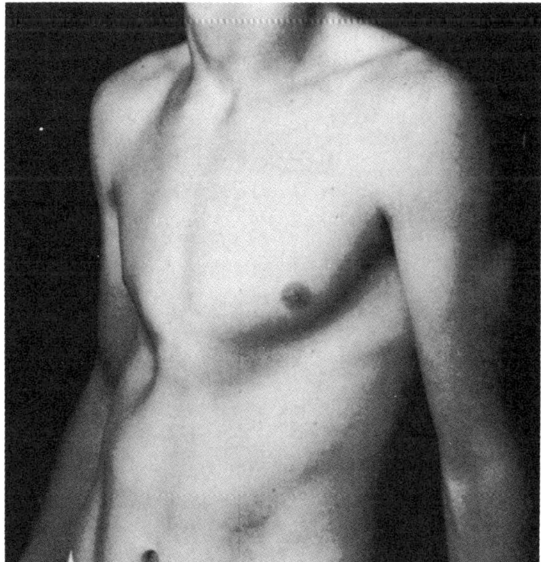

Figure 12–22. Pigeon breast (pectus carinatum) in a 16-year-old boy. Lateral depression of the ribs caused the elevated sternum. The deformity was satisfactorily corrected with surgery. (Reproduced by permission from Ravitch, M.: Disorders of the Chest. In Davis-Christopher Textbook of Surgery. [Sabiston, D., ed.] Philadelphia, W. B. Saunders Co., 1981.)

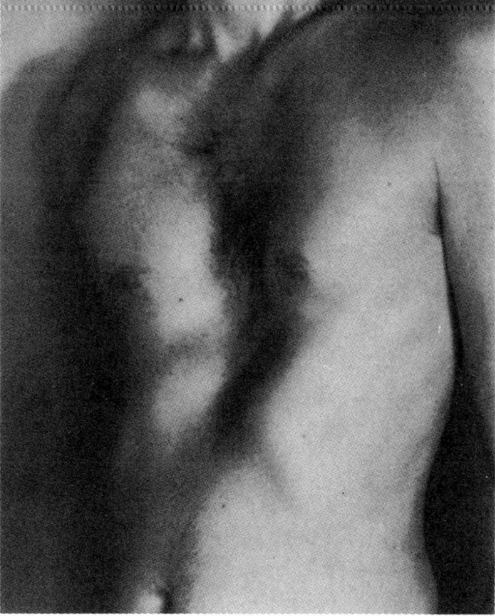

Figure 12–23. Funnel chest (pectus excavatum) in a 20-year-old man. Sternal depression displaced the heart posteriorly and was responsible for episodes of cardiac failure with fibrillation. Corrective surgery completely relieved symptoms. (Reproduced by permission from Ravitch, M.: Disorders of the Chest. In Davis-Christopher Textbook of Surgery. [Sabiston, D., ed.] Philadelphia, W. B. Saunders Co., 1981.)

it may be accompanied by heart sound abnormalities, such as murmur and increased splitting of the second heart sound. The majority of patients are symptom free and exhibit no signs of pulmonary impairment. Psychologic problems related to anxiety and the inability to cope effectively with a cosmetic deformity prompt some patients to undergo surgical correction. There is a need to screen these patients and others with severe chest deformities for possible body image problems. Psychologic needs may be overlooked because the patient has no significant impairment of cardiopulmonary function.

Spinal Deformities

Viewed from the side, the spine of the normal adult has three separate curves as follows: an *anterior curve of the neck* (cervical concavity), a *posterior curve of the midthoracic area* (thoracic convexity), and an *anterior curve of the lumbar* or *lower back area* (lumbar concavity) (Fig. 12–24). Alterations in these curves cause spinal deformities.

Common deformities of the lumbar spine, such as accentuation of the lumbar curve (e.g., lumbar lordosis) or straightening of the curve, rarely affect lung function. Severe deformity of the thoracic spine, however, can alter the configuration of the chest and cause severe restrictive pulmonary disease. The thoracic spinal deformities described hereafter include *kyphosis, angular kyphosis, scoliosis, kyphoscoliosis,* and *poker spine.*

Kyphosis. Kyphosis is an accentuation of the normal thoracic curve. The smooth, symmetric, convex curvature of the back gives the patient a hunched over or hunchbacked appearance (Fig. 12–25). Although usually associated with osteoporosis secondary to aging, it also occurs in other bone disorders. In spinal tuberculosis or Pott's disease, the vertebrae become inflamed and eventually ankylose the back in the kyphotic position. Kyphosis is also seen in patients with

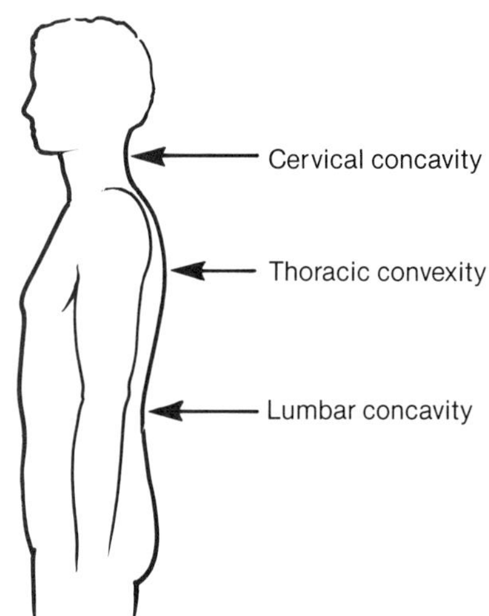

Figure 12–24. Curvatures of the normal spinal profile.

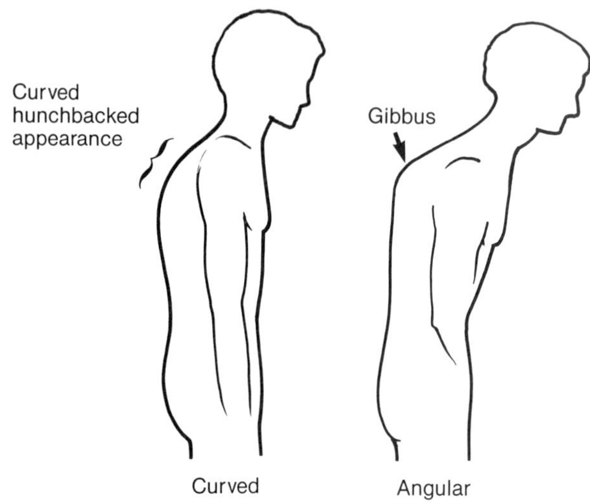

Figure 12–25. Curved and angular kyphosis.

Paget's disease, rheumatoid arthritis, acromegaly, and poor posture over a long period of time. Respiratory patients on long-term steroid medication may develop hunchback due to anterior wedging of the thoracic vertebrae from osteoporosis and frequent compression fractures. In kyphosis, cardiopulmonary problems do not develop until the angle of the thoracic curvature becomes greater than 20 degrees.

Angular Kyphosis. This is a variant of the curved kyphosis previously described. Instead of a smooth curve, the back exhibits a protruding angle caused by the collapse of one or more vertebral bodies. The protruding angle is called a *gibbus* (Fig. 12–25). Gibbus may result from tuberculosis or neoplasm of the vertebrae, syphilis, or compression fractures of the vertebrae from a variety of causes. Although the steroid-dependent respiratory patient loses calcium from bones and often develops compression fractures in end-stage disease, he becomes severely disabled and usually dies before a gibbus forms. Gibbus may cause marked rib crowding and anterior protrusion of the sternum into a type of pigeon breast deformity.

Scoliosis. Viewed from the back, the spinal column normally passes *midline* down the vertebral line. Scoliosis is *lateral* curvature of the thoracic spine. It develops as the result of irregular bone formation (e.g., congenital deformities), poor posture over a long period of time, compensatory mechanisms (e.g., thoracoplasty, shortened lower limb), or weakness or paralysis of back and abdominal muscles (e.g., neuromuscular disorders such as poliomyelitis and quadriplegia).

Mild scoliosis forms a single lateral curve, usually pointing to the right, in 75% of cases. Moderate to severe scoliosis exhibits two lateral curves pointing in opposite directions—a thoracic curve and a compensatory lumbar curve inferiorly located to complete the shape of the letter S or Ƨ when the thoracic curve points to the right. Sometimes the thoracic curve is so convex or curved that it forms a 90-degree angle when it swings back to form the second lumbar curve. In this abnormality, the spinous processes of the vertebrae involved always rotate medially towards the inside or concave side of the curve. This rotation causes three changes as follows: (1) *crowding of ribs* on the concave side of the curve; (2) *flaring (spreading) of ribs* on the opposite convex side; and (3) *elevated shoulder and lowered hip* to accommodate the expanded chest of the convex side (Fig. 12–26).

To identify mild scoliosis, ask the patient to lean over while you inspect and palpate the entire length of the spine. Pay particular attention to the thoracic area, noting any slight curvature to the right or left. Severe scoliosis (i.e., the S-shaped curve) is readily apparent in the upright position. Ask the patient to stand upright and to walk a few steps to check for the elevated shoulder, lowered hip, chest configuration, and gait problems. Carefully observe the chest from the side to check for any accompanying kyphosis and pigeon breast.

The physical finding of scoliosis is significant in respiratory assessment for three reasons. First, in scoliosis the bodies of the vertebrae rotate more than their spinous processes. Hence, the curvature detected by physical examination of the spinous processes is usually an under-representation of the degree of abnormality actually present. The patient's restrictive disease may be worse than you think.

Second, the flaring and crowding of ribs alters baseline chest assessment findings. Without previous knowledge of anticipated findings, it is difficult, if not impossible, to accurately assess the patient with scoliosis. With severe abnormality, breath sounds are typically louder over the flared ribs and more diminished over the increased density of crowded ribs. The crowded ribs limit expansion of the lungs and further contribute to decreased breath sounds on that side. This finding is true in spite of the fact that, theoretically, actual lung ventilation should be worse where ribs flare, owing to overinflated lungs on that side, and better where ribs crowd, owing to healthier underlying lung tissue. Because of these changes in baseline findings, it is crucial that nurses observe and chart initial assessments, especially breath sounds, to help others determine deviations from the patient's normal findings.

Last, severe scoliosis causes decreased chest wall compliance and restrictive pulmonary disease. It significantly compromises heart and lung function when the curvature is greater than 90 to 100 degrees, particularly when accompanied by kyphosis (kyphoscoliosis). Not only do crowded ribs restrict chest movement and lung expansion, but flared ribs encircle the chest posteriorly and flatten the chest anteriorly. Restricted lung expansion and heart contraction limit the patient's cardiopulmonary reserves. During exercise or any stressful event, the patient has a limited ability to increase minute ventilation or cardiac output to meet the demands of the body.

Kyphoscoliosis. Of all chest deformities discussed thus far, kyphoscoliosis produces the most physical impairment to the cardiopulmonary system. Etiologically, patients with this abnormality may be divided into three groups as follows (Fraser and Paré, 1979):

1. *Congenital anomaly group*—kyphoscoliosis constitutes only one part of the clinical picture, e.g., muscular dystrophy, Marfan's syndrome, neurofibromatosis, Friedreich's ataxia.
2. *Paralytic group*—scoliosis develops into kyphoscoliosis, most commonly secondary to poliomyelitis.
3. *Idiopathic group*—most patients fall into this group. More common in females, kyphoscoliosis is unassociated with congenital defects or other diseases.

Patients with severe kyphoscoliosis are severely disabled; the degree of disability is usually related to the increasing angle of scoliosis and the patient's age. Pulmonary hypertension develops into cor pulmonale

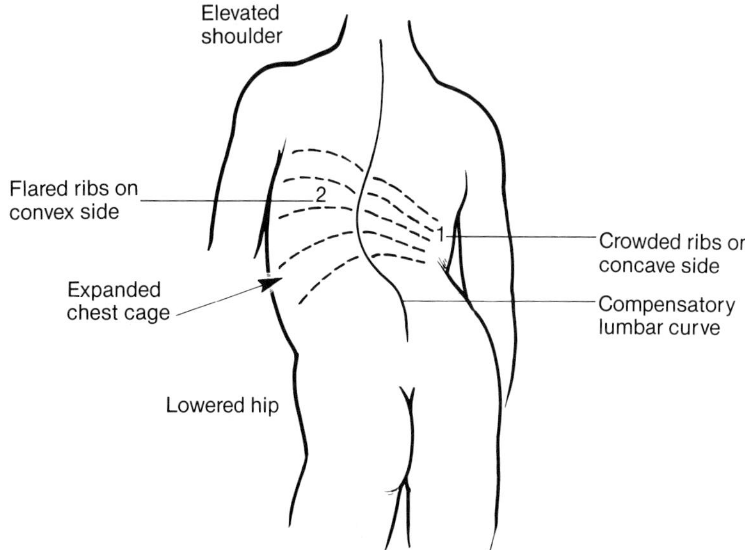

Figure 12–26. The effects of the S-shaped spinal curve in scoliosis (posterior view). In this case, the convex side of the thoracic curve points to the left.

and cardiac and respiratory failure by the time the individual is in his 40s or 50s. With the appearance of cardiopulmonary failure, the clinical course is gradually downhill, often precipitated by chest infections. Lung volumes (vital capacity and total lung capacity) are drastically reduced. Shallow respirations and unequal matching of ventilation and perfusion in the lung cause a low $Pa{O_2}$ and a high $Pa{CO_2}$. The gradual development of these changes may go unnoticed because the patient remains relatively asymptomatic until end-stage disease or until an accompanying underlying disease leads to hospitalization.

Poker Spine. The term *poker spine* refers to abnormal *straightening* of the thoracic curve of the spinal cord or abnormal *stiffness* of the back causing marked restriction of movement of the spine in all directions. Definitions differ owing to varying etiologies and clinical presentations. Actual straightening of the thoracic curve is rare except for the patient with a supporting spinal prosthesis to treat an orthopedic problem. Occasionally one might encounter a patient with congenital absence of the normal thoracic curve, known as *straight back syndrome*; this condition causes no significant impairment of pulmonary function. However, *stiffness* of the spine from rheumatoid arthritis. or, more commonly, ankylosing spondylitis can cause significant restrictive disease.

SKIN SURFACES

Moving from general observations to more specific ones, the nurse inspects the surface of the skin for *color, markings, bulges,* and *swollen areas.* The skin should appear smooth and supple, with the normal, symmetric distribution of hair on the surface. Although abnormalities on the skin's surface are more readily discovered and evaluated when inspection is used simultaneously with palpation, many abnormalities can be identified by inspection alone.

Skin surface findings commonly seen in respiratory patients are summarized in Table 12–1. Other abnormalities that might be encountered in the clinical setting are described hereafter.

The upper chest and neck areas are examined specifically for the presence of *edema, pallor, cyanosis,* and *dilated veins.* Tumors in the mediastinum, lung apex, or superior thoracic inlet may obstruct blood flow from the superior vena cava and produce these findings (Fig. 12–27). Enlarged lymph nodes from Hodgkin's disease, carcinoma, or tuberculosis can cause the same problem.

Other possible skin findings include birthmarks, telangiectasis, and spider nevi. *Telangiectasis* is superficial dilatation of capillaries and sometimes terminal arteries, producing a small, usually reddish spot. It may be a birthmark discovered in childhood; it may be due to several causes, including stomach problems, gallbladder disease, cirrhosis of the liver, tuberculosis, goiter, and infections. A *spider nevus,* common in patients with liver disease, is telangiectasis radiating from a central angioma in the skin, the *spider* effect. To differentiate spider nevi from petechiae, apply direct pressure to the abnormality; spider nevi blanch with direct pressure, whereas petechiae do not.

RESPIRATORY RATE AND BREATHING PATTERN

Normal Respiratory Rate

Respiratory rate, or breaths per minute, varies with the age of the individual, as shown.

Age	*Rate*
Newborn	30–60
Infant	20–40
Young child	15–25
Adolescent-adult	12–20

These rates are slower during sleep, down to 8 to 12 breaths per minute for the adult. The ratio of respira-

Table 12–1. COMMON SKIN SURFACE FINDINGS IN RESPIRATORY PATIENTS

Physical Findings	Clinical Implications
Increased pallor, cyanosis, dusky coloration	Central oxygenation problem
Diaphoresis	Acute anxiety, increased work of breathing, respiratory distress
Incisional scars	
Midsternal scar or scar running from the MSL around the lateral chest to the posterior chest	Thoracotomy
Small incisional scars	Old chest tube sites, thoracentesis, lung biopsy
Scars over deformed chest cage, upper anterior chest	Thoracoplasty for tuberculosis (operation used in the past, involving removal of portions of ribs and collapse of tuberculous lung tissue)
Reddish-purple markings in the center of the anterior chest	Radiation therapy to mediastinum for cancer involving the mediastinum
Small, red petechiae (dot-like purplish or red hemorrhagic spots)	Side effect of long-term steroid therapy
Skin rashes, urticaria	Hypersensitivity reaction in normal individuals or those with a history of atopy (hay fever, extrinsic asthma)
	Drug reaction; antibiotics or histamines such as Benadryl may be responsible
Erythema nodosum (red and painful nodules)	Streptococcal sore throat, tuberculosis, sarcoidosis, coccidioidomycosis
Infiltrative skin lesions or ulcers	Sarcoidosis, fungal infections, histiocytosis X
Swollen areas or bulges	Tumor, subcutaneous emphysema, lymphadenopathy, trauma
	Inserted cardiac pacemaker or phrenic nerve stimulator (immediately below skin in upper or lower chest areas)

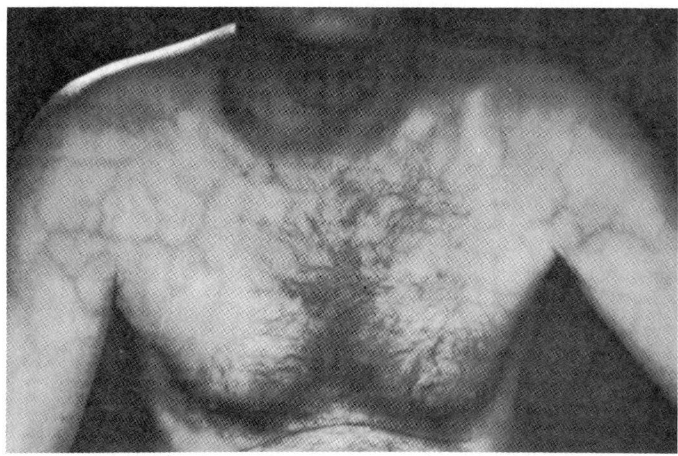

Figure 12–27. Obstruction of the superior vena cava from a lung tumor produces dilated jugular veins and visible veins over the chest and shoulder skin surfaces. The visible veins are the result of the development of subcutaneous collateral circulation. (Reproduced by permission from Delp, M. and Manning, R.: Major's Physical Diagnosis—An Introduction to the Clinical Process. Philadelphia, W. B. Saunders Co., 1981.)

tion to pulse is normally 1:4, and the ratio of respiration to temperature is 4:1 (four respirations for every 1° F over normal).

Normal Breathing Patterns

Adult respirations occur in a regular, even pattern with an occasional sigh or yawn every 5 to 10 minutes towards total lung capacity (Fig. 12–28). Respirations in the newborn, especially the premature infant, are normally irregular in pattern and uneven in depth (i.e., periodic breathing) during the first few weeks of life. This is caused by an immature respiratory center and has no pathologic significance.

Periodic breathing is more specifically defined as a change in respiratory rate, depth, or tidal volume, sometimes with periods of apnea (no breathing). In the newborn, periodic breathing becomes more marked during sleep. Sporadic brief apneic periods lasting no longer than 10 to 20 seconds and accompanied by no other alteration in body function are followed by a slightly elevated respiratory rate (i.e., physiologic hyperventilation). After the first few weeks of life, periodic breathing is abnormal as a baseline pattern. However, it normally may occur quite frequently during sleep.

In the adult, periodic breathing similar to that seen in the Cheyne-Stokes pattern (described hereafter) may normally occur during drowsiness and the lighter stages of sleep with brief apneic periods (lasting 5 to 15 seconds). Breathing becomes normal again once sleep is established, but in the last stage of sleep (rapid

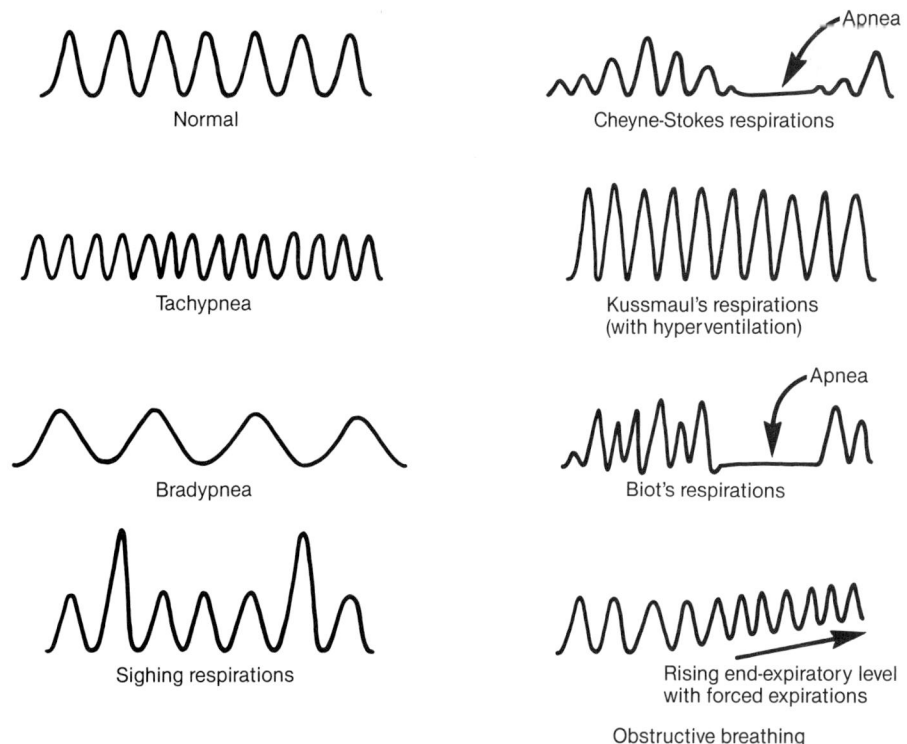

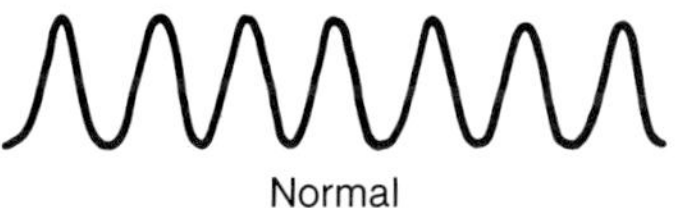

Apnea

Cheyne-Stokes respirations

Tachypnea

Kussmaul's respirations
(with hyperventilation)

Figure 12–28. Spirograms of types of breathing patterns.

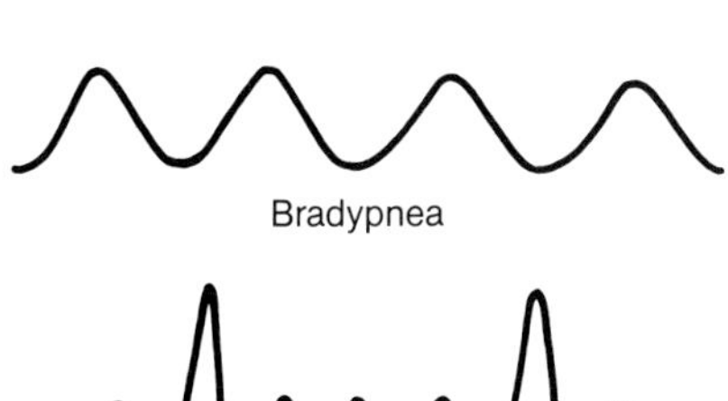

Apnea

Biot's respirations

Rising end-expiratory level
with forced expirations

Obstructive breathing

eye movement, or REM, sleep), when dreaming occurs, respirations may become periodic or irregular again with brief apneic periods.

Different patterns of periodic or irregular breathing are most likely to occur in normal persons over 40 years of age. They are universally present in persons sleeping at high altitudes and are most likely to occur in individuals with abnormal blood gases, particularly those who exhibit high $PaCO_2$ during the day. As a general monitoring parameter, apneic periods should never last longer than 15 to 20 seconds in adults and 10 seconds in healthy infants.

Abnormal Breathing Patterns

Alterations in the rate, quality, and depth of respiration produce the following abnormal breathing patterns (see Fig. 12–28).

Tachypnea. *Increased respiratory rate over 20 breaths per minute.* A nonspecific finding commonly due to pain, anxiety, fever, anemia, and blood gas disturbances from a variety of causes, this pattern allows the patient to increase minute ventilation to meet the greater oxygen demands of the body. It is commonly accompanied by shallow respirations.

Bradypnea. *Decreased respiratory rate under 10 breaths per minute.* Another nonspecific finding indicating severe abnormality, this pattern is due to a number of disorders as follows: brain disorders; administration of a sedative, narcotic, or tranquilizer; excessive alcohol intake; metabolic disorders; blood gas disturbances; overfatigue in the critically ill patient; and others.

Both bradypnea and tachypnea must be interpreted in light of other clinical findings. Although baseline respiratory rate itself can serve as a sensitive measurement of dysfunction, especially in infants and children, monitoring *change* in baseline rate is most important for nurses. Although tachypnea at 26 breaths per minute may be normal in a severe COPD patient and not of concern, any increase in rate may indicate the onset of acute bronchitis and bronchoconstriction. Sudden increases or decreases in rate indicate gross pathology, especially when accompanied by changes in vital signs and signs of respiratory distress.

Apnea. *Total cessation of air flow to the lungs.* Normal during sleep, as described previously, and pathologic when longer than 15 seconds, apnea is incompatible with life when extended beyond 2 minutes (i.e., *respiratory arrest*). Unless cardiopulmonary resuscitation measures restore respirations, respiratory arrest leads to *cardiac arrest*, and sometimes the two occur simultaneously, i.e., cardiopulmonary arrest. Respiratory arrest may occur from acute upper airway obstruction or damage or depression of the brain's respiratory center, as in head trauma, stroke, narcotic or anesthetic overdose, and alveolar hypoventilation. Brief apneic episodes may appear in periodic breathing patterns, e.g., Cheyne-Stokes or Biot's respirations. They disappear untreated over time or following treatment of the underlying disorder.

Brief apneic episodes, in addition to periodic breathing and hypopneas (described hereafter), occur normally at the onset of sleep and in REM sleep in healthy persons. In related studies, *sleep apnea* is frequently defined as a reduction of air flow of less than 20% of normal for at least 10 seconds (Nochomovitz and Cherniack, 1986). Hence, when the nurse reports apneic periods during sleep on physical examination, sleep apnea is suspected, but the medical diagnosis is actually based on measurements made during a sleep apnea study with special respiratory monitoring equipment. When apneic episodes are frequent and at least 10 seconds in duration, the *sleep apnea syndrome* is suspected (see Chapter 8).

Hyperpnea. *Increased depth of respiration.* Aside from normal occurrence with strenuous exercise, hyperpnea is rarely seen without a simultaneous increase in respiratory rate.

Hyperventilation. *Increased rate and depth of respiration.* This pattern is caused by fever, low PaO_2, and other disorders causing alveolar hyperventilation.

Hypoventilation. *Slow or irregular respiratory pattern with shallow respirations.* This pattern is commonly due to prolonged depression of the respiratory center from drug overdose, anesthesia, or splinting-type pain. It leads to alveolar hypoventilation and ventilatory failure in severe cases.

Hypopnea refers to *periods of hypoventilation during sleep.* Though it may be suspected during physical examination, the diagnosis is actually a medical one, requiring a formal sleep apnea study. During such a study, hypopnea is defined as an air flow of 20 to 50% of normal accompanied by a fall in oxygen saturation of at least 4% (Nochomovitz and Cherniack, 1986).

Most important, both hyperventilation and hypoventilation are nonspecific physical findings based on clinical impression. When either is suspected, an arterial blood gas study is always ordered to verify the presence and degree of *alveolar* hyperventilation or hypoventilation.

Most of the terms that follow are called "respirations" because they represent one or more respirations within a main breathing pattern, e.g., bradypnea with gasping respirations. However, they may represent the main breathing pattern in some cases.

Sighing Respirations. *Frequent sighs (more than 2 to 3 per minute) within a normal breathing pattern.* Seen in extremely anxious individuals, these respirations may be accompanied by dyspnea, chest tightness, and tingling in the extremities, as in the *hyperventilation syndrome*, defined as hyperventilation from psychologic causes. This syndrome may develop, for example, when a patient is informed of the diagnosis of his organic disease.

Cheyne-Stokes Respirations. *A cyclic pattern of progressively deeper respirations, followed by progressively shallower respirations and a period of apnea.* Each breathing cycle lasts 30 to 45 seconds and apneic periods up to 20 seconds. Since apneic periods may last longer with severe abnormality, they are always timed, and the physician is called when they become longer than 15 to 20 seconds. Disappearing and reappearing at random times, Cheyne-Stokes respirations indicate gross pathology due to brain disorders from trauma or disease to the cerebrum or conditions that increase cerebrospinal fluid pressure, renal failure, meningitis, or drug overdose. It may be observed in cardiopulmonary patients with congestive heart failure, presumably because of the blood's increased circulatory time to the brain (Cherniack and Cherniack, 1983). Pulmonary congestion and the inefficient failing heart account for the increased circulatory time and the central chemoreceptors' delay in responding to changes in blood gas tensions. Because of this delayed response, ventilatory response also lags behind changes in blood gases. The abnormal breathing pattern results. It disappears either after the heart failure has been effectively treated or spontaneously after the administration of oxygen.

Kussmaul's Respirations. *Deep, regular breaths, usually at a rate greater than 20 per minute.* Seen in those with diabetic ketoacidosis, renal failure, and other metabolic acidotic states, this pattern is suspected in the presence of obvious hyperventilation or increased respiratory rate. Sometimes, however, the pattern is barely noticeable, as in the patient on renal dialysis.

Biot's Respirations. *Irregular breaths of varying depths interrupted periodically by periods of apnea of varying lengths.* Occasional sighs may be interspersed throughout this pattern. The pattern is most frequently seen in patients with spinal meningitis and other neurologic disorders.

Gasping Respirations. *Deep breaths with spasmodic inspiratory effort.* The gasping breaths are accompanied by an increased respiratory rate and a regular or irregular breathing pattern or by bradypnea with apneic episodes in patients near death. The breaths are a sign of respiratory distress commonly seen in hospitalized patients experiencing severe pain, panic, acute airway obstruction, or acute pulmonary embolism.

Obstructive Breathing Pattern. *Gradual rise in end-expiratory level during forced rapid breathing* (Fig. 12–28H). This pattern occurs when retained secretions, wheezing, or upper airway obstruction causes respiratory distress. In ambulatory COPD patients, notably those with emphysema, it may appear with exertional dyspnea during activities of daily living or strenuous exercise. In each case, muscle fatigue, increased airway resistance, and mechanical obstruction prevent the complete expiration of air, causing a higher end-expiratory level with each successive breath and air trapping in the lungs.

Determination of Respiratory Rate and Breathing Pattern

The nurse watches the rise and fall of the chest cage or abdomen for 30 seconds to 1 minute, evaluating *respiratory rate per minute* and *breathing pattern* as well as *inspiratory-expiratory ratio*, *muscles of breathing*, and *chest movement*, described subsequently. For sedated patients or those in a deep sleep curled up to one side, it may be necessary to place the fingertips or hands on the chest wall to pick up subtle chest movements. In some cases, arousal and moving of the patient to a supine position may be necessary to verify the presence of respirations, to count respiratory rate, and to gather more specific baseline information on chest movements.

In the determination of breathing pattern, the nurse identifies the pattern that best approximates the patient's respirations and then, if necessary, describes other distinguishing features. Variations in the previously described breathing patterns and respirations commonly occur in the clinical setting. For example, conditions that slow the circulation of the blood to the brain (e.g., shock, hypothermia, and congestive heart failure) may produce slight variations in the Cheyne-Stokes respirations previously described. Frequent sighs may occur in the hyperventilation syndrome. Brain damage can produce a variety of irregular or periodic breathing patterns, depending on the pathology involved. In critically ill patients, respirations may wax and wane with changing blood gas disturbances.

The nonspecific nature of respiratory rate and pattern of breathing must be emphasized. They signal an abnormality affecting the respiratory system, but they do not indicate specifically *what* is wrong nor the *extent* of pathology. They may remain grossly insensitive to changing pathology.

INSPIRATORY TO EXPIRATORY (I:E) RATIO

Estimating *I:E ratio* in seconds is sometimes used to help identify restrictive versus obstructive pulmonary disease. Also, an abnormal ratio, when accompanied by other signs of distress, indicates respiratory distress.

The normal I:E ratio is about 1:2 seconds, with inspiration never longer than 2 seconds and expiration never longer than 4 seconds at rest. Restrictive disease produces a ratio of about 1:1, acute upper airway obstruction a ratio of 2:2 to 4:2 (i.e., prolonged inspiratory phase), and chronic obstructive disease a ratio closer to 1:4 (i.e., prolonged expiratory phase).

I:E ratio is commonly used to screen for the presence of COPD. The patient is asked to take a deep breath in and blow all his air out as fast as he can. In the presence of COPD, expiration lasts longer than 4 seconds, sometimes taking longer than 10 seconds in those able to complete the forced expiratory maneuver. Dyspneic COPD patients with severe disease who are unable to perform the maneuver may have a resting I:E ratio approaching 1:1. This ratio is a sign of severe air flow limitation, lung hyperinflation, and increased work of breathing.

MUSCLES OF BREATHING

Normal Breathing

As Chapter 6 points out, the diaphragm is the main muscle of breathing. During normal breathing, the upper abdomen and lower chest rise on inspiration as the lung bases fill with air, and they *passively* fall back to resting position on expiration. Variations in this pattern may be seen in normal individuals.

Though men are commonly labelled abdominal (i.e., diaphragmatic) breathers and women labelled chest breathers, research indicates that there are no major differences between men and women or between the young and the elderly (Sharp et al, 1975). During quiet breathing, most people are abdominal breathers when supine and chest breathers when upright. When chest movement predominates, actual intercostal muscle retractions should not be visible, unless the individual breathes deeply or develops labored breathing.

Labored Breathing

During labored breathing, a sign of increased work of breathing and respiratory distress, rib cage movement usually predominates over abdominal movement. However, as suggested in Chapter 6, the actions of both muscle groups are important because of their interactions to optimize the mechanical advantage of the diaphragm. The principal muscles of inspiration become more active; the intercostal muscles retract, and the abdomen and lower chest may expand more. Neck accessory muscles contract to elevate the sternum and slightly enlarge the chest. Shoulder and back muscles may also contribute to inspiratory and expiratory effort. In addition, expiration becomes active, as internal intercostals and abdominal muscles contract to help empty the lungs of air. (See Chapter 6 for a detailed description of muscles used during active breathing.)

Inspiratory accessory muscles are employed more than expiratory accessory muscles in patients with upper airway obstruction and those without obstructive disease. Also, inspiratory effort may become marked whenever abdominal protuberance or abdominal pain inhibits diaphragmatic movement.

In check-valve mechanical obstruction of the upper airway (i.e., air in but not out) or severe COPD, use of expiratory accessory muscles may predominate, with bulging of intercostal spaces during prolonged expiration.

Monitoring Muscle Groups

To facilitate monitoring, the nurse notes and charts the use of the following main accessory muscle groups: *shoulder muscles*, *neck muscles*, and *intercostal muscles*. The gentleman in Figure 7–13 is using all three muscle groups. This approach helps nurses on different shifts evaluate the progression of signs and symptoms and decide whether the patient's labored breathing is better, worse, or unchanged and whether the physician should be called for further medical evaluation.

CHEST MOVEMENTS

Chest Excursions

Chest excursion refers to the outward movement of the chest cage with each breath. *Minimal chest excursions* are normal for healthy adults at rest, but they indicate alveolar hypoventilation in the absence of periodic sighs (e.g., monotonous breathing pattern) or in the presence of maximal ventilatory effort (e.g., muscular effort). *Maximal chest excursions* at rest always indicate a ventilatory or oxygenation problem. More specifically, they indicate alveolar hyperventilation when auscultation of the lungs demonstrates normal or increased breath sounds, and hypoventilation when breath sounds are decreased or absent. Particularly in acute clinical settings, chest movement must be interpreted in light of auscultatory findings because maximal chest excursion may represent maximal muscular effort rather than maximal air movement or adequate alveolar ventilation, as in acute airway obstruction from aspiration of a foreign object.

Asymmetric Chest Movement

The nurse compares right and left sides of the anterior and posterior areas of the chest for *asymmetric chest movement*. Careful inspection during all phases of inspiration and expiration may identify slightly depressed or overexpanded areas not appreciated during general observations. By standing at the foot of the bed and observing the chest during quiet as well as deep breathing, the nurse may detect localized areas of the chest that do not follow the movement of the chest as a whole. When bilateral, such lags may indicate increased work of breathing and respiratory muscle fatigue. When localized unilaterally, a lag usually indicates underlying lung or pleural pathology.

Paradoxical Chest Movements

Paradoxical movement is present when the chest or part of the chest, abdomen, or both move inward instead of outward during inspiration and outward instead of inward during expiration. The chest and abdomen together may move paradoxically in a pattern exactly opposite that of normal respiration, or *asynchrony* may be present with chest and abdomen moving in opposite directions.

Open Pneumothorax. The patient with this disorder may present with paradoxical movement of air as well as paradoxical movement of the chest. Paradoxical movement of air occurs as follows: pleural pressures on the unaffected side are more negative than the near atmospheric pleural pressures on the affected side. Air is inspired into the normal lung from the semicollapsed lung (Fig. 12–29). During expiration, air from the

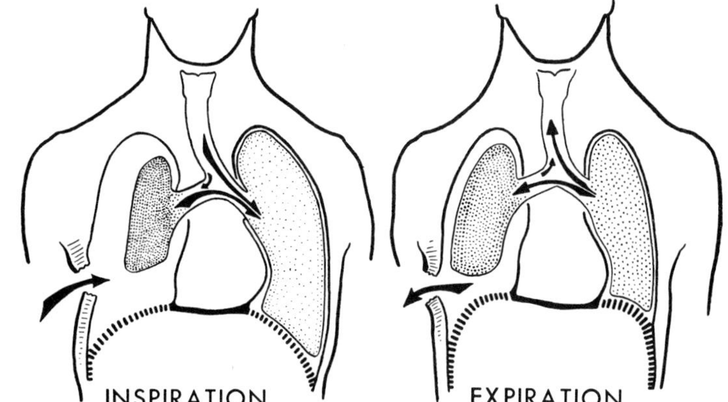

Figure 12–29. Paradoxical movement of air (Pendelluft) and mediastinal shift in open pneumothorax. (Reproduced by permission from Cherniack, R. and Cherniak, L.: Respiration in Health and Disease, 3rd ed. Philadelphia, W. B. Saunders Co., 1983.)

normal lung moves into the semicollapsed lung, causing it to expand slightly. The cycle continues as rebreathed air again is inspired into the normal lung, producing greater drops in blood oxygen levels. This paradoxical movement or shunting of air is called *Pendelluft.* In large pneumothoraces, Pendelluft may cause significant mediastinal shift, if the mediastinum is mobile and free of fibrous adhesions to permit it to swing back and forth with changing pleural pressures. The chest cage may remain relatively immobile on the affected side during the paradoxical movement of air.

Accompanying *paradoxical movement of the chest* on the affected side occurs as follows. In early inspiration, although the lung may begin to deflate as previously explained, the chest cage remains immobile or expands slightly as contraction of respiratory muscles on the affected side lowers pleural pressures, drawing more air into the pleural space. Increased air in the pleural space pushes the mediastinum even more towards the unaffected side. However, towards the end of inspiration, pressure in the pleural space in the affected side rises above atmospheric pressure, and air escapes from the pleural space out into the atmosphere through the opening in the chest. The chest cage falls inward as air escapes, and the mediastinum moves back towards midline position. This paradoxical movement of the chest may be very subtle, if it exists at all. It is often less noticeable than the hyperinflated, asymmetric chest on the affected side that exhibits minimal respiratory movement when compared with the opposite unaffected side. Furthermore, although paradoxical movement of the chest may appear minimal, paradoxical movement of air in the lungs may be quite significant. Open pneumothorax itself is a medical emergency. Paradoxical movement of the chest confirms the graveness of the situation.

Neuromuscular Disease. Paradoxical movement of the chest occurs in cervical cord injury with an intact phrenic nerve and diaphragm but a paralyzed rib cage. A sign of partial or complete diaphragmatic paralysis is paradoxical inward movement of the abdomen during inspiration, most evident in the supine position. This movement is typically accompanied by shallow, rapid respiration and complaints of disturbed sleep, morning headache, daytime fatigue, and shortness of breath. These findings indicate hypoventilation and can be greatly eased merely by placing the patient in the erect position, which minimizes upward movement of the diaphragm on inspiration. The supine position facilitates paradoxical inward movement of the abdomen and upward movement of the diaphragm because of displacement of the abdominal contents into the thorax.

Trauma and Flail Chest. Trauma patients are observed for *flail chest,* paradoxical movement of a segment of the chest wall. This occurs when fractured ribs are broken in at least two places. The resulting "floating" segment of chest cage moves inward during inspiration (i.e., pulled by negative intrathoracic pressures) and outward during expiration (i.e., pushed by more positive pressures) (Fig. 12–30). In the process, expired air from the affected lung may enter the unaffected lung (Fig. 12–30), producing the Pendelluft phenomenon already described. Intubation and mechanical ventilation may be necessary to stabilize the chest wall. With chest wall stabilization, flailing disappears or is barely noticeable. When breathing spontaneously during the weaning process, the patient is closely observed for the reappearance of the flail chest; the physician may decide to return the patient to mechanical ventilation for further chest stabilization.

Flail chest is also seen in postcardiac arrest patients resulting from sternal compressions. A correctly performed manual compression or one that is misplaced to the side may result in costal cartilage and rib fractures. Fractures may occur at *any* time during the arrest procedure, sometimes on the first compression in older patients or patients with hyperinflated chests.

Respiratory Failure. Patients in acute respiratory failure may exhibit all degrees of paradoxical movement of the chest, abdomen, or both with varying patterns of asynchronous breathing. In extreme cases, chest and abdominal movements may be completely asynchronous. Although clinicians may misinterpret the distorted breathing pattern as labored, laboratory measurements have actually documented the onset of expiration while the chest cage is still expanding (Pon-

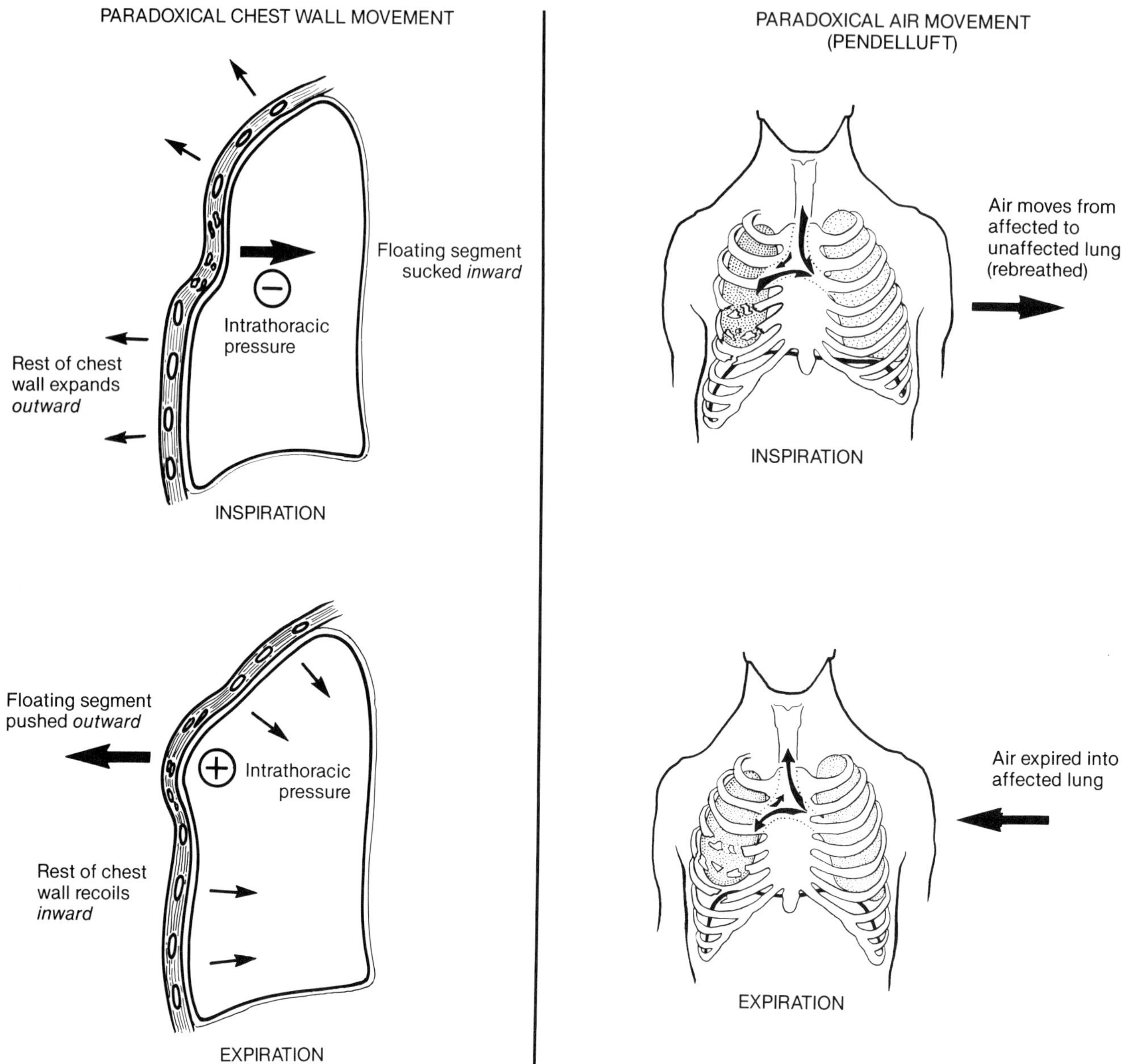

Figure 12–30. Flail chest with paradoxical chest wall movement (left) and paradoxical air movement (Pendelluft) (right). Right illustration reproduced and adapted by permission from Cherniack, R. and Cherniak, L.: Respiration in Health and Disease, 3rd ed. Philadelphia, W. B. Saunders Co., 1983.)

toppidan et al, 1972). Because of the inability to properly synchronize chest and diaphragmatic movements, the exact cause of the discoordination is unknown. This problem delays weaning from a ventilator until the pattern gradually improves over time.

COPD. Paradoxical movement of the abdomen may be seen in some patients with emphysema. Gilbert and associates (1979) studied 30 patients in all stages of emphysema. Respiratory movement during inspiration was normal. Expiratory chest movement, however, was paradoxical and somewhat spastic, as follows: at or near the start of expiration, the abdomen moves inward rapidly, followed immediately by a second outward movement much greater than that during inspiration. Then the abdomen moves inward again to complete expiration. Although most of the 13 patients exhibiting this paradoxical movement were on assisted ventilation, two were not, and one was ambulatory. Statistics from the study suggest that this abnormal pattern carries a grave prognosis for both disability and survival. More patients in the asynchronous breathing group eventually died when compared with those in the normal breathing group.

Postoperative Patients. The diaphragm's contribution to quiet breathing is greatly reduced during the first 24 hours after upper abdominal surgery. Little chest or abdominal movement may be observed. This change is accompanied by decreases in expiratory flow rates (FEV_1) and lung volumes (vital capacity), commonly leading to patchy areas of atelectasis on the chest x-ray (Ford et al, 1981).

One investigation (Catley et al, 1982) indicates that these and total hip replacement patients receiving regional anesthetic blocks or intravenous morphine during the first 16 hours postoperatively demonstrate numerous episodes of both central apnea, followed by hyperventilation, and obstructive apnea, followed by marked reductions in Pao_2. Apneic episodes were more numerous in those with morphine administration (i.e., 82 central and 27 obstructive), and sometimes the episodes lasted up to 2 minutes. Most important, in every case, drops in oxygen saturation were associated with paradoxical breathing. At the beginning of inspiration, the upper abdomen moved inward rather than outward, lagging behind thoracic chest movement. The conclusion of the study was that modest doses of intravenous morphine may produce paradoxical breathing during the postoperative stage, which, in some patients, results in potentially life-threatening drops in Pao_2.

Respiratory Alternans

This pattern refers to a cyclic one of breathing characterized by a series of abdominal breaths followed by a series of breaths effected by displacement of the rib cage. Respiratory alternans either accompanies the onset of paradoxical inward abdominal motion during inspiration or appears after sustained periods of abdominal paradox. Both respiratory alternans and abdominal paradox are signs of inspiratory muscle fatigue, especially when accompanied by tachypnea and increased $Paco_2$, and they may signal impending ventilatory failure (Cohen et al, 1982).

En Bloc Chest Movement

En bloc movement of the chest refers to the upward and downward movement of the *entire* chest cage with inspiration and expiration. Seen in severe COPD patients with hyperinflated chests from air trapping, mostly those with emphysema and severe chronic asthma, this movement is facilitated by the use of the accessory muscles of respiration. Barrel chest deformity and an obstructed breathing pattern usually accompany en bloc movement. Although the chest cage may appear to be quite mobile because of excessive respiratory muscle activity, *actual* chest excursion or movement is minimal, owing to lung hyperinflation.

Palpation

Palpation is the act of feeling the surface of the chest with the hands primarily *to identify areas of tenderness* and *to further assess abnormalities noted during inspection*. It has three other more specific purposes as follows: (1) to estimate lateral chest expansion, (2) to identify possible lung pathology by feeling for abnormal chest vibrations (i.e., fremitus), and (3) to help identify cardiac complications in respiratory disease.

This section of the chapter covers the following areas: general and fine palpation of the chest, palpation of the costal angle, lateral chest expansion, and fremitus. Aspects of the precordial examination that are easily integrated into inspection and palpation of the lungs and thorax are presented towards the end of this chapter.

GENERAL AND FINE PALPATION

The examiner uses both general and fine palpation techniques to palpate the chest. *General palpation* is performed with firm pressure applied to the palmar aspects of the fingers. It also may be done with firm pressure to the side of the hand with a closed fist. Both hands may be used at once, as shown in Figure 12–31A, to facilitate coverage of the entire chest in a short period of time. General palpation is used in combination with *fine palpation*, which is firm palpation with only a few fingertips. This technique is used to allow more thorough examination of localized areas of the chest or uneven chest surfaces, e.g., intercostal spaces (Fig. 12–31B).

To palpate the chest

1. *Sit the patient on the edge of the bed or examining table.*
2. *Use general palpation and screen the entire chest for areas of tenderness.* You can choose your own specific locations and methodology as long as you cover *all* chest areas down to roughly the fifth rib anteriorly and down to T10 to T12 posteriorly. Figure 12–42 can be used as a guide in developing a methodology, but remember to palpate the chest surfaces *between* the labelled areas and to cover lateral chest surfaces all the way up to the axillae. A few other points follow:
   a. Avoid bony structures, such as the clavicles and scapulae.
   b. Concentrate on areas where pain has been reported or where lesions are evident.
   c. When firm finger pressure is insufficient to elicit complaints of tenderness (e.g., individuals with thick chest walls), you may wish to modify your technique. Try tapping lightly once or twice on the chest with a closed fist. Some clinicians use this technique specifically when a chest wall abnormality is suspected.

   Tenderness usually indicates the presence of an inflammatory process or tissue trauma affecting bone, muscle, or underlying pleura. In the liver area at or slightly below the fifth rib anteriorly, it indicates liver disease or disorders affecting the liver, notably RV failure in the respiratory patient.

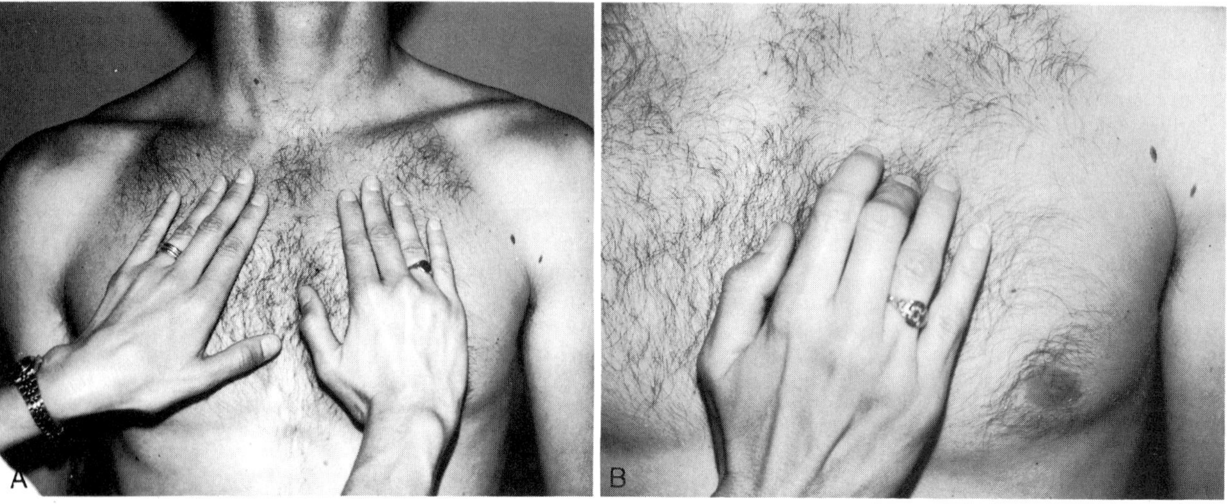

Figure 12–31. Technique for general palpation *(A)* and fine palpation *(B)* of the chest.

3. *Palpate the vertebral column from top to bottom using the closed fist technique* (i.e., ulnar aspect of a closed fist). Tap firmly one or two times in one location and move inferiorly in small ½-inch steps to avoid skipping any vertebrae or intervertebral spaces.

   Tenderness may indicate the presence of vertebral compression fractures from trauma, gross spinal deformity, or long-term steroid therapy.
4. *Switch from general to fine palpation to obtain more specific information.* Finely palpate the following areas:
   a. *Areas of tenderness, protuberances,* and *other abnormalities* discovered on inspection.
   b. *Ribs* as well as adjacent *intercostal spaces* to differentiate rib fractures or bone pain from muscle strain (i.e., ICS muscle pain).
   c. *Swollen areas* for *crepitation,* air under the skin. To detect crepitation, it may be necessary to "walk your fingers" in tiny steps along the chest's surface. A "crunching" or "crackling" is felt as the fingertips press down and displace subcutaneous air bubbles.

      For patients with new (1 to 3 days) tracheostomies, check for crepitation 1 to 2 inches around the stoma. Give attention to chest tube sites, infected subcutaneous tissues from gas gangrene, and surgical incisions. Patients at risk for crepitation include those with neck or thoracic surgery, barotrauma (e.g., pneumothorax and pneumomediastinum), any chest trauma, and those on mechanical ventilation with high peak inspiratory pressures. In postcardiac arrest patients, always check the anterior chest for signs of crepitation; if the patient develops a pneumothorax or pneumomediastinum (i.e., air in the mediastinum) from resuscitation procedures, air may dissect out to subcutaneous tissues to produce crepitation. The crepitation is usually worse in the ventilator patient than in the spontaneously breathing patient because ventilators deliver high positive pressures that can rapidly *push* air toward the periphery.
5. *During general and fine palpation, note the following skin characteristics: temperature, moisture,* and *skin turgor.*

   Warm, diaphoretic skin indicates fever from infection or overexertion from the increased work of breathing. *Dry skin* suggests dehydration, a serious problem in respiratory patients who need hydration to liquefy secretions and facilitate sputum production. To check for skin turgor, gently pinch the skin and watch it immediately return to normal resting position. A sluggish return to normal, called *poor skin turgor,* may indicate nutritional or fluid and electrolyte problems.

PALPATION OF THE COSTAL ANGLE

The nurse palpates the costal angle formed by the lower margin of the ribs with the xiphoid process. Healthy young adults have an angle of about 45 degrees. An angle that approximates 90 degrees is a sign of lung hyperinflation, as in COPD. Elderly individuals may demonstrate a wide costal angle from the aging process, but it never reaches 90 degrees.

LATERAL CHEST EXPANSION

The nurse palpates the lower lobes for lateral chest expansion, measuring it on a deep breath from the end of expiration to the end of inspiration. Measurement during a deep breath is necessary to pick up subtle differences in right and left expansion (excursion), particularly in patients with minimal chest excursions or fixed chest cage.

To measure lateral chest expansion

1. First, stand behind the patient.

2. Instruct the patient to take a *deep* breath in, as you grab the sides of the chest with your fingers and palmar aspects just above the diaphragm (T10 level), as shown in Figure 12–32A.

3. *As the patient expires completely, keep your fingers in the same position and move your thumbs to the midline position, gathering folds of skin in between* (Fig. 12–32B).

4. *As the patient takes another deep breath in, let your thumbs move outward with the lateral movement of the chest cage.* Encourage your hands to move *with* the chest by allowing your elbows to swing outward at the same time (Fig. 12–32C).

5. Now *visually estimate lateral chest expansion.* Measured from thumb to thumb, normal lateral chest expansion ranges from 2 to 3 in (5 to 8 cm) and up to 4 in (about 10 cm) in a young male adult with a large thorax.

This technique is used mostly to identify decreased expansion. An *equally bilateral decrease* is classically seen in COPD patients with lung hyperinflation and other patients with bilateral lung pathology.

A *unilateral decrease* in lateral expansion is usually from unilateral chest pathology, such as unilateral pneumothorax, pleural effusion, lobar pneumonia, pulmonary embolism or infarction, and lateral thoracotomy.

Since inspection during deep breathing identifies major areas with decreased expansion, this measurement is used to confirm suspected areas and to monitor the progress of the previously named restrictive processes. Unilateral decreases are measured or estimated from the vertebral column. An example of charting might be:

1. *Decreased rt. lateral chest expansion, only 2 cm from the vertebral column; left chest expansion 4 cm.*

If expansion is symmetrically equal, chart

2. *Lateral chest expansion symmetric, about 3 in* (8 cm), which is a normal measurement from thumb to thumb.

Although some clinicians estimate lateral chest expansion anteriorly, few actually use the technique as a routine monitoring parameter for any area except the lower lobes posteriorly.

Because visual measurements are subjective and actual measurements impractical and logistically difficult to make, since both hands are already on the chest, emphasis is *first* on the determination of normal

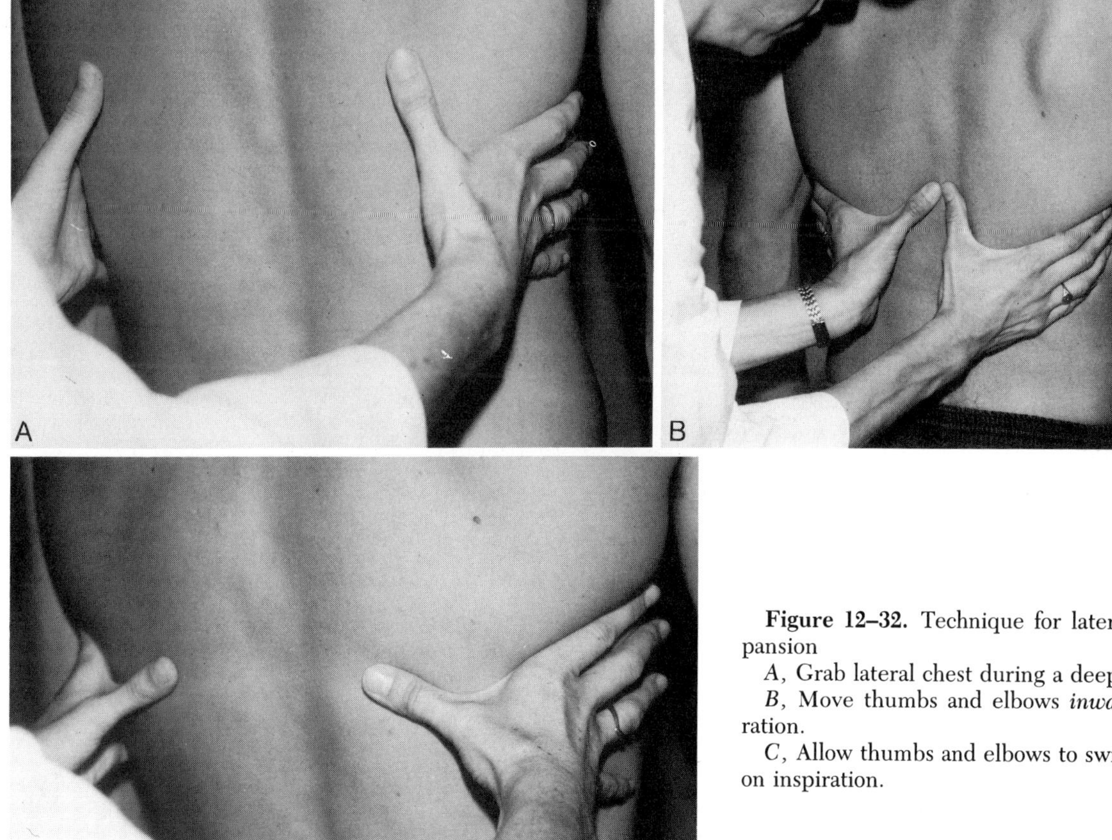

Figure 12–32. Technique for lateral chest expansion

A, Grab lateral chest during a deep breath.

B, Move thumbs and elbows *inward* on expiration.

C, Allow thumbs and elbows to swing *outward* on inspiration.

versus abnormal chest expansion and *second* on estimation in centimeters or inches. The technique is considered a general monitoring parameter.

FREMITUS

The nurse palpates the chest to feel for fremitus, abnormal vibrations on the chest wall. The three types of fremitus are *rhonchal fremitus*, *pleural rub fremitus*, and *vocal fremitus*.

Rhonchal Fremitus. This term refers to vibrations from secretions rumbling around in underlying large airways during breathing. It is less commonly produced by the passage of air through a stenotic trachea or major bronchus. In patients producing large amounts of mucus, place your hand on the anterior chest or over a consolidated segment of the lung to feel for mucus moving around. These patients usually need an intensive program of bronchial hygiene, coughing, deep breathing, and sometimes endotracheal suctioning or postural drainage. Rhonchal fremitus disappears with productive coughing.

Pleural Rub Fremitus. This vibration is a grating sensation created by the rubbing together of inflamed or roughened pleural surfaces (pleuritis). It is felt over areas where pleuritic pain is reported or a pleural friction rub is heard on auscultation.

To palpate the chest, place the hand firmly over the pathologic area and ask the patient to breathe deeply as you feel for the grating sensation. Pleural rub fremitus may feel like rhonchal fremitus, but it is different in that it usually occurs on inspiration and does *not* change at all with coughing. In contrast, rhonchal fremitus is usually inspiratory *and* expiratory, and it changes in intensity, timing during respiration, and location with vigorous coughing (i.e., mucus moving around in the chest).

Vocal Fremitus. This term refers to vibrations felt on the chest wall when the patient speaks. It is also called *tactile fremitus*, since the examiner must *touch* the chest to feel the voice vibrations.

Procedure. To elicit tactile fremitus

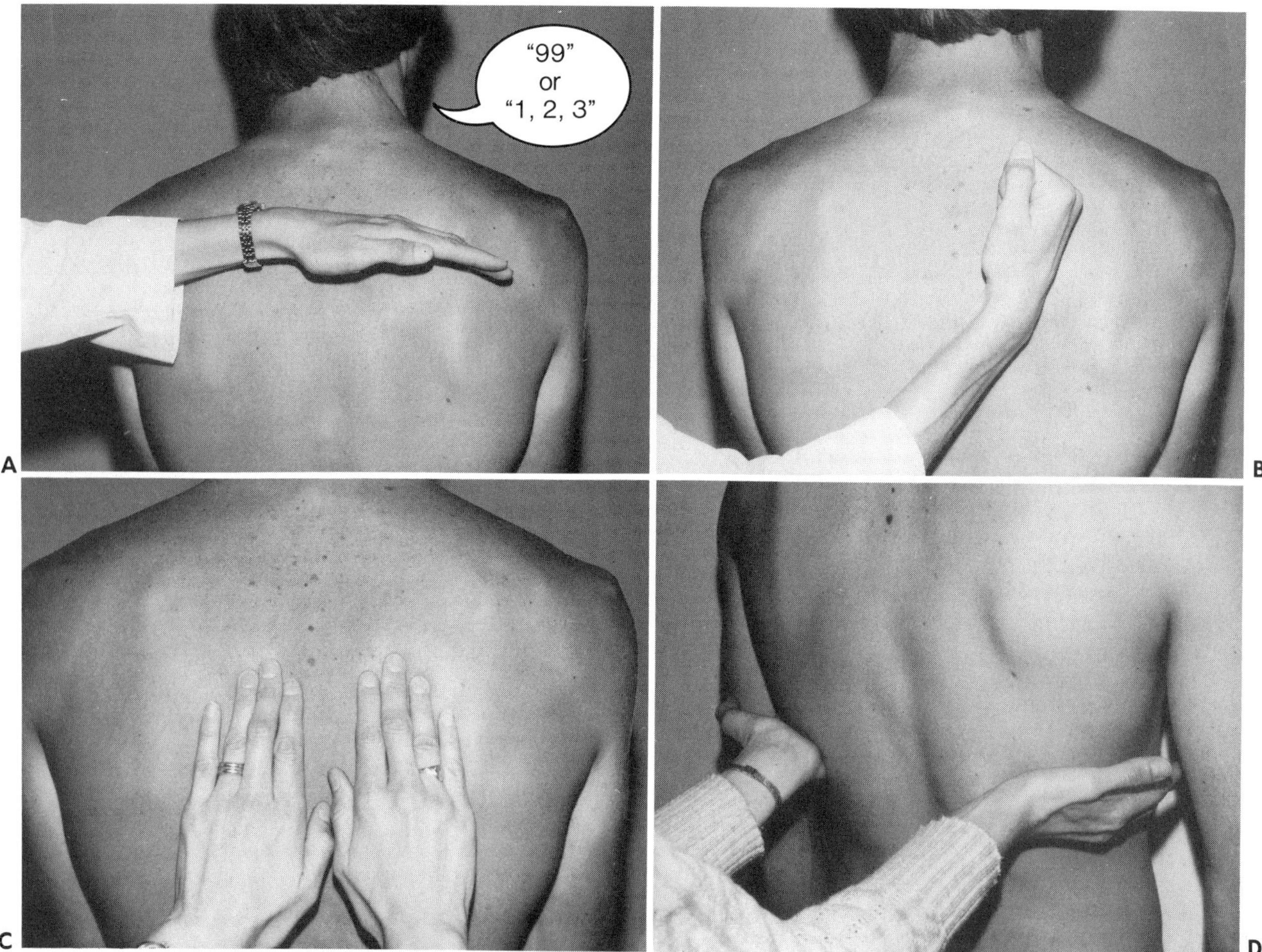

Figure 12–33. Different methods for detecting vocal (tactile) fremitus.
A, Ulnar aspect of hand.
B, Closed fist.
C, Fingertips, with both hands.
D, Ulnar aspects of hands for the lower lobes.

1. Sit the patient on the edge of the bed or examining table.

2. Firmly place the side of the hand against the chest in an ICS, as shown in Figure 12–33A.

The side of the hand is used because it is sensitive to touch, fits easily into ICSs, and permits coverage of a large area of chest in a short time span. Some clinicians prefer the palmar aspect of the fingers, closed fist, or fingertips. Any of these methods is acceptable (Fig. 12–33B, C, and D). Some clinicians vary their technique depending on the area and thoracic level under examination.

3. Ask the patient to say 99 or 1,2, 3 and feel for chest wall vibrations.

The spoken word instantly transmits voice vibrations from the larynx through the trachea, bronchi, lung tissue, pleura, and finally chest wall. The chest wall vibrations feel like the purr of a cat sounds and are present only when the patient speaks.

4. Place the hand in the same location on the opposite side of the chest and again ask the patient to say 99.

The intensity of the vibrations should be equal on both sides of the chest with the patient serving as his own control. The only exception is the upper lobes posteriorly. Intensity may be normally reduced over the left upper lobe posteriorly, owing to normal variations in chest anatomy.

If the vibrations are barely palpable, ask the patient to speak louder; a loud, forceful voice may make vibrations strong enough for detection and comparison.

5. Repeat this technique to palpate the rest of the chest. Palpate *at least* three areas anteriorly, two areas laterally, and four areas posteriorly, systematically moving across and down the chest, as illustrated by the arrows in Figure 12–42A, B, C, and D. Avoid the clavicles, scapulae, heart, and breast tissue.

Some clinicians prefer to screen patients by placing *both* hands in corresponding areas to simultaneously and more accurately compare chest vibrations at each horizontal level.

6. Always palpate previously identified areas of pathology more thoroughly.

7. Note specific areas of increased or decreased fremitus (vibration intensity) as well as any general trends, such as decreased fremitus throughout the chest or below a certain thoracic level.

Normal or Abnormal?—Consideration of Normal Variations. The clinician cannot decide whether fremitus is normal or abnormal without knowledge of normal increases and decreases in fremitus (Table 12–2). Generally, fremitus is normal if it is *about* the same as that found throughout the chest. In any individual, the intensity of the fremitus largely depends on the thickness of the chest wall, the pitch and quality of the patient's voice, and the variations in chest anatomy, producing a varying relation of the bronchi to the chest wall.

Fremitus also depends on whether the area under examination is located over central airways or over peripheral lung. It is normally increased over the sternum and between the scapulae and progressively decreases towards the lung periphery. Fremitus is decreased the most over the bases of the lower lobes. Deviation from this trend indicates abnormal fremitus.

Table 12–2 reviews causes of abnormal decreases and increases in fremitus. Usually only *gross* pathology produces perceptible changes in fremitus. Abnormal fremitus is a nonspecific finding and must be interpreted in light of other chest assessment findings and diagnostic test results. Some clinicians use fremitus, along with percussion, voice sounds, and breath sounds, *exclusively* to identify and differentiate lung consolidation (i.e., increased fremitus) from pleural effusion (i.e., decreased fremitus below the fluid level, as further described). Although abnormal fremitus does not identify (diagnose) specific diseases, it at least identifies the presence of disease and helps to determine its severity.

Decreased Tactile Fremitus. Decreased fremitus is caused by any condition interfering with the normal transmission of sound from the larynx to the chest's surface. Abnormalities between the lungs and the chest's surface increase the distance sound must travel and contribute to the varying mediums through which sound must travel. The combination of normal tissue and other tissue mediums, such as extra adipose tissue in obesity, muscle in a muscular athlete, tumors, fibrotic tissue in pleural thickening, or fluid in pleural effusion, slows and decreases the transmission of sound.

Decreased fremitus is found with any disease causing an increase in the amount of air in the lungs (lung hyperinflation) or in the pleural space (pneumothorax) because air is a relatively poor transmitter of sound. Also, the presence of air increases the distance sound must travel before it reaches the chest's surface.

A patient with atelectasis classically presents with decreased to absent fremitus, since collapsed or obstructed airways prevent the transmission of sound.

Increased Tactile Fremitus. Since a solid medium of uniform consistency conducts sound much better than air, conditions associated with an increased amount of solid medium in the lungs will produce *increased* tactile fremitus. This is true, however, *only* if nearby airways are patent to conduct the sound. Although increased fremitus is due more classically to lung consolidation or tumor, upon occasion it is due to atelectasis from lobar collapse, when a large amount of lung tissue presses together to produce an increase in solid medium.

Lung consolidation is defined as the *replacement of air in alveoli with a liquid or solid medium.* Although the term is commonly associated with lobar pneumonia when alveoli fill with fluid, mucus, and cellular debris from inflammation, lung consolidation is also used to refer to alveolar filling in other diseases, such as pulmonary tuberculosis and extensive pulmonary infarction. Lung tumor is not usually classified as lung consolidation per se because the tumor usually *compresses* rather than *fills* the alveoli and airways. Remember that although increased fremitus is a classic

Table 12–2. CAUSES AND LOCATIONS OF DECREASED, ABSENT, AND INCREASED TACTILE FREMITUS OR VOCAL RESONANCE

Normal Decrease (**Poor transmission of sound**)		**Normal Increase** (**Increase in transmission of sound**)	
Cause	***Location***	***Cause***	***Location***
	Peripheral lung tissue:		*Central airways:*
Thick chest wall, soft voice, high-pitched voice	Throughout the chest	Thin chest wall, loud voice, deep voice	Throughout the chest
Normal anatomy	Bases of lower lobes	Normal anatomy	Sternal area anteriorly Between the scapulae posteriorly
Normal anatomic variation	Left upper lobe posteriorly in some people		
Abnormal Decrease or Absence		**Abnormal Increase**	
Cause	***Location***	***Cause***	***Location***
Increased air in lungs (lung hyperinflation)		Increased solid medium in lungs with *patent* airways	
Severe asthma	Throughout the chest	*Lung consolidation*: (alveolar filling)	Area(s) of pathology
Emphysema	Throughout the chest, especially over bullae (air-filled cavities)	Lobar pneumonia	
		Pulmonary infarction	
		Tuberculosis	
Abnormality between lungs and chest surface		Pulmonary edema	ower (dependent) chest areas
Pleural disorders:		Lung tumor, atelectasis from lobar collapse	Area of pathology
Pleural thickening	rea of pathology		
Pleural effusion			
Pneumothorax		Diffuse interstitial fibrosis (severe)	Throughout the chest, especially lower lobes
Tumor			
Empyema		Extreme compression of lung tissue with patent airways	
Chest wall disorders:	Area of pathology	Severe abdominal or stomach distention, gross obesity	Just above resting level of diaphragm(s)
Tumors		Large pleural effusion	Just above pleural fluid level
Deformities			
Gross obesity	Throughout the chest		
Airway obstruction			
Atelectasis (closed airways)	Area of pathology		
Lung tumor, aspiration of foreign object, mucus plug	Peripheral to obstructive lesion		
Absence of underlying lung tissue			
Pneumonectomy	Affected hemithorax		
Elevated diaphragm:	Under resting level of diaphragm		
Large abdomen			
Stomach distention			
Paralyzed diaphragm			
Large lung resection			
Atelectasis			

sign of consolidation, if the patient has obstructed airways from mucus plugs, for example, he will *not* have increased fremitus; he will have *decreased* fremitus because the airway is blocked. This finding varies, depending on the degree of airway obstruction.

External compression of lung tissue causes increased fremitus because compressed tissue is less porous and more solid than normal lung tissue. The increased solid medium promotes sound transmission, providing nearby airways are patent. Lung tissue can become compressed from below (i.e., abdominal or stomach distention) or anywhere along the lung's costal surfaces. In pleural effusion, although fremitus is always decreased well below the fluid level, it may be increased near or just above the fluid level, owing to the compression of underlying lung tissue.

Interstitial Fibrosis. Many textbooks indicate that fremitus is classically increased in diffuse interstitial fibrosis. This may be so in many "pure" forms of the disease, but in reality patients who present with the disease may have increased, normal, or decreased fremitus, depending on the nature of the pathology involved.

Patients with *mild to moderate* disease demonstrate normal to increased fremitus due to generalized, relatively uniform thickening of interstitium and adjacent alveolar walls (i.e., increased solid medium) from inflammation and fibrosis. Increased fremitus tends to be more noticeable over the lower lobes of the lungs posteriorly. Diseases in this category may include sarcoidosis, idiopathic interstitial fibrosis, and pneumoconiosis.

Patients with *severe* diffuse interstitial fibrosis may demonstrate either increased fremitus *or* decreased to normal fremitus. Increased fremitus is most likely to occur in patients with *progressive massive fibrosis*

(PMF), as occurs in a very small percentage of patients with coal worker's pneumoconiosis and silicosis. However, any disease with small airway narrowing from fibrosis, a late finding in some interstitial diseases (see Chapter 8), may develop with decreased fremitus, particularly if a history of cigarette smoking is present. Physical findings produced by obstructive changes in cigarette smokers commonly dampen or eliminate any increases in fremitus resulting from severe interstitial disease, even if the chest x-ray shows severe interstitial disease. Also, fremitus is more likely to be decreased when alveolar thickening is not uniform, which is often the case.

Localized Fibrosis. In contrast, fremitus is decreased not increased over *localized* areas of lung fibrosis. Because of scarred tissue, fibrosis and decreased fremitus are present in patients recovering from lobar pneumonia or other inflammatory or infectious processes limited to specific areas. Sometimes decreased fremitus is present in the COPD patient in whom the chest x-ray shows interstitial markings, a finding indicating mixed chest pathology of approaching end-stage disease.

Summary. Tactile fremitus is another handy assessment tool, particularly in the absence of other available diagnostic tools, such as the chest x-ray. Since pulmonary patients often present with mixed or variable chest pathology, the determination of normal, increased, or decreased fremitus depends on careful consideration of expected findings for the specific pathology involved as well as other clinical findings.

Percussion

Percussion is the act of tapping on the surface of the chest (1) to evaluate the condition of underlying structures, (2) to identify the resting levels of the hemidiaphragms posteriorly, and (3) to measure diaphragmatic movement during breathing.

PERCUSSION OF LUNG FIELDS

Systematic percussion of the chest (i.e., lung fields) is an invaluable tool for routinely screening for lung disease as well as for monitoring disease progression on a day-to-day, week-to-week, or month-to-month basis. It is perhaps a more sensitive and reliable test than vocal fremitus because percussion notes are classified into separate categories, and the technique does not depend on the quality of the patient's voice.

In the acute care setting, percussion is best used selectively to help identify disorders that impair lung ventilation, notably *stomach distention, hemothorax from post-thoracotomy bleeding, lobar consolidation*, and *pneumothorax*. Although prompt recognition and treatment are critical, these conditions require refined physical assessment skills because the patient is usually comatose, sedated, or intubated and not fully able to report complaints that might help in disease recognition.

In any setting, percussion is most useful in the absence of background patient information, a recent chest x-ray, other diagnostic test results, and ready access to a physician for consultation.

Technique

Percussion involves use of the two middle fingers, one as the hammer, called the plexor, and the other as the anvil, called the pleximeter, as described.

1. *With the patient sitting, place the pleximeter finger firmly on the chest's surface in an ICS*, as shown in Figure 12–34A. *Elevate the palm of the hand and the other fingers slightly off the chest.*

   "Eyeball" the target area to be tapped, the chest area directly under the distal joint of the pleximeter finger. Many nurses with small hands prefer the medial joint because it is larger, conducts sound better because more bone is present, and often becomes less sore with frequent blows during the learning period.
2. Cock the wrist of the other hand and briskly strike the target area *twice* with the *tip* of the middle plexor finger, as shown in Figure 12–34B and C. During the strike, keep the plexor finger arched, and let it bounce off the pleximeter finger after each tap. Using only wrist movement, the two taps should be executed by two rhythmic motions of the hand.
3. *Listen to the sound of the percussion note, and feel the resulting vibrations under the pleximeter finger.* Experienced clinicians eventually can determine percussion notes just by the characteristics of the vibrations felt by the pleximeter finger.
4. Observe your percussion techniques for the following points:
   a. Firm pressure of only the target joint against the chest.
   b. Horizontal placement of the pleximeter finger in an ICS.
   c. Short fingernail of the striking finger; a long fingernail makes effective percussion impossible.
   d. Loose, flexible wrist movement with an arched plexor finger and a stable forearm.
   e. Two short, light taps in rhythmic succession.
   f. Production of a clear, normal resonant percussion note.

Five Types of Percussion Notes

Tapping on the chest causes vibrations that pass through underlying lung, heart, and chest wall tissue as well as through the air to your ears. The audible sound of the percussion note is largely determined by the characteristics of the tissues immediately underneath the pleximeter finger. Based on how sound travels through tissues of different densities, percussion notes are categorized into five different types:

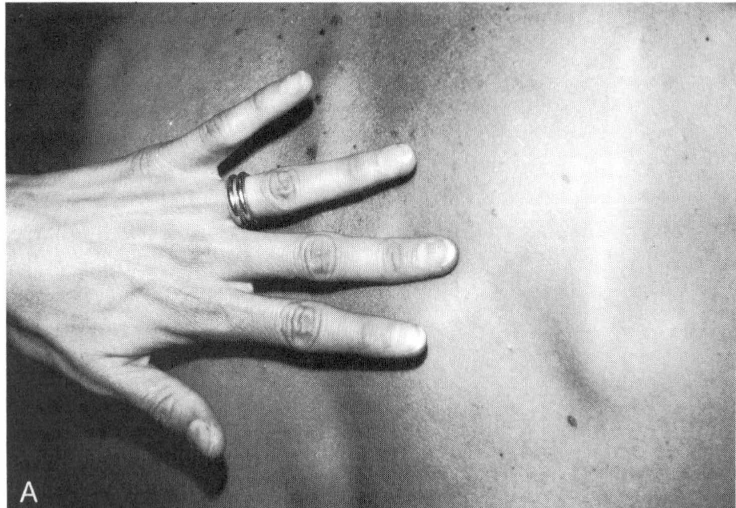

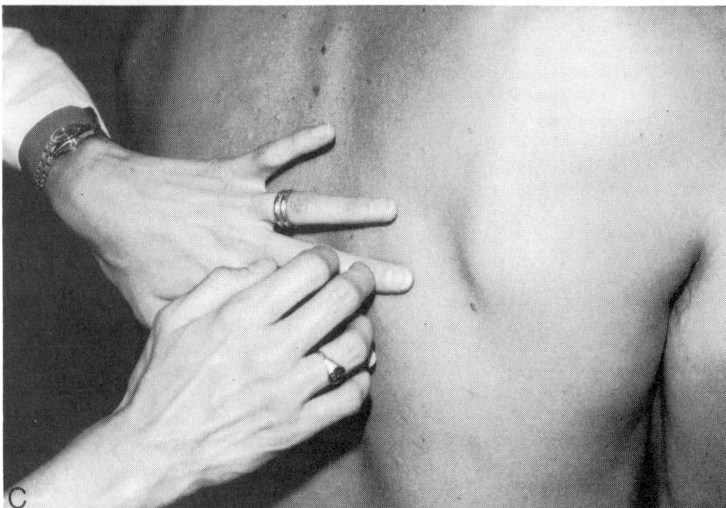

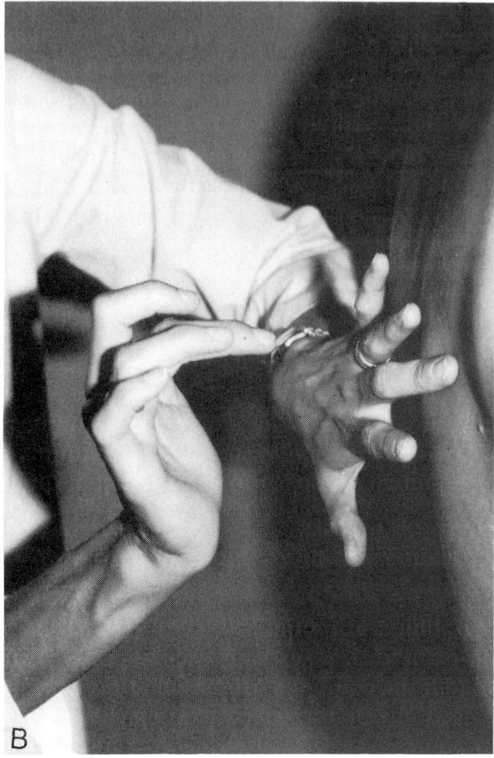

Figure 12–34. Technique for percussion of the chest.

A, Place middle pleximeter finger (distal joint) *firmly* on chest; elevate hand.

B, Cock wrist and arch middle plexor finger.

C, Strike *two* times. Each time, let plexor finger *bounce* off distal joint.

1. *Resonance* is produced by percussion over *normal* lung tissue.

2. *Dullness* is produced by percussion over tissue that is denser than normal lung tissue. Air is replaced by a solid medium, such as lung consolidation or tumor, that interrupts the transmission of vibrations. Abnormalities between the lungs and chest wall also increase the amount of solid tissue and block transmission, as in pleural effusion or pleural thickening.

3. *Flatness* is produced by the percussion of airless tissues, simulating the extremely dull note heard over the thigh. Lung diseases that produce a dull note may eventually produce a flat note if the patient worsens in spite of treatment.

4. *Hyperresonance*, a slightly musical note, is produced by an abnormal increase in the amount of air in the lungs or pleural space, as in emphysema or pneumothorax. Vibrations easily pass through a less dense medium such as air. Compression of lung tissue also causes hyperresonance, as in the area just above the fluid level of a pleural effusion. In this case, hyperresonance is probably due to hyperinflation of nearby alveoli and airways compensating for the underventilated, compressed lung tissue.

5. *Tympany* is produced by percussion of an enclosed, air-filled chamber or cavity, such as a large tension pneumothorax. Producing a pure musical sound unlike any of the other notes, tympany is loud and much higher pitched. Furthermore, its pitch and duration vary, depending on the amount of tension on the walls of the air-filled cavity. Pneumothorax or pulmonary cavitation from an infectious disease such as lung abscess or tuberculosis may produce a hyperresonant rather than tympanic percussion note if the large air-filled cavity is not under tension and, in the case of cavitation, if it is located peripherally in the lung.

For easy reference, normal locations and causes of abnormal percussion notes are summarized in Table 12–3.

Recognition of Percussion Notes

Beginners often have difficulty classifying percussion notes and distinguishing between "flat" and "dull" and "resonant" and "hyperresonant." Although notes are characterized in textbooks by intensity (loudness), pitch (high or low), duration (long or short), and quality

Table 12–3. NORMAL LOCATIONS AND CAUSES OF ABNORMAL PERCUSSION NOTES

Percussion Note	Normal Location	Abnormal Conditions	Explanation
Flatness	Thigh Under diaphragm posteriorly Shoulders Liver	Massive pleural effusions Lung collapse Pneumonectomy	Airless tissue
Dullness	Heart Border of liver Border of diaphragm	Pleural effusion Hemothorax Severe chest deformities Consolidation Pneumonia Pulmonary edema Lung abscess Tuberculosis Atelectasis Pulmonary fibrosis Tumors	Increase in solid tissue
Resonance	Normal lung in adults	Severe emphysema	Pathologic if the patient normally exhibits hyperresonance
Hyperresonance	Normal lung in children Thin adults on deep inspiration	Emphysema Acute asthmatic attack Pneumothorax	Increase in air content in lungs or pleural space
		Pleural effusion just above fluid level	Compression of lung tissue with overinflation of alveoli just above compressed area
		Gross obesity and severe abdominal distention just above resting levels of diaphragm	
Tympany	Gastric air bubble Puffed cheeks	Tension pneumothorax Large pulmonary cavity Emphysematous bullae under tension Gastric distention	Enclosed, air-filled chamber or cavity

(unique characteristics, musical or nonmusical), this classification requires subjective judgment and a knowledge of the qualities of resonance, the comparative baseline note.

Because perception rather than memorization of percussion note characteristics is involved, readers are urged to become familiar *first* with the sound of a clear, *resonant* note by percussing the anterior chest just below the clavicles (MCL). The sound of this basic note is then associated with the characteristics summarized in Table 12–4; loud in intensity, low in pitch, long in duration, and "muffled drum" sound.

Recognition of abnormal percussion notes is best learned by percussion of selected locations and patients, who typically present with unequivocal abnormal notes: flatness, the thigh; dullness, over the heart

Table 12–4. CHARACTERISTICS OF ABNORMAL PERCUSSION NOTES COMPARED WITH NORMAL RESONANCE

	Relative Intensity	Relative Pitch	Relative Duration	Quality
Flatness	Softest ↑	Highest ↑	Shortest ↑	Extreme dullness ↑
Dullness	Softer ↑	Higher ↑	Shorter ↑	Dull "thud" ↑
Resonance	*Loud* ↓	*Low* ↓	*Long* ↓	*A "muffled drum"* ↓
Hyperresonance	Louder ↓	Lower	Longer	"Hollow" drum Slightly musical ↓
Tympany	Loudest	Variable (usually highest)	Variable (usually longest)	Pure musical sound

or a lung consolidation; hyperresonance, over hyperinflated lung tissue of an emphysema patient; and tympany, over a puffed cheek or the gastric air bubble. With practice, the examiner eventually notices general trends in the characteristics of abnormal percussion notes *away* from resonance, the baseline sound. These trends are signified by the arrows in Table 12–4. Knowledge of these trends helps the nurse to anticipate and recognize abnormal percussion notes.

Procedure

For percussion of the anterior, posterior, and lateral chest, the nurse uses the same examination areas and method as those described for palpation of vocal fremitus (see Fig. 12–42A, B, C, and D). The main difference is that examination areas are vertically spaced *closer* together—*about 1½ in (4 cm) apart.* Other differences and important points are summarized as follows:

1. Avoid the scapulae, spine, clavicles, breast tissue, and heart.
2. *For the anterior area of the chest,* identify the upper border of the liver (i.e., level of fifth rib) by short percussion steps down the midclavicular line, starting at about the fourth rib. The change in percussion note from resonance to dullness marks the liver's border (Fig. 12–35 and Fig. 12–36).
3. Percuss the upper border of the gastric air bubble using the same technique, except listen for a different change in the percussion note, a change from resonance to tympany.
4. *For the posterior chest,* instruct the patient to flex his neck and place his arms forward in his lap to separate the scapulae and expose more lung. The examiner may need to step to one side to percuss the lower lobes with greater ease. Also, when approaching the bases of the lungs, "wing" out laterally (i.e., towards 5a and 5b in Figure 12–42B) to more thoroughly percuss underlying lung.
5. Percuss the resting level of the diaphragm (described in next section).
6. Percuss the apices, as illustrated in Figure 12–37. Normally about a 2-in (5-cm) band of resonance (Krönig's isthmus) is present between the neck and shoulder on each side. A narrowed band on one side indicates the presence of lung pathology.
7. *For the lateral area of the chest,* ask the patient to rest his hands on his head or arms across the bedside stand. This makes percussion in this area easier for both examiner and patient.
8. Be sure to percuss identified or suspected areas of abnormality more thoroughly, especially areas with abnormal vocal fremitus.

Limitations of Percussion

Although percussion is a worthwhile technique to learn and gradually integrate into clinical practice, it has its limitations. It is one of the most difficult physical assessment maneuvers to perform correctly, requiring time and practice with supervision to master. Even when mastered, the average nurse in clinical practice may have little use for it as a screening maneuver when skilled at inspection and palpation, both very sensitive parameters. In addition, percussion cannot detect abnormalities located medially because sound waves do not travel more than 4 to 5 cm below the chest's surface. Nor can percussion detect peripheral lesions less than 4 to 5 cm in diameter. The chest x-ray largely compensates for these limitations by detecting abnormalities discovered by percussion as well as those too deep to detect by percussion.

PERCUSSION OF DIAPHRAGM

During percussion of the posterior lower lobes, the nurse determines the *resting levels of the hemidia-*

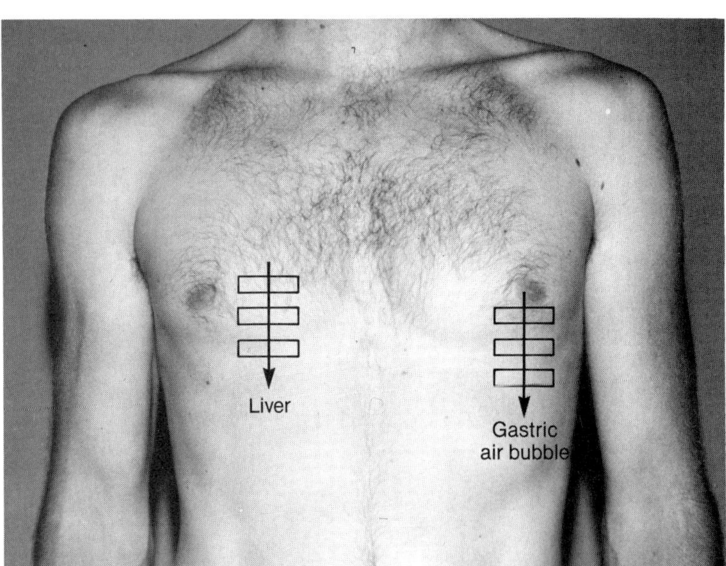

Figure 12–35. Downward percussion in small steps to the liver's upper border and to the gastric air bubble.

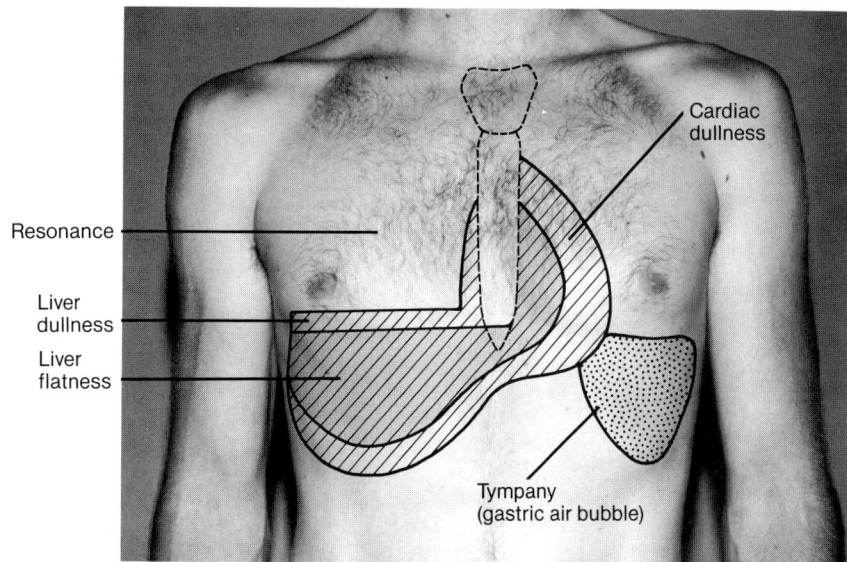

Figure 12–36. Percussion note variations in the normal chest. Most of the anterior chest region is resonant to percussion, except over the heart, liver, and stomach. The size of the gastric air bubble varies among individuals and at different times during the day.

phragms as well as *diaphragmatic excursions*, as described next.

Resting Diaphragmatic Levels

The resting level of each hemidiaphragm is determined with the patient breathing normally and with the use of the following technique:

1. *Starting at the T8 level, percuss downward in small (about 2 cm) steps until you hear resonance turn to dullness.* This point marks the resting level of the diaphragm (Fig. 12–38).
2. *Perform the same procedure on the opposite side of the chest.*
3. *Count the vertebrae along the spinal column to determine the vertebral level of the diaphragms.* Although the normal resting level of the diaphragm is at about T10, the right hemidiaphragm may be one ICS higher than the left because of displacement by the liver.
4. *Look for abnormality in resting diaphragmatic levels*: the unilaterally high diaphragm or bilaterally high or low diaphragm.

High Resting Levels. A high resting diaphragmatic level on one side of the chest indicates an elevated diaphragm from a variety of possible causes; denervation of the phrenic nerve that enervates the diaphragm, stomach distention (left side), hepatomegaly (right side), or significant atelectasis. In addition, lobectomy patients may exhibit unilateral elevation, especially in the immediate postoperative period. If an upper lobe is removed, the other lobes are pushed up from below by the diaphragm. If a small lobe (RML) is removed, the lungs hyperinflate to fill the entire chest cage again over a period of a few weeks to months.

Bilaterally high levels are seen in patients with elevated diaphragms from severe abdominal distention, gross obesity, or splinting respirations from pain.

If a high diaphragmatic level is identified, the nurse must rule out the possibility that the change in percussion note from resonance to dullness is due to some other condition that causes dullness, such as lung consolidation and the fluid level of a large pleural effusion. In these latter conditions, the percussed diaphragmatic level varies slightly or remains unchanged with deep breathing because one is actually percussing over pathologic areas of increased density rather than over an elevated diaphragm as it moves up and down with respiration. Suspected areas of lung consolidation or pleural effusion are confirmed by chest x-ray and other physical and laboratory findings.

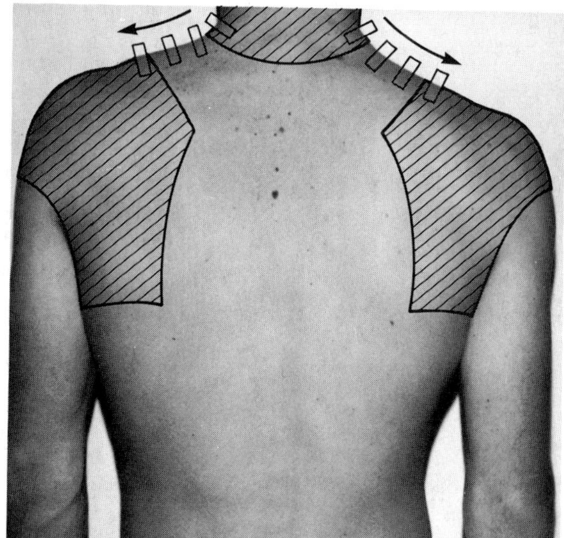

Figure 12–37. Percussion of the lung apices from the base of the neck to the shoulders. The slashed areas represent normal areas of dullness, when the arms are forward in the patient's lap. The normal band of resonance over the apices is about 5 cm wide.

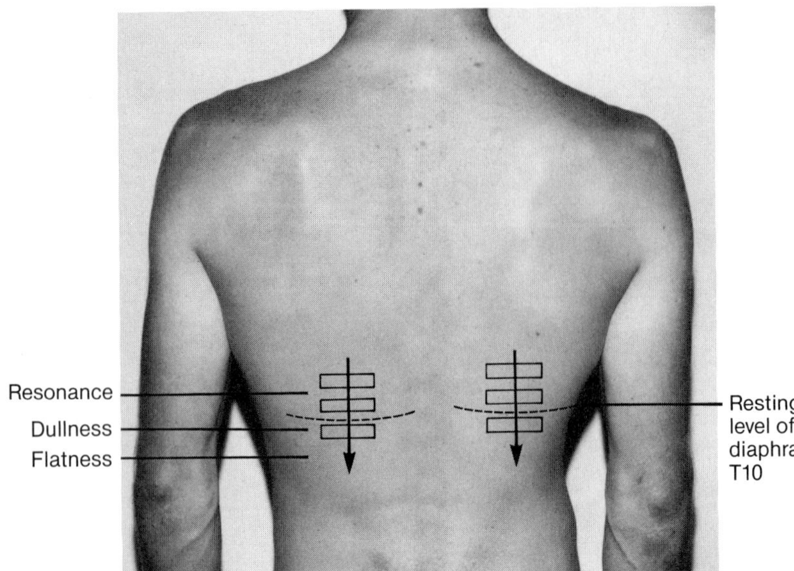

Figure 12–38. Percussion of resting diaphragmatic levels. The change in percussion note from resonance to dullness identifies the level on each side of the chest.

Low Resting Levels. A bilaterally low resting level indicates depressed diaphragms, usually from a severely hyperinflated chest. Patients with emphysema or acute asthma may exhibit resting levels down to T12. A unilaterally low resting level results from tension pneumothorax.

Diaphragmatic Excursion

Diaphragmatic excursion is the distance the posterior hemidiaphragms move with respiration. Percussion and measurement are executed during deep breathing rather than during quiet breathing because they are more sensitive assessment parameters at this time.

To percuss and measure diaphragmatic excursions

1. Stand behind the patient and slightly to the side to reach the bases of the lower lobes with greater ease.
2. Identify the resting diaphragmatic level on one side of the chest.
3. With your pleximeter finger still on the chest, ask the patient to take a deep breath in and expire fully, holding his breath for 3 to 5 seconds at the end of expiration.
4. As the patient begins to expire, move your pleximeter finger about 2 in *above* the resting diaphragmatic level and begin to percuss.
5. *Percuss downwards in short 1- to 2-cm steps until you encounter dullness at full expiration.* Be careful not to pass up the diaphragm by moving downwards too quickly. *Mark this point with a felt-tipped pen.*
6. *Now ask the patient to take a deep breath in and hold his breath for 3 to 5 seconds.*
7. At the beginning of inspiration, start to percuss downwards in the same manner (Fig. 12–39A) *until you encounter dullness at full inspiration. Mark this point with a pen.*

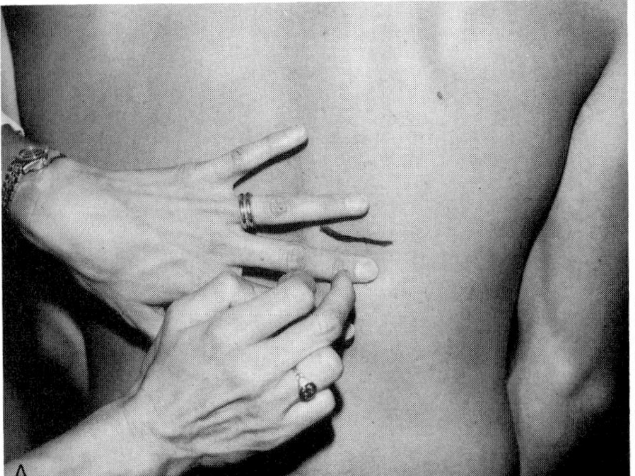

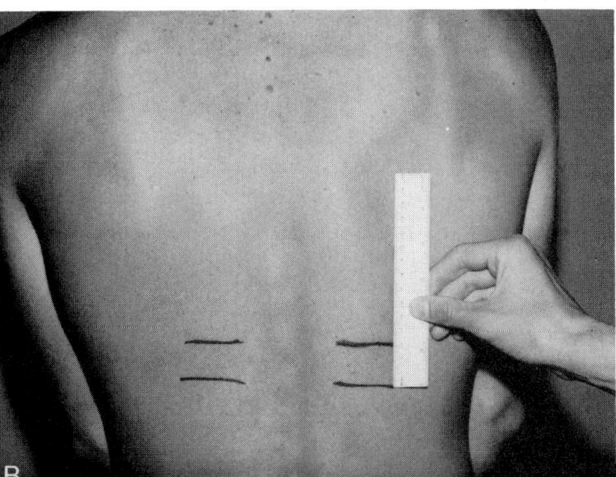

Figure 12–39. Percussion *(A)* and measurement *(B)* of diaphragmatic excursion from full expiration (top line) to full inspiration (bottom line).

8. *With a ruler, measure the distance between the two marks on the chest* (Fig. 12–39B). This distance between full expiration and full inspiration is the diaphragmatic excursion. Normal diaphragmatic excursion is *3 to 5 cm (1½ to 2 in)* bilaterally, although a healthy young male may have excursions up to *8 cm (3 in)*.

9. *Note the presence of unequal diaphragmatic excursions as well as any unilateral or bilateral decreases.*

Modification of the Technique. Although the technique described is perhaps the simplest way to learn to percuss the diaphragm, it is not practical for many clinical situations. Sick patients cannot hold their breath. A marking pen may not be available when needed. If a pen is available, you may not have time to mark the chest or find a ruler. Some patients may not want you to mark their backs. Therefore, once the technique is learned, modification is advised so that the nurse can eventually examine dyspneic patients without a marking pen or ruler.

To modify your technique, follow steps 1 through 4. Then, instead of marking the end-expiratory point with a pen, remember its location and identify it, if possible, by means of a nearby landmark, such as a freckle. With the point mentally identified, instruct the patient to breathe out. Percuss downwards until you encounter dullness at full expiration. Hold your pleximeter finger in position at this point, instruct the patient to relax while you estimate or measure the distance between the two identified points.

The key to success depends on remembering and implementing these following concepts:

1. Remember that the diaphragm moves up on expiration and down on inspiration.
2. Start with expiration.
3. Always percuss downwards.
4. Coordinate percussion with the patient's breathing. Talk to him *as* you percuss: "Deep breath in." "Hold." "Breathe all your air out." "Relax."

Interpretation of Findings. If diaphragmatic excursions are unequal, it is usually but not necessarily because diaphragmatic excursion on one side of the chest is decreased. Any patient with a significantly elevated diaphragm will have decreased excursions on the same side. However, frequently with lung disease in the lower lobes, one cannot measure excursions because lung consolidation or pleural fluid creates the same dull percussion note as that heard over the diaphragm. Measurement of diaphragmatic excursions is most practical in evaluating patients with clear chests; they have no lung consolidation or pleural disease to make identification of the diaphragm by percussion impossible. Unless other diagnostic tests are unavailable, measurement may not be necessary because it usually does not provide much more information than what one can deduce from other chest assessment findings. Radiologic techniques, such as chest x-rays at full expiration and full inspiration or fluoroscopy, can more effectively evaluate diaphragmatic excursions. Yet, to screen for pulmonary problems and to further assess abnormalities that specifically affect diaphragmatic movement, the physical assessment technique is useful to learn. Severe COPD typically decreases the movement of the diaphragms bilaterally. Neuromuscular patients with phrenic nerve damage typically present with elevated diaphragms and little to no diaphragmatic excursion on the affected sides.

SECTION IV—AUSCULTATION OF THE THORAX AND LUNGS

Auscultation is the act of listening to the chest with a stethoscope for normal voice sounds, breath sounds, and adventitious (extra) sounds. The purpose of auscultation is to assess air flow through the tracheobronchial tree; the presence of fluid, mucus, or obstruction in the air passages; and the condition of the surrounding lungs and pleural space. Many abnormalities not discovered by inspection, palpation, or percussion are identified by subtle changes in breath sounds, adventitious sounds, or both.

The Stethoscope—The Clinician's Basic Tool

PARTS OF THE STETHOSCOPE

Auscultation is performed with a stethoscope, ideally one with the following features (the numbers correspond to those in Figure 12–40):

1. *Appropriate eartips or earpiece tips.* Made of hard nylon or soft rubber, eartips should be of a shape and size that permit a comfortable and snug fit into the external auditory canal. Eartips that are too small or too large do not permit the necessary airtight system that excludes external noise. A common problem is large eartips, which cause the nurse to manually press the tips further into the ears to hear subtle findings. These tips can be easily replaced with smaller ones found at a medical supply shop.
2. *Appropriate binaurals (earpieces).* Eartips fit tightly into metal binaurals. Binurals should be long enough to clear the face and should curve inward and forward as one places the stethoscope into the ears.
3. *Metal brace.* A rigid spring or metal brace is located within or external to the Y-tubing between the binaurals. It permits the ends of the binaurals to cross each other in a resting position. A poor metal brace results in loosely fitted eartips and the poor transmission of sound to the ears.

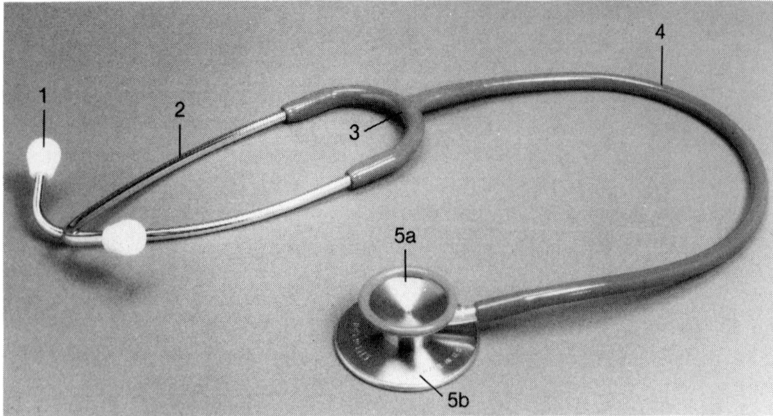

Figure 12–40. The popular Littman's *classic combination* type stethoscope. 1, *ear tip*; 2, *binaural*; 3, *metal brace* (under tubing); 4, *tubing*; 5a, *bell* of chest piece; and 5b, *diaphragm* of chest piece. (Courtesy of Medical Products Division/3M.)

4. *Tubing*. Stethoscope tubing should have a smooth inner surface and should be about ⅛ in diameter, thick enough to exclude outside noises and promote sound transmission. Lung sounds are more difficult to hear when using a stethoscope with thin, compressible tubing. In many cases, plastic tubing is more durable and provides better acoustic insulation than rubber tubing of the same thickness (Straight and Soukup, 1977).

Short tubing may prevent the nurse from reaching the patient with ease, whereas long tubing decreases sound transmission because of the extra distance to the ears. As a guideline, long stethoscopes should be cut to at least 17 in from metal brace to chest piece to permit both bedside maneuverability and sound detection and to 10 to 12 in for optimal auscultation of sounds. Cutting a good 3 to 4 inches off an extra long stethoscope may make the difference between hearing or missing a subtle finding, notably fine inspiratory crackles.

Unless tubing is thick and relatively short, one leading to the chest piece is better than two. Double tubing is more difficult to manipulate, as the two tubes tend to rub together and against clothing, creating extraneous sounds. Also, the extra length of tubing may hinder sound transmission.

5. *Chest piece*. The chest piece at the end of the tubing should have a diaphragm for high-pitched lung sounds and a smaller bell for low-pitched cardiac sounds. The *diaphragm* should never be larger than the traditional 4.4 cm (1¾ in) in diameter. Larger diaphragms cannot be used effectively on small chests, and they create and transmit more skin surface tension arising from tense muscles or hairy chests. Cracked diaphragms should be replaced to avoid the transmission of extraneous sounds. A *bell* is essential for auscultation of low-pitched cardiac sounds, such as gallops and some murmurs. It should be about 3.1 cm (1¼ in) in diameter and may have a rubber ring over the rim to facilitate an airtight seal with minimum pressure applied to the chest piece for gallops and to eliminate the chilling effect of a bare metal rim. Although not absolutely essential for lung auscultation, a bell comes in handy because it is small, and the application of firm pressure during use converts it into a diaphragm. Its use facilitates auscultation of small, more inaccessible areas of the chest, such as the apices above the clavicles and uneven chest surfaces, as in chest cage deformities or sunken intercostal spaces and prominent ribs from emaciation. With both bell and diaphragm, the nurse can switch to the bell to examine the chests of infants and children, thereby avoiding the need to invest in a smaller pediatric stethoscope or infantscope.

EVALUATING YOUR STETHOSCOPE

An appropriate stethoscope is a prerequisite to learning auscultation as well as integrating the skill into practice. The previously mentioned information provides suggestions as to how to improve the acoustic properties of your stethoscope. To find the limitations of your stethoscope, compare its performance with the performance of a stethoscope you know to be effective. Once you learn the basics of auscultation, comparing stethoscope performance in the process, you will discover your stethoscope's limitations; learn how to work around them, if possible; and master lung auscultation without unnecessary frustration.

If you need a new stethoscope, remember that low quality, cheap stethoscopes may be more than adequate to take blood pressures, but they usually miss subtle chest assessment findings or make it very difficult for you to learn to identify abnormal sounds. Medium to high quality, moderately priced stethoscopes with both diaphragm and bell are ideal. High quality, expensive electronic stethoscopes may be helpful in identifying different heart sounds, but the amplification system in many models creates a background "hum" that distracts some listeners from identifying lung sounds that are soft in intensity. If the nurse is well trained in auscultation of the chest, the expensive stethoscope often offers little advantage over the more moderately priced one with essentially the same features except for the amplification system.

Since ward stethoscopes tend to be designed for blood pressure measurements rather than for lung sounds, many pulmonary nurses find that they would rather buy their own stethoscopes than try to work around these limitations.

CORRECT USE OF THE STETHOSCOPE

The following points explain how to use the stethoscope:

1. *Perform auscultation in a quiet environment.* If necessary, ask patients to turn down their radios and televisions to allow full concentration and proper identification of low frequency sounds easily masked by outside noises.
2. *Place the stethoscope in your ears so that the ends of the binaurals curve forward* not backward. The eartip fit should be snug but not painful.
3. *Hold the chest piece between index and middle fingers underneath the rim of the bell,* as illustrated in Figure 12–41, or grab this site with your thumb and next two fingers. In some stethoscopes, handling the chest piece by the bell's rim wears out its soft rubber covering.
4. *Press the diaphragm firmly against the chest's surface.* Although excessive pressure may dampen sounds, usually nurses initially do not press firmly enough. Firm pressure eliminates external sounds and promotes the transmission of lung sounds.
5. *Avoid listening over chest hair.* Movement of hair against the diaphragm with respiration produces a sound similar to crackles. If avoidance of hair is impossible, wet hairy auscultation areas with water to help cut down on artifact.
6. *Do not listen over clothes or allow any part of the chest piece or tubing to touch clothes, bed sheets, or other objects.* To do so often creates decreased breath sounds or extraneous sounds that simulate crackles. Meticulous technique facilitates the correct identification of sounds. Dialysis unit nurses, visiting nurses, and emergency room nurses performing a quick examination may have difficulty working around the clothes of fully dressed patients, especially if there are no zippers or buttons on one-piece outfits. If necessary, remove or manipulate clothing, making sure you have clear access to key auscultation areas. When you are listening with the stethoscope underneath clothing, protect your chest piece with your hands and hold the tubing in an intermediate position between the clothes and surface of the patient's chest.
7. *Improvise in emergency situations.* Quickly listen over *any* accessible area of the chest—over clothes if necessary—to check for air movement, the critical variable.

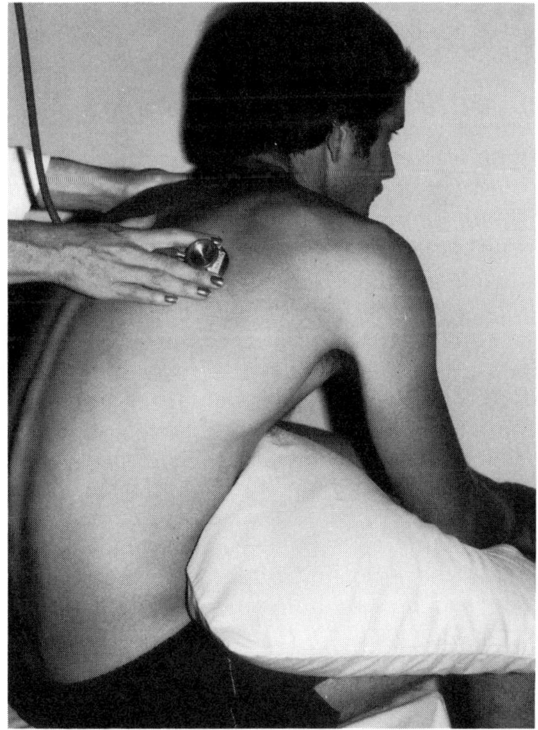

Figure 12–41. Correct use of the stethoscope. The chest piece is held between the index and middle fingers. The patient is sitting comfortably with arms pulled forward in the lap which moves the scapulae laterally and exposes more of the lung fields posteriorly.

Auscultation of Voice Sounds

The spoken voice heard by auscultation over lung tissue is called *vocal resonance* or *voice sounds.*

NORMAL VOICE SOUNDS

Normal voice sounds (vocal resonance) are present when spoken words sound muffled and only partially understandable when the patient is instructed to speak. Voice sounds transmitted from the patient's larynx, through the trachea, bronchi, lung tissue, and chest wall are normally less intense and distorted upon reaching the examiner's ears, especially when listening over more peripheral areas of the chest away from major airways. Over major airways, where one normally feels increased vocal fremitus, vocal resonance is also increased in intensity, but spoken words, especially whispered, are not transmitted clearly and distinctly. Essentially, normal vocal resonance varies within and between individuals in the same manner as vocal fremitus (review Table 12–2).

ABNORMAL VOICE SOUNDS

There are three different types of abnormal voice sounds. *Bronchophony* is an increase in the intensity and clarity of spoken sounds when the patient is instructed to say 99. *Egophony* is the selective transmission of the high frequency components of voice sounds. Normally, the E sounds like an E. When the spoken E becomes a loud, nasal sounding A (with a long ā), egophony is present. The high-pitched nasal quality of egophony has been likened to the bleating of a goat. *Whispered pectoriloquy* is an increase in the intensity and clarity of whispered voice sounds. Instruct the patient to whisper 99 or 1,2,3. These sounds normally are barely heard and hardly understood, depending on the pitch and loudness of the patient's voice. They are never clear and distinct.

TECHNIQUE

For general screening, the nurse checks *first* for bronchophony, egophony, or both, auscultating over the same palpation areas as those used for tactile fremitus. The technique is the same as that for tactile fremitus. In suspected or identified areas of pathology, especially over consolidated areas, the nurse checks for the presence of *all three* abnormal voice sounds, which is more thorough.

The test finding for abnormal voice sounds is *positive* when bronchophony, whispered pectoriloquy, or egophony is present. By definition, vocal resonance is increased when abnormal voice sounds are present because the spoken word sounds louder and clearer. Although vocal resonance theoretically is termed decreased when the spoken word is exceptionally muffled, most clinicians do not use voice sounds to identify and assess decreased vocal resonance. Instead, they may use tactile fremitus, because decreased vibratory sensations on the surface of the chest are usually easier to detect and assess than greatly muffled spoken words heard by auscultation.

INTERPRETATION OF FINDINGS

Conditions that cause an increase or decrease in vocal fremitus also cause an increase or decrease in vocal resonance, respectively. If necessary, review Table 12–2 with special attention to causes and locations of abnormal increases in the transmission of sound.

The presence of abnormal voice sounds does not always indicate pathology. For example, a normal individual might demonstrate negative test findings for bronchophony and whispered pectoriloquy with slight E to A changes over an area of the chest owing to a normal variation in anatomic structure. But *obvious E to A changes* and the clear, distinct transmission of voice sounds *always* indicate lung pathology when accompanied by increased tactile fremitus, dullness or hyperresonance to percussion, and bronchovesicular or bronchial breath sounds. These findings all indicate lung consolidation or compression of tissue.

For incompletely understood reasons, the three abnormal voice sounds may appear in varying combinations. In some cases, none of them may be present, even if the patient has extensive consolidation or compression of tissue. Whispered pectoriloquy is perhaps the most sensitive physical diagnostic test for lung consolidation—it may appear before bronchophony, egophony, and bronchovesicular or bronchial breath sounds. Egophony is commonly heard in the presence of a pleural effusion, heard just above the fluid level of the effusion.

In essence, a test for abnormal voice sounds is a relatively nonspecific and sometimes insensitive test. When one or more abnormal voice sounds are present, gross pathology is indicated; but this is true *only* when the finding is supported with other clinical evidence, such as other physical findings, abnormal chest x-rays, and other diagnostic tests.

Charting

When the test finding for abnormal voice sounds is negative, the nurse charts

Normal voice sounds or *negative for bronchophony, egophony, and whispered pectoriloquy.*

Positive findings might be charted as follows:

Negative for bronchophony and whispered pectoriloquy, slight E to A change RUL anteriorly, MCL, or *bronchophony, egophony, and whispered pectoriloquy are clearly present at the base of the LLL posteriorly.*

Auscultation of Lung Sounds

GENERAL PROCEDURE

1. *With the patient in the sitting position, ask him to open his mouth and breathe deeply. Explanation:* often while auscultating the chest, breath sounds suddenly become diminished; the patient starts to breathe through his nose or a half-opened mouth, or he tires and breathes more shallowly. Nose breathing does not produce clear breath sounds because of increased air turbulence, as air moves through nasal passages. A half-opened mouth is unsatisfactory because the sucking in of air around the teeth and tongue creates turbulence and extraneous sounds. The mouth must be *wide* open to allow the even flow of air to the back of the throat and down the trachea. Shallow breathing is inadequate because it does not allow ventilation and assessment of peripheral or diseased areas of the lungs, i.e., air moves to healthy, more accessible areas of the lungs where airway resistance is lowest. Patients with congestive heart failure or postoperative atelectasis may sound absolutely clear until prompted to take in a *very* deep breath to allow more air into peripheral and collapsed areas of the lungs.

The deep breathing pattern should appear relaxed with an active inspiration, a passive expiration, and a pause between breaths to avoid hyperventilation and dizzy spells. COPD patients especially must be encouraged to take relaxed deep breaths to avoid extensive use of accessory muscles and muscle tension, which creates artifact.

2. *Auscultate the anterior, posterior, and lateral chest areas from the apices to the diaphragm using the general auscultation areas indicated in Figure 12–42. Move across and down, always comparing one side of the chest with the other, at the same vertebral level.*

Explanation: after one or two deep breaths in one auscultation area, proceed to the other side of the chest, even if you are not sure of what you heard. The other side of the chest, serving as a control, will help you decide and describe what you heard. Prolonged breathing will also tire the patient, producing breath sounds of varying intensity and duration that are unsuitable for comparison.

Remember to examine symmetric areas of the chest. If you are 3 in from the spinal column, place the

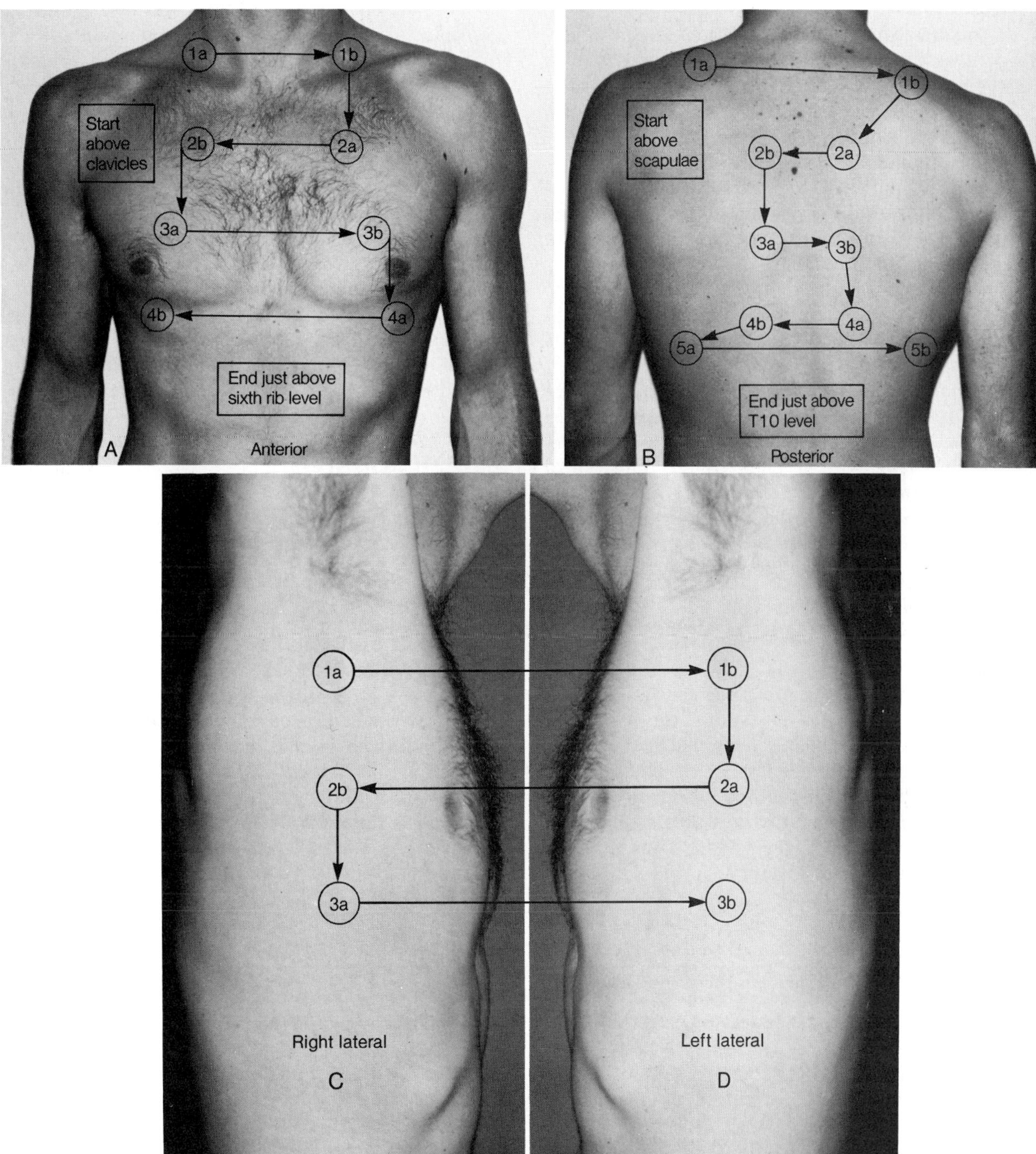

Figure 12–42. General areas and systematic method for *palpation, percussion,* and *auscultation* of the anterior (A), posterior (B), and lateral chest regions (C and D). These chest examination techniques involve systematic movement across the chest (from a to b) and down to the next horizontal level (numbered area). Other areas may be added at various horizontal (thoracic) levels, depending on the technique, chest size, and location of chest pathology.

diaphragm of the stethoscope 3—not 2 or 4—in from the spinal column on the other side. Asymmetric placement of the stethoscope on the chest causes the nurse to mistakenly identify decreased breath sounds on one side. Avoid auscultation of the scapulae, vertebral column, and breast tissue. Make sure you stay above the diaphragm (T10 level).

3. *As you move out laterally to auscultate the lower lobes, auscultate the sides of the chest in at least two areas—just above the diaphragm and 2 to 3 in below the axilla.*

4. *Auscultate identified or suspected areas of pathology more carefully by inching your stethoscope along the surface of the chest. Explanation:* for example, if fluid overload or atelectasis is suspected, search for adventitious sounds by inching your way further down to the diaphragm, posteriorly. Laboratory tests—the chest x-ray, particularly—and other chest assessment findings (e.g., minimal chest movement, flail chest, positive voice sounds) clue you in as to what areas should be examined more thoroughly.

5. *When checking the lower lobes posteriorly, ask the patient to pant or cough. Explanation:* the pant, cough, or deep breath just before the cough often elicits adventitious sounds not previously heard. Remember, *a chest is not considered clear unless it sounds clear with deep breathing and with a cough.* Panting is used when the patient has difficulty coughing, e.g., a neuromuscular patient with a poor cough reflex or a postsurgical patient splinting from pain. Specifically listen for a rhonchus or wheeze (described subsequently) right *with* not before or after the cough. The wheeze with a cough usually escapes the untrained ear.

Determination of Normal Versus Abnormal Lung Sounds

During auscultation, the examiner continually asks herself the following two questions to determine whether lung sounds are generally normal or abnormal: (1) Does the breath sound on this side of the chest sound *exactly* like that on the other side? Rationale: Unequal or "different" sounds suggest abnormal breath sounds. (2) Is the passage of air interrupted by any extra sounds? Rationale: Extra sounds indicate the presence of abnormal adventitious sounds.

In essence, if lung sounds are not equal in every way over corresponding areas of chest, abnormality is likely. Some clinicians learn to determine the presence of inequalities or abnormal sounds by noting differences in *overall passage of air* and specifics, such as the *duration of inspiration and expiration* and the *quality, pitch,* and *intensity* of sounds. Early attention to these specifics is most useful and less confusing to clinicians already familiar with auscultation and variations in breath sounds among individuals. Beginners are encouraged to refer to these two basic questions to determine abnormality and to gradually make their own associations about specifics, such as quality and pitch, as they gain experience in the clinical setting.

After the general determination of normal versus abnormal sounds, further analysis is necessary to classify sounds heard. Analysis focuses first on breath sounds, determining whether they are normal or abnormal, and then on adventitious sounds. This approach facilitates the sorting out of jumbles of confusing noises and eliminates the common error of concentrating on the more dominant adventitious sounds without regard for the underlying breath sounds.

BREATH SOUNDS

The four types of breath sounds are *normal, bronchial, bronchovesicular,* and *tracheal* (Table 12–5).

Normal Breath Sound

The most distinguishing characteristic of the normal breath sound is its *breezy* quality; air sounds as if it is moving in a very smooth, even laminar flow. A relatively low-pitched, breezy swish of air is heard during inspiration. The second most important characteristic is its long inspiratory phase, producing an audible inspiratory:expiratory ratio of 3:1. Note the audible I:E ratio is different from the actual I:E ratio of 1:2,

Table 12–5. TYPES OF BREATH SOUNDS

	Normal Location	Intensity	Pitch	Quality	I:E Ratio (audible)	Graphic Representation
Normal	Throughout chest except over central airways	Moderate	Low	Breezy	3:1	
Decreased	LUL posteriorly in some people	Soft	Low	Breezy	3:1	
Bronchial	Over manubrium	Loud	High	Hollow, tubular	2:3	
Bronchovesicular	Over large, central airways: sternal area, between scapulae, RUL posteriorly in some people	Moderate to loud	Medium to high	Hollow, breezy	1:1	
Tracheal	Over extrathoracic trachea (not usually auscultated)	Very loud	Very high	Hollow, harsh	5:6	

Figure 12–43. Breath sounds in the normal adult *anterior* region of the chest. The *bronchial* breath sound (B) is heard over the manubrium; the *bronchovesicular* breath sound (BV), over the body of the sternum; and the *normal* breath sound (NL) over the lung fields. The *tracheal* breath sound is heard normally over the extrathoracic trachea. The sound has the same hollow quality of the bronchial breath sound but seems much louder or "closer." The tracheal breath sound's location is not outlined in the illustration because it is of less clinical significance in comparision with the other breath sounds. The trachea is auscultated only in a few specific instances, e.g., in upper airway obstruction to evaluate stridor. Also, the tracheal breath sound is rarely auscultated over the chest; it is sometimes heard in atelectasis of the upper lobe when the collapsed region lies medially next to the mediastinum.

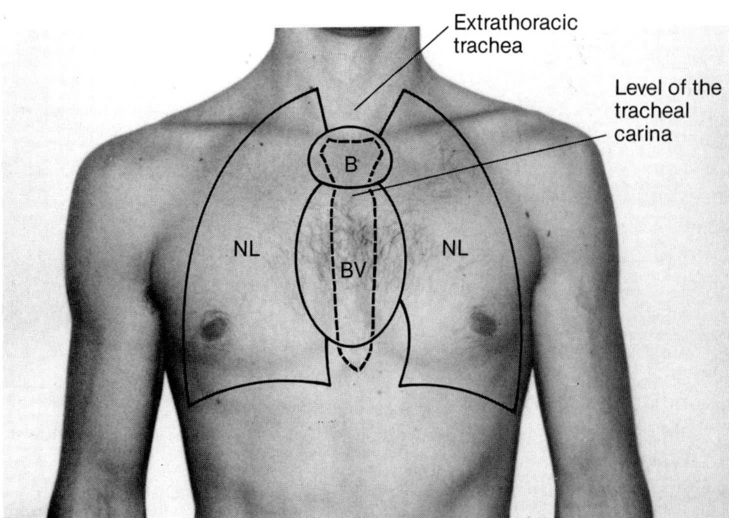

timed during chest inspection. Expiration is barely audible, except in thin-chested individuals and children. Normal breath sounds are heard throughout the chest, except in the middle of the chest anteriorly and posteriorly (Figs. 12–43 and 12–44).

Mechanism of Sound Production and Transmission. The physiologic mechanisms responsible for the production and transmission of normal and abnormal lung sounds are incompletely understood. The normal breath sound is believed to originate from gas vibrations in underlying large lobar and segmental airways. Gas vibrations are transmitted to the airway wall, through adjacent lung tissue, and finally to the chest's surface. This route is shorter and more direct compared with the airway route through the extensive network of peripheral airways.

During sound transmission, lung tissue acts as a low-pass filter. It filters out high-pitched sounds from large airways and passes only low-pitched sounds to the chest's surface (Murphy and Holford, 1980). Although most workers seem to agree that airborne sound traveling through peripheral airways contributes little, if anything, to the normal breath sound, Forgacs (1978a) indicates that peripheral areas may contribute to the normal breath sound when disease states produce irregular alveolar and bronchiolar air flow patterns. Airborne sound traveling in the other direction towards the mouth is readily heard at the mouth during deep breathing by any observer in close proximity. For accuracy, this text uses the term *normal* breath sound instead of *normal vesicular* breath sound. Forgacs (1978a) indicates that the term vesicular should be eliminated because it implies that sound is generated from alveoli, an incorrect assumption. Vesicular is from "vesicle," meaning a thin-walled cavity, such as an alveolus.

Variations in Baseline Normal Breath Sound. The normal breath sound may vary among individuals, depending on body build and other factors. Thin-chested, emaciated individuals may demonstrate an extremely loud baseline breath sound that takes the examiner by surprise. Patients with a mucus retention problem (e.g., diffuse lobular pneumonia) may have a normal breath sound that has a slightly harsh or raspy quality.

Patients on mechanical ventilation may lose some of the breezy quality of normal sound owing to the effects of mechanical ventilation through an endotracheal tube. In addition, mechanical ventilation causes the breath sound to become louder as flow rate is increased. The addition of positive end expiratory pressure (PEEP) has two effects at the same flow rate.

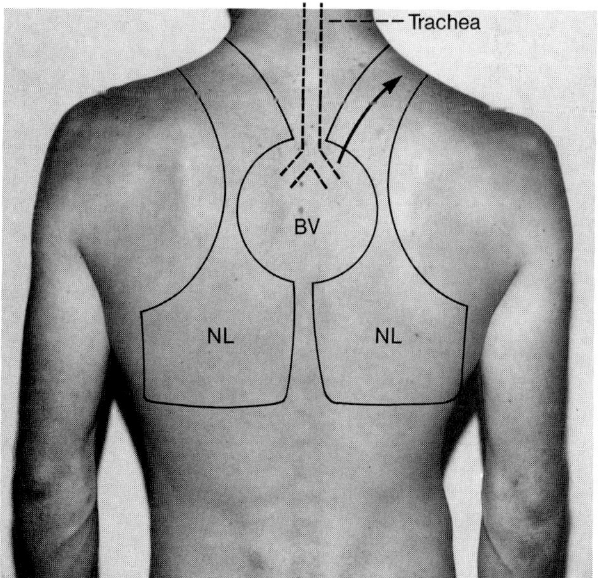

Figure 12–44. Breath sounds in the normal adult *posterior* region of the chest. The bronchovesicular breath sound (BV) is heard at the level of the tracheal carina in the middle of the back and may extend to the right apical area, as illustrated by the arrow. The normal breath sound (NL) is heard over the lung fields, away from central airways.

First, the intensity of the normal breath sound decreases. Second, sound intensity reaches its maximum earlier during inspiration (Krumpe, 1985).

In patients with advanced pulmonary disease, the normal breath sound may have a subtle or overt change in quality throughout the lungs or in localized areas, presumably due to differences in lung compliance, air flow patterns, or both. Lung sounds become louder or "closer" and less breezy, a quality described by clinicians as a "stiff" or "noncompliant" lung sound. Nurses caring for the critically ill patient with adult respiratory distress syndrome or the ambulatory patient with chronic cor pulmonale may hear variations of this sound throughout the chest or in localized pathologic areas. Although this sound indicates abnormality, it finds its way into the normal breath sound category by exclusion. It definitely does not sound like a bronchial breath sound. Sometimes it approximates the bronchovesicular breath sound, as in diffuse interstitial fibrosis. This type of sound is not categorized in medical literature because no objective means exist for its description. Yet, identification of localized decreases in the breezy quality of breath sounds is important because it may indicate underlying diseased lung tissue. In the presence of bronchitis and pneumonia, these diseased areas need to be carefully monitored for signs of retained mucus; diseased tissue is not as efficient at clearing mucus out of the lungs as healthy tissue.

Decreased Breath Sounds

The nurse notes any decrease in the intensity of normal breath sounds as a general trend throughout the chest or in localized areas.

With gross pathology, decreased or absent breath sounds are readily appreciated by focusing attention on the overall intensity of the breath sound. However, in patients with shallow breathing patterns, careful comparison of, first, the inspiratory phase and then the expiratory phase of respiration may be necessary to detect subtle decreases in breath sounds in localized areas. Although the actual I:E ratio may remain the same, the audible I:E ratio changes as one or both phases of respiration decrease in intensity and shorten in duration and as expiration becomes absent (inaudible). In equivocal cases, ask the patient to pant, cough twice, or take two *very* deep breaths as you quickly and carefully listen once on each side of the chest over corresponding auscultation areas.

A Normal Finding. Breath sounds are normally decreased over areas of the chest where tactile fremitus and voice sounds are normally decreased, notably *peripheral areas*, especially over the bases of the lower lobes near the diaphragm and the *left upper lobe posteriorly* above the scapula.

Slightly decreased breath sounds over the left upper lobe (LUL) areas are due to normal differences in lung anatomy among individuals. Two mechanisms may be involved. First, sound traveling through the left lung may be dissipated before reaching the LUL posteriorly because of the presence of the heart and great vessels on the left side of the chest. Second, the right main stem bronchus is normally shorter than the left main stem bronchus. Because sound has a shorter distance to travel to the right upper lobe (RUL) posteriorly, breath sounds may seem louder on the right side or less intense on the left side, depending on anatomic variations and the perceptions of the examiner. Although slight decreases in breath sound intensity are normal, large decreases are usually abnormal.

Last, generalized breath sounds throughout the chest are a normal finding in muscular individuals with thick chest walls. Also, the sounds may be present in elderly patients, owing to slight lung hyperinflation, redistribution of air in the aging lung, or both.

An Abnormal Finding. Decreased breath sounds may be an abnormal finding, occurring most frequently in association with decreased fremitus or decreased voice sounds. The physiologic mechanisms are the same as those for decreased fremitus, e.g., increased air content in the lungs (emphysema), abnormality between the lungs and chest surface (pleural effusion, pneumothorax), and airway obstruction or air flow limitation from mucus or fluid (pneumonia, left ventricular failure) or from collapsed areas of lung (atelectasis). Disorders commonly causing decreased breath sounds are summarized in Table 12–6.

Table 12–6. DISORDERS CAUSING DECREASED AND ABSENT BREATH SOUNDS

Decreased	Absent	Decreased or Absent
Hypoventilation	Respiratory arrest	Pleural effusion
Pleural thickening	Pneumonectomy	Hemothorax
Obesity	Elevated diaphragm	Pneumothorax
Chest cage deformity	Large abdomen	Empyema
Emphysema	Stomach distention	Malpositioned endotracheal tube
Pulmonary embolism	Paralyzed diaphragm	Partial to complete airway obstruction
Partial airway obstruction	Large lung resection	Tumor
Tumor	Atelectasis	Foreign object
Foreign object	Complete airway obstruction	Pneumonia
Left ventricular failure	Tumor	Upper airway obstruction
Pneumonia	Foreign object	Atelectasis
Atelectasis	Laryngeal spasm	Pulmonary cavitation
	Mucus plugs	
	Collapsed lung	

Perhaps the most common causes of *generalized decreased breath sounds* throughout the lungs are hypoventilation from sedation or tranquilizing drugs, chest pain, central nervous system depression, and pulmonary problems related to immobility. Untreated, alveolar hypoventilation leads to atelectasis, mucus retention, and further decreases in breath sounds.

In the patient with chronic pulmonary disease, a generalized decrease in breath sounds is a classic symptom of emphysema. With severe air flow limitation and lung hyperinflation, breath sounds are barely audible during deep breathing and absent during quiet breathing. In addition, intensity varies from one area of the chest to another, and sometimes it varies from one breath to another, presumably owing to changing regional differences in the production and transmission of breath sounds (Ploysongsang et al, 1981). This unevenness in intensity helps to distinguish the decreased breath sounds in emphysema from those in many normal chests. In the normal case, intensity remains unchanged throughout the chest and from breath to breath.

A *unilateral decrease* in breath sounds may indicate unilateral gross pathology, as in a large pneumothorax, but a malpositioned endotracheal tube should always be suspected in any patient recently intubated. The tip of an endotracheal tube should rest 5 cm (1½ to 2 in) above the carina, as confirmed by chest x-ray. Tube malpositioning into the right or left main stem bronchus may go unnoticed until a postintubation chest x-ray is taken. Or the tube may slip owing to improper positioning or taping. Malpositioning of a tube can arise at any time in any anxious or combative patient or in a patient with oral secretions that prevent adequate tape adhesion. Although the right main stem bronchus is more commonly intubated in error because of its more vertical orientation, the left main stem bronchus can be intubated if the advancing tube tip points directly to the left, with the angled lumen pointing downwards. Sometimes the tube is malpositioned at the carina. In this case, breath sounds change from breath to breath, from normal to decreased or absent, as the tube moves into a bronchus with neck extension. Oral rather than nasal endotracheal tubes are more apt to cause changing breath sounds when malpositioned because of their potentially more mobile position in the mouth and pharynx.

Absent Breath Sounds

Absent or inaudible breath sounds are confirmed by auscultation during deep breathing maneuvers, coughing, or change in position, if necessary. In the spontaneously breathing intubated patient, decreased to absent breath sounds may be difficult to detect in localized areas because of shallow breathing. When in doubt, if deep breathing, coughing, or a change in position does not stimulate deep breathing, briefly return the patient to mechanical ventilation or use a bedside resuscitation bag and auscultate suspicious areas during the first several deep breaths.

Generalized absent breath sounds indicate respiratory arrest in the absence of airflow at the mouth.

As a new finding, localized absent breath sounds indicate gross pathology requiring immediate medical evaluation to prevent further deterioration of pulmonary function. Sometimes absent breath sounds represent progressive disease, e.g., a small pleural effusion that has become massive, completely blocking the transmission of sound and compressing underlying lung, or mucus plugs that have further obstructed the airway. Other disorders causing absent breath sounds are listed in Table 12–6.

Monitoring the Intensity of Normal Breath Sounds

The following points should be kept in mind when monitoring the intensity of normal breath sounds. First, as intensity decreases, lung ventilation becomes more impaired. This change is most evident over localized areas of disease in the lung, such as over bullae, fibrosis, and atelectatic areas, the areas most likely to retain mucus and exhibit regional changes in ventilation.

Second, various patterns of decreased and absent sounds are characteristic of certain pulmonary disorders. For example, a patient with massive pleural effusion characteristically presents with absent breath sounds at the lung base. The intensity of the breath sound gradually increases towards the fluid level.

Third, in the absence of airflow limitation, an early sign of a dropping PaO_2 level is *increased* rather than decreased breath sounds. The intensity of inspiration and expiration increases with ventilatory effort and hyperventilation. Actual and audible I:E ratio approaches 1:1, as the patient becomes more tachypneic. Breath sounds become decreased much later, when general fatigue from the increased work of breathing causes hypoventilation or when an existing pathologic process begins to affect alveolar ventilation.

Last, COPD patients are monitored differently than individuals with normal lungs because their baseline normal breath sounds are different. The stable patient with moderate to severe airflow limitation has an audible I:E ratio approaching 1:4 rather than the normal 3:1. Unlike the normal individual with a faint expiratory phase, expiration in those with COPD is louder and more prolonged owing to accentuated airflow limitation during deep breathing and forced expiratory maneuvers. The onset of acute respiratory problems causes an increase in airflow limitation and a corresponding *decrease* in the intensity of expiration until this phase becomes absent altogether, as illustrated in Figure 12–45. Absent expiration with a short, faint inspiration is termed the "silent chest." It is a sign of a rising $PaCO_2$ and ventilatory failure. This finding explains why pulmonologists constantly remind

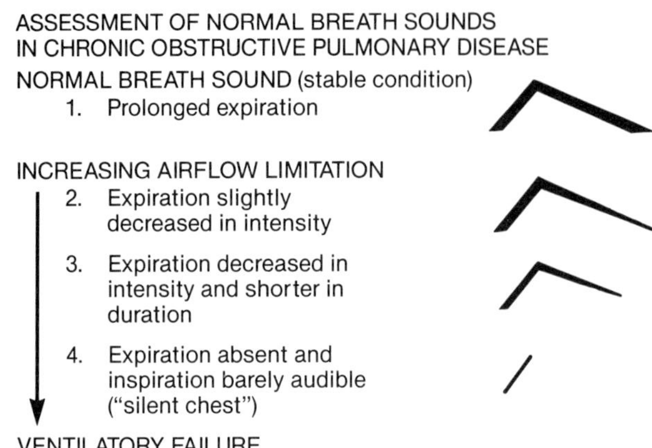

ASSESSMENT OF NORMAL BREATH SOUNDS
IN CHRONIC OBSTRUCTIVE PULMONARY DISEASE
NORMAL BREATH SOUND (stable condition)
1. Prolonged expiration
INCREASING AIRFLOW LIMITATION
2. Expiration slightly decreased in intensity
3. Expiration decreased in intensity and shorter in duration
4. Expiration absent and inspiration barely audible ("silent chest")
VENTILATORY FAILURE

Figure 12–45. Assessment of normal breath sounds in chronic obstructive pulmonary disease (COPD).

others that, particularly in emphysema, "it is not so much what you hear, but what you don't hear that is important" (Petty, 1979). Most important, monitoring for the disappearing expiratory phase of respiration is essential in *any* patient with airflow limitation.

Bronchial Breath Sound

The bronchial breath sound is dramatically different than the normal breath sound. Its loud, high-pitched, and extremely tubular quality sounds like air passing through a hollow tube. Although its end-inspiratory pause (see graphic representation in Table 12–5) may help distinguish the sound from the normal breath sound, the hollow quality during expiration is its most distinctive feature. Placing the stethoscope on the manubrium during expiration, especially during forced expiration, readily familiarizes the nurse with this sound. It is normally heard over the trachea in the area of the manubrium. The presence of the bronchial breath sound anywhere else is pathologic, indicating lung consolidation or compression of lung tissue.

Physiologic Mechanisms. As in abnormal voice sounds and increased fremitus, consolidation and compression of tissue produce a solid medium that conducts sound better than air-filled tissue. More specifically, the solid medium decreases the filtering effect of normal lung tissue such that sounds over peripheral areas sound similar to sounds directly over large airways (Murphy and Holford, 1980).

There is one crucial criterion for the transmission of the bronchial breath sound; *major airways must be open.* When airways are blocked by mucus or any obstructive mechanism, breath sounds are decreased or absent rather than bronchial, as illustrated in Figure 12–46. In this situation, decreased breath sounds represent a more severe condition than bronchial breath sounds.

Disorders. Generally, conditions that produce abnormal voice sounds and increased fremitus also produce the bronchial or bronchovesicular breath sound. *Pneumonia* is the classic example; the sound appears as alveoli fill with fluid and other by-products of inflammation.

Pulmonary cavitation produces varying breath sounds and adventitious sounds, depending on the underlying disease process, pulmonary complications (pneumonia is common), and clinical presentation. When lung consolidation is present, as in lung abscess, lung cancer, coccidioidomycosis, or tuberculosis, the bronchial breath sound may be heard, *if* lung cavities fill with fluid and adjacent airways remain patent to conduct the sound.

When air-filled or partially fluid-filled cavities are large and communicate with bronchi, a bronchial breath sound occurs with a quality similar to the sound made by blowing across the mouth of an empty bottle. Although this sound is slightly different from that produced over a typically consolidated area of lung, it is still classified as a bronchial breath sound.

In any case, the clinician should never rely upon physical findings for diagnosis of lung cavitation be-

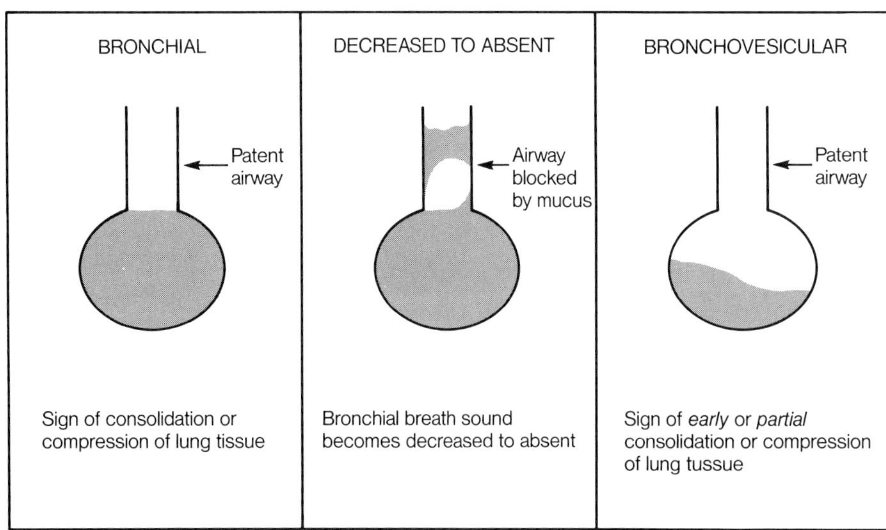

Figure 12–46. Role of airway patency in the transmission of bronchial and bronchovesicular breath sounds. A decreased to absent breath sound may be a more serious sign of disease than a bronchial or bronchovesicular breath sound.

cause they may be absent or inconclusive. A chest x-ray is always used for diagnosis and further evaluation. In equivocal cases, specialized x-rays (i.e., tomograms) are taken to more closely examine small areas of possible cavitation.

Pulmonary infarction produces lung consolidation as interstitial and alveolar spaces fill with blood and other cellular components. Similarly, *lung tumor* or, occasionally, a collapsed lobe of a lung, produces bronchial breath sounds providing the airway remains open. By compression of lung tissue from an outside source below the diaphragm, gross obesity, or abdominal distention can, in some cases, cause bronchial or bronchovesicular breath sounds just above the level of the diaphragm.

In processes that cause a significant loss of lung volume on one side of the chest (e.g., *massive atelectasis,* unilateral *pulmonary fibrosis*), the opposite lung hyperinflates to compensate for the loss of tissue available for gas exchange (Fig. 12–47). This process of hyperinflation is called *compensatory emphysema* and can usually be seen on the chest x-ray. If the hyperinflated lung crosses the midthorax, it compresses lung tissue on the other side and sometimes creates bronchial breath sounds there. Similarly, in patients with *long-standing pneumonectomy,* bronchial breath sounds may be heard near the midsternal line on the side of the pneumonectomy; the remaining lung hyperinflates, crosses the midthorax, and becomes compressed as its expansion is restricted by the fibrotic cavity on the pneumonectomy side. In acutely ill patients with massive atelectasis, the bronchial breath sounds in the midthoracic area may not be distinguishable from the bronchovesicular slightly hollow sounds normally heard in this area.

In *pleural effusion,* a bronchial breath sound is occasionally heard directly above the pleural fluid level, when the effusion is large and the underlying lung is compressed into airless tissue. It is accompanied by *egophony* and a *hyperresonant percussion note.* The latter is from compensatory hyperinflation of alveoli in the same general location. The former occurs because the thin layer of pleural fluid screens out low frequency sounds traveling to the chest's surface and transmits the high-pitched bronchial breath sound in addition to the high frequency formants of vowels. Hence, the E becomes an A with the nasal bleating quality so typical of egophony. These sounds are not heard below the fluid level because the thicker layer of pleural fluid blocks sound transmission.

With this knowledge, the pattern of breath sounds and other physical findings in pleural effusion discussed thus far can be summarized (Fig. 12–48). These findings vary depending on the depth and density of fluid in the pleural space at different thoracic levels. In small effusions, only decreased breath sounds, decreased voice sounds and fremitus, and dullness to percussion may be evident. Compare pleural effusion findings in Figure 12–48 with the classic findings for lung consolidation from pneumonia in Figure 12–49.

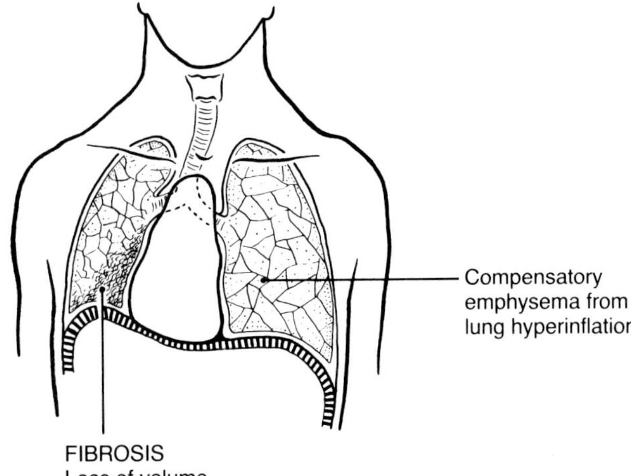

Figure 12–47. The loss of lung volume from severe unilateral fibrosis results in compensatory emphysema in the opposite normal lung. (Reproduced and adapted by permission from Cherniack, R. and Cherniak, L.: Respiration in Health and Disease, 3rd ed., Philadelphia, W. B. Saunders Co., 1983.)

Both disorders may present with the bronchial or bronchovesicular breath sound, but the pattern of breath sounds and presence of other physical findings helps to distinguish between the two disorders.

Bronchovesicular Breath Sound

The bronchovesicular breath sound is a cross between a normal (vesicular) and a bronchial breath sound. Its most distinguishing feature is its slightly hollow sound. Compared with the bronchial breath sound, it has a lower pitch, a longer inspiratory phase with an I:E ratio of 1:1 (see graphic representation in Table 12–5), and may sound "closer" to the ear.

It is normally heard over large central airways in the sternal area and between the scapulae, areas that correspond to the T4 level, where the trachea bifurcates. The general boundaries for the bronchovesicular sound in Figures 12–43 and 12–44 may vary, extending outward in thin individuals and inward in muscular or obese individuals. Sometimes the sound is identifiable only in the middle of the sternum.

Similarly, in the posterior chest (see Fig. 12–44), boundaries may extend to one or both apices especially the right apical area, where normal breath sounds are louder, depending on body build and normal anatomic variations.

Bronchovesicular breath sounds heard in areas in addition to the previously mentioned areas indicate *early* or partial lung consolidation or *early* compression of tissue; alveoli are not entirely filled, nor is compression as extensive as that of a bronchial breath sound (see Fig. 12–46). Hence, a breath sound becomes bronchovesicular and then bronchial as a pulmonary disorder worsens and vice versa as it improves. One

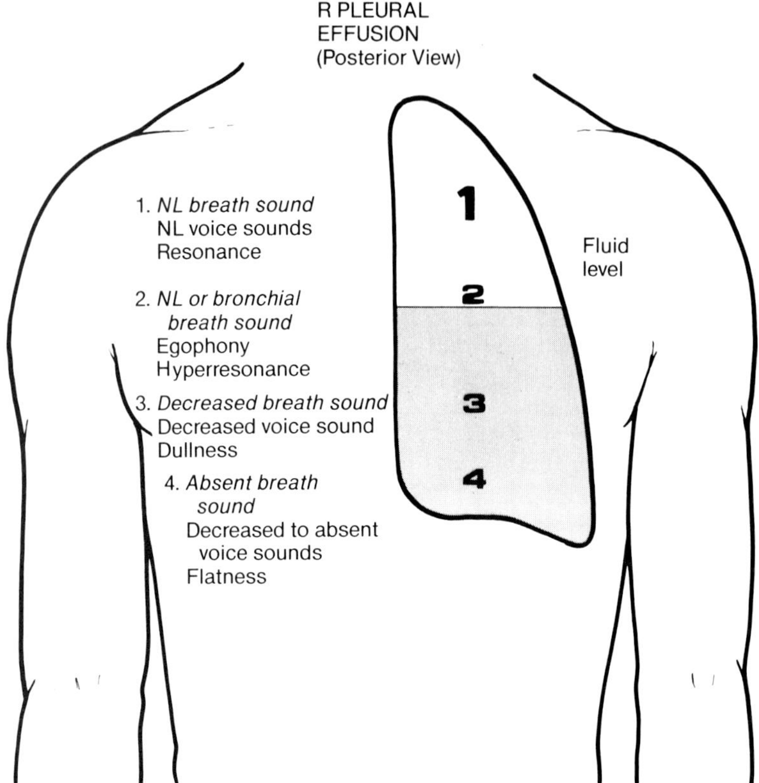

Figure 12–48. Breath sounds, voice sounds, and percussion notes at different thoracic levels in pleural effusion. The changes between levels two and three help determine the location of the fluid level. (NL = normal.)

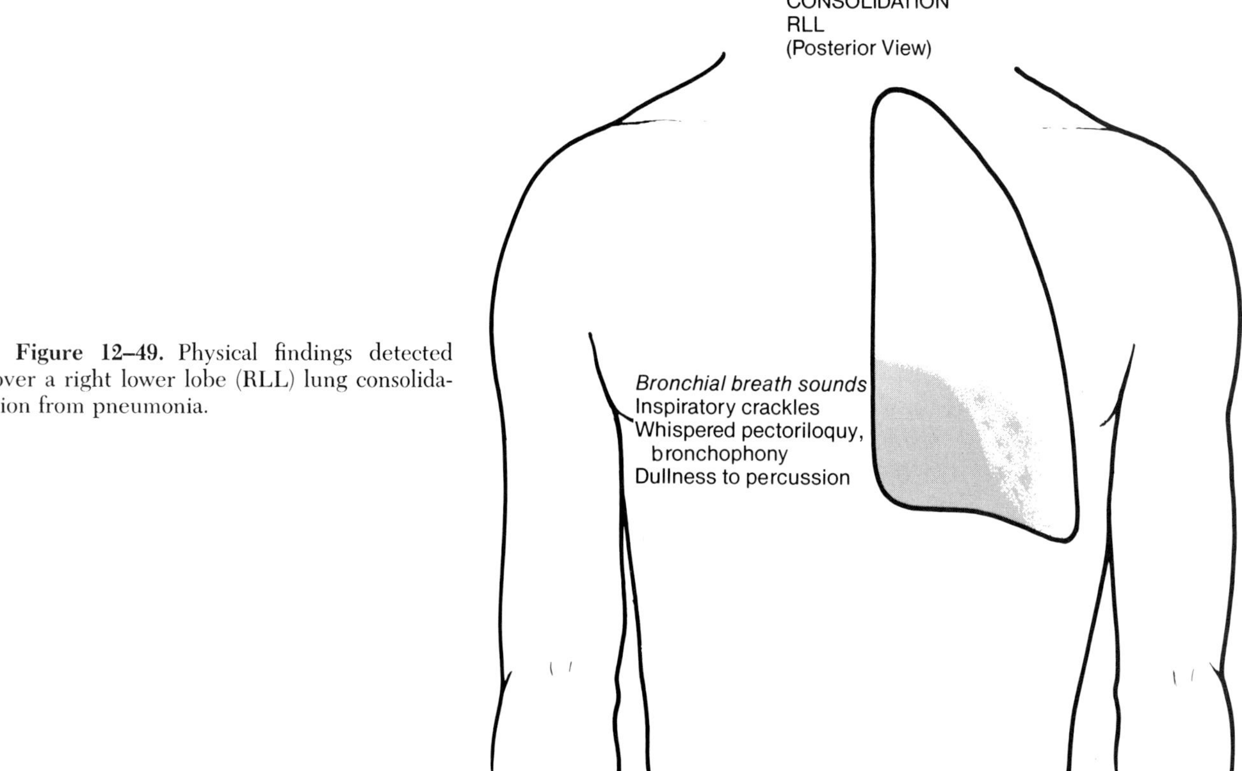

Figure 12–49. Physical findings detected over a right lower lobe (RLL) lung consolidation from pneumonia.

Table 12–7. DISORDERS CAUSING BRONCHIAL OR BRONCHOVESICULAR BREATH SOUNDS

Pleural effusion (at or just above fluid level)
Lung tumor
Collapsed lung
Pneumonia
Large pulmonary infarction
Pulmonary cavitation (with fluid-filled cavity)
Severe abdominal or stomach distention
Gross obesity
Compensatory emphysema
Severe interstitial fibrosis
*Pulmonary cavitation (from air-filled cavity in communication with bronchus)
†Pulmonary edema

*Bronchial sound only.
†Bronchovesicular sound only.

or both sounds may be present, depending on the severity, extent, and location of the pathology.

Disorders. Disorders causing both bronchovesicular and bronchial breath sounds are listed in Table 12–7. The only condition producing the bronchovesicular breath sound alone is pulmonary edema. Little has been documented regarding exactly how pulmonary edema produces bronchovesicular breath sounds. Usually, decreased breath sounds are evident as fluid bubbles into airways, blocking the transmission of sound. However, bronchovesicular sounds may occur when fluid remains predominantly interstitial (i.e., increased solid medium with a patent airway) and as fluid begins to fill alveoli on the all-or-none principle (i.e., partial consolidation).

Detection. Bronchovesicular breath sounds are easily missed in tachypneic patients or those with decreased breath sounds. A quick comparison of expiration over the pathologic area and corresponding normal area on the opposite side of the chest during forced expiration or panting may be necessary to bring out the slightly hollow sound. If secretions are present, auscultate after coughing or suctioning has eliminated or reduced interference from loud adventitious sounds.

Once an abnormal hollow sound has been identified, the question whether to classify it as bronchial or bronchovesicular arises. In this case, a guess is acceptable and may be necessary if the patient cannot tolerate extra breathing maneuvers to accentuate the sound. Whether an indication of early or late consolidation or mild or severe compression of tissue, *any* hollow sound in the periphery indicates gross pathology that requires immediate medical evaluation and further monitoring.

ADVENTITIOUS SOUNDS

Adventitious sounds are abnormal extra sounds superimposed on baseline breath sounds. They are the most readily detected indicators of lung pathology. Whereas normal breath sounds are believed to result from gas vibrations, adventitious sounds are believed to result from abnormal motions of airway walls and secretions or materials within airways during breathing.

The four main types of adventitious sounds include the *crackle (rale)*, *rhonchus*, *wheeze*, and *pleural friction rub*. The *mediastinal crunch* is also discussed in this section; the Joint Committee on Pulmonary Nomenclature (American College of Chest Physicians, 1975) lists it as a standard pulmonary term.

Crackles (Rales)

Crackles are commonly called *rales* in some textbooks and in those clinical settings that have not yet adopted the recently recommended American Thoracic Society nomenclature. Readers should be familiar with both terms, since they are commonly used interchangeably in the clinical setting; the change to the term *crackles* has been very recent in the United States. Of the two terms, crackles is preferable because it standardizes American terminology with that of Great Britain; it is more descriptive than rales; and it is less confusing, given the changing meanings of the term rales over the past century. (See subsequent discussion of controversy surrounding lung sounds.)

Crackles have two distinguishing features: they typically occur during inspiration, and they form a group of very discrete single sounds (see illustration in Table 12–8). Because they occur in brief bursts, they are labelled *discontinuous sounds*.

The crackling sound can be simulated by picking up a lock of hair with thumb and forefinger and slowly rubbing the strands together close to the ear. However, actual crackles in the chest may deviate greatly from this simulated sound, with pitch, quality, and occurrence during respiration varying, depending on the underlying physiologic mechanism and clinical disorder.

Types of Crackles. The American Thoracic Society divides crackles into *fine* and *coarse* categories based on sound waveforms (Murphy and Holford, 1980). *Fine crackles* are high in pitch, relatively soft in intensity, and short in duration compared with coarse crackles. They are heard in patients with atelectasis, fibrosis, early left ventricular failure, and pneumonia. *Coarse crackles* are low in pitch, loud, and may be longer in duration compared with fine crackles. They are heard in those with resolving pneumonia, pulmonary edema, and bronchitis.

This classification system serves as an excellent guideline in the description of crackles. However, particularly within the "fine" category, wide variations exist in the type of crackle heard at the bedside, ranging from the finest crackles of transient atelectasis to the more medium crackles of pneumonia and the more discrete "dry"-sounding crackles of interstitial fibrosis. These variations become quite evident as one gains experience in lung auscultation, sometimes causing the clinician to question the usefulness of the fine category.

Table 12–8. TYPES OF ADVENTITIOUS SOUNDS

Type	General Location	Associated Problem(s)	Characteristics	Graphic Illustration
Crackles (rales)	Peripheral airways and alveoli	Atelectasis Inflammation Excess fluid Excess mucus	Group of discrete crackles or popping sounds Discontinuous sound Usually inspiratory, may be inspiratory and expiratory	fine coarse
Rhonchi	Large airways	Inflammation Excess fluid Excess mucus	Coarse, low-pitched sonorous sounds Continuous sound Usually expiratory, may be inspiratory and expiratory Changes in quality and timing with coughing	
Wheeze	Large and/or small airways	Bronchoconstriction (airway narrowing) from bronchospasm, fluid, mucus, inflammatory by-products, obstructive lesion Airway instability	High- (sometimes low-) pitched musical sound Continuous sound Usually expiratory, may be inspiratory and expiratory	
Pleural friction rub	Pleural surfaces	Inflamed or roughened pleural surfaces (pleuritis)	Grating sound with continuous and discontinuous qualities May appear intermittently Variable duration; usually inspiratory, may be inspiratory and expiratory Sounds the same or louder with coughing	

The important point to remember when categorizing crackles either into the fine or coarse category (or into the fine, medium, or coarse category used by some clinicians) is *not* to quibble over precise categorization. In spite of the new development of waveforms to describe sounds, the clinical correlations of crackles and other lung sounds are imprecisely known. The most important goal in auscultation is to differentiate the crackle from the rhonchus, wheeze, and pleural friction rub.

Physiologic Mechanisms. At least two physiologic mechanisms are responsible for the sound of crackles. Crackles heard in patients with pulmonary edema probably result from *air bubbling through fluid.* Crackles heard in those with fibrosis, early left ventricular failure, and atelectasis are believed to result from the *sudden opening of airways* closed at the end of the previous expiration. The sudden release of stored energy produces a shower of crackling sounds as the lung expands. It is uncertain whether the crackles result from the sudden equalization of pressure between sites distal and proximal to the collapsed area or the bursting of airway surface film as the collapsed area opens.

Disorders. Generally, a patient with any condition that produces alveolar and small airway collapse (e.g., atelectasis) or fluid or mucus in small airways will present with crackles. The main disorders producing crackles are listed in Table 12–9 under specific causative physiologic mechanisms.

Atelectasis classically has fine crackles. They are most likely to occur in the conditions listed subsequently, particularly if more than one condition is present. Decreased breath sounds accompany crackles over crucial auscultation areas when ventilation to the region is significantly impaired.

Conditions	*Crucial Auscultation Areas*
Bed rest	Dependent areas, especially lower lobes
Post-thoracotomy	Incisional area, chest tube sites Axillary areas Anterior chest, particularly when patient "freezes" in a forward leaning position
Abdominal surgery	Bases of lower lobes
Immobile body or extremities	Dependent areas, especially lower lobes Axillary areas when arm range of motion is limited
Severe kypho-scoliosis	Lingular segments and right middle lobe (RML) Over "crowded" ribs posteriorly

More attention is being given to the presence of crackles in persons without lung disease. Normal persons may have fine end-inspiratory crackles in dependent lung regions after prolonged periods of recumbency and low volume breathing (Ploysongsang and Schonfeld, 1982). These crackles are usually heard in dependent lower lobes, and they disappear with a cough or few deep breaths. Workum and colleagues (1982) studied the presence and character of crackles in 56 normal young women in an upright seated position. Most subjects demonstrated fine mid to late

Table 12–9. PHYSIOLOGIC MECHANISMS RESPONSIBLE FOR ADVENTITIOUS SOUNDS

Physiologic Mechanism/ Clinical Disorder	Crackles (rales)	Rhonchi	Wheeze	Pleural Friction Rub
Excess fluid in the lungs				
Cardiogenic pulmonary edema Noncardiogenic pulmonary edema, e.g., adult respiratory distress syndrome Positive fluid balance Hypoalbuminemia	+	+	± Present from airway edema (cardiac asthma)	−
Airway inflammation and mucus secretion				
Pneumonia Bronchitis Bronchiolitis Bronchiectasis Asthma	+	+ May be present only with a cough	± Present with airway edema	− Present in pneumonia when pleura affected
Atelectasis due to				
Airway obstruction Partial: Large lung tumor Foreign object Mucus plug	+	± Present if airway disease or pneumonia develops	+	−
Complete:	−	−	−	−
Abnormal breathing pattern Immobility Use of sedatives, hypnotics, and tranquilizers Chest pain Postoperative chest	+	± Present if airway disease or pneumonia develops	−	−
Compression of lung tissue Gross obesity Acute abdomen Pleural effusion Large cavitary lesion (pneumatocele)	±	−	−	− May be present with small pleural effusion
Alveolitis				
Infectious Pneumonia	+	+ May be present only with cough	−	−
Noninfectious Diffuse interstitial fibrosis Hypersensitivity pneumonitis	+	−	−	−
Mediator release of bronchoactive substances				
Carcinoid tumor Byssinosis Asthma	−	−	+	−
Pleural inflammation				
Pulmonary embolus Tumor Pneumonia	+	± Present with airway disease or mucus retention	± Present with airway narrowing	+

KEY: + usually present
− usually absent
± may be present or absent

inspiratory crackles in the anterior bases after a full expiration. The crackles were faint and much easier to detect on a slow rather than rapid deep inspiration. They were thought to be due to the sudden opening of closed airways; airways normally close in dependent lung zones on maximum expiration. The predilection for anterior lung bases may be related to compression of the lung by the liver and spleen or to the slightly higher attachment of the diaphragm anteriorly. Before conclusions can be drawn, however, more research is needed to determine more precisely the prevalence, mechanism, and significance of crackles in normal persons.

Patients with *lobar pneumonia* classically present with fine to coarse crackles over the consolidated area. In contrast, those with *viral pneumonia* may present with only a few crackles to absent adventitious sounds with negative *or* positive chest x-ray findings. This type of pneumonia is characterized by discrepancies between physical and chest x-ray findings.

A patient with *pulmonary edema* presents with fine crackles in the lower lobes, as alveolar flooding begins. These sounds become coarse "popping" sounds, likened to the bubbling sound of a freshly opened bottle of a carbonated beverage, as overt pulmonary edema occurs. Generally, the greater the alveolar flooding, the more evident the crackles and the further up the posterior chest the crackles can be heard. However, pulmonary edema may worsen without *any* detectable change in crackles or other physical findings. The chest x-ray and hemodynamic measurements are more accurate indicators of the severity of pulmonary edema than physical findings.

A patient with *diffuse interstitial fibrosis* presents with crackles unlike any of those discussed thus far. They are "dry" rather than "wet" sounding, as in pulmonary edema. Sometimes called "cellophane" or "Velcro" crackles, the dry sound is likened to the sound heard when crumbling a piece of cellophane or peeling apart two pieces of Velcro. The crackles are high-pitched, usually end inspiratory, and more prevalent in the bases, where fibrosis begins. They extend up the posterior chest as fibrosis develops in upper lung regions. They are easiest to hear during a slow, deep inspiration after breath holding at low lung volumes. When their high-pitched, dry quality becomes "wet" sounding (e.g., less discrete and lower pitched), fluid retention from early left ventricular failure or mucus retention is suspected. However, unless the clinician is already familiar with the patient's typical lung sounds, this subtle change in quality may be difficult, if not impossible, to detect.

Bronchitis is observed with a few early inspiratory coarse crackles. They are easy to miss because only *one* or *two* soft pops may be auscultated as the patient starts to inhale. The crackles are heard only over a few small regions of a patient's chest. Intensity and number of crackles vary from region to region. When crackles are loud, they may be heard at the mouths of patients with significant airway disease.

The different presentations of crackles thus far discussed are summarized in Figure 12–50.

Detection and Interpretation. Since crackles are typically inspiratory, careful attention to the inspiratory phase of respiration is necessary for their detection. If the patient is on mechanical ventilation, it may be necessary to auscultate while pushing the ventilator's "sigh" button to detect crackles in dependent regions.

Timing during inspiration may help in the evaluation of crackles. As mentioned, patients with some disorders present with crackles at specific times during inspiration, e.g., bronchitis—early inspiration, and fibrosis and atelectasis—late inspiration. In the case of fluid retention, crackles are first end inspiratory. With disease progression, they start earlier during inspiration and are eventually heard throughout inspiration as well as expiration, as in pulmonary edema. A similar pattern occurs with a worsening mucus retention problem. In both cases, with effective deep breathing and coughing, mucus or fluid moves up into large airways. Many crackles disappear, and rhonchi dominate the chest until the patient expectorates secretions.

Furthermore, as with other adventitious sounds, the presence of crackles is always evaluated in light of the underlying breath sound. Lung ventilation is always worse when abnormal breath sounds are present.

Whenever the common finding of basilar crackles is detected, particularly in patients in the coronary care unit, the question arises, *"Are the crackles due to atelectasis, fluid accumulation in the lungs* (i.e., early left ventricular failure), *or mucus retention from bronchitis or pneumonia?"* This crucial question must be answered by looking at other physical findings and assessment parameters. Because the answer shapes the health care team's approach to the patient and the choice of medical, nursing, and respiratory therapy interventions, the clinician orients the patient assessment towards the gathering of data that will help answer the question, e.g., sputum changes, x-ray results, and recent pulmonary capillary wedge pressure measurements.

Charting. When charting crackles, the nurse notes timing during respiration, location, and exactly how far the crackles extend up the posterior chest. For example, *inspiratory crackles left lower lobe (LLL) posteriorly, extending to about T6.*

Transient crackles are also charted. Though usually not significant, their presence may indicate a potential ventilatory or fluid balance problem, particularly in the critically ill patient.

Rhonchi

Rhonchi are low-pitched sonorous sounds caused by mucus or fluid moving around in *large* airways. More specifically, when mucus is stuck to the bronchial wall, as in bronchitis, the mucus flap vibrates in the air stream, producing one or more *rhonchi.*

The most distinguishing features of rhonchi relate to quality and timing during respiration. Rhonchi have a coarse sound frequently associated with a smoker's cough. When friends report "He sounds so congested," undoubtedly the patient has rhonchi with deep breathing or at least with a cough. Auscultation with a

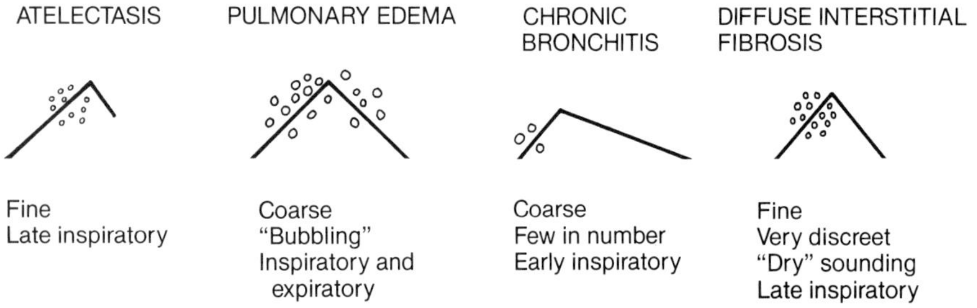

Figure 12–50. Different types of crackles (rales) in respiratory disease.

stethoscope reveals snoring or sonorous sounds that appear and disappear in a very disorganized pattern, sometimes changing slightly in quality and varying in location from minute to minute, hour to hour, and day to day, depending on the location of mucus or fluid in the chest. This pattern is in sharp contrast to the way in which crackles are heard, i.e., in a very organized cluster of discrete sounds during inspiration. In spite of the interrupted or disorganized pattern of the rhonchi, the rhonchus is still labelled as a continuous sound because it lasts much longer than a single crackle. Continuous sounds usually last longer than 0.25 second, although no established criteria exist for precise categorization.

Another distinguishing feature of the rhonchus is that it usually occurs during expiration, when the tracheobronchial tree normally narrows (see the graphic representation in Table 12–8). However, particularly in the presence of excessive secretions, it can occur at *any* time during the respiratory cycle, depending on the varying occlusion of the airway with mobile secretions. With a worsening mucus or fluid retention problem, expiratory rhonchi develop into both inspiratory and expiratory rhonchi, and rhonchal fremitus can be palpated on the chest's surface. Effective coughing loosens mucus from the inflamed bronchial walls, clears it from the lungs, and completely eliminates the adventitious sound during deep breathing, although it still may be heard along *with* the cough.

Disorders. Generally, rhonchi are anticipated in any disorder with *excess mucus,* usually from airway diseases such as bronchitis and bronchiectasis, or *excess fluid,* usually from inflammatory by-products, such as those in pneumonia or pulmonary edema. Other disorders that may present with rhonchi are listed in Table 12–9.

In *COPD,* it is bronchitis and not emphysema that causes secretions and rhonchi in the chest. As Chapter 7 points out, the stable emphysematous patient presents with a clear chest unless an acute asthmatic or bronchitic component develops to produce wheezing or crackles and rhonchi, respectively.

In *atelectasis,* the patient may develop rhonchi in addition to crackles, as alveolar ventilation decreases and secretions accumulate in the chest. Similarly, postoperative patients recovering from general anesthesia or patients on sedatives, hypnotics, or tranquilizers have depressed mucociliary escalators. Accumulation of thick secretions in the large airways or the oropharynx can potentially cause spontaneous airway occlusion and respiratory arrest unless secretions (i.e., rhonchi) are promptly cleared by deep breathing, coughing, and suctioning, if necessary.

A patient with pulmonary consolidation from *lobar pneumonia* presents with rhonchi but not until therapy has loosened alveolar secretions, and the patient begins to expectorate sputum. Recovery from lobar pneumonia is broken down into four conceptual stages (Fig. 12–51). The patient with severe consolidation presents with absent breath sounds to a barely audible inspiratory phase over the consolidated areas, no adventitious sounds, and normal breath sounds throughout the rest of the chest. The bronchus to the consolidated area remains blocked with one or more thick mucus plugs, or it may be completely consolidated, as in Figure 12–

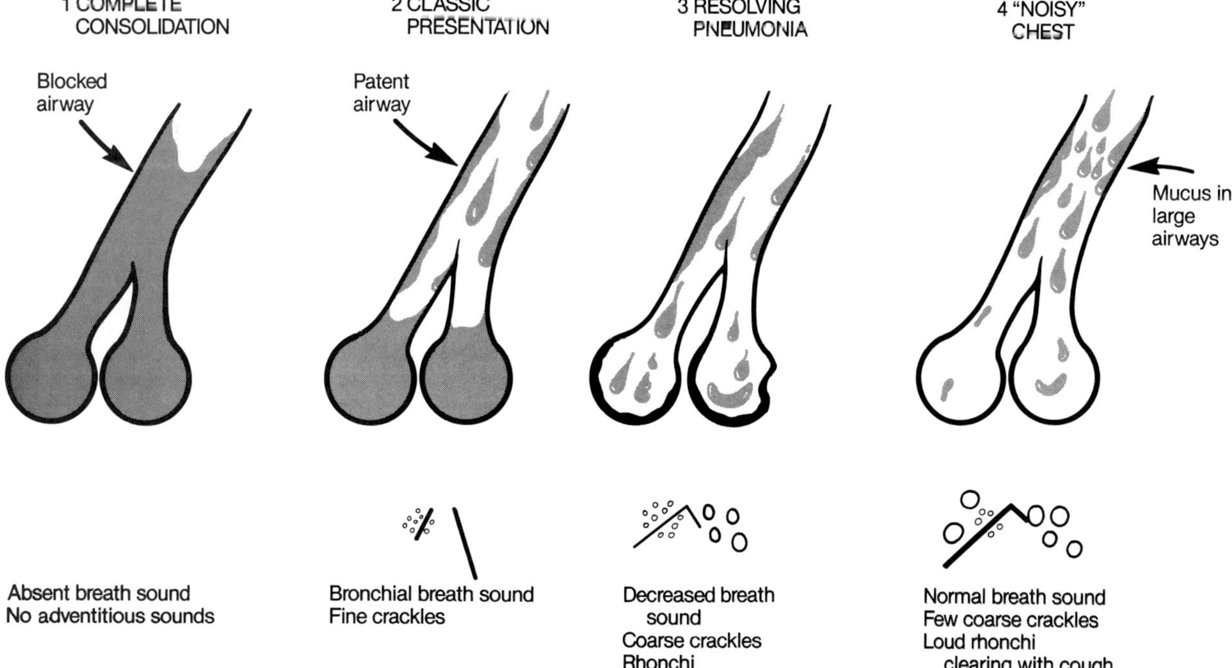

Figure 12–51. Conceptual stages for resolving lobar pneumonia with graphic illustrations of breath sounds and adventitious sounds.

51 (Stage 1). Since the advent of antibiotics and modern bronchial hygiene measures, complete consolidation is not as common as it used to be, but it does occur.

In most cases, the lobar pneumonia patient classically presents with bronchial breath sounds, a sign of consolidation, and inspiratory crackles over the consolidated area (Stage 2). A rhonchus is heard *only* with a cough. With further therapy, the bronchial breath sound becomes bronchovesicular (i.e., slightly hollow) and converts to a decreased normal vesicular breath sound shortly thereafter (Stage 3). As the breath sound changes, adventitious sounds become easier to hear. Inspiratory crackles may sound coarser and more numerous over the consolidated area. Expiratory rhonchi are heard over the affected lobe and, to a lesser degree, throughout the chest. At this time, or with further loosening of consolidated secretions, rhonchi dominate lung sounds throughout the chest, producing a "noisy" chest (Stage 4). The breath sound over the consolidated area is slightly decreased to normal, and a few inspiratory crackles may be heard, particularly after the patient rests in a supine position for a long time.

During these last two truly resolving stages, bedside personnel unfamiliar with lung sounds may become worried about the patient because "He sounds so congested." Most important, a "noisy" chest is a favorable sign, providing the underlying breath sound is normal and the patient is successfully coughing up sputum. In contrast, a chest that reverts to decreased to absent breath sounds and *no* adventitious sounds over the affected lobe is of more concern, because, most likely, purulent secretions have become consolidated again beyond the obstructed airways. If not already present, consolidation will develop as atelectasis beyond the obstruction promotes mucus retention.

Last, this sequence of lung sound changes varies from patient to patient, depending on the severity of the consolidation, the degree and extent of airway occlusion, and the presence of other chest diseases. With appropriate therapy, the chest of an otherwise healthy adult with a classic presentation of lobar pneumonia may become clear in a matter of days, except for a lingering rhonchus with a cough.

Detection and Interpretation. When present, rhonchi are readily evident during deep breathing. If the patient is on mechanical ventilation, be sure the tubing is emptied of condensed water before auscultation. Bubbling in the tubing may be heard during auscultation and may sound like rhonchi in the chest.

When rhonchi are absent during deep breathing, be sure to listen for a rhonchus along *with* the cough. The dehydrated patient with pneumonia may be entirely clear of adventitious sounds except for a rhonchus with a cough. Expiratory rhonchi develop as rehydration with intravenous or oral fluids liquefies secretions enough to permit them to flap around in the air stream.

Rhonchi in the chest along with sputum production are perhaps the easiest sign of a fluid or mucus retention problem to detect. As with crackles in undiagnosed patients, the nurse looks at other clinical findings to tentatively determine the etiology of the secretions. On the one hand, for example, rhonchi with neck vein distention, high central venous pressure, crackles, frothy pink sputum, and signs of respiratory distress indicate pulmonary edema. On the other hand, rhonchi with purulent sputum, early inspiratory crackles, and normal to decreased breath sounds *without* signs of respiratory distress indicate chronic bronchitis and, possibly, pneumonia.

In all patients, rhonchi and other lung sounds are monitored to help determine the effectiveness of therapy. With mucus retention, persisting rhonchi indicate a need to encourage routine bronchial hygiene measures, such as coughing, deep breathing, and incentive spirometry, or more aggressive measures, such as postural drainage or endotracheal suctioning, if routine measures fail to clear the chest of rhonchi. If rhonchi persist in a certain lobe, respiratory interventions should concentrate on that area, using extra measures, such as segmental chest expansion or chest percussion and vibration, if necessary. In any case, the important point is to *continue* to check for persisting rhonchi after treatments and to *continue* to alter interventions and consult the physician until an effective regimen is determined and lung sounds improve.

Charting. Examples of charting follow:

Inspiratory and expiratory rhonchi heard throughout the chest.

Expiratory rhonchi scattered throughout the chest, especially the base of LLL.

Chest clear except rhonchus with cough.

Wheeze

A wheeze is described as a musical, whistling, or "sibilant" sound produced by air movement through narrowed airways. Its musical quality is analogous to the sound quality produced by a reed instrument. Most nurses recognize the wheeze when asked to think of the high-pitched squeaking sound that an asthmatic produces when in respiratory distress. As the illustration in Table 12–8 shows, the wheeze is a continuous sound that usually occurs during expiration. It becomes both inspiratory and expiratory with severe airway narrowing.

Physiologic Mechanism. It was originally believed that the wheeze was generated in the same way as a note of a pipe organ, i.e., by the vibration of a column of air, with pitch depending on the length of the pipe and the density of the gas in the pipe. We now know that this observation is not true of wheezes in the chest. Wheezes are high-pitched or low-pitched, depending on several factors, including the varying tightness (i.e., compression) of airway walls and the rate of air flow through the constricted areas.

The physiologic mechanism believed responsible for the wheeze is summarized in Figure 12–52. In the lung unit on the far left, the arrow represents normal

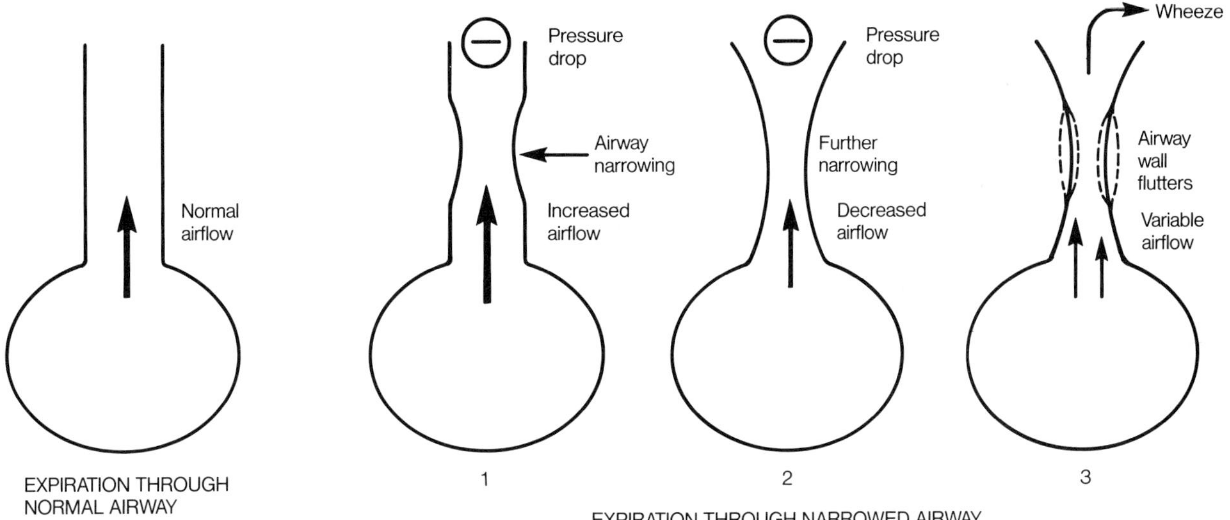

Figure 12–52. Postulated wheeze mechanism. (Adapted from Murphy, R. and Holford, S.: Lung sounds. *Basics of Respiratory Disease*, 8(4), 1980.)

airflow through normal airways during expiration. When the airway becomes narrowed by disease, as in 1, airflow must *increase* to move the same amount of air past the narrowed area. According to Bernouilli's principle (summarized in Chapter 22), the increased airflow produces a pressure drop across the constricted area. In 2, this pressure drop tends to collapse the airway and decrease expiratory airflow. As Murphy and Holford (1980) explain, when this occurs, pressure relationships reverse themselves, i.e., reduced airflow permits intraluminal pressures to rise, and the airway begins to open. However, as the expiratory phase of respiration continues, airflow increases, pressure drops, and the airway again narrows. This series of events causes the airway wall to oscillate or flutter back and forth, as in 3, producing the continuous sound of a wheeze.

Though airway narrowing is involved in the wheeze mechanism and is usually central to clinical interpretation of this adventitious lung sound, Cugell (1985) points out that flutter oscillations of bronchial walls may occur *without* airflow obstruction. The oscillations producing the wheeze depend on airway geometry, gas flow, and mechanical properties of vibrating tissue. The conclusion from this finding is that airway instability rather than airway narrowing may be the major factor contributing to the development of wheezing.

Disorders. Generally, a patient with any disorder with an asthmatic component may present with wheezing. However, airway narrowing from asthma does not always produce wheezing. Furthermore, when present, wheezing may not be from asthma. Airway narrowing (bronchoconstriction) may occur from a number of processes described in Table 12–9, e.g., edema, airway inflammation and mucus secretion, airway obstruction (i.e., mechanical), and mediator release of bronchoactive substances.

In *asthma*, wheezing ranges from an occasional, single, high-pitched squeak to a host of inspiratory and expiratory squeaks simulating different wind instruments, striking notes and chords to warm up for an evening performance. It is typically worse between 4:00 am and 4:30 am. The reason for increased symptoms at this time relates to changes in biologic circadian cycles affecting adrenal cortical functioning, ventilatory response to CO_2, catecholamine levels in the blood, and vagal tone. The wheezing is due to increased vagal tone, increased blood histamine levels, and decreased blood cortisol and epinephrine levels (Baughman and Loudon, 1985).

In bronchorrheal states, such as *chronic bronchitis* and *cystic fibrosis*, inspiratory wheezes are common (Waring et al, 1985).

In fibrosing diseases, such as *interstitial fibrosis* and *hypersensitivity pneumonitis*, a faint inspiratory wheeze may follow crackles in the same phase of respiration. The wheeze may be more prominent and simultaneous with the crackles, if considerable bronchiolitis is also present.

In *early left ventricular failure*, occasional single wheezes may be heard as the peribronchial interstitial space fills up with fluid and airways become edematous.

In *pulmonary edema*, airways narrow further owing to obstructive secretions. Sometimes airway compression from increased vasomotor nervous system stimulation to muscles around airways occurs, contributing to wheezing and *cardiac asthma*, a general term used to describe wheezing secondary to excess fluid in the lung.

Detection and Interpretation. The nurse determines whether the wheeze is high pitched or low pitched. High-pitched wheezing may be generated in central or peripheral airways, whereas low-pitched wheezing suggests large airway pathology.

Next, the nurse assesses the amount of wheezing

and its occurrence during the inspiratory and expiratory phases of respiration. Prominent wheezing suggests moderate to severe airway narrowing, airway instability, or both. Occasional wheezing suggests mild airway narrowing and instability.

Generally, expiratory wheezing favors the presence of an obstructive disease (except for the bronchorrheal states described previously). Inspiratory wheezing favors a restrictive disease. Moreover, if inspiratory wheezing is detected in an obstructive disease patient, it is a favorable sign because it predicts a significant response to bronchodilator medication (Stewart et al, 1985).

Wheezing that remains unchanged during both phases of respiration suggests fixed airway obstruction, e.g., mechanical obstruction by a tumor protruding into a bronchus. This wheezing is usually low pitched in quality.

In patients with asthma or an asthmatic component to mixed chest pathology, the nurse assesses wheezing more thoroughly to determine the degree of bronchoconstriction or bronchospasm. Although the degree of bronchospasm on physical examination does not always correlate with the degree of airflow limitation on the pulmonary function test, wheezing in the chest is sensitive enough for detection of general trends in bedside monitoring or outpatient management. It may be the only parameter readily available to determine whether bronchospasm is better or worse, whether a PRN bronchodilator should be given, or whether oral steroids are being tapered too quickly.

Based on the chest examination, bronchospasm is divided into mild, moderate, and severe categories, as shown in Figure 12–53. As *mild bronchospasm* develops, the patient demonstrates wheeze only with a cough, and then with cough as well as with panting and forced expiration. All these maneuvers may be necessary for detection. The most sensitive test for the wheeze is to listen anteriorly during panting or forced expiration with the patient in the supine position.

Moderate bronchospasm is present when wheezing becomes audible during expiration as well. The underlying breath sound remains normal to slightly decreased.

Severe bronchospasm is characterized by inspiratory and expiratory wheezing. At this late stage, assessment of the breath sound becomes crucial. If wheezes are barely audible because of decreased breath sounds, ventilatory failure may be present, regardless of whether or not other signs of respiratory distress are present. This presentation is more ominous than loud inspiratory and expiratory wheezes and a loud and clear normal breath sound, although in the latter case airway occlusion may occur at any moment in children. When wheezing stops and only a faint inspiratory phase is heard (i.e., silent chest, represented by 5 in Fig. 12–53), the calmed, overfatigued, and slightly dyspneic patient may appear to be resting comfortably when in fact ventilatory failure is imminent, if not already present.

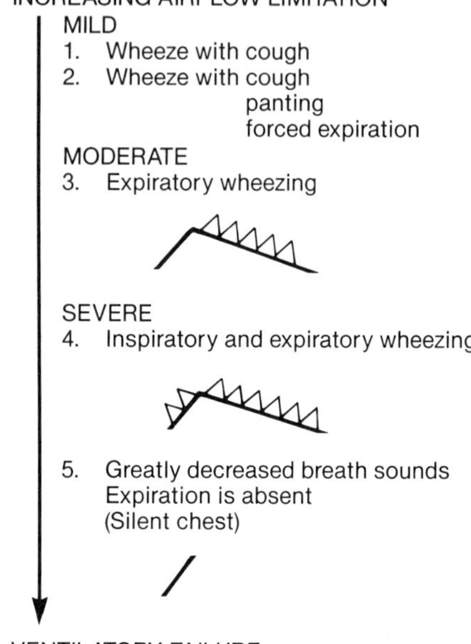

Figure 12–53. Assessment of bronchospasm in asthma.

Stridor. This loud musical sound of constant pitch may be classified under the wheeze category because of its musical quality. (See Chapter 7 and Table 14–3 for its physiologic mechanisms.) A sign of upper airway obstruction, stridor is commonly heard without a stethoscope in childhood croup (laryngotracheobronchitis). With extrathoracic upper airway obstruction, stridor is typically inspiratory and becomes inspiratory and expiratory as the airway becomes more obstructed by the pathologic process involved, e.g., foreign body aspiration, laryngeal tumors, and tracheal stenosis. In severe cases, stridor is accompanied by gasping respirations and use of accessory muscles of respiration. However, it also may be a subtle clinical finding in the comatose or sedated patient. To detect and differentiate stridor from wheezes in the lungs, the nurse auscultates the trachea below the Adam's apple on one side of the neck. Stridor sounds loudest in this location, whereas wheezing sounds loudest over chest areas.

Most important, when stridor is present, *never* use forced expiratory maneuvers to test for wheezing during the chest examination. Their use may precipitate bronchospasm and complete occlusion of the airway.

Charting. The presence of wheezing is charted in the same manner as that for rhonchi, with special attention to wheezing during cough, panting, or forced expiration as well as any changes after respiratory interventions, as follows:

Chest clear except loud wheeze with forced expiration.

Expiratory wheezes LLL, completely gone after aerosol treatment (Tx) with metaproterenol (Alupent).

Pleural Friction Rub

The pleural friction rub is a grating or scratching sound produced when irritated and inflamed visceral and parietal pleurae rub against each other during respiration. The friction from the roughened surfaces produces the sound. In the absence of inflammation, i.e., pleuritis, the two pleurae slide against their smooth lubricated surfaces with minimal friction and no adventitious sounds.

The grating quality of the pleural friction rub has been likened to the creak of shoe leather or an opening door. It has continuous and discontinuous qualities. Pleural friction rub may sound interrupted and jerky during at least half of inspiration and expiration; it may appear as a short late-inspiratory jerk or grate near full lung expansion.

Though usually inspiratory, friction rub may become inspiratory and expiratory when forced expiratory maneuvers further irritate the pleura. Upon occasion, a faint rub disappears after a few deep breaths, as pleural surfaces become better lubricated with fluid.

The pitch of rubs varies among individuals, ranging from a faint, high-pitched scratch to a louder, low-pitched grate that sometimes sounds exactly like a rhonchus.

Disorders. Pleuritis or any pulmonary disorder that happens to extend to pleural surfaces, such as *pneumonia, pulmonary infarction,* and *tumor,* may occur with pleural friction rub. Upon occasion, *pleural fibrosis* causes a rub, as fibrotic pleural surfaces rub against each other. In *pleural effusion,* a pleural friction rub is most likely when the effusion is small (e.g., dialysis in the renal patient), and roughened surfaces are still in contact with one another.

Detection. Detection largely depends on the clinician's ability to differentiate a rub from a rhonchus. When both are present in the same chest and both are low pitched and short in duration, they may sound identical. Whereas a rhonchus changes slightly in quality and greatly in timing and location, a pleural friction rub always occurs at *exactly* the same point during inspiration and its quality remains the same. If coughing does not accentuate the rub, firm pressure of the diaphragm against the chest wall accentuates it and often elicits an expiratory component, if not already audible. This maneuver works only if the patient tolerates the accompanying chest discomfort and is able to continue deep breathing during auscultation.

Detection of the rub also depends on knowing where to look for it. Mentally concentrate on inspiration and anticipate the rub over areas of pleuritic chest pain or possible pulmonary consolidation. By this time in the chest examination, such areas have already been identified by the patient's complaints, palpable pleural rub fremitus, decreased or bronchial breath sounds, dullness to percussion, or abnormal voice sounds. If no specific area has been identified, carefully listen where rubs are more frequently auscultated: over the lateral or anterolateral chest areas, the areas of greatest thoracic mobility.

Pleuropericardial Rub. The nurse suspects a *pleuropericardial rub* if a rub near the heart is synchronous with inspiration most of the time (i.e., pleural rub) and varies with the heart beat at other times (i.e., pericardial rub). Persisting between respirations and characterized by a to-and-fro grating sound, the pericardial component is a sign of *pericarditis,* which is inflammation of the pericardium around the heart.

Charting. Examples of charting friction rubs follow:

Inspiratory and expiratory pleural rub heard during coughing and deep breathing RLL at anterior axillary line (AAL). Slightly decreased chest excursions right lateral chest. Patient denies discomfort or chest pain.

Possible intermittent pleuropericardial rub heard sixth ICS, midclavicular line (MCL).

Difficult to assess because of loud rhonchi in same location.

Mediastinal Crunch

Although the mediastinal crunch is considered a pulmonary term, it is not a diagnostic sign. Mediastinal crunch is rarely heard in the clinical setting, except perhaps in trauma or emergency settings, and it is more likely to be detected during auscultation of the heart than the lungs. Nevertheless, knowledge of its existence can be helpful in bedside diagnosis, particularly in the assessment of patients with selected, life-threatening cardiopulmonary disorders.

The Joint Committee on Pulmonary Nomenclature (American College of Chest Physicians, 1975) describes the mediastinal crunch as "a coarse crackling sound or vibration synchronous with systole, heard over the precordium in the presence of mediastinal emphysema." All trauma patients and postcardiopulmonary resuscitation patients are candidates for possible mediastinal emphysema (i.e., air in the mediastinum), also called pneumomediastinum. The crunching or popping sound is thought to be due to air separating the visceral and parietal pericardia during the heart's contraction.

More recent literature states that although the mediastinal crunch, also called *Hamman's sign,* was thought to be diagnostic of pneumomediastinum, it is now thought to be associated more frequently with left pneumothorax (Fraser and Paré, 1979). The crunch results from the presence of gas in close contact with the heart, and it has been described as unusual, high-pitched "clicks" or "whoops," occurring in multiples throughout the cardiac cycle but influenced by respiration and the position of the patient. The sounds seem to appear more during inspiration. They may disappear completely if the patient moves from his left to his right side. The mediastinal crunch also may be heard in the elevation of the left hemidiaphragm in association with gas in the gastric fundus.

CLINICAL IMPLICATIONS OF ABNORMAL LUNG SOUNDS

Classification of lung sounds during bedside monitoring is crucial because each abnormal sound may indicate a completely different approach to respiratory intervention. Clinical implications of abnormal sounds are summarized in Table 12–10. Rather than covering all clinical implications discussed in the previous section, this table emphasizes main concepts and most frequently observed pathologic processes. In acute situations, it serves as a guide for immediate interpretation of lung sounds.

CONTROVERSY SURROUNDING CLASSIFICATION OF LUNG SOUNDS

It is ironic that, in spite of the clinical importance of correct identification of lung sounds, lung sounds are probably the most controversial subject in respiratory care. Clinicians and researchers continue to disagree on acceptable terms and categorization of sounds. Because of confusion over definitions, health educators wonder how to teach the subject, and some clinicians hesitate to chart lung sounds for fear of using the wrong label. As a result, the subject is glossed over with no clear link between specific sounds and implications for treatment.

Confusion on the topic has existed ever since Laennec listened to lung sounds over a century ago. He classified all abnormal lung sounds under the French word "râle" and added qualifying adjectives, such as crepitant (crackling), sibilant, and sonorous, to differentiate among sounds. To complicate matters, rale was translated into Latin as "rhonchus" and later into English as "wheeze." Through the years, clinicians continued to add qualifying adjectives to describe adventitious sounds and insure comprehension because of continued disagreement on uniform labelling. In some cases, qualifying adjectives have become

Table 12–10. CLINICAL IMPLICATIONS OF ABNORMAL LUNG SOUNDS

Abnormal Sound	Associated Problems	Implications for Treatment
Absent to decreased breath sounds	Impaired ventilation Hypoventilation Severe atelectasis, consolidation, or compression of tissue	More aggressive bronchial hygiene measures (e.g., coughing, deep breathing), frequent position changes, early ambulation.
Bronchial or bronchovesicular breath sound	Lung consolidation or compression of tissue	
Crackles (rales)	Impaired ventilation Atelectasis Mucus retention (small airways)	More aggressive bronchial hygiene measures, frequent position changes, early ambulation.
	Fluid retention (small airways) Fluid overload Left ventricular failure	Diuretics, fluid intake restrictions, low salt diet, and/or other measures to treat heart failure.
	Interstitial fibrosis ("dry" Velcro crackles)	None; sounds are from chronic disease. Important only when they increase in number or become "wet" sounding, as in early left ventricular failure.
Rhonchi	Fluid retention (large airways) Pulmonary edema	Immediate medical intervention with diuretics, cardiac drugs, morphine, aminophylline, rotating tourniquets, etc.
	Mucus retention (large airways) Bronchitis Pneumonia	Aggressive bronchial hygiene measures including postural drainage and endotracheal suctioning when ineffective cough is present. When wheezing is also present, bronchial hygiene measures may be ineffective unless bronchodilators are given simultaneously to open airways and facilitate expectoration.
Wheezes	Bronchoconstriction Bronchospasm (asthma)	Open airways with bronchodilators, relaxation exercises, psychological support. Determine etiology.
	Bronchospasm (cardiogenic, as in pulmonary edema)	Give aminophylline and morphine to decrease pulmonary vascular resistance and relieve bronchospasm and anxiety. Give diuretics to eliminate excess fluid in the lung.
	Mechanical obstruction of the airway (e.g., tumor, foreign object)	Medical evaluation to determine cause. Encourage deep breathing to improve lung ventilation. Push fluids to liquefy secretions and facilitate their removal past constricted area.
Pleural friction rub	Pleural inflammation (pleuritis)	Treat inflammatory process with antibiotics or drugs specific to underlying disease process. Encourage deep breathing to keep the lung expanded and prevent atelectasis.

repetitive and unnecessary, e.g., "crepitant rales" literally means "crackling crackles." In other cases, adjectives are misleading because they incorrectly prejudge the mode or origin of the sound, e.g., "vesicular" in normal vesicular breath sound, as previously described. Moreover, new terms have appeared to describe breath sounds, such as *cavernous*, *amphorphic*, and *cogwheel*. Most of these have no significant clinical implications and are no longer used.

In 1975, the Joint Committee on Pulmonary Nomenclature of the American College of Chest Physicians, American Thoracic Society, reclassified main adventitious sounds into two basic categories as follows: *rale* for discontinuous sounds, alternatively called crackle, and *rhonchus* for continuous sounds, alternatively called wheeze.

In 1980, the American Thoracic Society reclassified these sounds into the following three categories: (1) *crackles* (coarse and fine), (2) *wheeze*, and (3) *rhonchus*. Breath sounds were classified as *normal vesicular* and *bronchial* (Murphy and Holford, 1980). Classification was largely based on the analysis of lung sounds by their unique time-expanded waveforms.

Although this latest classification system is probably closest to what many clinicians have continued to use in practice, in spite of current medical literature, as Murphy and Holford point out, it cannot represent a definitive system. Clinical correlations of abnormal sounds are still largely unknown, owing to the paucity of controlled research studies on the topic. Clinicians must continue to rely heavily on their own experiences in making correlations.

This latest classification system has helped to standardize terms, however, it is limited in scope. The trend has been to eliminate categories, if existing objective measurements, such as waveform analysis, cannot define them with precision. For example, although Murphy and Holford recognize wide variations in normal and bronchial breath sounds among patients, they recommend elimination of the intermediate bronchovesicular category until its precise characteristics have been defined. Adherence to this suggestion has its drawbacks. First, it sometimes causes confusion or imprecise labelling when learners discover that hollow sounds over the manubrium and sternal area really do not sound the same and that *both* sounds must be classified as bronchial breath sounds. Second, when the bronchovesicular category is eliminated, respiratory assessment becomes less sensitive as clinicians look for the obvious bronchial breath sound, indicating consolidation, rather than the less hollow and more subtle bronchovesicular sound, a sign of *early* consolidation.

In spite of the usefulness of the bronchovesicular category, its elimination may be justified. Limitations of the teaching-learning situation, such as the limitation of time and the beginning level of the student, may require simplification of content. Also, elimination may not affect basic treatment, since basic interpretation of the two sounds is the same.

It is hoped that this discussion clarifies some of the issues clinicians and educators must face when implementing descriptions of lung sounds in clinical and educational settings. Categorization of the lung sounds in this text is consistent with the respiratory care terminology established for nursing practice by the American Lung Association (Boyce, 1976) and the American Thoracic Society's recent recommendations. However, similar to many other physical diagnosis textbooks, the bronchovesicular category has been retained because of its clinical usefulness in the monitoring of pulmonary patients.

The Need for Standardization of Terms

The previous discussion points out the need for all health care providers to take the time to standardize lung sound terminology in their specific settings. Terms should be consistent with the basic terms used in this text. When standard terms change—and undoubtedly they will since the "state of the art" has changed at least twice within 10 years—health care providers should scrutinize these proposals. Changing terminology requires careful consideration of the usefulness of proposed terms compared with the usefulness of terms already common. It also requires assessment of resources for effecting change; confusion over definitions will become worse instead of better unless educational programs and bedside rounds are planned to familiarize staff with terminology changes.

In any case, standardization of main terms is essential. Implementation of the chest examination in the clinical setting will not be totally successful unless lung sound labelling is consistent, and all members of the health care team can communicate their findings with as much precision and confidence as possible.

SECTION V—INTEGRATION OF THE PRECORDIAL EXAMINATION

Though normally considered part of a cardiovascular examination, the precordial examination is an important assessment parameter in pulmonary disease. A basic precordial examination is summarized here because many clinicians find it convenient and expedient to integrate at least some of its aspects with the complete chest examination. Brief inspection and palpation of the precordium along with the rest of the chest saves time and permits the early identification of obvious signs, such as abnormal cardiac impulses, pulsations, and thrills (palpable murmurs), that may help in the interpretation and further investigation of pulmonary signs already discovered. Most important, this approach facilitates the identification of obvious signs of pulmonary heart disease (e.g., cor pulmonale) and left ventricular failure. Cardiac auscultation may immediately follow inspection and palpation or may

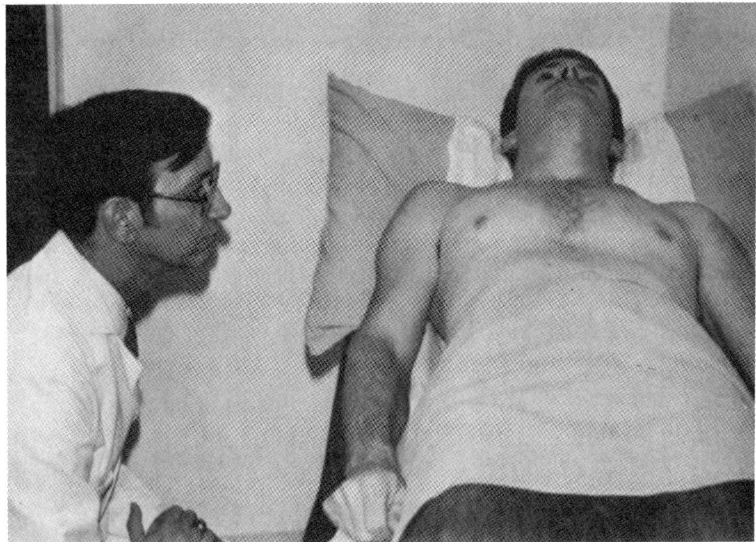

Figure 12–54. Tangential view by observer across the patient's chest makes precordial pulsations more conspicuous. (Reproduced by permission from Thompson, D.: Cardiovascular Assessment—Guide for Nurses and other Health Professionals. St. Louis, C. V. Mosby Co., 1981.)

be performed later with a complete cardiovascular examination.

Inspection is performed first, although usually it yields little, if any, data. Hyperinflated lungs from obstructive disease surround vascular structures, adding extra space between these structures and the chest wall, thus preventing the transmission of pulsations to the chest's surface. *To inspect the precordium,* the nurse either utilizes tangential lighting or sits at the level of the patient's chest and looks tangentially across the chest to notice slight pulsations (Fig. 12–54). Pulsations in any area and of any kind are important to note. Inspection and palpation concentrate mainly on certain areas (see the shaded areas in Figure 12–55) and on the identification of three pulsations as follows: (1) *left ventricular impulse,* (2) *right ventricular impulse,* and (3) *pulsations in the second ICS* (Erb's point). These pulsations in normal adults and in respiratory patients are reviewed in Table 12–11 and are further described.

Left Ventricular Impulse

This impulse, also called *apical impulse* or *point of maximal intensity* (PMI), is normally found in the apical area, overlying the left ventricle. *For palpation,* stand on the right-hand side of the bed, reach across the chest, and place your right hand over the apical area, as demonstrated in Figure 12–56. With firm pressure to the palmar aspect of the hand and fingertips, the impulse should feel like a light tap, lasting no longer than one third to one half of systole and covering an area no greater than 2 cm. Move your hand more medially or laterally towards the axilla, if you have

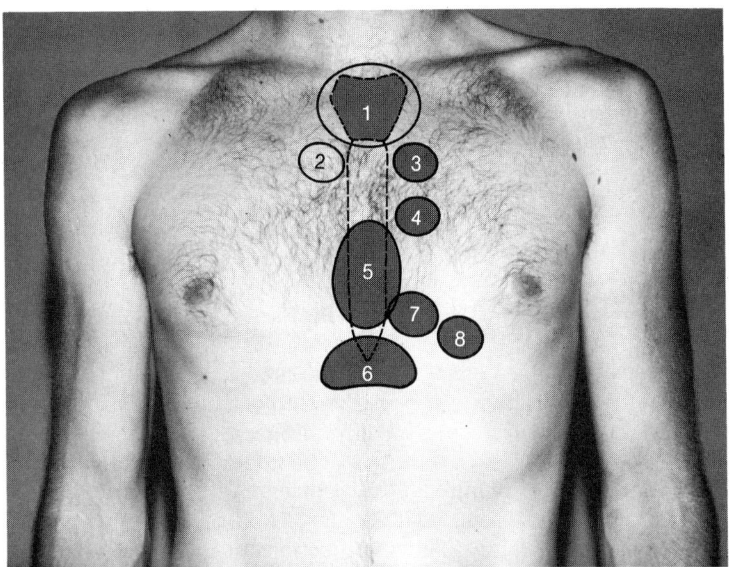

Figure 12–55. Key cardiac examination areas (numbered circles) in relation to the sternum (dotted lines). The shaded areas are emphasized in the assessment of respiratory patients. 1, *sternoclavicular*; 2, *aortic*—second RICS; 3, *pulmonic*—second LICS; 4, *Erb's point*—third LICS; 5, *lower parasternal* (also called *anterior precordium* or *right ventricular area*)—lower half of sternum, including adjacent intercostal spaces; 6, *epigastric*—just inferior to xiphoid process; 7, *tricuspid*—fifth LICS by sternum; and 8, *apical* (also called *mitral* area)—fifth LICS, at or slightly medial to MCL. (RICS = right intercostal space; LICS = left intercostal space; and MCL = midclavicular line.)

Table 12–11. PRECORDIAL PULSATIONS IN RESPIRATORY DISEASE

Pulsation	Description of Normal Pulsation in the Normal Adult	Description of Abnormal Pulsations Commonly Found in Respiratory Patients	Clinical Implications
Left ventricular impulse (apical impulse, PMI)	*Intensity*—Not visible or palpable in nearly half the adult population. When present, it is normally the *maximal* precordial impulse.	*Intensity*—Impulse absent or decreased in intensity along with other cardiac sounds.	Normal finding or sign of lung hyperinflation.
	Location—5th ICS at or just medial to MCL. Displaced to the left in obesity. Vertical orientation in tall, thin individuals. Normally displaced to the left AAL in the left lateral position.	*Location*–Displacement to the right or left with accompanying tracheal displacement (in same direction).	Pulmonary disorders causing mediastinal shift, e.g., tension pneumothorax, large pleural effusion, lung collapse.
		Displacement to the left and upward.	Conditions that elevate left hemidiaphragm, e.g., abdominal distention, pregnancy, partial or total denervation of left phrenic nerve.
	Presence or absence must be interpreted in light of other clinical findings.	Displacement to the left with a prominent sustained pulsation (left ventricular lift).	Pulmonary edema, left ventricular failure, left ventricular hypertrophy (from accompanying cardiac disease).
Right ventricular impulse	Usually absent, except pulsation at left sternal border in some persons with thin chests.	Parasternal lift or epigastric (subxiphoid) pulsation on palpation.	Pulmonary hypertension, acute or chronic cor pulmonale, mitral stenosis, pulmonic stenosis, left-to-right cardiac shunts, other high cardiac output states (e.g., hypervolemia); increased blood flow accentuates all precordial pulsations.
Pulsation(s) 2nd or 3rd left ICS	Usually absent, except for small pulsation in some persons with thin chests. Small pulsation may be present with anxiety, fever, anemia, hyperthyroidism, pregnancy.	Small or large pulsation.	Same as above.
		Palpable pulsations (not visible)— Brief shock from pulmonic valve closure (corresponds with loud P_2 on auscultation).	Pulmonary hypertension.
		Thrill—may radiate toward side of neck.	Pulmonary insufficiency or stenosis.

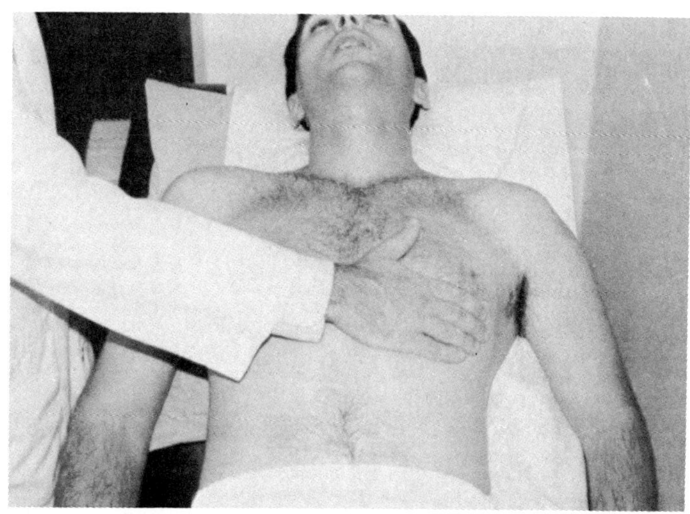

Figure 12–56. Palpating for the left ventricular impulse. (Reproduced by permission from Thompson, D.: Cardiovascular Assessment—Guide for Nurses and other Health Professionals. St. Louis, C. V. Mosby Co., 1981.)

difficulty finding the impulse. Once found, use fine palpation with fingertips in the ICSs to help determine its size and nature. A forceful, sustained, or diffuse impulse, covering two ICSs or more, is called a *left ventricular lift* or heave. Each heart beat *lifts* the chest outward and to the side. In COPD patients, rolling the patient far to the left side to compress the heart against the chest cage is necessary to find the impulse or lift, and even then the impulse is commonly absent owing to lung hyperinflation.

The nurse checks for *right* or *left shift* in the location of the left ventricular impulse. A shift in the direction of tracheal displacement is expected in pulmonary disorders that cause gross increases or decreases in lung or thoracic volume and a corresponding mediastinal shift, e.g., pneumothorax, large pleural effusion, gross atelectasis, and lung collapse. For example, in tension pneumothorax, the pleural air pushes the trachea, mediastinum, and heart within to the opposite side, simultaneously shifting the LV impulse in the same direction. A shift of the LV impulse always follows the direction of the mediastinal shift. The clue to the presence of possible mediastinal and LV impulse shift is lateral displacement of the trachea.

When checking for lateral displacement of the left ventricular impulse, the nurse must remember that rolling the patient far to the left during the examination results in the *normal* displacement of the impulse to the left *to* or *slightly past* the anterior axillary line (AAL). Hence, the actual determination of a left shift (displacement) may be difficult to make, unless the location of the impulse in the left lateral position was previously noted.

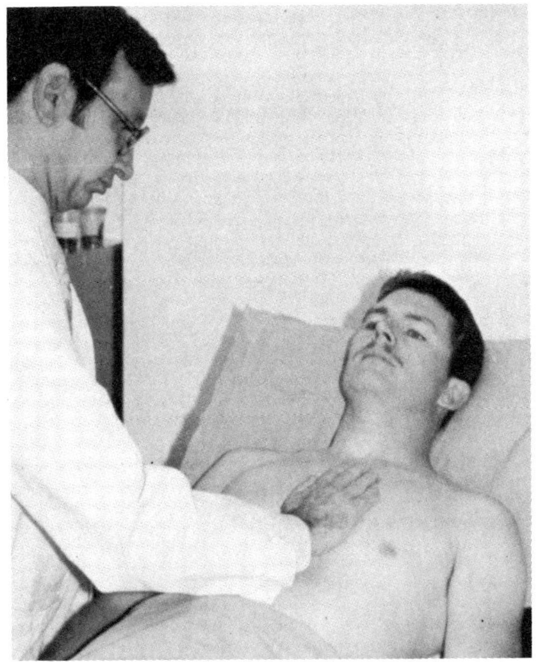

Figure 12–57. Palpating the lower parasternal area and left sternal border for a parasternal (right ventricular) lift. (Reproduced by permission from Thompson, D.: Cardiovascular Assessment—Guide for Nurses and other Health Professionals. St. Louis, C. V. Mosby Co., 1981.)

Right Ventricular Impulse

When palpable, this impulse is normally barely noticeable at the left sternal border and is less intense than the left ventricular impulse. Usually, it is absent.

To palpate, the nurse places the hand over the parasternal area with the heel of the hand at the xiphoid process and palpates in the same manner as that described for the left ventricular impulse, except the patient remains supine (Fig. 12–57). The impulse is more easily felt during expiration, when the lungs retreat laterally away from the sternum. If the impulse is not palpable with the palm of the hand, try palpating with the fingertips.

A sustained, outward thrust is called a *parasternal* or *right ventricular lift* (heave). As Chapter 9 indicates, it is a sign of right ventricular enlargement from acute cor pulmonale (RV dilatation), chronic cor pulmonale (RV hypertrophy), or both. It may also result from other disorders that increase blood flow through the heart or increase pulmonary pressures (see Table 12–11).

The sternum is lifted because the right ventricle normally lies immediately below this structure (Fig. 12–58). Also, in cor pulmonale the heart rotates in a counterclockwise direction, such that the left ventricle is located more posteriorly and the enlarged right ventricle more anteriorly towards the sternum.

To keep the parasternal lift in proper perspective, keep in mind that it usually, but not always, indicates right ventricular involvement; it may be from massive left atrial enlargement, usually from mitral stenosis or regurgitation. The posteriorly located enlarged left atrium expands during systole, forcing the heart forward towards the sternum. Because distinguishing between right atrial lift and right ventricular lift requires advanced assessment skills and even may be impossible, the left atrial lift is easily mistaken for a right ventricular lift.

In COPD patients, the RV impulse is more frequently felt in the epigastrium rather than in the parasternal area or left sternal edge, again because of the lung hyperinflation and fixed chest cage. *For palpation of the epigastrium,* slip two fingers up beneath the xiphoid process and gently press cephalad while the patient inhales. The presence of a downward epigastric pulsation indicates right ventricular enlargement. Upward pulsations against the palm of the hand are from the pulsating abdominal aorta.

Pulsations in the Second and Third ICSs

The nurse inspects and palpates the second and third intercostal spaces (ICSs) just to the left of the

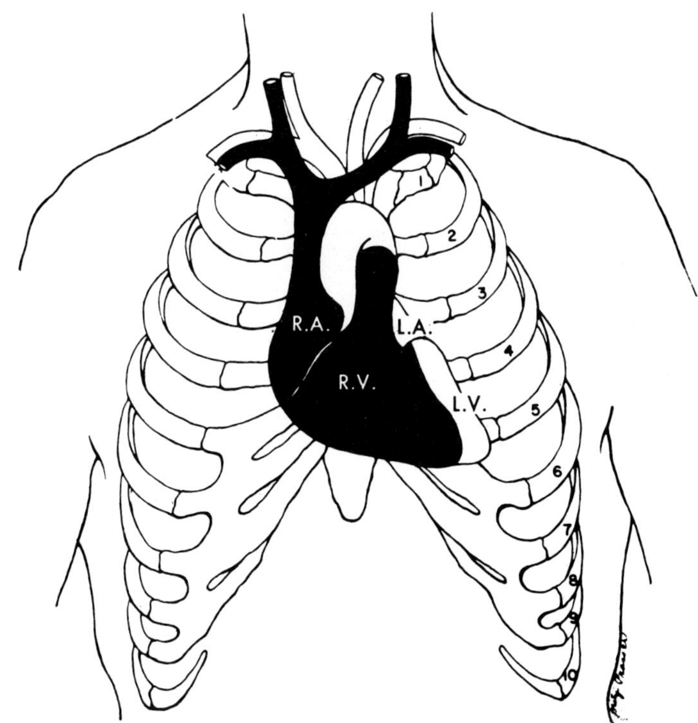

Figure 12–58. Topographical anatomy of the heart. R.A. = right atrium; R.V. = right ventricle; L.A. = left atrium; and L.V. = left ventricle. (Reproduced by permission from Prior, J., Silberstein, J., and Stang, J.: Physical Diagnosis—The History and Examination of the Patient, 6th ed. St. Louis, C. V. Mosby Co., 1981.)

sternum, with the palmar aspect of the fingers. Pulsations here may indicate an underlying dilated pulmonary artery and its branches, as in pulmonary hypertension and cor pulmonale, or increased pulmonary blood flow from high cardiac output states. Palpation may reveal a thrill (palpable murmur), from pulmonary insufficiency or stenosis, or a brief shock of pulmonic valve closure (i.e., loud P_2 on auscultation), a sign of moderate to severe pulmonary hypertension.

Cardiac Auscultation

This topic is beyond the scope of this text, but a few points may help clinicians apply the skill to respiratory patients.

First, when an abnormal impulse is detected on inspection and palpation, it is best auscultated immediately while still palpable and while the patient is resting comfortably. Slight pulsations may disappear with position changes, making it difficult or time consuming to relocate the site for auscultation later. The impulse site is important because auscultation normally begins with the stethoscope placed *exactly* over the site. In addition, a comfortable resting position is always best because deep breathing maneuvers later in the pulmonary examination may stimulate coughing and loosen secretions in the chest, producing distracting adventitious sounds that tend to mask cardiac sounds. Furthermore, in the presence of COPD, coughing and exertional dyspnea may promote air trapping in the lungs (i.e., lung hyperinflation) and decrease the intensity of cardiac sounds.

Second, the characteristic auscultatory finding in COPD is a *decrease* in the intensity of heart sounds. Lung hyperinflation may render all precordial pulsations and all heart sounds unappreciable. In this case, one must auscultate in the subxiphoid area where the right ventricular lift is palpated. Moreover, whenever auscultatory findings are absent or inconclusive, as is often the case, pulmonary signs and symptoms as well as vital signs become all the more crucial. Often a drop in PaO_2 is the only objective sign of impending heart failure.

Third, *right-sided* heart sounds—heard best at the left sternal border or epigastric area—must be differentiated from *left-sided* heart sounds, heard best in the apical area. This differentiation applies to murmurs, abnormal third heart sounds (S_3), fourth heart sounds (S_4), and other findings. Discussion of the right-sided and left-sided S_3 and S_4 emphasizes the significance of right versus left findings.

ABNORMAL S_3

The S_3 and S_4 are heard with very light pressure applied to the bell of the stethoscope. S_3 produces a gallop rhythm similar to the word Kentucky (Ken-tuck′-y), with the S_3 appearing after the S_2 in place of the y. The sound created by the rapid flow of blood into a dilated ventricle is a sign of heart failure. *Heard near the sternum,* the S_3 indicates *right* ventricular

Table 12–12. CAUSES OF ABNORMAL S_3 AND S_4 GALLOPS

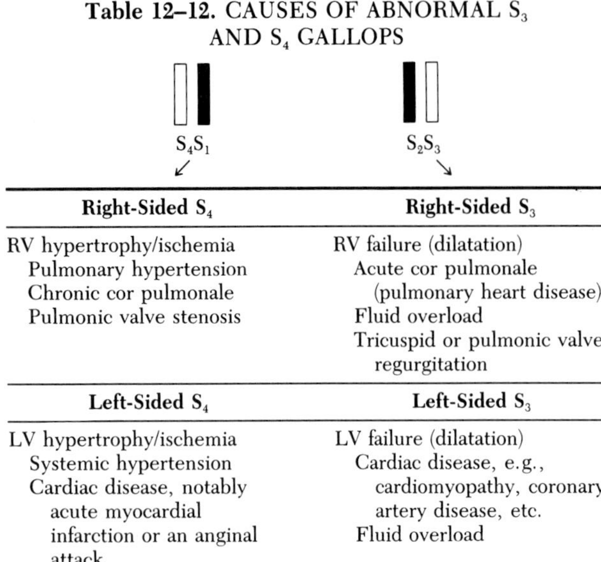

Right-Sided S_4	Right-Sided S_3
RV hypertrophy/ischemia Pulmonary hypertension Chronic cor pulmonale Pulmonic valve stenosis	RV failure (dilatation) Acute cor pulmonale (pulmonary heart disease) Fluid overload Tricuspid or pulmonic valve regurgitation
Left-Sided S_4	**Left-Sided S_3**
LV hypertrophy/ischemia Systemic hypertension Cardiac disease, notably acute myocardial infarction or an anginal attack	LV failure (dilatation) Cardiac disease, e.g., cardiomyopathy, coronary artery disease, etc. Fluid overload

failure (i.e., dilatation); *heard at the apex*, it indicates *left* ventricular failure (Table 12–12).

ABNORMAL S_4

Heard in diastole immediately before S_1, the S_4 produces a gallop rhythm similar to the word Tennessee (Ten-nes-see′), with the S_4 appearing in place of the first syllable. Usually one must imagine the presence of this sound before appreciating it. The sound is produced when atrial contraction pushes a volume of blood into a stiff ventricular wall. *Heard near the sternum or epigastrium*, the S_4 typically indicates *right* ventricular hypertrophy. However, it may occur with right ventricular ischemia *without* hypertrophy. *Heard at the apex*, it indicates *left* ventricular hypertrophy, ischemia, or both.

Right-Sided Versus Left-Sided Sounds

To help differentiate right-sided versus left-sided sounds, the nurse evaluates *intensity during respiration* as well as precordial location. The right-sided S_3 and S_4 increase during inspiration, owing to increased venous return to the right side of the heart. The left-sided S_3 and S_4 do not vary or decrease during inspiration, again owing to increased flow to the heart's right side, or they increase with expiration. When these sounds are difficult to hear, the patient is asked to cough a few times in the absence of hyperirritable airways, to do a few sit ups, or take a brief walk. Mild exercise should accentuate the sounds and make them easier to hear.

Associated Clinical Findings

The significance of right-sided and left-sided clinical findings depends on accompanying clinical findings. A right-sided S_4, for example, suggests cor pulmonale in the presence of pulmonary disease and signs of pulmonary hypertension. In the absence of confirming signs, it is not considered pathologic but a normal function of aging in the elderly.

Similarly, the significance of an S_3 always depends on the "company it keeps." Although almost always abnormal in adults over 40 years of age, it may not be pathologic. It is normal in children and young healthy adults and is termed a *normal* S_3.

As a general rule, the new appearance of an S_3 or S_4 indicates abnormality, heart failure in the first case and a stiff ventricle in the second. As a chronic finding, the S_3 indicates heart failure in the presence of other confirming signs. The clinician decides whether it is right-sided or left-sided (as described previously) and looks for signs of right and left ventricular failure.

Clinical Manifestations of Right Versus Left Ventricular Failure

Thorough familiarization with right ventricular (RV) versus left ventricular (LV) failure is essential in the detection and interpretation of both pulmonary and cardiac signs. Key clinical findings supporting right versus left ventricular failure are summarized in Table 12–13. Although RV failure *alone* is most likely in the pulmonary patient, biventricular failure is a possibility. In the general patient population, RV failure is most often caused by LV failure with secondary pulmonary hypertension.

SECTION VI—GETTING IT ALL TOGETHER—IMPLEMENTATION OF THE COMPLETE CHEST EXAMINATION

Previous sections have presented the extrathoracic examination and examination of the thorax and lungs

Table 12–13. KEY FINDINGS IN RIGHT VERSUS LEFT VENTRICULAR FAILURE

RV Failure	LV Failure
Parasternal lift	Left ventricular lift with shift of the LV impulse to the left
Right-sided S_3	Left-sided S_3
Elevated venous pressure and JVD	Absence of elevated venous pressure and JVD
Enlarged, tender liver	Liver normal in size; absence of tenderness
Absence of crackles in the lungs	New appearance of crackles in the lungs
Absence of white or pinkish foamy sputum	White or pinkish foamy sputum

Table 12–14. PATIENT SITUATIONS LEADING TO FALSE POSITIVE LUNG SOUNDS

Patient Situation	False Positive Lung Sound	Explanation	To Eliminate Sound
Mechanical ventilation	Rhonchi, usually expiratory	Water bubbling in ventilator tubings	Empty ventilator tubings before auscultation
Mechanical ventilation with PEEP (positive end-expiratory pressure)	Loud expiratory moan	Air moving through ventilator's expiratory tubing/valve	Ask respiratory therapist to adjust ventilator May be unavoidable in some set ups
Pursed lip breathing	Decreased breath sounds (expiration almost absent)	Mouth closed during expiration	Instruct patient to exhale with mouth wide open
Leaning on elbows	Bronchial breath sounds apices of upper lobes posteriorly	Compression of tissue	Instruct patient to relax shoulders and place arms and hands forward in lap
Nasogastric salem sump tube	High- or low-pitched squeak anterior chest	Varies with intermittent suction	Clamp nasogastric tube during auscultation
Chest hair	Crackles or other extraneous sounds	Hair moves against diaphragm during chest movement	Select areas free of hair or wet chest hair before auscultation
Stethoscope contact with patient's gown, bedsheets, etc.	Crackles or other extraneous sounds	Articles rub against stethoscope diaphragm or tubing	Do not listen over clothes or allow any part of stethoscope to touch articles of clothing
Muscle tension, as in Shivering Muscle twitching Pain Use of accessory muscles of respiration Tense individuals	Crackles or other extraneous sounds Decreased breath sounds	Increased surface tension Breathing is not free and easy	May be unavoidable Listen after sedation or pain medication Instruct tense patient to relax shoulders

in detail. The following points summarize methodology and emphasize a systematic approach to the patient.

1. *Start with extrathoracic structures*: the head, neck, and extremities. Then examine the thorax and lungs. Auscultate the heart whenever convenient, after chest palpation or later with the complete cardiovascular examination.

2. *Always mentally consider and execute the components of the complete examination in the same orderly fashion* as follows: *inspection, palpation, percussion,* and *auscultation.* Following this sequence prevents omission of important findings.

3. *Routinely work from the top down*—from the apices of the upper lobes down to the level of the diaphragm—as you execute each of the components of the examination.

4. *Work across the chest, comparing one side of the chest with the other side.* The patient serves as his own control. Pathology is suspected if abnormal findings are encountered or if findings on one side of the chest do not match findings on the other side at the same vertebral level. *Comparing sides is key.* You will not pick up subtle changes unless this continuous comparison takes place as you proceed down the anterior and posterior areas of the chest.

5. *Adapt your general approach to the clinical situation.* Time limitation, patient tolerance and cooperation, or a language barrier may necessitate modifications in methodology. If necessary, start with suspected areas of pathology or the most dependent areas of the lungs, the bases of the lower lobes. Thoroughly examine these areas with reference to the opposite side of the chest. Then, as the situation permits, routinely work *upward* towards the upper lobes. Use only inspection and auscultation, if the patient becomes overfatigued.

6. *Be on the alert for false positive lung sounds* (Table 12–14).

7. *Look for clusters of abnormalities that indicate pulmonary pathology.* Groupings of findings in certain areas of the chest localize pathology. Different presentations of findings help to diagnose pulmonary disease (Table 12–15)

8. *When in doubt, confirm abnormalities by reexamination.* Generally, the physical findings should be congruent with the patient's history, diagnosis, and previous chest assessment findings.

Although these points provide a framework for a systematic approach to the patient, in actual practice various structures or components may be omitted, depending on the purpose of the examination and on the individual patient situation. Also, some components may be performed at the same time (e.g., inspection and palpation), or the sequence of the examination may be mixed for expediency.

Emphasis on Inspection and Auscultation

In routine monitoring inspection followed by auscultation is the most expedient way to gather the most information in a short time period. Advanced skills, such as experienced palpation of lateral chest expansion and percussion, are helpful but take considerable time to learn well enough to implement selectively and effectively with the rest of the physical examination.

Table 12–15. MAIN PHYSICAL FINDINGS IN RESPIRATORY DISEASE

Disease/Disorder	Chest Excursions	Tactile Fremitus Vocal Resonance	Percussion Note	Breath Sounds	Adventitious Sounds
Acute asthma	↑; then ↓ with air trapping and fatigue	↓	Hyperrresonant	NL to ↓ with prolonged expiration	Wheezes
Chronic bronchitis	NL to ↑ ↓ with air trapping	NL to ↓	Resonant to hyperresonant	NL or ↓ with prolonged expiration	Rhonchi Early-insp. coarse crackles Wheeze with cough
Emphysema	↓ with en bloc chest movement	↓	Hyperresonant	↓ with prolonged expiration	None except rhonchus or wheeze with cough
Cystic fibrosis (severe)	↓ with en bloc chest movement	↓	Hyperresonant	NL to ↓ with prolonged expiration	Rhonchi Coarse crackles Wheeze with cough
Pneumothorax					
Small Less than 20% of lung	NL on affected side	NL to ↓	Resonant to hyperresonant	NL to slightly ↓	None
Large Greater than 20% of lung	↓ to absent on affected side Affected hemithorax may look overinflated	↓ to absent	Hyperresonant to tympanic	↓ to absent	None
Atelectasis	↓ on affected side Affected hemithorax may look depressed or smaller than the other side	↓	Dull	↓ to absent (with obstructed airway) Bronchial (with patent airway)	Fine late-insp. crackles Rhonchi or wheezes with airway obstruction
Pulmonary consolidation (e.g., lobar pneumonia)					
Severe (Classic presentation with patent airway)	↓ on affected side	↑	Dull	Bronchial	Fine crackles Rhonchus with cough
Resolving	NL	NL	Dull to resonant	Decreased to NL	Coarse crackles Loud rhonchi
Pulmonary cavitation (e.g., cavitary tuberculosis, lung abscess)	NL or slightly ↓ on affected side	*Large air-filled cavity in communication with patent airway* ↓	Resonant or hyperresonant	Bronchial	Variable, depends on disease process
		Large fluid-filled cavity (consolidation) in communication with patent airway ↑	Dull	Bronchial	
Right ventricular failure	NL	NL	Resonant	NL	None
Pulmonary edema	NL or ↑	Variable	NL to dull	NL to ↓ (alveolar flooding) Sometimes bronchovesicular (when fluid mostly interstitial)	Crackles Wheezes at times Rhonchi with cough
Pleurisy	NL to ↓ on affected side	NL	NL	NL to ↓	Pleural friction rub May have crackles from atelectasis
Small pleural effusion	NL to ↓	NL or ↓	Dull	NL to ↓	Pleural friction rub at times
Large pleural effusion (Fig. 12–48)	↓ on affected side		*At or just above fluid level*		None
		↑	Hyperresonant	Bronchial	Sometimes crackles from atelectasis
			Below fluid level		
		↓	Dull to flat	↓ to absent	
Pleural thickening	NL to ↓	↓	Dull	NL to ↓	None

Table 12–15. MAIN PHYSICAL FINDINGS IN RESPIRATORY DISEASE *Continued*

Disease/Disorder	Chest Excursions	Tactile Fremitus Vocal Resonance	Percussion Note	Breath Sounds	Adventitious Sounds
Diffuse interstitial fibrosis					
Mild to moderate	NL to ↓	NL to ↑	NL to slightly dull	NL to bronchovesicular	Late-insp. crackles (dry sounding)
Severe	↓	↑	Dull	Bronchovesicular to bronchial	Same

Note: This chart relates generalizations and trends to main physical findings. Because it assumes disease states *without* mixed pathology, it can only be used as a guide to learning.

KEY: ↑ = increased
↓ = decreased
NL = normal

Moreover, when used meticulously, inspection and auscultation are usually sensitive enough to pick up abnormalities, without necessitating palpation and percussion. For example, measuring lateral chest expansion is unnecessary when minimal chest excursions and decreased breath sounds have already documented a ventilatory problem.

Charting and Problem Identification

Implementation of the complete chest examination always involves the step of charting pertinent findings and problem identification. Beginners may chart all normal and abnormal findings to learn how to chart accurately and concisely. In clinical practice, however, charting is brief and systematic. It uses abbreviations whenever possible and emphasizes pertinent negative and positive findings for suspected respiratory problems. For example, the clinician might chart *"Chest clear on auscultation"* when examining a healthy adult and *"Chest clear on auscultation, even with a cough and forced expiration"* when examining a labile asthmatic. Similarly, in a patient with a history of recurrent pneumothoraces in the left lower lobe, the clinician anticipates abnormal findings and might rule them out by charting the following negative findings:

Normal breath sounds, normal tactile and vocal fremitus, and resonance to percussion LLL.

In essence, the aim of charting is to be brief but complete enough to rule out suspected problems, confirm others, and simultaneously establish baseline assessment findings to facilitate monitoring by all members of the health care team.

FORMAT FOR CHARTING

Clinicians develop their own format for charting, depending on the model or agency format used for data collection, personal adaptations, and the context of the situation, e.g., a complete versus a quick chest examination, simultaneous examination of other body systems. In any case, for the thorax and lungs, data collection and charting always follow the same sequence: inspection, palpation, percussion, and auscultation. The commonly used heading *General Appearance* represents first impressions, i.e., the view from the door. Extrathoracic or cardiac signs may fall under two separate headings, or they may be integrated into other headings, such as *Ear, Nose, and Throat* (ENT) and *Cardiovascular* (or Cor for heart), if a complete physical examination is performed.

RECORDING EXAMPLE

A recording example follows of the complete chest examination performed within the context of a complete physical examination.

Identifying Data

This is the fifth UCLA Hospital admission for this 82-year-old, widowed, retired, chronically ill white male of Hungarian descent, who is currently residing with his live-in housekeeper in an apartment in Los Angeles. Admitted 10/11 for pulmonary edema and respiratory failure, Mr. S. is now being followed on the general medical ward (4W) by Dr. S. Pinko. The patient appears to be capable of providing reliable history.

General Appearance

The patient is a disheveled, medium height, cachectic male. He appears to be in slight respiratory distress, with noticeable dyspnea at rest, obvious use of pursed lip breathing, and rigid body position hunched over his bedside stand. He is alert but lethargic and has no language difficulties. Now receiving supplemental oxygen at 3 L/min via nasal prongs.

Thorax and Lungs

Inspection—No extrathoracic signs of respiratory distress except for slightly blue-tinged mucous membranes of the lips. Chest appears symmetric and normal in configuration except for increased AP diameter. Costal angle about 90 degrees. Slight gynecomastia. No scars, masses, deformities, skin markings, or venous prominences. Skin is pale in color. Posteriorly, spine appears to be in normal alignment. Respiratory rate 28/min with an I:E ratio of 1:3. Normal rhythm. Bilaterally equal respiratory excursions with en bloc movement of the chest and little visible diaphragmatic motion. Some use of neck and shoulder accessory muscles with slight bulging of the intercostal spaces with pursed lip breathing.

Palpation—Trachea in midline position. Chest and spine demonstrate no areas of tenderness or pain. No palpable masses or structural abnormalities except for the 90-degree angle of the posterior ribs to the vertebral column. Lateral chest expansion of the lower lobes posteriorly is 4 cm. Normal tactile fremitus throughout the lung fields.

Percussion—Lungs resonant to percussion except for slight hyperresonance in both upper lobes anteriorly. Resting diaphragmatic levels: T10 on the left and T9 on the right. Diaphragmatic excursions 2 cm bilaterally.

Auscultation—Decreased breath sounds throughout the lungs, especially in the lower lobes posteriorly. Inspiratory crackles heard throughout the lower lobes posteriorly and laterally. Loud expiratory wheezing heard with a cough and after any exertional movements. Pronounced rhonchi heard with a cough. Negative findings for bronchophony, egophony, and whispered pectoriloquy.

Cor—No visible precordial pulsations. PMI palpable 5 ICS, 4 cm Lt of MSL. Pulse is slightly sustained and 2 cm in diameter in the left side-lying position. No palpable lifts or thrills. Apical heart rate 90/min, regular with occasional irregular beats and no pulse deficit. S_1 loudest at apex; S_2 loudest 2 ICS, LSB. Loud P_2 and pronounced physiologic splitting of S_2 in pulmonic area. No gallops, murmurs, pericardial friction rubs, or other heart sounds. Using external jugular vein, CVP estimated at 7 cm H_2O with HOB at 30 degrees. No JVD. Carotid pulse full and equal bilaterally without bruits.

Extremities

Obvious clubbing of the fingers with ridging of the fingernails and poor capillary refill. Fingers are slightly ruddy colored. Asterixis present. Feet appear normal except for bilateral 2+ pedal edema.

PROBLEM IDENTIFICATION

For this patient, the following problems can be documented based on listed definitive findings. (1) *Severe COPD*—Cachexia, increased AP diameter, costal angle 90 degrees, en bloc movement of chest, decreased diaphragmatic excursions, hyperresonance to percussion in upper lobes, decreased breath sounds throughout lungs. These findings are classic of the pink puffer (i.e., emphysema patient). (2) *Respiratory distress*—Cyanosis, dyspnea, and pursed lip breathing with slight bulging of ICSs and accessory muscles used in respiration. Irregular pulse and respiratory rate of 28/min may not be definitive; they may represent normal baseline findings for this chronic lung disease patient. (3) *Fluid and mucus retention*—Inspiratory crackles, possibly from acute bronchitis, pneumonia, left ventricular failure, or combination thereof. Absence of S_3 gallop and other positive cardiac findings does not support a left-sided heart problem, but a recent history of pulmonary edema indicates that all or some of the crackles may be from edema fluid. More information is needed. Bilateral 2+ pedal edema is a sign of right ventricular failure. (4) *Alveolar hypoventilation (high* Pa_{CO_2}*)*—Lethargy with asterixis and ruddy colored fingers. (5) *Impaired oxygenation*—Cyanosis on 3 L of O_2; signs of respiratory distress. (Patient may be receiving too much or too little O_2. Arterial blood gas is needed.) (6) *Possible pulmonary hypertension*—Loud P_2 in pulmonic area; pronounced splitting of S_2 due to delayed right ventricular ejection and possibly complete or incomplete right bundle branch block, a common ECG finding in advanced COPD. (7) *Possible chest infection*—No clear evidence but always suspect it, if rhonchi are present, until you observe sputum characteristics. (8) *Possible dependence on steroid medication*—slight gynecomastia in cachectic man.

SECTION VII—LEARNING CHEST ASSESSMENT

Learning Prerequisites

Chest assessment is relatively difficult to master because it is a "hands-on" topic and because many individual skills are involved. Successful implementation of skills in the clinical setting depends on the fulfillment of the following learning prerequisites.

Knowledge Base. This chapter provides an extensive knowledge base for the implementation of the complete chest examination.

Laboratory Experience on Normal Individuals. The chest assessment laboratory guide that follows facilitates the practice of basic skills on the normal adult.

Practice in the Clinical Setting. At the end of this chapter, the complete chest examination is reduced to a *quick chest examination*. It utilizes the components of inspection and auscultation and serves as a guide for the nurse to begin to implement basic skills. As experience and confidence are gained in the clinical setting, the nurse can gradually add other components and more advanced techniques to her repertoire of skills.

For nurses to learn all components of the complete examination at once, time limitations may necessitate refinements of one skill at a time, while going through the motions of all skills to learn basic methodology. In any case, *practice is a must!*

Supervision. Learning correct technique may become impossible or frustrating without supervision by a person trained in chest assessment. Supervision in laboratory experiences insures correct identification and labelling of lung sounds, correct methodology, and familiarity with individual variations of normal, bronchovesicular, and bronchial breath sounds. Supervision at the bedside is essential for verification and categorization of abnormal lung sounds and for an *initial* refinement of skills that often prove very difficult to perform on dyspneic patients with cardiopulmonary pathology or disabling illness. Since further refinement and integration of skills into clinical practice usually end as "on the job" activities, refinement and integration depend on reliance on an available physician, nurse, or respiratory therapist trained in chest assessment. At least one such resource person should be readily available to answer questions, to auscultate unfamiliar lung sounds *with* you, and to work out any methodologic difficulties that might arise.

Without this supervision and support, nurses and others rarely gain enough personal confidence or skill to chart all the chest assessment findings regularly observed in the clinical setting.

Personal Commitment and Patience. Successful implementation of skills requires a personal commitment to continue to practice on normal and abnormal individuals. A conscious effort to use selected skills and examine acclaimed cases of classic pathology (e.g., newly admitted patient with lobar pneumonia or pulmonary edema) is necessary before anticipation and ready recognition of abnormal findings are possible.

Personal commitment to practice must be combined with patience; it takes the average nurse about *2 to 3 months* to integrate the basic skills into her unique style of bedside nursing and to achieve a sufficient level of self confidence in the ready identification and interpretation of findings.

Role of Lung Sound Audiotapes. Lung sound audiotapes are commonly used in the learning process when normal and abnormal sounds are first introduced. This teaching tool helps learners formulate their own associations as to what the various lung sounds should sound like, thereby facilitating lung sound recognition. For maximum effectiveness, however, tapes should be used with discretion. They should *not* serve as a substitute for practice with clinical supervision, and lung sound labelling on the tapes should be consistent with terms used in the clinical setting. Most important, tapes are intended as teaching aides rather than the *sole* teaching device.

Chest Assessment Laboratory Guide

This guide is used for teaching and learning basic chest assessment skills on a normal adult.

OBJECTIVES

At the end of this session, the student will be able to do the following:

1. Identify and describe a normal breathing pattern.
2. Identify boundaries of the lobes of the lungs.
3. Identify and describe the sound of a normal, bronchial, and bronchovesicular breath sound.
4. Auscultate the lungs of a normal adult using correct technique.

INSTRUCTIONS TO INSTRUCTORS

1. Provide the students with disposable or borrowed patient gowns from the hospital.
2. Make sure you have a good stethoscope to loan to students having difficulty listening to sounds. It is most important that the student not only learn a new skill but also discover any limitations of his or her own stethoscope by comparing its performance with that of a good stethoscope.
3. Instruct students as they go along or mingle among them while they experiment on their own; ask examiners questions to be sure they are hearing what they are supposed to hear. If the student's description of the breath sounds is incongruent with theory, listen to the area in question. You will encounter variations in normal breath sounds that cause the student to make different associations with the sound. Give special attention to the correct placement of the stethoscope in appropriate auscultation areas.
4. If the student's partner happens to be very obese or very thin, make sure the student has the opportunity to listen to a normal adult whose findings more closely approximate the usual descriptions.
5. Ask if anyone is recovering from a cold; they may have a rhonchus or wheeze to auscultate. The smokers undoubtedly will have wheezes with coughs.
6. Allow at least 1 hour for this laboratory. Although the ideal instructor to student ratio is about 1:8, some instructors may be able to supervise 12 students (6 pairs) in some situations.

INSTRUCTIONS TO STUDENTS

1. Use the gown provided and your own stethoscope, if you have one.
2. Practice in pairs, one person acting as subject, and the other as examiner. After completing the laboratory procedure, change roles to allow the subject the time to practice under supervision.
3. During deep breathing, pause between breaths to avoid hyperventilation and dizziness.
4. Seek help if you are unsure of technique or chest assessment findings.

THE LABORATORY

Inspection

1. Observe the anterior and posterior thorax for general chest symmetry.
2. Answer the following questions with the subject breathing quietly at rest:

What muscles is he using for respiration?

Is he primarily a costal (i.e., using chest muscles) or diaphragmatic breather?

Is there any asymmetric chest movement?

Is the breathing pattern normal?

3. Ask the subject to breathe deeply and note any change in the breathing pattern, use of respiratory muscles, or chest symmetry. Particularly note any lag in chest movement in the lateral chest areas while observing the posterior thorax.

Identification of Breath Sounds

4. Place your stethoscope's diaphragm on the side of the throat over the trachea while the subject breathes deeply with an open mouth. Identify the *tracheal breath sound*. It is very loud and hollow because the trachea is the largest airway in the body, and it lies immediately below the chest piece.

5. As the subject continues to breathe deeply, move the stethoscope's diaphragm over the manubrium of the sternum just below the suprasternal notch. Note the *bronchial breath sound. What is the difference between this bronchial breath sound and the tracheal breath sound?* Compare pitch, intensity, and quality of the two sounds. Although both breath sounds sound hollow, the tracheal breath sound will sound "closer," louder, and harsher than the more "distant" bronchial breath sound. If you are unable to hear the difference between the two sounds, ask the subject to exhale forcefully as you listen again and compare exhalations at the two sites. Remember to use firm pressure of the stethoscope's diaphragm against the skin surface.

The bronchial breath sound is normally heard only over the area of the manubrium. It is abnormal, if heard anywhere else.

6. Listen over the middle of the sternum to identify the *bronchovesicular breath sound*. Compare pitch, intensity, and quality to determine the difference between the bronchial and bronchovesicular breath sounds. Careful listening during the expiratory phase helps to make the lower pitched, less hollow, and slightly breezy bronchovesicular sound more obvious.

The bronchovesicular breath sound is normally heard only over the sternal area and between the scapulae of the back. Heard anywhere else, it is abnormal.

7. To listen to an example of the *normal (vesicular) breath sound*, choose *one* auscultation area in the lateral or posterior chest area over a lower lobe. Compare pitch, intensity, and quality to determine the difference between the normal and bronchovesicular breath sounds. Differentiate the breezy quality of this sound with the hollowness of the bronchial breath sound. Also note whether expiration is audible throughout the expiratory phase (e.g., thin-build chest), whether it is present only during early expiration (e.g., medium-build chest), or whether it is absent (e.g., thick-build chest due to adipose tissue or muscle).

The normal breath sound is normally heard over peripheral areas of the lungs away from the central airways.

8. While listening to the normal breath sound, instruct the subject to close his mouth and breathe deeply through his nose. What happens to the intensity of the breath sound?

Do not proceed further unless you definitely can hear the difference among the normal, bronchovesicular, and bronchial breath sounds. Seek help if you are having difficulties.

Identification of the Lobes of the Lungs*

9. Identify the following *vertical imaginary lines:*

Midsternal line (MSL)
Midclavicular line (MCL)
Anterior axillary line (AAL)
Posterior axillary line (PAL)
Vertebral line (VL)

10. Identify the *sternal angle*, the bony protuberance where the manubrium joins the body of the sternum (see anatomy in Figure 1–10A and technique described on page 257). Then, palpate the second ICS and the third rib immediately below it. Be sure you know how to correctly count ribs and ICSs anteriorly.

11. Identify the fourth rib, right MCL, and the sixth rib, MCL, on both sides of the anterior chest area. Using these two landmarks and referring to Figure 12–5A, identify the following:

Right upper lobe (RUL)
Right middle lobe (RML)
Right lower lobe (RLL)
Left upper lobe (LUL)
Left lower lobe (LLL)

12. With the subject's neck flexed forward, palpate the spinous process of the *seventh cervical vertebra (C7)*, the *first* prominent spinous process in the neck. Palpate the spinal column down to the level of the spinous process of the *third thoracic vertebra* (T3), i.e., move from C7 to T1 to T2 to T3. Using T3 as a basic landmark and referring to Figure 12–5B, identify the following:

Right and left upper lobes
Right and left lower lobes

Note that the right middle lobe does not extend to the posterior thorax (see Fig. 12–5C).

Auscultation

Now you are ready to auscultate the chest.

13. Auscultate the upper lobes anteriorly and the lower lobes posteriorly, using the auscultation areas for the quick chest examination (see Fig. 12–60). If time permits, use auscultation areas for the complete chest examination to familiarize yourself with other areas used to examine patients more thoroughly (see Fig. 12–42). Remember to compare two auscultation areas at once. The areas must be on opposite sides of the chest, at the same vertebral level, and equidistant from the sternal or vertebral line. Spend no more than two to three breaths at each auscultation area.

14. Ask the subject to cough and listen for a wheeze or rhonchus right *with* the cough. If possible, compare the coughs of a normal subject, a smoker, and a subject recovering from a cold. Ask your instructor to confirm the absence or presence of adventitious sounds in your subject.

---

*Review Figs. 12–1, 12–2, and 12–3.

Protocol for the Quick Chest Examination

The following is a protocol for implementation of a quick chest examination in the clinical setting.* Since key information is in summary form, readers may need to refer to the beginning of this chapter or Chapter 8 for more detailed information or explanations.

The examination takes an experienced clinician no longer than 1 to 2 minutes to perform (Fig. 12–59). Because it is quick, it facilitates integration of pulmonary assessment findings into the overall nursing assessment in situations limited by time or patient tolerance.

I. The quick chest examination is performed to help the nurse and others quickly and efficiently assess patients with potential or diagnosed cardiopulmonary problems.

II. *Take the patient's vital signs*, or study the vital signs on flow sheets at the bedside or on the medical chart. Note any *gross changes* from signs taken during the last assessment as well as *general trends*, e.g., gradual increases or decreases in readings or signs over the past hours, days, or weeks. The following signs indicate a possible respiratory problem:
   - A. Increase or decrease in pulse, blood pressure, or respiratory rate
   - B. Irregular pulse
   - C. Cardiac arrhythmias on the monitor
   - D. Pulse deficit
   - E. Increased temperature

III. *Note changes in sensorium or behavior patterns* that might indicate a blood gas disorder:

Changes in Sensorium	*Changes in Behavior*
Lethargy with or without headache	Passive behavior
Drowsiness or coma	Combative behavior
Disorientation	Uncooperative behavior
Impaired judgment	Restlessness
Inability to concentrate	Anxiety
	Muscle uncoordination
	Mood swings

IV. *Note the presence of a weak or strong, productive or nonproductive cough. Check sputum* for the following:
   - A. *Amount*—minimal, small, moderate, or copious amounts with each episode of coughing. If possible, quantify in teaspoons, tablespoons, or cups. Observe the bedside sputum cup for amount every 24 hours.
   - B. *Color*—clear, white, yellow, green, red, or brown

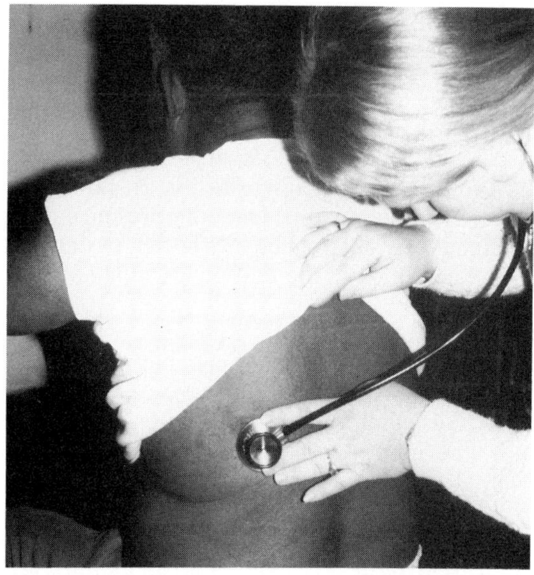

Figure 12–59. A home health nurse performs a quick chest examination to assess a mucus retention problem before deciding exactly how to implement postural drainage with percussion and vibration. Respiration interventions are continuously reevaluated and readapted, depending on changing assessment findings.

   - C. *Consistency*—thick, thin, or frothy
   - D. *Odor*—foul-smelling or other

V. *Inspect the head and neck, fingers, and chest for abnormalities.* Specifically note the pattern of breathing, chest symmetry, chest excursions, skin color, and any signs of respiratory distress. Look for the following main signs:

Extrathoracic Signs	*Thoracic Signs*
Increased pallor	Asymmetric chest
Cyanosis of lips	Minimal or maximal chest excursions
Poor capillary refill of nail beds	Abnormal breathing pattern or chest wall movement
Neck vein distention	Labored breathing with use of accessory muscles of respiration: neck muscles, shoulder muscles, intercostal muscles
Pronounced movement of Adam's apple with respiration	Prolonged expiration
Nasal flaring	
Facial tension	
Pursed lip breathing (i.e., COPD)	
Interrupted speech pattern	

VI. *Observe for signs of chronic obstructive pulmonary disease.* Prompt identification of COPD insures modification of standard emergency respiratory care procedures to the different needs of these patients. Also, the acute COPD patient has several chronic problems that need further attention. Observe the patient for these main signs of COPD as follows:
   - A. Obstructive breathing pattern
   - B. Productive cough or audible wheeze

---

*Portions of this protocol have been taken from the *Chest Examination Protocol* (1975 edition) developed and implemented by the author at Herrick Hospital and Health Center of the East Bay, Berkeley, California. These portions have been been adapted for publication by permission of the hospital and its pulmonary medicine department.

C. En bloc chest movement
D. Pursed lip breathing
E. Barrel chest or increased AP diameter
F. Cachexia or muscle wasting
G. Pack of cigarettes in pocket. Not a definitive sign, but it suggests air flow limitation.

VII. *Auscultate the lungs* to assess air flow through the tracheobronchial tree; the presence of fluid, mucus, or obstruction in the air passages; and the condition of the underlying lung and pleural space.
A. Sit the patient up, if possible.
B. Ask him to open his mouth and breathe *deeply*.
C. Auscultate at least two anterior areas (e.g., periphery of RUL and LUL) and four posterior areas (e.g., over the lower lobes of the lungs), as shown by the black circles in Figure 12–60A and B. These circles represent *basic* auscultation areas that are always auscultated during *any* examination. When choosing auscultation areas on the patient's chest, be sure that each group of two is at the same thoracic level and equidistant from the sternal or vertebral line, as shown in Figure 12–60.
D. When checking the lower lobes posteriorly, ask the patient to pant or cough and take a deep breath in. Often the lungs will sound clear until a cough elicits adventitious sounds.
E. Alter or extend auscultation areas, when necessary.
1. *Any patient with a recent history of cardiopulmonary problems or at an exceptionally high risk to develop such problems.* All of the auscultation areas in Figure 12–60A and B may be used (black circles and other circles). Use the same methodology as for the complete exami-

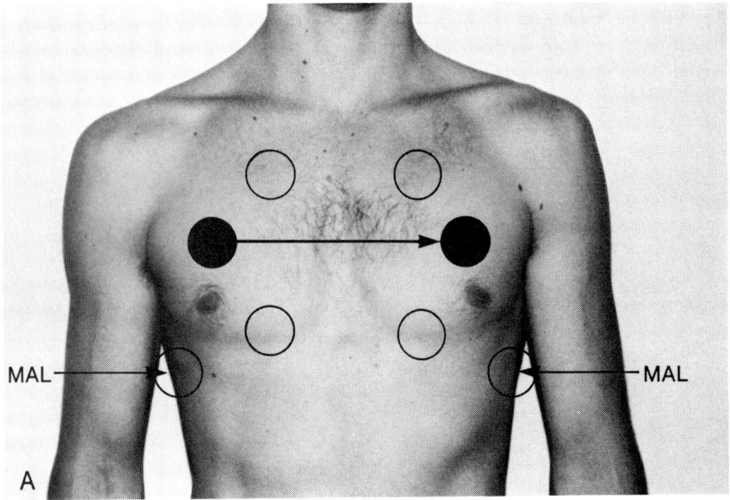

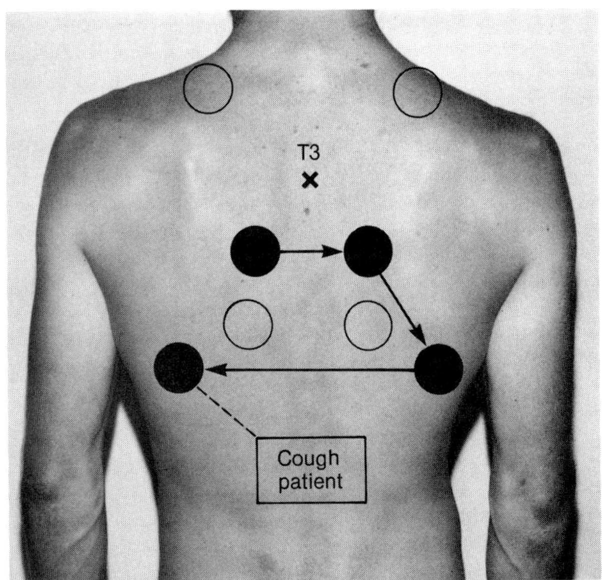

Figure 12–60. Auscultation areas for the quick chest examination or the anterior *(A)* and posterior *(B)* chest regions. The black circles indicate *basic* areas always auscultated during any chest examination. The other circles mark areas included as indicated by the specific situation. In the anterior region of the chest, the basic area is at or slightly *lateral* to the midclavicular line, to insure detection of bronchial breath sounds from right lower lobe consolidation. The patient's arms must be abducted to auscultate the lateral inferior area—at the level of about the sixth rib, midaxillary line (MAL) or posterior-axillary line for supine, critically ill patients. During auscultation of the posterior region of the chest, "coughing" the patient once or twice helps to elicit adventitious sounds.

nation, starting with the upper lobes and gradually working across and down the chest to the lower lobes.

2. *Immobile or acutely ill patients.* During the initial nursing assessment, use all of the auscultation areas for the anterior area of the chest in Figure 12–60A, moving back and forth across the chest in a systematic manner. Later, when help is available to position the patient forward a few inches, auscultate at least the basic areas over the lower lobes posteriorly. Auscultation with the patient in the lateral recumbent position is sometimes necessary but less than ideal because compression of lung tissue on the "down" side produces decreased or bronchial breath sounds; the "up" side has no opposite auscultation area to serve as a normal control.
3. *Thoroughly auscultate suspected areas of abnormality.*
   a. Areas of chest pain or tenderness
   b. Areas where the chest x-ray or a diagnostic test reports an abnormality
   c. Chest tube sites; auscultate over bandages if skin surfaces are unavailable.

VIII. *As you auscultate opposite sides of the chest, note the following:*

A. Equality of breath sounds: equal or unequal? Equality depends upon the overall passage of air and the duration of inspiration and expiration as well as the quality, pitch, and intensity of the breath sounds. To assess equality, ask yourself the following questions:
   1. Does the breath sound on one side of the chest sound exactly like that on the other side?
   2. Is the air passage interrupted by any extra (i.e., adventitious) sounds?

B. Identify normal breath sounds. Inspiration longer than expiration, low-pitched, soft, and breezy. This breath sound is normally auscultated throughout the lung periphery.

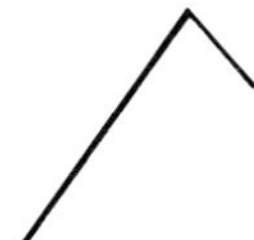

C. Identify and locate any of the following abnormal breath sounds.

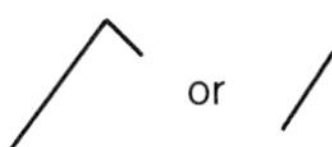

1. *Absent or decreased breath sounds.*
   a. Absent breath sounds are never normal; decreased breath sounds may be normal only if breath sounds are always decreased throughout the chest as a baseline normal finding for the patient in question.
   b. Sign of impaired ventilation; a medical emergency if other signs of respiratory distress are present, indicating an acute problem such as pneumothorax, bronchospasm, or upper airway obstruction.
2. *Bronchial breath sounds.* Expiration longer than inspiration, high-pitched, loud, and tubular like air passing through a hollow tube.

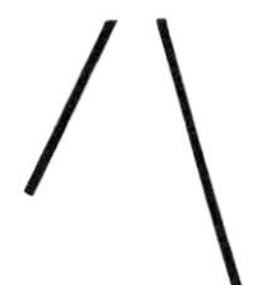

   a. Normally heard over manubrium of the sternum.
   b. Sign of consolidation or compression of lung tissue. Airway is patent.
3. *Bronchovesicular breath sounds.* I:E ratio of 1:1, medium in pitch and intensity, breezy-tubular quality.

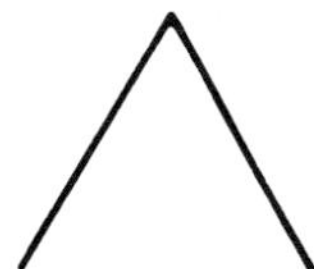

   a. Normally heard in the sternal area and between scapulae in back.
   b. Sign of early or partial consolidation or compression of tissue. Airway is patent.

D. Identify and locate any of the following adventitious (i.e., extra) breath sounds:
   1. *Crackles (rales)*: discrete crackles or pops caused by atelectasis, fibrosis, or secretions in alveoli and *small* airways. Usually inspiratory.

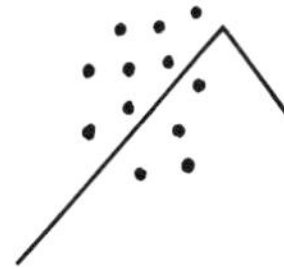

   2. *Rhonchi*: low-pitched, coarse, continuous sounds caused by bubbling secretions in *large* airways that have become narrowed by mucus, fluid, inflammation, or some other process. Usually more prominent during expiration.

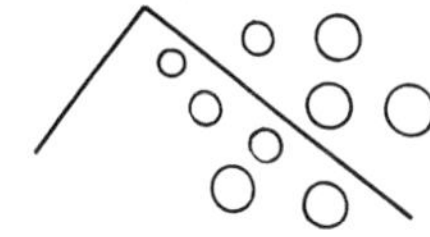

3. *Wheeze:* usually a high-pitched musical or squeaking sound produced when air passes through narrowed airways; typically heard in asthmatics. Usually more prominent during expiration.

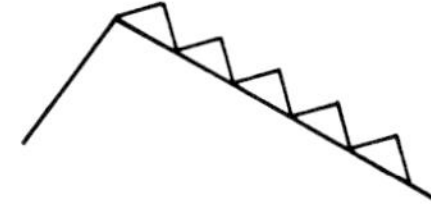

4. *Pleural friction rub:* interrupted grating or scraping sound commonly heard on inspiration in the anterolateral or lateral chest area. Unchanged with coughing.

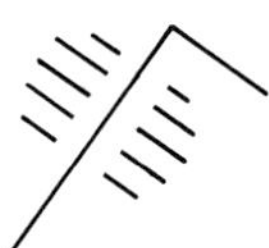

IX. While charting your overall nursing assessment, *chart your chest assessment findings* in the nurse's notes by stating positive and pertinent negative findings. Be brief and succinct, using abbreviations and headings whenever possible to help you recall and record appropriate data.

A. Examples of charting the entire quick examination:

1. A stable patient on a hospital ward: *Alert gentleman with stable vital signs, occasional strong, nonproductive cough, in no apparent distress. Lungs clear to auscultation.*
2. An acutely ill patient just admitted to an acute care unit: *Cooperative but drowsy elderly man, very slow to respond to questioning. Vital signs stable except for increased resp. rate of 30/min. Coughing up minimal amounts of thick yellow sputum.* ***Signs of respiratory distress****—labored breathing with use of neck, shoulder, and intercostal muscles. Neck veins distended. Lips do not appear pale or cyanotic, but poor capillary refill of nail beds is present. Extremities are pale and cool to touch.* ***Signs of COPD****—pack of cigarettes found in pocket, barrel chest.* ***Lungs****—on auscultation, breath sounds are greatly decreased throughout the chest. Pronounced wheeze and rhonchus with cough.*
3. *Discussion:* Note in this last example that the charting of information closely parallels the procedure of the quick chest examination. An alternative way to chart is to put appropriate data under two main headings, inspection and auscultation, the components used for data collection. Also note the following:
   a. The nurse charted the absence of cyanosis or pallor; the presence or absence of this sign may be crucial in deciding whether the patient needs oxygen immediately.
   b. Without auscultation during the cough, the nurse would have missed the presence of the wheeze and rhonchus.
   c. Charted findings clearly indicate a ventilatory and probably a mucus retention problem because of the yellow sputum production, rhonchus, and wheeze with cough, and greatly decreased breath sounds.

B. *Charting lung sounds:* Remember to chart the type of breath sound heard throughout the lungs in general as well as specific locations of abnormal breath sounds and adventitious sounds. Summarize diffuse findings and use comparative charting whenever possible to help assess whether the patient is worse, better, or unchanged. Some examples follow:

1. *Normal breath sounds with scattered expiratory rhonchi throughout the chest.*
2. *Lungs clear except for expiratory wheezing LLL.*
3. *Normal breath sounds. Inspiratory crackles RLL laterally, clearing with coughing.*
4. *Decreased breath sounds throughout the lungs, especially RUL anteriorly. Expiration sounds more decreased than yesterday; almost absent now over RUL. A few scattered expiratory wheezes throughout the chest.*

X. In coordination with other members of the health care team and within prescribed medical orders, *the nurse alters interventions according to chest assessment findings.*

Conclusion

This chapter has provided an extensive knowledge base for physical examination of the chest. Most of the presentation is devoted to breaking down the examination into small components so that the nurse thoroughly understands methodology and can selectively apply detailed information in the diagnostic process described subsequently in the text. After a brief discussion of integration of the precordial examination, the last part of the chapter returned the reader to the macrolevel. It described how to implement the complete chest examination in the clinical setting, emphasizing inspection and auscultation components for problem identification. To facilitate implementation, the section on learning chest assessment summarized learning prerequisites, laboratory practice, and finally clinical practice using the protocol for the quick chest examination.

In conclusion, performing a complete or quick chest examination can provide crucial pieces of objective data to confirm or rule out respiratory diagnoses. When an oxygenation, ventilation, or acid-base balance problem is suspected, these data are always interpreted in light of blood gas results and other findings.

REFERENCES

American College of Chest Physicians—American Thoracic Society: Pulmonary terms and symbols. *Chest,* 67(5):583–593, 1975.

Bates, B.: A Guide to Physical Examination and History Taking, 4th ed. Philadelphia, J. B. Lippincott Co., 1987.

Baughman, R. and Loudon, R.: Lung sound analysis for continuous evaluation of airflow obstruction in asthma. *Chest,* 88(3):364–368, 1985.

Boyce, B.: Respiratory Care Terminology. American Lung Association, no. 0014, 1976.

Burns, K. and Johnson, P.: The Chest and Pulmonary System. Health Assessment in Clinical Practice. Englewood Cliffs, New Jersey, Prentice Hall, Inc., 1980.

Burton, G.: Practical physical diagnosis in respiratory care. In: Respiratory Care—A Guide to Clinical Practice, 2nd ed. (Burton, G. and Hodgkin, J.–eds.) Philadelphia, J. B. Lippincott Co., 1984.

Catley, D., Thornton, C. et al: Continuous postoperative monitoring reveals oxygen desaturation associated with paradoxical respiration. *American Review of Respiratory Disease,* 125(4):105, 1982.

Catterall, J., Calverley, P. et al: Gas exchange, cardiac output, and pulmonary arterial pressure during transient nocturnal hypoxemia in "Blue and bloated" COPD. *American Review of Respiratory Disease,* 125(4): 91, 1982.

Cherniack, R. and Cherniack, L.: Respiration in Health and Disease, 3rd ed. Philadelphia, W. B. Saunders Co., 1983.

Cohen, C., Zagelbaum, G. et al.: Clinical manifestations of inspiratory muscle fatigue. *The American Journal of Medicine,* 73(3): 308–316, 1982.

Cugell, D.: Lung sounds: classification and controversies. *Seminars in Respiratory Medicine,* 6(3):180–182, 1985.

DeGowin, E. and DeGowin, R.: Bedside Diagnostic Examination, 4th ed. New York, MacMillan Publishing Co., 1981.

Delp, M. and Manning, R.: Major's Physical Diagnosis—An Introduction to the Clinical Process. Philadelphia, W. B. Saunders Co., 1981.

Desser, K. and Benchimol, A.: Clicks secondary to pneumothorax confounding the diagnosis of mitral valve prolapse. *Chest,* 71(4): 523–525, 1977.

Druger, G.: The Chest: Its Signs and Sounds. Los Angeles, Humetrics Corp., 1973.

Ford, G., Whitelaw, W. et al: Diaphragm function after upper abdominal surgery. *American Review of Respiratory Disease,* 123(4):186, 1981.

Forgacs, P.: Applied cardiopulmonary physiology—the functional basis of pulmonary sounds. From Brooke General Hospital, London, England. *Chest,* 73(3):199–405, 1978a.

Forgacs, P.: Lung Sounds. London, Baillière Tindall, 1978b.

Fraser, R. and Paré, J.: Diagnosis of Diseases of the Chest, Vol. 3, 2nd ed. Philadelphia, W. B. Saunders Co., 1979.

Gilbert, R. et al: Clinical value of observations of chest and abdominal motion in patients with pulmonary emphysema. *American Review of Respiratory Disease,* 119(2):155–158, 1979.

Glauser, F.: Signs and Symptoms in Pulmonary Medicine. Philadelphia, J. B. Lippincott Co., 1983.

Hinshaw, H. and Murray, J.: Diseases of the Chest, 4th ed. Philadelphia, W. B. Saunders Co., 1980.

Krumpe, P.: Practical applications of lung sounds research. *Seminars in Respiratory Medicine,* 6(3):229–237, 1985.

Leatham, A.: An Introduction to the Examination of the Cardiovascular System, 2nd ed. Oxford, Oxford University Press, 1979.

Leatham, A.: Auscultation of the Heart and Phonocardiography, 2nd ed. London, Churchill Livingstone, 1975.

Lehrer, S.: Understanding Lung Sounds. Philadelphia, W. B. Saunders Co., 1984.

Loudon, R. and Murphy, R.: State of the art—lung sounds. *American Review of Respiratory Disease,* 130(4): 663–673, 1984.

Murphy, R. and Holford, S.: Lung sounds. *Basics of Respiratory Disease,* 8(4), entire issue, 1980.

Netter, F.: The CIBA Collection of Medical Illustrations, Vol. 7, Respiratory System. New York, CIBA Pharmaceutical Co., 1979.

Newsom-Davis, J.: The diaphragm and neuromuscular disease. *American Review of Respiratory Disease,* 119(2):115–117, 1979.

Nochomovitz, M. and Cherniack, N. (eds.): Noninvasive Respiratory Monitoring. New York, Churchill Livingstone, 1986.

Petty, T.: Clinical evaluation of patients with chronic respiratory insufficiency. *Seminars in Respiratory Medicine,* 1(1):1–8, 1979.

Phillipson, E.: Breathing disorders during sleep. *Basics of Respiratory Disease,* 7(3):1–6, 1979.

Ploysongsang, Y., Paré, J. and Macklem, P.: Lung sounds in patients with emphysema. *American Review of Respiratory Disease,* 124(1): 45–49, 1981.

Ploysongsang, Y. and Schonfeld, S.: Mechanism of production of crackles after atelectasis during low-volume breathing. *American Review of Respiratory Disease,* 126(3):413–415, 1982.

Pontoppidan, H. et al: Acute respiratory failure in the adult. *New England Journal of Medicine,* 287(15):746, 1972.

Prior, J., Silberstein, J. and Stang, J.: Physical Diagnosis—The History and Examination of the Patient, 6th ed. St. Louis, C. V. Mosby, 1981.

Ravitch, M.: Disorders of the chest. In Davis-Christopher Textbook of Surgery. (Sabiston, D.–ed.) Philadelphia, W. B. Saunders Co., 1981.

Sharp, J., Goldberg, N., Druz, W. and Danon, J.: Relative contributions of rib cage and abdomen to breathing in normal subjects. *Journal of Applied Physiology,* 39(4):608–618, 1975.

Sherman, J. and Fields, S.: Guide to Patient Evaluation, 4th ed. Flushing, New York, Medical Examination Publishing Co., 1982.

Stewart, J., Ferguson, S., Bhola, R. and Wilson, A.: The significance of the timing of wheezes. *American Review of Respiratory Disease,* 131(4):A72, 1985.

Straight, P. and Soukup, S.: How to hear it right: evaluating and choosing a stethoscope. *American Journal of Nursing,* 77(9):1477, 1977.

Thompson, D.: Cardiovascular Assessment—Guide for Nurses and Other Health Professionals. St. Louis, C.V. Mosby, 1981.

Vanden Belt, R., Ronan, J. and Bedynek, J.: Cardiology—A Clinical Approach. Chicago, Year Book Medical Publishers, Inc., 1979.

Waring, W.: The history and physical examination. In Disorders of the Respiratory Tract in Children, 4th ed. (Kendig, E. and Chernick, V.—eds.) Philadelphia, W. B. Saunders Co., 1983.

Waring, W., Beckerman, R. and Hopkins, R.: Continuous adventitious lung sounds: site and method of production and significance. *Seminars in Respiratory Medicine,* 6(3):201–209, 1985.

Workum, P. et al: The prevalence and character of crackles (rales) in young women without significant lung disease. *American Review of Respiratory Disease,* 126(5): 921–923, 1982.

Blood Gases

13

Main Objectives

1. **Name at least three indications for ABG measurements.**
2. **Given a list of blood gas measurements, group them into oxygenation, ventilation, and acid-base balance categories for interpretation.**
3. **Define the following terms: blood pH, hypoxemia, hypoxia, oxygen saturation (%), respiratory failure, ventilatory failure, hypoxic drive to breathe, venous admixture, shunt-like effect, arteriovenous shunting, low V/Q ratio, and CO_2 narcosis.**
4. **Name and explain the four causes of hypoxemia. In your answer, clarify the following:**
   a. **The three different types of right to left intrapulmonary shunt.**
   b. **The use of the A-aO_2 gradient and a/A ratio in the clinical setting.**
   c. **The reasons why low V/Q ratios produce hypoxemia.**
   d. **The V/Q ratios in COPD.**
5. **Explain how to interpret the following measurements of tissue oxygenation: mixed venous**

Po_2 ($P\bar{v}o_2$) and arteriovenous oxygen content difference $C(a-\bar{v})o_2$.

6. **State the signs and symptoms of hypoxemia, hypoxia, and CO_2 narcosis.**
7. **For the hazards of oxygen (e.g., alveolar hypoventilation, absorption atelectasis, and pulmonary oxygen toxicity)**
   a. **Explain the physiologic mechanisms involved.**
   b. **Describe how to avoid adverse effects on the body.**
8. **For acute ventilatory failure**
   a. **Describe the physiologic chain of events leading to physical decompensation.**
   b. **List the accompanying clinical findings.**
   c. **Describe the monitoring of the patient at risk for ventilatory failure.**
9. **Explain how the four main acid-base disorders are described utilizing the Henderson-Hasselbalch equation.**
10. **Describe the changes in pH, $Paco_2$, and HCO_3^- that define the acute and chronic forms of the four basic acid-base disorders.**
11. **List three causes, three signs and symptoms, and three basic interventions for each of the following disorders and problems: respiratory acidosis, respiratory alkalosis, metabolic acidosis, and metabolic alkalosis.**
12. **Use a list of laboratory normal ranges to correctly interpret the set of ABG results at the end of this chapter.**

This chapter discusses blood gases, crucial parameters to consider in the assessment of problems related to oxygenation, ventilation, and acid-base balance. Initial focus is on the purpose of, the indications for, and the drawing of blood for a set of *arterial blood gases*, commonly called *ABGs* in the clinical setting. A set of ABGs is obtained from one arterial puncture. It consists of the following laboratory measurements: *blood pH, partial pressures* of *oxygen* and *carbon dioxide, oxygen saturation, base excess,* and *bicarbonate concentration.*

The main body of this chapter provides a theory base for interpretation of oxygenation, ventilation, and acid-base measurements. The theory base is an extension of physiologic content on oxygenation already presented in Chapter 3 and Chapter 5. The theory base is presented in sufficient depth to prepare the nurse for interpretation of both multiple and single measurements, as encountered in the clinical setting. A single measurement may be from a set of ABGs or from other parameters discussed in this chapter, such as mixed venous Po_2 and various shunt measurements. In other cases, it may represent a noninvasive measurement of Pao_2 (e.g., oximetry in Chapter 23) or $Paco_2$ (e.g., capnography in Chapter 28). Whatever the case may be, the ability to rapidly interpret a single measurement is becoming a crucial nursing function. When financial or situational constraints limit access to a full set of ABG results, the nurse may make decisions based on one or two measurements. Furthermore, the increasing use of noninvasive measurements of Pao_2 and $Paco_2$ has put an added responsibility on the nurse to use a limited series of single measurements for clinical decision-making.

The main theory base section of this chapter serves one more purpose. It links blood gas assessment directly to respiratory intervention. Assessment of oxygenation, for example, is not restricted to the assessment phase of clinical decision-making. Rather, it occurs almost continuously during respiratory nursing care. Hence, after presentation of each assessment parameter (e.g., oxygenation, ventilation, and acid-base balance), associated problems are discussed along with clinical recognition and implications for intervention. Emphasis is placed on the hazards of oxygen and ventilatory failure because of their close association with the respiratory component of acid-base balance.

Purpose and Indications

As a unit, the ABG results form an essential component of the complete pulmonary function test (PFT) (discussed in the next chapter). With other PFT measurements, ABG results help to assess the adequacy of lung function. Unlike other commonly used PFT measurements, however, ABGs provide the *only* objective means for assessing both the acid-base balance in the body and the adequacy of gas exchange in the lungs. Hence, though part of a more complete pulmonary function assessment, ABGs may be frequently obtained independent of PFTs to assess the changing condition of the patient and help modify respiratory interventions. ABGs are ordered for one or more of the reasons listed in the box on page 338.

Drawing the Arterial Blood Gas (ABG) Sample

When blood gases are ordered, an arterial puncture is assumed, unless a venous or mixed venous sample is specified. *Arterial* sampling is routinely performed by needle puncture into the radial or brachial artery. Also, sampling may occur via an indwelling arterial cannula or via the arterial side of an external shunt in a patient with renal disease. In contrast, a *venous* sample is taken via venous puncture or via a fistula in a patient with renal disease. A *mixed venous* sample is taken via a central line in the pulmonary artery.

PROCEDURE FOR ARTERIAL PUNCTURE

The following steps describe how to perform an arterial puncture without causing unnecessary patient discomfort and without introducing error into meas-

INDICATIONS FOR ABGs

To obtain baseline information about an individual in no apparent distress.

To determine the presence and severity of an oxygenation or CO_2 exchange problem.

To evaluate the progression of a disease, particularly acute exacerbations or episodes of respiratory distress, and to help determine a course of therapy.

To assess the effectiveness of respiratory interventions, particularly mechanical ventilation and weaning from mechanical ventilation in the acute care setting.

To assess acid-base balance in the body.

To document respiratory impairment, to substantiate the need for respiratory treatment at home (e.g., oxygen therapy), and to qualify an individual for related financial assistance.

urements. Avoidance of measurement errors is important because they lead to interpretation errors and sometimes to incorrect clinical assessments.

When an ABG is ordered the nurse follows these 15 steps as follows:

1. *Check respiratory therapy orders.* Place the patient on the ordered FIO_2 and respiratory therapy device. Wait 10 to 20 minutes for equilibration of gases within the lungs (Hess et al, 1985); wait 20 to 30 minutes for patients with severe V/Q mismatching, e.g., COPD patients. If the patient is already on the ordered FIO_2 and respiratory therapy device, a waiting period is still necessary if resting FIO_2 has been interrupted for any reason (e.g., suctioning, face mask removal, and exercise) within the last 20 minutes.

2. *Gather appropriate equipment.* If an ABG kit is not available (Fig. 13–1), obtain sterile 3- or 5-cc glass or plastic syringe; 1:1000 heparin solution; 21 to 22 gauge × 1 to 1½ in long needle for brachial artery; 22 to 25 gauge × 1 in long needle for radial artery; alcohol swabs; rolled towel; sterile gauze (2 × 2) or elastic bandage (Elastoplast); plug or cork to seal syringe; cup or small plastic bag with ice slush; and optional 1 to 2% lidocaine (Xylocaine) with 1-cc syringe with 25 gauge needle.

3. *Stamp a blood sample label and ABG laboratory requisition with the patient's name and billing number.* Fill out the requisition, providing the following information: FIO_2, mode of therapy with liter flow, basic ventilator information (optional), time of puncture, and current body temperature. Most laboratories correct results for temperature, if the patient's temperature deviates more than 1°C from normal; 37°C is considered a normal oral and axillary temperature; and 37.5°C, a normal rectal and intracardiac temperature. The intracardiac temperature is taken via a pulmonary artery catheter.

4. *Explain the procedure to the patient.* Stress why ABGs are needed. Answer questions and give appropriate reassurance.

5. *Choose an artery.* The radial artery (Fig. 13–2) is the first choice because it is the most accessible site and puncture is relatively pain free, provided the bony periosteum is avoided. Also, should vessel spasm, intralumenal clotting, or bleeding occur at the site, the ulnar artery usually provides adequate collateral circulation to peripheral tissues. If an adequate radial arterial pulse is present, the nurse uses *Allen's test* described in Figure 13–3 to be sure adequate collateral circulation exists. If both radial arteries appear to be good sites, always choose the artery with the strongest pulse or the site without nearby infected skin or other skin lesions.

The brachial artery in the antecubital fossa (see Fig. 13–2) is used when the Allen's test results are negative or when the radial pulses are weak, making successful puncture uncertain. This artery is larger than the radial artery, which increases the chances of successful puncture. However, careful technique is necessary to avoid inadvertent venous puncture and hematoma formation, since the artery lies close to large veins.

In most cases, a suitable radial or bracheal artery can be found. In some patients, such as those in shock or those with severe cardiovascular disease, pulses are fleeting, and the physician is then called to perform a femoral artery puncture. Though the femoral artery is large, it is always the puncture site of last resort because obstruction endangers blood flow to the entire lower extremity. Also, there is increased risk for venous puncture, hematoma formation, and hemorrhage, particularly if the patient is on anticoagulants or has a low platelet count.

6. *Assess need for a local anesthetic.* A local anesthetic is optional and is usually unnecessary, unless the patient is extremely anxious. Anxiety reactions may lead to breath holding or hyperventilation, potentially introducing errors into ABG results. When a need exists and when an anesthetic is ordered by the physician, the clinician injects about 1 ml of 1% or 2% lidocaine (Xylocaine) into the dermis, subcutaneously above the artery, and then on either side of the artery. The needle should enter the skin at a 25-degree angle, and a 25-gauge needle should be used. Care is taken to avoid the artery itself and to aspirate before the injection to be sure that the needle is not in the blood vessel. After a small wheal is made, the clinician waits several minutes for the anesthetic to take effect.

7. *Heparinize the ABG syringe.* This step prevents clotting of the blood sample. The nurse draws 0.5 cc of 1:1000 heparin, pulls back on the plunger to lubricate the entire syringe, and ejects excess heparin

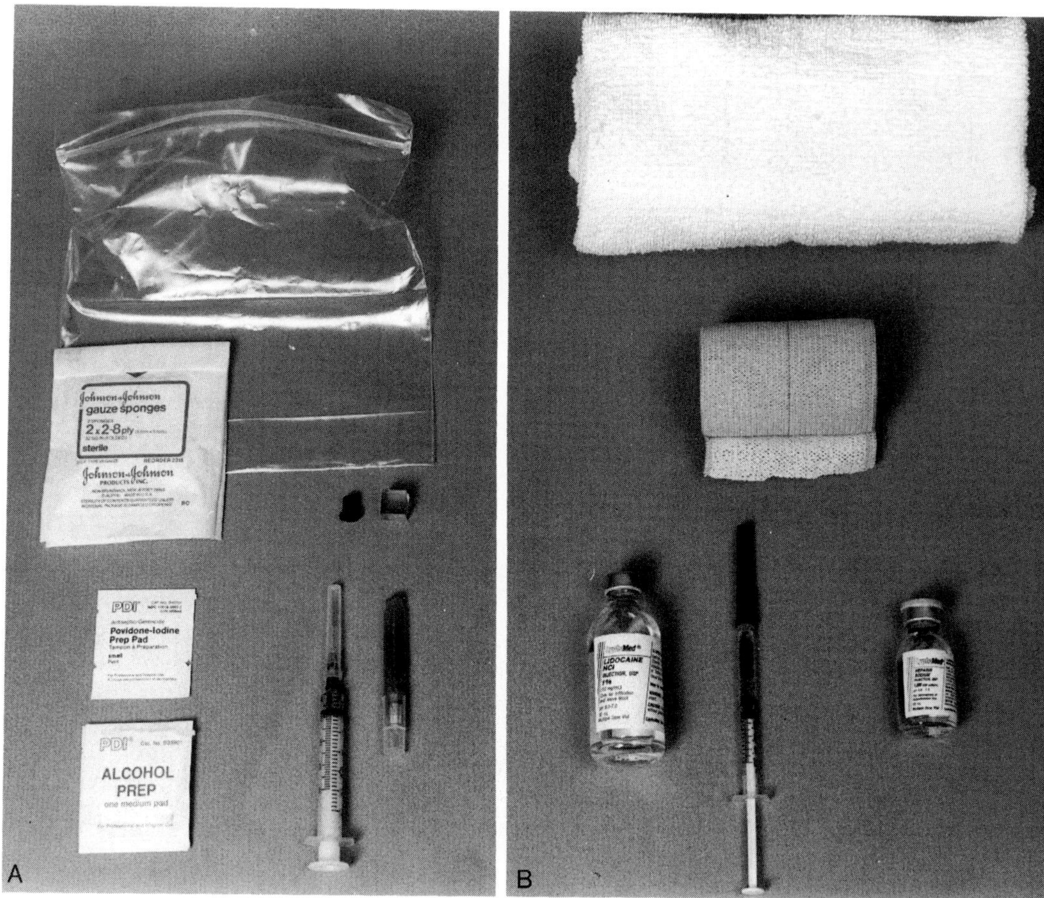

Figure 13–1. Equipment for arterial puncture. *A*, Items typically found in an ABG kit. Note that alcohol, povidone-iodine (Betadine) swabs, or both may be used for skin preparation. The syringe is preheparinized. *B*, Other items, excluding ice slush for the plastic bag.

Figure 13–2. Brachial, radial, and femoral arteries for arterial puncture. This illustration also shows collateral circulation. *a*, Deep brachial, superior, and inferior ulnar collateral arteries usually provide sufficient flow to the radial and ulnar arteries if the brachial artery is obstructed. *b*, The palmar arches usually provide adequate flow to the hand and fingers when either the ulnar or radial arteries are obstructed. *c*, The deep femoral artery is the only collateral source of flow to the lower extremity—it usually originates well below the level of the inguinal ligament; thus, obstruction to flow in the femoral artery above this point leaves the lower extremity without arterial blood flow. *d*, The arterial arches that provide blood flow to the feet and toes are usually supplied by both the dorsalis pedis and the posterior tibial arteries. (Reproduced by permission from Shapiro, B. et al. Clinical Application of Blood Gases, 3rd ed. Chicago, Year Book Medical Publishers, 1982.)

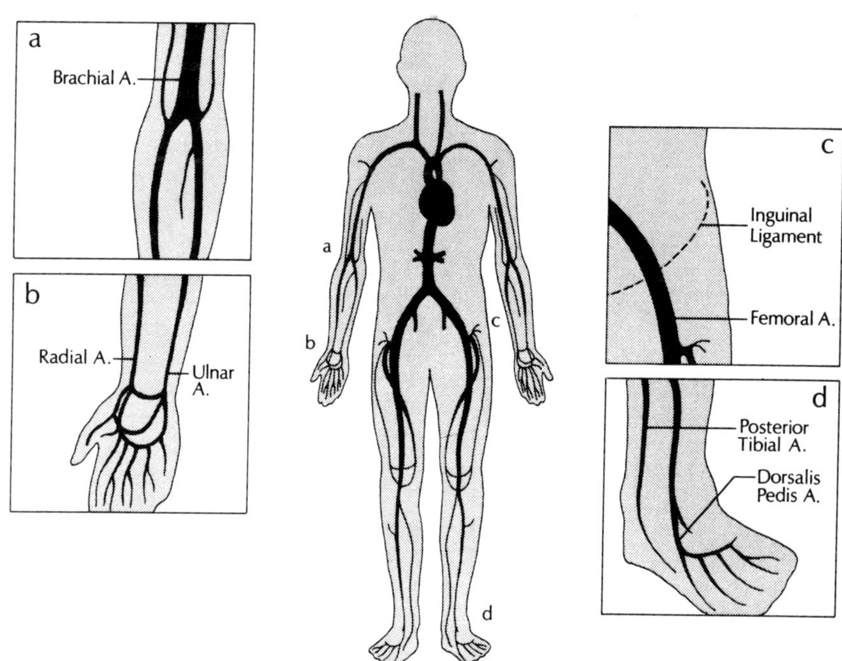

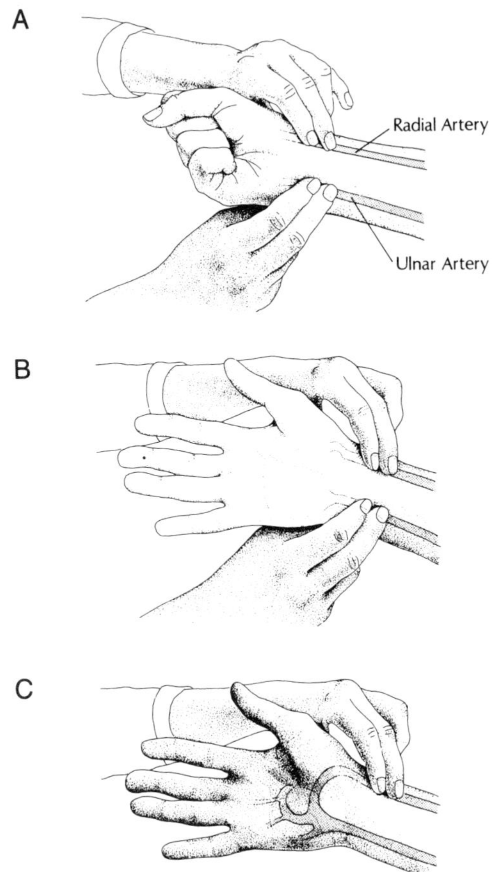

Figure 13–3. Allen's test.

1. Ask the patient to make a fist. This action forces blood from the hand.
2. Apply pressure over the radial and ulnar arteries, as shown in A.
3. Tell the patient to release the fist and relax the hand, while you maintain pressure over the arteries. Note the blanched appearance of palm and fingers (B).
4. Remove pressure from the ulnar artery. The hand should become flushed within 15 seconds, as blood from the ulnar artery refills the capillary bed (C).
5. A flushed hand indicates a *positive Allen's test* finding and a suitable radial artery for puncture. A hand with incomplete to absent capillary refill indicates a *negative Allen's test* finding—puncture of the radial artery is contraindicated.

(Reproduced by permission from Shapiro, B., Harrison, R., and Walton, J.: Clinical Application of Blood Gases, 3rd ed. Chicago, Year Book Medical Publishers, 1982.)

before blood sampling. Once a glass syringe is heparinized, it is held with the needle down to prevent the plunger from sliding back and letting in air.

A glass syringe is better than a plastic syringe because it freely fills from arterial pressures; it facilitates inspection and removal of air bubbles; and it permits minimal contamination and loss of gases (Clausen, 1984).

Disposal of excess heparin from the syringe is important because too much heparin can introduce artifacts into the ABG results. The value affected the most is $Pa{CO_2}$—increased amounts of heparin or small quantities of blood decrease $Pa{CO_2}$ (Bageant, 1975). For this reason, heparin-filled stopcocks are not routinely inserted between needle and syringe to simultaneously draw blood for other laboratory tests. Similarly, preheparinized scalp vein needles (i.e., butterfly infusion sets) are never used for "difficult sticks," unless the heparin in the dead space is allowed to drip out before blood is aspirated into the syringe.

Most commercial ABG kits contain a plastic preheparinized syringe, e.g., Omnistik ABG syringe (Petty and Bailey, 1981). This type of syringe is preheparinized with dry or lyophilized heparin and vented to facilitate bubble-free, anaerobic blood sampling. While this syringe eliminates the problem of heparin dilution, it may not be as effective in preventing clot formation (Clausen, 1984).

8. *Position the patient.* Hyperextend the patient's arm on a table or bed. *For a radial stick,* dorsiflex the patient's wrist about 30 degrees and place a small rolled towel underneath the wrist for support. *For a brachial stick,* rotate the patient's hand outward with the wrist hyperextended. Place a rolled towel under the elbow. *For a femoral stick,* the leg is rotated outward slightly. Put on gloves if the patient's blood is positive for hepatitis, AIDS, or other disorders communicated by blood contact. Sit down so that you can comfortably relocate the artery and perform the puncture.

9. *Relocate the artery.* For a radial stick, palpate the wrist and identify the site where the arterial pulse is maximal.

10. *Cleanse the area with an alcohol swab.*

11. *Secure the artery* along the artery's course, with one finger (Fig. 13–4) or with two fingers about 3 cm apart (Fig. 13–5). Apply gentle pressure—excessive pressure will occlude blood flow. For a fleeting pulse, rotate the wrist slightly or adjust hyperextension until a better pulse is palpable.

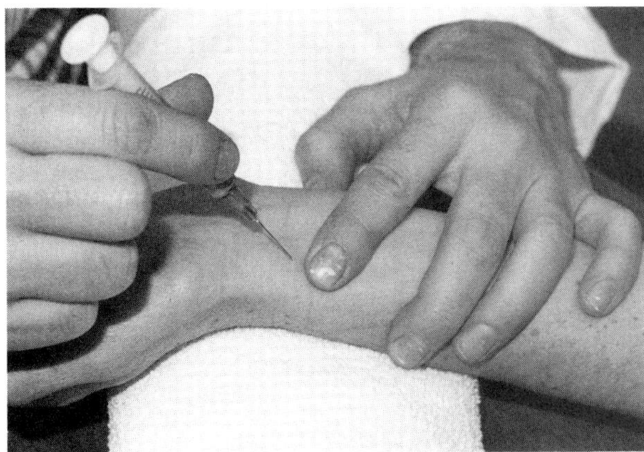

Figure 13–4. Radial arterial puncture. The index finger of one hand palpates the radial artery to determine artery location, while other fingers help to stabilize the forearm. The other hand holds the syringe and needle and punctures the artery, maintaining a 45-degree angle at the skin surface.

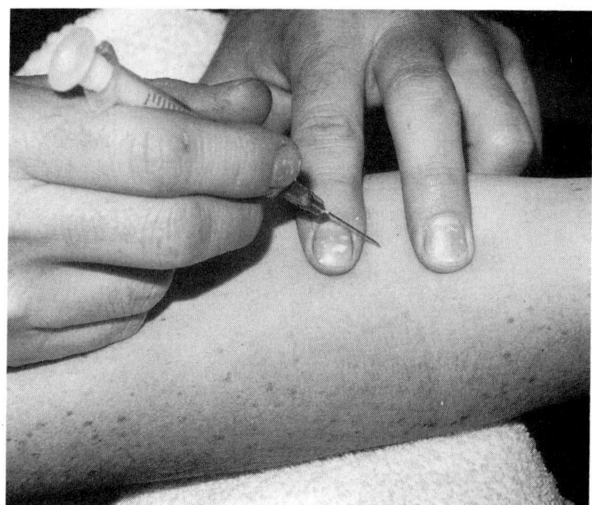

Figure 13–5. Brachial arterial puncture. Two fingers of one hand localize and immobilize a section of the brachial artery. The puncture is performed between the two fingers, maintaining a 45-degree angle at the skin surface.

12. *Perform the puncture.* With the needle's bevel facing up, insert the needle between the two fingers, parallel to the artery's course, and at a 45-degree angle with the skin surface. Puncture the skin slowly, constantly watching the needle's hub for the appearance of blood. If blood appears, stop the needle's advancement and allow the blood to flow freely into the syringe. For plastic syringes, you may need to pull back gently on the plunger to start blood flow and obtain enough blood. If the puncture is unsuccessful and the needle passes through both walls of the artery, slowly withdraw the needle until the tip reenters the artery and blood flows into the hub. If the attempt is still unsuccessful and a good pulse is still present, withdraw the needle a few millimeters and redirect it to the right or left, or wherever the pulse is maximal. If the pulse disappears, *immediately withdraw the needle*—the artery is probably in spasm; a puncture at a different site is required. The physician is called to draw the ABG after two unsuccessful arterial punctures.

13. *Obtain a 2 to 5 ml blood sample.* For serial ABGs, try to consistently collect the same amount of blood to avoid different heparin dilutional effects.

14. *Care for the puncture site.* Immediately after needle withdrawal, apply direct pressure to the puncture site for 3 to 5 minutes—10 minutes for patients on anticoagulants or those with low platelet counts or other clotting disorders. If the site continues to bleed, apply pressure for an additional 3 minutes or until oozing stops. Apply a Band-Aid or Elastoplast (optional), when bleeding has been excessive. In 5 to 10 minutes, check the site for the presence of a pulse and the absence of bleeding.

15. *Prepare the blood sample for the laboratory.* Immediately after sampling, ask another health team member to hold the puncture site while you prepare the blood sample. With the needle pointed up, express all air bubbles, using 2×2 or 4×4 gauze to catch spilled blood. Stick the needle into a rubber stopper or remove the needle and apply a rubber plug to seal the sample. Roll the syringe between your fingers to evenly distribute the heparin. Label the syringe. Place the syringe in a cup or a plastic bag containing ice slush. Samples stored at room temperature result in misleading ABG results, unless analysis is performed immediately after collection. Clausen (1984) reports that as long as a glass syringe with a close-fitting plunger is used, and the $PaCO_2$ of the blood sample is less than 150 mmHg, a sample may be stored in ice for up to 2 hours without significant changes in ABG results. Since these requirements are not always met, samples should be analyzed as soon as possible or within 45 minutes. Prompt analysis is most important when PaO_2 is greater than 150 mmHg, as in shunt studies, or when plastic syringes are used.

ARTERIAL LINE AND MIXED VENOUS BLOOD SAMPLING

Arterial puncture is unnecessary when a patient has an indwelling arterial cannula for serial blood sampling and continuous arterial pressure monitoring. In brief, *to draw an ABG from an arterial line,* the nurse aspirates diluted blood from a stopcock proximal to the cannula and discards it. Then, the nurse draws the blood sample with a preheparinized syringe (Fig. 13–6) and flushes the line after sampling.

Steps for drawing a mixed venous blood gas sample are presented in Chapter 29.

Interpretation of Blood Gas Measurements

In hospital and outpatient settings, ABG results are relayed by telephone to the nurse or physician ideally within 1 hour of the arterial puncture. Interpretation of arterial and other blood gas results occurs in two ways. First, the nurse utilizes previous knowledge and experience to interpret selected values, such as PaO_2 and SaO_2, on the spur of the moment. Second, the nurse may use a more systematic method, such as the one presented at the end of this chapter, for a more detailed and complete interpretation. Both of these approaches require knowledge of normal ranges as well as the grouping of measurements into basic categories to facilitate interpretation (Table 13–1).

LABORATORY NORMAL RANGES FOR ABGs

The normal range for arterial measurements will vary slightly, depending on each laboratory's estab-

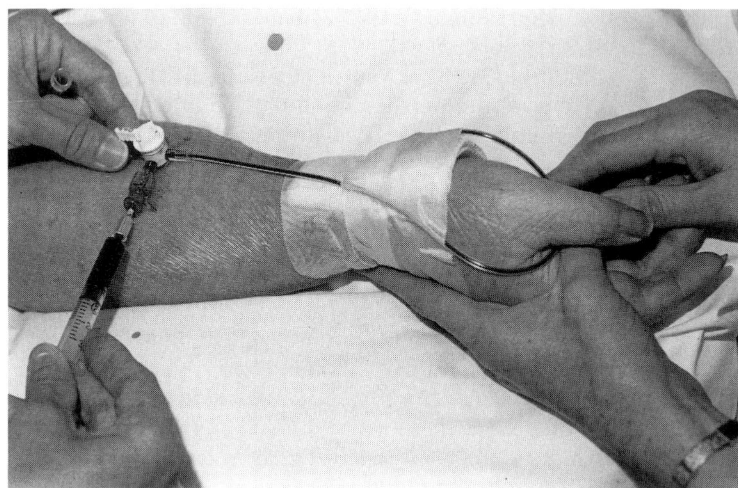

Figure 13–6. Blood sampling from an arterial line. One nurse draws the blood from a proximal stopcock. Another person's touch provides psychologic support while stabilizing the hand and wrist.

lished normal range. The normal ranges are determined by statistical analysis of a large representative population. Hence, in different practice settings, the nurse preferably should interpret ABG results using the range determined by the local laboratory where the patient's blood was analyzed.

Note in Table 13–1 that two ranges are given for $PaCO_2$ and pH (a measure of hydrogen ion concentration in the blood). This text consistently uses the first range without the parentheses. Since other sources may use other ranges, a brief explanation will help clarify why both ranges are acceptable and why incongruities still remain between medical sources and clinical settings.

The narrow pH range of 7.38 to 7.42 and the narrow $PaCO_2$ range of 38 to 42 mmHg represent the first standard deviation (1 SD) from the mean values of 7.40 and 40 mmHg respectively. The broader pH range of 7.35 to 7.45 and the $PaCO_2$ range of 35 to 45 mmHg represent the second standard deviation (2 SD) from the mean. Variability in normal biologic function and normal range is inevitable in large diverse populations. The 2 SD values are commonly used because they statistically represent "normal" for 95% of a given population. The narrower ranged 1 SD values represent "normal" for only about 66% of a given population. Clinicians who use the broad range state that although it may not detect abnormality in some patients, minor variations from normal are seldom therapeutically significant. Those using the narrow range, including many pulmonary specialists, believe it is more sensitive. One can detect subtle changes in $PaCO_2$ and pH that often signal the beginning of clinical deterioration or improvement. Also, if the less sensitive broad range of normal is used, patients with values at the lower or higher limits of normal may already show early clinical signs of an acid-base disorder.

GROUPING OF MEASUREMENTS FOR INTERPRETATION

To avoid confusion and simplify interpretation, the nurse can mentally regroup blood gas measurements in the chart into three assessment categories as follows: (1) oxygenation, (2) ventilation, and (3) acid-base balance. The first pertains to the assessment of the oxygenation status of the patient. The second pertains to the adequacy of alveolar ventilation. The third helps the nurse assess the nature and severity of respiratory and metabolic disorders.

Since blood gas measurements are easily confused and blood gas interpretation and associated problem identification depend on the ability to constantly think in terms of oxygenation, ventilation, and acid base balance, most measurements will be repeated in summary form throughout the remainder of this text. The particular parameter under discussion at the moment is oxygenation (see the box). Note that specific measurements are listed. Problems that the measurements assess are also listed.

Assessment of Oxygenation

OXYGENATION

MEASUREMENTS	***PROBLEMS***
Arterial: PaO_2, SaO_2	Hypoxemia
Intrapulmonary shunt: A-aO_2 gradient, a/A, $\dot{Q}_S/\dot{Q}_T$	Hypoxia
Venous: $P\bar{v}O_2$, $C(a-\bar{v})O_2$	

ABG interpretation begins by assessing PaO_2 and SaO_2 measurements, because when these values are subnormal, the patient has an immediate need for oxygen therapy and other interventions to correct the hypoxemia, hypoxia, or both.

HYPOXEMIA

Remember (see Chapter 3) that *normal* PaO_2 is 80 to 100 mmHg or 60 to 80 mmHg in the elderly.

Table 13–1. MEASUREMENTS OF OXYGENATION, VENTILATION, AND ACID-BASE BALANCE

Measurement	Definition	Normal Range or Values
Oxygenation		
PaO_2	Partial pressure of oxygen in arterial blood	80 to 100 mmHg
SaO_2*	Percent saturation of hemoglobin with oxygen in arterial blood	Greater than 95%
A-aO_2 gradient	Oxygen pressure difference between alveoli and arterial blood; also written as P(A-a)O_2, and A-aDO_2.	5 to 20 mm Hg
a/A ratio	Partial pressure of oxygen in arterial blood divided by alveolar oxygen partial pressure or PaO_2/PAO_2.	Greater than or equal to 0.80
CaO_2	Content of oxygen in arterial blood expressed as ml per 100 ml blood or vol %.	16 to 20 ml/100 ml blood
$\dot{Q}_S/\dot{Q}_T$	Shunted cardiac output (L/min) divided by total cardiac output (L/min), expressed as a percent.	5% to 10%
$P\bar{v}O_2$	Partial pressure of oxygen in mixed venous blood drawn from a pulmonary artery catheter.	35 to 40 mmHg
$C(a-\bar{v})O_2$	Difference in oxygen content between arterial blood and mixed venous blood, expressed in ml per 100 ml blood; also written as $CaO_2 - C\bar{v}O_2$ (vol %).	3.5 to 5 ml/100 ml blood
Ventilation		
$PaCO_2$	Partial pressure of carbon dioxide in arterial blood	38 to 42 mmHg or 35 to 45 mmHg
Acid-Base Balance		
pH	Hydrogen ion concentration in the blood	7.38 to 7.42 or 7.35 to 7.45
$PaCO_2$	Partial pressure of carbon dioxide in arterial blood	38 to 42 mmHg or 35 to 45 mmHg
HCO_3^-	Plasma bicarbonate concentration	24 to 30 mEq/L
BE	Base excess	+2 to −2 mEq/L
Anion gap	Estimate of unmeasured cations minus unmeasured anions	12 to 16 mEq/L

*See Chapter 29 for $S\bar{v}O_2$ − Percent saturation of hemoglobin with oxygen in mixed venous blood. Normal = 60 to 80%.

Hypoxemia is defined as PaO_2 of less than 80 mmHg. Reductions in PaO_2 are assessed based on two factors as follows:

1. Whether the reduction occurs at the top of the oxyhemoglobin dissociation curve, where both PaO_2 and SaO_2 are high. 2. Whether the reduction occurs towards the bottom of the curve—in the critical zone (PaO_2 below 60 mmHg)—where a small reduction in PaO_2 results in a proportionately larger reduction in SaO_2.

The second case is more likely to result in life-threatening hypoxemia. If these concepts are unfamiliar, take time to review oxygenation in Chapter 3 before reading further in this chapter.

Pulmonary and extrapulmonary causes of hypoxemia are presented in Chapter 3. The four pulmonary causes of hypoxemia are (1) alveolar hypoventilation, (2) right-to-left intrapulmonary shunting, (3) diffusion defect, and (4) ventilation perfusion abnormality.

Alveolar Hypoventilation as a Cause of Hypoxemia

Alveolar hypoventilation is defined as a $PaCO_2$ level *above* the normal range of 38 to 42 mmHg or 35 to 45 mmHg, if 2 SD values are used, as previously explained. *Ventilatory failure* is present when $PaCO_2$ increases *above 50 mmHg.*

Hypoxemia occurs simultaneously with alveolar hypoventilation because of the following rule:

RELATIONSHIP BETWEEN $PaCO_2$ AND PaO_2 ON ROOM AIR

A change in $PaCO_2$ causes an equal and opposite change in PaO_2 and vice versa.

For example, if a patient's $PaCO_2$ increases from 40 mmHg to 60 mmHg, the PaO_2 simultaneously decreases by 20 mmHg. Conversely, if PaO_2 increases by 20 mmHg, $PaCO_2$ decreases by 20 mmHg.

This rule does not apply to individuals receiving supplementary oxygen because supplementary oxygen alters normal pressure relationships in the lungs. Also, the relationship may not apply to renal dialysis patients. During dialysis, a portion of CO_2 produced by the tissues is cleared by the dialysis machine, resulting in a *decreased* respiratory drive to breathe, *decreased* lung ventilation, and *decreased* PaO_2. However, arterial hydrogen ion concentration and $PaCO_2$ remain within *normal* limits.

Right-to-Left Intrapulmonary Shunting

Right-to-left intrapulmonary shunting, also called total *physiologic shunt*, is present when blood passes from the right side of the heart through the lungs to the left side *without* participating in gas exchange with alveolar air. Physiologic shunt is divided into three parts as follows: (1) *anatomic shunt*, (2) *capillary shunt*, and (3) *venous admixture*.

Anatomic Shunt. Oxygenated blood supplying the lung's bronchial circulation returns unoxygenated to the left side of the heart. This 2 to 5% of the total cardiac output is *normal anatomic shunt*. *Pathologic anatomic shunt* may be pulmonary or cardiac in origin. A right-to-left anatomic *intrapulmonary* shunt results from bronchiectasis, a large vascular lung tumor, or an intrapulmonary fistula permitting blood to pass directly into pulmonary veins without alveolar contact (Fig. 13–7 shows resulting V/Q ratio). Fistulas may be congenital or arise from chest trauma or disease. An *intracardiac* shunt usually arises from a congenital

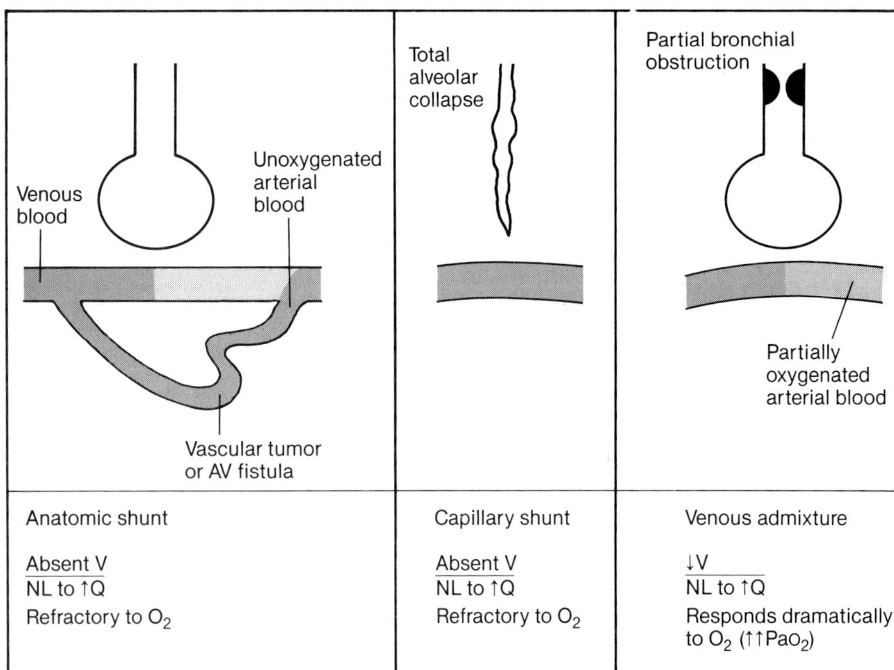

Figure 13–7. Absolute shunt (anatomic and capillary) versus venous admixture.

heart disease, e.g., in atrial septal defect, unoxygenated blood completely bypasses the lungs and moves directly from the right atrium into the left atrium.

Capillary Shunt. Capillary shunting results from pulmonary capillary blood in contact with *totally* unventilated alveoli (Shapiro et al, 1982). Blood passes through pulmonary capillaries without becoming oxygenated, as in the case of total bronchial obstruction from mucus consolidation, tumor, or total collapse of a lobe of a lung.

The sum of anatomic and capillary shunts is called *true* or *absolute shunt.* It is called absolute because oxygenation does *not* significantly improve when the hypoxemic individual receives oxygen therapy.

Venous Admixture. Venous admixture is defined as *perfusion in excess of ventilation;* it occurs when alveolar ventilation becomes decreased—*but not totally absent*—as in the case of capillary shunt. Venous admixture may occur in any chest disorder characterized by unevenness in the distribution of ventilation and perfusion, particularly the former. Examples include obstructive lung diseases (e.g., bronchitis, asthma, and bronchiectasis) and interstitial lung disorders. In partial bronchial obstruction (see Fig. 13–7), the alveolus is patent, but alveolar ventilation (V_A) is decreased though not absent, since the exchange of old air for new fresh air is impaired. The Pao_2 approaches Pvo_2 with increasing airway obstruction.

Essentially, venous admixture is an example of a ventilation perfusion abnormality. Its clinical significance is that unlike absolute shunt, *venous admixture responds dramatically to oxygen therapy.* A small increase in the concentration of inspired oxygen results in a large increase in Pao_2. The clinician often cannot differentiate hypoxemia due to absolute shunt from that due to venous admixture until FIo_2 is increased and the different Po_2 responses are observed. Hence, the combined effects of absolute shunt and venous admixture are sometimes casually referred to as venous admixture or shunt-like effect (Murray, 1983).

The concept of right-to-left intrapulmonary shunting is an important one because shunting is a common cause of hypoxemia. In all the aforementioned types of intrapulmonary shunting, the degree of oxygen supply impairment depends on the extent of the anatomic abnormality, the degree of desaturation of shunted blood entering the left side of the heart, the total blood O_2 content, and most important the ability to increase cardiac output. Cardiac output indirectly affects degree of hypoxemia by altering oxygen delivery and the Po_2 of shunted blood. With a stable metabolic rate, an increased cardiac output improves oxygen delivery. This results in a decrease in the amount of oxygen extracted from any given volume of blood and increases the Po_2 of venous blood and the amount of hemoglobin still saturated with oxygen.

Measurement of Intrapulmonary Shunting. One or more of the methods described subsequently may be used to estimate intrapulmonary shunting.

The A-ao_2 Gradient. The *alveolar to arterial pressure gradient,* the previously mentioned PAo_2-Pao_2 pressure gradient, abbreviated *A-ao_2 gradient,* is perhaps the most commonly used parameter for estimation of hypoxemia and intrapulmonary shunting. It is also known as the *A-a oxygen difference* (A-aDo_2). To obtain an A-ao_2 gradient

1. Note FIO_2. The A-aO_2 gradient can be measured on any oxygen concentration, but Shapiro and associates (1982) recommend an FIO_2 no greater than 0.50 to 0.60. Wait 15 to 30 minutes, if FIO_2 changed recently.
2. Obtain an arterial blood gas sample.
3. Calculate the gradient using the formula in the box to the right.

The normal range for the A-aO_2 gradient is 5 to 20 mmHg—the amount due to normal anatomic shunt. A value *over 20 mmHg* indicates *increased shunting.*

The A-aO_2 gradient is particularly useful in two situations. *First,* it helps the physician determine the presence of primary lung disease. For example, consider an undiagnosed individual with a low PaO_2 and a high $PaCO_2$. If the gradient is found to be *normal,* then respiratory problems are of *extracardiopulmonary origin.* If the gradient is *above normal,* cardiopulmonary disease is present. Provided congenital heart disease and intracardiac shunt have been ruled out, the individual's abnormal blood gases are a manifestation of a primary lung disease.

Second, the A-aO_2 gradient helps determine how much physiologic shunt is due to venous admixture from underventilated alveoli. A dramatic decrease in gradient with the administration of a higher FIO_2 suggests pathology is due to venous admixture rather than absolute shunt.

Measurement of the A-aO_2 gradient has its limitations. It gives only an estimate of the degree of intrapulmonary shunting, because the measured value changes with different cardiac outputs and inspired oxygen concentrations. In the latter case, although increasing FIO_2 will improve shunting due to venous admixture, it may aggravate capillary shunting by causing absorption atelectasis (to be described subsequently). Moreover, for any given degree of absolute shunting, the A-aO_2 gradient will increase with greater FIO_2. The increase in shunting may be dramatic in respiratory patients with already underventilated but perfused lung areas.

For the aforementioned reasons, the *PaO_2/PA_{O_2} ratio,* abbreviated *a/A ratio,* may be utilized along with the A-aO_2 gradient to either compensate for FIO_2 changes or help diagnose pulmonary disease (see steps 5 and 6 in the previous box). The normal ratio is about 0.80; the value decreases as intrapulmonary shunting increases. Some clinicians may use related ratios for the same purpose, e.g., A-a_{O_2} gradient/PAO_2 (Fromm, 1979); PaO_2/FIO_2 (Pierson, 1983; and Cohen et al, 1983).

The $\dot{Q}_A/\dot{Q}_T$ Shunt Equation. The $\dot{Q}_S/\dot{Q}_T$ equation is another method of determining shunt. It measures the fraction of total cardiac output (Q_T) that is not oxygenated during passage through the lungs (see the next box for calculations). While this equation is a more specific measure of intrapulmonary shunting than the A-aO_2 gradient, and hence is considered more accurate, it is not always used because it requires a mixed

---

CALCULATION OF THE ALVEOLAR-ARTERIAL (A-a) OXYGEN GRADIENT AND A-aO_2 GRADIENT RATIO

1. Check ABG results for arterial oxygen pressure (PaO_2) and carbon dioxide pressure ($PaCO_2$) values.
2. Determine the alveolar oxygen pressure (PA_{O_2}) by means of the following alveolar air equation:

$$PA_{O_2} = [(FIO_2) \times (P_B - 47)] - \frac{PaCO_2}{R}$$

FIO_2 = fractional concentration of inspired oxygen.

B_B = barometric pressure (760 mmHg at sea level).

R = respiratory exchange ratio of 0.8 that remains relatively stable in health and even in severe lung disease (Demers and Irwin, 1979).

EXAMPLE

Individual breathing room air with a PaO_2 of 90 mmHg and $PaCO_2$ of 40 mmHg.

$$PA_{O_2} = [(0.21) \times (760-47)] - \frac{40}{0.8}$$
$$= 150 - 50$$
$$= 100 \text{ mmHg}$$

3. A-a oxygen gradient equals PA_{O_2} minus PaO_2.

EXAMPLE

100 mmHg − 90 mmHg = 10 mmHg (normal value)

4. The normal range for A-aO_2 gradient is 5 to 20 mmHg. In the supine position, A-aO_2 gradient increases about 4 mmHg (3 mmHg in the upright position) per decade above the age of 20 years, starting at 5 mmHg, the value for healthy 20-year-old nonsmokers breathing room air (Demers and Irwin, 1979).
5. Calculate the PaO_2/PA_{O_2} (a/A) ratio, if the patient is breathing a high FIO_2 (greater than 0.60).

EXAMPLE

$$\frac{PaO_2}{PA_{O_2}} = \frac{80 \text{ mmHg}}{100 \text{ mmHg}} = 0.80 \text{ (normal)}$$

6. An a/A ratio of less than 0.80 suggests the presence of primary lung disease; the value decreases as intrapulmonary shunting increases.

venous blood sample. This type of blood sample must be drawn through an indwelling pulmonary artery catheter, an invasive monitoring device not always present in the patient.

CALCULATION OF $\dot{Q}_S/\dot{Q}_T$ (Q_S = SHUNTED CARDIAC OUTPUT AND Q_T = TOTAL CARDIAC OUTPUT)

CLASSIC SHUNT EQUATION

$$\frac{Cc\text{O}_2 - \text{CaO}_2}{\text{Cc}\text{O}_2 - \text{C}\bar{\text{v}}\text{O}_2}$$

CcO_2 = pulmonary capillary oxygen content
CaO_2 = arterial oxygen content
$\text{C}\bar{\text{v}}\text{O}_2$ = mixed venous oxygen content

The following calculations are made after the patient has been placed on 100% oxygen for 15 to 20 minutes. Arterial and mixed venous blood samples are drawn and sent to the laboratory for PaO_2, PaCO_2 and $\text{P}\bar{\text{v}}\text{O}_2$ analyses.

1. Calculate CcO_2.
   a. Pulmonary capillary oxygen tension is assumed equal to alveolar oxygen tension. $\text{PA}_{\text{O}2}$ is derived from the alveolar air equation as follows:

$$\text{PA}_{\text{O}_2} = [(\text{FIO}_2) \times (\text{P}_\text{B} - 47)] - \frac{\text{PaCO}_2}{\text{R}}$$

   b. Calculate CcO_2 utilizing information on page 46.

$$(\text{HgB} \times 1.34) + (\text{PA}_{\text{O}2} \times 0.0031)$$

2. Calculate CaO_2: (Hbg × 1.34 × SaO_2) + (PaO_2 × 0.0031)
3. Calculate $\text{C}\bar{\text{v}}\text{O}_2$: (Hbg × 1.34 × $\text{S}\bar{\text{v}}\text{O}_2$) + ($\text{P}\bar{\text{v}}\text{O}_2$ × 0.0031)
4. Insert appropriate numbers into the $\dot{Q}_S/\dot{Q}_T$ shunt equation. The normal value for a healthy subject is 5% (0.05) to 10% (0.10). The value increases as intrapulmonary shunting increases.
5. The following *clinical shunt equation* is sometimes used instead of the classic equation because it is simpler and can be used with FIO_2 values lower than 1.0. However, it is less accurate and must be employed with patients who have stable cardiovascular status, normal metabolism, and fully saturated hemoglobin. It is best with an FIO_2 of 1.0, when shunt is less than 30% and PaO_2 is greater than 100 mmHg.

$$\frac{\dot{Q}_S}{\dot{Q}_T} = \frac{(\text{PA}_{\text{O}2} - \text{PaO}_2)\ (0.0031)}{(4.5 \text{ vol }\%) + (\text{PA}_{\text{O}2} - \text{PaO}_2)\ (0.0031)}$$

A 4.5 vol % is the assumed normal A-$\bar{\text{v}}\text{O}_2$ gradient.

Shunt Estimation. In some situations, clinicians may prefer to omit calculations of A-aO_2 gradient and Q_S/Q_T and estimate shunt as follows: As long as FIO_2 is at 1.0 and PaO_2 is 100 mmHg or greater, *add 5% shunt for every 100 mmHg below 700 mmHg.* For example, for a PaO_2 of 500 mmHg on 100% O_2, the patient has a 10% shunt. This method is adequate for general assessment.

Diffusion Defect

Diffusion defect refers to the impairment of gas diffusion across the alveolar-capillary membrane owing to diseases such as emphysema and interstitial fibrosis. In these and other diseases, the obliteration of capillaries and alveoli reduces the surface area available for gas exchange. This loss of surface area is responsible for the diffusion defect (see Chapter 14).

By itself, diffusion defect is a rare cause of hypoxemia. However, under certain conditions (e.g., exercise, low FIO_2), it may be the main cause. In disease states, diffusion defect becomes a factor only in the presence of other severe abnormalities, such as V/Q abnormality and decreased red blood cell transit time past the alveolar capillary membrane.

Ventilation-Perfusion Abnormality

The main cause of hypoxemia is ventilation-perfusion abnormality, specifically a *low V/Q ratio* for regional areas of lungs.

Almost all chest diseases are associated with V/Q abnormality, particularly when disease is severe or pathology is distributed unevenly throughout the lungs. Moreover, intrapulmonary shunting is actually considered an extreme form of V/Q abnormality, with ventilation totally absent rather than merely decreased.

Why Low V/Q Ratio Produces Hypoxemia. Chapter 5 introduced the concept of low V/Q ratio. A low PaO_2 results when high V/Q lung regions cannot compensate for low V/Q regions with respect to O_2 exchange. A brief explanation will help the nurse understand exactly why patients with low V/Q ratios become hypoxemic.

In Figure 13–8, blood from high and low V/Q regions mixes, producing new blood gases for arterial blood. In the example on the left, alveolar ventilation decreases due to a chest disease, such as emphysema and partial bronchial obstruction. Alveolar PCO_2 is high (50 mmHg), and alveolar PO_2 is extremely low (40 mmHg). Perfusion remains normal and V/Q ratio low, as summarized.

$$\frac{\downarrow \text{V}}{\text{NL Q}} = \downarrow \text{V/Q ratio}$$

The patient compensates by increasing ventilation to healthy lung units, in an attempt to reduce PCO_2 and increase PO_2. On the right side of Figure 13–8, the increased ventilation drastically lowers $\text{PA}_{\text{CO}2}$. It

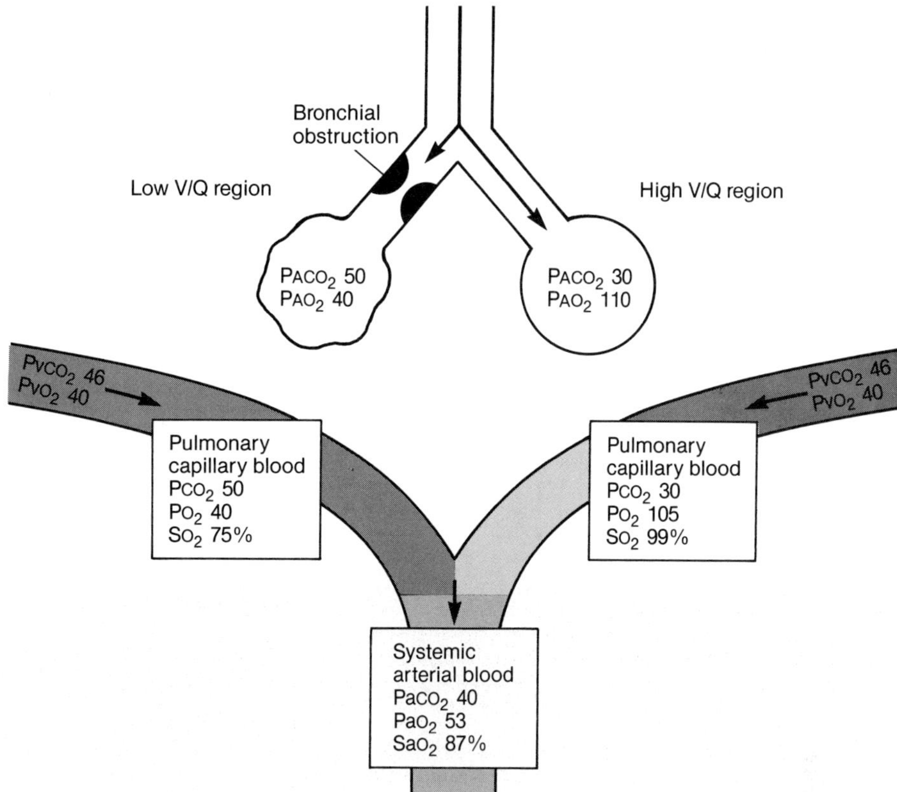

Figure 13–8. Hypoxemia due to a low V/Q ratio. High V/Q regions cannot compensate for low V/Q regions with regard to O_2 exchange.

has a great impact on arterial PCO_2, returning it to normal (40 mmHg). Note that averaging the pulmonary capillary PCO_2 values from high and low V/Q regions results in an arterial PCO_2 value that lies exactly between the two extremes. Averaging is appropriate because the relationship between CO_2 tension and content is linear.

However, compensatory hyperventilation cannot remedy the markedly oxygen desaturated blood flowing past diseased low V/Q regions. The reason is related to the curved as opposed to the linear shape of the previously described oxyhemoglobin desaturation curve. At the flat top of the curve, increasing PaO_2 to over 100 mmHg will not improve SaO_2, because the hemoglobin is already fully saturated with oxygen. Hence, in high V/Q regions, alveolar hyperventilation will increase P_{AO_2} and PaO_2 but not SaO_2, the most important determinant of oxygenation. With this information in mind, when equal proportions of blood from high and low V/Q regions are mixed, the following conclusions hold true:

1. Arterial PO_2 is determined by *first* averaging pulmonary capillary oxygen saturations (not PaO_2s) from involved lung regions. In Figure 13–8, the average of 75% and 99% is 87% SaO_2. The value for PaO_2 (53 mmHg in this case) is then read from the oxyhemoglobin dissociation curve.
2. Arterial PO_2 increases to a level only slightly above that of the low V/Q region.
3. When regional mismatching is great, SaO_2 remains below normal, and the patient remains hypoxemic.

Furthermore, two factors tend to exacerbate V/Q mismatching between high and low V/Q regions and limit the ability to normalize ABGs. First, most high V/Q units (regions) are located at the top of the lungs, where perfusion is normally reduced. These units have a relatively small impact on PaO_2 because they contribute a relatively small volume of blood to the systemic circulation compared with the well-perfused units at the lung bases. Second, though attempts may occur to compensate for a low V_A by increasing cardiac output, the increase in perfusion to low V/Q regions promotes V/Q mismatching, as the following ratio shows:

$$\frac{\downarrow V_A}{\uparrow Q} = \downarrow\downarrow \frac{V}{Q} \text{ ratio}$$

The lower V/Q ratio worsens existing hypoxemia.

V/Q Ratios in COPD. Asthma, bronchitis, and emphysema alter V/Q ratios and produce hypoxemia in certain classic situations, e.g., acute asthmatic and blue bloater with chronic bronchitis (see Chapter 7). These ratios and the extent of hypoxemia vary in each patient, depending on the type and extent of pathology and degree of mixed chest disease.

Consider the following different types of emphysema. In the usual type of emphysema (centrilobular), the irregular destruction of alveolar capillary units and accompanying bronchial disease create uneven ventilation and many low V/Q regions in the lungs. The low V/Q regions are responsible for the hypoxemia that occurs commonly and relatively early in the course of the disease.

V/Q abnormality is different in the classic but much rarer panlobular type of emphysema. The pink puffer patient demonstrates the uniform destruction of alveolar capillary units throughout the lungs with little in the way of bronchial disease (see Chapter 7). The relatively uniform pathology results in matched decreases in ventilation and perfusion where alveolar septa are destroyed, such that

$$\frac{\downarrow V}{\downarrow Q} = \text{normal } \frac{V}{Q} \text{ ratio.}$$

The pink puffer is able to maintain normal oxygenation and alveolar ventilation until late in the disease course because high V/Q regions counterbalance low V/Q regions in the lungs, and the V/Q ratio for the lungs as a whole remains normal.

As disease becomes extensive, $Paco_2$ remains normal, since high V/Q regions are still able to compensate for any impairment of CO_2 exchange caused by the low V/Q areas. However, Pao_2 gradually falls, because these high V/Q regions can no longer compensate with respect to O_2 exchange.

With mixed chest pathology (e.g., emphysema with bronchospasm), the dramatic increase in low V/Q regions and decrease in alveolar Po_2 result in profound hypoxemia, worsened by alveolar hypoventilation.

Signs and Symptoms of Hypoxemia

The nurse identifies a possible oxygenation problem by noting the presence of any of the signs and symptoms listed in the box. Then, an ABG sample is drawn to diagnose hypoxemia with certainty and to further evaluate this problem.

Signs and symptoms of hypoxemia vary in number and severity, depending on the type and stage of chest disease, the individual response to illness, and the degree of hypoxia present. On the one hand, when circulation to body tissues is impaired and hypoxia severe, the critically ill or debilitated patient demonstrates most of the manifestations listed in the box, along with a drastically reduced Pao_2. On the other hand, the patient with adequate cardiopulmonary reserves and the same degree of pathology may demonstrate mild hypoxemia (i.e., borderline, low Pao_2) and few clinical signs of hypoxemia. Hypoxemia remains mild because he is able to increase blood flow to compensate for the lack of oxygen.

The four following points are important to remember when monitoring for signs of hypoxemia:

1. *Extent of clinical signs does not always correlate with severity of hypoxemia.* For example, a nurse may encounter a COPD patient who walks into a chest clinic for a routine checkup with no complaints of dyspnea. He may lack clinical signs of hypoxemia, except for slightly blue-tinged lips. Although he states he feels fine, the ABG results reveal a Pao_2 of 40 mmHg, a 15 mmHg drop from baseline value of 55 mmHg. In contrast, an extremely anxious individual may emotionally overreact to mild dyspnea and demonstrate many clinical signs of hypoxemia in spite of a normal Pao_2. Because of this wide variation in response to illness, reporting *any* possible signs of hypoxemia is crucial. Usually, changes in oxygenation precede changes in $Paco_2$ and ventilatory failure.

2. *Cyanosis is a late sign of hypoxemia and is an unreliable index of the state of arterial oxygenation.* Skin color changes depend on the individual's skin thickness and natural pigmentation, capillary density, and effect of external lighting. Also, the development of cyanosis depends on the amount of *reduced hemoglobin* in the blood. Reduced hemoglobin is the oxygen-free form of hemoglobin produced as the result of oxyhemoglobin decomposition. Cyanosis is correlated with the presence of 5 gm or greater reduced hemoglobin per 100 ml blood. Anemic individuals with hypoxemia may never become cyanotic; polycythemic individuals may become obviously cyanotic with mild hypoxemia because they are already slightly blue tinged from the increased amount of reduced hemoglobin in the blood. Under normal circumstances of 15 gm hemoglobin per 100 ml blood, individuals do not become cyanotic until Sao_2 drops to about 80%.

3. *Presenting signs of hypoxemia may be different*

SIGNS AND SYMPTOMS OF HYPOXEMIA

RESPIRATORY
- Dyspnea
- Tachypnea

CARDIOVASCULAR
- Increased heart rate (HR)
- Increased pulmonary vascular resistance
- Cardiac arrhythmias
- Acute hypertension with increased HR (sympathetic response)
- Hypotension with decreased HR
- Paleness or cyanosis

CENTRAL NERVOUS SYSTEM
- Impaired judgment
- Disorientation
- Restlessness
- Combativeness
- Motor incoordination
- Personality change or paranoia
- Delirium
- Coma

OTHER
- General fatigue
- Gradual increase in blood hemoglobin and hematocrit values

than those previously listed. Variations in presenting signs may relate to the individual's response to illness, the presence of ventilatory failure, or the disorders affecting other body organs in addition to the heart and lungs.

4. *Asymptomatic individuals with normal PaO_2s at rest may develop hypoxemia during physical exercise.* PaO_2 during exercise is a more sensitive indicator of hypoxemia and chest disease than clinical signs at the bedside *or* the routinely measured *resting* PaO_2. PaO_2 during exercise is measured in the pulmonary function laboratory.

HYPOXIA

Hypoxia is the lack or insufficient amounts of oxygen in the tissues. Causes are explained in Chapter 3 in relation to the four main types: hypoxemic, circulatory, anemic, and histotoxic hypoxia.

Measurements

Perhaps the quickest way to assess oxygenation of peripheral tissues is to assess *cardiac output,* a major determinant. Indirectly and noninvasively determined signs of an adequate cardiac output include warm well-perfused skin; good urine output; normal pulse pressure, suggestive of normal cardiac stroke volume and heart rate; and normal sensorium. If a pulmonary artery catheter is in place (see Chapter 29), the nurse monitors for a drop in cardiac output and cardiac index, suggestive of decreased oxygen transport to peripheral tissues and possible hypoxia.

Mixed Venous PO_2 ($P\bar{v}O_2$). $P\bar{v}O_2$ is determined directly from a mixed venous blood sample drawn from the pulmonary artery catheter or indirectly from a sample of expired gas. *The normal range is 35 to 40 mmHg.* A value below 30 mmHG indicates tissue hypoxia due to one or more factors, including increased tissue oxygen consumption, decreased PaO_2, and decreased cardiac output. Below the so-called *threshold* or *critical* level of 27 mmHg, tissues turn to anaerobic metabolism, causing lactic acid formation, *increased blood lactate* levels, and lactic acidosis.

Arteriovenous Oxygen Content Difference $C(a-\bar{v})O_2$. The $C(a-\bar{v})O_2$ is *the average amount of oxygen extracted by the tissues per unit volume of blood.* It is determined by calculating the O_2 content of arterial blood (CaO_2) and subtracting the O_2 content of mixed venous blood (CaO_2). A $C(a-\bar{v})O_2$ of about 5 ml/100 ml indicates adequate tissue oxygenation to meet metabolic needs (Zagelbaum and Paré, 1982). A widening (i.e., increased value) of the arteriovenous oxygen difference indicates increased tissue extraction of oxygen due to decreased cardiac output or increased oxygen consumption. A narrowing (i.e., decreased value) for $C(a-\bar{v})O_2$ may be due to septic shock, increased cardiac output, anemia, or increased oxygen affinity (i.e., left shift of the oxyhemoglobin dissociation curve) (Wilkins et al, 1985).

Serial measurements of $P\bar{v}O_2$ and $C(a-\bar{v})O_2$ help assess subtle changes in cardiopulmonary status, as shown in the following example. With the onset of acute illness, the heart compensates by automatically increasing cardiac output. More oxygenated blood reaches peripheral tissues. When well supplied with oxygen, tissues extract less oxygen from capillary blood, and $P\bar{v}O_2$ increases. This increase results in a *decrease* in arterial-venous oxygen content.

A reduction in cardiac output to normal signals cardiac decompensation. $P\bar{v}O_2$ falls, producing an *increase* in the arterial-venous oxygen content difference. It is important to remember that these findings may be observed *before* PaO_2 falls. Hence, in certain situations, the $P\bar{v}O_2$ and $C(a-\bar{v})O_2$ measurements may be more sensitive to cardiopulmonary change than the PaO_2 measurement.

Limitations of $P\bar{v}O_2$. $P\bar{v}O_2$ is best used with other variables to assess tissue oxygenation because of the following limitation: a normal $P\bar{v}O_2$ indicates adequate tissue oxygenation *only* when circulation is intact and tissue oxygen uptake is unimpaired. $P\bar{v}O_2$ may not accurately reflect changes in tissue oxygenation or cardiac output in the presence of histologic hypoxia (e.g., cyanide poisoning) or poor perfusion states (e.g., septic shock, adult respiratory distress syndrome, hemorrhagic shock, congestive heart failure, and various febrile states). In septic shock, for example, a portion of arterial blood bypasses poorly perfused areas of the systemic capillary bed. This *arteriovenous shunting* and the decreased tissue oxygen consumption result in a normal to increased $P\bar{v}O_2$. The areas of poor perfusion contribute little venous blood to total venous blood return, and hence $P\bar{v}O_2$ does not drop to reflect the drastically low $P\bar{v}O_2$ in these regions. Instead, it may increase to represent primarily the well-oxygenated shunted blood (Nelson et al, 1983). For this reason, the accuracy of $P\bar{v}O_2$ is questioned whenever a normal or high value is associated with either a PaO_2 of less than 60 mmHg or an abnormal systemic vascular resistance, or whenever a metabolic acidosis exists.

Signs and Symptoms of Hypoxia

Unless a $P\bar{v}O_2$ measurement is available, it may be difficult if not impossible to assess or identify hypoxia by observation at the bedside. In most cases, if PaO_2 is already low, then any new signs of hypoxemia combined with extreme paleness or cyanosis indicate the presence of hypoxia.

TREATMENT OF HYPOXEMIA

The following two sections present an overview of the treatment of hypoxemia and point out the monitoring considerations to aid in the prevention and early identification of the hazards of oxygen, a powerful drug. This information helps the nurse realize the implications for intervention involved in the identification of hypoxemia or hypoxia as a respiratory problem.

The treatment of hypoxemia consists of oxygen administration; the treatment of the cause of the hypoxemia; and, in selected cases, hyperbaric oxygenation.

Oxygen Administration

The main treatment of hypoxemia is oxygen administration that provides adequate oxygenation at the lowest possible concentration. In some situations, the physician may not treat patients with borderline low Pa_{O_2} values between 55 and 60 mmHg.

The following terms may be used when oxygen is prescribed. (See Chapter 23 for discussion of short-term and long-term oxygen therapy.)

1. *Intermittent* oxygen—less than 24 hours per day.
2. *Continuous* oxygen—24 hours per day or at least 15 to 18 hours per day.
3. *Short-term* oxygen—administered for 30 days or less.
4. *Long-term* oxygen—administered for more than 30 days.
5. *Low-flow* oxygen—via nasal cannula at 1 to 3/L min or via 24% to 28% Venturi mask.

The COPD patient usually requires low flow oxygen, since his baseline Pa_{O_2} is normally low—between 60 to 70 mmHg, and sometimes in the high 50's. Also, hypoxemia is usually due to V/Q abnormalities that are corrected with small amounts of oxygen.

Treatment of the Cause of Hypoxemia

Relief of hypoxemia may be temporary unless the cause is treated simultaneously. In the case of mucus retention, unless the patient coughs, breathes deeply, and expectorates retained secretions, oxygen administration will only partially and temporarily reverse hypoxemia. In fact, if mucus plugs cause extensive airway obstruction, Pa_{O_2} will continue to decrease rather than increase to a therapeutic level.

Hyperbaric Oxygenation

Hyperbaric oxygenation is the administration of a high concentration of oxygen (usually 100%) in an environment of increased atmospheric pressure (usually 2 to 3 atmospheres). This form of oxygen therapy can cause a 22-fold increase in P_{AO_2}. The resultant increase in dissolved oxygen in the blood enhances tissue oxygenation above that which can be achieved at normal atmospheric pressure. Hyperbaric oxygen treatments are performed in single- or multiple-occupancy chambers and are indicated in specific situations. Patients may be critically ill and severely hypoxemic, as in the cases of carbon monoxide poisoning and gas embolism, after a serious underwater diving accident. Except for decompression sickness (i.e., the bends) and gas embolism from underwater diving, hyperbaric oxygenation is used more as an adjunct to medical or surgical intervention to enhance tissue oxygenation. It is not considered to be the primary intervention. In disorders such as burns, compromised skin flaps and grafts, gas gangrene, and skin ulcers, patients may demonstrate tissue hypoxia in the absence of any respiratory problems; hyperbaric treatments serve to promote the healing of injured or hypoxic tissues.

HAZARDS OF OXYGEN

In the treatment of hypoxemia, oxygen is considered a potent drug that must be titrated in precise amounts, according to ABG results. Too little oxygen may worsen hypoxemia; too much may cause alveolar hypoventilation, absorption atelectasis, retrolental fibroplasia, or oxygen toxicity. (See Chapter 23 for hazards associated with oxygen therapy.)

Alveolar Hypoventilation

Oxygen may cause alveolar hypoventilation in patients with COPD. As the COPD patient adjusts to a chronically high Pa_{CO_2} level, the chemoreceptors located in the carotid body and medulla of the brain no longer or minimally respond to changes in Pa_{CO_2}. The remaining stimulus to breathe is hypoxemia. The administration of too much oxygen eliminates this life-sustaining *hypoxic drive* to breathe, which is normally prominent at oxygen tensions of up to 60 mmHg. Hence, for treatment of hypoxemia, COPD patients typically require low flow oxygen, as previously described.

CASE STUDY

Alveolar hypoventilation can occur with small increases in F_{IO_2}. The following case example illustrates this point.

A 65-year-old cachectic man is admitted to an emergency room in acute respiratory distress. The physician recognizes the presence of severe COPD and orders low flow oxygen via nasal cannula at 2 L/min to correct hypoxemia. ABG results (Set A in Table 13–2) indicate that the patient is, in fact, hypoxemic with a Pa_{O_2} of 51 mmHg. He is in ventilatory failure because the Pa_{CO_2} level is above 50 mmHg. The physician wishes to correct the hypoxemia to a Pa_{O_2} level of at least 55 to 60 mmHg but is concerned that the increase in oxygen will eliminate the patient's hypoxic drive to breathe and worsen the ventilatory failure. Subsequent ABG results confirm the physician's concerns. With administration of O_2 at 4 L/min (see ABG results in set B in Table 13–2), oxygenation improved as evidenced by an increased Pa_{O_2} and Sa_{O_2}. However, since the ventilatory failure worsened, i.e., Pa_{CO_2} increased to 65 mmHg, and the patient was becoming more lethargic, the oxygen was titrated to

3 L/min (ABG results in set C of Table 13–2) and finally to 2½ L/min (ABG results in set D of Table 13–2).

Important clinical implications related to this case are summarized as follows:

1. When both $Pa{CO_2}$ and $Pa{O_2}$ are in the 50's, as in the so-called *50/50 COPD patient*, determination of a therapeutic oxygen tension is difficult because of the danger of worsening ventilatory failure while correcting hypoxemia.

2. Though $Pa{O_2}$ and $Pa{CO_2}$ tend to rise about 7 to 10 mmHg/L O_2 administered by nasal cannula, this rule does not apply in all cases. ABG results are unpredictable in individuals with extreme sensitivity to oxygen and those whose A-aO_2 gradients and V/Q abnormalities change to varying degrees with oxygen administration.

3. *Oxygen is a powerful drug!* Increases or decreases in $FI{O_2}$ are carried out with great precision. Calibrated flow meters with quarter (¼, ½, ¾) L/min gradations should be used for COPD patients with hypoxic drives.

4. When COPD patients receive oxygen—and especially when $FI{O_2}$ is increased—the nurse checks for signs and symptoms of *CO_2 narcosis*, the term that describes a patient's clinical condition when alveolar hypoventilation, also called *hypercapnea* and *hypercarbia*, is severe enough to cause respiratory and CNS depression.

Signs and Symptoms of CO_2 Narcosis. Signs and symptoms of CO_2 narcosis are listed in the box.

SIGNS AND SYMPTOMS OF CO_2 NARCOSIS

SYMPTOMS

- Headache
- Lethargy→Drowsiness→Coma

SIGNS

- Papilledema from increased cerebral blood flow
- Redness of skin, sclera, and conjunctiva from increased cutaneous blood flow
- Sweating
- Hypertension and increased heart rate
- Tremulousness or asterixis
- Inappropriate response or lack of response to verbal questioning
- Blank stare into space

Most signs and symptoms are attributed to CO_2's anesthetic effect; its potent cerebral vasodilating effect, which increases cerebral blood flow; and the body's sympathetic response. Many times, the only signs of CO_2 retention are vague complaints of headache, lethargy, and drowsiness. Untreated, these progress to coma, as ventilatory failure becomes worse. Loss of alertness generally occurs when $Pa{CO_2}$ is greater than 70 mmHg, but exceptions to this rule exist. Upon occasion, one encounters a patient with chronic lung disease who engages in appropriate conversation even though the $Pa{CO_2}$ level has climbed to 70 and even to 90 mmHg.

Table 13–2. ABG CHANGES IN A COPD PATIENT WITH HYPOXIC RESPIRATORY DRIVE (ABGs ON NASAL CANNULA)

	Set A	Set B	Set C	Set D
ABG Results	**O_2 at 2 L/min**	**O_2 at 4 L/min**	**O_2 at 3 L/min**	**O_2 at 2½ L/min**
PH	7.39	7.30	7.36	7.37
$Pa{CO_2}$ (mmHg)	55	65	60	57
$Pa{O_2}$ (mmHg)	51	70	58	55
HCO_3^- (mEq/L)	33	34	34	33
$Sa{O_2}$	86%	92%	89%	88%

Absorption Atelectasis

Patients receiving high concentrations of oxygen develop absorption atelectasis, particularly patients with previously compromised lung function. With the administration of 100% O_2, nitrogen is completely washed out of the lungs. This eliminates the large partial pressure of nitrogen (573 mmHg, room air) that normally helps to maintain patent airways and alveoli. What remains is primarily oxygen with small amounts of carbon dioxide and even smaller amounts of water vapor. Alveoli collapse as oxygen is rapidly absorbed into the pulmonary circulation.

Clinical Implications. In emergency or critical situations, mechanical ventilation or manual bagging with 100% oxygen is necessary to treat hypoxemia or to avoid increased risk of hypoxemia. High concentrations are mandatory in order to improve tissue oxygenation. In other situations, however, the administration of 100% oxygen may unnecessarily impair ventilation, particularly if the patient already has adequate ABGs on a much lower $FI{O_2}$ (e.g., 0.21 to 0.25) and does not need the extra oxygen. In normal subjects breathing 100% oxygen, absorption atelectasis occurs within 1 hour, as evidenced by an increased A-aO_2 gradient (Pierson, 1983). In the clinical setting, absorption atelectasis may occur within 3 to 20 minutes, particularly in patients with diseased lung regions with low ventilation in relation to perfusion (Baun and Flones, 1984).

Retrolental Fibroplasia

High concentrations of oxygen may cause a retinopathy in the neonate called *retrolental fibroplasia* that leads to blindness. When $Pa{O_2}$ is increased to levels over 80 mmHg, retinal vessels constrict, causing hemorrhage, retinal detachment, and eventually blindness. Extent of damage is related to degree of prematurity of the newborn, length of exposure to high FIO_2, and degree of PaO_2 elevation. The severity of retrolental fibroplasia may be decreased by the administration of oral vitamin E. After recovery, the infant is at increased risk to develop the chronic pulmonary disorder bronchopulmonary dysplasia.

Oxygen Toxicity

Too much oxygen may cause oxygen toxicity. There are two common manifestations of oxygen toxicity; *CNS toxicity* and *pulmonary oxygen toxicity.*

CNS toxicity. Symptoms of CNS toxicity include *nausea; anxiety; numbness; visual disturbances; muscular twitching,* especially around the eyelids and lips; and *grand mal seizure* (Norkool, 1979). Though pulmonary patients on high concentrations of oxygen breathing at atmospheric pressure may experience some of these symptoms, CNS toxicity is primarily an entity in hyperbaric oxygenation. The physiologic mechanism is not fully understood, but seems to be related to subtle neuronal and biochemical changes that alter the electric activity of the CNS. Avoidance of toxicity is achieved by the administration of 100% oxygen at pressures no greater than 2 atmospheres and by the provision for short periods of breathing of room air during long hyperbaric treatments.

Pulmonary Oxygen Toxicity. The second manifestation of oxygen toxicity is *pulmonary oxygen toxicity,* an entity seldom seen in hyperbaric oxygenation because exposure is intermittent rather than continuous. Prolonged administration of high FIO_2 causes an *oxygen-induced lung injury* that leads to adult or infant respiratory distress syndrome, bronchopulmonary dysplasia, or both (see Chapter 8).

Phases of Acute Lung Injury. The following pathologic changes occur when alveoli are exposed to high oxygen concentrations in the acute care hospital setting. Changes are in two phases, exudative and proliferative. *The exudative phase* occurs after 1 to 4 days of exposure. *During the first 6 hours* of exposure to 100% oxygen, decreased tracheal mucus flow, decreased macrophage function, and tracheobronchitis are observed, while pulmonary function remains normal. *After 6 hours,* vital capacity (i.e., volume exhaled after a full inspiration) begins to decrease. This change is due to (1) poor lung expansion from the substernal chest pain, (2) retained lung water from endothelial cell damage, and (3) progressive atelectasis from rapid absorption of oxygen-rich gas from poorly ventilated alveoli (Jenkinson, 1983). *After 30 hours,* the diffusion of gases across the alveolar capillary membrane becomes progressively more impaired. Loss of surfactant occurs owing to the inactivation of plasma components and the loss of type II alveolar cell function. Atelectasis becomes worse, since incomplete lung expansion prevents renewal of surfactant activity to keep alveoli expanded. Eventually, the classic pathologic features of the exudative phase of oxygen toxicity begin to appear. These features include intra-alveolar, interstitial, and perivascular edema and hemorrhage with necrosis of type I alveolar cells. Protein and fibrin exudates begin to form hyaline membranes, and the clinical picture resembles that of ARDS (see Chapter 8).

The subacute or chronic *proliferative phase* of oxygen-induced injury becomes most prominent on the 12th day of high oxygen exposure. This phase is characterized by progressive resorption of exudates, cellular swelling, and thickening of alveolar septa or blood-air interface due to hyperplasia and hypertrophy of type II alveolar cells. Lungs with these changes are very edematous and heavy, as observed on gross examination at autopsy. Mortality is high in pulmonary oxygen toxicity. Persons who survive demonstrate permanent changes in lung structure and function due to diffuse scarring.

Chronic Oxygen Toxicity. Mild proliferative and fibrotic changes occur in 40 to 50% of COPD patients receiving low-flow (FIO_2, 0.24 to 0.28), long-term oxygen therapy at home (Findley et al, 1983). However, since the benefits of oxygen therapy usually far outweigh any of the minor cell changes that have been reported from autopsy findings, the small degree of toxicity is not of clinical significance.

Monitoring the Patient. The nurse can help monitor for possible signs of toxicity by *first* identifying those patients at increased risk for both absorption atelectasis and pulmonary oxygen toxicity. These include individuals receiving high FIO_2 via the following: mechanical ventilation, breathing devices attached to nebulizers set at high oxygen concentrations, partial rebreathing oxygen masks that deliver up to 60% $oxygen_2$, and nonrebreathing masks that deliver up to 90% oxygen.

Recent blood gas results (PaO_2 and SaO_2) should be available to substantiate the need for a high oxygen concentration. In ARDS of any etiology, daily or hourly ABGs or noninvasive measurements may be necessary to adjust FIO_2 to a level that prevents hypoxemia and, at the same time, minimizes as much as possible oxygen toxicity and absorption atelectasis. The oxygen dilemma encountered in ARDS is summarized in Figure 13–9.

The nurse monitors the high risk patient for early signs of oxygen toxicity, including nonproductive cough and substernal chest pain from tracheobronchitis. Other symptoms may include general malaise, fatigue, and nausea and vomiting. If the patient is unconscious or unable to communicate owing to the presence of an endotracheal tube, the nurse observes for early signs of ARDS as follows: a sudden drop in PaO_2 and a change in vital signs or chest assessment findings indicating respiratory distress.

How Much Oxygen is too Much? Exactly how much oxygen will cause pulmonary oxygen toxicity is a controversial matter now under investigation. The presence and extent of toxicity seems to be governed by a

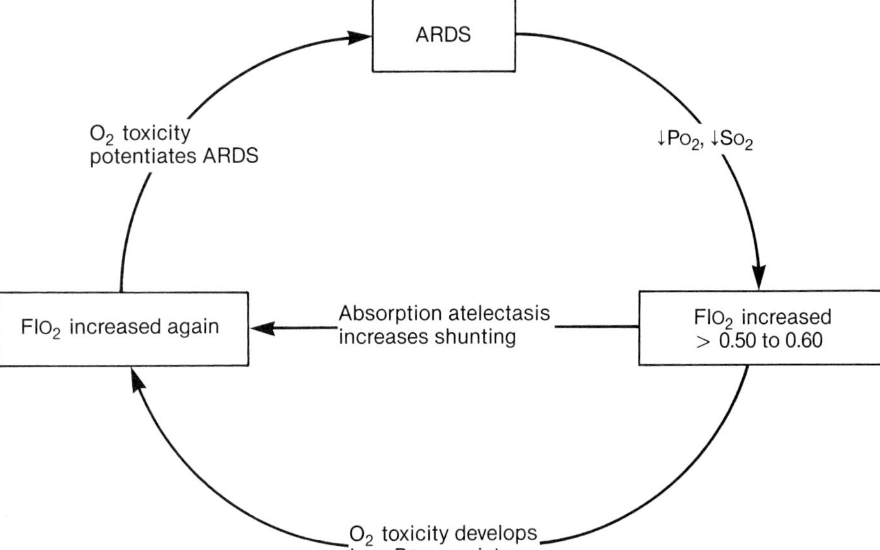

Figure 13–9. The oxygen dilemma in adult respiratory distress syndrome (ARDS). This vicious circle of events exacerbates acute lung injury and necessitates close blood gas monitoring in an effort to reduce FIo_2 to safe levels below 0.50.

number of variables, including inspired oxygen concentration, exposure time, preexisting lung disease, age, metabolic and nutritional status, and exposure to other compounds capable of causing related damage to the lungs.

As a general guideline, *oxygen concentrations greater than 50% for more than 24 to 48 hours continuously may damage the lungs and worsen respiratory problems* (Frank and Massaro, 1979). *An oxygen concentration of 100% is regarded as safe for up to 24 hours.* Beyond these statements, other guidelines vary depending on the source and tend not to be supported by reliable, valid research.

Because oxygen toxicity is incompletely understood and because there is great individual variation in susceptibility and resistance to lung injury, clinicians in the acute care setting make every effort to implement these following two basic interventions:

1. Reduce FIo_2 to as low as possible, maintaining an adequate Pao_2 of 70 to 100 mmHg or no greater than 60 to 70 mmHg (e.g., in the COPD patient).
2. Reduce exposure to 24 hours or less.

Assessment of Ventilation

Oxygenation
Pao_2, Sao_2
$A\text{-}ao_2$ gradient, a/A ratio, $\dot{Q}_S/\dot{Q}_T$
$P\bar{v}o_2$, $C(a-\bar{v})o_2$

VENTILATION

MEASUREMENT	***PROBLEMS***
$Paco_2$	Alveolar hyperventilation Alveolar hypoventilation Ventilatory failure

$Paco_2$ is the best measurement of alveolar ventilation. Normal alveolar ventilation is present when $Paco_2$ is within the normal range of 38 to 42 mmHg. *Alveolar hyperventilation* is present when $Paco_2$ is below normal. *Alveolar hypoventilation* occurs when $Paco_2$ increases above normal.

Acid-base changes associated with alveolar hyperventilation and hypoventilation are best explained subsequently in relation to pH, the Henderson-Hasselbalch equation, and principles of CO_2 transport.

Assessment of ventilation largely focuses on the monitoring for early signs of ventilatory failure, a major cause of morbidity and mortality in pulmonary patients.

OVERVIEW OF VENTILATORY FAILURE

Ventilatory failure is a pulmonary function disorder with serious acid-base consequences. The content presented here emphasizes pulmonary function aspects and changes in $Paco_2$ and Pao_2 that occur with increasing alveolar hypoventilation. Acid-base consequences are introduced and are elucidated in the next section on acid-base balance.

Definition

Ventilatory failure is present when $Paco_2$ rises above 50 mmHg. However, many clinicians set the limit at a $Paco_2$ greater than 45 mmHg for adults with normal lungs (Spragg and Moser, 1982). Shapiro and coworkers (1985) state that ventilatory failure is the condition in which the lungs are unable to meet the metabolic demands of the body as far as carbon dioxide homeostasis is concerned. Because of lung disease or some other serious illness, the body becomes unable to excrete the CO_2 produced in the tissues. Most important, ventilatory failure cannot be diagnosed without a $Paco_2$ level, a parameter obtained from an ABG or from a special rebreathing technique in the pulmonary function laboratory.

Acute and Chronic Forms

Acute and chronic ventilatory failure are defined according to the ABG values in the box.

ACUTE VENTILATORY FAILURE

$PaCO_2$ greater than 50 mmHg
pH less than 7.30

CHRONIC VENTILATORY FAILURE

$PaCO_2$ greater than 50 mmHg
pH greater than 7.30

In the chronic form, pH typically remains near normal (7.30 to 7.40), assuming normal compensatory mechanisms and absence of other independent acid-base disorders.

Severity of Illness

The severity of ventilatory failure depends on (1) the *degree of accompanying acidemia* (defined as a blood pH of less than 7.38) and (2) the *suddenness of the change in pH.* Cellular function becomes more disrupted by sudden changes in pH rather than by gradual changes. Hence, acute ventilatory failure is more life-threatening than chronic ventilatory failure. If acuteness and chronicity are difficult to determine because of the presence of mixed disorders, *sensorium* is frequently used as an indicator. Acute changes are more likely to cause loss of alertness and coma. These changes are thought to be due to the lowering of pH of cerebrospinal fluid (CSF) in which the central chemoreceptors are located. Chronic changes can produce a clear sensorium at very high $PaCO_2$ levels since only a few days are necessary for the accumulation of HCO_3^- in CSF and the correction of its pH towards normal.

Ventilatory Versus Respiratory Failure

Some clinicians inadvertently use the terms ventilatory failure and respiratory failure interchangeably, probably because of varying definitions in the medical literature. Yet, the distinction between the two terms is an important one. *Ventilatory failure* is diagnosed base on laboratory measurement of $PaCO_2$ greater than 50 mmHg. *Respiratory failure* is a broad, nonspecific clinical diagnosis, defined as *failure of the pulmonary system to provide adequate gas exchange.* The two entities are contrasted next.

Ventilatory Failure	*Respiratory Failure*
Laboratory diagnosis based on $PaCO_2$ level.	*Clinical* diagnosis based on deteriorating signs and symptoms, e.g., cyanosis and other signs of respiratory distress. The signs and symptoms suggest progressive deterioration in ABGs and clinical condition.
$PaCO_2$ is greater than 50 mmHg.	Subsequent ABG indicates PaO_2 less than 50 mmHg or $PaCO_2$ greater than 50 mmHg.
Indicates a ventilation problem (e.g., alveolar hypoventilation).	Cause is nonspecific—it may be a problem in oxygenation, ventilation, or both. Alveolar hypoventilation or hyperventilation may be present.
Requires immediate intervention to avoid cardiopulmonary arrest.	Requires immediate intervention to avoid cardiopulmonary arrest.

In both conditions, a STAT ABG is absolutely necessary to diagnose the presence and extent of hypoxemia, ventilatory failure, and acid-base disorders. Initial treatment usually includes oxygenation, ventilation, or both along with interventions specific to the disorder causing the respiratory or ventilatory failure.

ACUTE VENTILATORY FAILURE

All nurses, regardless of their specializations, must be familiar with *acute ventilatory failure* (AVF); AVF can occur as a result of any disorder, if it is severe enough or if the patient has limited cardiopulmonary reserves. This type of ventilatory failure occurs in healthy individuals with normal lungs as well as in ill individuals with chronic respiratory acidosis or chronic ventilatory failure from pulmonary disease. AVF is most likely in individuals with poor respiratory efforts and ineffective coughs and in those with disorders typically leading to AVF during acute illness (see Table 13–4 on page 362).

Common precipitating events in pulmonary patients include respiratory infection from bronchitis or pneumonia, congestive heart failure, pneumothorax, oversedation, and excessive oxygenation. In COPD patients, cardiac decompensation from hypoxemia or myocardial infarction is a common cause.

Physiologic Chain of Events

The two physiologic causes of AVF are *decreased CO_2 elimination* and *increased tissue CO_2 production.* The main causes of decreased CO_2 elimination include the following:

1. Decreased ventilation due to depressants, muscle relaxants, and so forth.
2. V/Q abnormality from severe diffuse airway disease, e.g., chronic bronchitis and asthma.
3. Increased dead space ventilation from emphysema, vascular disease, and pulmonary restriction.

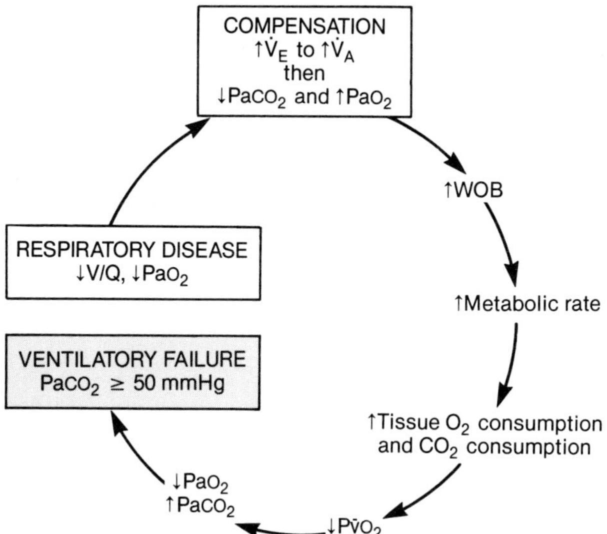

Figure 13–10. Physiologic events in acute ventilatory failure with hypoxemia.

Increased tissue CO_2 production is a cause of AVF but only when impaired lung function prevents compensation. The patient is unable to compensate owing to the increased work of breathing associated with decreased lung and chest wall compliance or one of the previously listed causes of decreased CO_2 elimination.

Hypoxemia, by itself, does not cause ARF, but the increased work of breathing induced may cause a marginally ventilated patient to decompensate.

Figure 13–10 and the subsequent discussion summarize physiologic events in the common type of ARF with hypoxemia. Keep in mind that events listed do not apply to all cases of ARF, particularly in those patients already receiving oxygen.

Consider a COPD patient with acute bronchitis breathing room air. Initially, retained mucus in the lungs decreases regional ventilation (↓ V/Q). A right-to-left intrapulmonary shunt (i.e., venous admixture) exists because perfusion is in excess of ventilation. The severity of the shunt determines how low PaO_2 will fall. The body responds to the decrease in V/Q and hypoxemia by increasing minute ventilation ($\dot{V}_E$) in an effort to better ventilate alveoli. With adequate cardiopulmonary reserves, compensation is possible—$PaCO_2$ decreases, reflecting hyperventilation, and PaO_2 increases correspondingly to an acceptable level.

The low $PaCO_2$ level is an indicator of *increased work of breathing.* To meet the demand for more energy, the body's metabolic rate increases, causing a rise in tissue O_2 consumption and CO_2 production. As more O_2 is extracted at the tissue level, the partial pressure of venous blood ($P\bar{v}O_2$) falls. This drop is followed by a drop in arterial PO_2. Arterial PCO_2 falls also, unless the patient is unable to increase minute ventilation even more to compensate. With further increased work of breathing, $PaCO_2$ rises to 50 mmHg, producing ventilatory failure.

Signs and Symptoms. These physiologic changes in an individual with a normal preexisting $PaCO_2$ can produce obvious signs of CO_2 narcosis and respiratory distress by the time a $PaCO_2$ of 50 mmHg is attained. In an individual with preexisting hypercapnia, however, these changes may produce only mild signs and symptoms, such as mild dyspnea, restlessness, slightly increased heart rate, and drowsiness. This observation is especially true in the case of a COPD patient whose $PaCO_2$ is normally about 45 mmHg.

Physical Decompensation

Three main factors determine a patient's ability to compensate for a rising $PaCO_2$ level as follows: (1) *cardiac reserve*—a failure of the heart to maintain cardiac output to peripheral tissues and vital organs can interrupt the physiologic chain of events at any point and cause physical deterioration; (2) *kidney function and presence of buffer substances*—an inadequate supply of buffers and failure of the kidneys to excrete H^+ acid and conserve HCO_3^- base can prevent pH normalization; and (3) *ventilatory reserve*—an individual with decreased ventilatory reserve decompensates when the increased minute ventilation required to maintain gas exchange dramatically increases the work of breathing to an intolerable degree, as explained next.

Ventilatory Reserve. A decreased ventilatory reserve is present when the ability to increase alveolar ventilation to meet gas exchange requirements is limited. Under such circumstances, the work of breathing and related oxygen consumption are inappropriately elevated. Clinical signs include use of accessory muscles of breathing; tachypnea; diaphoresis; and, in the case of COPD, an active and prolonged expiratory phase of respiration.

Shapiro and coworkers (1982) state that *vital capacity* (VC) is a gross indicator of ventilatory reserve. A decrease in VC indicates a decrease in ventilatory reserve because the individual is less able to increase tidal volume and minute ventilation without greatly increasing the percentage of total body oxygen consumption being used for breathing.

Increased Work of Breathing. In pulmonary patients without cardiac complications, it is the increased work of breathing during a sustained acute illness that leads to physical decompensation (Fig. 13–11). A brief discussion of work of breathing facilitates comprehension of the physiologic chain of events during decompensation.

In a healthy resting adult, less than 5% of the total 250 ml/min of oxygen consumed by the body is used for work of breathing. About 90% of the energy expended for this work is lost as heat within ventilatory muscles, and only 10% is actually used for moving gas in and out of the lungs. From this perspective, energy utilization for breathing is amazingly inefficient normally.

In pulmonary disease, the percentage of total body

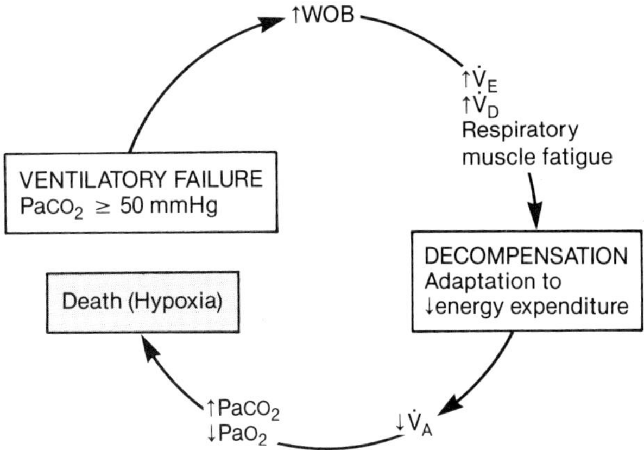

Figure 13–11. Physical decompensation in acute ventilatory failure.

oxygen consumption used for breathing increases as respiratory rate and minute ventilation increase, resulting in increased dead space ventilation ($\dot{V}_D$) (see Chapter 5). This percentage of total body oxygen consumption also dramatically rises with increases in airway resistance from obstructive processes as well as with decreases in compliance from restrictive processes, such as pneumonia and atelectasis. Because COPD patients tend to have increased respiratory rates and inefficient breathing from preexisting changes in lung mechanics, they are more likely to decompensate when acute illness demands even higher minute ventilations to improve alveolar ventilation. This tendency towards decompensation is especially prominent in a emphysematous patient whose chest disease is characterized by increased work of breathing in a stable state.

Increased $\dot{V}_E$ and $\dot{V}_D$. Patients with high dead space ventilation or markedly reduced compliance may demonstrate minute ventilations up to 10 to 12 L/min or twice the normal minute ventilation. Respiratory rates over 30 to 40/min and a $\dot{V}_E$ greater than 10 to 12 L/min may lead to decompensation within hours due to respiratory muscle fatigue. In some cases, breathing becomes so shallow and rapid that the patient manages only to ventilate anatomic dead space.

At this point, if not before, intubation and mechanical ventilation are indicated to decrease the work of breathing, the $\dot{V}_D$, and the respiratory muscle fatigue, and to normalize ABGs. In COPD, however, nonventilator or conservative management is recommended, unless the patient becomes apneic or comatose. Once such a patient with severe lung dysfunction is mechanically ventilated, the likelihood of successful weaning becomes reduced, and mortality rate becomes increased (Rhodes, 1979).

Decompensation. Physical decompensation develops when respiratory muscle fatigue leads to ineffective work of breathing for CO_2 gas exchange requirements (see Table 28–5). Simultaneously, a reduction in oxygen supply may occur, as oxygen gained by a high minute ventilation is completely consumed by ventilatory muscles, leaving little oxygen for other body tissues.

At the point of decompensation in Figure 13–11, the body's adaptive responses are to decrease rather than increase alveolar ventilation ($\dot{V}_A$) and to expend less energy, in an effort to conserve oxygen and improve work efficiency. The patient shows clinical signs of body fatigue, decreased breath sounds on auscultation, and barely audible or absent adventitious sounds. Instead of appearing distressed, the patient may appear less dyspneic and almost serene, as if he has decided to give up his struggle for life. $PaCO_2$ quickly climbs upward, PaO_2 drops, and the patient slips into coma.

In the chain of events shown in Figure 13–11, decreased PaO_2 and hypoxia are in parentheses as a reminder that decompensation and death can occur independently of oxygen need and utilization. Though hypoxia may be a contributing factor and eventually the end result, initial decompensation stems primarily from the ventilatory problem rather than the oxygenation problem.

MONITORING THE PATIENT

The chain of events in ventilatory failure may occur over a few hours in patients with acute illness or over days and weeks in patients with underlying chronic lung disease. Since no precise, practical, or reliable indicators of ventilatory reserve exist, clinicians cannot anticipate physical decompensation with absolute certainty. Hence, ongoing monitoring of the patient's ventilatory status is crucial.

Monitoring focuses on ongoing assessment of $PaCO_2$ (alveolar ventilation), pH (acid-base balance), and signs and symptoms indicating increased work of breathing and accompanying hypoxemia. In addition, familiarity with specific causes of ventilatory failure helps the nurse identify persons who are likely to develop the disorder. For quick reference, summary of causes,

Assessment of Acid-Base Balance

Oxygenation
- PaO_2, SaO_2
- $A\text{-}aO_2$ gradient, a/A ratio, $\dot{Q}_S/\dot{Q}_T$
- $P\bar{v}O_2$, $C(a-\bar{v})O_2$

Ventilation
- $PaCO_2$

ACID-BASE BALANCE

MEASUREMENTS	*PROBLEMS (ACID-BASE DISORDERS)*
pH	Respiratory acidosis
Respiratory: $PaCO_2$	Respiratory alkalosis
Metabolic: HCO_3^-, base excess, anion gap	Metabolic acidosis
	Metabolic alkalosis

signs and symptoms, and interventions is found in Table 13–4.

Assessment of oxygenation and ventilation alone, particularly in acute situations, may lead to the initiation of appropriate intervention, such as oxygen therapy or mechanical ventilation. Eventually, however, assessment of acid-base balance is required to determine more precisely the nature and severity of illness.

This last section of the blood gas theory base describes basic acid-base principles, including the derivation of the blood pH measurement, the relationship of pH to Pa_{CO_2} and bicarbonate measurements, and the derivation of the main acid-base disorders from the Henderson-Hasselbalch equation.

BLOOD pH

Blood pH is a crucial measurement; it describes the acid-base balance in the body and it helps in the assessment of the severity of hypoxemia, ventilatory failure, and any acid-base disorder.

As an indicator of overall clinical condition, pH determines whether the body is too acid or too alkaline. More specifically, it reflects *hydrogen ion (H^+) activity* in the body, one of the most important determinants of cellular metabolism. The amount of H^+ activity is determined by the interrelationship of blood acids, blood bases, and buffer substances, as described subsequently.

Acid

An *acid* is a substance that donates hydrogen ions to a solution. There are two types of acids in the body—*volatile* and *nonvolatile*. A volatile acid can chemically change between liquid and gaseous states. The major blood acid is carbonic acid (H_2CO_3), the substance that transports the metabolite CO_2 so that it can be excreted via the lungs.

All other sources of hydrogen ions are considered nonvolatile or *fixed* acids. They cannot change to a gaseous state for excretion by the lungs—they *must* be excreted by the kidneys. Main sources of nonvolatile acids are *organic* and *inorganic acids* from dietary intake; *lactic acid*, which accumulates in the absence of oxygen; and *keto acid*, which is produced in the absence of glucose, insulin, or both. Although the liver is a major organ of metabolism for nonvolatile acids, the kidneys still control their excretion from the body.

When compared with the large amounts of CO_2 produced and excreted by the lungs—20,000 to 25,000 mM/day—the kidneys excrete relatively small amounts of nonvolatile acid each day—50 to 100 mEq normally and up to 1000 mEq in acidotic states. Therefore, the lungs clearly regulate more acid than the kidneys.

Base

A *base* is a substance that accepts hydrogen ions, thereby removing them from solution. The major blood base is plasma *bicarbonate* (HCO_3^-); it is regulated primarily by the kidneys. The presence of the enzyme *carbonic anhydrase* in renal tubular cells allows this reaction to take place.

$$H_2O + CO_2 \longleftrightarrow H_2CO_3 \longleftrightarrow HCO_3 + H^+$$

(carbonic anhydrase acts at the first step)

This reaction shifts to the right as carbonic acid (H_2CO_3) is converted to HCO_3^-. If there is too much HCO_3^- in the body, some is excreted by the kidneys, and some is converted to carbonic acid and ultimately excreted by the lungs in the form of CO_2—the chemical reaction shown in the box shifts to the left. The reaction shifts to the right or left depending on whether CO_2 (acid) or HCO_3 (base) needs to be saved or excreted from the body.

Buffers

The formation of acid and base is largely governed by *buffer* substances. A buffer prevents extreme increases or decreases in H^+ concentration so that cellular metabolism continues unimpeded. When acid is added to the body, buffers act in the same manner as bicarbonate—they accept hydrogen ions, thus reducing the great changes possible in body acidity.

There are two main buffer systems in the body as follows: (1) the *bicarbonate* buffer system and (2) the *nonbicarbonate* buffer system composed of *hemoglobin*, which accounts for 80 to 90% of nonbicarbonate buffering; *phosphate*; and *serum protein*. Bicarbonate is the most important extracellular buffer, accounting for 60 to 90% of extracellular buffering of a fixed acid load (Simmons, 1974). Hence, bicarbonate is used to analyze the body's acid-base balance.

The Henderson-Hasselbalch Equation

This equation defines pH in terms of the relationship between carbonic acid and bicarbonate.

$$pH = pK + \log \frac{[HCO_3^-]}{[H_2CO_3]}$$

The term pH stands for the negative log of hydrogen ion concentration ($-\log[H^+]$). The pK is a constant equal to 6.1. (A mathematic explanation of this formula and actual calculation of pH are beyond the scope of this text.) It is most practical for the nurse to understand the carbonic acid–bicarbonate relationship and how fundamental acid-base disorders arise from changes in this relationship.

The clinical form of the Henderson-Hasselbalch equation is written as follows:

$$pH = pK + \log \frac{[HCO_3^-]}{s \times Pa_{CO_2}}$$

The *s* is carbon dioxide's solubility coefficient of 0.03. The s × Pa_{CO_2} is substituted for carbonic acid (H_2CO_3). The following discussion of the Pa_{CO_2} measurement and CO_2 transport in the body helps explain the reason for this substitution.

Pa_{CO_2} and CO_2 Transport. The following equation describes the formation of carbonic acid in blood plasma. The dCO_2 stands for dissolved carbon dioxide. It is the same as the measurement of Pa_{CO_2}.

$$H_2O + dCO_2 \longrightarrow H_2CO_3 \longleftrightarrow H^+ + HCO_3^-$$
$$dCO_2:H_2CO_3$$
$$1000:1$$

This reaction *readily* occurs in red blood cells and in kidney tubular cells because of the presence of the catalyzing enzyme carbonic anhydrase. Owing to the *absence* of this enzyme in blood plasma, this reaction is slowed there. This fact explains why little H_2CO_3 exists in plasma and why the $dCO_2:H_2CO_3$ ratio is 1000:1.

Note that although this amount of dCO_2 is large when compared with the amount of H_2CO_3 present, *it is only a very small portion of the total amount of CO_2 in the blood.* When CO_2 leaves peripheral tissues and enters blood plasma, most of it enters red blood cells. Here, CO_2 is rapidly buffered by bicarbonate, hemoglobin, and other proteins (e.g., carbamino compounds), and transported to the lungs for excretion. Yet, similar to dissolved O_2, *this small amount of dissolved CO_2 in plasma is critical.* Its small partial pressure determines the pressure gradient by which CO_2 enters or leaves the blood.

Simplification of the Henderson-Hasselbalch Equation

The Henderson-Hasselbalch equation may be simplified as follows:

$$pH = \frac{[HCO_3^-]}{Pa_{CO_2}} \text{ or } \frac{\text{metabolic component}}{\text{respiratory component}} \text{ or } \frac{\text{kidneys}}{\text{lungs}}$$

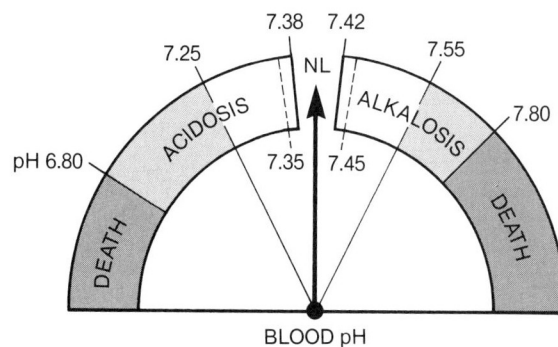

The simplification emphasizes this concept: pH reflects the *ability of the kidneys to alter HCO_3^-* through metabolic processes and the *ability of the lungs to alter Pa_{CO_2}* through respiration. Moreover, though HCO_3^- is derived from CO_2 and H_2CO_3, it is primarily determined by kidney function.

Another version of the same formula shows that the normal ratio of bicarbonate to carbonic acid is 20:1, assuming normal laboratory values for HCO_3^- and Pa_{CO_2}.

$$pH = \frac{[HCO_3^-]}{[H_2CO_3]} = \frac{[HCO_3^-]}{s \times Pa_{CO_2}} = \frac{24 \text{ mEq/L}}{0.03^* \times 40 \text{ mmHg}} = \frac{20 \text{ parts base}}{1 \text{ part acid}}$$

*H_2CO_3 is always 3% of Pa_{CO_2}.

More important than the calculation of values is the concept of maintenance of normal pH that requires a *balance* between base and Pa_{CO_2}-related carbonic acid. The body strives to maintain the normal 20:1 ratio to keep pH near its normal slightly alkaline value of 7.40. On the pH scale of 1 to 14, a pH of 7.0 is electrochemically neutral.

MAIN ACID-BASE DISORDERS

Main acid-base disorders are derived from various unbalanced relationships between Pa_{CO_2} and bicarbonate. In the beginning, many students frequently become confused and easily disheartened by the task of truly understanding acid-base balance and acid-base disorders. The intricacies of the Henderson-Hasselbalch equation are difficult to understand for many health professionals, including nurses. However, detailed knowledge is not necessary to understand and apply basic related principles to clinical practice. When one understands how changes in Pa_{CO_2} and bicarbonate alter pH, one understands the derivation of main acid-base disorders.

This section presents basic definitions and shows how to derive disorders by applying simple arithmetic to the Henderson-Hasselbalch equation. Once this crucial subject matter is mastered, supplementary information is easier to understand and hence is presented in more concise table form later in this chapter.

Derivation of Disorders from the Henderson-Hasselbalch Equation

Normal pH rarely is 7.4 in the clinical setting. The normal range is 7.38 to 7.42 with allowance for ± 0.02 error in either direction (Fig. 13–12).

Acidemia and Acidosis. *Acidemia* is defined as a blood pH of *less than* 7.38. *Acidosis* is a process causing the acidemia, e.g., diabetic ketoacidosis. Refer again to these relationships as follows:

$$pH = \frac{[HCO_3^-]}{Pa_{CO_2}} \text{ or } \frac{\text{metabolic component}}{\text{respiratory component}} \text{ or } \frac{\text{kidneys}}{\text{lungs}}$$

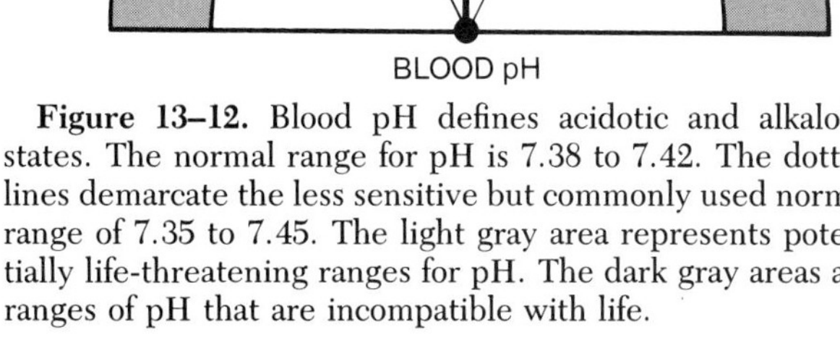

Figure 13–12. Blood pH defines acidotic and alkalotic states. The normal range for pH is 7.38 to 7.42. The dotted lines demarcate the less sensitive but commonly used normal range of 7.35 to 7.45. The light gray area represents potentially life-threatening ranges for pH. The dark gray areas are ranges of pH that are incompatible with life.

Mathematically, there are only two ways, which follow, to decrease the pH value to cause acidemia:

1. Decrease the numerator, HCO_3^-—by definition, the presence of a low HCO_3 value is called a *metabolic acidosis*.

2. Increase the denominator, $Paco_2$—the presence of a high $Paco_2$ value is called a *respiratory acidosis*, alveolar hypoventilation, or hypercapnea. All these terms have the same meaning.

Alkalemia and Alkalosis. *Alkalemia* is defined as a blood pH *greater than* 7.42. *Alkalosis* is a process causing alkalemia. As with acidosis, there are only two ways, which follow, to increase the pH value and cause alkalemia:

1. Increase HCO_3 in the HCO_3:$Paco_2$ ratio—the presence of a high HCO_3 is called *metabolic alkalosis*.

2. Decrease $Paco_2$ and cause *respiratory alkalosis*, also referred to as alveolar hyperventilation or hypocapnea.

Thus far, by looking at the bicarbonate and carbonic acid relationship in the Henderson-Hasselbalch equation, we have identified all the main acid-base disorders in the body. Note, for primary disorders, whenever HCO_3^- is altered, the acid-base disorder is metabolic. Conversely, whenever $Paco_2$ is altered, the disorder is always respiratory.

These generalizations may still hold true when combined respiratory and metabolic changes occur simultaneously. For example, in the first case, while some HCO_3^- is always generated or removed by changes in $Paco_2$, most HCO_3^- reflects metabolic rather than respiratory changes. However, with large $Paco_2$ changes, *actual* (combined respiratory and metabolic) *bicarbonate* may reflect primarily respiratory changes. In this and other cases, separating metabolic and respiratory components may be difficult, especially since most diagnostic laboratories use the actual bicarbonate measurement and may not include the *standard bicarbonate* measurement. The standard bicarbonate measurement normalizes the respiratory component, calculated at a $Paco_2$ equilibrated to 40 mmHg, and serves as a better index of metabolic changes.

Compensatory Processes

Once pH is altered by a primary acid-base disorder, the body immediately uses compensatory processes to bring pH back to normal. For example, a *primary* metabolic acidosis (decreased HCO_3^- base) will cause a *compensatory* respiratory alkalosis (decreased $Paco_2$ acid) to return pH to its normal near neutral value.

The lungs compensate for diseased kidneys or metabolic disorders by changing $Paco_2$ through alveolar hypoventilation or hyperventilation. Compensation begins in a matter of seconds. In contrast, the kidneys compensate for respiratory disorders by retention or excretion of bicarbonate and hydrogen ion. Renal compensation, however, exerts no noticeable influence for 12 to 24 hours. *Partial compensation* defined as *slight or incomplete change in pH towards normal*, may be evident in 12 to 24 hours, but *full compensation*, the *return of pH to the normal range*, takes up to 2 days (Schrier, 1980).

Based on this knowledge, a respiratory acidosis or alkalosis is defined as *acute* if the kidneys have not compensated for the disorder and the HCO_3^- value remains normal. If HCO_3^- has changed, renal compensation is present, and the process is defined as *chronic*.

Now one can fully appreciate the important roles of the lungs and kidneys in maintaining homeostasis. The body has an amazing capacity to compensate for chronic acid-base disorders as well as mildly acute ones. However, gross changes in pH are life-threatening, as illustrated in Figure 13–12. Moreover, it should be evident that patients with *both* kidney and lung disease are at increased risk to develop severe acid-base disorders from loss of both renal and respiratory compensatory mechanisms. These patients can become critically ill, if mild acid-base disorders are not promptly recognized and treated.

Quick Recognition of Main Disorders

Quick recognition of the main disorders requires thorough familiarity with changes in pH, $Paco_2$, and HCO_3^- that define acute and chronic processes. For review and study, Table 13–3 summarizes this information. The table also provides tips for interpretation of main and *mixed* acid-base disorders, when more than one primary disorder is present.

Further Assessment of the Metabolic Component

Though this text focuses on the use of HCO_3^- to assess the metabolic component of acid-base balance, *base excess* or *anion gap* may help to assess this component.

Base Excess. Base excess is another measurement in addition to HCO_3^- that reflects the concentration of bicarbonate in the body. It is a true nonrespiratory measurement; whereas a change in nonvolatile or fixed acid concentration does affect it, a change in carbonic acid concentration does *not* affect it. More specifically, base excess is a *measure of deviation of fixed acids from normal*, defined as zero for blood with a pH of 7.4 and Pco_2 of 40. The normal range is +2 to −2 mEq/L. *Minus* values indicate deficiency in base or excess fixed acid; plus values indicate excess base or a deficiency of fixed acid.

A base excess value is not mandatory for ABG interpretation because the HCO_3^- value gives sufficient information about metabolic status. Yet, many clinicians routinely employ it because of its easy-to-remember normal range and its greater accuracy in quantifying metabolic changes in the body. More specifically, base excess reflects activity of all buffer systems in the body not just the bicarbonate system. Base excess is not influenced by changes in hemoglobin

Table 13–3. RECOGNITION OF MAIN ACID-BASE DISORDERS (HCO_3^- = STANDARD BICARBONATE)

	Respiratory Acidosis (Alveolar Hypoventilation)	Respiratory Alkalosis (Alveolar Hyperventilation)	Metabolic Acidosis	Metabolic Alkalosis
Acute	pH ↓ $Paco_2$ ↑ HCO_3^- Normal	pH ↑ $Paco_2$ ↓ HCO_3^- Normal	pH ↓ $Paco_1$ Normal to ↓ (beginning compensation) HCO_3^-	pH ↑ $Paco_2$ Normal to ↑ (beginning compensation) HCO_3^-
Chronic	pH Normal $Paco_2$ ↑ HCO_3^- ↑ Compensatory metabolic alkalosis	pH Normal $Paco_2$ ↓ HCO_3^- ↓ Compensatory metabolic acidosis	pH Normal to ↓ $Paco_2$ ↓ Compensatory respiratory alkalosis HCO_3^- ↓	pH Normal to ↑ $Paco_2$ ↑ Compensatory respiratory acidosis HCO_3^- ↑
Tips for interpretation	*Ventilatory failure* is present if $Paco_2$ is greater than 50 mmHg.	In *acute* respiratory alkalosis, for every 10 mmHg decrease in Pco_2, pH will increase by 0.10-units. HCO_3^- remains within a normal range, but small changes may be evident; HCO_3^- falls 2 mEq/L for each 10 mmHg fall in $Paco_2$.	Maximal respiratory response takes hours to days, usually 12 to 48 hours, because central chemoreceptors respond slower to changes in pH than peripheral arterial chemoreceptors in the aortic-carotid area. Except in the case of very mild acidosis, respiratory compensation is never complete, and pH is never restored to the preexisting normal level.	In *chronic* metabolic alkalosis, with rare exception, $Paco_2$ will not increase above 50 *mmHg*, regardless of the severity of the metabolic alkalosis. If $Paco_2$ is greater than 50 mmHg, the respiratory acidosis is due to both normal respiratory compensation *and* accompanying pulmonary disorder, causing ventilatory failure.
	In *acute* respiratory acidosis, for every 10 mmHg increase in $Paco_2$, starting at $Paco_2$ of 40 mmHg, pH will decrease by 0.10 units. HCO_3^- remains within a normal range, but small changes may be evident; HCO_3^- rises 2 mEq/L for each 10 mmHg rise in $Paco_2$.	In *chronic* respiratory alkalosis, compensatory HCO_3^- falls 5 mEq/L for each 10 mmHg falls in $Paco_2$.		
HCO_3^- = actual bicarbonate	In *chronic* respiratory acidosis, if HCO_3^- is greater than 35 mEq/L, suspect an additional metabolic alkalosis unrelated to the one compensating for the respiratory acidosis. For each 10 mmHg increase in $Paco_2$, compensatory HCO_3^- rises by 4 mEq/L, with a range of 4 mEq/L in either direction. Note blood pH remains above 7.25, even with chronic $Paco_2$ elevations to 110 mmHg.	Remember to look at Pao_2; respiratory alkalosis is produced by many stimuli, including hypoxemia, which may be obscured by a rise in Pao_2, resulting from hyperventilation.		

content, which do influence HCO_3^- estimates. Finally, correcting actual bicarbonate for PCO_2 effects to estimate metabolic changes is unnecessary, since base excess is by definition a pure metabolic assessment parameter.

Anion Gap. The *anion gap* is an estimate of unmeasured cations minus unmeasured anions in the blood. In the following formula, anion gap represents those anions, other than chloride and bicarbonate, required to counterbalance sodium's and potassium's positive charge. Note that potassium (K^+) may be omitted from the formula to simplify calculations.

$$(Na^+ + K^+) - (Cl^- + HCO_3^-)$$
$$(140 \text{ mEq/L} + 4.0 \text{ mEq/L}) - (101 \text{ mEq/L} + 28 \text{ mEq/L}) = 15 \text{ mEq/L}$$

Hence, the anion gap is considered a measure of *undetermined anions*, e.g., negatively charged proteins, phosphates, sulfates, and organic anions. The normal range is 12 to 16 mEq/L. This parameter is used to assess metabolic acidosis and differentiate conditions with an *increased* anion gap, e.g., renal failure, diabetic ketoacidosis, and other disorders (see those with asterisks in Table 13–4), from conditions with a *normal* anion gap, e.g., diarrhea, pancreatic fluid drainage, ammonium chloride ingestion, acetazolamide therapy, renal tubular acidosis, and occasionally pyelonephritis.

Guidelines for a Systematic Approach to ABG Interpretation

The preceding content on the interpretation of individual blood gas measurements provides a foundation for the following systematic approach to ABG interpretation.

For any set of ABG results, use of the guide in the box will always lead to correct ABG interpretations. To gain experience in such interpretations, the reader is encouraged to apply this guide and Table 13–3 to the sets of ABG results at the end of this chapter. Practice in the clinical setting then will refine interpretation skills and will facilitate problem identification in patients in the nurse's care.

GUIDE TO ARTERIAL BLOOD GAS INTERPRETATION

LABORATORY NORMAL RANGES

pH	7.38 to 7.42 (7.35 to 7.45, 2 standard deviations from the mean).
$PaCO_2$	38 to 42 mmHg (35 to 45 mmHg, 2 standard deviations from the mean).
PaO_2	80 to 100 mmHg
Base Excess	+2 to −2 mEq/L
HCO_3^-	24 to 30 mEq/L
O_2 Saturation	Greater than 95%

QUESTIONS FOR INTERPRETATION

Adhere to the given order for a correct ABG interpretation.

PaO_2 and O_2 Saturation

1. *Is the PaO_2 and O_2 saturation normal?*
   A reduction in PaO_2 and O_2 saturation indicates hypoxemia.

2a. *Is the pH within normal limits?*
   If the pH is normal, the set of blood gases is either normal or full compensation has occurred for a blood gas disorder.
   If the pH is abnormal, the amount of deviation from normal helps to determine the severity of the blood gas disorder and the degree of partial compensation.

2b. *Is the pH on the acid or alkaline side of 7.40?*
   A pH on the acid side of 7.40 (less than 7.40) indicates that the primary or initiating disorder is an acidosis.
   A pH on the alkaline side of 7.40 (greater than 7.40) indicates that the primary or initiating disorder is an alkalosis.
   Analysis of $PaCO_2$ and HCO_3^- determines the type of acidosis or alkalosis present.

$PaCO_2$

3. *Is $PaCO_2$ high (respiratory acidosis), low (respiratory alkalosis), or normal?*
   An abnormal $PaCO_2$ with a normal HCO_3^- indicates an *acute* respiratory acidosis or alkalosis without metabolic compensation by the kidneys.

HCO_3^-

4. *Is HCO_3^- high (metabolic alkalosis), low (metabolic acidosis), or normal?*
   Remember, as a compensatory mechanism, a change in HCO_3^- takes up to 2 days.
   Optional: What is the base excess? Values over +2 confirm a metabolic alkalosis: values less than −2 confirm a metabolic acidosis.

5. *What are the primary and compensatory (if present) acid-base disorders?*
   The primary disorder has already been identified. In mixed disorders the other respiratory or metabolic disorder is the compensatory process.

Example: Primary respiratory acidosis with a compensatory metabolic alkalosis.

6. *What is the final interpretation?*
   Indicate whether the disorder is acute or chronic and whether compensation is partial or full.

Examples: Acute respiratory acidosis assumes the absence of metabolic compensation. Chronic partially or fully compensated respiratory acidosis assumes that compensation is metabolic.

Note: For prolonged illnesses or complicated cardiopulmonary problems, a series of blood gas results is necessary to fully evaluate respiratory and metabolic components.

Table 13–4. SUMMARY OF ACID-BASE DISORDERS

Acid-Base Disorders	Causes
Respiratory acidosis and ventilatory failure	Any severe physiologic disorder, particularly disorders characterized by
	Upper airway obstruction
	Lower airway obstruction
	Bronchial asthma, bronchitis, emphysema, and cystic fibrosis
	Respiratory muscle weakness
	Poliomyelitis, Guillain-Barré syndrome, myasthenia gravis, spinal cord trauma, and cervical vertebral fracture
	Decreased chest wall compliance
	Rib fracture with flail chest, rheumatoid spondylitis, and severe kyphoscoliosis
	Decreased lung compliance
	End-stage interstitial disease, severe pneumonia, lung collapse, pulmonary edema, cardiogenic left ventricular failure, ARDS, smoke inhalation, massive pulmonary embolism
	Respiratory depression
	Analgesic, sedative, or tranquilizer overdose, cerebrovascular accidents, head trauma, sleep apnea syndrome, primary hypoventilation
	Ineffective coughing and deep breathing due to poor effort or pain
	Hypoxemia sufficiently severe to induce respiratory center failure
	Metabolic alkalosis
	Note this causes a respiratory acidosis *without* ventilatory failure.
Respiratory alkalosis†	Hypoxemia
	From chronic or acute pulmonary disease or from undetermined cause
	Metabolic acidosis
	Central nervous system stimulation of respiration from nonpulmonary causes
	Anxiety, neurosis, psychosis, head trauma, brain tumor, vascular accidents, salicylate overdose, and fever
	Peripheral stimulation of medullary respiratory center from low Po_2, stimulation of pain receptors or lung stretch receptors
	High altitude, postoperative pain, pulmonary emboli, heart failure, interstitial lung diseases, "stiff" lungs without hypoxemia, pneumonia, atelectasis, and pneumothorax
	Mechanical hyperventilation
	Prolonged manual bagging, inappropriately set mechanical ventilator
	Therapeutic measure in brain injury patients to produce cerebral vasoconstriction
	Others
	Anemia, hepatic insufficiency, gram-negative sepsis
Metabolic acidosis	Respiratory alkalosis
	Gastrointestinal loss of HCO_3^-
	Diarrhea
	Loss of small bowel, biliary, and pancreatic drainage from tubes or external fistulas
	Ureterosigmoidostomy, obstructed ileal loop conduit
	Anion-exchange resins (e.g., cholestyramine)
	Renal loss of HCO_3^-
	Carbonic anhydrase inhibitors
	Renal tubular acidosis
	Increased acid production*
	Diabetic ketoacidosis, lactic acidosis from shock and anaerobic metabolism, starvation, alcoholic ketoacidosis, nonketotic hyperosmolar coma, inborn errors of metabolism
	Ingestion of toxic substances*
	Salicylate overdose, paraldehyde poisoning, methyl alcohol ingestion, and ethylene glycol ingestion
	Failure of acid excretion
	Acute or chronic renal failure, shock
	Other
	Hyperalimentation acidosis, administration of hydrochloric acid, ammonium chloride, or acetazolamide (Diamox); rapid administration of a solution lacking HCO_3^- (e.g., isotonic saline)

Table 13–4. SUMMARY OF ACID-BASE DISORDERS *Continued*

Signs and Symptoms	Interventions
Slight increase in Pa_{CO_2} Mild dyspnea, increased heart rate, or drowsiness; otherwise, few if any signs and symptoms may be present. *On auscultation:* slight decrease in air movement (lung ventilation); unchanged or increased adventitious sounds Ventilatory failure (Pa_{CO_2} greater than 50 mmHg) Signs of hypoxemia, if Pa_{O_2} is low, including restlessness, tachypnea, and dyspnea Signs of respiratory distress and increased work of breathing Signs of CO_2 narcosis, including headache, hypertension, increased heart rate, marked lethargy, and drowsiness Body fatigue *On auscultation:* progressive decrease in ventilation and adventitious sounds Loss of alertness and coma Bedside measurements Change in minute ventilation, though it is an unreliable indicator of V_A. V_D/V_T greater than 0.55 Reduced expiratory flow rates	The following interventions are for ventilatory failure. Interventions for mild respiratory acidosis are basically the same, except extreme measures are unnecessary. ***Life Saving Interventions*** 1. Give oxygen to correct hypoxemia, if present. For the COPD patient, add oxygen to provide a Pa_{O_2} of at least 50-55 mmHg without pH falling below 7.25. The pH rather than Pa_{CO_2} is used as the ultimate guide because an acceptable pH is associated with a better prognosis (Warren et al, 1980). Also, PO_2 should not exceed 60-70 mmHg to preclude further hypoventilation. 2. Give a ventilatory stimulant, such as doxapram, to increase V_A (used rarely in specific instances of respiratory depression or COPD). 3. Implement mechanical ventilation to relieve obstruction, decrease work of breathing, stabilize the chest wall (flail chest), and improve V_A. Note, nonventilator treatment is recommended for COPD patients. 4. Bypass upper airway obstruction or decrease dead space ventilation by tracheostomy. ***Other Interventions*** Goals To determine the causes and precipitating factors for the ventilatory failure To implement therapy to reverse underlying problems. 1. Control infection with antibiotics. 2. Administer bronchodilators and other pulmonary medications, as needed. Avoid use of narcotics, sedatives, and tranquilizers. 3. Administer diuretics, if in heart failure or if oxygen, bed rest; and treatment of infection do not reverse salt and water retention secondary to hypercapnea.‡ 4. Reverse metabolic alkalosis. 5. Maintain a program of bronchial hygiene: Coughing and deep breathing Endotracheal suctioning Frequent change in body position and early ambulation Adequate hydration Humidification and mist therapy Postural drainage with percussion and vibration 6. Order serial blood gases until the patient is stable. 7. Encourage cessation of smoking. 8. For patients with chronic lung disease, provide counseling and education to help them understand and adapt to the limitations of their disease. Assess for participation in a pulmonary rehabilitation program.
Signs and symptoms tend to be vague. They may include Hyperventilation Dizziness Perioral and extremity numbness, prickling and tingling (parasthesia) Muscle cramps Tinnitus Tetany, seizures, and increases in deep tendon reflexes Cardiac arrhythmias Loss of alertness	1. Treat the disorder causing the hyperventilation. 2. Give oxygen to correct hypoxemia. 3. If the patient is on a ventilator, decrease minute ventilation or add mechanical dead space. In severe cases, the physician will order sedative or a paralyzing drug; set the ventilator on controlled ventilation, and repeat blood gases.
Kussmaul breathing—prominent when HCO_3^- is less than 15 mEq/L Lethargy Nausea and vomiting Hypotension Cardiac arrhythmias Signs of tissue hypoxia Loss of alertness and coma Blood tests Decreased total CO_2 content reflects the decreased HCO_3^-. Normal to increased potassium concentration; K^+ shifts to the extracellular space.	1. Give sodium bicarbonate infusion until HCO_3^- increases to 15 mEq/L. The patient with chronic renal disease may be on daily oral doses of sodium bicarbonate. 2. Correct fluid and electrolyte imbalances. 3. Avoid rapid correction of the acidosis. 4. Use hemodialysis for renal failure and removal of toxic substances, if the acidosis is severe. 5. Treat the underlying disease.

Table continued on following page

Table 13–4. SUMMARY OF ACID-BASE DISORDERS *Continued*

Acid-Base Disorders	Causes
Metabolic alkalosis	Respiratory acidosis In COPD with chronic ventilatory failure, implementation of mechanical ventilation may result in overventilation. Rapid decrease in $Paco_2$ leaves HCO_3^- elevated, thus unmasking the metabolic alkalosis. A lack of chloride (Cl^-) perpetuates metabolic alkalosis. The kidneys cannot begin to excrete HCO_3^- unless ample chloride is present to replace it. Alkalosis may be severe enough to cause seizures and further suppression of respiratory drive. Loss of gastric acid (Cl^-) Vomiting, drainage of gastric fluid via nasogastric suction, gastrostomy tube, or external fistula Volume depletion with subsequent concentration of HCO_3^- Renal excretion of H^+, K^+, and Cl^- Profound potassium depletion (hypokalemia) Diuretic therapy—loss of Na^+, K^+, and Cl^+ with volume depletion Cystic fibrosis—marked loss of Cl^- in sweat Cushing's syndrome, corticosteroid therapy, and hyperaldosteronism—stimulation of renal reabsorption and excretion of H^+ and K^+ Administration of HCO_3^- Milk-alkali syndrome from administration of large amounts of antacids containing calcium absorbable alkali Hypercalcemia from metastatic bone lesions or multiple myeloma The destruction of bone causes the release of buffers.

AVOIDANCE OF INTERPRETATION ERRORS

Use of the Clinical History and Serial ABGs

To avoid errors, remember that interpretation of a mixed disorder usually requires a clinical history in addition to a series of ABGs over hours, days, or weeks. The following example illustrates this point. Look at this set of ABG values.

pH = 7.58
$Paco_2$ = 47 mmHg
HCO_3^- = 44 mEq/L

The laboratory interpretation indicates a chronic partially compensated metabolic alkalosis. Yet, knowledge of the patient's history leads to a different clinical interpretation. His original or primary problem was actually not a metabolic alkalosis—it was a respiratory acidosis. He has a history of severe COPD and chronically high $Paco_2$ values, causing a primary respiratory acidosis with a compensatory metabolic alkalosis. Since HCO_3^- is excessively high (over 35 mEq/L) and pH grossly elevated, the patient has an additional nonrespiratory metabolic alkalosis. He retained bicarbonate, and pH climbed to 7.58 because he overdosed with diuretic medication at home. Since diuretics cause a loss of chloride (Cl^-), Cl^- is not available to exchange with HCO_3^-. Hence, HCO_3^- cannot be excreted, and it accumulates in the body. In this way, the accumulation of base (i.e., HCO_3^-) in the body masked the underlying primary, respiratory acidosis. Without a clinical history, comparison of this set of ABGs with a set drawn prior to the diuretic overdose would unmask the true primary disorder and help the physician determine appropriate treatment for both respiratory and metabolic problems.

Other Tips for Interpretation

Two other tips help the nurse avoid interpretation errors related to faulty blood sampling and laboratory processing.

First, remember that in normal adults, the Pvo_2 is dramatically less than the Pao_2 (see Part One). *Whenever blood gases from a clinically stable state show a Pao_2 as low as 40 mmHg with an elevated $Paco_2$, the nurse should suspect the blood sample was venous rather than arterial.* The physician is notified, and a repeat ABG is usually ordered to insure arterial rather than venous sampling.

Second, remember that at the alveolar level, the sum of PAO_2 (100 mmHg) and $PACO_2$ (40 mmHg) equals 140 mmHg (see Fig. 3–2). *Generally, the sum of Pao_2 and $Paco_2$ should never be greater than 140 mmHg when the patient is breathing room air.* A total greater than 140 mmHg indicates either laboratory error in the measurement of one of these values or inadvertent administration of oxygen during or immediately prior to arterial sampling. This rule does not apply to individuals receiving supplementary oxygen.

Monitoring Patients for Acid-Base Disorders

The nurse's role in monitoring patients for acid-base disorders is summarized as follows:

1. Report any abnormal laboratory values to the physician immediately.
2. Report signs or symptoms indicative of a possible disorder (Table 13–4). If signs or symptoms are mild or vague and vital signs and chest assessment findings unchanged, note subtle signs and symptoms in your notes and monitor closely for a change in status.

Table 13–4. SUMMARY OF ACID-BASE DISORDERS *Continued*

Signs and Symptoms	Interventions
Signs and symptoms are relatively nonspecific; they usually include one or more of the following: Muscle cramps or weakness Hypertension (hyperaldosteronism) Hyperactive reflexes Tetany Blood tests Increased total CO_2 content Decreased serum Cl^+ Decreased serum K^+ Mild increase in urea nitrogen, creatinine, and hematocrit from volume depletion Signs and symptoms are more pronounced if hypocalcemia is present.	1. Give fluids to correct volume depletion. 2. Provide ample chloride so the kidneys can excrete bicarbonate. 3. Give K^+ (usually KCL) to correct potassium depletion. 4. Give other medication as needed, e.g., HCL to replace H^+, Diamox to increase renal HCO_3^- excretion, or spironolactone to decrease mineralocorticoid activity. 5. Treat the underlying disorder. 6. With the implementation of mechanical ventilation, the clinician *slowly* lowers $Paco_2$ to the pulmonary patient's stable outpatient level. This, in addition to correction of hypochloremia, will prevent the development of *severe* alkalemia due to the *sudden* lowering of $Paco_2$.

*Causes an increase in unmeasurable anions and hence an *anion gap metabolic acidosis*.
†Adapted from Schrier, R. (ed.): Renal and Electrolyte Disorders, 2nd ed. Boston, Little, Brown, & Co., 1980.
‡Adapted from Rhodes, M. Acute respiratory failure in COLD. *Critical care quarterly*, 1(4): 1–13, 1979.

3. If you are certified to do so, draw a PRN ABG when signs and symptoms of hypoxemia, alveolar hypoventilation, or respiratory distress appear. If you are not certified, call the physician, respiratory therapist, or technician to draw the ABG.
4. Whenever possible, utilize noninvasive measurements of Pao_2 and $Paco_2$ until an ABG sample can be drawn and results are available for interpretation (see Chapters 23 and 28).
5. Interpret blood gas results in light of the patient's clinical history and other assessment findings. Remember, a set of ABG results represents only one assessment parameter.
6. Implement appropriate interventions to relieve hypoxemia and resolve the acid-base disorder. Basic interventions are summarized in Table 13–4. Specific interventions are discussed later in other chapters of this text.

Conclusion

This chapter provides a comprehensive theory base for assessment of oxygenation, alveolar ventilation, and acid-base balance in the body as well as specific guidelines for interpretation of a set of ABGs in the clinical setting. This knowledge will enable the nurse to diagnose problems, such as hypoxemia, ventilatory failure, and acidemia or acidosis, and promptly intervene with measures that enhance health and may save the patient's life. Moreover, when considered with pulmonary function test interpretation (see Chapter 14), ABG interpretation adds key information to a patient's data base. Its judicious utilization can make respiratory care more efficient and effective and reduce the phenomenal amounts of time and energy expended in the prevention and treatment of disorders such as ventilatory failure.

Arterial Blood Gas Problems

DIRECTIONS:

Assume that the patient is breathing room air and interpret the following ABG results, using the interpretation guide on page 361 (with the narrow 1 SD range for pH and $Paco_2$). The answers to these problems are in Appendix II.

I. A.

pH	7.25
$Paco_2$	63 mmHg
Pao_2	55 mmHg
BE	+2 mEq/L
HCO_3^-	27 mEq/L
O_2 sat.	81%

Answer: ____________

B.

pH	7.39
$Paco_2$	63
Pao_2	55
BE	+11
HCO_3^-	38
O_2 sat.	87%

Answer: ____________

II. A.

pH	7.54
$Paco_2$	28 mmHg
Pao_2	37 mmHg
BE	−2 mEq/L
HCO_3^-	24 mEq/L
O_2 sat.	78%

Answer: ____________

B.

pH	7.42
$Paco_2$	28
Pao_2	37
BE	−5
HCO_3^-	18
O_2 sat.	72%

Answer: ____________

III. A.

pH	7.35
$Paco_2$	35 mmHg
Pao_2	80 mmHg
BE	−5 mEq/L
HCO_3^-	19 mEq/L
O_2 sat.	94%

Answer: ____________

B.

pH	7.38
$Paco_2$	32
Pao_2	83
BE	−5
HCO_3^-	19
O_2 sat.	96.1%

Answer: ____________

IV. A.		*B.*	
pH	7.50	pH	7.43
$PaCO_2$	42 mmHg	$PaCO_2$	47
PaO_2	70 mmHg	PaO_2	65
BE	+9 mEq/L	BE	+5
HCO_3^-	33 mEq/L	HCO_3^-	31
O_2 sat.	95.6%	O_2 sat.	93%
Answer: ________		*Answer:* ________	

REFERENCES

Bageant, R.: Variations in arterial blood gas measurements due to sampling techniques. *Respiratory care*, 20(6):565–570, 1975.

Baun, M. and Flones, M.: Cumulative effects of three sequential endotracheal suctioning episodes in the dog model. *Heart & lung*, 13(2):148–154, 1984.

Clausen, J.: Pulmonary Function Testing Guidelines and Controversies. Orlando, Florida, Grune & Stratton, Inc., 1984.

Cohen, A., Taeusch, H. W., and Stanton, C.: Usefulness of the arterial/alveolar oxygen tension ratio in the care of infants with respiratory distress syndrome. *Respiratory care*, 28(2):169–173, 1983.

Demers, R. and Irwin, R.: Management of hypercapnic respiratory failure: a systematic approach. *Respiratory care*, 24(4):328–335, 1979.

Findley, L., Whelan, D. and Moser, K.: Long-term oxygen therapy in COPD. *Chest*, 83(4):671–674, 1983.

Frank, L. and Massaro, D.: The lung and oxygen toxicity. *Archives of internal medicine*, 139(3):347–350, 1979.

Fromm, G.: Using basic laboratory data to evaluate patients with acute respiratory failure. *Critical care quarterly*, 1(4):43–51, 1979.

Fuchs, P.: Getting the best out of oxygen delivery systems. *Nursing 80*, 10(12):34–43, 1980.

Hess, D., et al: The validity of assessing arterial blood gases 10 minutes after an FIO_2 change in mechanically ventilated patients without chronic pulmonary disease. *Respiratory care*, 30(12):1037–1041, 1985.

Jenkinson, S.: Oxygen toxicity in acute respiratory failure. *Respiratory care*, 28(5):614–617, 1983.

Keyes, J.: Fluid, Electrolyte and Acid-base Regulation. Belmont, California, Wadsworth, Inc., 1985.

Morrison, M.: Respiratory Intensive Care Nursing, 2nd ed. Boston, Little, Brown and Co., 1979.

Murray, J.: Pathophysiology of acute respiratory failure. Respiratory care, 28(5):531–540, 1983.

Narins, R. and Emmett, M.: Simple and mixed acid-base disorders: a practical approach. *Medicine*, 59(3):161–187, 1980.

Nelson, R., Wilkins, R., Jacobsen, W., and Sheldon, R.: Supranormal PvO_2 in the presence of tissue hypoxia: a case report. *Respiratory care*, 28(2):191–194, 1983.

Norkool, D. M.: Current concepts in hyperbaric oxygenation and its application in critical care. *Heart & lung*, 8(4):728–735, 1979.

Petty, T. and Bailey, D.: A new, versatile blood gas syringe. *Heart & lung*, 10(4):672–674, 1981.

Pierce, A.: Oxygen toxicity. *Basics of respiratory disease*, 1(2), 1972.

Pierson, D.: The toxicity of low-flow oxygen therapy. *Respiratory care*, 28(7):889–897, 1983.

Pierson, D.: Weaning from mechanical ventilation in acute ventilatory failure: concepts, indications, and techniques. *Respiratory care*, 28(5):646–662, 1983.

Rhodes, M.: Acute respiratory failure in COLD. *Critical care quarterly*, 1(4):1–13, 1979.

Risser, N.: Preoperative and postoperative care to prevent pulmonary complications. *Heart & lung*, 9(1):57–67, 1980.

Rogers, R. and Juers, J.: Physiologic considerations in the treatment of acute respiratory failure. *Basics of respiratory disease*, 3(5), 1975.

Rose, B.: Clinical Physiology of Acid-Base and Electrolyte Disorders, 2nd ed. New York, McGraw-Hill Book Co., 1984.

Schrier, R. (ed.) Renal and Electrolyte Disorders, 2nd ed. Boston, Little, Brown & Co., 1980.

Shapiro, B., Harrison, R., and Walton, J.: Clinical Application of Blood Gases, 3rd ed. Chicago, Year Book Medical Publishers, 1982.

Simmons, D.: Blood gases. In Guide to Pulmonary Medicine (Tashkin, D. and Cassan, S.—eds.) New York, Grune & Stratton, Inc., 1978.

Simmons, D.: Evaluation of acid-base status. *Basics of respiratory disease*, 2(3), 1974.

Slonim, N. and Hamilton, L.: Respiratory Physiology, 4th ed. St. Louis, C.V. Mosby Co., 1981.

Spragg, R. and Moser, K.: Respiratory Emergencies, 2nd ed. St. Louis, C.V. Mosby Co., 1982.

Sue, D.: Measurement of shunt in respiratory failure. (Letter to the editor.) *Chest*, 78(6):898–899, 1980.

Warren, P., Millar, J., Flenley, D., and Avery, A.: Respiratory failure revisited: acute exacerbations of chronic bronchitis between 1961–68 and 1970–76. *Lancet*, 1(8166):467–471, 1980.

West, J.: Respiratory Physiology—The Essentials, 3rd ed. Baltimore, Williams & Wilkins, 1985.

White, K.: Completing the hemodynamic picture: $S\bar{v}O_2$. *Heart & lung*, 14(3):272–280, 1985.

Wilkins, R., Sheldon, R., and Krider, S.: Clinical Assessment in Respiratory Care. St. Louis, C.V. Mosby Co., 1985.

Zagelbaum, G. and Paré, J.: Manual of Acute Respiratory Care. Boston, Little, Brown & Company, 1982.

Pulmonary Function Tests

14

Main Objectives

1. Name four indications for pulmonary function tests (PFTs).
2. Explain the relevance of PFTs for nursing.
3. Name the four components of the complete PFT.
4. Define the terms *predicted* value, *observed* value, *percent predicted* value, and *percent change after bronchodilator* value.
5. Define and state the significance of the following:
Vital capacity (VC)
Forced vital capacity (FVC)
Residual volume (RV)
Total lung capacity (TLC)
Residual volume/total lung capacity (RV/TLC)
Forced expiratory volume in 1 second (FEV_1)
FEV_1% (FEV_1/FVC)
Forced mid-expiratory flow ($FEF_{25-75\%}$)
Diffusing capacity of the lung (DL)
6. Use observed FEV_1 to define mild, moderate, and severe degrees of respiratory impairment for obstructive disease.
7. Correctly identify spirometry tracings of individuals with normal lung function, obstructive disease, and restrictive disease.
8. Identify the following flow-volume loop patterns: normal, obstructive disease, restrictive disease, and upper airway obstruction. Explain the significance of reduced expiratory air flow at low lung volumes.
9. Describe the nurse's role in scheduling the PFTs, preparing the patient, and obtaining the bedside PFTs.

10. Explain how to systematically analyze PFT results and make a basic interpretation with emphasis on the following:
   a. The identification of normal and grossly abnormal PFT results.
   b. Differentiation between a purely obstructive and a purely restrictive disease.
   c. Determination of disease reversibility.
   d. Determination of general progression of disease.

Pulmonary function tests (PFTs) are perhaps the least understood and most underutilized of all assessment parameters. The reasons in part are a lack of knowledge of chronic airflow limitation and its progression and detection and possible ways of altering its course before serious symptoms occur. Also, only recently have the PFTs been used for detection and prevention of chronic airflow limitation rather than solely for the identification of obvious disease in symptomatic individuals.

This chapter discusses the main components of the complete PFT and provides knowledge for the basic interpretation of the laboratory or bedside PFT results. Interpretation is emphasized because the PFT, along with the physical examination, is the main source of objective data for evaluation of physiologic nursing diagnoses.

Review of basic pathophysiologies of obstructive and restrictive diseases in Chapters 7 and 8 will enhance comprehension of the patterns of abnormal lung function discussed in this chapter.

Purpose and Indications

The purpose of PFTs is to assess the integrity and functioning of the lungs, specifically the airways, vascular system, and interstitium.

Four main indications are described.

1. *To determine the presence of lung disease or an abnormality of lung function.* The PFT may confirm evidence of disease found during the physical examination or the history taking or on the chest x-ray film, or it may detect a functional disorder in the patient with no signs or symptoms of disease. Some researchers are using PFTs for the mass screening of populations for pulmonary disease (Detels et al, 1982).

   A special test called the *bronchial inhalation challenge* or the *bronchial provocation test* is used to detect airway hyperreactivity (hyperresponsiveness) and to determine the effect of various fumes, chemicals, and drugs on pulmonary function. As introduced in Chapter 7, testing consists of administration of an aerosolized cholinergic agent (i.e., methacholine, carbachol, or histamine) in increasing concentrations and measurement of pulmonary function before and after administration. The administration of a suspected antigen rather than a cholinergic drug may be used in the evaluation of occupational asthma, for hyposensitization therapy, or for equivocal allergy testing results.
2. *To determine the degree of respiratory impairment and overall progression of disease.* A PFT is necessary to determine the presence and degree of *respiratory impairment*, defined as *deviation from normal lung function.* The physician must document respiratory impairment before ordering various home respiratory care treatments, such as oxygen administration or a respirator or compressor nebulizer setup. Also, the degree of impairment determines the disability and the amount of financial assistance or worker's compensation insurance a disabled person may receive. Though medical and legal definitions of the term disability are not in total agreement, *disability* refers to *being unable to perform a particular job*; if the person is capable of work duties, he does so only "at the expense of undue distress" (Morgan, 1979).

   Along with other assessment parameters, the PFT helps to label the patient's condition as better, worse, or status quo. For example, serial PFTs may be used to determine whether the pulmonary function of a chest trauma patient is in fact returning to normal. In a patient with chronic obstructive pulmonary disease (COPD), the tests may identify acute exacerbations and remissions while monitoring the overall gradual decline in pulmonary function over many years and decades.
3. *To determine a course of therapy in the treatment of disease.* A PFT may be ordered to determine the effectiveness of pulmonary medications and other bronchial hygiene measures or to help answer specific clinical questions, such as the following:
   a. Is the patient fully bronchodilated?
   b. Has pulmonary function deteriorated as much as other clinical findings suggest?
   c. Should the clinician adjust a medication dosage or give a PRN medication more frequently?
   d. Should various respiratory interventions be increased or decreased in intensity, frequency, or both?
   e. Is a nonpulmonary medication, such as a beta blocking agent (i.e., propranolol or atenolol), causing adverse pulmonary side effects (e.g., bronchoconstriction)?
4. *To determine risk for postoperative pulmonary complications.* A preoperative PFT helps to identify persons at risk to develop postoperative pulmonary complications. It is usually required for resectional lung surgery; it is indicated for thoracic-upper abdominal surgery or prolonged gen-

eral anesthesia, when other risk factors, such as over 40 years of age, obesity, history of smoking, chronic pulmonary disease, cough, or dyspnea, are present.

Relevance for Nursing

In most situations, a technician, not a nurse, conducts the complete PFT and calculates the values; a pulmonary physician makes the formal detailed interpretation for the chart. Nevertheless, a working knowledge of PFTs is highly relevant to nursing for several reasons. First, in the hospital and some home settings, it is the nurse who prepares the patient for test administration and then afterwards must cope with the fatigued, dyspneic patient upon his return from the laboratory. The nurse cannot fully counsel the patient without a basic knowledge of how and why PFT measurements are made.

Second, knowledge of PFTs helps one understand how both restrictive and obstructive diseases of varying severity alter lung function.

Third, knowledge of pulmonary function terminology and related physiologic principles facilitates communication with physicians on medical or physiologic aspects of care. Such communication is likely to promote more comprehensive assessments of patient needs, more realistic patient goals, and more comprehensive plans for intervention.

Last, in some situations, the nurse measures basic PFT values. PFTs have become an integral part of respiratory care in acute care and ambulatory settings, and their role needs to be expanded in the home setting. The recent development of reliable portable devices for measuring volumes, flow rates, and pressures permits more frequent use of bedside PFTs to monitor respiratory status and help determine the appropriateness of various maneuvers, such as change in body position, return to mechanical ventilation, or trial of a new breathing technique to enhance aerosol deposition in the lungs.

The Complete Pulmonary Function Test (PFT)

There are four components to a routine complete PFT: *lung volumes, mechanics of breathing, diffusion,* and *arterial blood gases.* The first three components are discussed in this chapter. Arterial blood gases are discussed in Chapter 13.

GENERAL PROCEDURE

The test takes 1 1/2 to 2 hours to complete. Although most measurements are obtained by single breath maneuvers, lung volumes involve rebreathing gases through a mouthpiece for several minutes. The technician spends a great deal of time explaining exactly how to perform the desired breathing maneuvers. Forced expiratory maneuvers are performed at least three times to insure valid and reliable results. Because test results are useless without maximum patient effort and cooperation, the technician may have to continually coach and sometimes raise his voice at the patient to elicit a smooth and continuous forced exhalation without any hesitation. After lung volumes and mechanics of breathing measurements are taken, mechanics of breathing measurements are again taken after inhalation of a bronchodilator medication. Diffusion of gases is measured on a single breathholding maneuver.

DETERMINATION OF PREDICTED, OBSERVED, AND PERCENT PREDICTED VALUES

Looking at a pulmonary function report can be very confusing, especially since laboratories in various hospitals organize the data differently and the results of specialized tests are sometimes mixed with results of routine PFTs. Although organizations may differ slightly, data for lung volumes, mechanics of breathing, and diffusion are always divided into columns for *predicted, observed* or measured, and *percent predicted* values.

Predicted values are anticipated normal values determined from nomograms based on the patient's sex (males have larger lung volumes than females), age (volumes decrease with age), and height (volumes are larger in tall individuals than in short individuals). Recently, nomograms have been developed to correct for race; lung volumes of blacks, American Indians, and orientals are as much as 12 to 14% lower than those for whites (Foley et al, 1977; American College of Chest Physicians, 1983).

Separate nomograms exist to determine predicted values for children because of their constantly changing rates of growth and development (Polgar and Promadhat, 1971).

Observed values are the values the patient actually achieved on the test.

A *percent predicted* value is equal to the observed value divided by the predicted value. To scan PFT results, the nurse focuses on the percent predicted column. *As a general rule, all percent predicted values should fall between 80 and 120% of predicted.* Hence, 122% predicted is abnormally high, 75% is abnormally low, and 105% is normal. Since statistical lower limits of normal vary from one pulmonary function laboratory to another, this general rule must be used only as a guide to help the nurse make a basic interpretation of results. If serial PFTs are available, then normality and abnormality are more accurately determined by comparing past and present observed values and con-

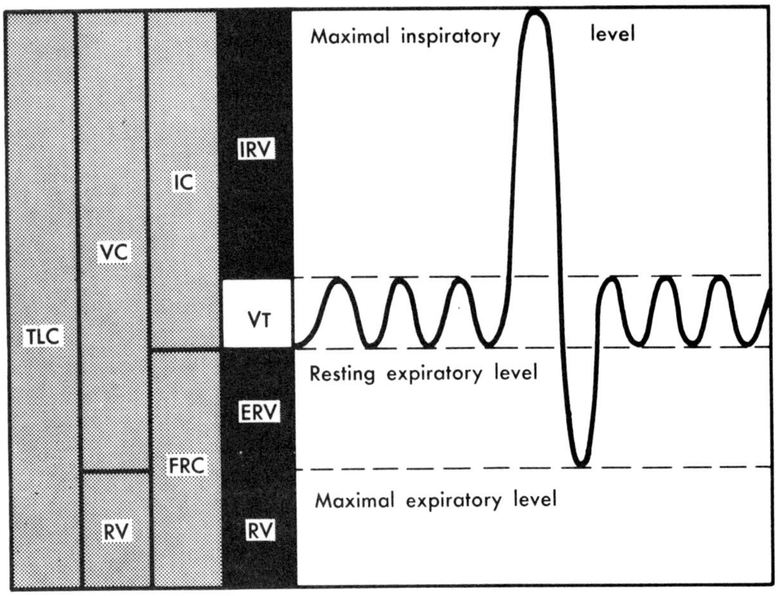

Figure 14–1. Lung volumes and capacities. Diagrammatic representation of various lung compartments, based on a typical spirogram. *TLC*, Total lung capacity; *VC*, vital capacity; *RV*, residual volume; *FRC*, functional residual capacity; *IC*, inspiratory capacity; V_T, tidal volume; *IRV*, inspiratory reserve volume; *ERV*, expiratory reserve volume. Shaded areas indicate relationships between the subdivisions and relative sizes as compared to the TLC. The resting expiratory level should be noted, since it remains more stable than other identifiable points during repeated spirograms, and hence is used as a starting point for FRC determinations, etc. (Reproduced by permission from Ruppel, G. Manual of Pulmonary Function Testing, 4th ed. St. Louis, C. V. Mosby, 1986.)

sidering PFT results in relation to other clinical findings.

LUNG VOLUMES AND CAPACITIES

Basic lung volumes and capacities (i.e., combinations of lung volumes) are introduced in Chapter 5 in relation to lung ventilation. The many volumes and capacities listed on a complete PFT report and selectively referred to in the clinical setting are defined hereafter and shown diagrammatically in Figure 14–1.

Lung Volumes

expiratory reserve volume (ERV)—the maximal volume of air exhaled after a normal exhalation. A decreased ERV occurs in those with restrictive processes, such as gross obesity, ascites, pregnancy, or other processes that cause elevation of the diaphragm.

inspiratory reserve volume (IRV)—the maximal volume of air inhaled after a normal inspiration.

residual volume (RV)—volume of air left in the lungs after maximal expiration. This is the only volume that cannot be measured directly. It is increased in COPD from air trapping in the lungs and in acute obstructive processes (e.g., bronchospasm, airway edema) from premature airway closure during expiration.

tidal volume (TV or V_T)—volume of air inhaled or exhaled with each breath during quiet breathing. V_T may not vary significantly, even with severe disease. In the complete PFT, it is recorded graphically but not measured for interpretation. It is primarily a bedside assessment parameter.

Lung Capacities

functional residual capacity (FRC)—volume of air left in the lungs at the end of normal expiration.

inspiratory capacity (IC)—the maximal volume of air inspired after a normal exhalation.

residual volume/total lung capacity (RV/TLC)—the ratio of residual volume to total lung capacity, expressed as a percentage (%). It is determined by dividing RV by TLC and multiplying by 100. The nurse looks in the "predicted" column to determine the normal percentage for the patient in question. If "less than 33%" is predicted (the usual normal value for most individuals), this means that any percentage below 33% is normal. In other words, no more than 33% of TLC should be made up of RV. Increased RV/TLC indicates air trapping, as in severe COPD, asthma, or sometimes bronchial obstruction. When the percentage is increased, the nurse checks separate RV and TLC values to determine which value changed the most and altered the overall RV/TLC percentage.

total lung capacity (TLC)—total volume of air in the lungs after maximal inspiration. A decreased TLC indicates restrictive disease; an increased TLC indicates lung hyperinflation and obstructive disease.

vital capacity (VC)—total volume of air exhaled after a maximal inspiration. Nonspecific in nature, VC measures the presence and progression of pulmonary disease. A decreased VC might indicate increasing airway obstruction, increasing respiratory muscular weakness (e.g., from neuromuscular disease and body fatigue), or decreasing lung or chest wall compliance (e.g., atelectasis, pulmonary edema, and kyphoscoliosis). Since this measurement is taken on a slow and relaxed exhalation as opposed to a forced one, it is sometimes called slow vital capacity (SVC).

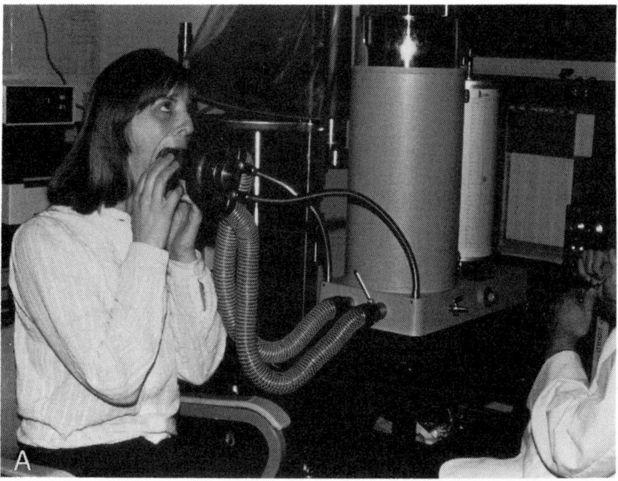
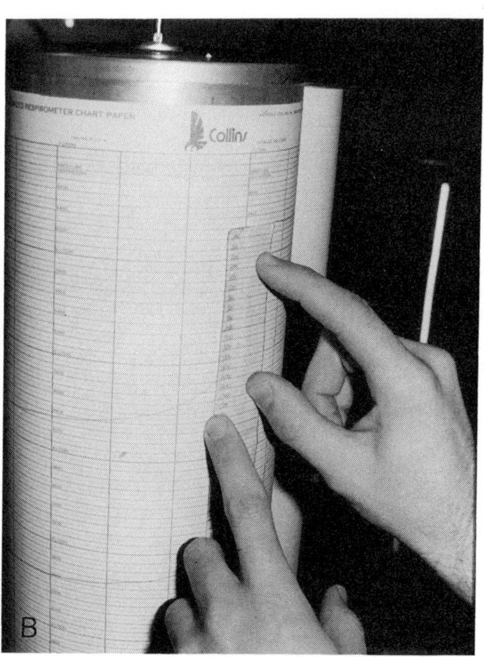

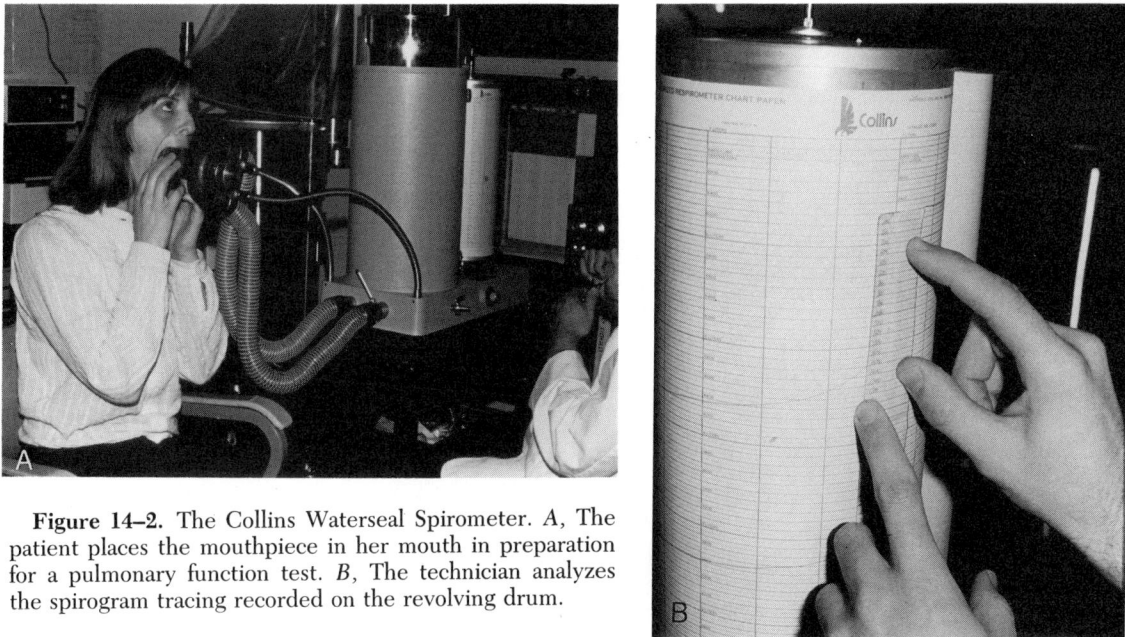

Figure 14–2. The Collins Waterseal Spirometer. *A*, The patient places the mouthpiece in her mouth in preparation for a pulmonary function test. *B*, The technician analyzes the spirogram tracing recorded on the revolving drum.

Measuring Lung Volumes and Capacities

Lung volumes and capacities as well as some mechanics of breathing are measured with a spirometer. Until recently, the traditional standard spirometer in the pulmonary function laboratory had been the *waterseal spirometer* (Fig. 14–2A). A cylindric bell floats in a metal container filled with water. The bell moves up and down with respiration while a pen attached to it writes on a rotating drum to record the patient's spirogram (Fig. 14–2B). A *spirogram* is a graphic tracing of lung volume measurements. Now, however, most laboratories have replaced these manual spirometers with more sensitive waterless spirometers, and many laboratories use electronic computerized equipment to facilitate data collection, calculations, and interpretation (Fig. 14–3).

Spirograms will vary slightly in appearance, depending on paper speed and position and the nature of the recording device. For example, some devices record in dotted lines (Fig. 14–4), whereas others record in solid lines. Some record from right to left and others from left to right. A spirogram from a portable spirometer looks upside down compared with a tracing from a laboratory waterseal spirometer. In spite of these relatively minor differences, basic patterns are the same, regardless of the spirometer used.

Most volumes and capacities, except residual volume (RV) and functional residual capacity (FRC), are easily measured by a standard spirometer and simple breathing maneuvers. Measurement of RV and FRC is more complicated because additional breathing maneuvers and equipment are required to measure RV, the volume in the lungs after a vital capacity maneuver. Measurement involves first determining FRC by either the nitrogen washout method or the helium dilution method described hereafter. Then, RV is determined by simple arithmetic as follows: FRC − ERV = RV.

Nitrogen Washout Method. Different types of nitrogen washout methods exist to measure FRC, other lung volumes, and gas distribution within the lungs. In the rebreathing method, the patient breathes 100% oxygen (O_2) starting at the end of a tidal volume and ending when practically all the nitrogen (N_2) is "washed out" of the lungs. Equilibration normally occurs within a 7-minute period. For a normal person breathing room air, 80% of the lung volume consists of N_2. When N_2 is washed out with 100% O_2, the volume of N_2 washed out of the lungs is proportional to the person's lung volume (FRC).

Helium Dilution Method. In this more commonly used method, the patient breathes a known concentration of helium (He) until the concentration of He in the lungs and in the spirometer equilibrates. At this point, FRC is calculated from the change in He concentration in the spirometer. The more diluted the He in the spirometer, the larger the patient's lung volume. The higher the He concentration, the smaller the patient's lung volume.

A major problem with both the N_2 washout and the He dilution methods pertains to the length of time required for gas equilibration. Although the N_2 may be washed out and the He concentration equilibrated in 3 to 4 minutes in a healthy person, this process may take as long as 7 to 20 minutes in patients with severe COPD with air trapping in the lungs. Some alveoli may never be washed out, and values for FRC and RV may be underestimated.

Body Plethysmograph Method. The *body plethysmograph*, nicknamed the *body box*, is the fastest and

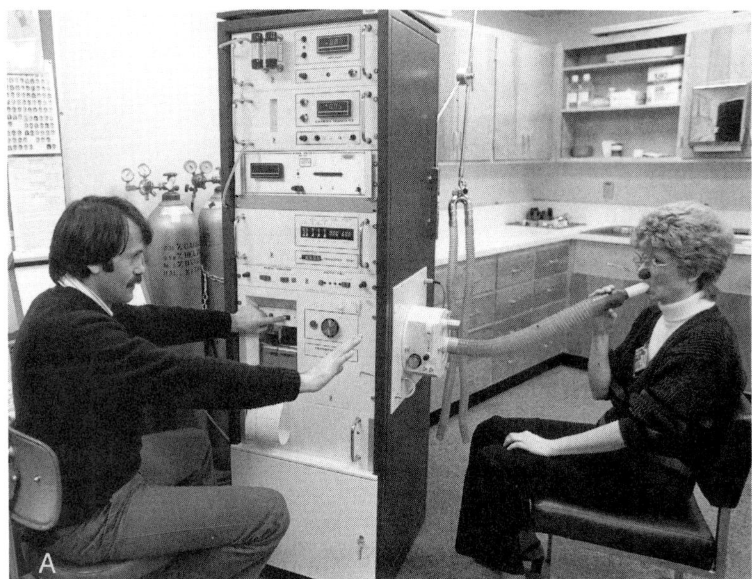

Figure 14–3. A computerized pulmonary function system. *A*, Testing with equipment in a pulmonary function laboratory. *B*, Spirograms and graphic results. Left, prebronchodilator (solid line) and postbronchodilator (dotted lines) flow-volume loops. Upper right, predicted and observed lung volumes. Lower right, forced vital capacity (FVC) spirogram.

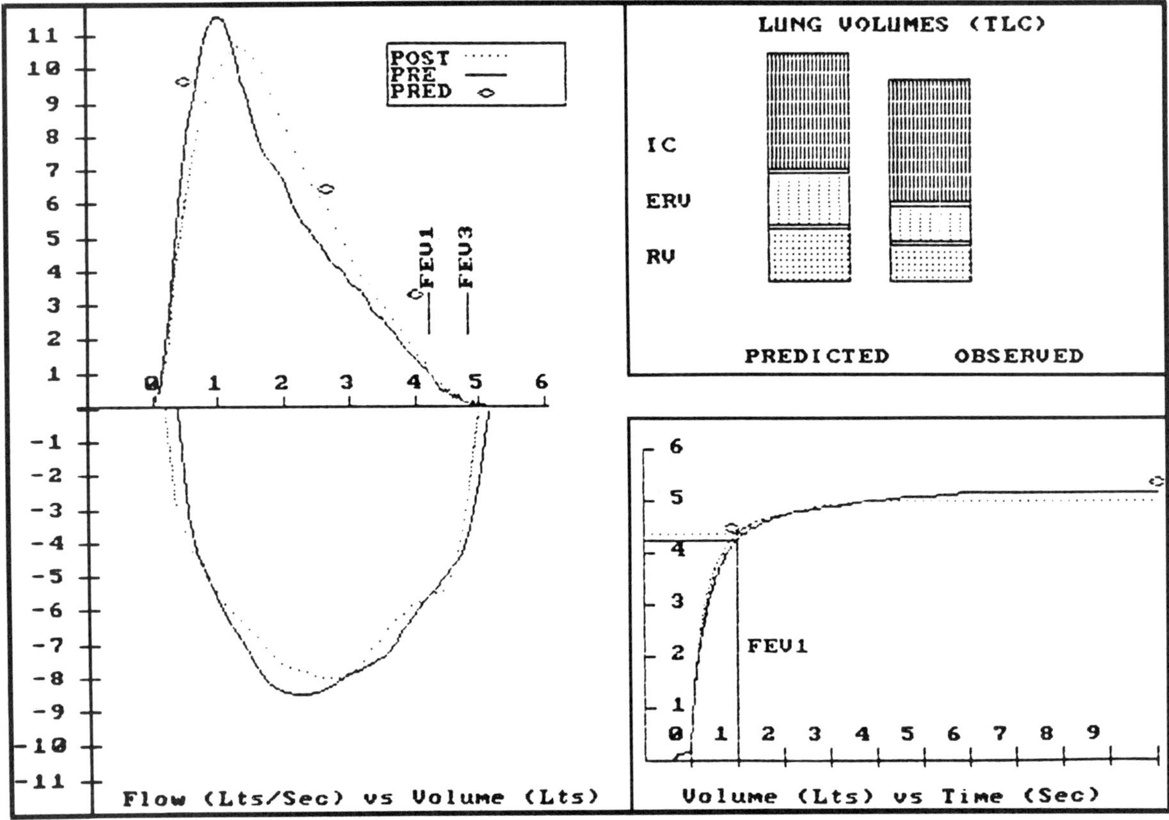

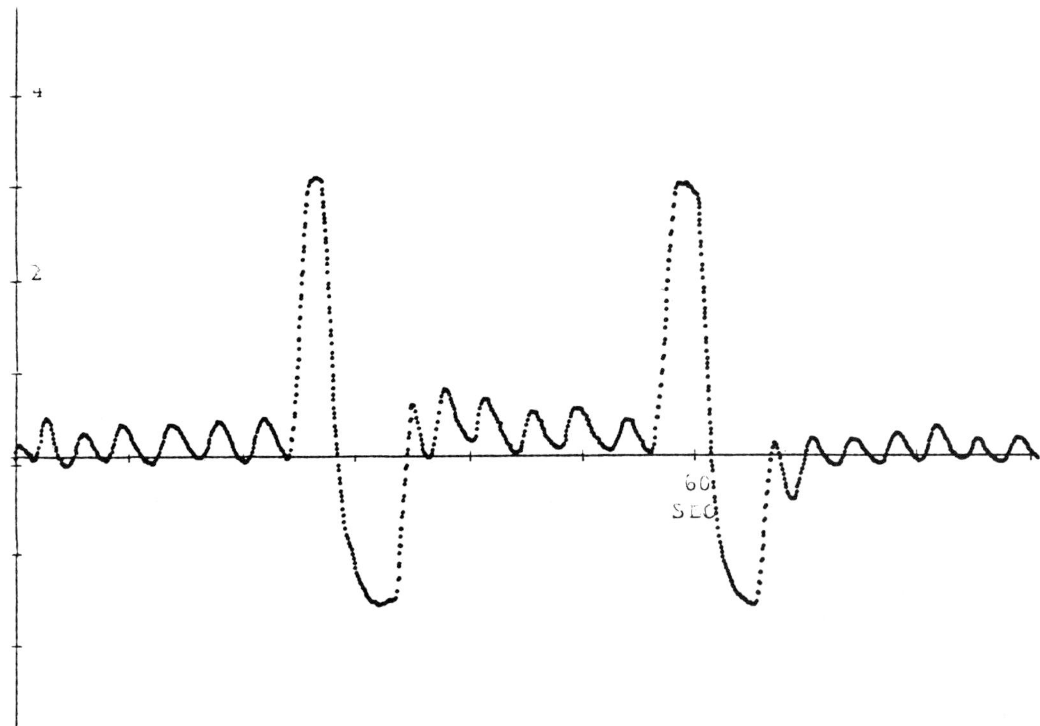

Figure 14–4. Normal spirogram recorded by an electronic computerized spirometer. Normal tidal volumes are interrupted by two forced vital capacities. (The vertical axis indicates the volume in liters, and the horizontal axis indicates the time in seconds.)

most accurate method of measuring lung volumes. The subject sits in an airtight box with his mouth over a mouthpiece (Fig. 14–5). During a panting maneuver against an occluded mouthpiece, changes in box pressure reflect changes in thoracic volume. By this method, *thoracic gas volume* (TGV) at FRC is measured and compared with FRC obtained by the He dilution or N_2 washout method. In healthy individuals, the two FRCs are about equal (± 300 cc). In those with obstructive disease, the *body box FRC* may be higher, and the difference between the two measurements estimates the degree of air trapping or the volume of poorly ventilated regions in the lungs.

In addition, the body box may be used for other useful measurements, such as airway resistance. However, the cost and complexity of the equipment usually restricts its use to large medical centers. Also, some patients cannot be tested by this method because they cannot execute the panting maneuver. Others do not tolerate the feeling of being in the closed and confining environment of the box; intravenous lines, infusion pumps, and other equipment interfere with test administration.

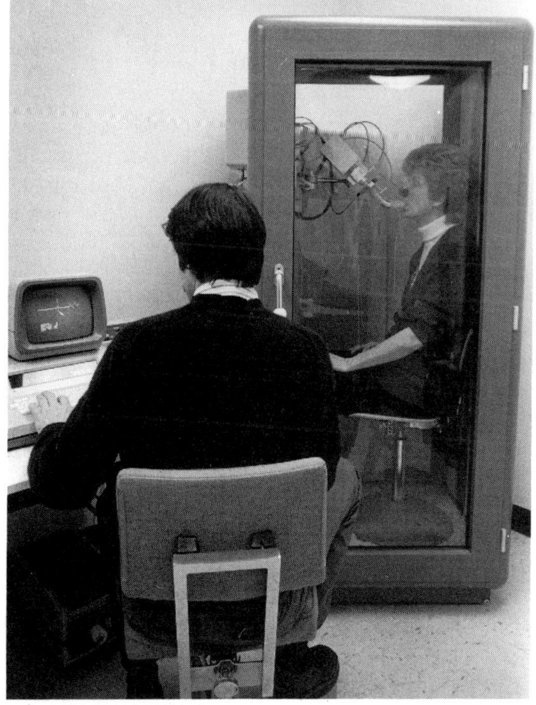

Figure 14–5. Whole body plethysmograph with the patient enclosed in the box. This system may be used for evaluation of basic spirometry, lung volumes, airway resistance, and clinical response during bronchial provocation studies.

Lung Volumes in Restrictive Versus Obstructive Disease

Figure 14–6 compares the normal pattern for TLC and its subdivisions with patterns for obstructive and restrictive diseases. Restrictive disease is characterized by a decrease in TLC and all volumes in general. Obstructive disease is characterized by an increase in

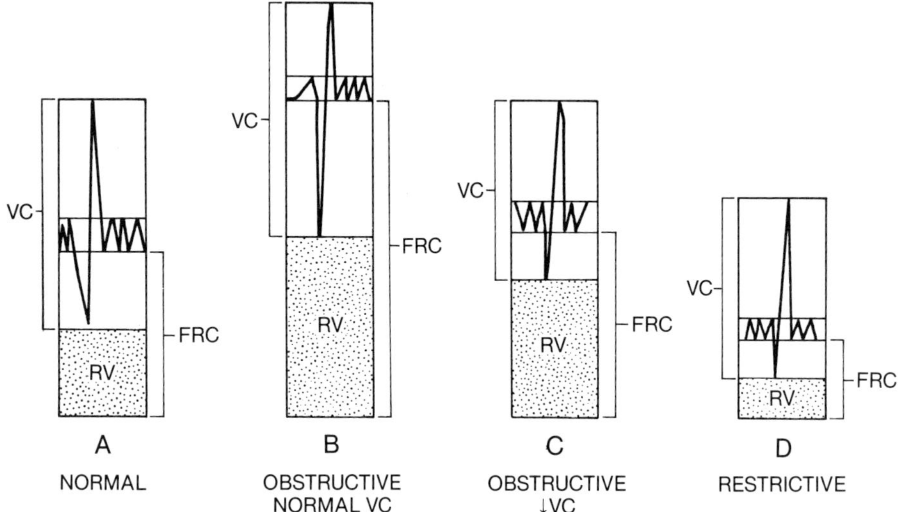

Figure 14–6. Total lung capacity (TLC) and its subdivisions in normal, obstructive, and restrictive patterns. The dotted areas represent residual volume in the lung after full exhalation.

RV, FRC, and TLC. It must be emphasized that VC may be normal (Fig. 14–6B) or reduced (Fig. 14–6C), and TLC may be increased or normal. It is not uncommon for an individual with severe COPD to present with a *normal* TLC and signs of lung hyperinflation on the chest x-ray film. (Lung hyperinflation must be severe before TLC increases significantly.) An elevated TLC is most characteristic of lung diseases, such as emphysema and cystic fibrosis, that produce severe lung hyperinflation.

MECHANICS OF BREATHING

Mechanics of breathing is the second component of the complete PFT. It assesses the flow of gas in and out of the lungs and helps determine whether altered respiratory muscle strength, lung and chest wall compliance, or airway and lung tissue resistance has significantly altered lung function. Test results confirm the diagnosis of restrictive disease made on the basis of a decreased TLC. Mechanics of breathing results are crucial in determining the severity and nature of airway obstruction in obstructive disease.

Essentially, test values are flow rates during forced breathing maneuvers, usually forced exhalation, measured in *volumes per unit of time* (*liters per minute* or *liters per second*). The lung volume at which flows are measured largely influences test results. Maximum flow rates at high lung volumes are greater than flow rates at lower lung volumes. Similarly, a healthy adult with a TLC of 6 L will generate much higher flow rates than a restrictive disease patient with a TLC of 3.5 L. Also, the degree of lung recoil as well as airway diameter largely determines expiratory air flow. Diseases with *decreased lung recoil* (e.g., emphysema) or *decreased airway diameter* (e.g., asthma, acute bronchitis) cause reduction in flow rates at any given lung volume. Diseases with *increased lung recoil* (e.g., mild interstitial fibrosis, interstitial pulmonary edema) may cause an elevation in flow rates.

Basic Measurements

Forced Vital Capacity (FVC). *Vital capacity is performed rapidly and with maximal effort throughout expiration.* FVC is reduced in restrictive disease and may be reduced in obstructive disease when severe airway obstruction is present.

FVC is compared with *slow* vital capacity (SVC). Observed values are identical (± 20 cc) in normal individuals and those with restrictive disease. Great variations in the two values are commonly seen in patients with obstructive disease or hyperirritable airways. FVC may be 50 to 100 cc less than SVC owing to increasing bronchospasm or blockage of airways with secretions on any forced expiratory maneuver.

Figure 14–7 shows a normal FVC spirogram. Note that the first 25% of FVC is totally effort dependent, whereas the last 75% of FVC is effort independent. This means that flow rates measured in early expiration near TLC vary with the degree of force exerted by the patient. Unless maximal effort is exerted, they are less reliable and valid than flow rates measured in the mid or late portions of the curve.

Forced Expiratory Volume in 1 Second (FEV_1). *The volume of air exhaled during the first second of the FVC* (Fig. 14–8). FEV_1 reflects air flow in *large* as opposed to small airways. A decreased value indicates the presence of airway obstruction. FEV_1 is decreased in restrictive disease, when lung volumes are severely reduced.

FEV_1 is perhaps the most useful mechanics of breathing parameter for evaluating degree of respiratory impairment and disease progression in pure obstructive disease. The following clinical guidelines are relatively easy to remember:

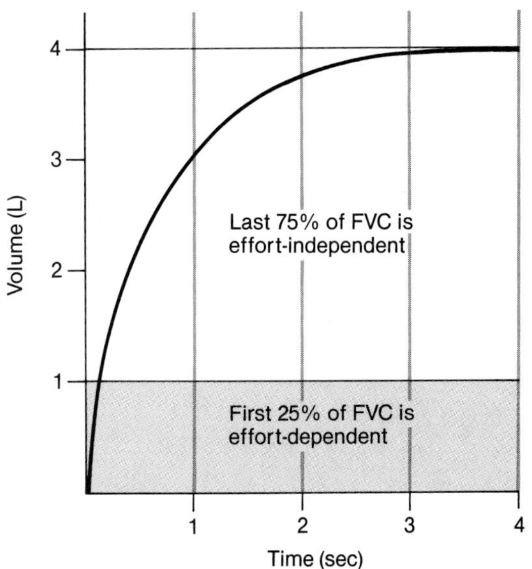

Figure 14–7. Normal FVC spirogram showing effort-dependent and effort-independent sections of the curve. (Adapted from Ruppel, G.: Manual of Pulmonary Function Testing. St. Louis, C. V. Mosby Co., 1986.)

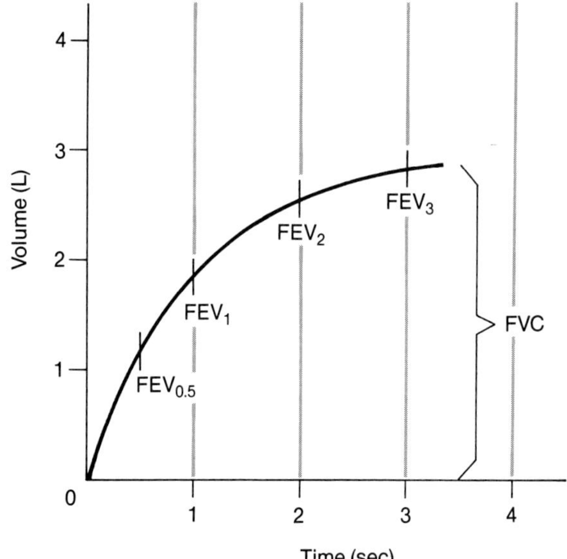

Figure 14–8. A spirogram of a forced vital capacity (FVC) maneuver with forced expiratory volume (FEV) labelled at various time intervals. The FEV at 1 second (FEV_1) is the most important measurement.

$FEV_1 < 1.0$ L—severe obstruction
$FEV_1 = 1.0$ to 2.0 L—moderate obstruction
$FEV_1 > 2.0$ L to normal—mild obstruction

The expected decline in FEV_1 in adults over 20 years of age is as follows:

Normal adults—20 to 50 ml/yr (Fletcher and Peto, 1977). Progressive decline in pulmonary function from aging may not begin until the mid 30s in some individuals.
Adults with COPD—50 to 80 ml/yr (Petty et al, 1973). A more rapid annual rate of decline in FEV_1 (> 90 ml/yr) and a rapid decline in FVC (≥ 75 ml/yr) are associated with a low probability for survival (Kanner and Renzetti, 1984).

Other timed forced expiratory volumes (FEV_t), such as $FEV_{0.5\ sec}$, $FEV_{2\ sec}$, and $FEV_{3\ sec}$ (labelled in Fig. 14–8), may be used with the FEV_1 to further evaluate mechanics of breathing.

FEV_1/FVC (%). *The percentage of FVC exhaled in 1 second.* This measurement may be written as *FEV_1%*. It is calculated as follows:

$$FEV_1\% = \frac{FEV_1}{FVC} \times 100$$

Although the predicted value varies with age, about 75% of the FVC should be out of the lungs in 1 second, as illustrated in Figure 14–9A.

A *decreased FEV_1/FVC* indicates airway obstruction. A slightly reduced value in light of a normal FVC indicates early airway obstruction. A greatly reduced value with a spirogram that is flat, long, and drawn out, such as the one in Figure 14–9B, indicates moderate to severe obstructive disease. In the obstructive pattern, FEV_1/FVC is reduced because the FEV_1 (i.e., the numerator) is reduced. The patient usually has adequate lung volume (i.e., normal FVC), but he cannot expire it within the 3- to 4-second time period a normal person can expire it.

An *increased FEV_1/FVC* of over 80 to 90% indicates restrictive disease, provided the patient exerts full effort during the expiratory maneuver. Note the smallness of the spirogram in Figure 14–9C as well as the steepness of its slope. In this restrictive pattern, both FEV_1 and FVC are decreased owing to the overall decrease in lung volume. However, FEV_1 is never decreased as much as FVC. The reason for the proportionally higher FEV_1 value relates to the restrictive patient's increased lung elastic recoil (see Chapter 8) and the absence of airway obstruction. The lungs empty rapidly and completely on exhalation.

The FEV_1/FVC helps to evaluate prognosis and the likelihood of progressive deterioration of pulmonary function. One study reported that patients with values less than 60% had an increased death rate and a more rapid reduction in lung function compared with those with values over 75% (Petty et al, 1973). Similarly, those within a range of 60 to 75% had a higher than normal loss of lung function over time.

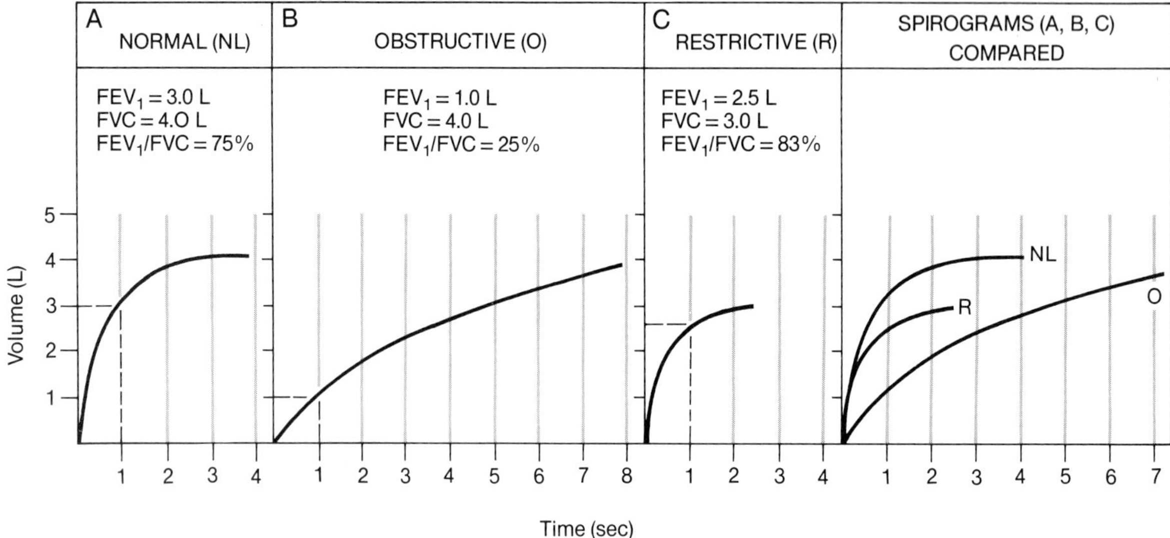

Figure 14–9. Examples of spirograms and flow rates for normal lungs (NL), obstructive disease (O), and restrictive disease (R). Spirograms represent one forced vital capacity breathing maneuver.

Forced Midexpiratory Flow ($FEF_{25-75\%}$). *Mean rate of air flow over the middle half of the FVC* (Fig. 14–10). This value was previously called the *maximal midexpiratory flow rate* (MMFR).

The $FEF_{25-75\%}$ reflects flow in *small* (less than 2 mm in diameter) peripheral airways as opposed to large airways. A *slightly reduced* value in light of an otherwise completely normal PFT indicates minimal to mild airway obstruction. As obstructive disease progresses, the FEV_1 gradually decreases as air flow becomes limited in large airways as well.

An *elevated* $FEF_{25-75\%}$ may be found in mild restrictive disease owing to increased lung elastic recoil. On expiration, the stiff lungs rapidly recoil to resting position in a manner similar to the recoil action of stiff springs. Subsequently, the mid flow rate gradually decreases to below normal, as lung volumes decrease with progressive restrictive disease.

The $FEF_{25-75\%}$ is one of the best indexes of airway resistance because it is sensitive to early airway obstruction, and because it is measured in midexpiration in the effort-independent portion of the FVC curve. Nevertheless, use of $FEF_{25-75\%}$ as a screening measurement remains controversial. Because of the way it is calculated from FVC, a spuriously low value may result from an unusually vigorous initial effort exerted by some young persons during testing (Chan-Yeung et al, 1985). In addition, in some cases, FEV_1/FVC may be just as useful as $FEF_{25-75\%}$ in the detection of mild obstructive disease. For obstructive disease only, if FEV_1/FVC is equal to or greater than 75% and normal, the $FEF_{25-75\%}$ will be normal and its measurement unnecessary. An obstructive process is suspected when FEV_1/FVC is less than 75%, though not always outside predicted limits (Gelb et al, 1983). In this case, full spirometry is indicated for further evaluation.

Other Measurements

The following flow rates are also commonly seen on a complete pulmonary function test.

Forced Expiratory Flow ($FEF_{200-1200cc}$) or Maximum Expiratory Flow Rate (MEFR). *Average flow rate measured at the beginning of expiration between 200 and 1200 cc of FVC.* This value is greatly influenced

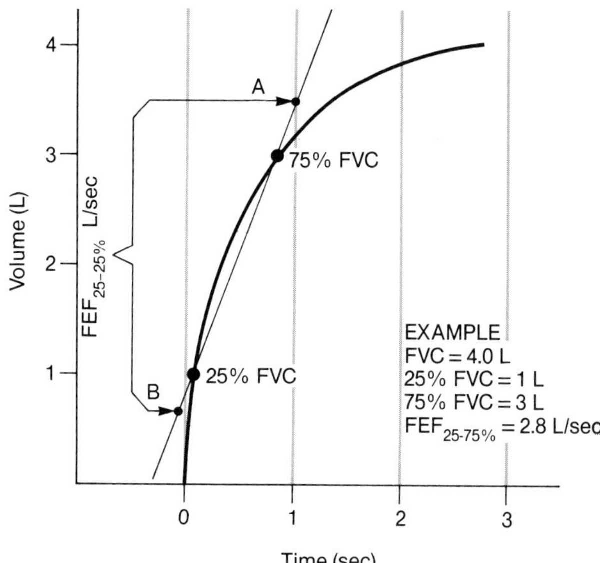

Figure 14–10. Spirogram of the forced midexpiratory flow ($FEF_{25-75\%}$) from 25% of forced vital capacity (FVC × 0.25) to 75% of FVC (FVC × 0.75). The $FEF_{25-75\%}$ is determined by first extending the line between these two points to the vertical, 1-second time lines (points A and B). The volume between A and B (2.8 L in this case) is read directly as the $FEF_{25-75\%}$ in L/sec.

by patient effort and the size of the lungs. It is most useful for serial evaluation of PFTs.

Maximum Inspiratory Flow Rate (MIFR). *Beginning near residual volume, the flow rate is measured between 200 and 1200 cc of rapid forced inspiration.* The normal value is 300 L/min or greater. Although a reduced value is found in those with neuromuscular disorders, poor effort, and extrathoracic upper airway obstruction, the most common cause of a reduced value is poor patient cooperation. This value is totally effort dependent.

Maximum Voluntary Ventilation (MVV) or Maximum Breathing Capacity (MBC). *Maximum volume of air a person can ventilate over 1 minute.* The patient is asked to breathe as deeply and rapidly as possible, setting his own respiratory rate and moving more than tidal volume but less than vital capacity with each breath. The test is performed over a specific time interval of 10, 12, or 15 seconds, and then the volume expired, as measured by a spirometer, is multiplied by a factor of 6, 5, or 4, respectively, to obtain flow rate in L/min. When the test is performed in the PFT laboratory, inspiration and expiration are recorded, yielding spirographic tracings typical of those of normal lung function, restrictive disease, and obstructive disease. Note the obstructive pattern in Figure 14–11. The tracing moves above the baseline level as forced breathing increases air trapping in the lungs. A large reduction in MVV indicates obstructive disease. Normal values vary by as much as 30% from the mean because the breathing maneuver is largely effort dependent. MVV is strikingly normal or near normal in pure restrictive disease.

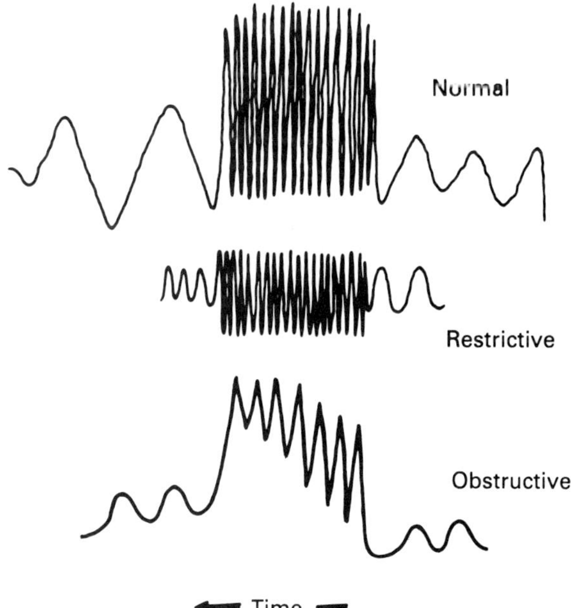

Figure 14–11. Maximum voluntary ventilation spirograms for normal lungs and restrictive and obstructive diseases. In the obstructive pattern, note the rising end-expiratory level indicative of air trapping. (Reproduced by permission from Burton, G. and Hodgkin, J. Respiratory Care—A Guide to Clinical Practice, 2nd ed. J. B. Lippincott Co., 1984.)

The MVV has limited usefulness because it is so effort dependent. Nevertheless, it may help evaluate respiratory muscle strength in neuromuscular patients. Also, in acute cases, it may be used with other PFT measurements to evaluate the ability of respiratory muscles to sustain spontaneous breathing. Because patient cooperation, motivation, and physical stamina are required to produce an MVV greater than 80 %, some clinicians use the MVV to help identify patients at high risk to develop postoperative pulmonary complications due to ineffective coughing and deep breathing. Patients with an MVV of less than 45 L/min are prone to postoperative pulmonary complications leading to death or undue disability (Arabian et al, 1982).

The MVV may be estimated by multiplying the observed FEV_1 by 35. A discrepancy between the observed MVV and the estimated MVV based on FEV_1 indicates poor patient effort and invalid test results (American College of Chest Physicians, 1983).

Response to Bronchodilator

Mechanics of breathing is again measured after inhalation of 2 to 15 puffs of a bronchodilator such as isoproterenol (Isuprel) or isoetharine via a compressor-driven or hand-bulb nebulizer device or a metered cartridge inhaler. The clinician waits 5 to 20 minutes for maximal response to the agent before repeating measurements. The waiting period varies depending on the drug used and its strength.

On the PFT report, there are separate columns for the postbronchodilator (post BD) *observed (measured)* and the *percent predicted* values and on some, the calculated *percent change* value, defined as *the percentage change of the postbronchodilator observed value compared with the prebronchodilator (pre BD) observed value.* The formula is as follows:

$$\%\ \text{change} = \frac{\text{observed post BD value (L)} - \text{observed pre BD value (L)}}{\text{observed pre BD value (L)}}$$

Consider the example of a patient whose FEV_1 improves from 1.0 L before bronchodilator to 1.2 L after bronchodilator. There is a 0.2 L (200 cc) improvement in value (1.2 − 1.0). The percent change is 20%: $\frac{0.2}{1.0} = 0.20$ or 20%.

Normal Response. Measurements before and after bronchodilation are the same in normal individuals as well as in persons with pure restrictive disease. The percent change is zero.

Response in Obstructive Disease. Pre BD and post BD values vary in obstructive disease. The primary purpose of measuring response to a bronchodilator is to determine the reversibility of airway obstruction. *Reversible airway obstruction is said to be present when percent change is 15% or greater in at least two of the following three values: FVC, FEV_1, and $FEF_{25-75\%}$* (Snider et al, 1974). For a pulmonary patient with obstructive disease, a 15% change is highly favor-

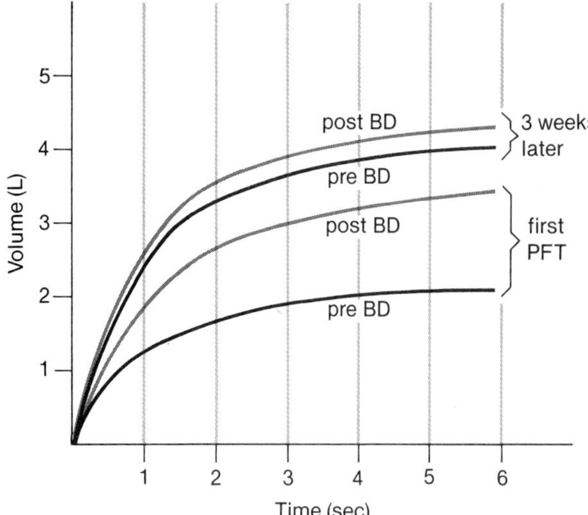

Figure 14–12. Spirograms of an individual recovering from acute asthmatic bronchitis. The first PFT shows a large difference between prebronchodilator and postbronchodilator measurements. After 3 weeks of bronchodilator medication and bronchial hygiene measures, the patient is almost fully bronchodilated. Prebronchodilator and postbronchodilator spirograms are almost the same. (BD = bronchodilator and PFT = pulmonary function test.)

able; it confirms the diagnosis of asthma or identifies an asthmatic or reversible component in mixed chest pathology. The higher the value above 15%, the more reversible the disease. Clinical improvement is expected once the patient starts daily bronchodilator medication. Subsequent progress is monitored, and the effectiveness of various regimens is evaluated by serial PFTs over days, weeks, and months. The goal of therapy is to increase pre BD values to post BD values. As flow rates improve, the spirogram tracing approaches a normal pattern, as illustrated in Figure 14–12.

No response to the bronchodilator (0 to 5% change) is an unfavorable sign, suggesting the presence of irreversible lung disease (e.g., emphysema). Although no response identifies individuals who are most likely to experience little benefit from clinical bronchodilator therapy, percent change does not always measure potential subjective and objective clinical improvement. The emphysematous patient may experience dramatic improvement in symptoms with minimal objective improvement in PFTs after a few weeks of bronchodilation and recently added corticosteroid therapy. The bronchitic patient demonstrating minimal or no improvement (i.e., less than 12 to 15% change) may begin to respond better to bronchodilators once he gives up smoking and the airways begin to heal. Furthermore, other factors may be responsible for the lack of response to bronchodilators, such as the persisting effect of bronchodilators administered earlier in the day and the development of resistance to the particular bronchodilator administered. Because disease reversibility is not entirely determined by response to the bronchodilator on the PFT, some pulmonary physicians may broadly interpret a percent change of less than 15% as "some significant response" rather than "no response," without suggesting the presence of irreversibility. This approach gives the patient benefit of the doubt, and it discourages the labelling of a patient's condition as irreversible and hopeless without full consideration of other clinical parameters. The nurse will find that criteria for a significant versus an insignificant response to bronchodilator may vary greatly among PFT interpreters, clinical settings, and related sources of literature.

DIFFUSION

The third major component of the complete PFT is diffusion, formally called *diffusing capacity of the lung* and abbreviated DL or DL_{CO}. Actually, DL measures gas transfer not a lung capacity. In technical terms, it measures the *milliliters of carbon monoxide (CO)*, the test gas, *transferred per minute for each mmHg pressure difference for CO across the lung.* It is expressed as ml/min/mmHg. The normal predicted DL varies, depending on height, age, and hematocrit value, but it usually ranges from *30 to 35* (young males) to *20 to 25* (males over 50 years of age) *ml/min/mmHg.*

More specifically, the DL measurement determines *how well the test gas carbon monoxide diffuses across the alveolar-capillary membrane and combines with hemoglobin in pulmonary capillary red blood cells.* CO is used because its affinity for hemoglobin is about 210 times. Hence, when the patient breathes CO, all alveolar CO binds with hemoglobin, and none remains in blood plasma. The plasma partial pressure of CO equals zero, and the gradient for gas diffusion becomes equal to the measured alveolar concentration of CO. Under these conditions, any alteration in gas diffusion is attributed to altered lung function and not CO, the test gas, provided the patient's hemoglobin is normal. An altered DL is clinically correlated with an altered diffusing capacity for oxygen.

DL measurements aid in diagnosing chest diseases when other clinical manifestations are absent. A *slightly reduced* DL may be the earliest detectable abnormality in pulmonary vascular diseases or restrictive diseases, such as sarcoidosis and asbestosis. In mixed chest pathology (e.g., COPD), DL helps to identify the irreversible emphysematous component.

In addition, *serial DLs* help in the evaluation of disease progression as well as response to therapy in patients with chronic disease and those recuperating from acute diseases, such as multiple pulmonary emboli and adult respiratory distress syndrome (ARDS). Some clinicians use serial DLs to evaluate pulmonary hemorrhage (Weinberger et al, 1980). The presence of fresh intra-alveolar blood is associated with an increased DL. In most acute situations, however, measurement of DL is impractical and not indicated, because obvious signs (e.g., hemoptysis) are present to justify the appropriate intervention indicated.

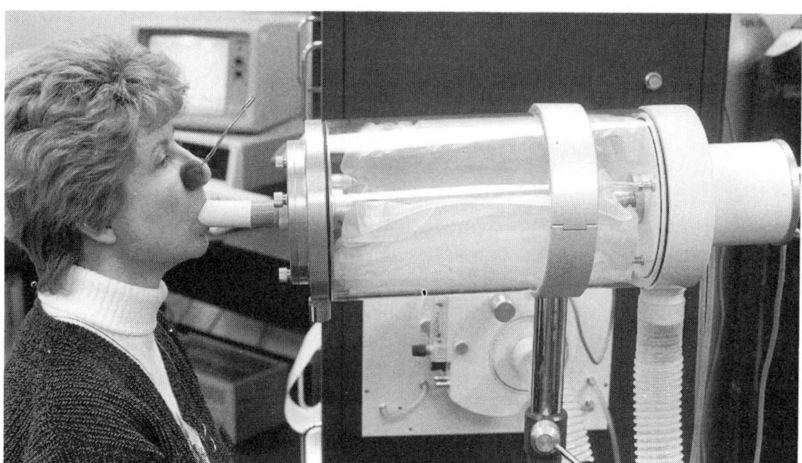

Figure 14–13. Use of a diffusion module for measurement of diffusing capacity of the lung (DL).

Measuring DL

DL is usually measured using a single breath method. The patient inhales maximally from a bag in the diffusion module containing a mixture of gases (Fig. 14–13); he holds his breath for 10 seconds to allow time for the CO to leave the alveoli and enter the blood; then he exhales. A separate collection bag in the diffusion module collects a sample of midexpiratory gas for analysis. The rest of the exhaled gas is automatically vented to the room.

Even though the DL measurement is a valuable assessment parameter, it is not always reported on the complete PFT for a variety of reasons. First, DL is not always ordered because it is considered a periodic rather than a routine test for clinical monitoring. Second, some laboratories do not perform the test because of the expensive equipment required. Also, administration problems may preclude its use on selected individuals. For example, the test cannot be administered to dyspneic persons who cannot hold their breath for the required 10 seconds. In acutely ill patients and those with severe chronic diseases, poor effort may yield a submaximal inspiration on the test, a relatively low lung volume, and a low DL value that does not necessarily indicate pathology. Hence, even if the test is ordered by the physician, the technician may not be able to complete it.

Factors Influencing DL

Two main factors influencing DL measurement are *blood hemoglobin level* and *alveolar-capillary surface area*. The causes of an abnormal DL (Table 14–1) are discussed below in relation to these and other factors. Keep in mind that an *increased* DL indicates increased gas diffusion across the alveolar-capillary membrane. In contrast, a *decreased* DL indicates the presence of a *diffusion defect*, a general term referring to impairment of gas diffusion.

Blood Hemoglobin. The quantity of hemoglobin per unit volume of blood alters DL by altering the number of hemoglobin molecule sites available for CO uptake. Polycythemia increases DL because more sites are available for CO uptake. Anemia decreases DL about 7% for each gm% of hemoglobin deficit. However, most laboratories use correction factors in DL determinations to account for varying hemoglobin levels.

Alveolar-Capillary Surface Area. In the past, diffusion defects were largely attributed to a thickened interstitium from fibrosis or edema (i.e., interstitial fibrosis or interstitial pulmonary edema) or to a thickened capillary membrane (i.e., pulmonary vasculitis or primary pulmonary hypertension). Fluid or thickened tissue was believed to reduce DL by lengthening the pathway for gas diffusion. While these factors may contribute to a reduced DL, researchers now have established that *the main cause of a reduced DL is the loss of alveolar-capillary surface area available for gas exchange*. The loss of surface area may be due to surgical resection or pathologic destruction of lung tissue. Alveoli, interstitium, and capillaries are lost in emphysema. Thickening of the alveolar walls and interstitium is accompanied by the destruction of nearby

Table 14–1. COMMON CAUSES OF AN ABNORMAL DIFFUSING CAPACITY (DL)

Increased DL	Decreased DL
Polycythemia	Anemia
Hypervolemia	Emphysema
Acute asthma (some cases)	Hypovolemia
Left ventricular failure (early)	Diffuse interstitial disease: fibrosis (idiopathic or as in scleroderma, sarcoidosis, asbestosis); interstitial pneumonia
Pulmonary hemorrhage	Pulmonary vascular disease (multiple pulmonary emboli, primary pulmonary hypertension)
Congenital heart defects with increased pulmonary blood volume (i.e., atrial septal defect)	Pulmonary resection
Exercise	

capillaries in diffuse interstitial fibrosis. In multiple pulmonary emboli, capillaries become blocked and adjacent alveoli become nonfunctional or ineffective because O_2 and CO_2 exchange does not take place. As Comroe and associates (1962) have stated, ". . . the critical area for diffusion is neither of the alveoli nor of the pulmonary *capillaries*, but of the *functioning alveoli in contact with functioning capillaries.*" When capillaries are obstructed or obliterated (e.g., emphysema, interstitial fibrosis), DL may decrease even further, owing to a reduced pulmonary capillary blood volume.

In contrast, an increased DL is often due to an *increased alveolar-capillary surface area* from an increased pulmonary capillary blood volume, as in physical exercise (i.e., capillaries are recruited), in hypervolemia, and in left ventricular failure. In asthma, DL is usually normal, but it may be greater in acute states due to higher perfusion of the lung apices and higher pulmonary capillary blood volume from negative intrathoracic pressures, increasing venous return to the heart and lungs (Weinberger et al, 1980). With mucus plugging and further impaired ventilation, DL decreases, but in this situation, the test is not needed or indicated for assessment and intervention.

Other Factors. Other factors, including *rate of intra-capillary gas transfers and chemical associations, degree of hypoxemia,* and *presence of intra-alveolar blood* from pulmonary hemorrhage, may contribute to an abnormal DL. Moreover, all of these factors may be involved to varying degrees, or one factor may counterbalance another to produce a normal DL value.

In a few cases, physicians cannot account for normal or abnormal DL values. For example, the patient with classic signs and symptoms of diffuse interstitial fibrosis may present upon rare occasion with a normal rather than a decreased DL.

Diffusion Defects and Hypoxemia

Patients with diffusion defects are not hypoxemic at rest unless pathology is extensive, as evidenced by a severely reduced DL below 40 to 50%. The administration of oxygen reverses the hypoxemia in the absence of intrapulmonary shunting from disorders such as pulmonary edema, pneumonia, and atelectasis.

Though the patient with a moderately reduced DL may maintain normal oxygenation at rest, PaO_2 typically drops during exercise. The hypoxemia is due to the loss of alveolar-capillary surface area and the shortened red blood cell (RBC) transit time, as explained hereafter. First, the destruction of capillaries by fibrosis, emphysema, or pulmonary vascular disease reduces the number of healthy capillaries available for recruitment during exercise. When the limited number of unperfused capillaries are fully recruited, blood flow increases because of the limited size of the pulmonary capillary bed. Hypoxemia occurs mainly because of the limited number of sites available for O_2–CO_2 exchange. Also, the increased blood flow shortens red blood cell transit time past alveolar-capillary units. It decreases equilibration time for gas exchange and thus contributes to hypoxemia.

Generally, the greater the loss of alveolar-capillary surface area, the greater the drop in PaO_2 during exercise. Also, the drop in PaO_2 during exercise and at rest will be more dramatic when fever or other high cardiac output states further shorten RBC transit time.

THE FLOW-VOLUME LOOP

The *flow-volume loop* is a graphic display of the relationship between air flow and volume during a forced expiration (FVC) followed by a forced inspiration. It is usually part of the complete PFT, though it is also used as a sole PFT monitoring parameter in the outpatient setting. Its primary usefulness lies in the detection and further evaluation of lower and upper airway obstruction.

The flow-volume loop is recorded with a device called an *x-y recorder* (Fig. 14–14). A normal loop is shown in Figure 14–15. During forced expiration, air flow peaks early in the first 20 to 30% of FVC, the effort-dependent portion of the curve. The peak marks the *peak expiratory flow rate* (PEFR). The characteristic straight curve between the PEFR and end-expiration at residual volume represents the linear relationship between reductions in air flow and volume in normal lungs. An automatic timing device permits the marking of $FEV_{0.5}$, FEV_1, and FEV_3 as shown in Figure 14–15 by the three dips in the expiratory curve.

In addition, forced expiratory flow (FEF) measurements may be determined at various lung volumes along the expiratory curve. The most important FEF measurement is the $FEF_{50\%}$, also called the $\dot{V}_{max\ 50}$. It represents air flow at 50% of forced vital capacity, as shown in Figure 14–16. $FEF_{50\%}$ may be correlated with the midflow rate ($FEF_{25-75\%}$) obtained during routine spirometry.

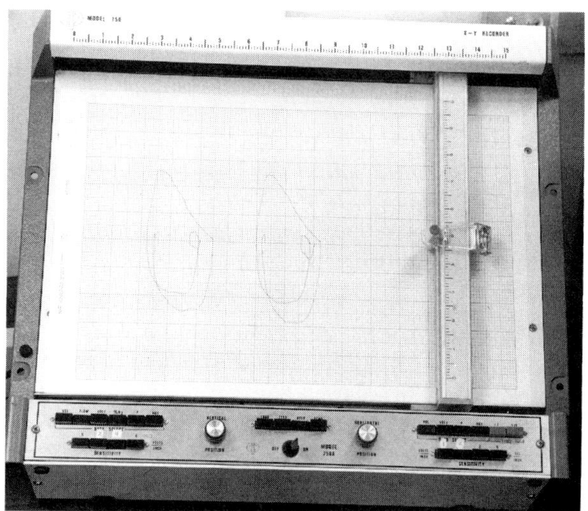

Figure 14–14. An x-y recorder for determination of the flow-volume loop.

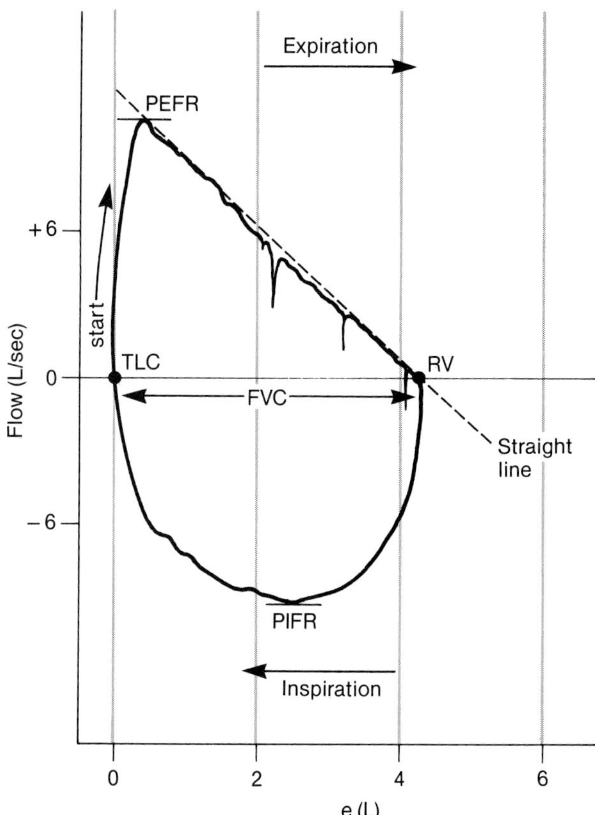

Figure 14–15. *The normal flow-volume loop.* After a period of quiet breathing, the patient is instructed to inhale as rapidly and as forcefully as possible (to total lung capacity or TLC), to hold his breath 1 to 2 seconds, and to exhale as rapidly, forcefully, and completely as possible. This expiratory maneuver is represented by the top half of the loop. When residual volume (RV) is reached and expiratory flow equals zero, the patient is instructed to inhale rapidly to TLC, as the lower half of the curve is recorded. The three short dips in the expiratory curve are time markers for $FEV_{0.5}$, FEV_1, and FEV_3. (PEFR = peak expiratory flow rate; TLC = total lung capacity; FVC = forced vital capacity; PIFR = peak inspiratory flow rate.)

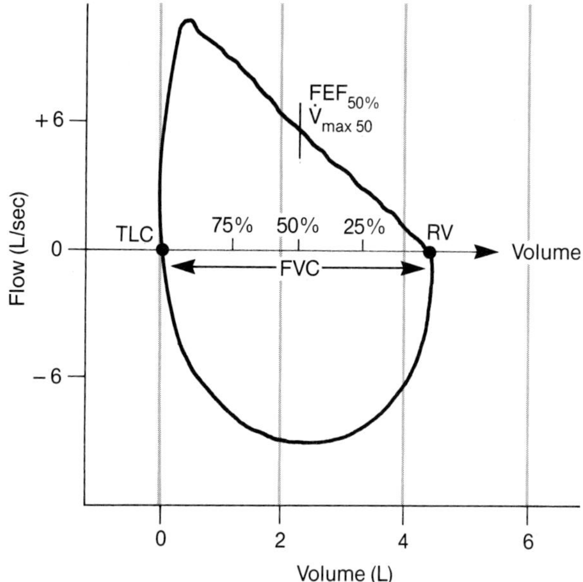

Figure 14–16. Forced expiratory flow at 50% of forced vital capacity ($FEF_{50\%}$ or $\dot{V}_{max\ 50}$), as shown in a normal flow volume loop.

The normal inspiratory loop begins at residual volume (RV). Air flow increases to its maximum at 50% of forced vital capacity and decreases to 0 at total lung capacity (TLC). The point of maximum inspiratory air flow is called the *peak inspiratory flow rate* (PIFR).

Obstructive and Restrictive Disease

The flow-volume loop pattern for obstructive disease is as follows: in minimal to mild small airway obstruction, the complete PFT may be normal, except for a slight "scooping" at the end of expiration on the flow-volume loop, as shown in Table 14–2. This scooping is referred to as *reduced expiratory air flow at low lung volumes.* As airway obstruction becomes worse, the scooping along the expiratory curve becomes more marked, and peak flow rates more reduced. The airway obstruction is said to be reversible, if the scooping reverts to normal (see the dotted lines) after the administration of a bronchodilator. In severe obstructive disease (e.g., emphysema), the sudden collapse of airways during early expiration produces an expiratory loop shaped like an index finger, as shown in Table 14–2.

The flow-volume loop pattern for restrictive disease looks relatively normal except for the small size (see last illustration, Table 14–2).

Upper Airway Obstruction

The flow-volume loop is crucial in upper airway obstruction (UAO) because symptoms and routine spirometry often mimic characteristic features of lower airway obstruction.

Upper airway lesions are divided into *fixed* and *variable* types based on the mobility of the airway at the site of obstruction and the representative flow-volume loop pattern. In *fixed upper airway obstruction*, the lesion remains stiff and immobile throughout the respiratory cycle. Airway diameter does not change. Regardless of the lesion's extrathoracic or intrathoracic location, the flow-volume loop demonstrates both inspiratory and expiratory plateaus, as shown in the second column of Table 14–3.

In variable UAO, the lesion's pliable nature is responsible for variable airway mobility and variable changes in airway diameter during respiration. Table 14–3 explains in detail how airway obstruction occurs during different phases of respiration, depending on the lesion's intra- or extrathoracic location. For *extrathoracic lesions* (e.g., vocal cord paralysis), airway narrowing develops during inspiration to produce the

Table 14–2. FLOW-VOLUME LOOP PATTERNS FOR OBSTRUCTIVE AND RESTRICTIVE DISEASE*

	Patterns	*Explanation*
Normal Pattern	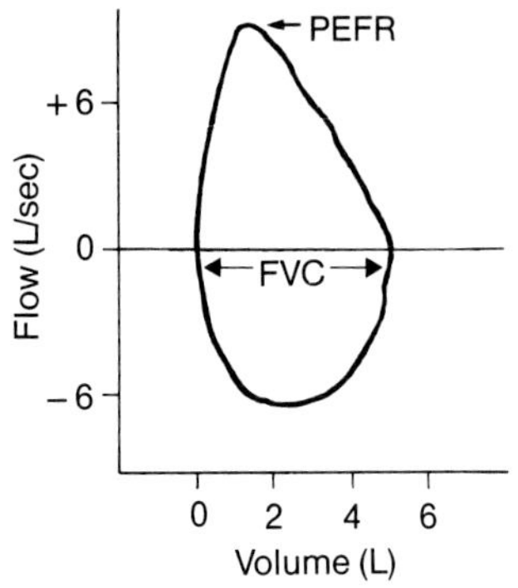 PEFR; +6; 0; −6; Flow (L/sec); FVC; 0 2 4 6; Volume (L)	The expiratory curve shows a straight line decrease in flow after peak flow (PEFR). The inspiratory curve has a normal rounded pattern.
Obstructive Pattern	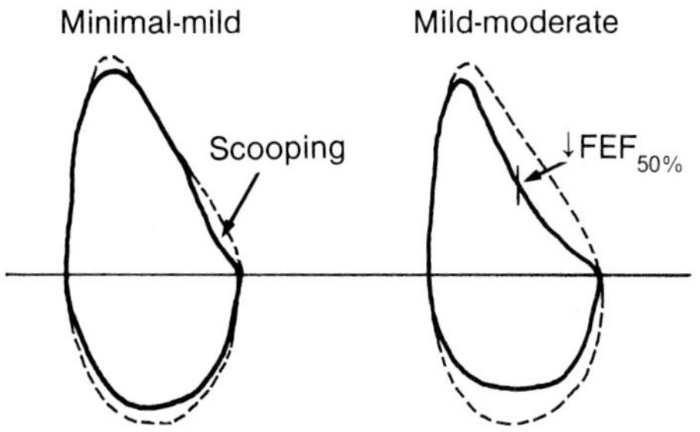 Minimal-mild: Scooping; Mild-moderate: ↓$FEF_{50\%}$	The expiratory curve shows scooping at low lung volumes (minimal to mild obstruction). As obstruction increases, the scooping becomes more marked and is accompanied by a decreased $FEF_{50\%}$ (mild to moderate obstruction).
	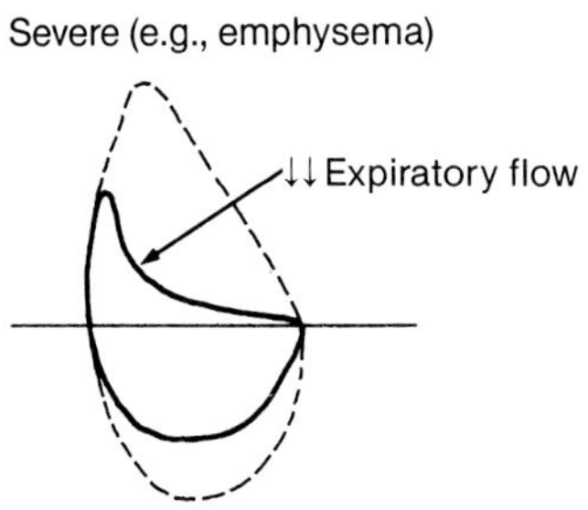 Severe (e.g., emphysema): ↓↓ Expiratory flow	The expiratory curve shows a sudden decrease in PEFR in an "index finger" pattern, followed by a nearly horizontal line. The inspiratory curve is normal, except for absolute decreases in flow rates.
Restrictive Pattern	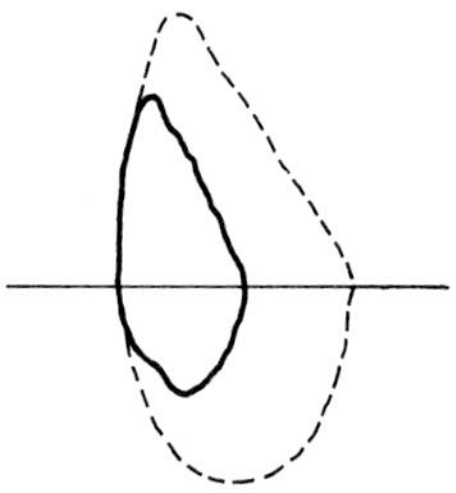	The entire loop resembles a miniature normal flow-volume loop. The FVC is markedly reduced. The expiratory curve shows a straight line decrease in flow with decreasing lung volumes. Peak flow rates may be normal, increased, or decreased, depending on the degree of respiratory impairment.

*The dotted lines represent the boundaries of the normal flow-volume loop.

characteristic inspiratory plateau on the flow-volume loop. For *intrathoracic lesions*, airway narrowing is observed during expiration rather than inspiration, and the flow-volume loop has an expiratory plateau instead of an inspiratory plateau.

Moreover, the plateaus in Table 14–3 correspond with the timing of accompanying musical sounds (e.g., stridor and wheezes) heard on auscultation. Musical sounds help in the diagnosis and differentiation of various types of airway obstruction. They are present as long as increasing airway obstruction and decreasing breath sounds do not develop into a silent chest, an ominous clinical sign.

LIMITATIONS OF THE COMPLETE PFT

The complete PFT without the flow-volume loop has its limitations. The absence of abnormality does not necessarily indicate the absence of disease. For example, a COPD patient with a 20-pack-year history of cigarette smoking may have normal PFT values, including a normal $FEF_{25-75\%}$. Although the $FEF_{25-75\%}$ measures air flow in small airways, remember that only 20% or less of total airway resistance in the lungs is attributed to small airways less than 2 mm in diameter. These peripheral airways are low resistance structures. Considerable alveolar and small airway disease must be present before airway resistance rises to produce detectable abnormal lung function and pulmonary symptoms.

The physician may order specialized tests to further study possible small airway disease. Yet, the additional tests available (e.g., whole-body plethysmography, frequency-dependent compliance, He isoflow) require specialized equipment not always available in the typical clinic or hospital. When available, the tests are usually not crucial to assessment and intervention, and they often involve unnecessary cost to the patient.

The limitations of the complete PFT have contributed to the rising popularity of the flow-volume loop as perhaps the most sensitive and practical single PFT parameter in the assessment of obstructive disease. In many cases, the first sign of airway obstruction is scooping along the loop's end-expiratory portion and a reduced $FEF_{50\%}$, whereas the complete PFT, including the $FEF_{25-75\%}$, remains normal. In addition, the flow-volume loop has other advantages. Test administration is relatively easy, requiring only three forced expiratory maneuvers. (Only one loop is chosen for analysis.) Numerous parameters are obtainable from a single loop, including $FEF_{50\%}$, FVC, FEV_1, and peak flow rates. Most important, the nurse can analyze loop patterns and quickly make basic interpretations without complicated calculations.

The Nurse's Role in PFTs

The nurse's role in PFTs focuses on scheduling laboratory tests at an appropriate time, preparing the patient, and obtaining bedside PFTs as indicated by the situation. Interpretation of test results, another role, is discussed in the next section.

SCHEDULING PFTS

When the physician orders "PFTs in the am," the nurse checks whether a complete PFT or routine spirometry is desired. A *complete PFT* includes all four components described here and in Chapter 13 as follows: lung volumes, mechanics of breathing measurements, diffusing capacities, and arterial blood gases (ABGs). *Routine spirometry* includes only a few basic measurements, such as SVC, FVC, FEV_1, and a mid-flow rate (i.e., $FEF_{25-75\%}$ from the usual FVC spirogram or $FEF_{50\%}$ from the flow-volume loop). The order should specify whether post BD measurements are desired. Several other points to keep in mind when scheduling PFTs follow:

1. For patients with early morning cough and sputum production, schedule PFTs in the late morning or early afternoon, after routine bronchial hygiene measures and postural drainage have cleared airways of obstructive secretions.
2. If the patient becomes acutely ill, check with the physician regarding the cancelling of the PFT and the ordering of bedside spirometry, ABGs, or both.
3. In the case of the ambulatory patient undergoing pre-employment or periodic surveillance, postpone the PFT if the patient becomes ill for any reason. Also postpone the test if the patient has had an upper or lower respiratory tract infection within the last 3 weeks.
4. In the case of an infectious disease, such as tuberculosis or pneumonia, the test should be cancelled and rescheduled after resolution of the infectious disease. However, when testing is mandatory (e.g., preoperative evaluation of the high risk patient), the PFT laboratory is notified of the infection ahead of time, so that appropriate infection control precautions can be implemented.
5. For patients in reverse (i.e., protective) isolation, spirometry may be performed at the bedside with disinfected equipment.

PREPARING THE PATIENT

Bronchodilator medications are usually withheld prior to testing, assuming that the purpose of the test is to verify the presence and extent of pulmonary disease. In some cases, however, bronchodilators are not withheld when the primary purpose of the PFT is to evaluate clinical response to a particular bronchodilator regimen.

The guidelines for withholding bronchodilators are as follows: 6 hours for inhaled sympathomimetics, 12 hours for short-acting theophylline drugs, and 24 hours for long-acting theophylline drugs (Clausen, 1984). The patient is cautioned to avoid taking a PRN puff from

Table 14-3. Flow-Volume Loop Patterns and Pathophysiology of Upper Airway Obstruction

Type of Upper Airway Obstruction	Flow-Volume Loop Pattern (solid lines)*	Pathophysiology/Corresponding Lung Sounds†	Comment
Fixed (extrathoracic and intrathoracic) obstruction (e.g., tumor, foreign object)	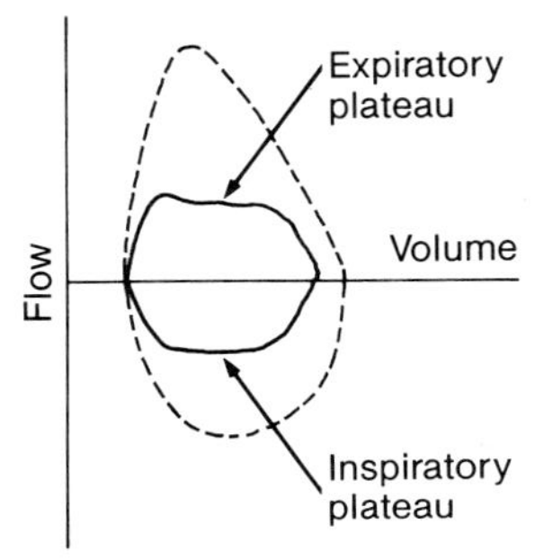 Flow; Volume; Expiratory plateau; Inspiratory plateau	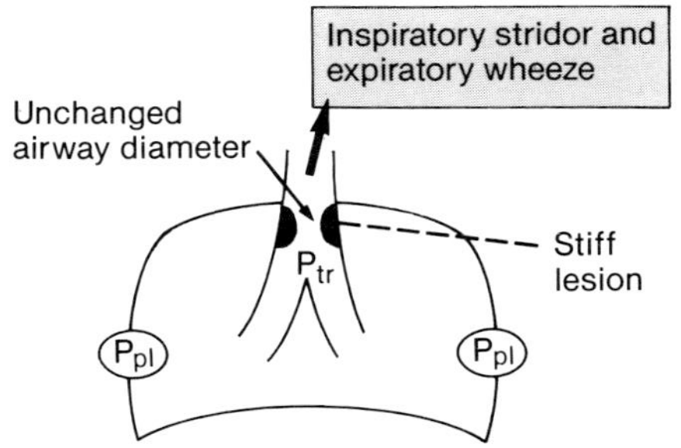 Unchanged airway diameter; Inspiratory stridor and expiratory wheeze; Stiff lesion; P_{tr}; P_{pl}; P_{pl}	*Explanation* Because the lesion is stiff, airway diameter at the site of the obstruction remains unchanged throughout the respiratory cycle, even though pleural pressure (P_{pl}) and tracheal pressure (P_{tr}) may vary greatly (see Chapter 1, mechanics of breathing). Inspiratory and expiratory plateaus on the flow-volume loop correspond to inspiratory and expiratory "musical" sounds (stridor and wheezes).
Variable extrathoracic obstruction (e.g., vocal cord paralysis)	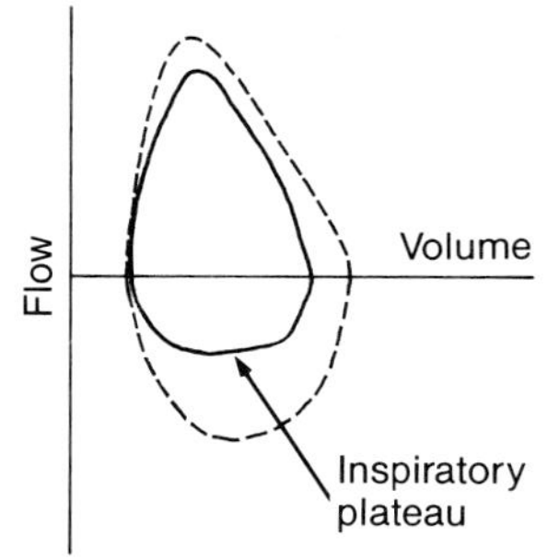 Flow; Volume; Inspiratory plateau	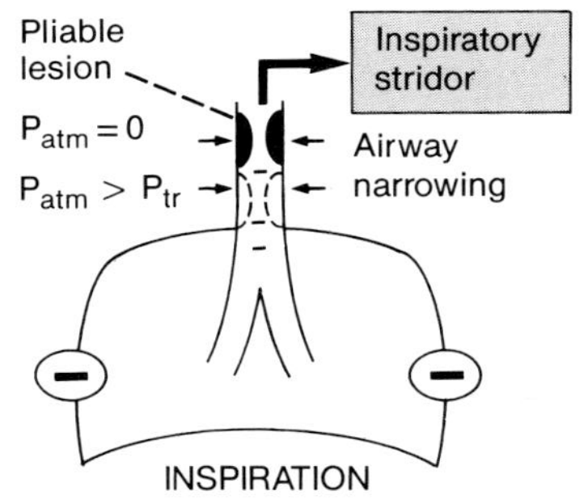 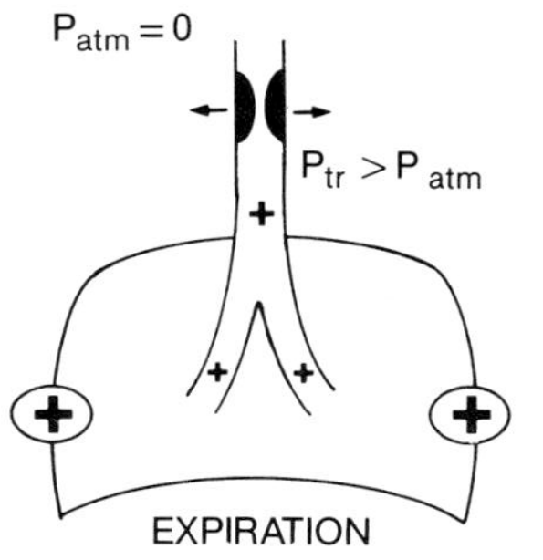 Pliable lesion; Inspiratory stridor; $P_{atm} = 0$; $P_{atm} > P_{tr}$; Airway narrowing; INSPIRATION $P_{atm} = 0$; $P_{tr} > P_{atm}$; EXPIRATION	*Summary* Airway narrowing occurs during inspiration to produce inspiratory stridor in the patient and an inspiratory plateau on the flow-volume loop. *During inspiration*, nagative pleural pressure transmitted to the trachea is greater than atmospheric pressure, such that $P_{atm} > P_{tr}$. The site of obstruction tends to collapse inward. As air is inspired past this mechanical obstruction, a pressure drop occurs across the lesion to produce dynamic compression of the airway (dotted lines) and further airway narrowing. *During expiration*, the patient generates positive pleural pressures to move sufficient air past the obstruction. The airway tends to move outward, since tracheal pressure (P_{tr}) is now greater than P_{atm}.

Variable intrathoracic obstruction (e.g., tumor)

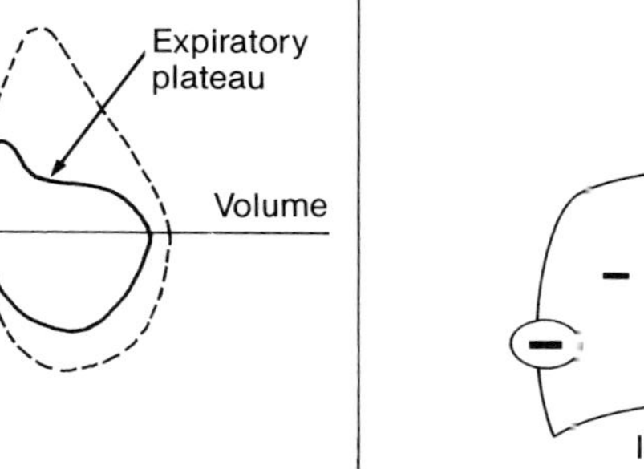

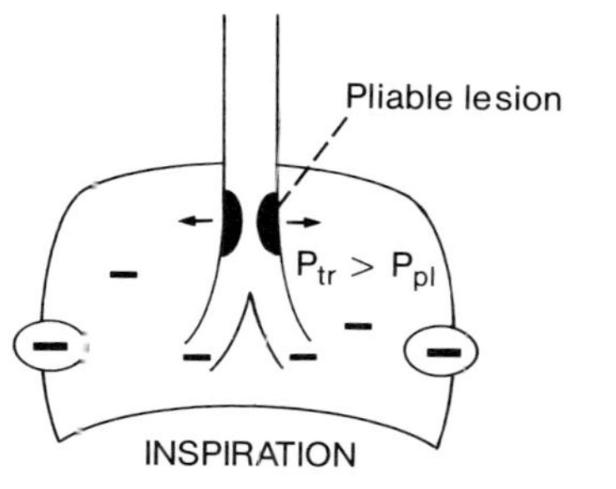

Summary
Pressure relationships are the reverse of those just described. Airway narrowing occurs during expiration rather than inspiration, producing a prominent expiratory wheeze in the patient and an expiratory plateau on the flow-volume loop.

During inspiration, upper and lower airways distend outward, as negative pleural pressure normally opens airways and alveoli. P_{tr} is greater than P_{pl}, a normal pressure relationship.

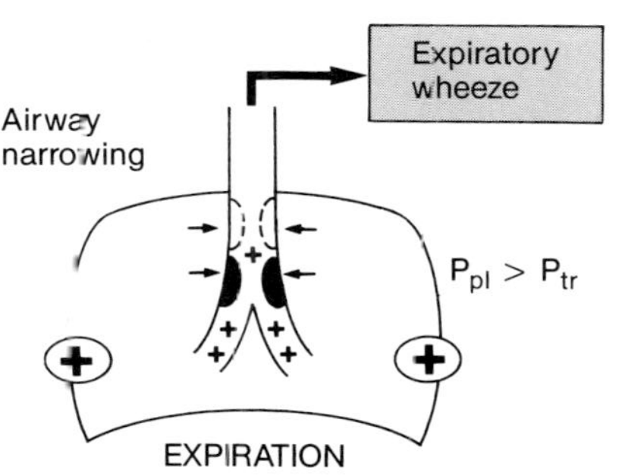

During forced expiration, pleural pressure becomes much greater than tracheal pressure as the patient tries to force air past the obstruction. This action produces a positive transmural pressure — pressure outside the airway exceeds pressure inside the airway. Mechanical obstruction occurs, as the airway collapses at the site of the lesion. In addition, tracheal pressure on the oral side of the lesion may be significantly reduced, owing to increasing air turbulence and decreasing air flow at this site. When P_{tr} at the lesion becomes much less than P_{tr} distal to the lesion, the pressure drop across the lesion may cause dynamic compression of the airway (dotted lines), increased obstruction, and barely audible breath sounds,
an ominous clinical sign.

*The dotted lines represent the normal flow-volume loop pattern.
†Tinted gray

his bedside or pocket-metered inhaler until after the test. If the patient is on a q4–6h aerosol bronchodilator, the bronchodilator given during the PFT is considered as a treatment, and the next treatment is scheduled for 4 to 6 hours after the test.

Educating the patient about the PFT beforehand is also important. It helps to alleviate any anxiety, facilitate test procedure, and provide an opportunity for the patient to ask questions and communicate concerns. After stating the scheduled time, duration, and purpose of the PFT, the nurse may describe the laboratory, its equipment, the general procedure, and the laboratory personnel. This information is best obtained by visiting a local hospital or clinic laboratory and familiarizing yourself with these aspects. During the educational process, the nurse discusses with the patient the following precautions:

1. *Refrain from smoking* for about 12 hours before a PFT or at least 4 hours before the DL test; carboxyhemoglobin in the blood may alter DL results.
2. *Wear loose clothing* for breathing comfort.
3. *Avoid the ingestion of alcohol, a heavy meal, or a large quantity of liquid* prior to test time. These precautions increase the likelihood of maximal breathing effort during the test.
4. *Arrive at the laboratory rested and relaxed.* Energy-consuming activities should be postponed until after the test. A rushed trip to the PFT laboratory should be avoided because a fatigued patient may become tense, irritable, and more bronchoconstricted before the test begins. In this situation, patient cooperation is difficult to elicit, and PFT values may not truly represent resting pulmonary function values.

Some other points to keep in mind when preparing the patient for a PFT are as follows:

1. The nurse should accompany children, anxious individuals, the elderly and those with learning difficulties to the laboratory if possible to help explain procedures, elicit cooperation, and give emotional support.
2. Children may benefit from visiting the laboratory ahead of time and watching another child take a PFT. Also, involving a play therapist may help allay the fears of an overly anxious child.
3. For patients on continuous oxygen, provisions must be made for portable oxygen during transport to the laboratory.
4. The patient with a tracheostomy must be sent to the laboratory with the cuff inflated. The technician may measure lung volumes through the tracheostomy tube during slow breathing maneuvers. However, mechanics of breathing may be impossible to measure owing to air leakage around the cuff during forced breathing.
5. For a patient with a recently discontinued tracheostomy tube, the PFT is best performed after complete stomal closure. If necessary, however, pressure over an occlusive stomal dressing may prevent air leakage and permit PFT testing.

OBTAINING BEDSIDE PFTS

Whether taken at the bedside or in ambulatory or home settings, the term *bedside PFTs* refers to spirometry and other measurements taken by portable devices outside the PFT laboratory.

Bedside PFTs supplement the more expensive and elaborate complete PFT. They are used for periodic ward, clinic, and home monitoring. When used judiciously, they can eliminate many unnecessary trips to the PFT laboratory for spirometry.

Measurements such as V_T, VC, and minute ventilation ($\dot{V}_E$) are routinely monitored and recorded on bedside flow sheets for all acutely ill patients on mechanical ventilation. Most ventilators have spirometers attached to the expiratory lines of the ventilator circuits to facilitate monitoring. As described further in Chapter 28, these and other bedside PFTs help assess the patient's readiness for weaning from me-

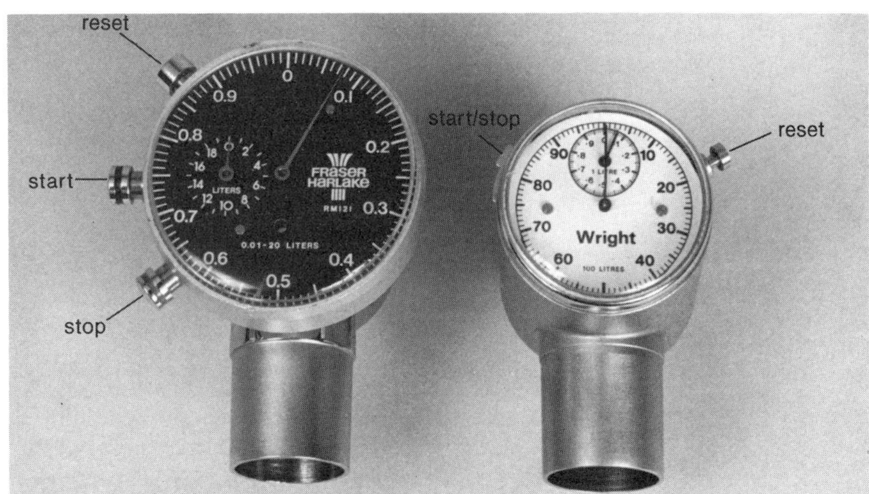

Figure 14–17. The Wright (right) and Fraser-Harlake (left) respirometers.

chanical ventilation as well as the progress during the weaning process.

When intermittent positive pressure breathing (IPPB) is ordered for a patient, the clinician may periodically measure exhaled volumes to be sure the patient is receiving adequate volumes and to coach him to take deeper breaths during the treatment.

Spontaneous PFT parameters include the following measurements: VT (V_T), breathing rate per minute (f), $\dot{V}_E$, VC, maximal voluntary ventilation (MVV), maximal inspiratory and expiratory pressures (MIP and MEP), and peak expiratory flow rate (PEFR). Volumes are measured with a hand-held respirometer (spirometer), such as the Wright respirometer (Fig. 14–17).

Mechanics of breathing measurements are taken as soon as the patient is well enough to perform forced breathing maneuvers. Maximal inspiratory and expiratory pressures are measured with special devices (Fig. 14–18). Other measurements, including FVC, FEV_1, FEV_1/FVC, and $FEF_{25\%-75\%}$, are taken with an x-y recorder (i.e., flow volume loop); with a portable dry, rolling seal type of spirometer, such as the SMI I spirometer (Fig. 14–19); or with another type of portable spirometer.

When portability, ease of operation, and ease of computation of results are of concern, health professionals may use smaller models than the ones presented thus far for monitoring purposes. For example, the Respiradyne spirometer (Fig. 14–20) is pocket sized and has immediate visual displays of results for clinical decision-making.

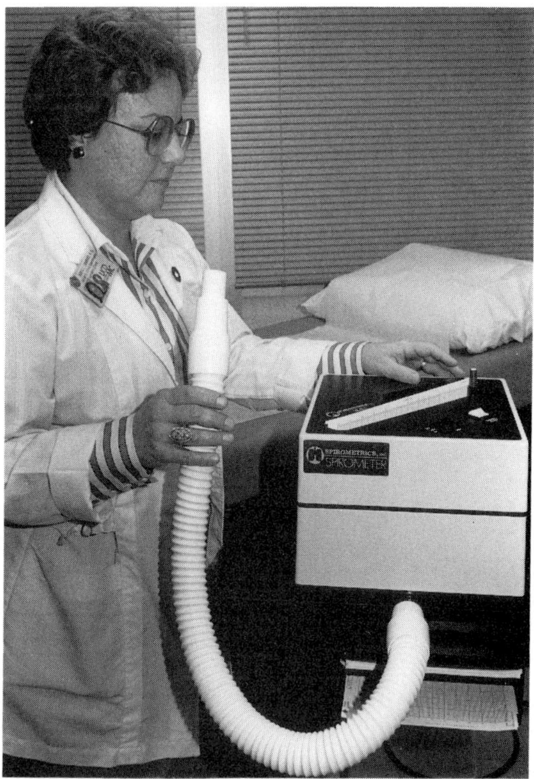

Figure 14–19. A clinic nurse prepares for pulmonary function testing using the SMI I spirometer (Spirometrics, Inc.). The device measures the following: FVC, FEV_1, FEV_t (selected time), $FEV_1/FVC_{\%}$, $FEF_{25-75\%}$, maximal voluntary ventilation, and VC.

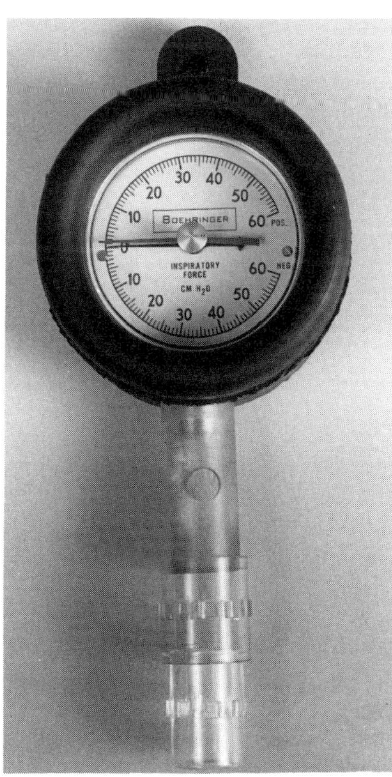

Figure 14–18. An inspiratory force meter (Boehringer).

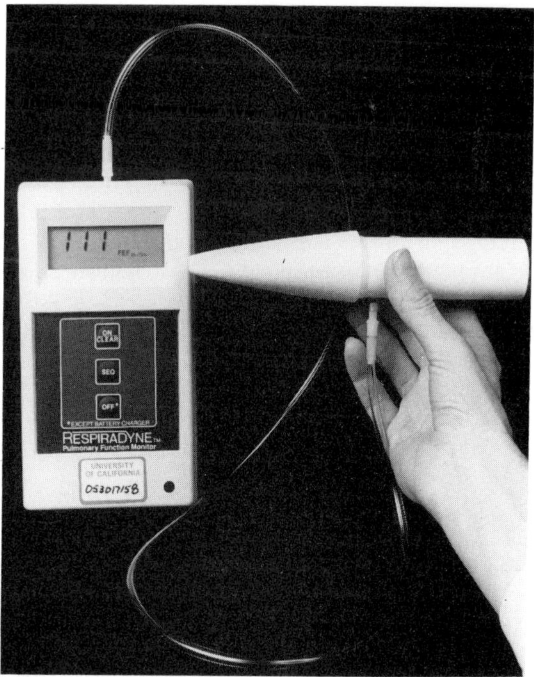

Figure 14–20. Respiradyne spirometer (Sherwood Medical). The device provides sequential digital display of the following measurements: FVC, FEV_1, PF, $FEF_{25-75\%}$, FEF_1/FVC, and $Vol_{extra\ \%}$ (i.e., percent extrapolated volume).

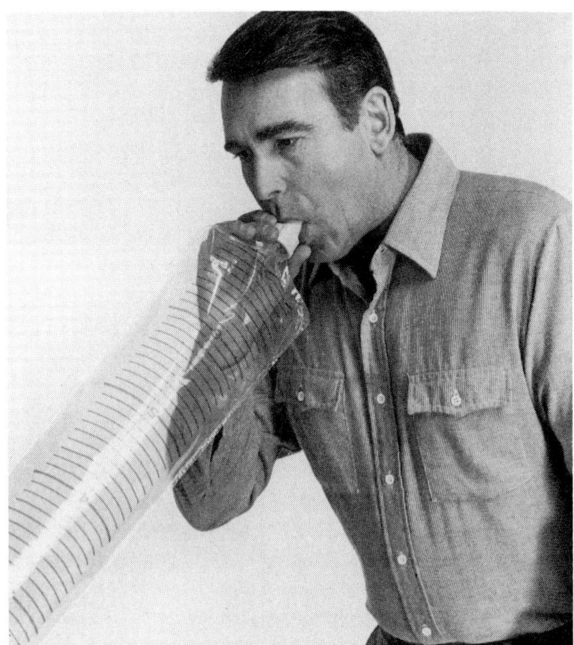

Figure 14–21. Use of the Vitometer for measurement of forced vital capacity. *To take an FVC*: (1) ask the patient to exhale maximally into the bag, as shown. The mouthpiece has a one-way valve to prevent gas from escaping; (2) manually compress the trapped gas in the bag to the least space possible; (3) read the FVC from the numeric gradations on the bag. (Courtesy of HealthScan Inc., Cedar Grove, New Jersey.)

When cost is a major consideration, the nurse may use a plastic bag device to obtain at least one objective measure of pulmonary function in clinic, office, or home setting. The Vitometer (Fig. 14–21) simply and accurately measures FVC (Anders et al, 1984).

In most situations, only a few PFT parameters are needed to assess pulmonary function and guide clinical decision-making. The parameters chosen depend upon equipment availability and the patient's ability and willingness to perform the required maneuvers. The clinician might monitor a few basic measurements, such as VC, FVC, and FEV_1, and a periodic ABG to assess ventilation, oxygenation, and acid-base balance. These parameters are considered in light of other assessment parameters, e.g., chest x-ray film, physical examination, motivational assessment, and clinical impressions based on past experience.

Measurement

The role of the nurse in measuring pulmonary function varies depending on the available equipment and the roles of the nurse and respiratory therapist in different clinical settings. Whereas some nurses have sole responsibility for measurements, other nurses share responsibility with respiratory therapists and take measurements only in the absence of therapists when increased ventilatory impairment is suspected.

General Methology. Body position is important in the measurement of PFTs. A sitting or standing position is acceptable, though forced expiratory volumes and vital capacity tend to be significantly greater in the standing position, probably because subjects take slightly larger inspirations in this posture (Townsend, 1984). Adults are usually tested in the sitting position because they feel more comfortable and relaxed in the sitting position. Children are optimally tested in the standing position, the position that results in the greatest vital capacity. Patients with ventilators are tested in the Fowler's or semi-Fowler's position, as tolerated. Most important, testing position should be indicated in the chart and consistently maintained during serial PFTs.

For single breath maneuvers, the clinician performs each test three times, as tolerated by the patient, and records the highest value. After each test, the patient is immediately placed back on the ventilator for at least 30 seconds. Similarly, the spontaneously breathing patient is allowed to rest to avoid shortness of breath and hypoxemia. Noseclips may be applied during testing to avoid the leakage of air through the nose.

Respiratory Rate, Tidal Volume and Minute Ventilation. *To obtain f, V_T, and $\dot{V}_E$*, the clinician instructs the patient to breathe normally with teeth and lips over the respirometer's mouthpiece. Continue to measure exhaled volumes for 1 minute, simultaneously counting respirations. The volume read off the dial is minute ventilation ($\dot{V}_E$). Determine V_T by dividing the measured $\dot{V}_E$ by the respiratory rate. The same procedure may be followed for a patient with a ventilator, except the spirometer is connected to the exhalation line of the ventilator's circuit. All measurements are taken after and not before suctioning or other bronchial hygiene measures.

Tidal volume and minute ventilation may be measured with a plastic bag device (Hudson) when a respirometer is unavailable.

Maximum Voluntary Ventilation. *To take an MVV*, the clinician instructs the patient, as described previously in this chapter. Supplementary oxygen is provided during and for a few minutes after the test for patients who are likely to develop dyspnea or hypoxemia. For charting, the respiratory rate per minute (f) is recorded in a subscript, i.e., MVV_{70} = 66 L/min or MVV_{110} = 170 L/min.

Slow and Forced Vital Capacities. *To take a slow vital capacity* (SVC), instruct the patient to inhale as deeply as possible and to exhale as slowly and completely as possible. Coach the patient by calling out "A little more, a little more" until you feel he has exhaled to residual volume.

To take a forced vital capacity (FVC), instruct the patient to inhale as deeply as possible and exhale as rapidly, forcefully, and completely as possible. Since exhalation should start without hesitation, it may be necessary to shout, "Blow! Blow!" to elicit peak flow and to continue exhalation to residual volume. The

FVC should be sustained for 6 seconds and be free of coughing for valid results (Clausen, 1984). If the measuring device records a spirogram, the clinician can coach the patient to continue exhalation until the tracing approaches an actual or estimated baseline level.

An FVC is required only when mechanics of breathing (i.e., flow rates) are desired. If a bedside vital capacity is ordered, a slow rather than a forced measurement is usually taken. A slow unforced maneuver prevents early airway closure on expiration in COPD patients and is more suitable for commonly used respirometers, such as the Wright respirometer. High peak flow rates, exceeding 300 L/min, generated during forced expiratory maneuvers may damage the rotor blade in this sensitive and expensive device made to measure volume rather than flow. For hand-held respirometers, the slow vital capacity (SVC) is read directly off the respirometer's dial.

If an FVC spirogram is obtained, the clinician measures the FVC on the graph paper and determines flow rates according to operating manual instructions and American Thoracic Society guidelines (1979). Observed values are compared with predicted values obtained from nomograms for normal lung function (Fig. 14–22).

Pressure and Flow Measurements. Table 14–4 summarizes bedside pressure and flow measurements. Of those listed, *maximal inspiratory pressure* (MIP) is the most important test of inspiratory muscle strength.

Peak expiratory flow rate (PEFR) is commonly used to monitor pulmonary function because the test is simple and easy to administer to both children and adults (Fig. 14–23 and Fig. 14–24). It does not require full expiration to residual volume. Also, an educated patient can measure his own PEFR every morning at home, interpret the results, and adjust the bronchodilator medications appropriately. In spite of its usefulness, however, the PEFR has the disadvantage of being effort dependent. Because accuracy depends upon maximal patient effort, a periodic flow-volume loop is recommended for comparison. The PEFR measured by the peak flow meter should correspond with the flow-volume loop's PEFR (see Fig. 14–15). Submaximal patient effort and test inaccuracy are most readily identified by looking at the flow-volume loop tracing. Submaximal effort is present when the early expiratory portion of the loop lacks a sharp peak. This finding may be described as *decreased flow rates at high lung volumes*.

The FEV_1, *FVC* and $FEV_1\%$ are other bedside measurements considered in the assessment of air flow and mechanics of breathing. They have been described.

It is hoped that further integration of these pressure and flow measurements into nursing practice will greatly sharpen respiratory assessment skills and facilitate the use of simple measuring devices in home and ambulatory care settings in particular.

Guide to Basic PFT Interpretation

When contact with the patient is brief or when disease is mild, interpretation of bedside spirometry results alone may be adequate for clinical decision-making. However, a basic interpretation of a complete PFT is always needed at some point in time to understand the nature of any underlying chronic lung disease and to begin the plan for comprehensive and continuing care. Moreover, understanding how to clarify a complete PFT makes interpretation of bedside results simpler and probably more meaningful because of a broader context. Hence, this section on basic PFT interpretation focuses on the complete PFT and serves to summarize important information presented in this chapter.

As with interpretation of blood gas measurements, a systematic approach to the interpretation of PFT values is essential because of the array of results displayed on bedside flow sheets, hospital PFT reports, and lengthy computerized read-outs. The nurse must learn how to sift through data, select a few crucial parameters, and make a basic interpretation in a reasonable amount of time.

The guide to basic PFT interpretation in the box on page 395 summarizes how to look at a PFT report and what test values to analyze. The following points help in basic interpretation:

1. Determine whether the results are normal or abnormal.
2. Determine whether the results indicate obstructive or restrictive disease. Table 14–5 summarizes the patterns of pulmonary function abnormality seen in obstructive and restrictive disease. For purely obstructive or restrictive disease, use Table 14–6 to estimate the degree of respiratory impairment in acute states represented by worst values as well as in stable states before hospitalization represented by best values.
3. *Determine the reversibility of the abnormality.*
4. *Look at serial PFT values* in light of the pulmonary history and physical examination to determine progression of disease.
5. *Suspect invalid test results when signs of poor patient effort are present.* These signs include complaints of excessive fatigue or dyspnea during testing, decreased VC, decreased flow rates at high lung volumes, decreased MVV, and uneven or notched spirogram tracings. The optimal spirogram is one that is highly reproducible with repeated testing.

Experience in PFT interpretation is necessary before the clinician gains confidence in the ability to identify gross abnormalities in pulmonary function. To solidify methodology and facilitate learning, use the PFT guide as well as Tables 14–5 and 14–6 to interpret the PFT tests at the end of this chapter. Then, these learning aids may be copied and used in the clinical setting to

Text continued on page 395

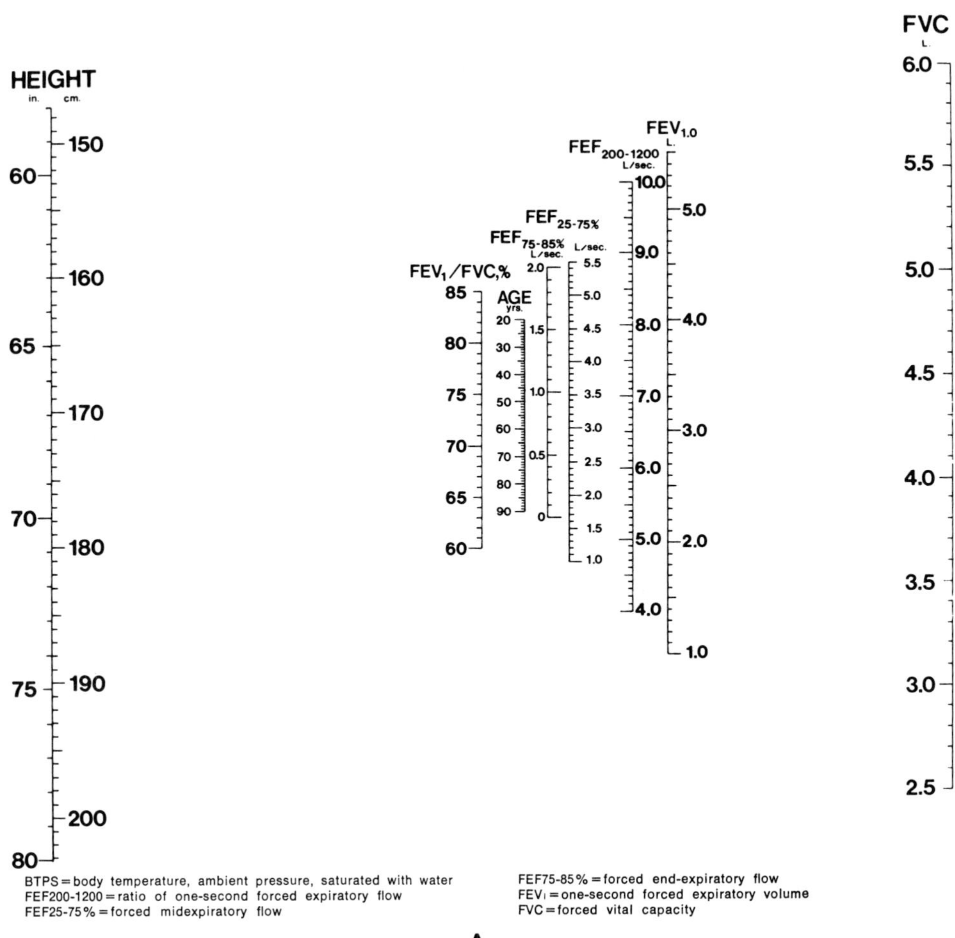

Figure 14–22. Nomograms for predicting normal mechanics of breathing values on the pulmonary function test. *A*, Nomogram for males.

Illustration continued on opposite page

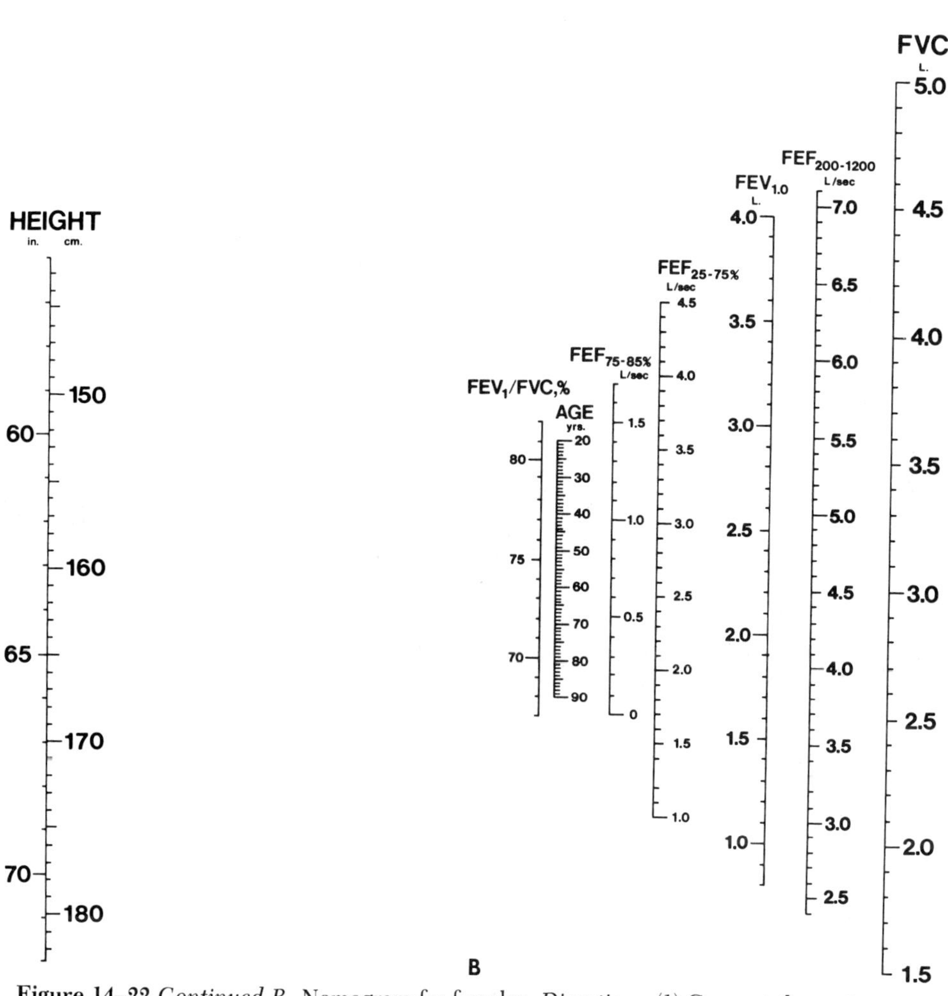

Figure 14–22 *Continued B,* Nomogram for females. *Directions:* (1) Connect the patients age and height with a straight edge. (2) Read the normal predicted values where the straight edge intersects each scale. (Reproduced by permission from Morris, J. Spirometry in the evaluation of pulmonary function. *The Western Journal of Medicine,* 125(2):110–118, 1976.)

Table 14–4. BEDSIDE PRESSURE AND FLOW MEASUREMENTS

Pulmonary Function Test	Main Purposes	Measurement	Guidelines for Interpretation
Maximal inspiratory pressure (MIP) Also called: Peak inspiratory pressure (PIP) Negative inspiratory force (NIF) Negative inspiratory effort (NIE) Peak inspiratory force (PIF)	To test inspiratory muscle strength or diaphragmatic function in neuromuscular patients and other patients with impaired diaphragmatic function. To assess readiness for weaning from mechanical ventilation.	Connect the patient to a pressure gauge or inspiratory force meter (Fig. 14–18) via a mouthpiece or adaptor. Attach noseclips. Instruct the patient to expire to residual volume and make a maximal inspiratory effort for 3 to 5 seconds. During exhalation, occlude the pressure gauge's safety port and note the maximum inspiratory pressure produced *after* the initial 1-second period. Disregard needle overshoots.	Normal is greater than −80 to −100 cmH_2O. A pressure more negative than −20 to −25 cmH_2O indicates readiness for weaning from mechanical ventilation.
Maximal expiratory pressure (MEP)	To test respiratory muscle strength in neuromuscular patients. To test ability to cough (contract abdominal muscles against a closed glottis).	Connect the patient to a pressure gauge via a mouthpiece. Attach nose clips. Instruct the patient to inspire to TLC. Occlude the gauge's safety port (or close a three-way valve) and instruct the patient to expire with maximal expiratory effort. Note the maximal pressure produced for 2 to 3 seconds, ignoring initial needle overshoot.	Normal is greater than +80 to +100 cmH_2O. A pressure greater than +40 cmH_2O is needed for an effective cough.
Peak expiratory flow rate (PEFR) Also called: Maximum expiratory flow rate (MEFR)	To monitor general progress and response to bronchodilator in persons with obstructive disease. To monitor progress in patients with neuromuscular disease, e.g., Guillain-Barré syndrome.	Use a peak flow meter (see Fig. 14–23 or other pulmonary monitor). Instruct the patient to place teeth and lips over the mouthpiece, take a deep breath in, and exhale as fast and hard as possible into the flow meter. Note the peak flow rate on the dial or flow gauge.	Normal is determined from nomograms (Fig. 14–24) but is usually between 400 L/min and 700 L/min in adults. *Decreasing* values indicate increasing air flow limitation. In asthma, if PEFR does not improve after bronchodilator aerosol, epinephrine or terbutaline is given by injection, and more aggressive therapy may be indicated. *Increasing values* indicate clinical improvement; PCO_2 will not be higher and a repeat ABG is usually unnecessary (Williams, 1979). PEFR in L/min multiplied by 9 gives a close approximation FEV_1 in ml.
Forced expiratory volume in 1 second (FEV_1) Forced vital capacity (FVC) FEV_1/FVC (%)	To evaluate degree of respiratory impairment, disease progression, and response to bronchodilators. To help differentiate obstructive from restrictive disease.	Use a portable dry rolling seal spirometer (e.g., SMI I and Vitalograph spirometer) or an x-y recorder (flow-volume loop). Instructions are the same as those described for the PEFR, except the patient is encouraged to continue exhalation to residual volume.	*In normal lungs:* FEV_1 and FVC are determined from nomograms (see Fig. 14–23). FEV_1 declines 20 to 50 ml/yr owing to aging. *In obstructive disease:* Both FEV_1 and FEV_1 % are decreased. An FEV_1 of less than 1.0 L indicates severe impairment. FEV_1 is expected to decline 50 to 80 ml/yr in COPD. Obstruction is reversible when the postbronchodilator % change is 15% or greater for FVC and FEV_1. *In restrictive disease:* FEV_1 and FVC are decreased, but the FEV_1 % is increased over 80 to 90%.

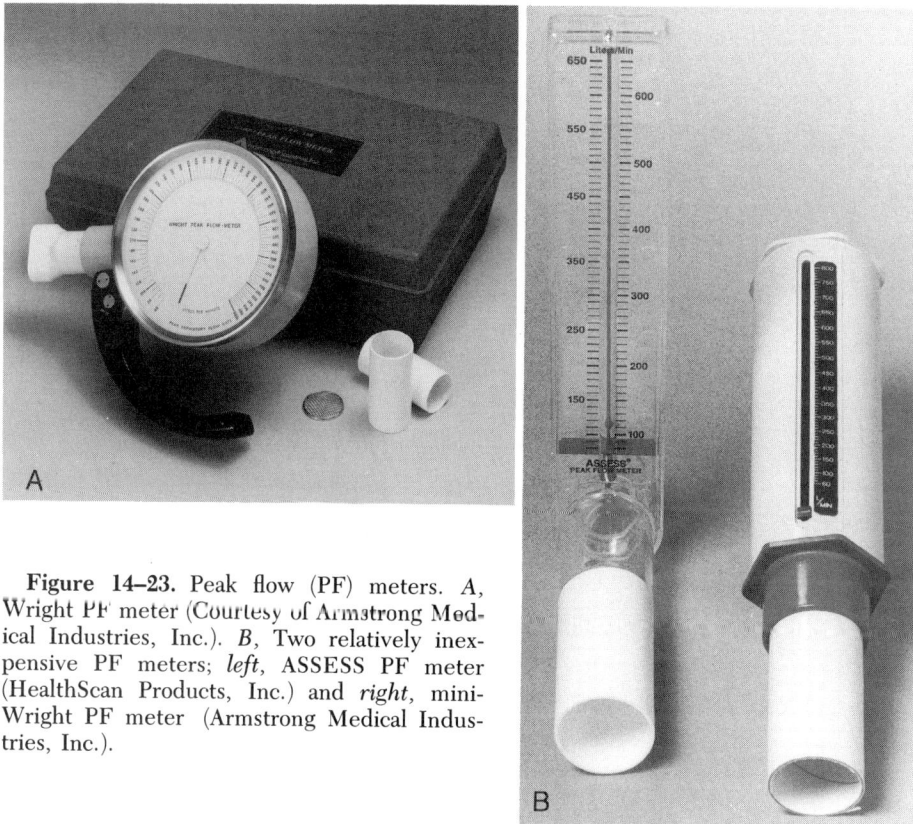

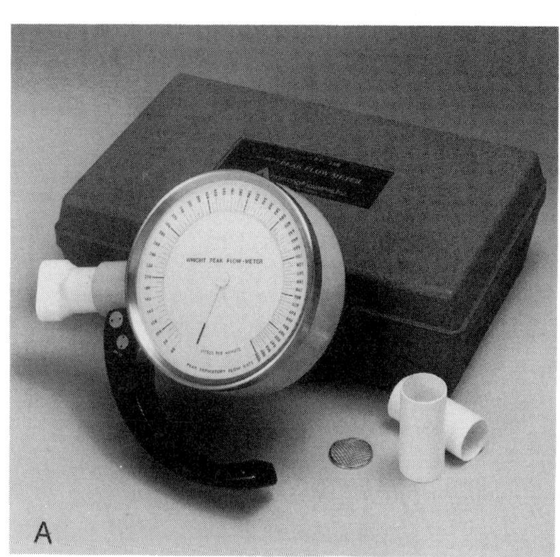

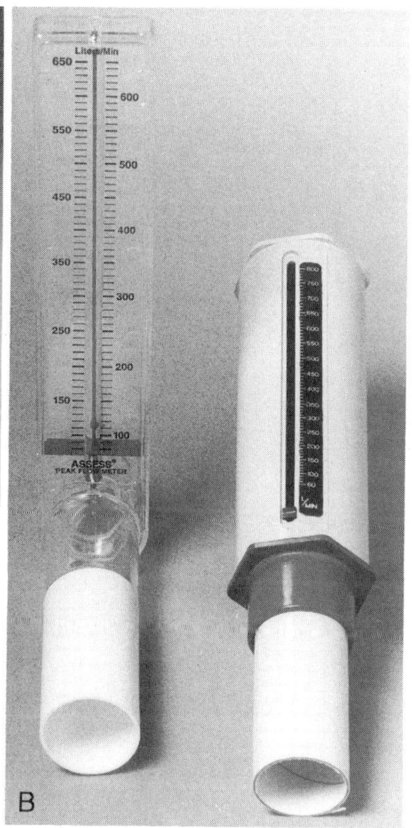

Figure 14–23. Peak flow (PF) meters. *A*, Wright PF meter (Courtesy of Armstrong Medical Industries, Inc.). *B*, Two relatively inexpensive PF meters; *left*, ASSESS PF meter (HealthScan Products, Inc.) and *right*, mini-Wright PF meter (Armstrong Medical Industries, Inc.).

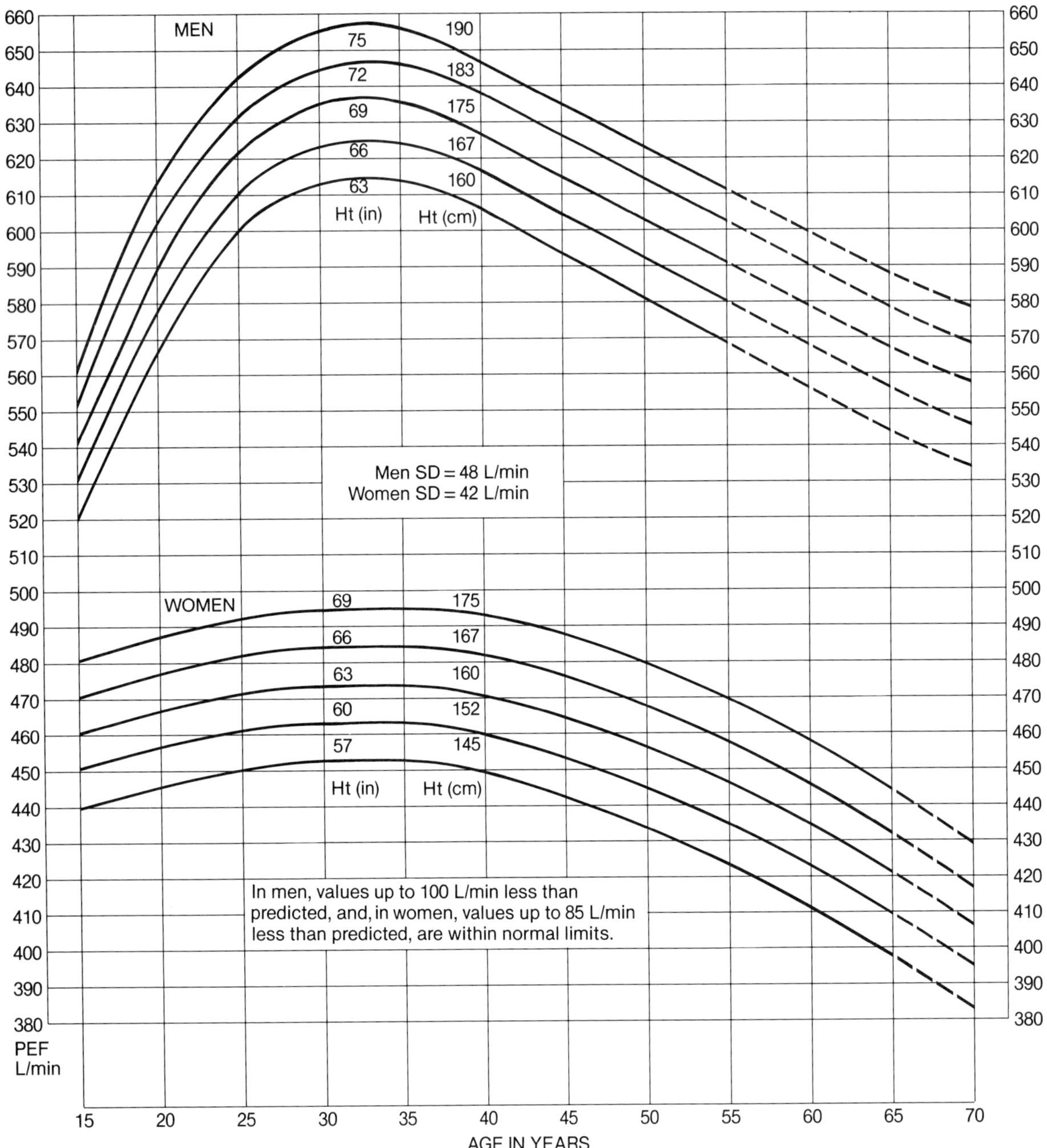

Figure 14–24. Normal values of peak expiratory flow for men (top) and women (bottom). *Directions:* (1) Locate the patient's age on the horizontal scale on the bottom of the graph. (2) Locate the height in inches (in) or centimeters (cm) on the appropriate height curve. (3) Starting with age, draw a vertical line upwards, stopping at the appropriate height curve. (4) Follow the height curve to the left or right to read PEF L/min. (Courtesy of Armstrong Medical Industries, Inc.)

GUIDE TO BASIC PFT INTERPRETATION

I. Note identifying data (e.g., age, weight, medical diagnosis) for clues regarding the presence and nature of lung disease.
II. Concentrate on percent predicted columns; normal percent predicted values fall between 80 and 120%.
III. Look at *lung volumes.*
   A. Vital capacity.
   B. RV/TLC (%). Normal is less than 33%. Look at separate values for RV and TLC to see what values changed to make RV/TLC abnormal.
      1. RV.
      2. TLC.
IV. Look at *mechanics of breathing* (note both observed and percent predicted values).
   A. FEV_1. Reflects air flow in large airways.
   B. FEV_1/FVC (%). Look at separate values for FEV_1 and FVC to see what values changed to make FEV_1/FVC abnormal.
   C. FVC.
   D. $FEF_{25-75\%}$ (also called MMFR). Reflects air flow in small airways.
   E. Forced vital capacity (FVC) compared with *slow* vital capacity (VC or SVC). If FVC is significantly less than VC, air trapping is present.
   F. Post BD values. Reversibility is defined as greater than 15% improvement in observed values in two of the following: FEV_1, FVC, and $FEF_{25-75\%}$.
   G. Examine spirograms, particularly the *flow-volume loop tracing.*
      1. Look at $FEF_{50\%}$ (corresponds with $FEF_{25-75\%}$).
      2. Check for scooping along the expiratory curve that indicates lower airway obstruction.
      3. Check for decreased inspiratory flow rates or an inspiratory plateau that suggests upper airway obstruction.
V. Look at *diffusing capacity* (DL or DL_{CO}).
VI. Look at *arterial blood gases* to assess ventilation, oxygenation, and acid-base balance.
VII. Compare the present PFT with the last PFT. Also, compare the PFT with values obtained before the onset of acute illness.
VIII. Make a *conclusion,* indicating the type of pulmonary disease (i.e., restrictive versus obstructive), severity (i.e., mild, moderate, or severe), response to bronchodilator, and degree of hypoxemia or alveolar hypoventilation or hyperventilation if abnormal ABGs are present.

gain more experience. When you are uncertain of a correct interpretation, look at the pulmonary physician's more detailed PFT interpretation and check the results of specialized tests for additional information on the patient's condition.

Finally, one must realize that all the necessary data for this type of comprehensive approach may not be readily available. The nurse gathers data from both bedside and laboratory PFTs. Sometimes, the nurse must check an old PFT report or a physician's progress notes for measurements only periodically performed (e.g., TLC and DL).

Conclusion

This chapter describes the complete pulmonary function test as well as bedside measurements, with emphasis on interpretation of results. Though this assessment parameter is largely underutilized by health professionals, it is hoped that nurses will be assisted in the integration of important concepts and methodologies into nursing practice in general and especially into the realm of home health care, the most neglected area. More specifically, knowledge of the contents of this chapter prepares the nurse to use the PFT as a main source of objective data in the identification and assessment of respiratory problems. For example, the degrees of respiratory impairment indicated in Table 14–6 may be used to identify different degrees of airflow limitation and to establish an unquestionable need for many of the interventions described in this book.

Pulmonary Function Test Problems

Directions: Use the interpretation guide on pages 389 to 395 to interpret the following two PFTs. The answers to these problems are in Appendix II.

PFT 1: Mr. R., a 58-year-old, 120-lb Asian male.

Lung Volumes and Capacities BTPS		Pre-dicted	Ob-served	% Pre-dicted	After Broncho-dilator	% Pre-dicted
Vital capacity (VC)	(L)	3.59	3.08	86		
Inspiratory capacity (IC)	(L)	2.41	1.70	71		
Exp. Res. Vol. (ERV)	(L)	1.19	1.38	117		
Residual volume (RV)	(L)	2.13	3.35	157		
Total lung cap. (TLC)	(L)	5.72	6.43	112		
Residual vol./TLC	(%)	<33	52			
Funct. resid. cap. (FRC)	(L)	3.31	4.73	143		
Mechanics of Breathing						
Forced expir. vol. (1 sec) (FEV_1)	(L)	2.52	0.70	28	0.87	35
% expir in 1 sec (FEV_1/FVC)	(%)	>70	26		27	
Forced vital capacity (FVC)	(L)	3.59	2.66	74	3.26	91
Forced mid expir. flow 25–75%	(L/min)	164	9	5	14	9
Max. vol. vent. (MVV)	(L/min)	89	24	27		
Max. expir. flow rate (200–1200)	(L/min)	390	20	5	27	7
Max. inspir. flow rate (200–1200)	(L/min)		102			

Diffusion		Pre-dicted +	Ob-served	% Pre-dicted
Pulm. diffusing cap. (DL_{CO}) (ml/min/mmHg) (single breath CO)		20.6	16.3	
Pulm. diffusing cap. (DL_{CO}) corrected for Hgb (ml/min/mmHg)		20.6	17.2	84
Alveolar volume (single breath)	(L)	=	4.25	
Hemoglobin (Hgb)	gm %	=	13.5	
+ Predicted according to Ogilvie based on body surface area		=	23.4	
+ Predicted based on alveolar volume and age		=	20.6	
Arterial Blood			***Air***	$\boldsymbol{O_2}$
pH	(units)	7.38–7.42	7.42	
CO_2 tension (measured) pCO_2	(mmHg)	38–42	40	
O_2 tension pO_2	(mmHg)	80–100	80	
Base excess	(units)	±2	+1	
HCO_3 calculated—plasma	(mEq/L)	24–28	25	
CO_2 content—blood	(mM/L)	20.5–23.1	26	
O_2 saturation	(%)	96–99	96	
Hemoglobin	(gm %)	15.0		
Hematocrit	(%)	45		

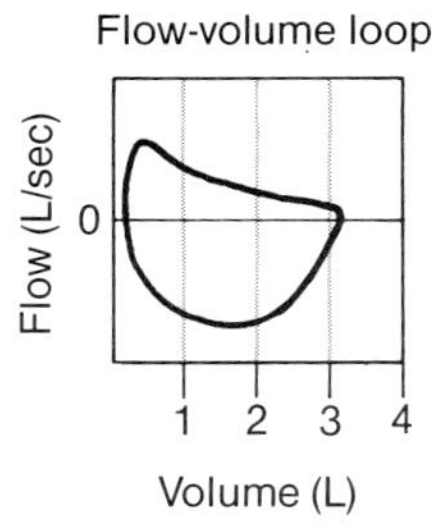

Flow-volume loop

Flow (L/sec)

0

1 2 3 4

Volume (L)

PFT 2: Mr. W., a 66-year-old, 158-lb white male.

Lung Volumes and Capacities BTPS		Pre-dicted	Ob-served	% Pre-dicted	After Broncho-dilator	% Pre-dicted
Vital capacity (VC)	(L)	3.59	2.65	74		
Inspiratory capacity (IC)	(L)	2.40	2.18	91		
Exp. Res. Vol. (ERV)	(L)	1.18	0.47	4C		
Residual volume (RV)	(L)	2.37	0.95	4(		
Total lung cap. (TLC)	(L)	5.96	3.60	60		
Residual vol./TLC	(%)	<33	26			
Funct. resid. cap. (FRC)	(L)	3.55	1.42	4)		
Mechanics of Breathing						
Forced expir. vol. (1 sec) (FEV_1)	(L)	2.41	2.11	37		
% expir. in 1 sec (FEV_1/FVC)	(%)	>67	84			
Forced vital capacity (FVC)	(L)	3.59	2.52	70		
Forced mid expir. flow 25–75%	(L/min)	168	210	125		
Max. vol. vent. (MVV)	(L/min)	93	80	86		
Max. expir. flow rate (200–1200)	(L/min)	377	165	44		
Max. inspir. flow rate (200–1200)	(L/min)		168			

Diffusion		Pre-dicted +	Ob-served	% Pre-dicted
Pulm. diffusing cap. (DL_{CO}) (ml/min/mmHg) (single breath CO)		14.8	17.1	
Pulm. diffusing cap. (DL_{CO}) corrected for Hgb (ml/min/mmHg)		14.8	13.2	89
Alveolar volume (single breath)	(L)	=	3.28	
Hemoglobin (Hgb)	gm %	=	15.6	
+ Predicted according to Ogilvie based on body surface area		=	27.9	
+ Predicted based on alveolar volume and age		=	14.8	
Arterial Blood			***Air***	***O_2***
pH	(units)	7.38–7.42	7.37	
CO_2 tension (measured) pCO_2	(mmHg)	38–42	41	
O_2 tension pO_2	(mmHg)	80–100	68	
Base excess	(units)	±2	−2	
HCO_3 calculated—plasma	(mEq/L)	24–28	23	
CO_2 content—blood	(mM/L)	20.5–23.1		
O_2 saturation	(%)	96–99	93	
Hemoglobin	(gm %)	15.0		
Hematocrit	(%)	45		

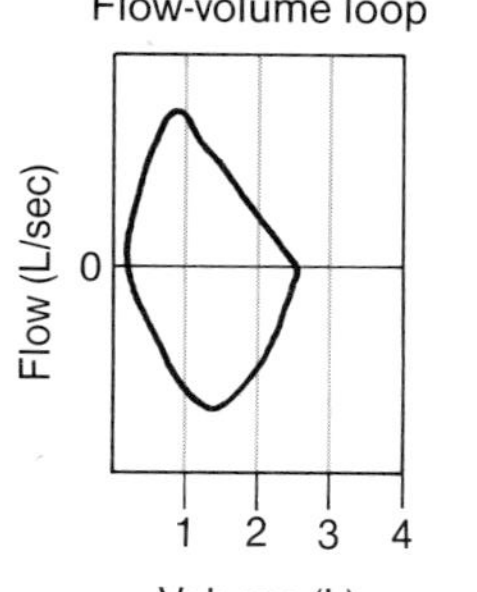

Table 14–5. PATTERNS OF PULMONARY FUNCTION ABNORMALITY IN OBSTRUCTIVE RESTRICTIVE DISEASE

Assessment Parameters	*Bronchial Asthma*	Obstructive Disease *Chronic Bronchitis*	*Emphysema*	Restrictive Disease
VC	NL to ↓	↓	NL to ↓	↓
RV	NL to ↑	↑	↑	↓ or NL
TLC	NL	NL	NL to ↑	↓
RV/TLC	NL to ↑	↑	↑	NL
Expiratory flow rates	NL to ↓	NL to ↓	NL to ↓	NL (or ↑ $FEF_{25-75\%}$ mild disease ↓ moderate to severe disease
FEV_1/FVC (%)	NL to ↓	↓	↓	NL to ↑ (greater than 80 to 90%)
Response to bronchodilator (% change)	Great response (>15% change)	Some to no response (0 to 15% change)	No response	No response
Diffusing capacity	NL to ↑ ↓ during acute severe attack	NL to ↓	↓	NL or ↓ (depends on type of disease)
Pa_{O_2}	NL ↓ during acute attack	↓	NL until very advanced disease; then ↓	NL or ↓
Pa_{CO_2}	NL First ↓ and then ↑ during acute attack	↑	NL until very advanced disease; then ↑	NL or ↓; ↑ in very advanced disease

Combined Restrictive/Obstructive Abnormalities

1. VC and TLC are reduced, but RV/TLC is elevated from the obstructive component.
2. Flow rates are reduced, but the reduction in flow (FEV_1) is proportionally greater than the reduction in volume (TLC).
3. The FEV_1/FVC% approaches normal; it is not as high as one expects in a purely restrictive disease, nor is it as low as one expects in a purely obstructive disease.

NL = normal
↑ = increased
↓ = decreased

Table 14–6. DEGREES OF RESPIRATORY IMPAIRMENT

Basic PFTs	*FEV_1 (L/min) % Predicted**	*FEV_1/FVC %*	*VC and TLC (% Predicted)*
Normal Lung Function	*Predicted Value or >80%*	*Predicted Value or >75%*	*>80%*
Degrees of Impairment	**Obstructive Disease**		**Restrictive Disease**
mild	>2 L/min or 65–80%	60–75%	65–80%
moderate	1–2 L/min or 50–65%	40–60%	50–65%
severe	<1 L/min or <50%	<40%	<50%

*After Morris, J. Spirometry in the evaluation of pulmonary function. *The western journal of medicine,* 125(2):110–118, 1976.

For more specific criteria, see Cary, J., Huseby, J., and Culver, B. Variability in interpretation of PFTs. *Chest,* 76(4): 389–390, 1979; Morgan, W. K. Pulmonary disability and impairment can't work? Won't work? *Basics of respiratory disease,* 10(5):entire issue, 1982.

REFERENCES

Acres, J. C. and Kryger, M. H.: Clinical significance of pulmonary function tests—upper airway obstruction. *Chest*, 80(2): 207–211, 1981.

American College of Chest Physicians: Statement on spirometry—a report of the section on respiratory pathophysiology. *Chest*, 83(3): 547–550, 1983.

American College of Chest Physicians—American Thoracic Society: Pulmonary terms and symbols. *Chest*, 67(5): 583–593, 1975.

American Thoracic Society: ATS statement—Snowbird workshop on standardization of spirometry. *American review of respiratory disease*, 119(5): 831–838, 1979.

American Thoracic Society: Guidelines for bronchial inhalation challenges with pharmacologic and antigenic agents (position paper). *ATS news*, 6(2): 11–19, Spring, 1980.

Anders, A., Baidwan, B., and Petty, T. An evaluation of the vitometer, a simple device for measuring vital capacity. *Respiratory care*, 29(11):1144–1146, 1984.

Arabian, A., Spagnolo, S. and Rohatgi, P.: Evaluation and therapy of pulmonary problems in surgical patients. *Clinical notes on respiratory diseases*, 21(3): 3–14, 1982.

Ayers, L., Whipp, B. and Ziment, I.: A Guide to the Interpretation of Pulmonary Function Tests. New York, Projects in Health, Inc., 1974.

Cary, J., Huseby, J., and Culver, B.: Variability in interpretation of PFTs. *Chest*, 76(4): 389–390, 1979.

Chan-Yeung, M., Lam, S. and Enarson, D.: Pulmonary function measurement in the industrial setting. *Chest*, 88(2): 270–275, 1985.

Cherniack, R.: Pulmonary Function Testing. Philadelphia, W. B. Saunders Co., 1977.

Cherniack, R.: Pitfalls in pulmonary function testing. *Respiratory care*, 28(4): 434–441, 1983.

Clausen, J.: Pulmonary Function Testing Guidelines and Controversies. Orlando, Grune & Stratton, Inc., 1984.

Comroe, J., et al: The Lung—Clinical Physiology and Pulmonary Function Tests, 2nd ed. Chicago, Year Book Medical Publishers, Inc., 1962.

Conrad, S., Kinasewitz, G., and George, R.: Pulmonary Function Testing—Principles and Practice. New York, Churchill Livingstone, Inc., 1984.

Detels, R., Tashkin, D. et al: The UCLA population studies of chronic obstructive respiratory disease. 5. Agreement and disagreement of tests in identifying abnormal lung function. *Chest*, 82(5): 630–638, 1982.

Fletcher, C. and Peto, R.: The natural history of chronic airflow obstruction. *British medical journal*, 6077, 1645–1648, 1977.

Foley, M., Tomashefski, J., and Underwood, E.: Pulmonary function screening tests in industry. *American journal of nursing*, 77(9): 1480–1485, 1977.

Gazioglu, K. and Israel, R.: The pulmonary function test. In Problems in Pulmonary Medicine for the Primary Physician. Philadelphia, Lea & Febiger, 1982.

Gelb, A., Williams, A., and Zamel, N.: Clinical significance of pulmonary function tests—spirometry FEV_1 vs FEF_{25-75} percent. *Chest*, 84(4): 473–474, 1983.

Goddard, R., Klein, W., and Smith, R.: A simple office spirometer for the pediatrician. *Annals of allergy*, 44(4): 206–211, 1980.

Hodgkin, J. E.: Routine Pulmonary Function Tests and Specialized Pulmonary Function Tests. In Respiratory Care—A Guide to Clinical Practice, 2nd ed. (Burton, G. and Hodgkin, J.—eds.) Philadelphia, J. B. Lippincott Co., 1984.

Hudson, L., et al: Clinical evaluation of a new office spirometer. *Journal of the american medical association*, 240(25): 2754, 1978.

Kanner, R. and Renzetti, A.: Predictors of spirometric changes and mortality in the obstructive airway disorders. *Chest*, 85(6): 155–195, 1984.

Lazarus, A.: Pulmonary function tests in upper airway obstruction. *Basics of respiratory disease*, 8(3): entire issue, 1980.

Morgan, W. K.: Clinical significance of PFTs—disability or disinclination? *Chest*, 75(6): 712–715, 1979.

Morgan, W. K.: Pulmonary disability and impairment can't work? Won't work? *Basics of respiratory disease*, 10(5): entire issue, 1982.

Morris, J.: Spirometry in the evaluation of pulmonary function. *The western journal of medicine*, 125(2): 110–118, 1976.

Nadel, J.: Pulmonary function testing. *Basics of respiratory disease*, 1(4): entire issue, 1973.

Petty, T.: Office Spirometry for the Assessment of Pulmonary Disease. New York, Breon Laboratories, Inc., 1980.

Petty, T., Hudson, L., and Neff, T.: Methods of ambulatory care. *Medical clinics of north america*, 57(3): 751–762, 1973.

Polgar, G. and Promadhat, V.: Pulmonary Function in Children: Techniques and Standards. Philadelphia, W. B. Saunders Co., 1971.

Ruppel, G.: Manual of Pulmonary Function Testing. St. Louis, C. V. Mosby, 1986.

Snider, G., et al: American College of Chest Physicians. Committee report—criteria for the assessment of reversibility in airways obstruction. *Chest*, 65(5): 552–553, 1974.

Townsend, M.: Spirometric forced expiratory volumes measured in the standing versus the sitting posture. *American review of respiratory disease*, 130(1): 123–124, 1984.

Wade, J.: Comprehensive Respiratory Care: Physiology and Technique, 3rd ed. St. Louis, C. V. Mosby Co., 1982.

Weinberger, S., Johnson, T., and Weiss, S.: Clinical significance of PFTs—use and interpretation of the single-breath diffusing capacity. *Chest*, 78(3): 483–488, 1980.

Williams, M. H.: Evaluation of asthma. *Chest*, 76(1): 3–4, 1979.

Wyka, K.: Techniques for the detection of small-airways disease. *Respiratory therapy*, 10(1): 50–52, 1980.

Chest Roentgenology

15

Main Objectives

1. **Name four indications for a chest roentgenogram (chest x-ray film).**
2. **Define the following terms: radiolucency, radiopacity, film underpenetration, film overpenetration, artifact, air bronchogram sign, silhouette sign, air-fluid level, and hilum.**
3. **Name and give examples of the four basic roentgen densities.**
4. **Define and explain the clinical uses of the following types of chest x-ray films: posteroanterior (PA), anteroposterior (AP), left lateral, decubitus, lordotic, oblique, inspiratory and expiratory, tomograms, and bronchograms.**
5. **Explain how the nurse can help the technician take an optimal portable film.**
6. **Describe a systematic method for examining chest x-ray films.**
7. **Correctly identify all of the curves of the normal mediastinal profile as well as the general location of the right ventricle.**

8. **Describe normal anatomic relationships among the central pulmonary arteries, tracheobronchial tree, and aorta. Also, describe how the spatial orientation of the right and left pulmonary arteries affects the position of these vessels on the normal chest x-ray.**
9. **Identify the location of the lobes of the lungs on frontal and lateral films.**
10. **Recognize and localize gross pathology on frontal and lateral films, using knowledge of the segmental and lobar anatomy, the silhouette sign, and the mediastinal compartments.**
11. **Name and explain the significance of radiologic signs that help to differentiate interstitial from alveolar chest disease.**
12. **Name radiologic signs typical of these following pathologic states: lung hyperinflation, lung collapse, pleural effusion, pneumothorax, pneumonia, diffuse interstitial fibrosis, chronic bronchitis, emphysema, cor pulmonale, and cardiogenic left ventricular failure.**

The focus of this chapter is the *chest roentgenogram* or *chest x-ray*, another parameter used to assess respiratory problems.

The first part of this chapter discusses the basic concepts of chest roentgenology as well as the nurse's role in taking an optimal portable film.

The second part presents a systematic method for viewing a chest x-ray. It is written primarily for those in advanced nursing practice and other health professionals who view chest x-ray films in clinical settings. However, nurses who do not usually view chest x-ray films will also benefit from this section. The terminology and concepts presented prepare all nurses to (1) understand the radiology report in the chart; (2) selectively use key radiology findings in the overall patient assessment; and (3) integrate the chest radiology findings into respiratory interventions, e.g., counseling the patient, determining key postural drainage positions, readjusting endotracheal tube position, and referring the patient to a physician for immediate medical attention.

In addition, the second part of this chapter benefits others who seek a deeper understanding of normal cardiopulmonary anatomy and abnormal physical findings of the chest. The study of chest roentgenology may be the best possible way of truly understanding pulmonary anatomy short of the observation of cardiothoracic surgery or cadaver dissection.

Purpose and Indications

The physician orders a chest x-ray for one or more of the following reasons:

1. *To help diagnose chest disease or disorders.* When chest x-ray findings are positive for pathology, the information provided may be the key to the diagnosis and evaluation of various disorders, such as lung tumors and heart failure. However, when findings are negative, a pathologic disorder is not automatically ruled out. For example, a person with a normal chest x-ray may demonstrate tumorous lymph nodes at surgery. The patient who has chronic bronchitis with cough and increased sputum production may continue to have normal chest x-ray findings in spite of dramatic worsening of pulmonary signs and symptoms, leading to hospitalization for acute bronchitis.

2. *To assess changes in lung pathology.* The chest x-ray helps determine the severity and progression of respiratory problems, such as mucus retention, pulmonary consolidation from pneumonia, atelectasis, and cor pulmonale.

3. *To locate foreign bodies in the chest.*

4. *To identify the location of monitoring lines, pacemaker lines, endotracheal tubes, and other tubes in the chest.*

Basic Concepts

THE NATURE OF X-RAYS

X-rays are a form of radiant energy similar to light in two important ways as follows:

1. Both x-rays and light rays radiate from their source in all directions.

2. Only a few rays are absorbed by air as both beams pass through the atmosphere, whereas all rays are absorbed by metal as the beams attempt to pass through a sheet of metal.

X-rays are fundamental to the science of radiology because of the following unique characteristics:

1. Their wavelength is shorter than that of ultraviolet light.

2. They penetrate opaque objects that are not penetrated by light.

3. They are invisible and cause fluorescence on the surfaces receiving the x-ray beams.

THE CREATION OF IMAGES ON THE CHEST FILM

Before a chest x-ray is taken, a photographic film is placed in a *cassette* or film holder (Fig. 15–1*A*). In the cross-sectional view of a modern cassette (Fig. 15–1*B*), the film in the middle consists of an acetate sheet coated on both sides with a photographic emulsion. When the radiograph is taken, x-rays are flashed directly onto the film, initiating a photochemical process. Metallic silver is precipitated in fine particles within the gelatin emulsion on the film. Since x-rays precipitate silver on a photographic film much slower than light rays, the cassette has a fluorescent screen next to the film to speed up the process of silver

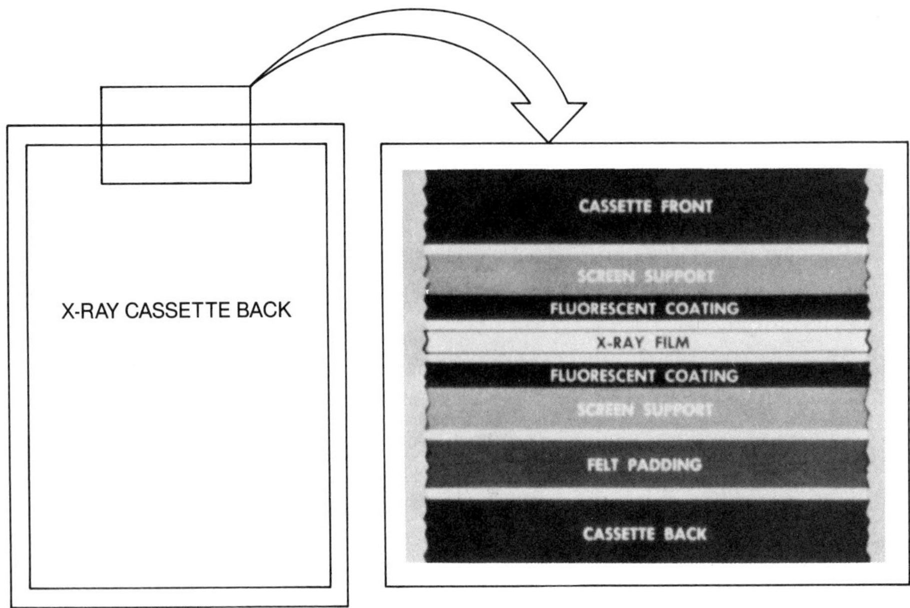

Figure 15–1. *A*, Modern x-ray cassette. *B*, Cross-sectional view. (Courtesy of Eastman Kodak Company, Rochester, NY.)

precipitation and reduce exposure time necessary for production of an adequate chest radiograph. This fluorescent screen emits light rays after activation by x-rays. It is the photochemical effects of light rays emitted from this screen in addition to the x-rays themselves that create images on the film in the cassette.

Radiolucency

When nothing lies between the cassette and x-ray source, x-rays completely penetrate the atmosphere and strike the film and fluorescent screen. Silver readily precipitates on the film, rendering the film *black* or *radiolucent*. Radiolucent areas on the chest film are areas of *blackness* or *radiolucency (i.e., transparency)*.

Radiopacity

When an object lies between the cassette and beam of x-rays, it absorbs some and disperses most of the x-rays. Few rays actually reach the cassette to trigger silver precipitation. Hence, the film becomes *radiopaque*; radiopaque areas on a chest x-ray are areas of *whiteness* or *increased density*.

Four Basic Roentgen Densities

When a patient's chest is radiographed, the images on the film represent different degrees of x-ray penetration and silver precipitation, which in turn depend on the relative radiodensities of tissues that compose the chest. Every image on the film is made up of one or more of these four basic roentgen densities, listed in the next box in order of increasing density and illustrated in Figure 15–2.

DENSITY	*DESCRIPTION*	*EXAMPLES*
Gas (air)	Black, radiolucent	Lung tissue, trachea, bronchi, gas in stomach or intestine
Fat	Gray, less radiolucent	Soft tissue around muscle
Water	Whitish, slightly radiopaque	Heart, blood vessels, muscle, diaphragm
Metal	All white, radiopaque	Calcium of ribs, vertebrae, scapulae, clavicles, other bones, prostheses, contrast media

Note from the descriptions and the examples on the normal chest x-rays that these densities represent different degrees of radiolucency (blackness) and radiopacity (whiteness) (Fig. 15–3 and Fig. 15–4). Color becomes progressively lighter as tissues become denser, starting with the *black* of air-filled lungs and ending with the *white* metal density of bones.

THE OPTIMAL FILM

To take a chest x-ray, the technician positions the patient against the cassette. These positions are described in the next section. The technician then situates the x-ray beam source about 6 ft away from the

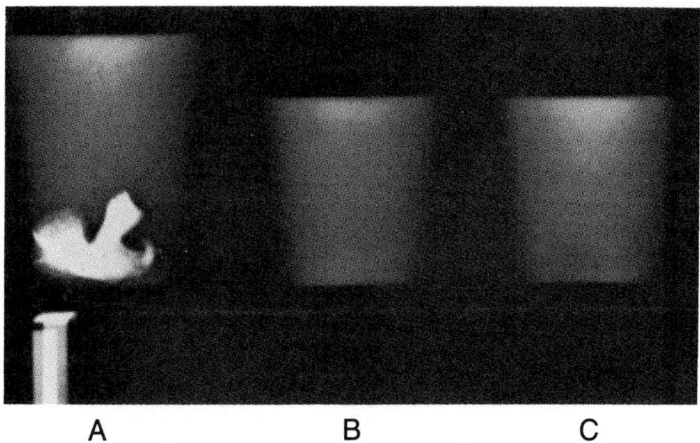

Figure 15–2. Radiograph of three paper cups partly filled with water, each containing a piece of tissue. The black area surrounding the cups is air density. The piece of bone at the bottom of cup A is metal density. The piece of muscle in cup B is invisible because both muscle and water are water density. The piece of fat in cup C is fat density. The paper cups themselves cast no roentgen image. (Reproduced by permission from Squire, L. F., et al: Chest, Abdomen, Bone and the Total Patient. Philadelphia, W. B. Saunders Co., 1981.)

patient and flashes the x-ray beam perpendicular to the patient's chest. This procedure produces the *optimal film*—one with least magnification, optimal sharpness, and minimal angular distortion.

Magnification and Sharpness

The chest film is taken at a distance of 6 ft to reduce magnification and enhance sharpness. The following experiment illustrates this concept:

1. Project the shadow of your hand on a wall with a flashlight. *Application:* The flashlight represents the x-ray beam and the wall, the film cassette.
2. With the flashlight stationary, move your hand closer to the wall. Note, as your hand moves closer to the wall, the shadow becomes less magnified, smaller, and sharper. *Application:* In a standard frontal chest x-ray, the cassette is situated next to the anterior chest area, and the x-ray beam travels through the posterior chest area to the cassette in front. Anatomic structures closest to the cassette (e.g., heart) are clearer on the x-ray film than structures more distant to the cassette (e.g., lesions in the posterior chest area).
3. Now with your hand stationary, gradually move the flashlight farther away. Note that the shadow of your hand becomes gradually smaller and sharper. *Application:* In chest roentgenology, the least magnification occurs with the patient 20 ft away from the x-ray source, but because of the unsafe dispersion of x-rays, the patient is placed closer at a distance of 6 ft.

Angle of the X-ray Beam

The angle at which the x-ray beam strikes the chest and cassette also determines the accuracy of the film image. The optimal 90-degree angle minimizes distortion but often is difficult to achieve in so-called portable films because of equipment limitations and patient immobility. When the beam's angle is less than 90 degrees, the oblique angulation of the beam through many structures may shorten or lengthen images on the film and change the normal radiodensity expected for a specific area of the chest. Alterations in normal images may lead to interpretation difficulties.

X-ray Penetration

The technician adjusts x-ray beam penetration through the chest to produce a film with *ideal exposure* or *optimum penetration.* Ideal exposure allows faint visualization of the thoracic spine and intervertebral spaces through the heart and clear visualization of lung markings behind the heart; it lies between an *underpenetrated* and *overpenetrated* film.

The *underpenetrated film* appears radiopaque and lacks the contrast and sharpness of an adequately penetrated normal chest film (Fig. 15–5). Few x-rays reach the film in the cassette to blacken it. Most of the x-rays hit the patient and are reflected outward in the form of *scattered radiation.* The scattered radiation produces the radiopaque blurring of images on the chest x-ray.

Underpenetration prevents adequate visualization of superimposed dense structures, such as the sternum, mediastinal structures, and thoracic spine; it is a common problem in grossly obese individuals who have dense tissues in general. Sometimes underpenetration is compensated for by adjusting x-ray equipment and increasing exposure factors. At other times, scattered radiation is reduced by use of a *Bucky grid* placed between patient and film. This grid absorbs the oblique rays of scattered radiation and allows only perpendicular rays to pass through the grid to the film underneath. This technique makes the chest x-ray more radiolucent, the anatomic structures more distinct, and the chest x-ray easier to read. The *overpenetrated chest film* appears more radiolucent than the normal chest film (Fig. 15–6). Most of the x-rays reach the film in the cassette to blacken it. Although overpenetration is usually undesirable, it is used intentionally in the following three situations:

1. To locate the tips of endotracheal or tracheal tubes, central venous pressure catheters, nasogastric tubes, and pulmonary artery catheters.
2. To verify placement of pacemakers and other devices.
3. To provide clearer detail to dense anatomic or pathologic areas that appear obscure and radiopaque on the chest film.

Text continued on page 408

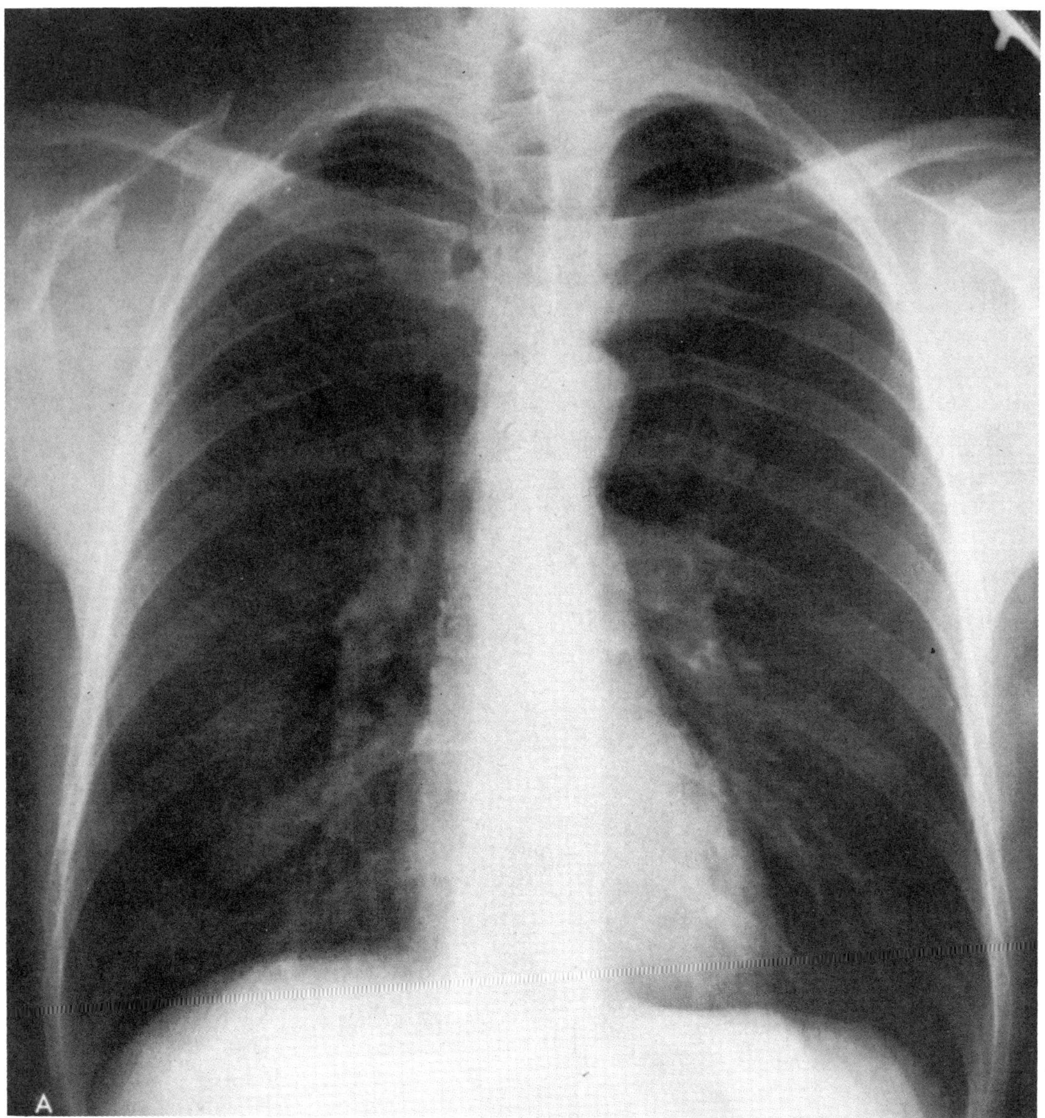

Figure 15–3. Normal chest roentgenogram, posteroanterior projection. *A*, A roentgenogram of the chest in the erect position of an asymptomatic 26-year-old man.

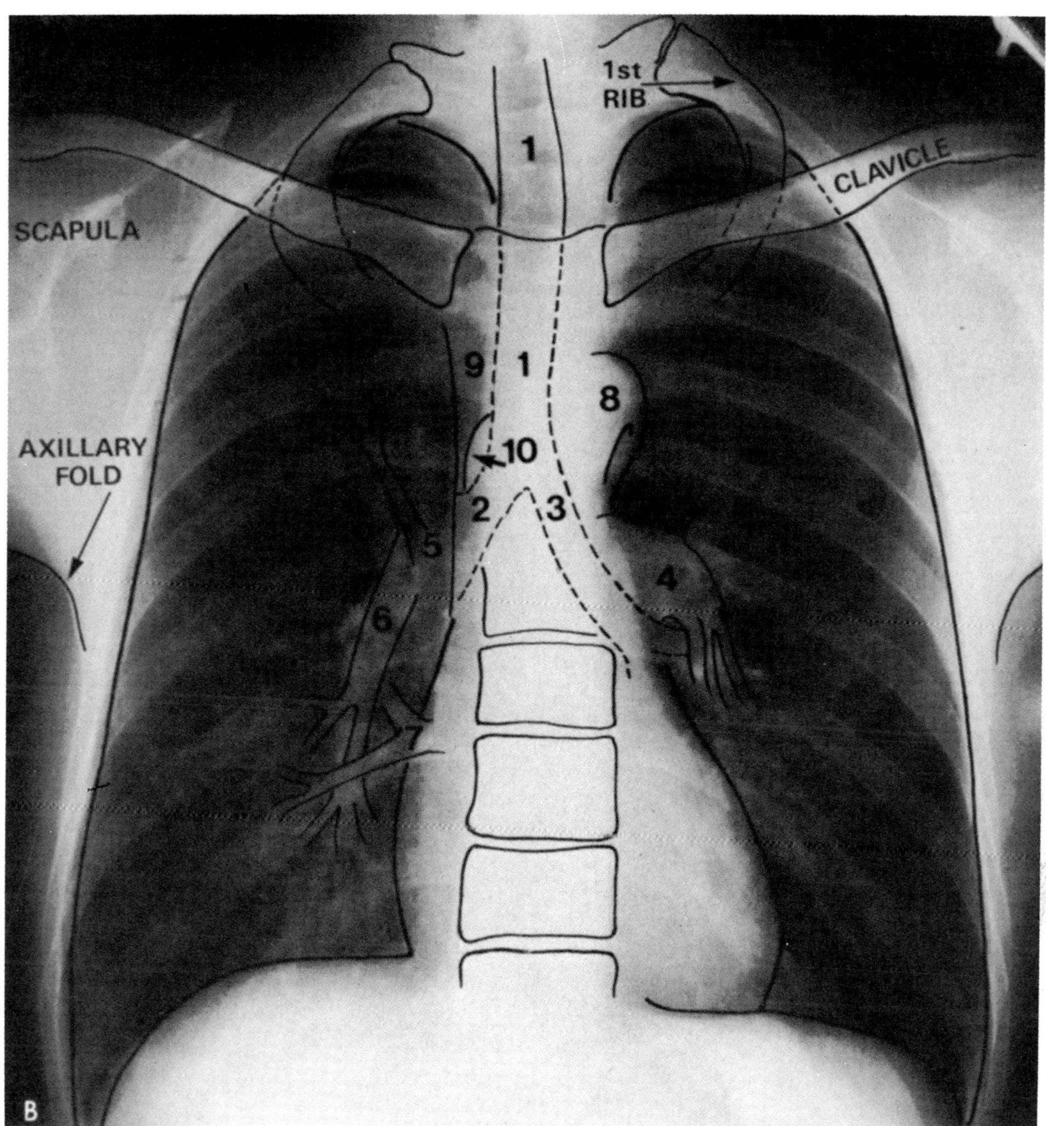

Figure 15–3 *Continued B*, A diagrammatic overlay shows the normal anatomic structures numbered or labelled; (1) trachea, (2) right main bronchus, (3) left main bronchus, (4) left pulmonary artery, (5) right upper lobe pulmonary vein, (6) right interlobar artery, (7) right lower and middle lobe vein, (8) aortic knob, and (9) superior vena cava. (Reproduced by permission from Fraser, R. G. and Paré, J. A.: Diagnosis of Diseases of the Chest, vol. I, 2nd ed. Philadelphia, W. B. Saunders Co., 1977.)

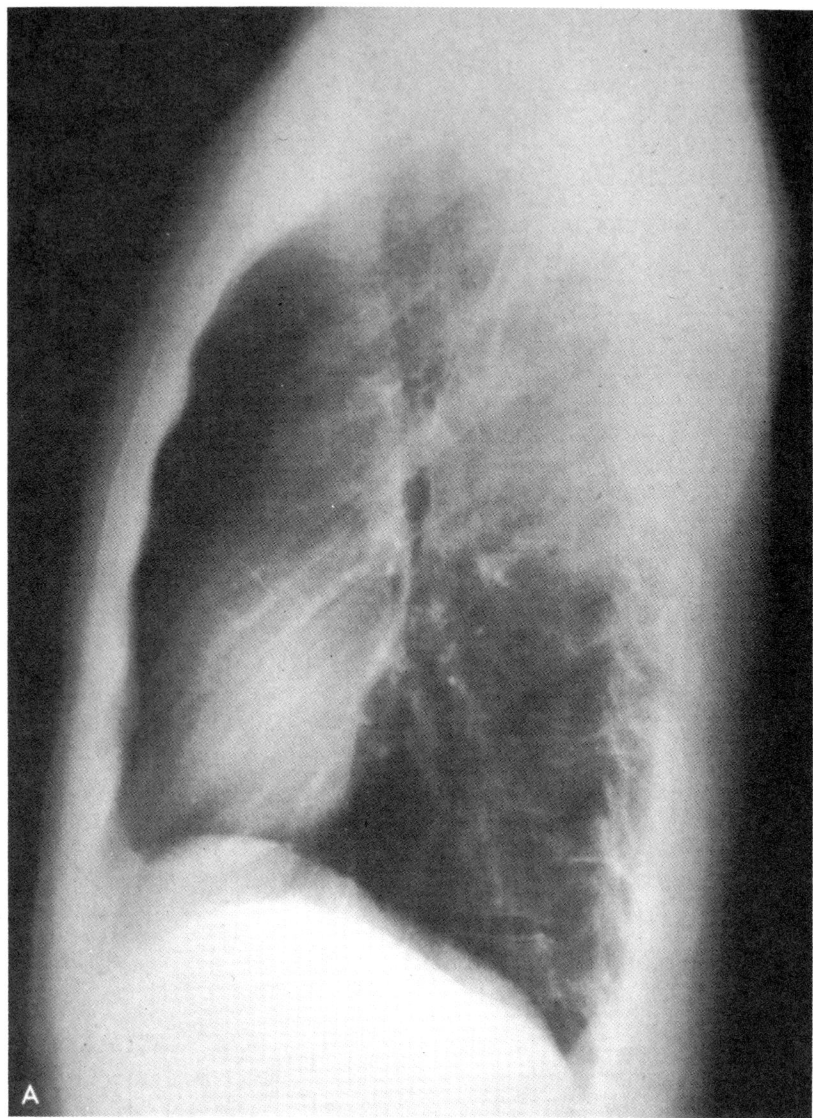

Figure 15–4. Normal chest roentgenogram, lateral projection. *A*, A roentgenogram of the chest in the erect position of an asymptomatic 26-year-old man.

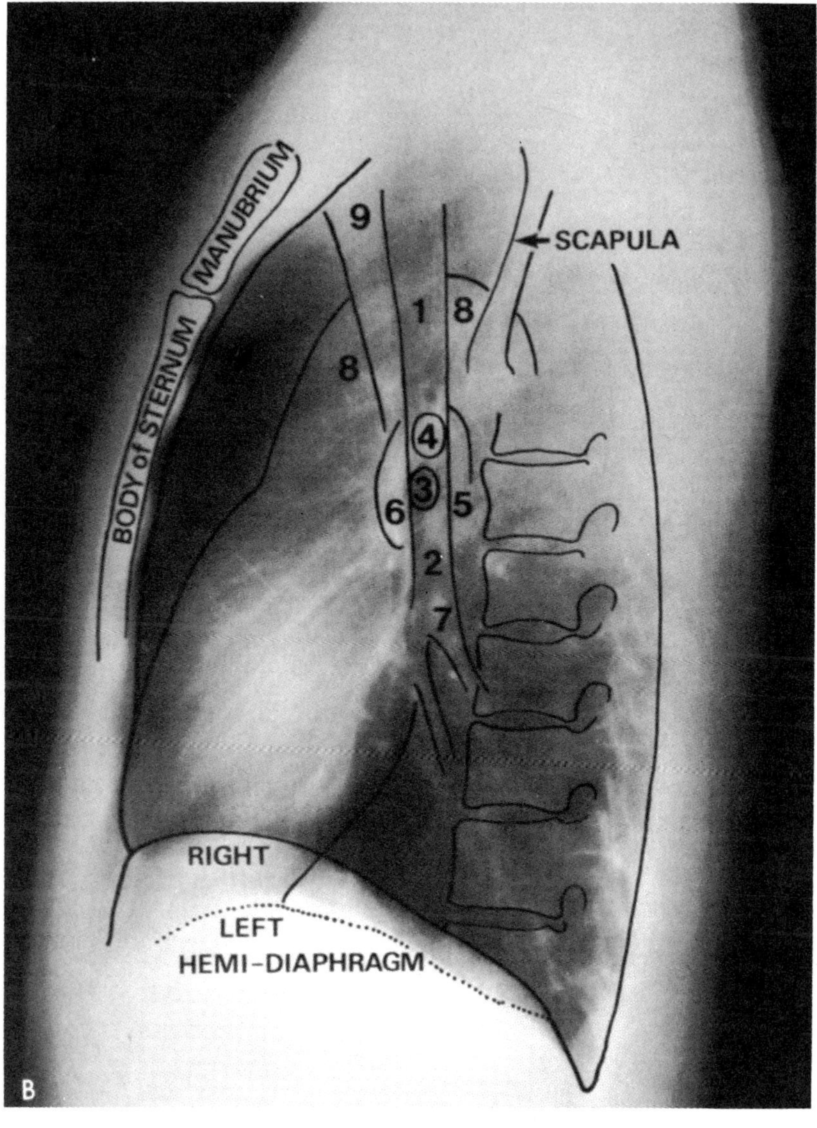

Figure 15–4 *Continued B,* A diagrammatic overlay shows the normal anatomic structures numbered or labelled; (1) tracheal air column, (2) right intermediate bronchus, (3) left upper lobe bronchus, (4) right upper lobe bronchus, (5) left interlobar artery, (6) right interlobar artery, (7) confluence of pulmonary veins, (8) aortic arch, and (9) brachiocephalic vessels. (Reproduced by permission from Fraser, R. G. and Paré, J. A.: Diagnosis of Diseases of the Chest, vol. I, 2nd ed. Philadelphia, W. B. Saunders Co., 1977.)

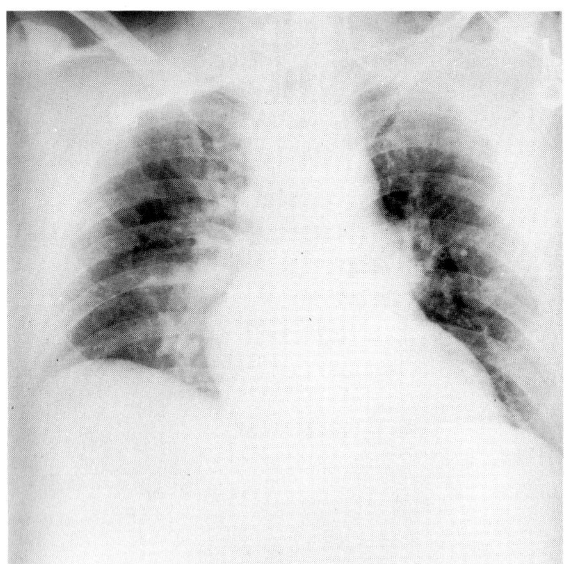

Figure 15–5. Example of an underpenetrated chest x-ray film.

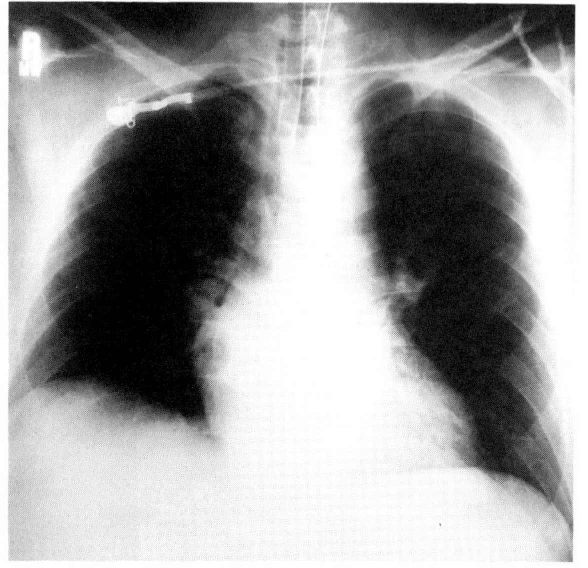

Figure 15–6. Example of an overpenetrated chest x-ray film.

BASIC VIEWS OF THE CHEST

The most commonly ordered views of the chest are the *frontal* and *lateral* views. Basic frontal and lateral views are described subsequently and shown in Figure 15–7, Figure 15–8, and Figure 15–9 for comparison. The relationship of the chest to the cassette is illustrated underneath each x-ray. In the drawings, the arrow indicates the direction of the x-ray beam to the cassette.

Posteroanterior (PA) View

The *posteroanterior (PA) teleoroentgenogram,* called the *PA teleo* or the *PA chest x-ray,* represents the standard frontal view of the chest. The term postercanterior refers to the direction the x-ray beam travels—from the posterior to the anterior areas of the chest. This type of film can only be taken in the radiology department. It is taken with the patient standing and pressing the shoulders and anterior chest area as close to the x-ray cassette as possible.

Lateral View

Most medical evaluations require a PA view and a *lateral view,* the next most commonly ordered view of the chest. The lateral view is taken with the patient standing upright with the hands held above the head. The *left lateral view* is taken with the left side of the chest against the film cassette, and the *right lateral view,* with the right side against the film cassette.

The left lateral view is routinely preferred over the right lateral view because the former produces a sharper image of the heart and surrounding lung parenchyma than the latter. However, when pathology is present, the view that places the lesion closest to the cassette is always used.

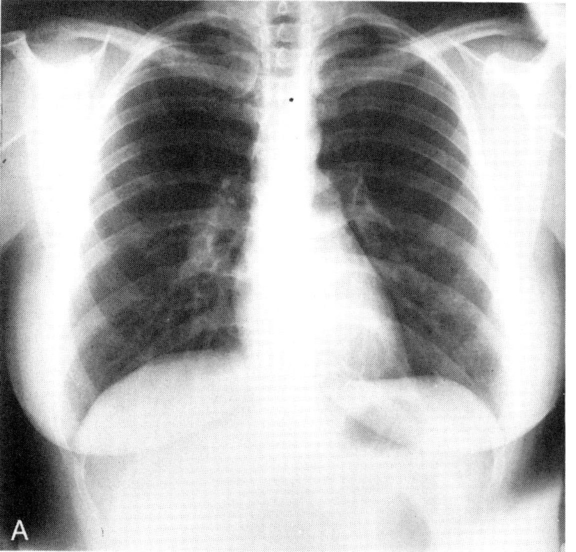

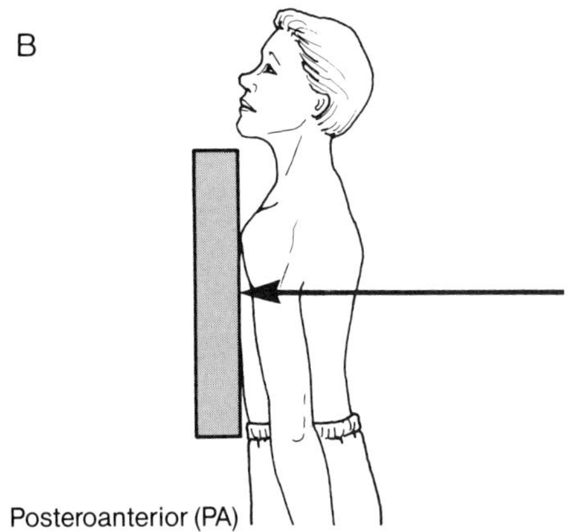

Figure 15–7. Posteroanterior view of the chest. *A,* Normal chest x-ray film of a healthy 30–year–old woman. *B,* The x-ray beam travels from posterior to anterior chest areas until it reaches the cassette.

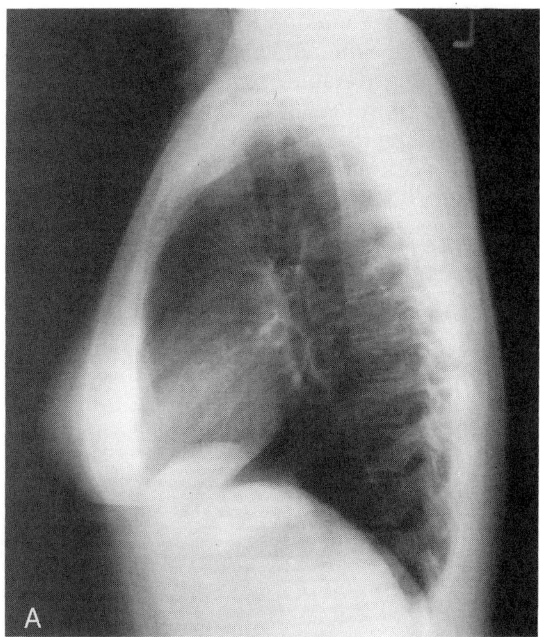

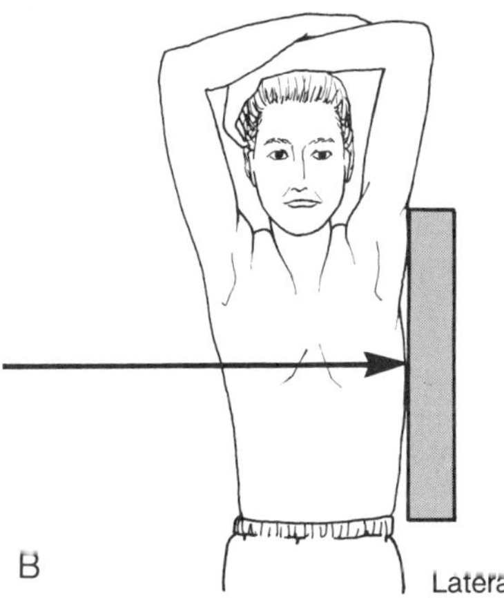

Figure 15–8. Left lateral view of the chest. *A*, Normal chest x-ray film of a healthy 30–year–old woman. *B*, The left side of the chest is closest to the cassette. The x-ray beam travels through the side of the chest.

The lateral view exposes areas that cannot be seen on the frontal view, such as the areas behind the heart and the posterior lung bases. The lateral view helps differentiate anterior from posterior structures, and it helps locate lesions by mediastinal compartment or involved lung segments.

Anteroposterior (AP) View

In the *anteroposterior* (AP) frontal view, the x-ray beam passes through the patient from anterior to posterior. This view represents the routine portable chest films taken in the acute care setting, the operating suite, or the patient's room with the patient sitting *upright* or lying *supine*. The supine AP view is also used in the radiology department for very sick patients, infants, and young children.

The AP view is less desirable than the PA view for several reasons. First, it produces more magnification; the film is taken at shorter distances, about 3 ft for supine films and 6 ft for upright films. Also, anterior structures are magnified because they do not lie closest to the x-ray cassette. The heart appears larger (compare Fig. 15–7 with Fig. 15–9), making evaluation of cardiomegaly more difficult. Second, maximum x-ray energy necessary for clear images may not be possible with portable x-ray equipment. Third, optimal positioning is difficult to achieve, especially for patients who are critically ill, attached to ventilators, EKG monitors, and intravenous lines, and unable to maintain the upright position for the portable film.

When the supine position is used instead of the upright position, interpretation of the film becomes even more difficult because of the following changes:

1. Hemidiaphragms are elevated, owing to the reduced vital capacity in the supine position.
2. The heart and mediastinum appear larger.
3. Pulmonary blood flow redistributes to the upper lobes.

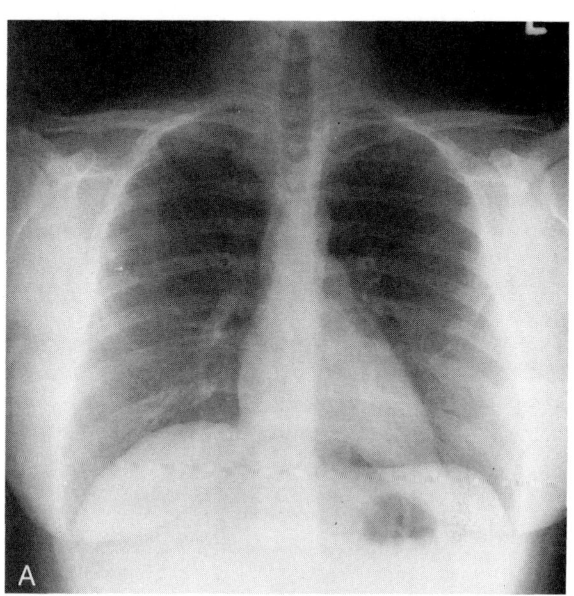

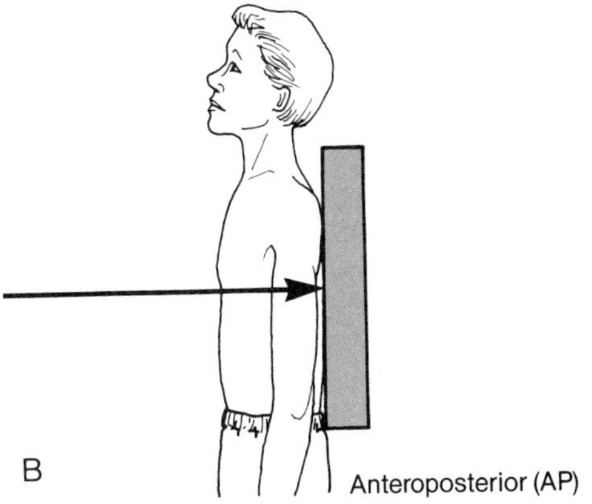

Figure 15–9. Anteroposterior view. *A*, Normal chest x-ray film of a healthy 30–year–old woman. *B*, The x-ray beam travels from anterior to posterior chest until it reaches the cassette.

4. Gravitational effects may change the appearance of disease processes; e.g., the fluid level of a large pleural effusion shows on an upright film but is replaced by water density throughout the whole lung in the supine position.

5. The angle of the clavicles may change.

OTHER CHEST X-RAY VIEWS AND SPECIAL STUDIES

Expiratory View and Fluoroscopy

Most chest x-rays films are inspiratory—they are taken at the peak of a maximum inspiration. When both inspiratory and expiratory films are ordered, the *expiratory film* is taken at the end of a maximum expiration (i.e., slow vital capacity maneuver) (Fig. 15–10). Differences in general appearance are readily appreciated when the two films are viewed side by side. The clear inspiratory film with radiolucent lung fields and normal heart size contrasts dramatically with the "cloudy" expiratory film. In the latter case, the heart looks larger, and the elevated hemidiaphragms have reduced the size of the lung fields.

Expiratory films have four main uses. First, small pneumothoraces absent on the inspiratory film may be evident on the expiratory film. During expiration, the lung contracts its volume, allowing the intrapleural air to spread out more within the pleural space. Second, the expiratory film is used to demonstrate generalized air trapping (e.g., emphysema) or localized air trapping (e.g., bronchial obstruction from aspiration of a foreign object or from an endobronchial tumor). Third, when viewed with the inspiratory film, the expiratory film is used to assess diaphragmatic movement during respiration. When more thorough assessment of changes during respiration is needed, *fluoroscopy* is ordered. Fluoroscopy is a roentgenographic procedure providing constant imaging of anatomic structures during respiration. Fourth, an expiratory film may be used to confirm the presence of a lung lesion—it becomes more visible on the expiratory film because of its change in position relative to ribs and intercostal spaces.

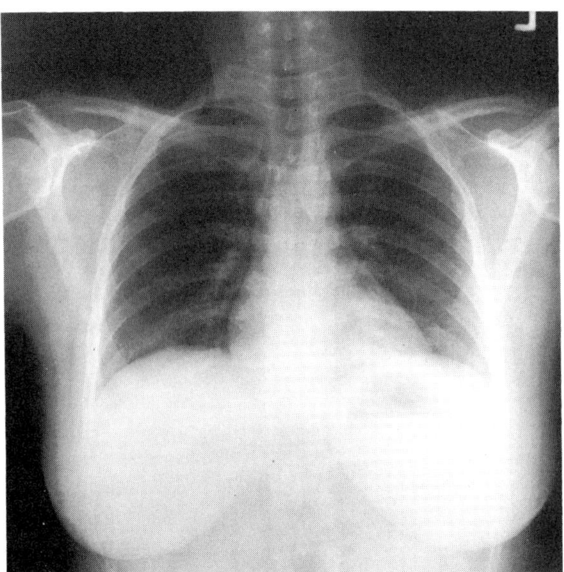

Figure 15–10. Posterior-anterior film of a healthy 30–year–old woman taken at the end of a maximum expiration. Compare this expiratory film with the inspiratory film in Figure 15–7A.

Other chest x-ray views include the decubitus, lordotic, and oblique, as described next.

Decubitus View

A *decubitus view* is a PA or AP view taken with the patient lying down, i.e., prone, supine, or on the right side (the *right lateral decubitus*) or on the left side (the *left lateral decubitus* (Fig. 15–11). A decubitus

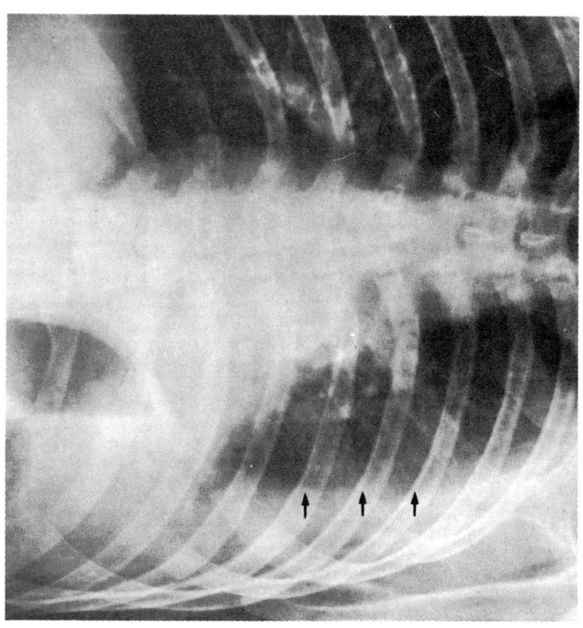

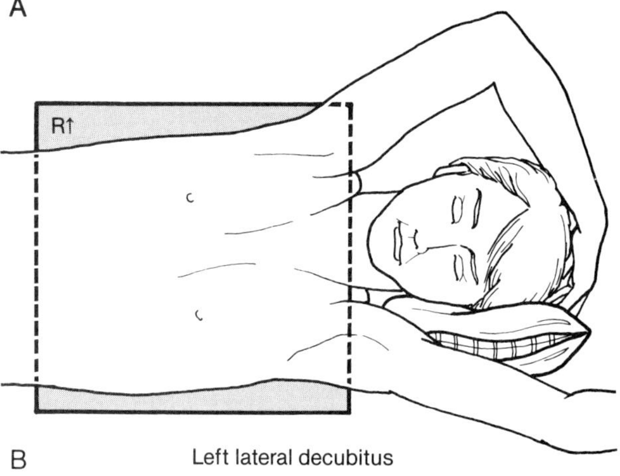

Figure 15–11. Left lateral decubitus view. *A*, Abnormal chest x-ray film showing a layer of fluid (arrows) lying against the left lateral thoracic wall. *B*, The film is taken with the patient lying on the left side with the film cassette placed against the back. (*A* reproduced by permission from Felson, B. et al: Principles of Chest Roentgenology. Philadelphia, W. B. Saunders Co., 1965.)

view is ordered to confirm the suspicion of an air-fluid level in the lungs, a small pneumothorax, or a small pleural effusion. As little as 50 to 100 ml of fluid is seen in the pleural space in the lateral decubitus view. In comparison, about 350 ml of fluid must be present for an effusion to be demonstrated on the frontal upright view. In addition, this type of view is used to evaluate the mobility of a mediastinal mass and to shift pleural fluid so that the underlying lung can be better radiographed and thus visualized.

Lordotic View

A *lordotic view* is a PA or AP upright film taken with the x-ray beam penetrating at an oblique angle (Fig. 15–12A). The x-ray tube is lowered and angled upward, as shown in Figure 15–12B. The patient may be tipped backward slightly to better project the clavicles above the lung apices on the film. The uses of the lordotic view are as follows:

1. It allows better visualization and evaluation of apical regions. The oblique angle of the beam superimposes anterior and posterior aspects of the same ribs and projects the clavicles above the apices rather than on top of them, as in the PA or AP film.
2. It is used specifically to screen for pulmonary tuberculosis, since this disease typically manifests itself in apical regions.
3. It is used to better visualize disease in the right median lobe (RML) or lingular segments of the left

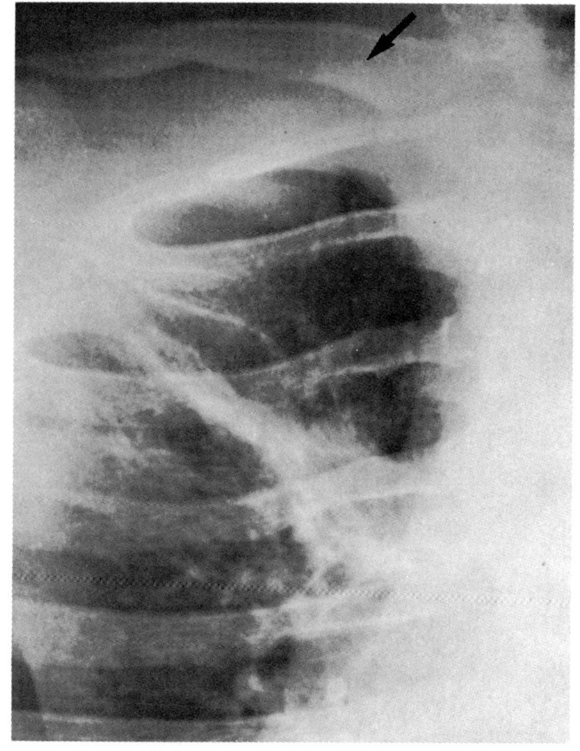

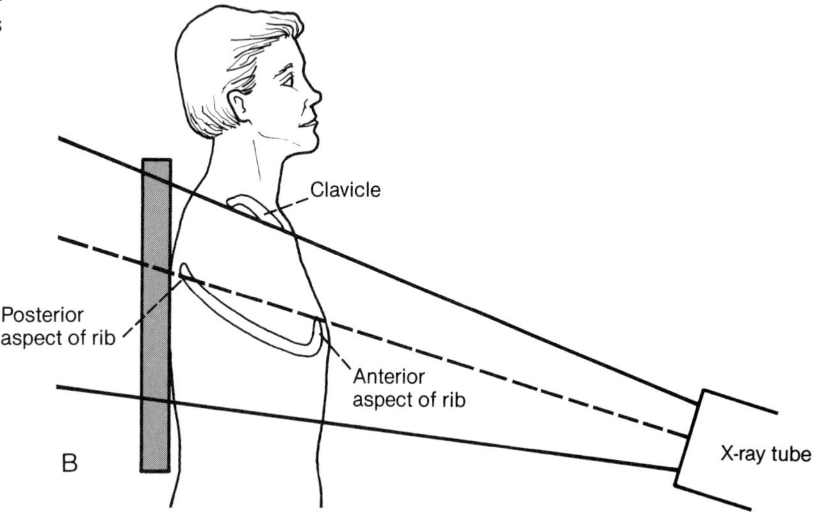

Figure 15–12. Lordotic view. *A*, In this chest x-ray film, the clavicle (arrow) is raised above the lung apex, and the anterior and posterior ribs are superimposed on each other. The result is better exposure of the tuberculous lesion in the right upper lobe. Compare this x-ray with the apical area in the PA view shown in Figure 15–3*A*. *B*, The x-ray beam travels upwards at an oblique angle to superimpose anterior and posterior ribs and to better expose the lung apices. (*A* reproduced by permission from Felson, B. et al: Principles of Chest Roentgenology. Philadelphia, W. B. Saunders Co., 1965.)

upper lobe (LUL). The beam moves obliquely along the longest axis of the RML and lingula. Pneumonia or lung collapse is more radiopaque than in the PA view because the beam traverses through more diseased lung tissue.

Oblique View

An *oblique view* is a frontal film taken with the patient standing diagonally at an angle of 45 to 60 degrees to the x-ray cassette (Fig. 15–13A). Oblique views include the following:

1. *Right anterior oblique* (RAO)—the right anterior area of the chest rests against the cassette in front (Fig. 15–13B).
2. *Left anterior oblique* (LAO)—the left anterior chest area is positioned closest to the cassette in front.
3. *Right* and *left posterior oblique* (RPO and LPO)—the right or left side of the back is positioned against the cassette.

In all the oblique positions listed, the x-ray beam passes through the chest at an angle, "spreading out" previously superimposed organs or lesions. For example, in the RAO view, structures in the left thorax are spread out to allow better visualization.

The oblique views may be ordered for one or more of the following reasons:

1. To better visualize the carina.
2. To localize the lesions visible on the PA view but not on the lateral view.
3. To view the heart, great vessels, and other cardiovascular structures and to evaluate enlargement of individual chambers of the heart.

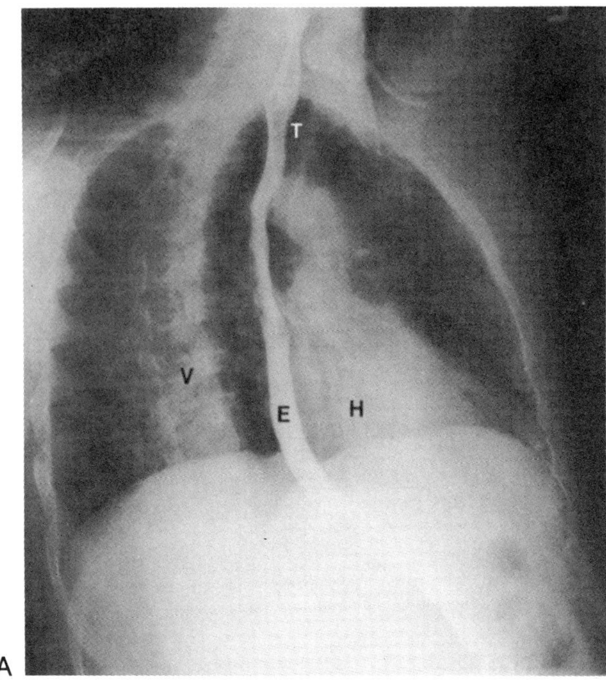

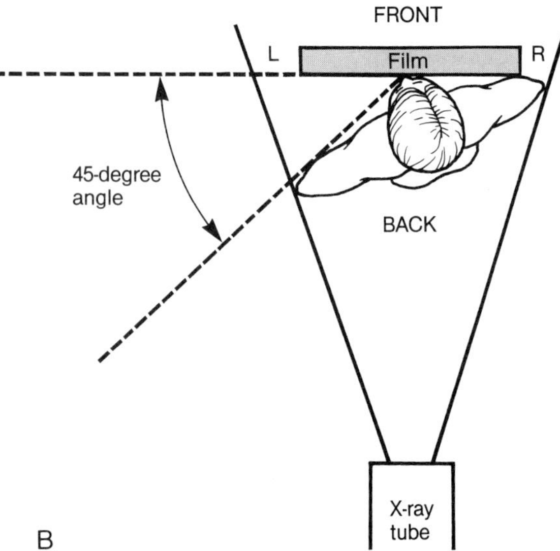

Figure 15–13. Right anterior oblique view. *A*, In this chest x-ray film, the heart and entire left side of the chest are spread out by the oblique angle created by patient positioning. T = trachea; E = esophagus visualized during a barium swallow; V = vertebrae; H = heart. *B*, The right anterior chest rests against the cassette in front. The x-ray beam travels from posterior to anterior chest areas. (*A* reproduced by permission from Rau, J. and Pearce, D.: Understanding Chest Radiographs. Denver, Colorado, Multimedia Publishing, Inc., 1984.)

4. To identify and evaluate peripheral lesions and structures, e.g., lateral aspects of the ribs and pleura.

The RAO and LAO views are used routinely to detect the pleural thickening associated with asbestosis and asbestos-related diseases.

Tomograms

Tomograms and bronchograms are both special radiologic studies. A *tomogram* is a body section radiograph that may also be referred to as a *laminogram* or *planigram* (Fig. 15–14A). It is made by simultaneously moving the x-ray source and film plate in opposite directions, so that the axis of rotation identifies a particular plane of focus or horizontal body section to be x-rayed (Fig. 15–14B). Several tomograms are taken in succession, each representing a different horizontal body slice and each labelled with a number representing the distance in centimeters from the x-ray table top (Fig. 15–14C). The procedure for obtaining tomograms is referred to as *tomography*.

Tomograms provide a detailed examination of the lung parenchyma, hilar areas, and mediastinum. Tomography is localized to the area of pathology in the case of a solitary nodule, calcification, endobronchial lesion, or obscure mass suspected or identified on the PA view. Full chest tomography, i.e., from right to left and front to back, is used to detect and evaluate metastatic lung disease.

Bronchograms

A *bronchogram* is a chest x-ray taken after intrabronchial instillation of a contrast medium (Fig. 15–15). After a topical anesthetic is applied, the contrast medium is instilled via a nasotracheal or other catheter. With careful patient positioning, the contrast medium coats the tracheobronchial tree, permitting visualization of all or select bronchial anatomy and pathology. Procedural complications are uncommon but may include anaphylactic or toxic reaction to the topical anesthetic or contrast medium, fever, and chemical-induced pneumonia.

Bronchography is ordered to evaluate the severity and distribution of bronchiectasis. Bronchiectasis is divided into three classifications based on bronchographic patterns, as explained in Chapter 7. When this disease is present and surgical resection is under consideration, all 19 bronchopulmonary segments are visualized and radiographed on several bronchogram films.

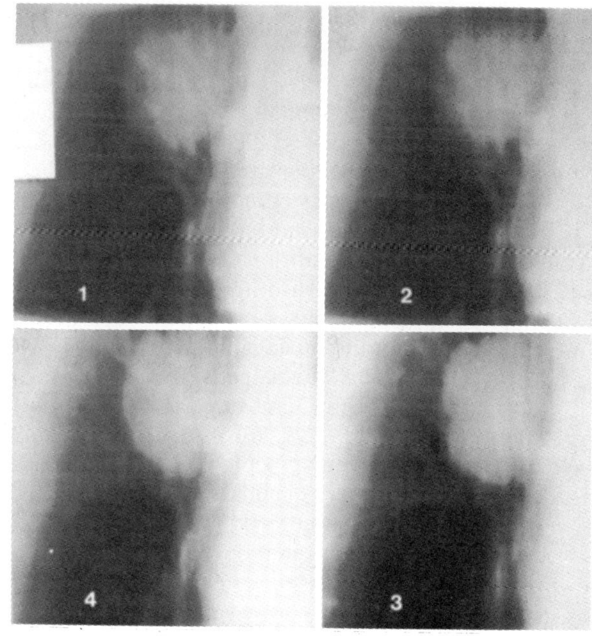

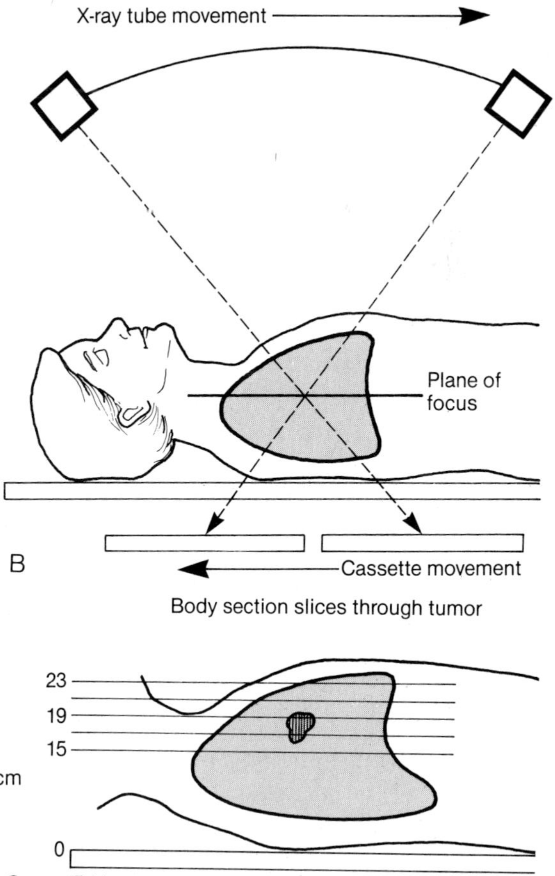

Figure 15–14. *A*, A series of four tomograms used to visualize a right upper lobe density. (*A* reproduced by permission from Rau, J. and Pearce, D.: Understanding Chest Radiographs. Denver, Colorado, Multimedia Publishing, Inc., 1984.) *B*, A tomogram is made by simultaneous movement of the x-ray source and film cassette in opposite directions. *C*, Each tomogram represents a body section slice identified by distance in centimeters from the x-ray table top.

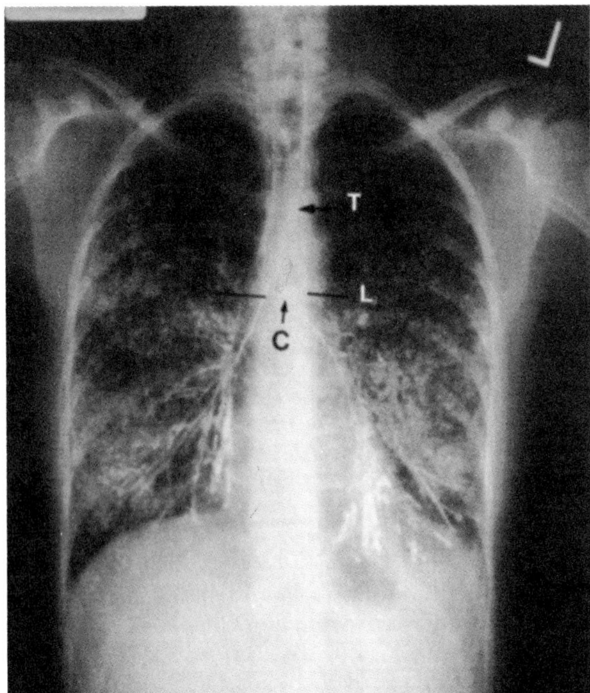

Figure 15–15. PA view of a bronchogram. T = trachea; C = carina; R = right main stem bronchus; L = left main stem bronchus. (Reproduced by permission from Rau, J. and Pearce, D.: Understanding Chest Radiographs. Denver, Colorado, Multimedia Publishing, Inc., 1984.)

Other Studies

Other radiologic studies used to supplement frontal and lateral chest x-rays are summarized in Table 15–1.

The Nurse's Role in Taking an Optimal Chest Film

At least for portable films, the nurse shares responsibility with the x-ray technician for taking an optimal chest film, one that provides optimum visualization of anatomic structures. Following the suggestions provided will help insure the taking of an optimal film without exposing patient and staff to excess irradiation.

1. *Encourage the patient to take a maximum inspiration.* For a normal inspiratory film, the technician asks the patient to take a deep breath and to hold it, while the technician takes the x-ray. Shallow breathing or poor inspiratory effort results in a poor inspiratory film that may look like an expiratory film.

2. *Whenever possible, use the erect rather than the supine position.* If necessary, place tape across the forehead of a comatose patient to maintain the erect position or put on a protective lead apron and hold the patient in place.

3. *Help the technician position the patient with the back flat against the x-ray cassette and the arms and shoulders arranged symmetrically.* The head of the bed is elevated until the x-ray beam is anticipated to strike the chest at a perpendicular angle. Avoid any rotation. If the patient is turned only a few degrees to one side, the clavicles will demonstrate marked asymmetry on the chest film, and the obliquely radiographed heart and mediastinum may appear enlarged and distorted.

4. *Eliminate artifacts and pull ventilator tubes, monitoring wires, and other tubes away from the chest area.* To eliminate *artifacts* (i.e., images on the film that have no anatomic basis), the nurse helps remove all extraneous objects and items from the surface of the chest, e.g., extra clothing in addition to the patient's gown; jewelry; safety pins; long hair or braids; chest binders, but check with the physician first; and other devices that can be temporarily removed. Relocate EKG electrodes if they lie over an anticipated area of pathology. Reposition ventilator tubing above the shoulder and away from the chest. Similarly, carefully pull away other lines and tubes, taping or pinning them to the bed sheet, if necessary.

5. *Elicit patient cooperation.* The technician or nurse explains the procedure to the patient and answers questions to maximize cooperation and allay anxieties related to the taking of the x-ray film. Breathing instructions are repeated, if necessary. Emphasis is placed on not moving during the taking of the film—movement causes the blurring of images on the chest x-ray film.

6. *Protect patient and staff from the hazardous effects of irradiation,* e.g., erythema, hematopoietic injury, induction of malignant tumors, and sterility. With proper use of portable equipment and adherence to basic precautionary measures, roentgen exposure is kept to safe levels, and hazardous effects are unlikely. The technician traditionally shouts "X-ray!" before taking a film to warn others of possible exposure. At this time, all persons should leave the room or wear protective aprons during the 1 to 2 seconds of exposure. In addition, the selective ordering of chest films helps reduce x-ray exposure as well as cost to the patient. Chest x-rays are reduced in frequency or discontinued when an acute disease stabilizes or when a recurrent pattern, such as in pulmonary edema, is recognized and monitored by other means. For the screening of asymptomatic disease, routine chest x-rays are not indicated, unless the history, physical examination, or specific diagnostic test results suggest possible chest disease (American Thoracic Society, 1984).

7. *Whenever possible, send the patient to the radiology department when a PA view is ordered.* The portable AP view is more likely to result in a suboptimal film, several retakes, and interpretation difficulties.

8. *Write the patient's diagnosis and reason for the chest film on the radiology requisition.* The location of pathology is important because it informs the technician of the key area that requires optimum visualiza-

Table 15–1. OTHER RADIOLOGIC STUDIES

Study	Description	Main Indications
Lung perfusions and ventilation scintiscans	In the perfusion scan, the patient is injected intravenously with a radiotracer. In the ventilation scan, the patient breathes a radioactive gas (xenon) through a closed system. Absent or uneven radioactive uptake on the x-ray film locates a perfusion or ventilation defect in the lung. The size and distribution of such a defect is further evaluated.	Suspected abnormality in lung perfusion, e.g., pulmonary embolism. Preoperative evaluation for lung resection. Right-to-left shunt evaluation.
Computerized axial tomography (CAT) of the chest	The patient is supine while a beam scans horizontal slices of the chest, and computerized equipment synthesizes a cross-sectional image for analysis. A contrast medium may be injected intravenously beforehand. This method provides anatomic detail and quantifies radiographic tissue density.	Detection and evaluation of mediastinal pathology: metastases to the lungs, especially when the chest x-ray findings are negative, and chest wall or pleural pathology.
Ultrasonography of the chest	With the patient erect, ultrasonic energy scans the chest, making an image for graphic display.	Ultrasonography has limited usefulness, since the lung reflects rather than transmits ultrasonic energy. Assessment of diaphragmatic motion Location of free pleural fluid in the chest and loculated pleural fluid for biopsy or removal (thoracentesis), when the routine chest x-ray cannot be used for this purpose.
Pulmonary angiography	Under fluoroscopy, a catheter is passed through the femoral artery and into the pulmonary artery. Contrast medium is injected, while sequential scintigraphic images are obtained to evaluate blood flow through the lungs and heart. Intralumenal filling defects or abrupt pulmonary vessel cutoffs indicate pulmonary embolism.	Suspected pulmonary embolism, especially when the ventilation-perfusion scan is equivocal.
Barium swallow	The patient swallows barium and is observed in various positions fluoroscopically. When a chest x-ray is taken, the metal density of the barium in the esophagus is in sharp contrast to the water density of nearby structures, thus facilitating visualization and evaluation.	Esophageal pathology, e.g., stricture, tumor, neuromuscular dysfunction leading to aspiration, esophageal foreign body. Mediastinal masses in the middle mediastinal compartment. Assessment of heart chamber enlargement.

tion. As previously described, the technician adjusts the degree of x-ray beam penetration, depending on whether the film is ordered to assess pathology or to check endotracheal tube, monitoring line, or pacemaker wire placement.

Systematic Method for Viewing a Chest X-ray

The remainder of this chapter describes how to systematically view a chest x-ray film, mainly the frontal view; how to recognize basic positive radiologic signs; and how to interpret their significance.

While studying films and anatomic relationships, the reader is encouraged to constantly think in three sets of dimensions—right and left, inferior and superior, anterior and posterior—even though each film presents only two sets of dimensions. For frontal films, always check the lateral film for the "missing" anterior-posterior dimension. This approach facilitates the recognition of the anatomic bases for normal and abnormal findings.

PLACING THE FILM ON THE VIEW BOX

The first step in viewing a film is to place it correctly on the view box. Frontal views are labelled in the upper corners with a right mark (R), left mark (L), or both to indicate the patient's right and left sides. Place the film on the view box so that the *patient's left side* or the film's left mark is on *your right side*. Unless the patient has reversed internal organs (i.e., dextrocardia or situs inversus), the arch of the aorta and the shadow of the heart normally mark the patient's left side.

Place the left lateral view marked with a left mark on the view box as though the patient's left side were facing you. The situation is reversed for the right lateral view—the patient's right side should be facing you.

Serial films are viewed in chronologic order from earliest to latest to identify changes from the patient's normal baseline film and to evaluate the progression of chest disease. Frontal films are placed in one row, and lateral films in another row directly below corresponding frontal views. This arrangement facilitates film comparisons and the identification of subtle changes over time.

INITIAL IMPRESSIONS

The clinician stands back from the view box at least 6 to 8 ft for an initial general impression. Does the chest x-ray appear normal or abnormal? Does anything appear asymmetric or out of place? What looks hazy, ambiguous, or obviously abnormal?

Abnormalities suspected from general impressions indicate where to search more carefully at closer distances (2 to 4 ft) during the subsequent systematic examination.

SYSTEMATIC EXAMINATION

A systematic method of examination is mandatory for the interpretation of chest films. Such a method may serve as the beginner's main tool for the detection of abnormality or the experienced radiologist's final check after a free-search method of scanning films. Some systems, such as the one described here, begin with the soft tissues on the outside of the chest and work inward to the bony thorax, pleura, mediastinum, and lungs. Other systems, such as the one described by Rau and Pearce (1984), start with the mediastinum and work outward, toward the soft tissues. Though the form may vary, each clinician must learn a system and then gradually make adaptations to improve interpretation efficiency and accuracy. Even experienced radiologists have an astonishingly high rate of intraobserver and interobserver error—3 to 31% and 9 to 24% respectively, as reported by Paré and Fraser (1983).

The systematic method discussed here consists of examination of the following anatomic structures, as listed in the box.

STRUCTURES IN SEQUENCE

Soft tissues
Trachea
Bony thorax
Intercostal spaces
Diaphragm and area below the diaphragm
Pleural surfaces
Mediastinum
Hila
Lung fields

Structures in Sequence

Examination of each of the listed structures is described here. Review of relevant content in Part One of this book—the lungs within the chest cage, the mediastinum, the pulmonary circulation, and the interstitial space—facilitates the comprehension of anatomic relationships. Periodic study of normal PA and lateral views (see Fig. 15–3 and Fig. 15–4) in relation to illustrations on subsequent pages also helps orient the reader to the normal appearance of structures on the chest x-ray. Chest x-rays illustrating abnormalities are limited in number because of space considerations, and because many x-ray details reproduce poorly. Nevertheless, descriptive content presented enables the clinician to more readily recognize and interpret an abnormality, when it appears in the clinical setting.

SOFT TISSUES

Soft tissues consist of skin and subcutaneous fat. Their fat density blends into the water density of underlying muscles, such as the pectoralis major and sternocleidomastoid.

The clinician scans one side of the thorax and then the other side (gray areas in Fig. 15–16), inspecting the soft tissues of the neck, superior shoulder, axillary area, and breast. The two sides should appear symmetric and of the same density.

As you view the soft tissues, note the following, as listed in the box.

SOFT TISSUE VISUALIZATION

1. Cutaneous lesions or areas of increased density within soft tissues.
2. Structures that protrude from the skin's surface, e.g., warts and neurofibromas.
3. Air density in subcutaneous tissues or between muscles from surgery, chest trauma, esophageal or tracheal perforation, or pneumothorax. Figure 15–17 illustrates the appearance of subcutaneous emphysema.
4. Paucity of soft tissues along the sides of the chest from recent weight loss or cachexia.
5. Increase in soft tissues along the sides of the chest from weight gain or obesity.
6. Any increase or decrease in density in and around the axillary areas. Slightly increased density on one side of the chest may be due to well-developed muscles from being right or left handed. Bilateral increased density occurs in men with heavy muscular development in general.
7. Absence of one or more breasts in a woman. Suspect mastectomy if one lung looks more radiolucent than the other.
8. Presence or absence of nipples and areoli in males—they are commonly absent. A unilateral nipple shadow may represent a lesion.

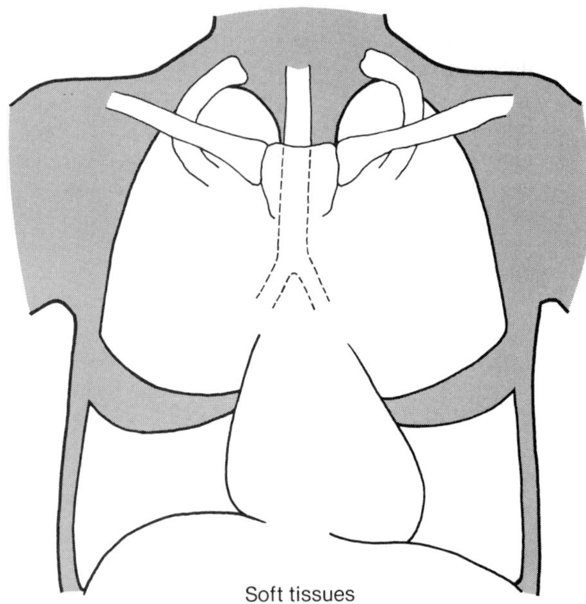

Figure 15–16. Soft tissues are shaded gray. (The gray areas extending inwards towards the heart represent breast tissue.)

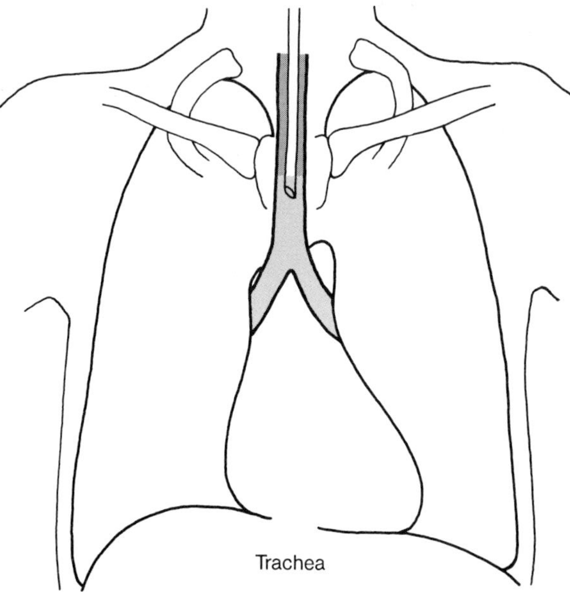

Figure 15–18. Trachea with an endotracheal tube in place. The dark gray area is readily visible on the chest x-ray. The light gray area may not be easily appreciated or may be completely replaced by radiopacity.

TRACHEA

The column of radiolucency readily visible above the clavicles represents the air density of the trachea (Fig. 15–18). This column normally lies midline over the spine. However, Felson (1973) reports that 2% of normal chest x-rays demonstrate slight deviations of the trachea to the right or left of this midline position.

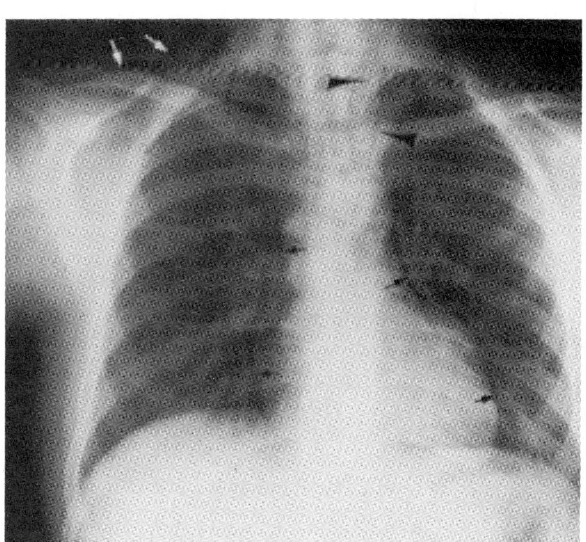

Figure 15–17. Mediastinal emphysema, subcutaneous emphysema. Streaks of air around the mediastinum (black arrows) have dissected outwards to the soft tissues of the neck (black arrowheads) and shoulder (white arrows), where they now represent subcutaneous emphysema. (Reproduced by permission from Teplick, J. and Haskin, M.: Roentgenologic Diagnosis, 3rd ed. Philadelphia, W. B. Saunders Co., 1976.)

The most common cause of tracheal deviation is chest rotation. Pathologic deviation may be due to a large tumor pushing the trachea to one side, or it may be due to a mediastinal shift—a large right pneumothorax pushes the trachea to the left, or a collapsed right lung pulls the trachea to the right (Fig. 15–19).

Normally, the radiolucency of the trachea below the clavicles and the beginning of the right and left main bronchi are visible on the frontal view. On some films, however, these structures are invisible—they are lost in the radiopacity of superimposed mediastinal structures, especially if these films are underpenetrated.

To identify indistinct airways, the clinician views at a distance of 6 ft, to locate the carina and to trace the outside margins of the bronchi. Location of the carina is particularly important if the patient has an endotracheal tube in place. Proper tube placement in the trachea is determined by noting the distance of the tube's tip from the carina. The tip should rest 5 cm (± 2 cm) above the carina with the head in the neutral position.

BONY THORAX

The clinician notes the general size, shape, and symmetry of the chest cage or bony thorax on the frontal view. The size of the chest cage indicates general body build (e.g., small, medium, and large). Asymmetry or abnormal shape indicates the presence

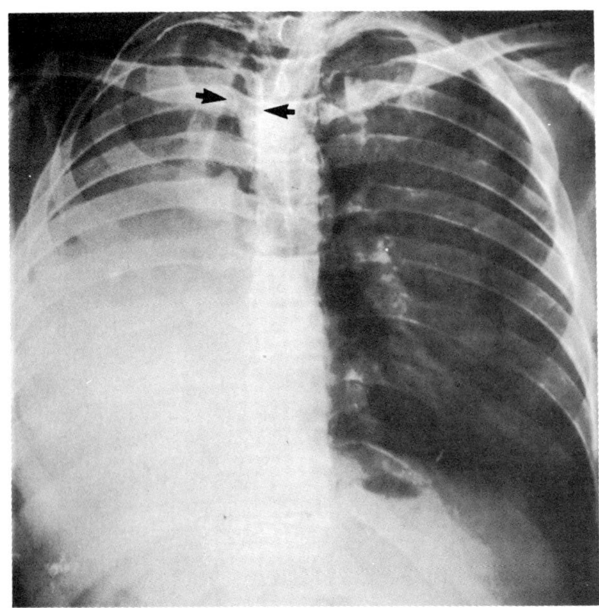

Figure 15–19. Tracheal deviation and mediastinal shift to the right due to collapse of the entire right lung. The lung collapse was from a fractured right bronchus. The arrows identify the tracheal borders. (Reproduced by permission from Felson, B. et al: Principles of Chest Roentgenology. Philadelphia, W. B. Saunders Co., 1965.)

of a chest wall deformity or an abnormal chest configuration. Some abnormal chest configurations are readily visible on the frontal view e.g., scoliosis. Others, such as increased AP diameter, funnel chest, and pigeon chest, are best appreciated on lateral views.

The clinician looks more carefully at the scapulae, clavicles, ribs, humeri, and thoracic spines (Fig. 15–20).

Humerus

The head of the humerus articulates with the scapula. It may not be clearly visible on the routine PA view because its image is mixed with the radiopacity of other shoulder bones. In the case of a large body build, it is not present on the film because the large chest cage takes up all the space.

Scapulae

The triangular-shaped scapulae are relatively easy to identify. On the PA film, the medial aspect is lateral and outside the lung fields, since the arms are positioned above the head. However, on the AP view, the medial aspect appears radiographically as a vertical or an oblique line within the lung field. This line may be mistaken for a lung marking.

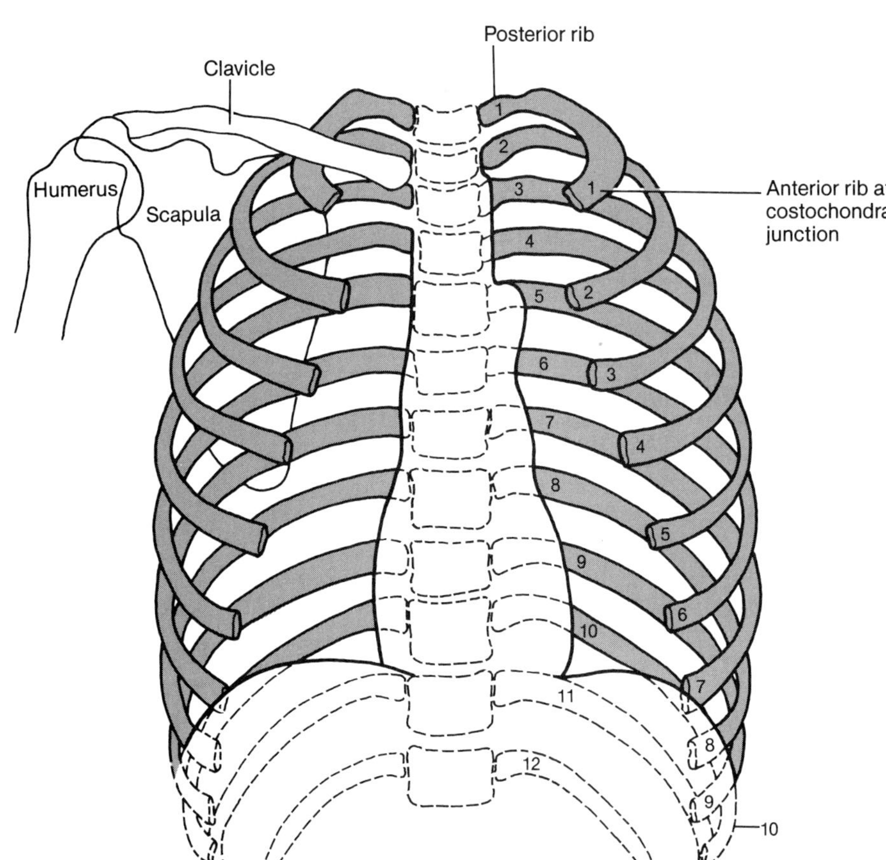

Figure 15–20. The bony thorax. Ribs that are readily viewed on the chest film are shaded gray. On the anteroposterior (AP) film, the medial and inferior borders of the scapula may be viewed within the field as shown.

Clavicles

The clavicles should appear symmetric and similar to those shown in Figure 15–3. Asymmetry indicates abnormality or presence of chest rotation, except in a few cases. For example, an irregular notch or indentation in the inferior medial aspect of the clavicle is a normal finding. The indentation is called a *rhomboid fossa* (Fig. 15–21A). Also, the clavicles may have a *companion shadow*, 2- to 3-mm fat density shadow parallel to the superior aspect (Fig. 15–21B). Absence of a shadow on one side may be normal, or it may suggest supraclavicular lymph node enlargement or some other process, if other abnormalities are present.

Spine

The thoracic spine is straight on the frontal view and gently convex posteriorly on the lateral view. Scoliosis is best demonstrated on the frontal view, whereas kyphosis is best demonstrated on the lateral view.

On the lateral view, the roentgenographic density of the spine decreases uniformly from top to bottom.

Decreased density of the spine, ribs, and other bones represents the loss of calcium from bones, as occurs in various bone diseases and long term steroid dependency.

Ribs

Count the posterior aspects of the thoracic ribs to determine whether the film is a normal or poor inspiratory film. A *normal inspiratory film* is one in which *nine to ten ribs* are visible on the frontal projection. The clinician counts the posterior rather than anterior aspect of the ribs, as shown in Figure 15–20. The last rib counted should touch or lie proximal to the lateral aspect of the diaphragm. An *expiratory* or *poor inspiratory film* is one in which *eight ribs or less* are visible.

During this examination, trace the course of each rib from the spine and the rib's posterior aspect, along its lateral curvature, as far as possible anteriorly.

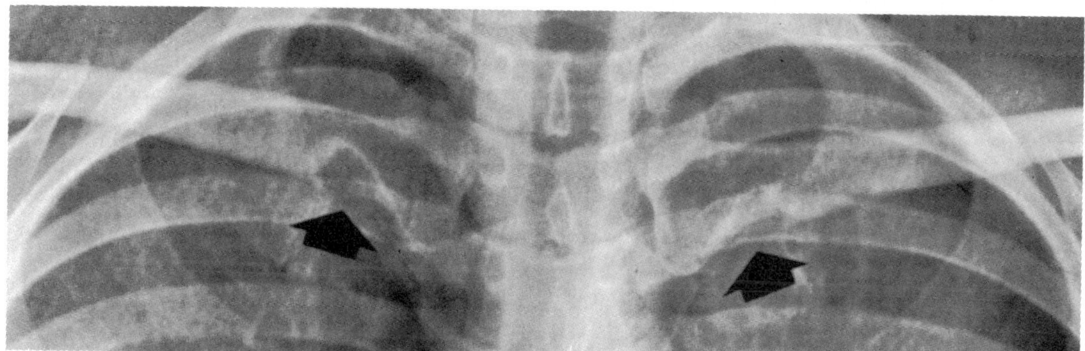

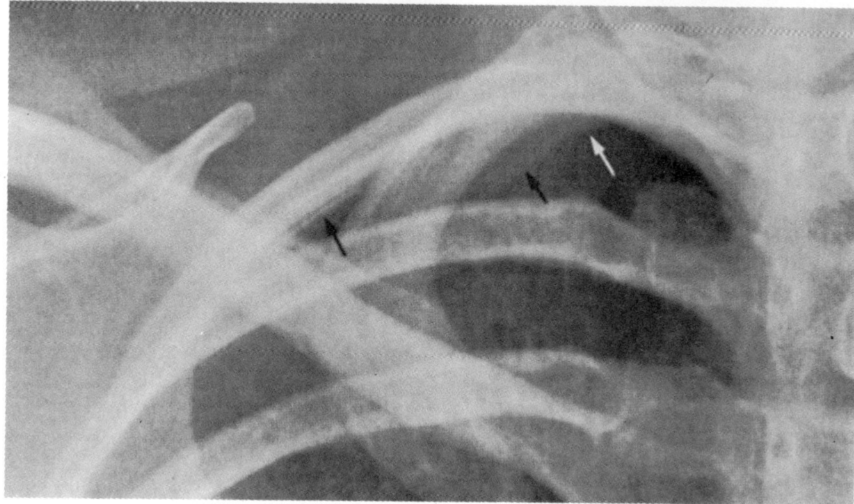

Figure 15–21. Normal clavicles. *A*, Rhomboid fossae. An irregular notch or indentation is present in the inferior aspect of both clavicles about 2 cm from their sternal end (arrows). These fossae give origin to the costoclavicular or rhomboid ligaments. *B*, Companion shadows. The clavicle may have a companion shadow parallel to its superior aspect. In addition, companion shadows are present parallel to the inferior surfaces of the first and second ribs (arrows). These companion shadows are caused by visualization in tangential projection of a combination of parietal pleura and soft tissues immediately external to the pleura. (Reproduced by permission from Fraser, R. and Paré, J.: Diagnosis of Diseases of the Chest. 2nd ed. Philadelphia, W. B. Saunders Co., 1977.)

Compare ribs on one side of the chest with ribs on the other side, noting asymmetry or areas of increased or decreased density. Keep the following points in mind:

1. In young adults, anterior aspects of the ribs become invisible before they join the sternum, as bone turns into costal cartilage. In the elderly, the anterior aspects may be clearly visible, owing to bone ossification associated with the aging process.

2. Fractured ribs commonly occur in the lateral chest area (Fig. 15–22). Carefully check the lateral curvature of each rib for discontinuities.

3. Unilateral or, more commonly, bilateral cervical

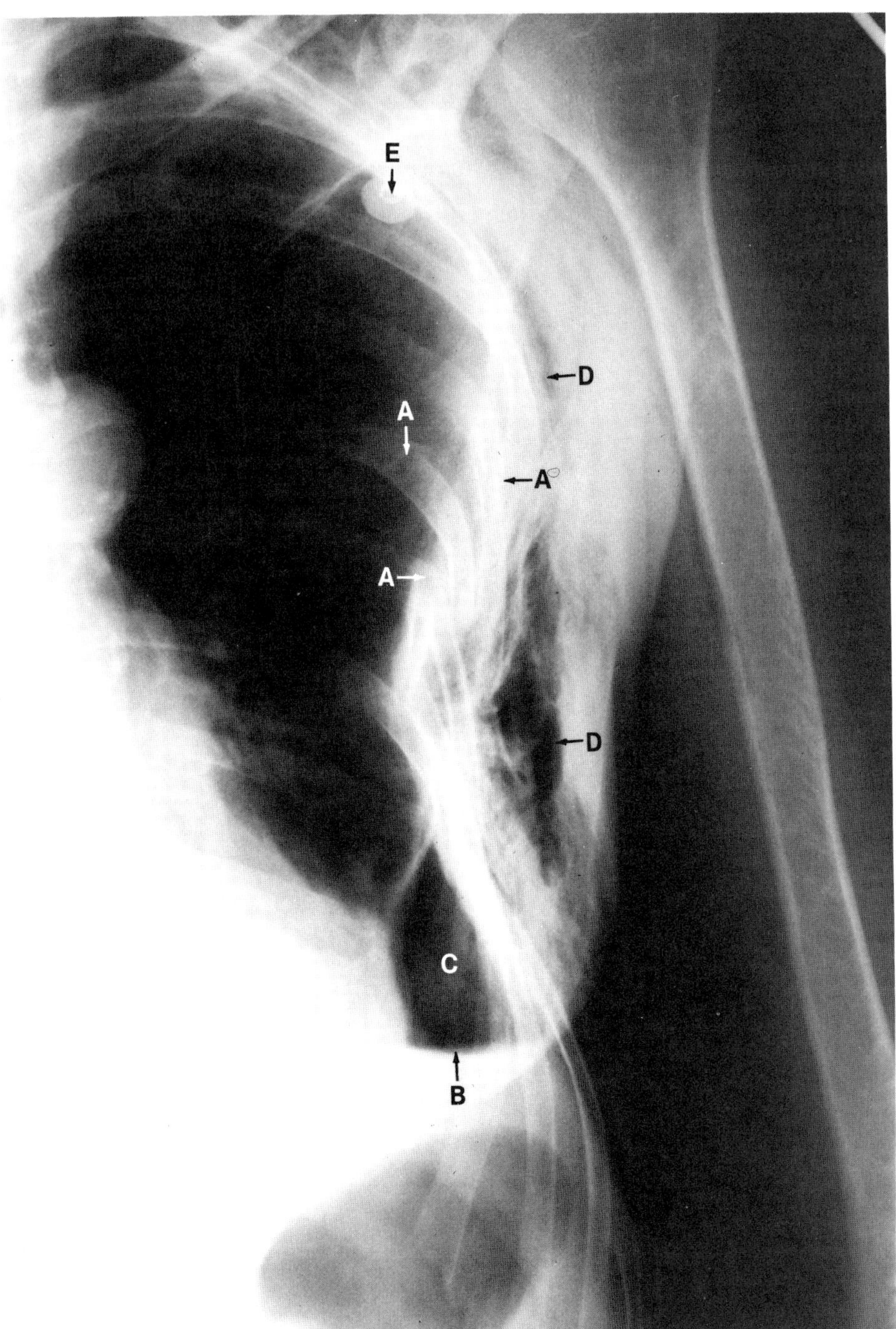

Figure 15–22. Multiple rib fractures with associated hemopneumothorax. A = rib fractures; B = gas fluid level (note a gas fluid level associated with acute trauma indicates hemopneumothorax); C = pneumothorax; D = subcutaneous emphysema; E = metal density of an ECG electrode (artifact). (Reproduced by permission from Levy, R., Hawkins, H., and Barsan, W.: Radiology in Emergency Medicine. St. Louis, The C. V. Mosby Co., 1986.)

ribs arising from the seventh cervical vertebra (above T1) are occasionally found in normal individuals.

4. Companion shadows normally may be found parallel to the inferior and inferolateral margins of the first and second ribs and along the axillary portions of the lower ribs. These shadows are formed by the tangential radiographing of parietal pleura and more superficial soft tissues.

5. Absence of a rib usually indicates a past thoracotomy procedure.

6. Watch for *rib notching,* defined as localized indentations along the surface of a rib. As a normal finding, it usually is mild and occurs along the inferior border of the medial half (posterior aspects) of one or more ribs. Pathologic rib notching is more marked, more extensive, and more lateral, near the midclavicular line (Fig. 15–23). It is most commonly due to dilated and tortuous intercostal arteries from coarctation of the aorta.

INTERCOSTAL SPACES (ICSs)

Similar to the physical examination, the intercostal spaces (ICSs) are numbered according to the rib above, e.g., the sixth ICS lies below the sixth rib. Both ribs and ICSs help the interpreter describe the location of lesions or other abnormalities on the chest film (e.g., 2 cm in diameter water density lesion noted sixth ICS, mid-clavicular line (MCL).

The clinician examines intercostal width in a systematic fashion, viewing each hemithorax from top to bottom and then both together, noting any increase or decrease in ICS width. The best way to become familiar with normal ICS width is to study normal chest x-rays.

Widened intercostal spaces occur in conditions that increase lung or thoracic volume, such as chronic obstructive pulmonary disease (COPD), large pneumothorax, and large pleural effusion. With severe lung hyperinflation, the *costovertebral angle,* i.e., the angle of the ribs to the spine, is increased to 90 degrees. The normal angle is about 45 degrees (Fig. 15–24).

Narrowed intercostal spaces are found in conditions that decrease lung volume, e.g., atelectasis and severe interstitial fibrosis.

DIAPHRAGM AND AREA BELOW THE DIAPHRAGM

Diaphragm

Each hemidiaphragm is water density and dome-shaped with distinct margins (Fig. 15–25). The right hemidiaphragm is normally 1 to 3 cm above the left hemidiaphragm, owing to the inferiorly located liver on the right side.

Slight alterations in shape are normal. However, alterations due to diaphragmatic elevation, depression, or abrupt interruptions in contour are always abnormal. *Abrupt interruptions* may be from penetrating wounds of the abdomen or hiatus hernia, as the stomach penetrates the mediastinal cavity.

Diaphragmatic elevation may be present when fewer than nine to ten ribs show, using the lateral aspect of the diaphragm as a reference point. Also, elevation of the diaphragm is present when some alteration in the 1- to 3-cm difference in hemidiaphragmatic levels appears or when the convex curvature appears accentuated. Elevation may be due to abdominal or stomach distention, phrenic nerve paralysis, or lung collapse (Fig. 15–26).

Diaphragmatic depression is present when 11 to 12 thoracic ribs are visualized on the frontal view. It is most common in emphysematous individuals from

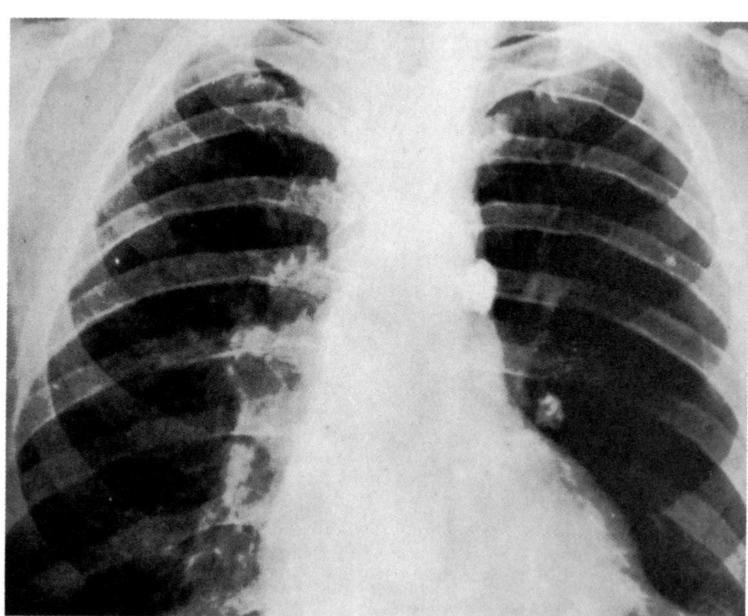

Figure 15–23. Rib notching due to coarctation of the aorta. The notching or scalloping is seen along the inferior medial aspects of the ribs. (Reproduced by permission from Felson, B. et al: Principles of Chest Roentgenology. Philadelphia, W. B. Saunders Co., 1965.)

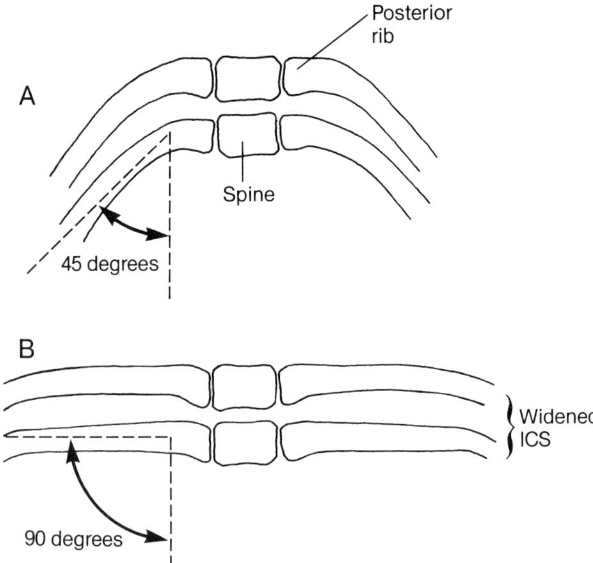

Figure 15–24. Costovertebral angle and intercostal space (ICS) width. *A*, Normal compared with *B*, lung hyperinflation.

severe air trapping; however, this finding alone is unreliable because some normal individuals may demonstrate diaphragmatic depression to the level of the eleventh rib. The most reliable chest x-ray sign of lung hyperinflation is the *flattening* of the diaphragmatic domes. In adults, severe diaphragmatic depression with bilateral concave hemidiaphragms is a sure sign of emphysema (Fraser and Paré, 1979).

Area Below the Diaphragm

The area below the diaphragm remains water density, except for the air density of the gastric bubble just below the left hemidiaphragm. This bubble represents air in the stomach. It frequently is observed with a *fluid level*, also called an *air-fluid level*, defined as *the horizontal interface between fluid and air* (see Fig. 15–25). The top margin of the gastric bubble normally lies within 1 to 2 cm of the dome of the left hemidiaphragm. The bubble may be barely visible or invisible, owing to low position in the stomach, inadequate penetration of the film, improper patient positioning and stomach decompression from nasogastric suction. In the last case, a thin radiopaque line (i.e., nasogastric tube) descends down the center of the chest and into the stomach.

PLEURAL SURFACES

The visceral and parietal pleurae appear intermittently as a thin hair-like line along the apices and lateral area of the chest, where the x-ray beam penetrates several millimeters of pleurae (Fig. 15–27). When present and not obscured by the superimposition of the lateral ribs, it remains the same thickness along all lung surfaces.

Pleural thickening from scarred tissue is present where the pleural line becomes thicker than normal (Fig. 15–28) or where the lateral chest wall or superior apical margins appear thicker compared with the opposite side of the chest.

A pneumothorax is present when the pleural line (i.e., visceral pleura) deviates medially away from the chest wall and is seen within the lung fields. The area peripheral to the line is more radiolucent or absolutely black because the pleural space is filled with air instead of lung tissue. The area medial to the pleural line contains the collapsed lung. The more extensive the lung collapse, the more radiopaque the lung's image.

Costophrenic and Cardiophrenic Angles

The lateral hemidiaphragms curve downward to form *lateral costophrenic angles* with the chest wall (Fig. 15–28A). Both right and left angles form a distinct point inferiorly. They appear to be about the same size and depth. Hemidiaphragms are clearly visible in males; they may be hazy or obscure in females owing to overlying breast tissue.

The medial aspects of the hemidiaphragms curve downward to form *cardiophrenic angles* with the heart borders, as shown in Figure 15–27.

On the lateral view, the diaphragm curves backward to form the *posterior costophrenic angle* and forward to form the *anterior costophrenic angle* by the heart.

Figure 15–27 also demonstrates a few basic anatomic relationships that help the clinician understand find-

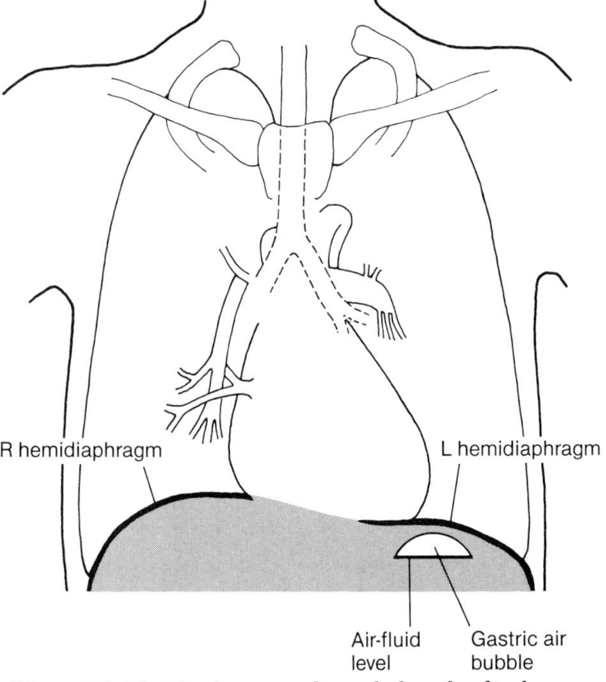

Figure 15–25. Diaphragm and area below the diaphragm.

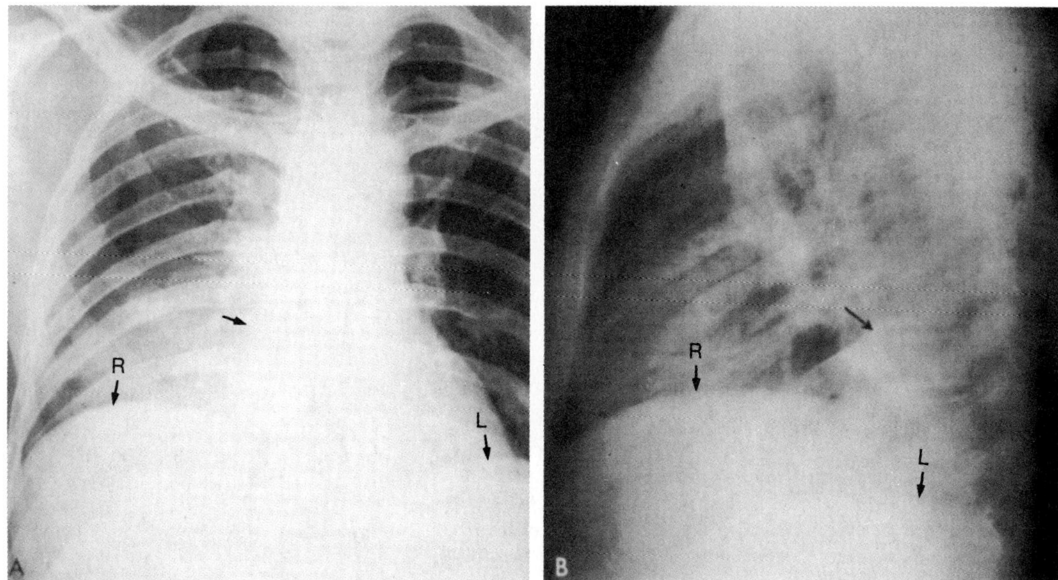

Figure 15–26. Postoperative collapse of the right lower lobe. *A*, The frontal view shows preservation of the right heart border (arrow) and elevation of the right hemidiaphragm (R). *B*, The right lateral view shows backward displacement of the major fissure, which becomes lost at the level of the arrow. The right hemidiaphragm (R) is elevated far above the left hemidiaphragm (L). (Reproduced by permission from Felson, B.: Chest Roentgenology. Philadelphia, W. B. Saunders, 1973.)

ings that involve the diaphragmatic and costophrenic angles.

1. On the frontal view, the domes, i.e., the uppermost part, of the hemidiaphragms lie in the posterior chest, not the anterior chest area.

2. The inferior border of the diaphragm and pleural cavity lies well *below* the dome and lateral angles (see Fig. 1–5).

3. The posterior costophrenic angle is deeper than all the other angles. When a small amount of fluid is present here, it is not visible or only partially visible on the frontal projection, because structures below the dome are radiopaque.

A *dulled* (shallow) or *obliterated* angle suggests pleural thickening, if the change occurred over several months or years (Fig. 15–28B). It suggests an acute process, such as atelectasis, pneumonia, and pleural effusion, if changes are recent.

The presence of a horizontal *fluid level* indicates pleural effusion. However, if fluid freely moves around

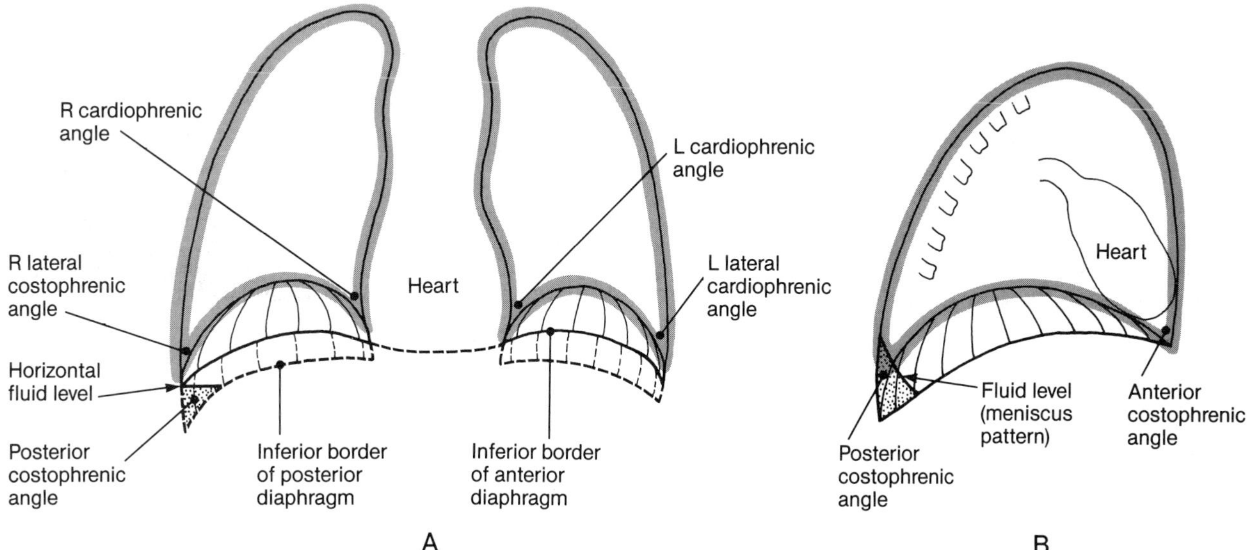

Figure 15–27. Costophrenic and cardiophrenic angles. Frontal *(A)* and right lateral *(B)* views. The dots represent fluid in the posterior costophrenic angle. The gray outline represents lung surfaces where pleura (thin black line) may be seen on the normal chest x-ray.

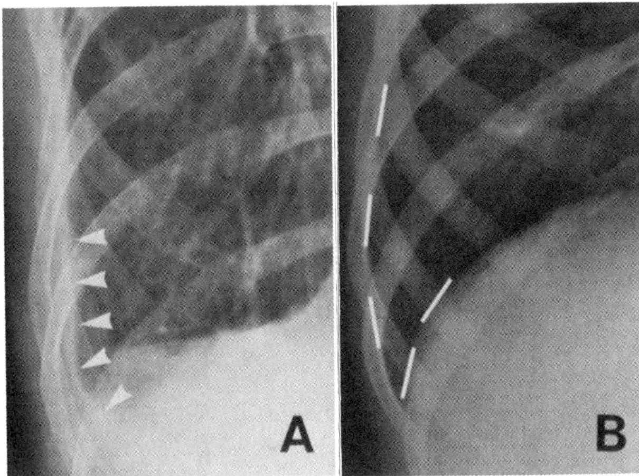

Figure 15–28. Normal and abnormal pleurae. In *A*, pleural thickening causes a dulled angle. In *B*, the dotted lines along normal pleura form a clear lateral costophrenic angle. (From Eastman Kodak Company, *Medicine Radiography and Photography*, 23:54–56, 1952.)

the pleural space, the shape of the fluid level may form a *meniscus* or crescent-shaped pattern, with the lateral concave border rising higher than the medial concave border, as shown in Fig. 15–27B. Moreover, if pleural adhesions restrict the movement of fluid within the pleural space, the fluid may become loculated in one place, forming a *pseudotumor*, a water density shape, resembling a lesion or tumor.

In congestive heart failure, pleural effusions are common. They are almost always on the right side. If they are bilateral, the right effusion is typically larger than the left effusion (Felson, 1965).

Interlobar Fissure

The term *interlobar fissure* refers to a thin radiopaque line that marks contact surfaces between pulmonary lobes. It is sometimes more correctly referred to as an *interlobar septum*. Technically, the x-ray beam radiographs the *septum*, defined as a divider formed by two adjacent visceral surfaces, and not the *fissure*, the potential space in between the surfaces. However, the terms are used interchangeably in the clinical setting.

The clinician checks the frontal and lateral views for the presence and proper positioning of minor and major fissures.

The *minor fissure*, also called the *horizontal fissure*, separates the right middle lobe from the right upper lobe. It is visible on the frontal view at about the level of the fourth rib, but it can intersect the lateral chest area anywhere between the anterior aspects of the second to sixth ribs (Fig. 15–29A).

Two *major fissures*, also called *oblique fissures*, separate the upper and right middle lobes from the more posteriorly located lower lobes. Depending on the angle of the x-ray beam, they are seen on the lateral view as one or two parallel radiopaque lines running obliquely downward from T4 or T5 to just behind the anterior costophrenic angle (Fig. 15–29B).

Both minor and major fissures may be absent or visualized only intermittently along their long axes. Several factors account for visualization difficulties. First, a fissure is difficult to radiograph because it is

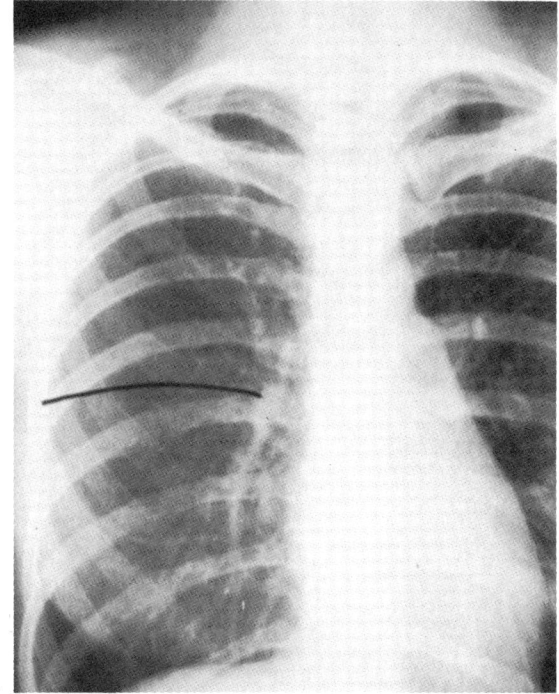

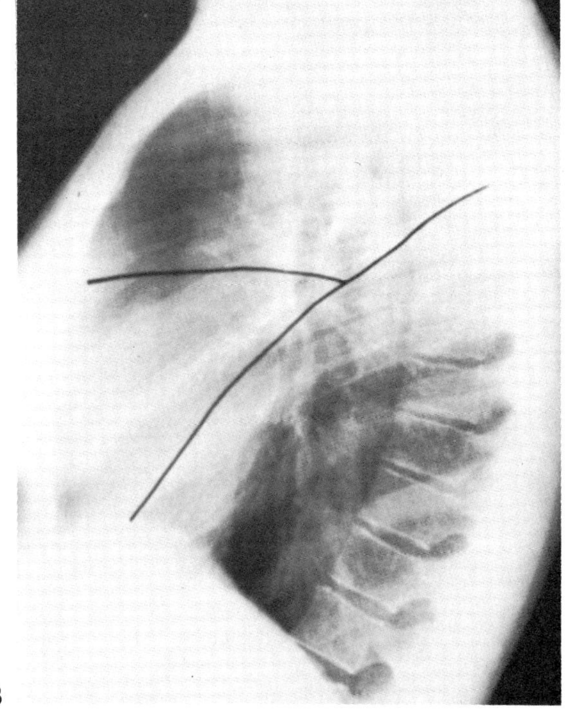

Figure 15–29. *A*, Minor horizontal and, *B*, major oblique fissures. (Reproduced by permission from Felson, B., Weinstein, A., and Spitz, H.: Principles of Chest Roentgenology. Philadelphia, W. B. Saunders Co., 1965.)

less than 1 to 2 mm thick, and the x-ray beam must strike exactly parallel to the fissure for it to show up on the film. Also, contrary to the straight lines presented in some basic textbooks to help identify lobar boundaries, fissures have an S-configuration of varying depth, as shown in Figure 15–30. Their curved surfaces and thinness decrease the likelihood of the beam striking parallel to the fissure. Moreover, though the minor fissure may be appreciated on both frontal and lateral projections, major fissures are not normally seen at all on the frontal view because anatomically, their long axes do not lie parallel to the x-ray beam, as shown in Figure 15–31. The beam strikes the fissures at an angle, and hence is not radiographed.

The two main fissure abnormalities seen on the chest film are as follows:

1. *Fissure displacement*—medially or laterally—upwards or downwards—indicates an increase or a decrease in lung volume. It is the most reliable sign of lung collapse from disorders such as atelectasis and pneumothorax. The direction of fissure displacement is towards the collapsed lung segment, or away from the hyperinflated lung or other compressing organs.
2. *Increased thickness* may be due to pleural thickening, pleural fluid, tumor, or pseudotumor (Fig. 15–32).

MEDIASTINUM

The borders of the mediastinum are outlined in Figure 15–33.

General Appearance

The size of the mediastinum normally varies—it may be short and wide in short, stocky persons and long and narrow in tall, thin persons. However, general shape should resemble that of the normal mediastinum in Figure 15–3.

Because of overlapping structures, the mediastinum is varying degrees of water density, except for the

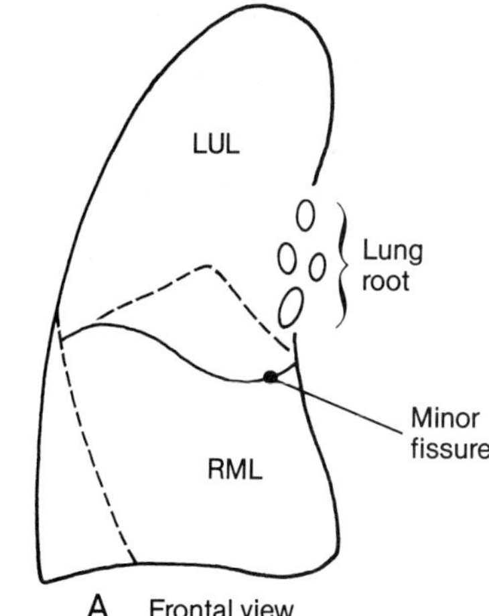

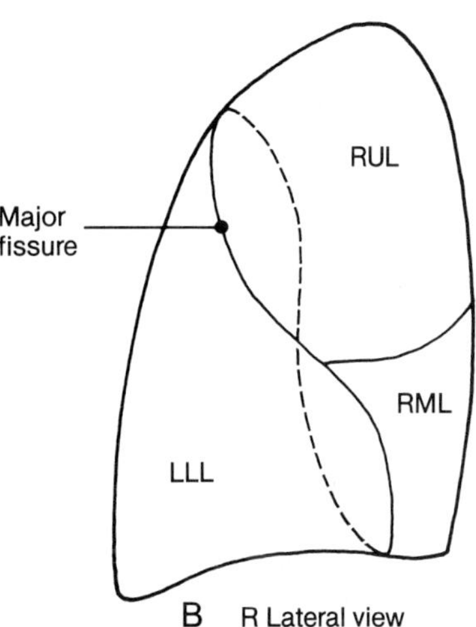

Figure 15–30. Anatomy of interlobar fissures. *A*, The minor fissure forms a shallow S-shaped curve. Its horizontal plane forms a triangle with the apex in the middle of the chest. *B*, Major fissures are also S shaped on their lateral borders. Their surfaces are shaped like an airplane propeller. They face forward and slightly outward in their top half and forward and slightly medial in their bottom half.

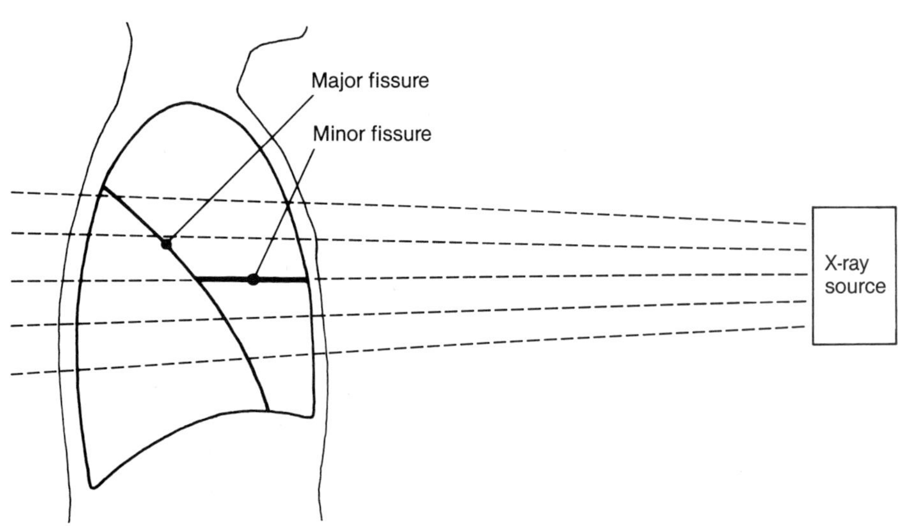

Figure 15–31. The radiography of fissures, frontal view. The minor fissure is demonstrated radiographically because it is parallel with the x-ray beam. The major fissure does not show up on the film because it lies at an angle to the x-ray beam.

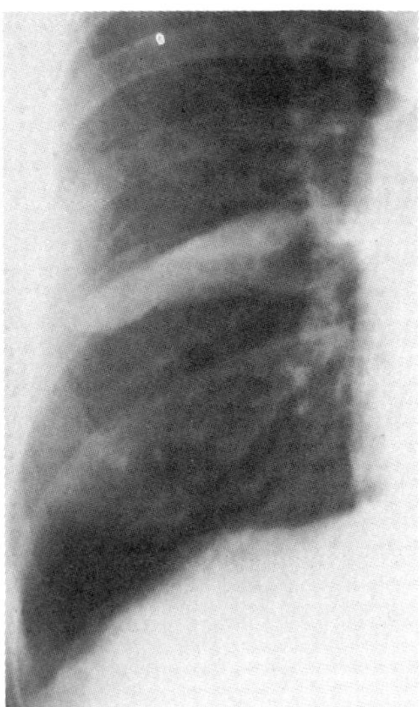

Figure 15–32. Interlobar pleural fluid. This sausage-like density in the minor fissure represents pleural fluid. Its interlobar location becomes more readily apparent on the lateral view (not shown). (Reproduced by permission from Teplick, J. and Haskin, M.: Roentgenologic Diagnosis, 3rd ed. Philadelphia, W. B. Saunders Co., 1976.)

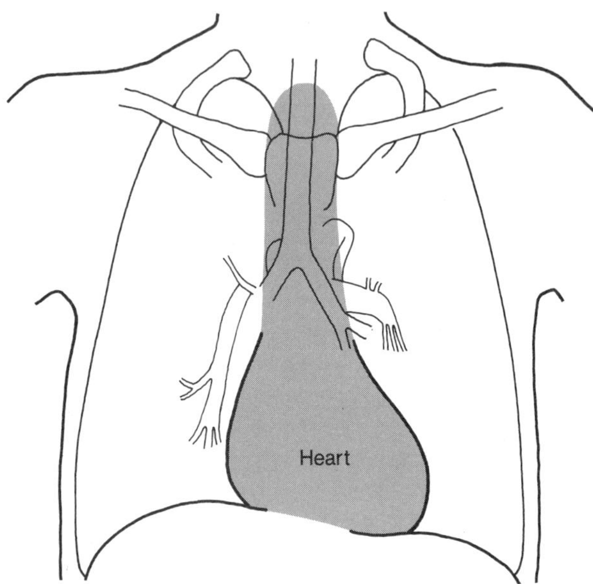

Figure 15–33. The mediastinum containing the heart is shaded gray.

radiolucent trachea and the right and left main bronchi when visible.

The heart's shadow spans the entire width of the mediastinum's base. It may be centrally located over the spine. In most cases, however, most of the heart lies in the left thorax, and only a small segment of right heart border—no more than one third the heart's transverse diameter—extends into the right thorax. In rare instances, the right heart border will exactly coincide with the spine.

While viewing the general appearance, the clinician checks for these specific abnormalities.

1. *Mediastinal widening* may indicate the presence

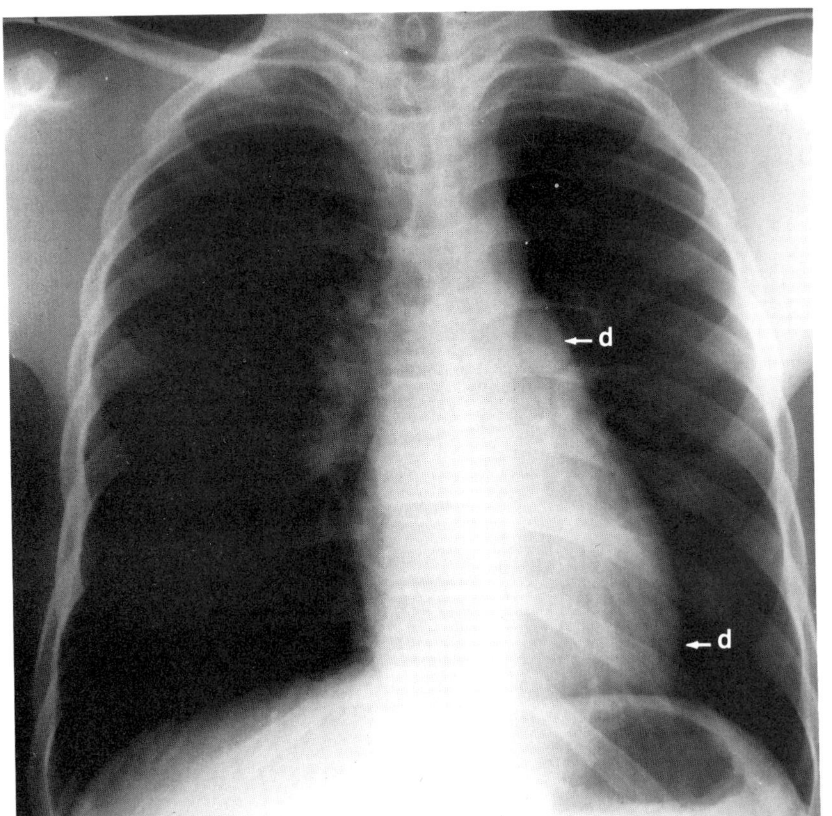

Figure 15–34. Foreign body aspiration. *Left*, PA view of the chest on inspiration. The mediastinum is in normal position (d). The foreign body is not seen because it is not radiopaque.

of tumor, enlarged lymph nodes, cardiomegaly, inflammation (e.g., mediastinitis), hemorrhage, or vascular aneurysms.

2. *Mediastinal shift* is present when the *trachea, aortic arch* (described subsequently), or *right heart border* shifts to the right or left (Fig. 15–34). Previous films may need to be viewed to detect change in position.

3. *Areas of gas density* or radiolucency may indicate the presence of a hernia that is esophageal in origin or a mediastinal abscess with a fluid level.

4. *Areas of metal density* may mark the location of surgical clips or sternal wires from past surgery, cardiac valves with metal parts, pacemaker wires, or electrocardiographic electrodes and wires. When an area of metal density cannot be accounted for by treatment modalities, it is most likely from *calcifications.* Mediastinal calcifications may occur within cysts or tumors or along aneurysms, dilated vessels, or tortuous aortas of aged individuals.

Mediastinal Profile

The *normal mediastinal profile,* frontal view, is shown in Figure 15–35A. Abnormality is present when any of the curves become distorted, blurred, or obliterated.

Study of the series of illustrations in Figure 15–35 will help you understand the anatomic basis for each curve in the mediastinal profile. The following list summarizes further important points:

1. The right atrium forms the right heart border and the lower right mediastinal profile (Fig. 15–35A and B).

2. The right ventricle is not visible on the frontal view because it is centrally located between right and left heart borders (see Fig. 15–35B).

3. The inferior vena cava (i.e., curve 4 in Fig. 15–35A) may not be visible, depending on body build, diaphragmatic level, and presence of a cardiac fat pad in the cardiophrenic angle. A *cardiac fat pad* is a thin layer of fat, lying along the inner surface of the parietal pericardium (see Fig. 15–35F).

4. The ascending aorta normally curves laterally and posteriorly before it descends in front of the spine (Fig. 15–35C). Here, the oblique radiographing of the aortic arch forms the *aortic arch* or *aortic knob* (curve 6) on the chest film (see Fig. 15–35A).

5. Below the aortic knob, curve 7 (see Fig. 15–35A) represents the main pulmonary artery just before it divides into right and left pulmonary arteries. This curve becomes more convex and prominent in pulmonary hypertension.

6. The right pulmonary artery lies posterior to the ascending aorta and anterior to the right bronchus (Fig. 15–35D). It is horizontal and always relatively lower than the left pulmonary artery. The left pulmonary artery passes immediately anterior to the left

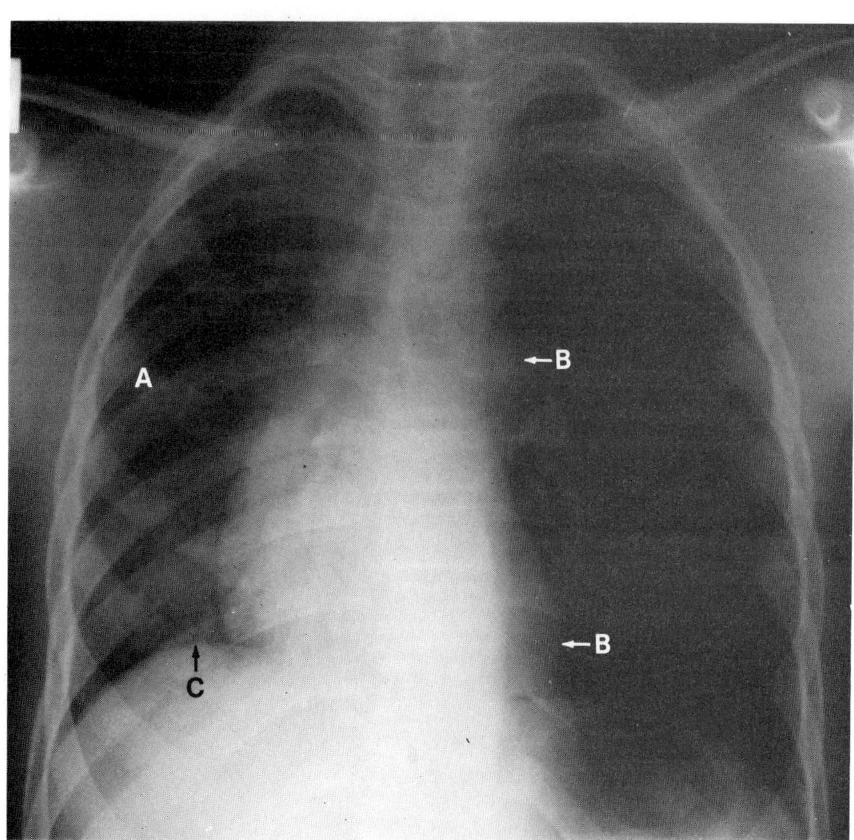

Figure 15–34 *Continued Right,* PA view of the chest on expiration. Note the asymmetric density of the lung fields (A). The left lung field is more radiolucent because the foreign body is acting as a check valve—air enters the left lung but is incompletely expelled owing to the obstruction. The mediastinum shifts to the right (B). Asymmetric hemidiaphragm elevation (C) occurs owing to the differential pulmonary aeration. (Reproduced by permission from Levy, R., Hawkins, H., and Barsan, W.: Radiology in Emergency Medicine. St. Louis, The C. V. Mosby Co., 1986.)

1. Superior vena cava
   a. as in a young adult
   b. as in the elderly
2. Ascending aorta
   a. as in a young adult
   b. as in the elderly
3. Right atrium
4. Inferior vena cava when visible
5. Left subclavian vein and artery; left common carotid artery
6. Aortic arch (knob)
7. Main pulmonary artery
8. Left atrium when visible
9. Left ventricle
10. Cardiac fat pad when present

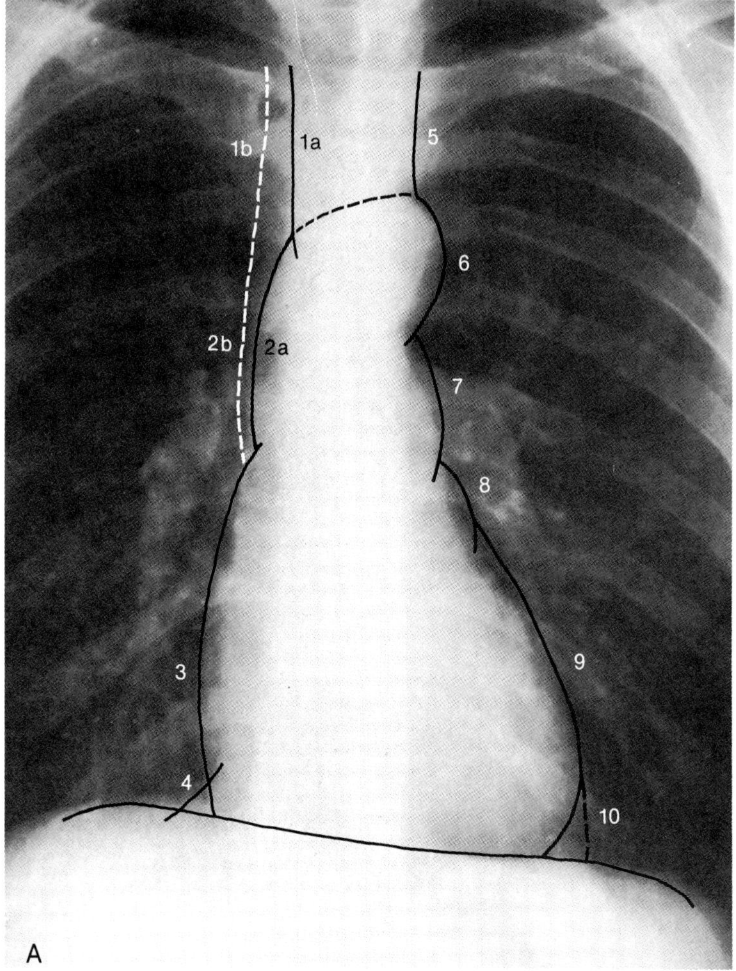

Figure 15–35. Anatomy of the mediastinal profile. *A*, Normal mediastinal profile, frontal view.

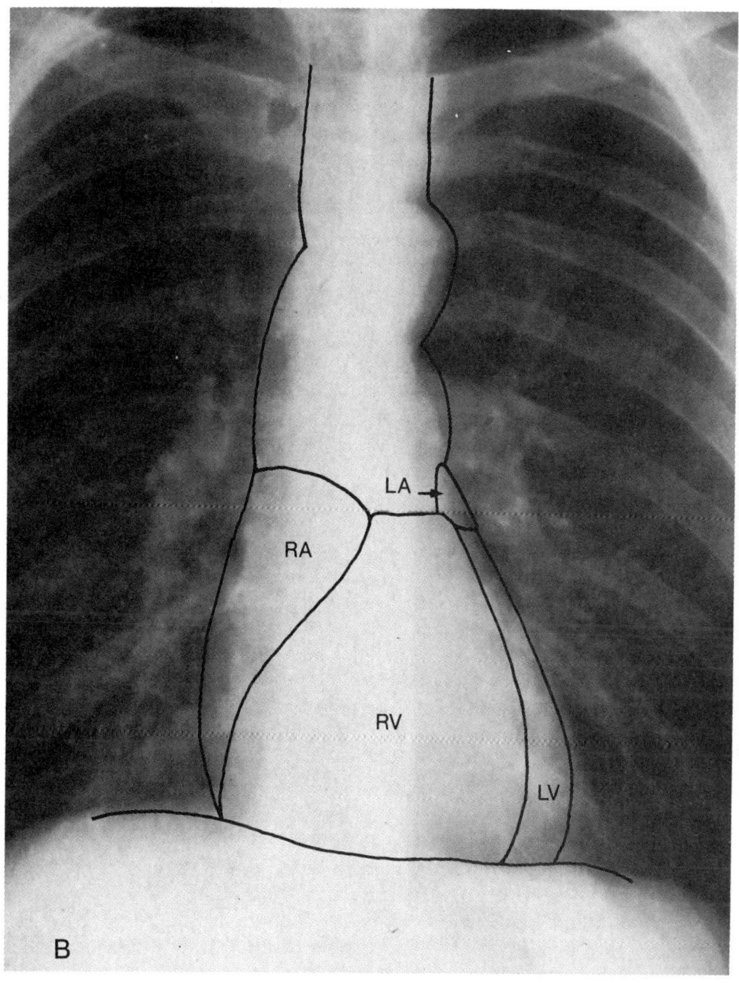

Figure 15–35 *Continued B*, Chambers of the heart, frontal view. (RA = right atrium; LA = left atrium; RV = right ventricle; LV = left ventricle.)

Illustration continued on following page

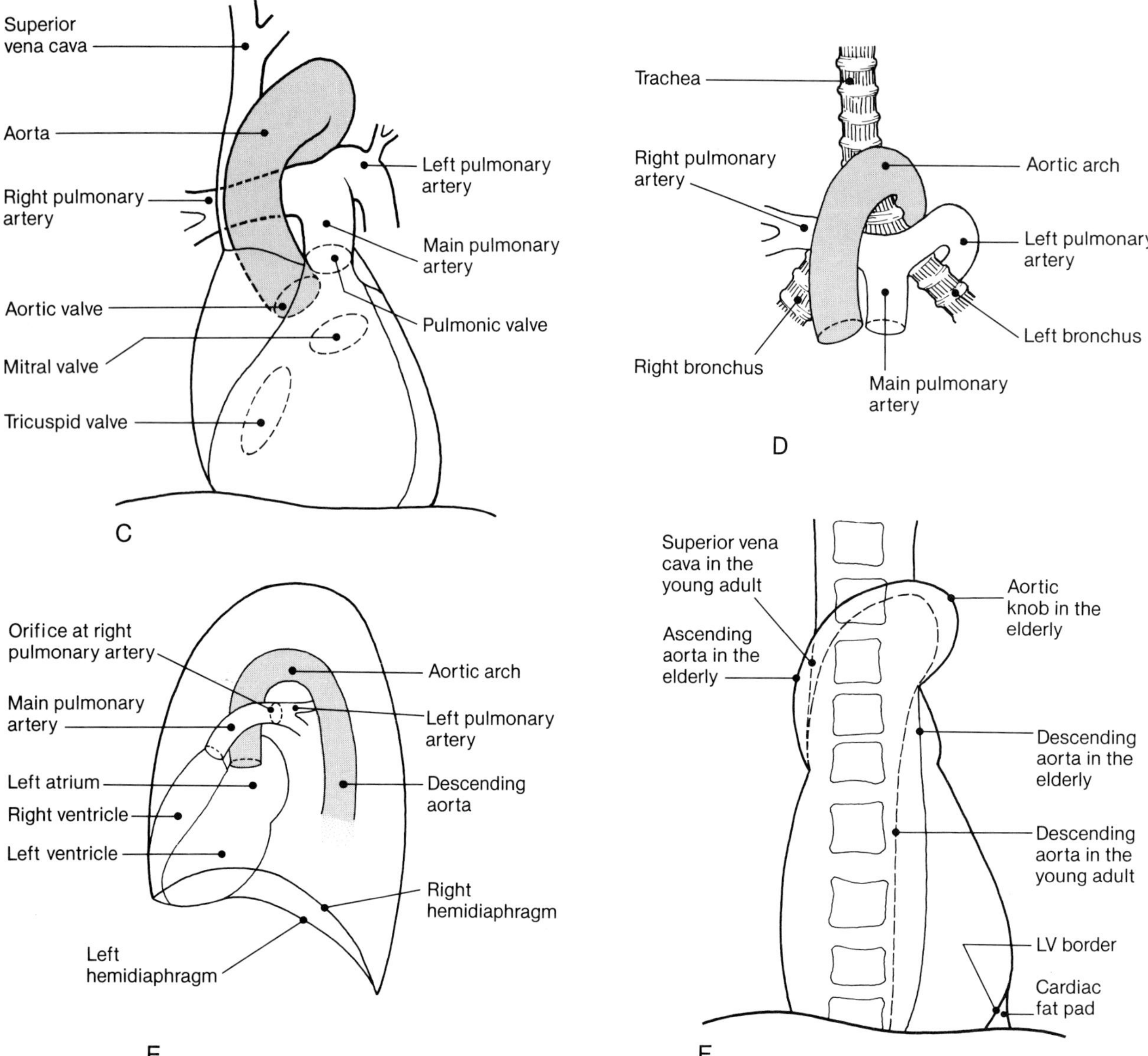

Figure 15–35 *Continued C*, Heart, great vessels, and cardiac valves, frontal view. The aorta is shaded gray to help differentiate vessels. *D*, Anatomic relationship among pulmonary arteries, aorta, and tracheobronchial tree. *E*, Heart and great vessels, left lateral view. Different sections of the aorta (gray) serve as important anatomic landmarks. *F*, Descending aorta and cardiac fat pad. The pad is seen through the normal heart shadow.

bronchus and then curves sharply upward and backward toward the posterior chest area. Its anteroposterior orientation shows up on the film in the lateral view (Fig. 15–35E).

7. The left atrium and left ventricle form the left heart border. Although the atrial curve (curve 8) (see Fig. 15–35A) is convex for illustrative purposes, it is usually flat and indistinguishable from the left ventricular border. In an individual with a barrel chest, it is not part of the mediastinal profile because the atrial chamber is rotated more posteriorly. A convex curve indicates congenital enlargement of the atrial appendage, herniation of the appendage through a pericardial defect, or atrial enlargement from cardiopulmonary disease.

8. The left ventricular border normally becomes convex, forming an apex before meeting the diaphragm (see Fig. 15–35A). It may meet the diaphragm more laterally if a cardiac fat pad is present in the cardiophrenic angle. Cardiac fat pads are more common on the left rather than the right side of the heart, and they commonly may be absent.

9. Age alters the normal mediastinal silhouette. In the elderly, the aorta unfolds, thus altering the position of the ascending aorta, aortic knob, and descending aorta, as shown in Figure 15–35F. In the young adult, the superior vena cava forms the upper right mediastinal profile, and the descending aorta cannot be seen behind the heart, when it descends exactly in front of the spine.

Heart Size

To assess overall heart size, the clinician determines the *cardiothoracic (C-T) ratio,* defined as *the widest heart diameter compared with the widest thoracic diameter,* or AB compared with CD in Figure 15–36. In adults, normal C-T ratio is less than 1:2.

The radiologist more thoroughly evaluates heart size using a ruler to measure distances, by studying serial or oblique films, and by using nomograms based on height, weight, and body surface area to determine normal versus enlarged heart chambers.

When cardiomegaly is present, the clinician checks for signs of right and left ventricular enlargement. In *right ventricular enlargement* (e.g., from right ventricular (RV) hypertrophy and cor pulmonale), the enlarged right ventricle pushes the right atrium outward, increasing the convexity of the right heart border. The pulmonary arteries enlarge, and the profile of the main pulmonary artery appears more convex. On the lateral view, the right ventricle becomes more convex anteriorly, and it appears to "climb" upward along the sternum as it enlarges, encroaching on the retrosternal air space.

In *left ventricular enlargement,* from left ventricular hypertrophy, dilatation, or both, the left heart border sags—its contour becomes more rounded and distended in the apical area. The left heart border extends more to the left, and the left diaphragm may be depressed. If the increased convexity lies above the apex of the left cardiac profile, it is due to *right* not left ventricular enlargement. On the lateral view, the left ventricle enlarges posteriorly into the retrocardiac space and downward into the left diaphragm. Its border is convex. In severe cases, the ventricle completely fills the retrocardiac space and eliminates it.

Locating Mediastinal Lesions

An area of increased or decreased density may represent a mediastinal lesion. Lesions and other abnormalities within the mediastinum are localized by compartment to facilitate description and to aid in medical diagnosis. Most lesions tend to occur in a specific mediastinal compartment, as shown in Table 15–2.

The boundaries for mediastinal compartments on the chest x-ray differ from those based strictly on anatomic dissection (see Chapter 1). Felson (1973) divides the mediastinum into anterior, middle, and posterior compartments, as shown in Figure 15–37.

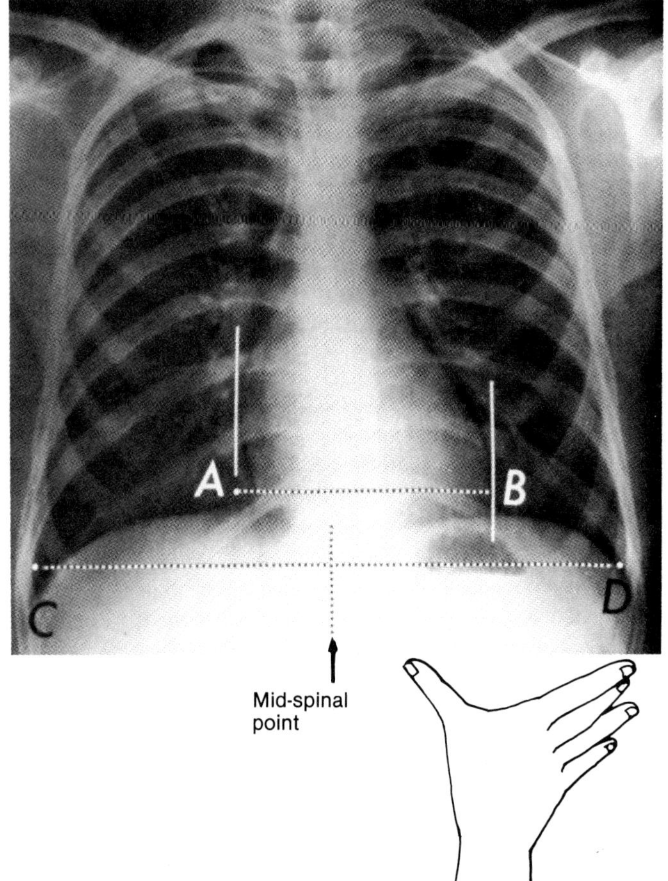

Figure 15–36. Determination of cardiothoracic ratio. For a quick assessment, the clinician may use the hand to compare segment AB with segment MD (Mid-spiral point to D). Heart enlargement is *not* present in this chest x-ray because AB is less than MD. The C-T ratio is less than 1:2 (normal). (Adapted courtesy of Eastman Kodak Company and Dr. H. Forsyth, Jr., Rochester, New York.)

Table 15–2. MEDIASTINAL LESIONS BY MEDIASTINAL COMPARTMENT*

Anterior	Middle	Posterior
Thyroid enlargement and tumor	Thyroid enlargement and tumor	Neurogenic tumors neurilemmoma neurofibroma ganglioneuroma Schwann's cell tumor
Teratoma	Tracheal tumor	Paraspinal lesions
Thymoma†	Bronchogenic or pericardial cysts	Bone and cartilage tumors
Thymic cyst	Lymphadenopathy	Aneurysm or descending aorta
Lymphadenopathy	Lymphoma, metastatic cancer	Esophageal lesions
Lymphoma	Mediastinitis	
Enlargement of ascending aorta (aneurysm), pulmonary artery, or superior vena cava	Cardiomegaly	
	Hematomas	
	Vascular dilatation or aneurysm	
	Esophageal lesions	
	Hiatus hernia	

*Partial listing.

†Thymoma is a tumor orginating in the epithelial tissues of the thymus gland. It is seen in 15% of individuals with myasthenia gravis. About 50% of thymomas are malignant.

HILA

As described in Chapter 1, the hila form the root of the lungs at the level of T4 or T5. The *hila* or *hilar areas* are shaded gray in Figure 15–38. On the chest film, shadows within these areas consist mostly of large pulmonary arteries and upper lobe veins that extend outward from the mediastinal profile on either side of the heart. The main bronchi are invisible here, outside the mediastinum, because they are air density. Similarly, lymph nodes are present in hilar areas, but they are normally too small to produce an image on the film.

With distance viewing, the two hila appear symmetric and about the same size and density. The right hilar vessels may appear to extend out farther than those on the left, but this observation is largely because the left hilum is obscured by the heart's shadow.

Upon closer examination, the hila are relatively ill-defined, blotchy areas of varying radiopacity. The blotchiness is due to the different numbers and thicknesses of superimposed vessels in the hilar areas and the varying angles that the x-ray beam strikes each vessel.

Major vessels that leave the mediastinal profile are shown in Figure 15–3. The right pulmonary artery is not seen projecting outward from the profile because it lies entirely within the pericardial sac until it bifurcates. In contrast, the left pulmonary artery is usually observed projecting outward because it lies outside the pericardial sac.

To detect gross hilar abnormality, the clinician assesses hilar position, density, and size.

Position

The relative positions of right and left hila are important to note. Position refers to the horizontal level where the right or left main pulmonary artery leaves the mediastinal profile. In most normal individuals, the left hilum is a few centimeters higher than the right hilum (Fig. 15–39A). In rare cases, the two hila are at the same level. The reason for an anatomically higher left hila pertains to the superior-posterior course of the left pulmonary artery over the left main bronchus, as illustrated in Figure 15–35D.

Hilar displacement, elevation, or depression in the level of a hilum is the most important indirect sign of lung collapse (i.e., loss of lung volume). Hilar *elevation* is always present in upper lobe collapse, while *depression* is common in lower lobe collapse (Fig. 15–39B). Displacement is absent in RML or lingular collapse. In addition, hilar displacement toward the diseased lobe occurs in other restrictive processes, such as tuberculosis and interstitial fibrosis, where loss of volume is typical.

Density

Increased water density of one hilum compared with the other indicates abnormality in the hilum or lung anterior or posterior to it. The presence of *metal density* may represent calcifications in lymph nodes or tumors.

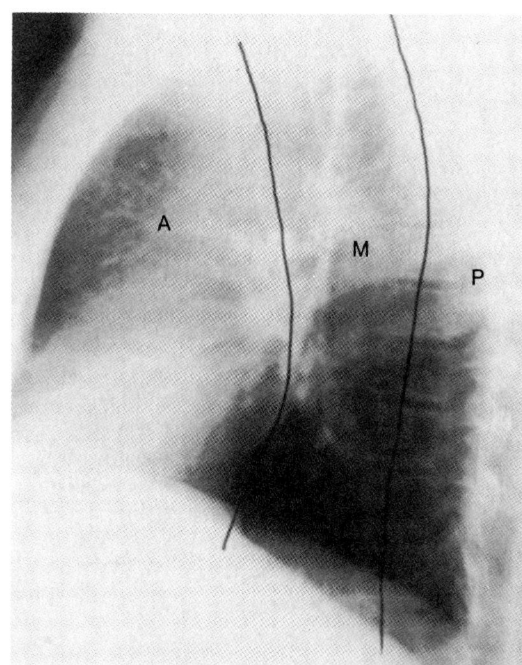

Figure 15–37. Mediastinal compartments on the lateral chest x-ray. The line between *anterior* (A) and *middle* (M) compartments extends along the anterior trachea and the posterior heart border. The line between the *middle* and *posterior* (P) compartments extends down the spine about 1 cm behind its anterior border. This posterior compartment includes the vertebral gutter or paravertebral zones, areas not included in the anatomic classification described in Chapter 1. (Reproduced by permission from Felson, B.: Chest Roentgenology. Philadelphia, W. B. Saunders Co., 1973.)

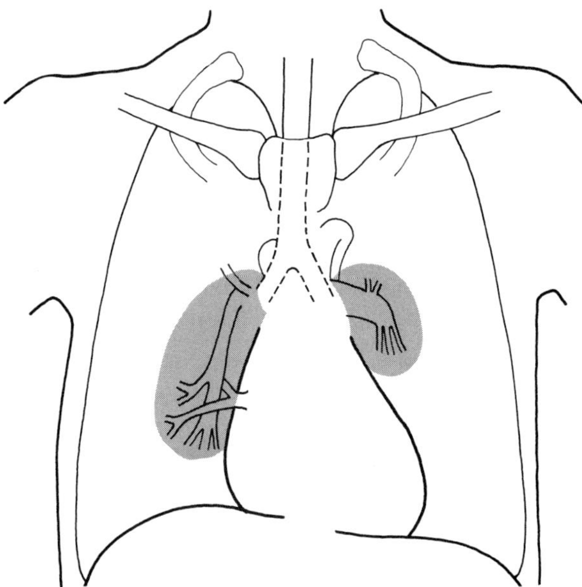

Figure 15–38. The hilar areas. The left hilum is slightly higher than the right hilum.

Size

Hila may be unilaterally or bilaterally *small* or *enlarged* (Fig. 8–18B). Associated disorders are listed in Table 15–3. In congestive heart failure, the hila enlarge; borders becomes indistinct, producing *hilar clouding*, as fluid moves out of the vascular space and into the interstitium.

Table 15–3. DISORDERS ASSOCIATED WITH SMALL AND ENLARGED HILA

Chest X-ray Finding	Unilateral	Bilateral
Small hilum	Congenital absence or hypoplasia of a pulmonary artery Pulmonary embolism Tumor Lobar collapse, with the hilum displaced behind the heart	Congenital heart disease tetralogy of Fallot tricuspid atresia truncus arteriosus transposition of the great vessels
Enlarged hilum	Lymphadenopathy Tumor Herniation of the pulmonary artery through a congenital pericardial defect Pulmonary embolism Vascular aneurysm Valvular pulmonary stenosis	Vascular dilatation from LV failure, cor pulmonale, congenital left to right cardiac shunts, mitral valve disease Pulmonary hypertension Lymphadenopathy Tumor

THE LUNG FIELDS—TOOLS FOR ASSESSMENT

The lung fields are the largest areas on the chest film and often the most impressive areas when gross pathology is present (Fig. 15–40).

Knowledge of lobar and segmental anatomy and the important radiologic silhouette sign is essential before learning how to view and assess lung fields.

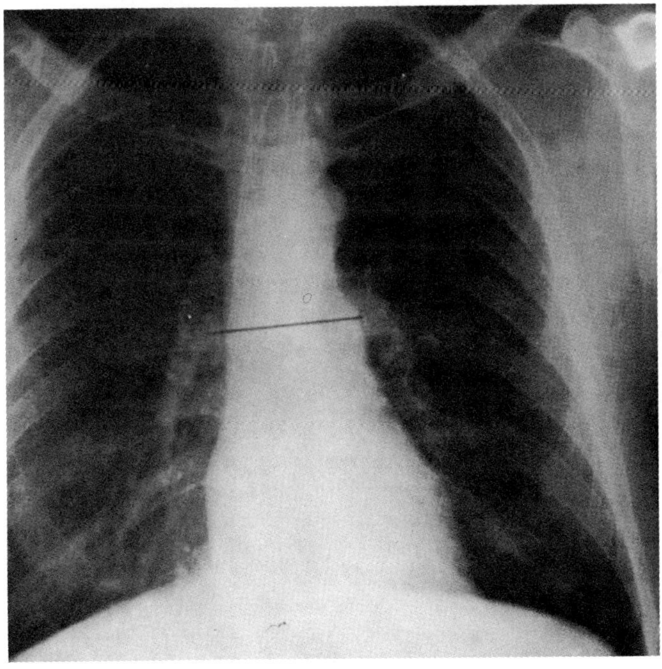

A

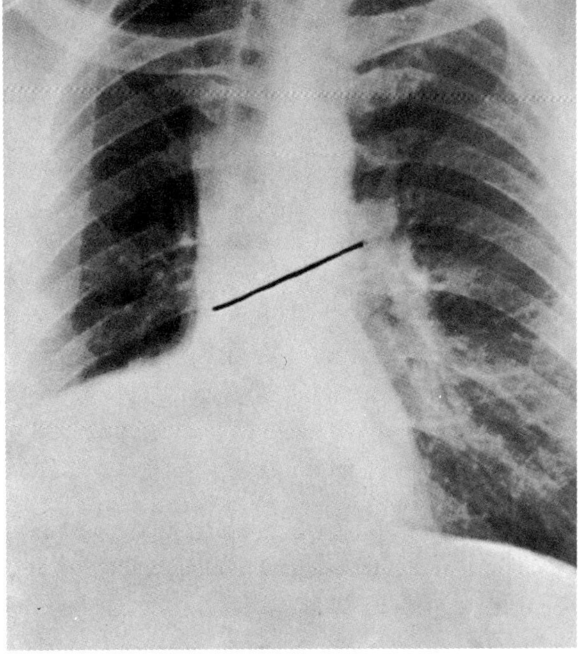

B

Figure 15–39. The position of the hila. *A*, The normal relationship of the hila (line) with the left hilum slightly higher than the right hilum. *B*, Downward and medial displacement of the right hilum in postoperative collapse of the right median lobe (RML) and right lower lobe (RLL). (Reproduced by permission from Felson, B. et al: Principles of Chest Roentgenology. Philadelphia, W. B. Saunders Co., 1965.)

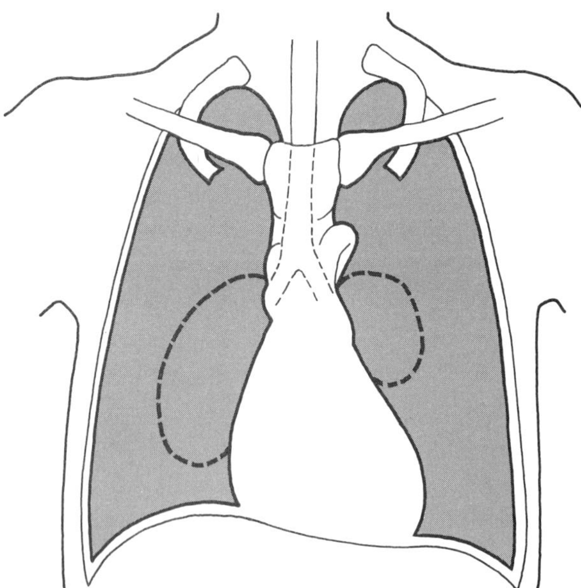

Figure 15–40. The lung fields. The heavy dotted lines mark the hilar borders.

Lobes and Segments on the Chest X-ray

The general boundaries of major lobes and segments of the lungs are shown in Figure 15–41. These boundaries represent approximations that may differ greatly among individuals, owing to normal variations in segments and fissures, chest rotation, and varying angles that the x-ray beam strikes the chest. The illustrations do not account for overlapping parts of lung, in some cases. The key lobes and segments illustrated serve as landmarks to help the beginning interpreter describe the location of densities within or near their boundaries. While studying the four chest x-rays presented, concentrate on the following relationships. (See Fig. 2–10B for a review of segmental anatomy.)

1. *The location of pulmonary lobes on the frontal view as compared with their location on the lateral view.* Which lobes are superimposed on each other on the lateral view?
2. *The location of lobes and segments in relation to the major and minor fissures.* Which lobes and segments lie immediately above and below each of these fissures?
3. *The location of lobes and segments in relation to the mediastinal profile,* frontal view. Noting the following relationships will help the reader understand the silhouette sign described next.
   a. The RML is in anatomic contact with the right heart border. On the other side of the chest, the lingular segments of the left upper lobe (LUL) are in contact with the left heart border.
   b. The anterior segment of the right upper lobe (RUL) is in contact with the ascending aorta and the upper right heart border.
   c. The anterior segment of the LUL is in anatomic contact with the upper left heart border. This contact is limited to only a very small area by left atrial and main pulmonary artery curves.
   d. The apical-posterior segment of the LUL is in anatomic contact with the aortic knob.
   e. Remember that the diaphragm is a posteriorly located structure on the frontal film. The right and left hemidiaphragms are in contact with the right and left lower lobes, respectively.

Silhouette Sign

To differentiate anterior from posterior on frontal films and right from left on lateral films, the clinician looks for the presence of the *silhouette sign,* a roentgenologic sign used to localize normal and abnormal structures on the chest film. The sign is explained here as it relates to the localization of lung lesions, but the concept applies to the localization of pleural and mediastinal abnormalities as well.

The term *silhouette sign* refers to the loss of the normal roentgen silhouette. It is present when ". . . water density in anatomic contact with another water density obliterates the existing interface" (Felson, 1965). To understand this concept, consider two water-filled balloons situated side by side, as shown in Figure 15–42A. When they are radiographed, the demarcation between balloons disappears (Fig. 15–42B), because the touching balloons are both water density. No contrast in density (i.e., air) exists to make their touching edges visible on the x-ray; a silhouette sign is present.

Now suppose one of the two water balloons is moved several inches posteriorly and another x-ray is taken. The silhouette sign is absent (Fig. 15–42C), because a contrast medium (i.e., air) is present between the two water densities to make the edges of the two balloons clearly visible.

In short, when evaluating two touching water density images, the presence of a silhouette sign indicates that the two structures touch each other in the chest. Absence of this sign indicates that overlapping structures do not touch each other—usually lung tissue (air density) separates their surfaces.

In the application of this concept to lung lesions, one water balloon might represent a typical lung lesion, such as an area of pneumonia or collapsed lung, a hematoma, a tumor, or an enlarged lymph node near a hilum. The other water balloon may represent an anatomic structure, such as part of the mediastinal profile, descending aorta, or hemidiaphragm. The following steps along with Table 15–4 help the clinician determine the location of the water-density lung lesion.

Text continued on page 439

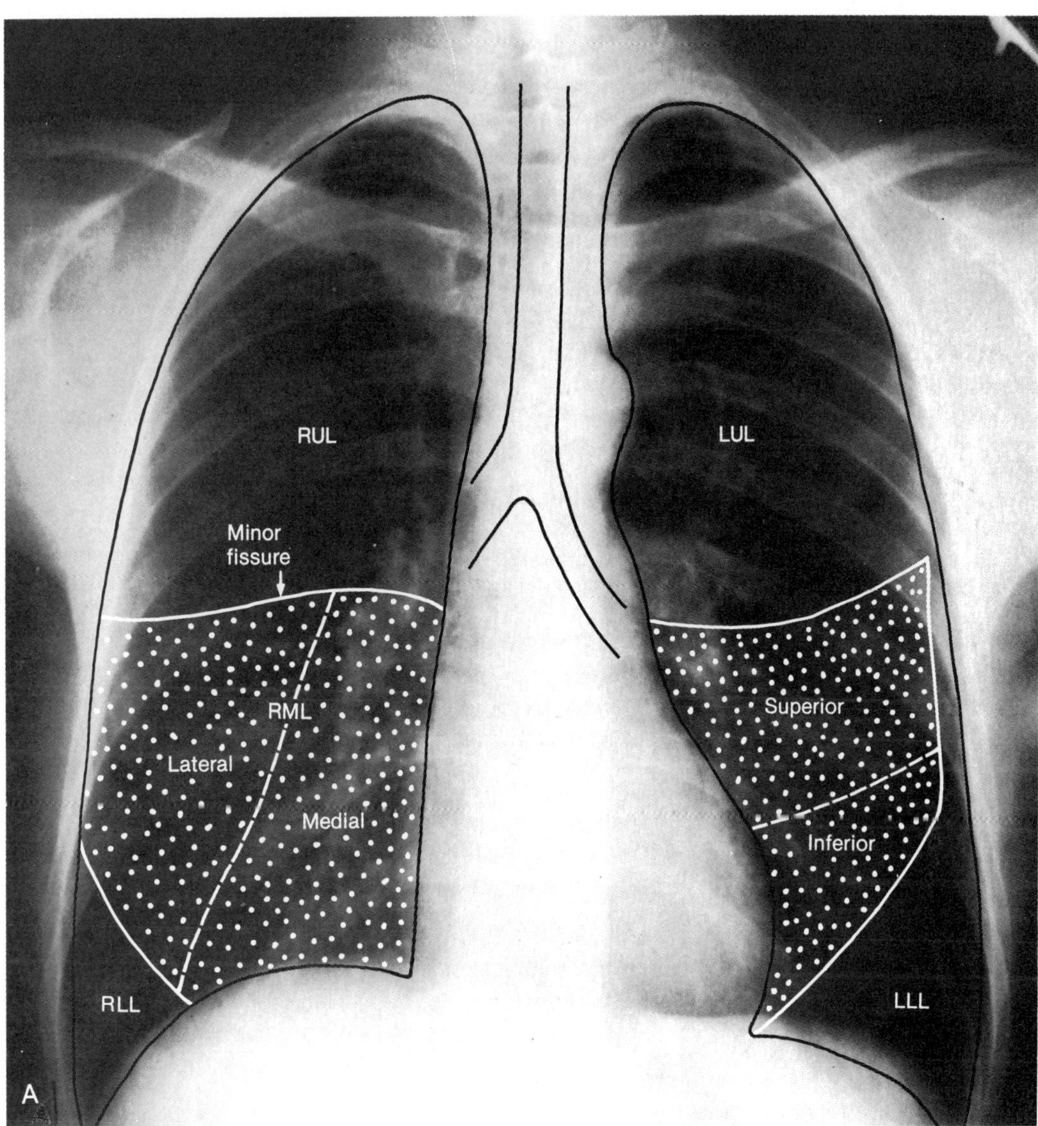

Figure 15–41. Key lobes and segments of the lungs on the chest x-ray. *A*, Right middle lobe and lingular segments of the left upper lobe, frontal view. (RUL = right upper lobe; LUL = left upper lobe; RML = right middle lobe; LLL = left lower lobe; RLL = right lower lobe.)

Illustration continued on following page

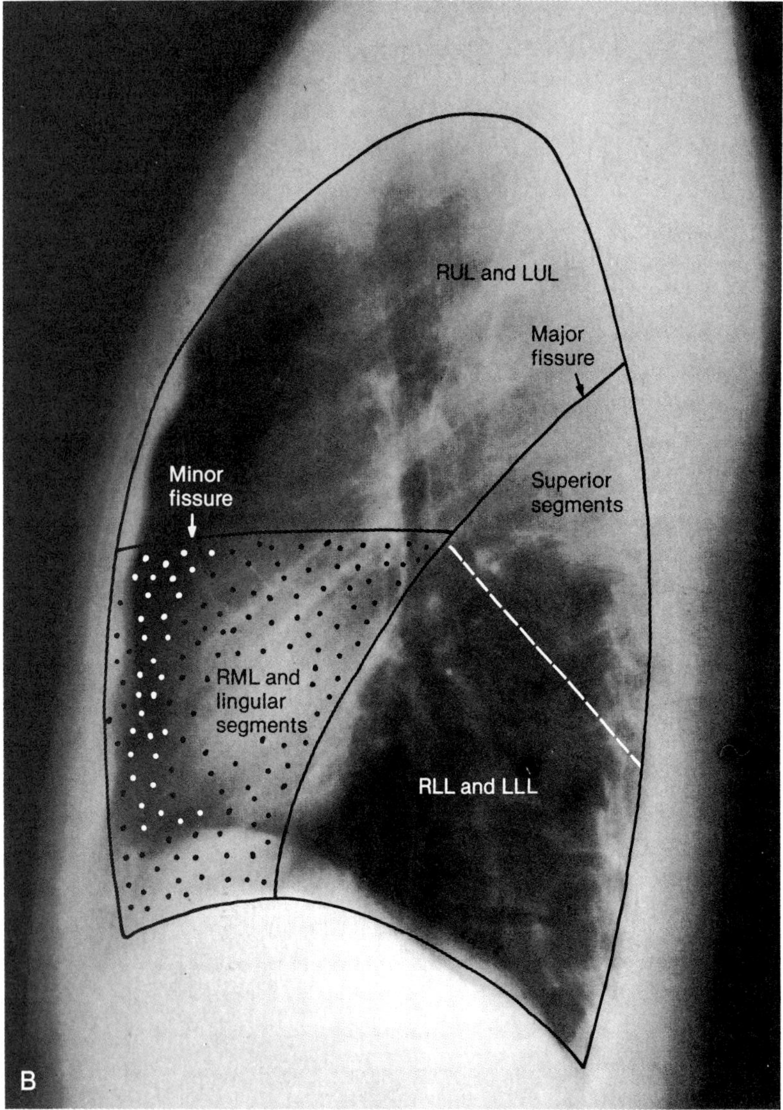

Figure 15–41 *Continued B*, Right middle lobe and lingular segments of the left upper lobe, lateral view. (RUL = right upper lobe; LUL = left upper lobe; RML = right middle lobe; LLL = left lower lobe; RLL = right lower lobe.)

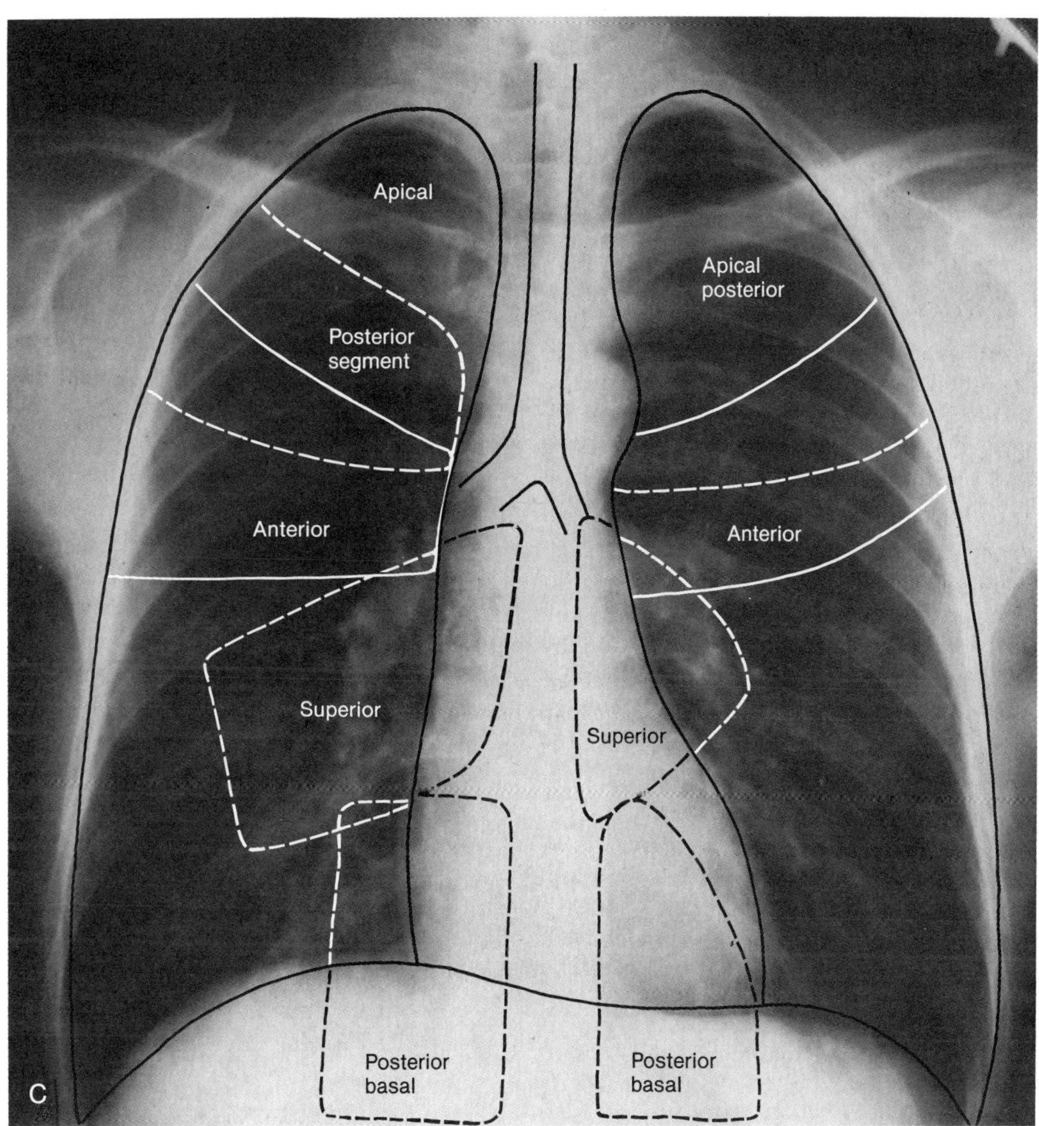

Figure 14–41 *Continued C,* Key upper and lower lobe segments, frontal view. The lower lobes are distinguished from the upper lobes by the dotted lines (except posterior portions of upper lobes).

Illustration continued on following page

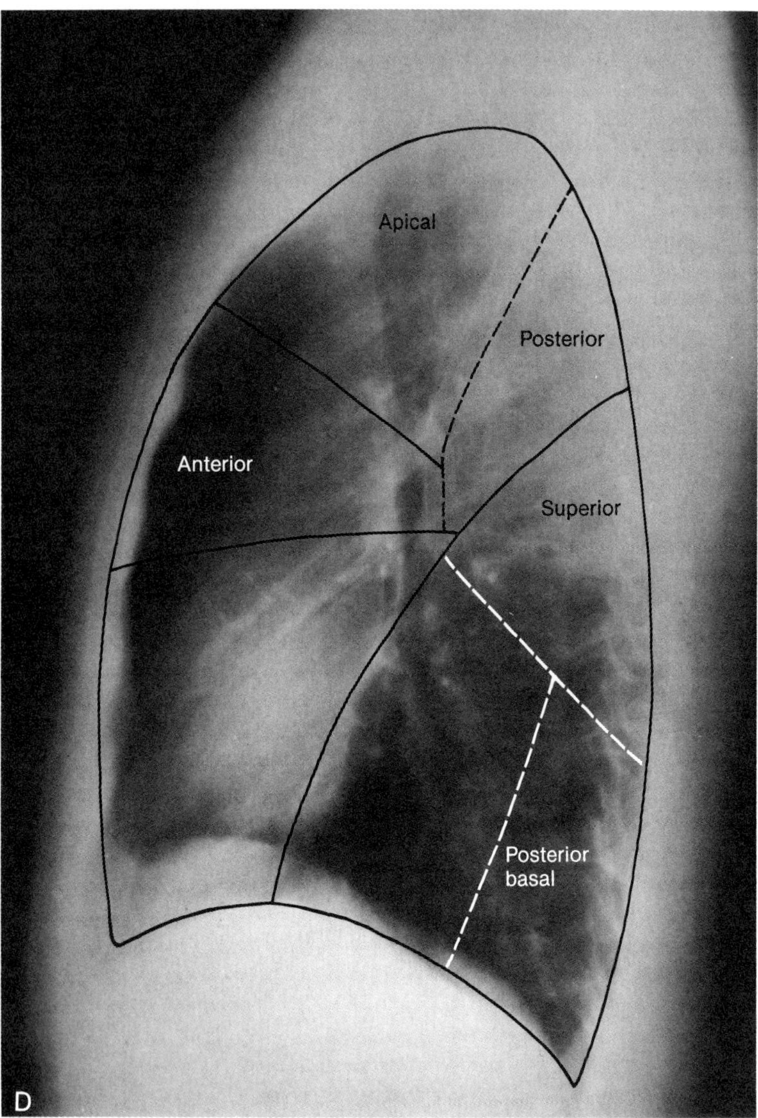

Figure 15–41 *Continued D,* Upper and lower lobe segments, lateral view.

1. Observe which anatomic structure the density appears to be touching.
   Example
   An area of water density in the lung fields is touching the right heart border on a frontal film.
2. Check Table 15–4 to determine whether the anatomic structure is located anteriorly or posteriorly in the chest.
   Example
   The right heart border is an anterior border.
3. Observe whether the density obliterates or merely overlaps the border of the anatomic structure.
4. If the structure's border is obliterated, a silhouette sign is present. One observes the loss of the normal roentgen silhouette in that area. The abnormal density is located in the lobe and segment *immediately adjacent* to the anatomic structure.
   Example
   Obliteration of the right heart border indicates the presence of a silhouette sign and localizes the density immediately adjacent to this border. Since this border is located anteriorly in the chest, the density must be located anteriorly in the RML rather than posteriorly in the RLL (Fig. 15–43A).
5. If the structure's border is still visible—the water densities merely overlap—the silhouette sign is absent. The abnormal density lies at a distance from the anatomic structure, in the opposite side of the chest or just a few inches anteriorly or posteriorly.
   Example
   When the right heart border is clearly visible, the abnormal density is located posteriorly in the RLL (Fig. 15–43B).

The silhouette sign does not help localize a lesion that lies in the middle of the lung field, without anatomic contact with water-density structures, such as the aorta and hemidiaphragms.

The silhouette sign is sometimes used to localize normal structures. For example, when a gastric air bubble is not visible on the lateral view to help localize the left hemidiaphragm, the clinician looks for the silhouette sign at the anterior aspects of the hemidiaphragms. Its existence marks the right hemidiaphragm's contact with the heart and thus helps differentiate right from left hemidiaphragm.

THE LUNG FIELDS—SYSTEMATIC EXAMINATION

The clinician examines the lung fields from top to bottom, comparing sides for general symmetry and

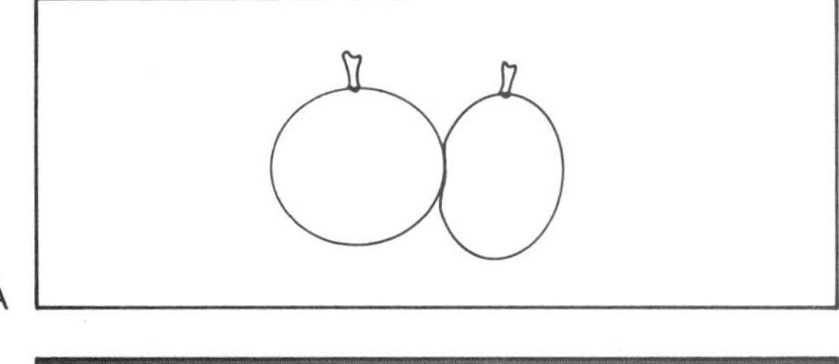

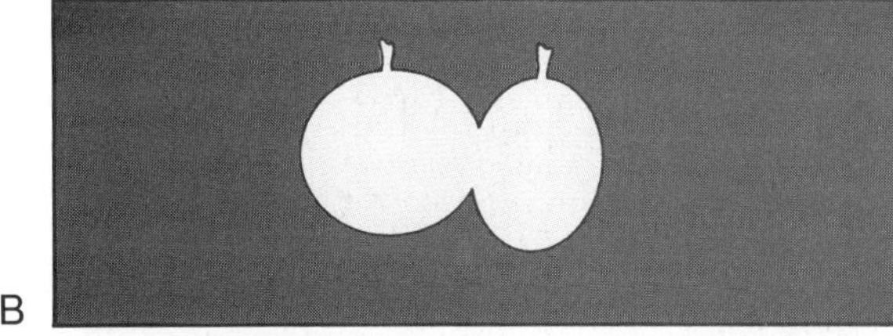

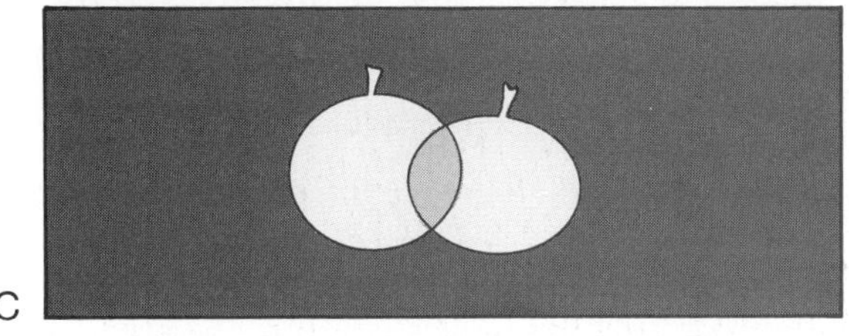

Figure 15–42. An example of the silhouette sign. *A*, Two adjacent water balloons. *B*, X-ray image with silhouette sign. *C*, X-ray image without silhouette sign.

equal roentgen density. Special attention is given to *bronchovascular markings* and *lung parenchyma.*

Bronchovascular Markings

Bronchovascular markings refer to airways and hilar vessels that branch and taper to the periphery of the lung fields. Airways outside the mediastinum are normally invisible because of their thin walls and air density. Hence, on the normal chest x-ray, bronchovascular markings consist only of pulmonary arteries and veins. For this reason, they are frequently referred to as *vasculature* or *vascularity.*

General Pattern. The clinician examines the general pattern of markings throughout the lung fields. The characteristics of normal bronchovascular markings are itemized as follows:

1. They branch out in all directions from the hilar areas.
2. They gradually taper, as they approach the lung periphery.
3. They disappear in the outer third of the lung fields. When visible in this area, they are seldom well defined.
4. They appear larger on the expiratory film compared with the inspiratory film because vessels increase in size during expiration.

Roentgen Density. Next, the clinician looks at roentgen density. Though all lung fields are air density, shades of air density are visible on the film in the normal pattern described as follows:

1. The lungs become more radiolucent or blacker,

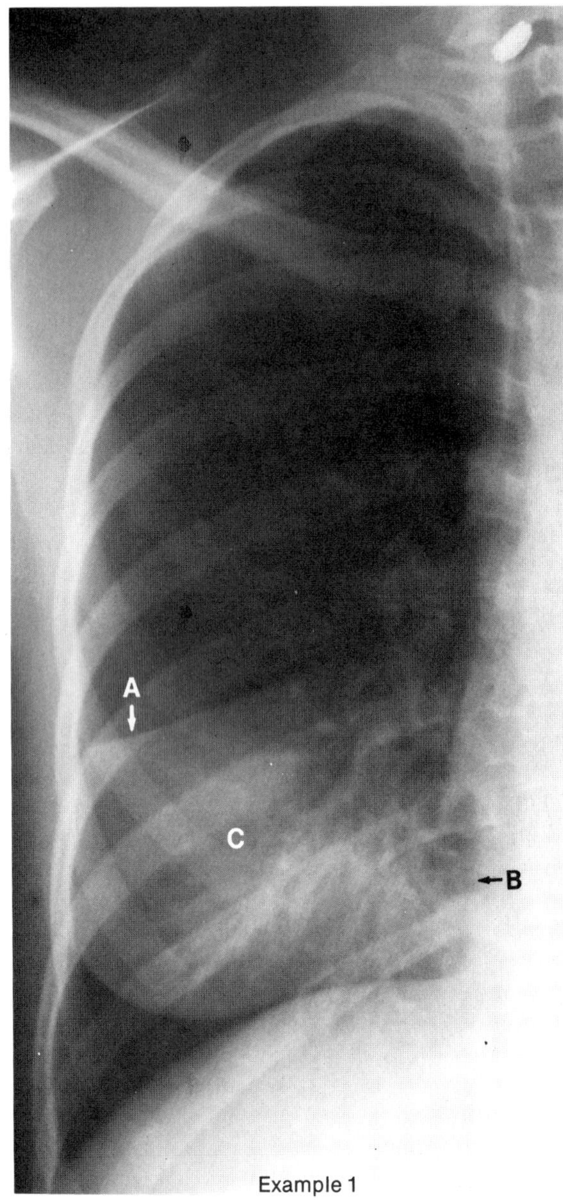

Figure 15–43. Use of the silhouette sign to assess the location of pneumonia. *Example 1,* The density (C) is most likely localized in the right middle lobe (RML) because of the obscured right heart border at B (silhouette sign) and because of the clearly visible right hemidiaphragm, a posterior structure. The downward displacement of the minor fissure (A) is due to partial collapse of the RML.

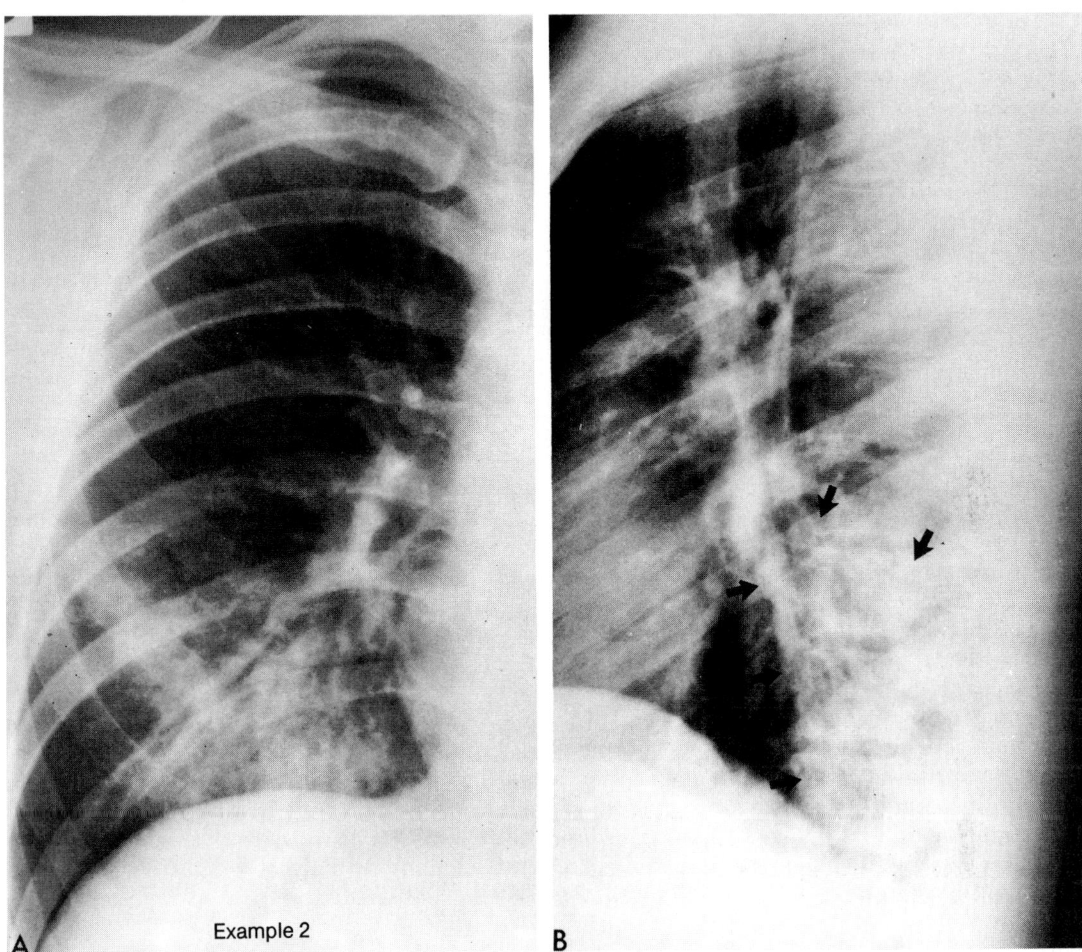

Figure 15–43 *Continued Example 2,* On the frontal projection (A), the absent silhouette sign by the right heart border indicates that the patchy density in the lower lung field lies in the right lower lobe (RLL) not in the RML. On the lateral projection (B), the same density is seen in the posterior basal segment of the RLL (arrows). The density's distal location from the hemidiaphragm explains why the hemidiaphragm was not obscured on the frontal projection. The patient had acute bronchopneumonia from *Streptococcus pyogenes.* (*Example 1* reproduced by permission from Levy, R., Hawkins, H., and Barsan, W.: Radiology in Emergency Medicine. St. Louis, The C. V. Mosby Co., 1986. *Example 2* reproduced by permission from Paré, J. and Fraser, R.: Synopsis of Diseases of the Chest. Philadelphia, W. B. Saunders Co., 1983.)

Table 15–4. USE OF THE SILHOUETTE SIGN TO LOCALIZE LUNG LESIONS ON FRONTAL FILMS

Anatomic Structure in Contact with Lung Lesion	Anterior Posterior Location of Structure in Chest	Location of Lesion (if Silhouette Sign is Present)	Likely Location of Lesion (if Silhouette Sign is Absent)
Right heart border	Anterior	Right median lobe (RML)	Right lower lobe (RLL)—superior segment if midportion of heart border is involved.
Upper right heart border and ascending aorta	Anterior	Anterior segment of left upper lobe (LUL)	Superior segment of RLL
Left heart border	Anterior	Lingular segments of LUL	Left lower lobe (LLL)—superior segment if midportion of heart border is involved.
Upper left heart border (main pulmonary artery and left atrial mediastinal curves)	Anterior	Anterior segment of LUL	Superior segment of LLL
Aortic knob	Posterior	Apical-posterior segment of LUL (posterior aspect)	Apical posterior segment of LUL (anterior aspect) *or* Apical-posterior segment of LUL *far* posterior aspect, or superior segment of LLL
Descending Aorta	Posterior	LLL	Anterior or lingular segments of LUL *or* LLL, *far* posterior aspect
Right hemidiaphragm (medial two-thirds portion)	Posterior	RLL	RML
Left hemidiaphragm	Posterior	LLL	Lingular segments of LUL

as bronchopulmonary markings become smaller and approach the periphery.

2. Right and left lung fields appear about the same roentgen density, when areas equidistant to the spine and at the same vertebral level are compared.

3. The upper lobes normally appear more radiolucent than the lower lobes, because the lung is thinner in apical areas.

4. The lung fields appear less radiolucent (i.e., more radiopaque) on expiratory films. Lung density is inversely proportional to the amount of air in the lungs.

Alterations in the aforementioned normal pattern may occur, owing to individual variation in bronchopulmonary markings, film quality, body build, and age.

Abnormal Markings. Using serial films to compare general pattern and caliber of markings, the clinician looks for *increased markings*, *decreased markings*, *unequal markings* between lung fields, and *rapid tapering of markings* toward the periphery, as described in Table 15–5.

Increased markings is a classic sign of venous dilatation from pulmonary vascular congestion and the most reliable sign of impending left ventricular failure (see Chapter 8). The following chest x-ray findings are observed with worsening pulmonary congestion:

1. *General increase in the caliber of pulmonary vessels*—first veins dilate and then arteries, as congestion backs up toward the right ventricle.

2. *Redistribution of pulmonary blood flow to the*

Table 15–5. ABNORMAL BRONCHOPULMONARY MARKINGS

Chest X-ray Finding	Description	Common Causes
Increased markings	Markings are prominent and extend to the periphery of the lung fields.	Pulmonary vascular congestion (impending left ventricular failure).
Decreased markings (*oligemia*)	Markings are notably decreased in caliber and number, such that the lung fields appear abnormally radiolucent.	Pulmonary arterial undercirculation and decreased blood flow, e.g., cyanotic congenital heart disease, notably with pulmonic stenosis, and right-to-left shunt. Increased pulmonary vascular resistance, as in emphysema, pulmonary embolism, and primary pulmonary hypertension. Unilateral oligemia: hypoplasia or thromboembolism of right or left pulmonary artery, tumor, unilateral emphysema.
Unequal markings	Markings are slightly different between lungs	Tetralogy of Fallot Left-to-right cardiac shunts
Rapid tapering of markings	Markings taper rapidly and end before reaching the outer third of the lung fields. Sometimes a vessel ends abruptly, forming a "prune-tree" appearance, when a major artery is obstructed.	Increased vascular resistance with severe pulmonary arterial hypertension, e.g., emphysema, interstitial fibrosis, cor pulmonale, left ventricular failure, congenital heart disease with increased pulmonary blood flow.

upper lobes—lower lobe vessel constriction and upper lobe vessel dilatation account for the increased caliber of LUL vessels (Fig. 15–44). The exact physiologic mechanism for this change is not clear.

3. *Change in the distinctiveness of vessel borders*—the borders become hazy or blurred, as fluid begins to move outward into interstitial spaces. As failure worsens, hilar vessels are affected, and hilar clouding begins.

These three early signs of left ventricular failure are not always sequential or associated with specific pulmonary artery pressures. The signs occur to varying degrees in different persons, when pulmonary artery (PA) wedge pressure rises significantly above normal. Changes may be acute or chronic, and the absence of signs does not necessarily indicate normal PA wedge and left atrial pressures.

Increased markings due to chronic bronchitis may appear in a diffuse pattern, with those that are prominent as well as irregular in contour and indistinct in definition. This presentation is nicknamed the "dirty chest," because of the cluttered, hazy appearance of the lung fields (Fig. 15–45).

Decreased markings throughout the lung fields may be accompanied by signs of lung hyperinflation. This presentation is the so-called *arterial deficiency* pattern of emphysema (Fig. 15–46).

Lung Parenchyma

The lung parenchyma surrounds bronchopulmonary markings in the lung fields. Because it consists of 92% air and only 8% tissue and capillary blood, lung parenchyma represents the least dense or most radiolucent area visible inside the chest wall. Its normal density is best appreciated in the outermost 2 cm on the lung fields, where bronchopulmonary markings are absent.

Lung Lesions. To detect a lung lesion, the clinician systematically scans each lung field for the presence of any abnormal density that interrupts bronchopulmonary markings or alters the normal roentgen density of the lung fields.

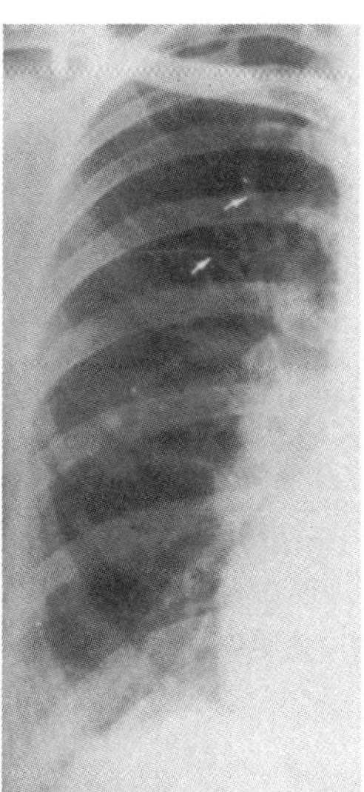

Figure 15–44. Redistribution of blood flow. Increased venous pressures cause the vessels in the upper lung fields to become more prominent and somewhat enlarged (arrows). The vascular shadows in the lower lung fields are smaller than usual. These findings are significant only when present on erect films. (Reproduced by permission from Teplick, J. and Haskin, M.: Roentgenologic Diagnosis, 3rd ed. Philadelphia, W. B. Saunders Co., 1976.)

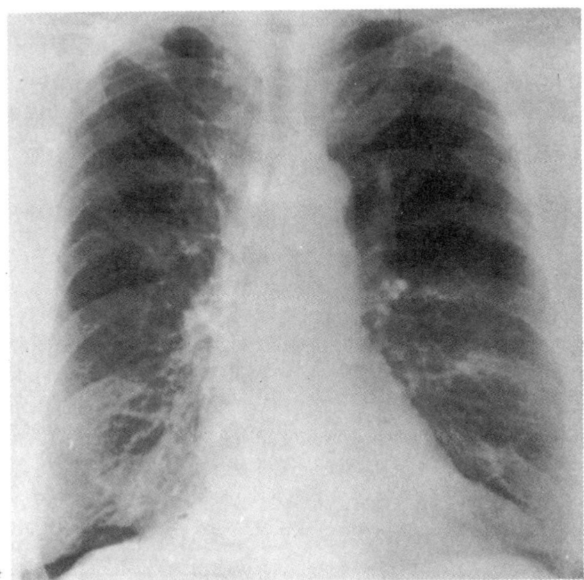

Figure 15–45. Chronic bronchitis—the "dirty chest." Bronchovascular markings are accentuated throughout both lung fields. Lung hyperinflation is also present. (Reproduced by permission from Fraser, R. and Paré, J.: Diagnosis of Diseases of the Chest, 2nd ed. Philadelphia, W. B. Saunders, 1977.)

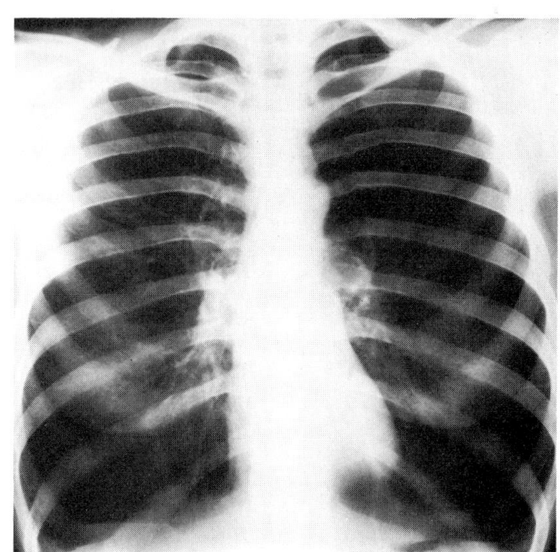

Figure 15–46. Arterial deficiency pattern (oligemia) with lung hyperinflation. (Reproduced by permission from Paré, J. A. and Fraser, R.: Synopsis of Diseases of the Chest. Philadelphia, W. B. Saunders Co., 1983.)

Table 15–6 describes lesions commonly observed when viewing the chest films of pulmonary patients. Also, it familiarizes the reader with the roentgenographic terms usually employed to describe lung abnormalities on chest x-ray reports.

When an unfamiliar image is seen on a film, the clinician describes it with attention to *roentgen density, size, shape, nature of its borders* (e.g., poorly versus well defined), *specific location,* and *general distribution* in the case of multiple lesions (e.g., scattered throughout the lung fields, situated centrally versus peripherally, and distributed in specific lobes or segments).

Roentgenographic Patterns. Next, the clinician examines the lung fields for abnormal roentgenographic patterns. The two main patterns are *alveolar* and *interstitial.* They may occur diffusely throughout the lung fields, in specific areas, or in combinations, with one pattern predominating.

Alveolar Pattern and the Air Bronchogram Sign. Radiopaque confluent densities are characteristic of the *alveolar pattern,* also called the *acinar pattern.* This pattern has been likened to "fluffy white clouds" in the lungs. The analogy is accurate except margins are more ill defined than those of the cumulous clouds in the sky. Pattern distribution is localized, diffuse, or central, depending on the disease process. Localized areas tend to be segmental or lobar in distribution and may represent tumor or localized infectious processes. Localized disease may progress to diffuse disease and a diffuse alveolar pattern, as in aspiration pneumonia. A central perihilar distribution that spares the lung

Table 15–6. RADIOLOGIC SIGNS OF COMMON LUNG LESIONS

Radiologic Sign	Characteristics	Exemplary Disease Prosesses
Air-filled cavity (cavitation) or bulla	Radiolucent center Walls of the cavity are partially or completely visible. Cavity is greater than 2 cm in diameter.	Emphysema Complicated acute staphyloccoccal pneumonia (mostly children and infants)
Confluent density — RUL pneumonia —Tumor	Homogeneous area of increased density Margins often are well defined, if density is lobar or segmental in distribution. Tumor or other single lesion may have well or poorly defined (hazy) margins	Lung consolidation, e.g., pneumonia, mucoid impaction, lung abscess, tumor or mass of unknown etiology
Cavitation with a fluid level*	Cavitation is usually within an area of consolidation. Fluid level sharply delineates interface between radiolucent top and radiopaque bottom of cavity.	Infectious process, e.g., active tuberculosis, lung abscess, staphylococcal pneumonia
Linear or plate-like atelectasis	Linear lines of increased density at lung bases Horizontal orientation 1 to 3 mm in thickness and several cm long	Alveolar hypoventilation and decreased diaphragmatic excursions, as in post-operative atelectasis after thoracoabdominal surgery
Lung collapse (loss of lung volume)† Collapsed RML LATERAL VIEW FRONTAL VIEW	Well-outlined area of increased density Often triangular in shape Change in position of fissures, hilum, mediastinum Individual lobes and segments collapse in characteristic directions, e.g., right median lobe collapses cephalad and medially.	Atelectasis from bronchial obstruction, e.g., RML collapse. Lateral view shows change in position of fissures and the triangular "pancake" of tissue. Collapse may not be evident on the frontal view except for a silhouette sign along the right heart border.

Table 15–6. RADIOLOGIC SIGNS OF COMMON LUNG LESIONS *Continued*

Radiologic Sign	Characteristics	Exemplary Disease Prosesses
Coin lesion	Small round area of increased density about the size of a small coin	Granulomatious lesion, early malignant tumor, hamartoma, adenoma, exudate, or blood vessels radiographed on end.
Calcification "Eggshell" calcification around lymph node periphery (silicosis) Irregular calcification within granulomatous lesion	Metal density Size, shape, and location depends on disease process. Occurs within granulomatous lesions, tumors (hamartoma and others), and lymph nodes	Indicates a benign lung lesion, except in rare cases Usually associated with healing infectious processes, e.g., histoplasmosis and tuberculosis Combination of a peripheral granulomatous lesion (Ghon's lesion) and a central calcified lymph node (a Ranke's complex)
Hampton's hump Infarcted tissue Pruned hilar vessels Decreased vascular markings	Rounded, wedged shaped density of infarcted lung tissue peripheral to obstructed vessels Located in or near lateral costophrenic angle when visible on frontal film Convex surface (hump) faces medially towards pruned hilar vessels. Distal end may be obscured by pleural fluid and elevated diaphragm.	Pulmonary embolism with infarction

*See Figure 8–16.
†Arrows show direction of collapse.

periphery is characteristic of the so-called *bat wings* or *butterfly* radiographic presentation of pulmonary edema (Fig. 15–47).

The alveolar pattern indicates the presence of an alveolar pathologic process, e.g., alveolar pneumonia, alveolar pulmonary edema, and others (Table 15–7). Replacement of air in alveoli or acinar units with edema, mucus, blood, tumor, or inflammatory by-products changes roentgen density from the normal air density to water density. Lung radiolucency is replaced with radiopacity, as shown conceptually in Figure 15–48A and Figure 15–48B.

The presence of an *air bronchogram sign* on the chest x-ray is pathognomonic of alveolar disease. Defined as *visualization of air in an airway,* an air bronchogram develops when a bronchus becomes surrounded by water density, as in pneumonia. In Figure 15–48C, the mucus-filled alveoli immediately adjacent to the airway provide a contrast medium. The air bronchogram is visible as a radiolucent column of air.

Table 15–7. BASIC ROENTGENOGRAPHIC PATTERNS OF CHEST DISEASES

Alveolar Pattern	Interstitial Pattern (Reticular)	Nodular Pattern	Ground-Glass Pattern (Granular)
Alveolar pneumonia and bronchopneumonia Alveolar pulmonary edema Pulmonary embolism with infarction Pulmonary hemorrhage Goodpasture's syndrome pulmonary hemosiderosis systemic lupus erythematosus *Pneumocystis* carinii (late stage) Aspiration pneumonia Adult respiratory distress syndrome	Interstitial pneumonia Interstitial pulmonary edema Idiopathic diffuse interstitial fibrosis Sarcoidosis Scleroderma Metastatic carcinoma *Pneumocystis carinii* (early stage) Silicosis Asbestosis Cystic fibrosis (late stage)	Miliary tuberculosis Coccidioidomycosis Histoplasmosis Varicella pneumonia Sarcoidosis Silicosis Metastatic carcinoma Bronchogenic spread of tuberculosis Pulmonary hemosiderosis (late stage) Alveolar microlithiasis	*Early* interstitial disease miliary tuberculosis asbestosis berylliosis rheumatoid lung idiopathic interstitial fibrosis

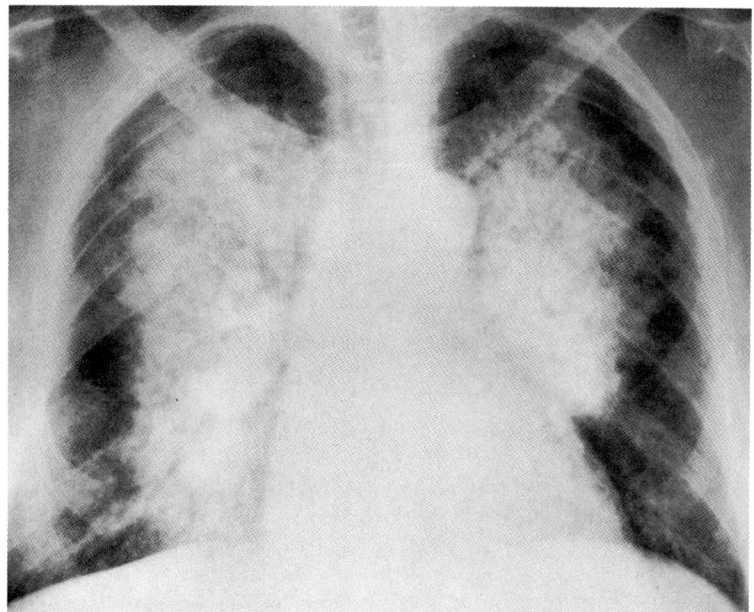

Figure 15–47. The "bat's wing" pattern of pulmonary edema. (Reproduced by permission from Fraser, R. and Paré, J.: Diagnosis of Diseases of the Chest, vol. II, 2nd ed. Philadelphia, W. B. Saunders Co., 1978.)

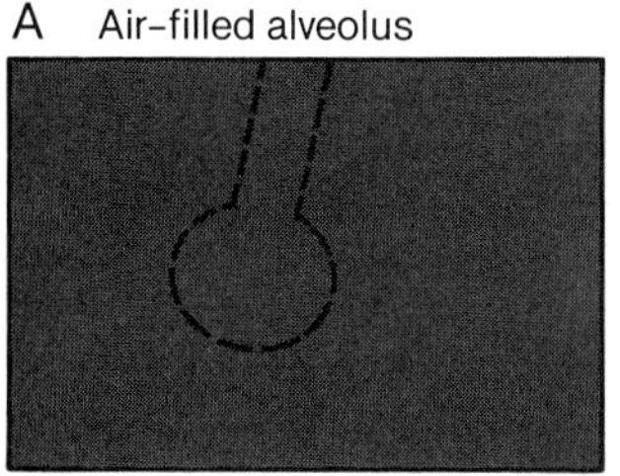

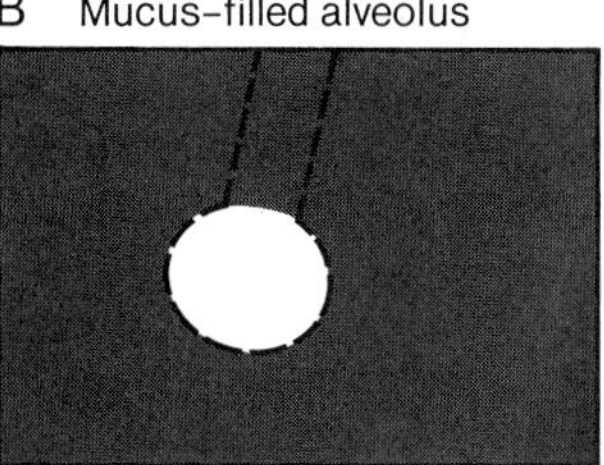

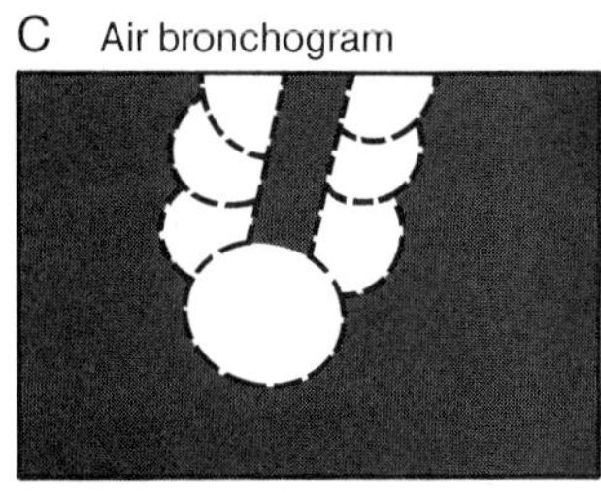

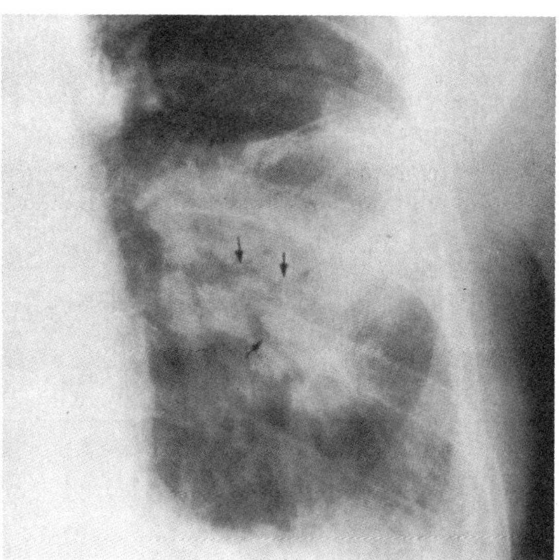

Figure 15–48. The alveolar pattern and air bronchogram sign. *A*, The air-filled alveolus is invisible on the chest x-ray. *B*, The accumulation of mucus in the alveolus produces a radiopaque area. *C*, The airway surrounded by mucus-filled alveoli produces a radiolucent column of air, called an air bronchogram sign. *D*, Several air bronchogram signs are seen as branching linear areas of hyperlucency within the irregular area of radiopaqueness. Their presence confirms the alveolar nature of an infiltrate. (*D*, Reproduced by permission from Teplick, J. and Haskin, M.: Roentgenologic Diagnosis, 3rd ed. Philadelphia, W. B. Saunders Co., 1976.)

When one thinks in three dimensions, it helps in the understanding of the anatomic basis for this sign—acinar units extend in *all* directions, similar to a bunch of grapes.

Interstitial Pattern. The *interstitial pattern*, also called the *reticular pattern*, is the visualization of the lung interstitium thickened by one or more of the following interstitial processes:

1. *Fibrosis*, as in diffuse interstitial fibrosis.
2. *Fluid*, as in interstitial pulmonary edema.
3. *Inflammatory by-products*, as in interstitial pneumonias.
4. Other processes represented by the diseases listed in Table 15–7.

This pattern is illustrated in Figure 15–49. The effect of a thickened alveolar interstitial space is the formation of thin-walled cystic spaces *less than 10 mm* in diameter and sometimes barely noticeable without a magnifying lens. Many experts divide the reticular pattern into three subcategories—*fine*, *medium*, and *coarse*—based on the degree of interstitial thickening and the size of the cystic spaces. Generally, the thicker the interstitium and the larger the cystic spaces, the coarser the reticular pattern and the more severe the interstitial disease. The fine-to-medium reticulations in Figure 15–49A represent the typical pattern found in most acute and many chronic interstitial diseases (Fig. 15–50).

When reticulations become coarse, forming cystic spaces *greater than 5 mm* in diameter, *honeycombing* is said to be present. This particular term is used because the network formed appears similar to the comb built by honeybees. This analogy helps one remember the general appearance of the interstitial pattern, but it has its limitations. The coarse reticular pattern is actually more irregular than the structure of a honeycomb; the interstitium is not uniformly thickened, and cystic spaces vary in size. Moreover, the term honeycombing is used to refer to coarse reticulations shown in Figure 15–49B and not the fine or medium reticulations shown in Figure 15–49A. Honeycombing is the most reliable sign of interstitial fibrosis; it is associated with the severe interstitial fibrosis of end-stage pulmonary disease.

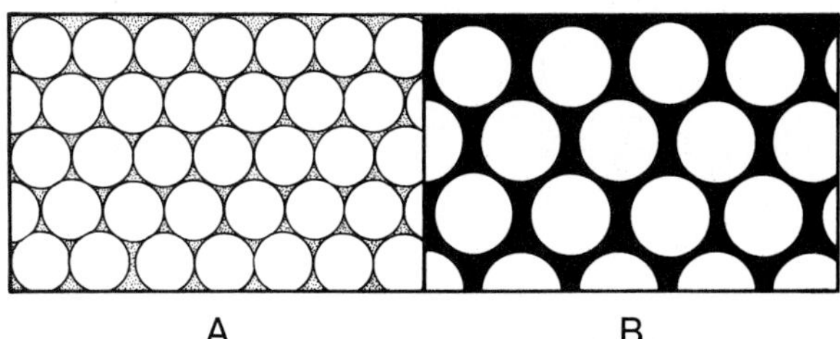

Figure 15–49. Conceptual illustrations of interstitial (reticular) patterns. *A*, Interstitial pattern with fine to medium reticulation (light gray). *B*, Honeycombing with coarse reticulation (black).

Other Signs of Interstitial Disease. The interstitial pattern is often accompanied by other signs of interstitial disease, such as *peribronchial cuffing*, which is a radiopaque ring or cuff around a bronchus. The anatomic basis for this sign is shown in Figure 15–51. In Figure 15–51A, fluid from edema or tissue from fibrosis extends into the bronchovascular interstitial space called the peribronchial or perivascular interstitial space (see Chapter 2). On the chest x-ray (Fig. 15–51B), the thickened interstitium is visible as a radiopaque ring or cuff around the radiolucent bronchus. This sign is present only when the airway is radiographed on end, as shown in the illustration.

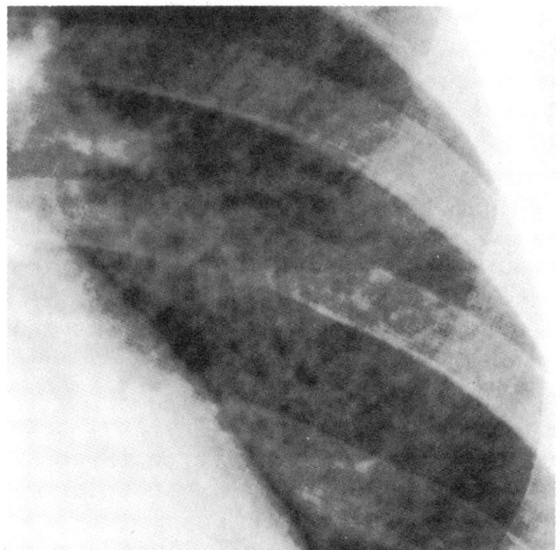

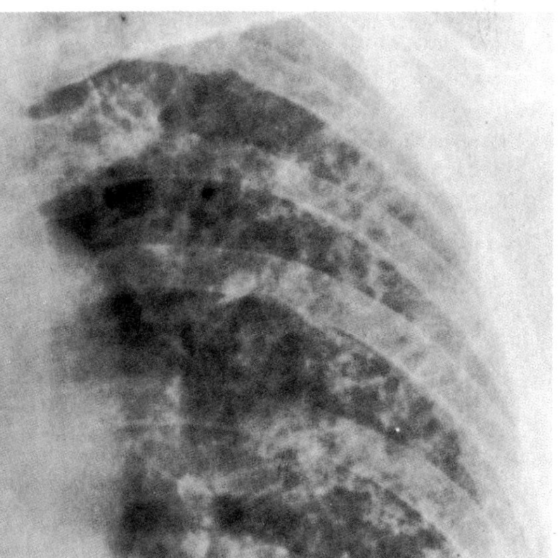

Figure 15–50. Medium and coarse interstitial reticular patterns. In this medium pattern (A), the patient's diagnosis was pulmonary hemosiderosis with fibrosis secondary to recurrent pulmonary edema. In the coarse or honeycomb pattern (B), the patient's diagnosis was advanced histiocytosis X, a restrictive pulmonary disease. Note the irregular cystic spaces with their relatively thick walls. (Reproduced by permission from Fraser, R. and Paré, J.: Diagnosis of Diseases of the Chest, 2nd ed. Philadelphia, W. B. Saunders Co., 1977 and 1978.)

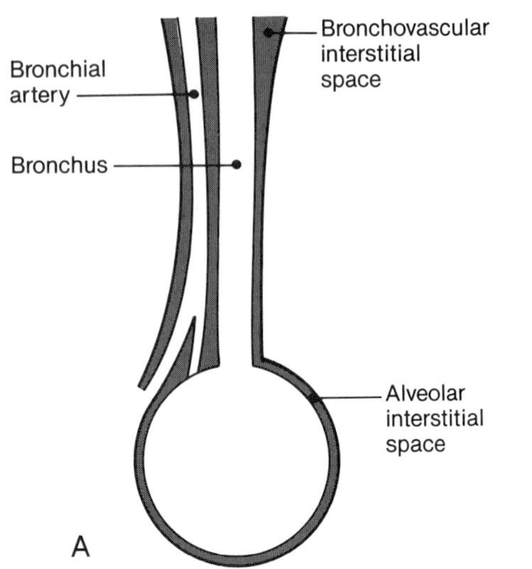

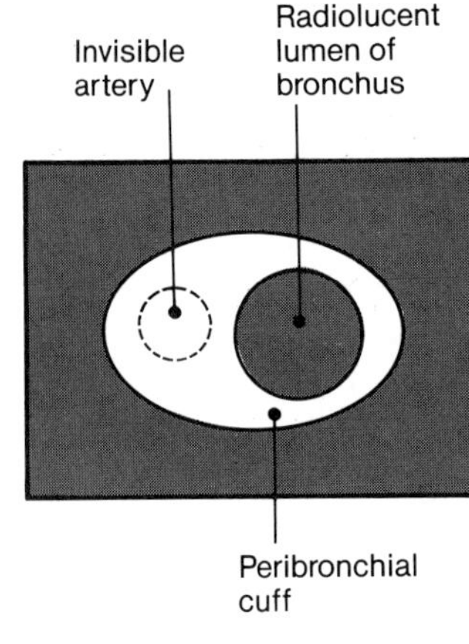

Figure 15–51. Pathophysiology of peribronchial cuffing. *A*, Conceptual illustration of increased fluid or tissue (gray) in bronchovascular and alveolar interstitial spaces. *B*, View of the airway in *A* radiographed on end. The artery is invisible, since it is the same density as the adjacent fluid or tissue. The increase in fluid or tissue forms a radiopaque ring or cuff around the bronchus.

Table 15–8. OTHER RADIOLOGIC SIGNS OF INTERSTITIAL DISEASE

Sign	Description	Location	Significance	Illustration
Kerley's A line	Linear density 2 to 6 cm long and less than 1 mm thick Oblique orientation Perpendicular to nearest pleural surface	Upper lobes	Increased tissue, fluid, or both within perilymphatic interstitial tissue	
Kerley's B line	Short, thin linear density Less than 2 cm long and 1 mm thick Horizontal orientation (lines never touch)	Lung periphery near lateral costophrenic angles	Increased tissue, fluid, or both in interlobar septa (chiefly perilymphatic interstitial tissue)	
Peribronchial cuffing	Radiopaque cuff or ring around a bronchus x-rayed on end Radiolucent center (bronchial lumen) Seldom larger than 5 mm	Usually near hilar areas where airways are large	Increased tissue, fluid, or both in perivascular or peribronchial interstitial space	

Table 15–8 summarizes and illustrates peribronchial cuffing as well as two other radiologic signs of interstitial pathology, *Kerley's A lines* and *Kerley's B lines.*

Kerley's lines, referred to as *septal lines,* are interlobular septa that have become visible on the chest film, owing to thickening from edema, infection, hemorrhage, neoplasm, or other processes. The lines are commonly seen in congestive heart failure and interstitial pulmonary edema and disappear rapidly once diuretics and other agents rid the body of excess fluid. However, similar to peribronchial cuffing, septal lines may represent an irreversible finding, as in diffuse interstitial fibrosis, lymphangitic spread of neoplasm, and chronic mitral valve disease.

Kerley's A and B lines are the main septal lines or linear densities found on chest films. Kerley's C and D lines are described in the medical literature; they are not discussed here because their significance and existence as separate entities are controversial.

Mixed Alveolar-interstitial Pattern. The chest x-ray may show a mixed alveolar-interstitial pattern (Fig. 8–20C), particularly when mixed chest pathology is present. In acute disease, such as left ventricular failure, the mixed pattern may represent only the transition between interstitial and alveolar pulmonary edema. In chronic disease, mixed patterns usually represent an acute alveolar process superimposed on a chronic interstitial process, e.g., alveolar pneumonia in the patient with idiopathic interstitial fibrosis.

Other Patterns. Two other roentgenographic patterns are the *ground-glass* and *nodular.* They are common in chronic interstitial diseases.

The ground-glass or *granular* pattern appears as a homogeneous clouding or haze over both lung fields. It is indicative of early interstitial disease. Examination of the film with a magnifying glass may reveal tiny nodules or opacities, as in early miliary tuberculosis, or fine reticulations, as in early asbestosis.

In the nodular pattern, the aforementioned nodules grow in size to produce the *miliary nodular pattern,* as in miliary tuberculosis. The small discrete nodules are less than 5 mm in size and are distributed uniformly throughout both lung fields (see Fig. 8–17). In contrast, the patient with the nodular pattern in metastatic carcinoma to the lung presents with larger nodules that are less uniform in distribution than the small punctate opacities in miliary tuberculosis.

Patients with other diseases present with other pattern combinations, such as the *reticulonodular pattern,* a combination of the reticular (interstitial) and nodular patterns (see Fig. 8–18B).

Examination of Serial Films

Finally, the clinician examines serial films to identify changes in lesions, bronchovascular markings, and roentgenographic patterns over time, and to determine whether changes are acute or chronic. On the one hand, the films of a patient with left ventricular failure may progress from a normal chest x-ray pattern to an interstitial and finally alveolar pattern in a period of minutes, hours, or days. On the other hand, the slow development of an interstitial pattern over months to years most likely represents fibrosis, a chronic irreversible process.

Areas of Focus

Learning to identify gross pathology on the chest film is a time-consuming process for the beginning interpreter, especially when one considers the number and scope of possible radiologic signs. The following areas of focus, however, will help the beginner get started on viewing chest x-ray films.

1. *Always apply a systematic method.* The procedural guide summarizes the system presented in this chapter (see the box). It can be photocopied and brought to the laboratory or the clinical setting to serve as a learning aid. Initially, the clinician may wish to concentrate on the four following structural areas of the chest:
   a. Ribs and intercostal spaces
   b. Diaphragm
   c. Heart and mediastinum
   d. Lung fields
2. *Look for the clustering of radiologic signs* or, more specifically, the following:
   a. Any increase or decrease in lung volume (Table 15–9).
   b. Alveolar disease versus interstitial disease (Table 15–10).
   c. Radiologic signs of main chest diseases (Table 15–11).
3. *When in doubt, always return to your first impression* of the films.

Table 15–9. RADIOLOGIC SIGNS OF INCREASE AND DECREASE IN LUNG VOLUME*

Increase in Lung Volume (Lung Hyperinflation)	Decrease in Lung Volume (Atelectasis; Segmental, Lobar, or Entire Lung Collapse)
Flat hemidiaphragms	Plate-like atelectasis
Widened intercostal spaces	***Direct Signs of Lung Collapse***
Costovertebral angle of 90 degrees	Increased radiopacity of lung fields
Tenting (visualization of costophrenic muscle slips by diaphragm)	Crowding of bronchovascular markings
	Fissure displacement
Increased size of retrosternal air space (lateral view)	***Indirect Signs of Lung Collapse***
	Hilar displacement
	Elevation of diaphragm
Increased arteroposterior diameter (lateral view)	Mediastinal shift
	Narrowed intercostal spaces
Lung hyperlucency (oligemia)	Compensatory emphysema

*Adapted from Felson, B., Weinstein, A., and Spitz, H.: Principles of Chest Roentgenology—A Programmed Text. Philadelphia, W. B. Saunders Co., 1965.

Table 15–10. RADIOLOGIC SIGNS SUPPORTING ALVEOLAR VERSUS INTERSTITIAL DISEASE

Alveolar Disease	Interstitial Disease
Roentgenographic Pattern	***Roentgenographic Pattern***
Alveolar (acinar)	*Interstitial* (reticular), reticulonodular, granular, or miliary nodular
Bat wing or butterfly appearance	diffuse symmetric involvement of both lungs
Lobar or segmental in distribution	
Rapid change in appearance over hours or days except in a few cases (e.g., alveolar proteinosis and alveolar cell carcinoma)	slow change in appearance over weeks, months or years (except in a few cases, e.g., acute interstitial pneumonia, interstitial pulmonary edema)
Other Signs	***Other Signs***
Air bronchogram	Absence of air bronchogram
	Honeycombing
	Septal lines (Kerley's A and B lines)
	Peribronchial cuffing

4. *Whenever possible, view chest x-ray films with a person experienced in their interpretation.* Such a person can validate your interpretations, answer your questions, and provide crucial or more detailed information not presented in this chapter.

GUIDE FOR VIEWING A CHEST X-RAY

I. Correctly place the chest x-ray on the view box.

II. Stand back 6 to 8 ft for an initial impression. What appears abnormal?

III. Observe the following structures:

A. *Soft tissues*—neck, shoulder, chest wall, axillary area, breast tissue.
Abnormalities: skin or chest wall lesions, unilateral nipple shadows, subcutaneous emphysema, weight gain, weight loss, mastectomy.

B. *Trachea*
Abnormalities: tracheal deviation, stenosis, or dilatation; malpositioned tracheal or endotracheal tube.

C. *Bony thorax*—humeri, scapulae, clavicles, spine, and ribs.
Abnormalities: clavicular asymmetry, scoliosis, kyphosis, increased AP diameter, chest wall deformities, loss of calcium from bones, absence of ribs, rib fractures, rib notching.

D. *Width of intercostal spaces* (ICS)—compare both sides of the chest; apical and basilar areas.
Abnormalities: widened ICS due to increase in lung or thoracic volume, e.g., COPD, large pneumothorax, and large pleural effusion; *narrowed* ICS due to decrease in lung volume, e.g., atelectasis and severe interstitial fibrosis.

E. *Diaphragm and area below diaphragm*
Abnormalities of diaphragm—abnormal shape due to tumor, cyst, fluid, tenting, or scalloping; *elevation* due to abdominal or stomach distention, phrenic nerve paralysis, lung collapse, or subpulmonary pattern of pleural effusion; *depression* due to large pneumothorax or severe lung hyperinflation from COPD or aspiration of foreign object.
Abnormalities below diaphragm—gastric distention, subdiaphragmatic air or fluid, calcifications or plaques. Check for presence of nasogastric tube.

F. *Pleural surfaces*—costophrenic angles and interlobar fissures.
Abnormalities: tumor within the pleura, pleural thickening, medial deviation of pleural line (e.g., pneumothorax), dulled or obliterated costophrenic or cardiophrenic angles, fissure displacement or thickening.

G. *Mediastinum*—heart and great vessels. (Observe frontal and lateral projections.)
Abnormalities: mediastinal widening or shift, presence of silhouette signs, accentuated mediastinal curves (note which ones), *small heart* from lung hyperinflation, *enlarged heart* from pericardial effusion, cardiac dilatation, and hypertrophy; dextrocardia; tumor; calcifications.

H. *Hila*
Abnormalities: enlargement due to lymphadenopathy, tumor, pulmonary hypertension; *hilar clouding* from heart failure; bilaterally *small hila* from congenital heart disease; *increased density* from fluid, tumor, or calcifications.

I. *Lung fields*—compare both sides of the chest for general symmetry and equal roentgen density.

1. *Bronchovascular markings*—note absence, presence, paucity, prominence, haziness of borders, overall distribution, tapering towards lung periphery.
2. *Lung parenchyma*
   a. *Lesions*—cavities, bullae, confluent densities (check for air bronchogram and silhouette signs), air-fluid levels, linear markings (plate-like atelectasis, Kerley's lines), calcifications, and possible areas of lung collapse.
   b. *Roentgenographic pattern*—normal, interstitial, or alveolar pattern.

Table 15–11. RADIOLOGIC SIGNS OF MAIN CHEST DISEASES

Acute asthma	Signs of lung hyperinflation Bulging intercostal spaces Maintenance of normal caliber and tapering of peripheral bronchovascular markings Normal to small heart size
Atelectasis	Signs vary, ranging from a confluent density in the lung fields (lobar collapse) to plate-like atelectasis in the bases without other signs (subsegmental collapse). Signs of loss of volume, including narrowed intercostal spaces, diaphragmatic elevation, and mediastinal shift.
Cardiogenic left ventricular failure *Stage I*—pulmonary congestion	Distention of pulmonary veins (vascular markings) Redistribution of blood flow to upper lobes Blurring of the margins of pulmonary vessels Kerley's B lines may begin to appear in lung bases. Left ventricle may look enlarged.
Stage II—interstitial pulmonary edema	Interstitial pattern in lung fields Peribronchial cuffing, Kerley's B and A lines are rare. Vascular structures become more blurred. Costophrenic angles may become dulled or obliterated from pleural effusions. Right hemidiaphragm may be elevated from liver engorgement.
Stage III—alveolar pulmonary edema	Alveolar pattern in lung fields. Bat wing or butterfly appearance is diagnostic. Hilar clouding Air bronchogram signs Marked left ventricular enlargement
Chronic bronchitis	Increased bronchovascular markings ("dirty chest" appearance) with some signs of lung hyperinflation, enlarged hila from pulmonary hypertension, normal to enlarged heart, and *no bullae.* Some may have patterns similar to the arterial deficiency patterns of emphysematous patients.
Cor pulmonale	Signs of pulmonary hypertension Right ventricular enlargement
Cystic fibrosis	Signs of lung hyperinflation, increased bronchovascular markings, and enlarged hila from adenopathy. Peribronchial cuffing and reticular pattern; in some areas, cysts, or bullae. Other changes often include confluent densities (e.g., abscess, mucoid impaction) and loss of lung volume (atelectasis), particularly in the right upper lobe. Bronchogram shows cylindric and sometimes cystic bronchiectasis.
Diffuse interstial fibrosis	Interstitial pattern in lung fields Loss of lung volume may be present. Other signs depend on disease process involved.
Emphysema	Bullae Signs of lung hyperinflation called the arterial deficiency pattern when diffuse as in panlobular emphysema. Some patients may have an increased markings pattern similar to that of patients with chronic bronchitis. Signs may be localized or generalized.
Pleural effusion (greater than 350 ccs)	Area of increased density Blunted costophrenic angle Horizontal or meniscus-shaped fluid level Fluid in an interlobar fissure A lateral decubitus film may be ordered to differentiate pleural fluid from pneumonia.
Pneumonia	Alveolar pattern: confluent densities restricted to a lobe or segment (alveolar pneumonia) or patchy densities without a segmental or lobar distribution (bronchopneumonia) Air bronchogram Interstitial pattern (interstitial pneumonia) Look for a silhouette sign to help localize pathology.
Pneumothorax	Visceral pleura clearly visible within lung field. Absolute radiolucency between chest wall and visceral pleura; it increases in size on an expiratory film. Increased density of collapsed lung. In tension pneumothorax: invisible lung (100% collapse), signs of lung hyperinflation, and mediastinal shift towards the opposite lung.
Pulmonary hypertension	Distention of main, right, and left pulmonary arteries Abrupt tapering or "pruning" of hilar vessels Decreased bronchovascular markings in peripheral lung fields
Right ventricular failure	Normal lung fields Enlargement of azygos vein greater than 4 mm in diameter. This is normally invisible, or small vein sits in the shoulder of the trachea and right upper lobe bronchus. Enlargement of the right atrium, right ventricle, and superior vena cava may be present.

Conclusion

The chest roentgenogram is an important and sometimes crucial assessment parameter in comprehensive respiratory care. This chapter has covered basic radiologic concepts, logistics of taking an optimal portable chest x-ray film, and a systematic method for viewing a chest x-ray film.

Although this chapter has provided tools for making a basic interpretation of a chest x-ray, it does not describe how to gain skill and confidence in a final interpretation. (Making a final interpretation is beyond the scope of this text.) A final interpretation is best achieved by viewing numerous films in laboratory and clinical settings, where one can gradually develop a perception for normal and abnormal images. This chapter, hopefully, has provided an extensive knowledge base to facilitate the development of perception skills and the learning of interpretation skills during laboratory and clinical experiences.

REFERENCES

American Thoracic Society: Chest x-ray screening statements. *American thoracic society news,* 10(2):14, 1984.

Bein, M. E.: Approach to Chest Radiographic Interpretation. In Guide to Pulmonary Medicine (Tashkin, D. and Cassan, S., eds.). New York, Grune & Stratton, 1978.

Canobbio, M.: Chest x-ray film interpretation. *Focus on critical care,* 11(2):18–24, 1984.

Chen, J.: The Chest Roentgenogram. In The Heart, Arteries and Veins, 5th ed. (Hurst, J. W., ed.). New York, McGraw-Hill Book Co., 1982.

Conway, N.: An Atlas of Cardiology—Electrocardiograms and Chest X-rays. Chicago, Yearbook Medical Publishers, Inc., 1977.

Felson, B.: Chest Roentgenology. Philadelphia, W. B. Saunders Co., 1973.

Felson, B.: The chest roentgenologic workup—What and Why? Conventional methods. *Basics of respiratory disease,* 8:5, 1–5, 1980.

Felson, B., Weinstein, A., and Spitz, H.: Principles of Chest Roentgenology—A Programmed Text. Philadelphia, W. B. Saunders Co., 1965.

Fraser, R. G. and Paré, J. A.: Diagnosis of Diseases of the Chest, vol. I, 2nd ed. Philadelphia, W. B. Saunders Co., 1977.

Fraser, R. G. and Paré, J. A.: Diagnosis of Diseases of the Chest, Vol. II, 2nd ed. Philadelphia, W. B. Saunders Co., 1978.

Fraser, R. G. and Paré, J. A.: Diagnosis of Diseases of the Chest, vol. III, 2nd ed. Philadelphia, W. B. Saunders Co., 1979.

Griffiths, H. and Sarno, R.: Contemporary Radiology—An Introduction to Imaging. Philadelphia, W. B. Saunders Co., 1979.

Guenter, C. and Welch, M.: Pulmonary Medicine, 2nd ed. Philadelphia, J. B. Lippincott Co., 1982.

Herman, P. G.: The chest roentgenogram—its role in evaluating cardiomegaly and COPD. *Chest,* 71(6):689–690, 1977.

Keen, G.: Chest Injuries, 2nd ed. Bristol, England, John Wright & Sons, 1984.

Levy, R., Hawkins, H., and Barson, W.: Radiology in Emergency Medicine. St. Louis, C. V. Mosby Co., 1986.

Meschan, I.: Synopsis of Analysis of Roentgen Signs in General Radiology. Philadelphia, W. B. Saunders Co., 1976.

Netter, F.: The CIBA Collection of Medical Illustrations, vol. 5, Heart. New Jersey, CIBA Pharmaceutical Co., 1971.

Netter, F.: The CIBA Collection of Medical Illustrations, vol. 7, Respiratory System. New Jersey, CIBA Pharmaceutical Co., 1979.

Paré, J. A. and Fraser, R.: Synopsis of Diseases of the Chest. Philadelphia, W. B. Saunders Co., 1983.

Proto, A.: Conventional chest tomography. *Basics of respiratory disease,* 9(1):1–2, 1980.

Rau, J. and Pearce, D.: Understanding Chest Radiographs. Denver, Colorado, Multimedia Publishing, Inc., 1984.

Schapiro, R. L. and Musallam, J. J.: A radiologic approach to disorders involving the interstitium of the lung. *Heart and lung,* 6:4, 635–643, 1977.

Schooley, E.: An Introduction to X-rays of the Cardiopulmonary System (Learning module). Baltimore, Williams & Wilkins, 1976.

Shanks, S. C. and Kerley, P.: A Textbook of X-ray Diagnosis. Philadelphia, W. B. Saunders Co., 1972.

Squire, L. F.: Fundamentals of Radiology, 3rd ed. Cambridge, Massachusetts, Harvard University Press, 1982.

Squire, L. F., et al: Exercises in Diagnostic Radiology—Chest, Abdomen, Bone, and the Total Patient. Philadelphia, W. B. Saunders Co., 1981.

Teplick, J. and Haskin, M.: Roentgenologic Diagnosis, 3rd ed. Philadelphia, W. B. Saunders Co., 1976.

Tinker, J.: Understanding Chest X-rays. *American journal of nursing,* 76:1, 54–58, 1976.

Victor, L.: An Atlas of Critical Care Chest Roentgenology. Rockville, Maryland, Aspen Systems Corp., 1985.

Warwick, R. and Williams, P.: Gray's Anatomy (36th British Edition). Philadelphia, W. B. Saunders Co., 1980.

Patient Motivation

16

Main Objectives

1. **Name two main purposes and three indications for motivational assessment.**
2. **Describe the psychophysiologic effects of emotional *states of action* and *states of nonaction* in pulmonary patients.**
3. **Name the three psychologic coping mechanisms of COPD patients.**
4. **Define and discuss at least two theories of motivation including clinical applications of major concepts.**
5. **Name at least four features of noncompliant patients based on the Health Belief Model (HBM) of health behavior.**
6. **List four appropriate times for motivational assessment and intervention.**
7. **Name the four components of the motivational model presented in this chapter, then describe how to use the model for assessment and intervention in the clinical setting.**
8. **Identify the causes and signs of burnout in pulmonary nurses. Discuss four ways to prevent its occurrence or reduce its incidence.**

It is not unusual for the patient with chronic pulmonary disease to demonstrate a lack of motivation to participate in respiratory care. His overtly unappreciative behavior, anger, depression, or anxiety limits his capacity to develop motivation. When he refuses care or continually blocks efforts to involve him in self care, the nurse and others may become frustrated and label the patient as "difficult" or "noncompliant." Both family and staff wonder what to do about the patient's lack of motivation.

This chapter describes the motivational states of respiratory patients, motivational theory, and a motivational model for helping the patient to develop this needed motivation. It assumes that motivation is developed primarily from within and cannot be instilled extrinsically by a health professional, whose goal is to give prescribed treatments or follow a predetermined plan of care. Because facilitation of the motivational process is emotionally and physically draining for nurses who constantly work with respiratory patients, the problem of "burnout" is briefly addressed at the end of the chapter.

Importance of Motivational Assessment

Motivational assessment is important for four reasons. First, since behavior is always motivated in some way, psychosocial and physiologic problems must be analyzed within the context of the patient's motivational state.

Second, the recent incorporation of self-care concepts into nursing theoretic frameworks has placed more emphasis on the role of motivation in the nursing process. In Orem's self-care model, motivation in addition to knowledge and skill is a key factor in the practice of self care (Joseph, 1980).

Third, motivation is regarded as basic in the rehabilitation of respiratory patients, especially those with chronic obstructive pulmonary disease (COPD). Studies have shown that overall improvement in a patient's condition is associated with high levels of morale and motivation (Rosillo et al, 1971). The nurse coordinating a rehabilitation program routinely assesses motivation because it is a criterion for admission into the program. Nurses in acute and extended care settings are looking increasingly at motivational assessment because pulmonary rehabilitation is no longer restricted to the ambulatory setting. Patient education and self-care strategies are gradually introduced during recovery from acute illness when the patient indicates physical and psychologic readiness to learn.

Fourth, motivational assessment is important because it helps the nurse focus on key subjective information and motivational factors that affect patient goals, alternatives, and outcomes. This approach keeps the focus on the patient rather than on the staff and their frustrations and beliefs about what the patient needs based solely on consideration of objective data and medical diagnosis.

Purposes and Indications

The main purposes of motivational assessment are as follows:

1. To identify intrinsic motivational factors within the patient and extrinsic motivational factors outside the patient that promote or hinder health-seeking behavior.
2. To facilitate the motivational process so that the patient wants to and is able to participate in respiratory care.

Certain types of patients benefit more than other patients from motivational assessment, as it is presented in this chapter. Those who demonstrate many of the characteristics of an unmotivated patient are candidates for a thorough motivational assessment (Table 16–1). Moreover, with an acute exacerbation of a disease process, these characteristics may become more prominent. For example, the patient with a low energy level at home may regress to a passive dependent role in the hospital, even after the acute illness has stabilized. Similarly, the patient who has difficulty solving problems at home may become less evaluative and more unrealistic in the acute care setting. These regressive behaviors may normally occur in those with respiratory failure, congestive heart failure, alkalosis, acidosis, and other conditions that interfere with brain functioning, orientation, mood stability, impulse control, perception, and level of consciousness (Strain, 1978). These behaviors are adaptive when they facilitate physical recovery from the acute episode, e.g., the patient in the passive dependent role conserves energy for the work of breathing. Once the acute illness has stabilized, however, regressive behaviors hinder rehabilitative care.

In addition, motivational assessment is indicated for patients with numerous psychosocial problems or few *psychosocial assets*, defined as qualities or conditions that promote health-seeking behavior, such as high

Table 16–1. CHARACTERISTICS OF MOTIVATED VERSUS UNMOTIVATED PATIENTS

Motivated Patients	Unmotivated Patients
High expectations	Low expectations
Goal-oriented behavior	Lack of personal goals
High level of interactions with environment	Low level of interactions with environment
High energy level	Low energy level
Desire for personal growth and a full life	No desire for personal growth or change May see no hope
High level of awareness and perception	Unaware of alternatives; may see self as subject to fate
May have high cognitive capacities	May have strong beliefs or traditions contradicting proposed health-seeking behavior
Few, if any, psychosocial problems	Psychosocial problems often present, e.g., hostility, anxiety, depression, denial, social isolation

self esteem, adaptability, a strong support system, and so on. The patient with few psychosocial assets is less likely to cope effectively with pulmonary disease than the motivated patient with many psychosocial assets. The former type of patient requires a thorough assessment with input from the physician, social worker, and psychologist to determine the nature and extent of problems and the potential for rehabilitation.

Furthermore, motivational assessment helps the nurse identify and analyze *noncompliance*, defined as patient nonadherence to prescribed preventive and curative treatments. Low compliance rates have been well documented in ambulatory patients. Windsor and coworkers (1980) reviewed the literature and reported that failure to take prescribed medications may occur among 25 to 50% of persons with chronic disease. Becker and Maiman (1975) report that at least one third of the patient population in most studies fails to follow physician recommendations. Noncompliance may be in excess of 60% in low-income clinic populations. To complicate matters, physicians are known to underestimate patient noncompliance (Windsor et al, 1980), and some patients may not realize they are not complying with therapy, owing to ignorance or misunderstanding about instructions. Although no studies have been done specifically on respiratory patients, noncompliance levels may be higher for COPD and asthmatic patients than for those with other medical diagnoses. COPD and asthma are the most commonly reported medical problems in the United States. The 1975–1976 National Ambulatory Medical Care Survey reported that respiratory disease constituted 14% of all office visits to physicians during that 2-year period. Most of the complaints represented new rather than continuing problems.

Motivational States of Respiratory Patients

The basic concepts of pulmonary psychophysiology in this section of the chapter represent one way of explaining the motivational states of respiratory patients, specifically COPD patients and others with moderate to severe pulmonary disease.

In moderate to severe COPD, psychologic or emotional *states of action*, such as anxiety, anger, or excitement, are associated with increased energy expenditure, elevated lung ventilation, high oxygen consumption, and skeletal muscle tension.

Question: *What happens when the COPD patient with compromised ventilatory function becomes anxious, angry, or overly excited about some event?*

Answer: His respiratory rate goes up, but, owing to limited ventilatory reserves, he cannot adequately increase lung ventilation and oxygen supply to meet the increased psychologic and physiologic demands of the body. With increased work of breathing and increased oxygen consumption, Pa_{O_2} goes down, and Pa_{CO_2} climbs upward. The worsening arterial blood gases (ABGs) are accompanied by uncomfortable symptoms, such as increasing dyspnea, cough, and mucus production. Brief episodes of anxiety or anger may precipitate acute dyspnea and a panic reaction. A persisting state of action may cause acute ventilatory failure and hypoxemia.

In comparison, psychologic or emotional *states of nonaction*, such as apathy, depression, sadness, and deep relaxation, are associated with reduced energy expenditure, decreased lung ventilation, low oxygen consumption, and skeletal muscle relaxation.

Question: *What happens when the COPD patient becomes depressed?*

Answer: He reduces physical activity and breathes very shallowly and more slowly. This hypoventilation causes a decreased Pa_{O_2} and an elevated Pa_{CO_2}. The decreased lung ventilation is greater than the reduction in body metabolism. Over days and weeks, ABGs may gradually worsen until the patient goes into chronic ventilatory failure.

In both the action and nonaction patterns, the basic physiologic defect relates to the pulmonary system's inability to supply O_2 and remove CO_2. The appearance of dyspnea tends to produce more psychologic reactions (e.g., anxiety, fear of suffocation, depression), which in turn worsen ABGs and lead to physical decompensation. In Figure 16–1, note how emotional reactions to dyspnea aggravate symptoms and create a vicious circle of events. In this circle, past experience in controlling dyspnea and coping with psychosocial problems largely determines the nature and extent of emotional reactions and worsening of pulmonary symptoms.

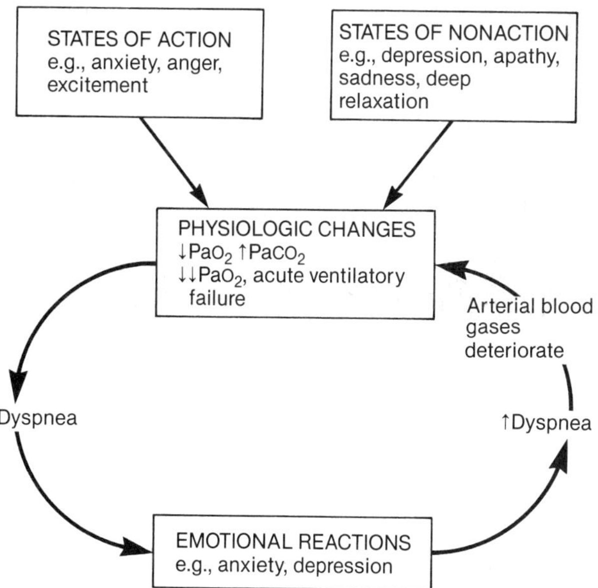

Figure 16–1. Pulmonary psychophysiologic consequences of states of action and nonaction.

PSYCHOLOGIC COPING MECHANISMS

The patient copes with states of action and nonaction by being in what Dudley and associates (1973) call an emotional "straightjacket." The patient avoids emotional reactions because they may lead to pulmonary symptoms and physical decompensation. Furthermore, both physical and psychologic sensory inputs are typically dealt with through one or more of the following coping mechanisms: isolation, depression, denial, and repression.

Isolation and Depression. The patient tends to isolate himself from others physically and socially. To avoid psychologic stimulation, he rarely leaves the house or exposes himself to situations where he might learn to control emotional reactions and accompanying dyspnea. The increasing pulmonary symptoms may cause him to revert to a passive approach or complete avoidance of sexual activity. All of these behaviors perpetuate existing emotional and interpersonal problems among family members. Also, they may prevent the patient from developing a support system outside the home. When increasing anger, frustration, and despair lead to hopelessness, the patient reverts to a dependent role in the family, even though he could lead a more active life if he were to participate more in his own care.

Self-imposed social isolation is a sign of depression, especially when accompanied by verbal or nonverbal expressions of helplessness and hopelessness. The prevalence of depression in moderate to severe COPD patients is about 50% (Light et al, 1985).

Denial and Repression. These two coping mechanisms are so interrelated that they may be impossible to differentiate. In general, the patient cannot face the truth about his diagnosis, express his fears or feelings, or deal with his interpersonal conflicts without risking acute exacerbation of the disease process. The patient may repeatedly insist, "Everything is fine," regardless of his physical state. This behavior represents denial; the patient refuses to recognize worsening pulmonary symptoms. It also represents repression when the patient recognizes symptoms and feelings but suppresses them for fear of alienating the key staff and family members whom he depends upon for respiratory care. In other situations, the patient may deny pulmonary symptoms but become preoccupied with minor somatic complaints related to other systems. He may become defensive, superficial, or labile in emotional response. With end-stage disease, the patient may unrealistically expect and even demand a cure for his illness, while gradually becoming more debilitated and dependent. The patient with few psychosocial assets may use denial to the very end and refuse to talk about death with close family members, physicians, or pulmonary nurses who have coordinated his respiratory care over the past years.

DECREASED ABILITY TO LEARN

When the patient resorts to the previously mentioned psychologic coping mechanisms, altered perceptions and limited interactions with family friends and health professionals contribute to a limited ability to learn. Perception is altered because of the patient's way of processing information. He methodically conceives (i.e., takes into one's mind) information. However, he may not perceive (i.e., understand and become aware of) key concepts for personal application.

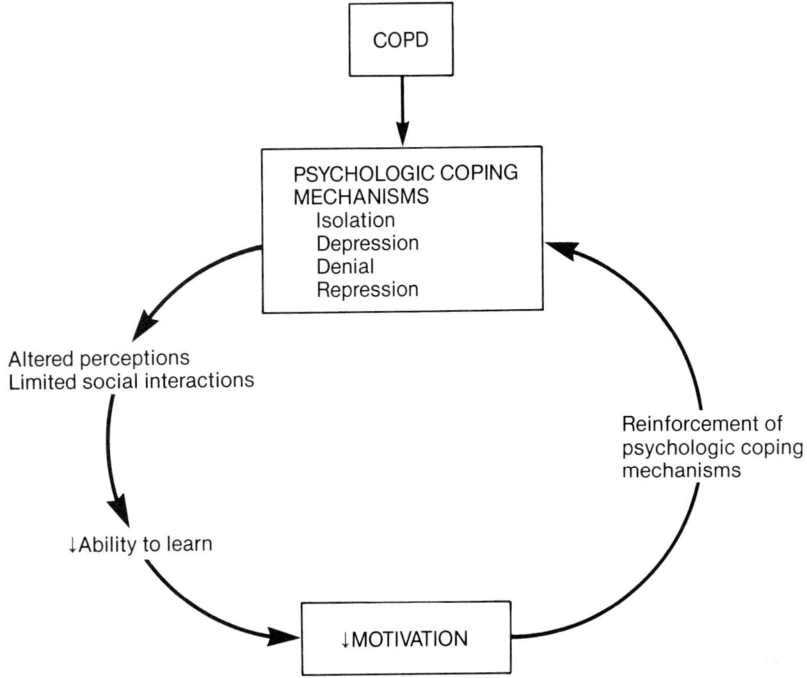

Figure 16–2. Effects of psychologic coping mechanisms in chronic obstructive pulmonary disease (COPD).

Even when he verbally agrees to participate in a teaching-learning situation, he tends to avoid energy-consuming problem-solving activities that may increase the risk of intrapersonal and interpersonal conflict. Hence, though the patient has access to health information and support persons, he limits interactions with those who might help him learn. When interactions do occur, he either disregards key information or selectively processes information to reinforce his psychologic coping mechanisms. The resulting decrease in motivation reinforces the isolation, depression, denial, and repression, as shown diagrammatically in Figure 16–2. This cycle of events accelerates when brain hypoxia and vasodilatation from a high $PaCO_2$ alter brain functioning and limit perception.

HOSPITAL SETTING

Admission to the hospital often precipitates a change in the patient's motivational state, making him more willing to participate in respiratory care. In many situations, fright and fear of suffocation associated with acute dyspnea force him to reconsider the seriousness of his illness and the need for rehabilitative care. In other cases, the recalcitrant home patient becomes exceedingly cooperative in the hospital, where his compliant behavior is rewarded by continual attention by a highly accessible staff. In addition, the family, relieved of the burden of caring for the disabled patient, is often more willing and able to examine coping patterns that promote or hinder health-seeking behavior.

In the acute care setting, motivation and cooperation may wax and wane with the patient's physical state. When the patient is in an unstable respiratory state, motivation is low, as frequent respiratory treatments, medication administrations, and vital sign assessments interrupt sleep and overfatigue the patient. Unless the patient receives continual psychologic support and interventions are grouped at intervals to facilitate undisturbed sleep, the patient may consider his state hopeless and may physically decompensate.

Perhaps the most common and challenging encounter with the unmotivated, acutely ill COPD patient pertains to the gradual weaning from mechanical ventilation. Weaning is a threatening event for the patient because it represents the loss of full emotional expression and the loss of a sense of well being. Consider the patient's predicament; for years, he adapted to chronic pulmonary disease and abnormal ABGs by living in the previously described emotional straightjacket. Once intubated and ventilated by a respirator, energy previously exerted in the work of breathing is channelled toward full emotional expression. Breathing is accomplished with less energy and without the threat of decompensation. The patient feels better psychologically and physically.

With the gradual withdrawal of mechanical support, more and more energy is again channelled towards the work of breathing, leaving less energy for social interactions and other activities. As PaO_2 decreases and $PaCO_2$ slightly increases, the patient may become angry and frustrated with the accompanying loss of full emotional expression and decreased sense of well being. He may become violent and demand to be reattached to the ventilator, thus eliminating the threat of decompensation. Helplessness may prevail until ABGs stabilize, and the weaning process is complete. The patient once again adapts to the emotional straightjacket of chronic pulmonary disease, as shown in Figure 16–3.

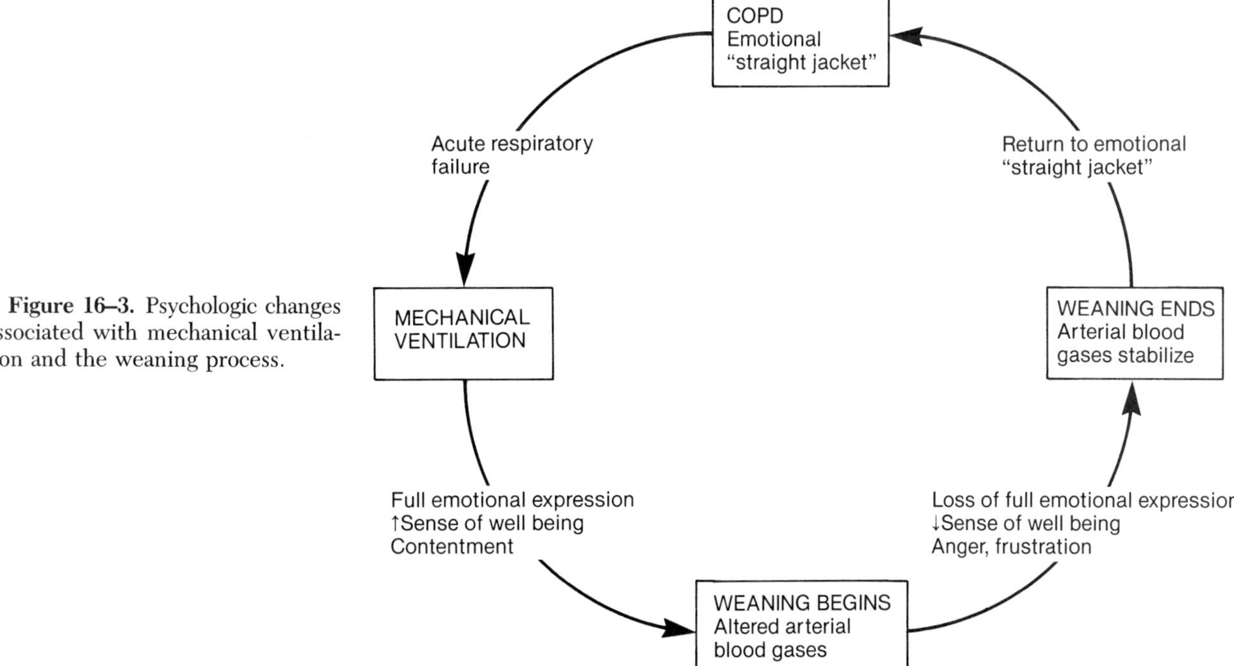

Figure 16–3. Psychologic changes associated with mechanical ventilation and the weaning process.

RESPECT FOR PSYCHOLOGIC COPING MECHANISMS

Throughout motivational assessment, it is essential that the COPD patient's psychologic coping mechanisms be respected and even protected until intervention becomes appropriate. As the previous discussion points out, there is a physiologic basis for these coping mechanisms. The isolation, denial, and repression represent the patient's only ways of limiting sensory inputs, maintaining stable ABGs, and preventing feared pulmonary symptoms.

During acute illness, respect for coping mechanisms involves encouraging the patient to freely verbalize feelings, concerns, and fears. The nurse who is in near constant attendance at the bedside may be overwhelmed with the task of listening to an anxious, angry patient, while seeing to his physical care needs. Chapter 28 discusses how to give psychologic support to the patient during the stages of weaning from mechanical ventilation. The motivational model discussed subsequently explains how to approach the patient.

Motivational Theory with Clinical Applications

This section of the chapter discusses motivational theory with clinical applications; the theory base for the motivational model is discussed in the next section.

Because motivation is an internal experience that cannot be studied directly, there are many theories of motivation today. None empirically defines the motivational process, but some, particularly the stimulus-response learning theory from which behavioral theory is derived, are useful in predicting health-related behavior and levels of therapy compliance. Many theories emphasize the importance of personal awareness and personal goals in the development of motivation.

PERSONAL AWARENESS

According to Vernon (1969), motivation involves awareness and prompt reaction to particular features in the environment, i.e., it requires an environmental stimulus.

In the case of the COPD patient, environmental stimulus is key because his defense mechanisms serve to limit his personal awareness and consideration of change. Until the patient successfully tries self-care strategies on his own, family, friends, community support persons, and health professionals are necessary to influence his perceptions of sensory inputs and provide support throughout the rehabilitative process.

The role of health professionals is especially important. Windsor and colleagues (1980) report that the physician's ". . . success in motivating patient behavior has been found to be strongly associated with the effort, client orientation, and empathy of the physician toward his or her client." Habenger and coworkers (1971) documented the COPD patient's psychologic disabilities and stated that motivation provided by an aggressive team is the major component in rehabilitation.

The problem facing the rehabilitation team is how to increase the COPD patient's personal awareness about his condition and the effects of treatment when he often imperceptibly becomes what he is by drifting into a set behavior pattern. To increase awareness of his present state, it is helpful to ask the patient to review the course of his disease, with special emphasis on health habits; related beliefs, attitudes, and feelings; and what he considers to be effective and ineffective coping behaviors. If time permits, much of this subjective data can be gathered during the nursing history. In any case, refined communications skills plus allotment of ample time for exploration are required so that the patient will feel comfortable verbalizing these feelings. Past experiences are contrasted with present ones so that the patient becomes personally aware of the ramifications of his present condition and can see progress from day to day, week to week, or month to month.

During the review of past experiences, the patient frequently asks the nurse questions. Sometimes misconceptions about his disease and its treatment arise. For example, the patient may think that all pulmonary medications are "no good" because his beclomethasone inhaler never effectively reduced acute dyspnea. Misconceptions are clarified by providing information, e.g., the patient is told that beclomethasone prevents dyspnea but cannot reduce dyspnea once it occurs. In this case, the altered personal awareness facilitates the motivational process and the teaching of new ways to control acute dyspnea.

Confrontation may be necessary, if the review of past experiences does not provide an opportunity to alter awareness. *Confrontation* is defined as *directing the patient's attention to the bare factual content of his actions or statements or to a coincidence which he has perceived but has not, or professes not to have, registered* (Devereux, 1951). Confrontation is a manipulation of attention; it consolidates content in past conversations and stimulates new insights. However, confrontation must be used cautiously. The decision to confront the patient with facts depends upon the following two factors (Johnson, 1981):

1. *The quality of the nurse's relationship with the patient.* A strong relationship based on trust favors confrontation. When the nurse has had brief contact with the patient and family, confrontation is less effective and sometimes inappropriate until a later time when the relationship is stronger.

2. *The perceived ability of the patient to act upon the confrontation.* Confrontation is eliminated or the strength of wording decreased when the patient is anxious or physically unstable, and his capacity to perceive and act on the confrontation is limited. For

example, consider the patient who decided to start smoking again after failing his employee physical examination and losing his job. Upon hospital admission, the nurse decides to wait until his episode of acute asthmatic bronchitis stabilizes before confronting the patient with the problem of smoking. In this and other situations, the nurse may direct health teaching primarily to supportive family members until the patient's psychologic and physiologic condition improves, and the threat of physical decompensation is lessened.

PERSONAL GOALS

Lazarus (1966) defines motivation as the psychologic representation of goals and routes to goals. If goals are important, the person has strong motivation to attain them, whereas weaker goals are sacrificed.

Setting and maintaining goals are perhaps the most crucial aspects of the motivational process. It is not unusual for a patient with severe COPD to be aware of his condition but have no personal goals when asked about them in an interview situation. The inability to even imagine the future is understandable in light of his defense mechanisms, his more frequent state of being out of touch with his body and thinking, the irreversibility of his disease, and his periodic fears of suffocation and death.

Motivation develops and is sustained when the patient identifies personal goals. These goals, whether they relate directly to respiratory care or to other aspects of life, such as completing a project or going to the movies once a week, must be encouraged and incorporated into the overall care plan.

Lack of motivation develops when personal goals are absent or unrealistic or when patient and staff do not agree on at least one mutually satisfying goal.

Absence of Goals

The following factors may account for the absence of personal goals:

1. Despair and hopelessness due to the disabling nature of pulmonary disease.
2. Lack of knowledge regarding the disease process and potential for improvement.
3. Focus on long-term rather than easily attainable short-term goals.
4. Repeated failures with prescribed treatments.
5. Absence of positive reinforcement for health-seeking behaviors.
6. Inability to imagine an improved respiratory status.

In spite of counseling and patient education, the patient may still demonstrate difficulty in goal setting. Application of May's theory of motivation (1969) may help the patient begin to think about the future and a possible goal. In May's theory, wish leads to will and eventually decision and responsibility, as shown.

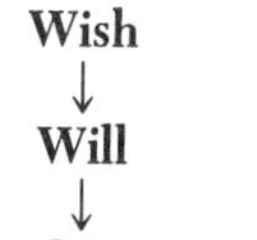

Decision and Responsibility

Wish is the imaginative playing with the possibility of some act occurring. The patient is asked to disregard beliefs about what he perceives he is capable of accomplishing. He is instructed to relate how he wishes he could feel. His response—usually relating to the reduction in dyspnea or other symptom—serves as a starting point for discussion.

Will is more concrete. It pertains to a definite intent to accomplish some act. Will may be developed by providing information, clarifying misconceptions, and encouraging the patient to set short-term goals that are more likely to guarantee success and avoid feelings of despair and hopelessness. Successful experiences reinforce health-seeking behavior. The greater the success, the more the patient raises his aspiration level.

The *decision and responsibility* for health-seeking behavior lie with the patient and not the health professional. These qualities may be strengthened by helping the patient work towards a goal. In some cases, however, the patient goes only as far as wishing he were in a better physical condition. Faced with a terminal illness and totally convinced of the impossibility of feeling better, he remains unable to identify a personal goal. In this case, the nurse may counsel the patient in one of two ways. First, the patient may be encouraged to maintain the status quo to accomplish some outside goal, such as seeing a grandchild graduate from high school or an elderly spouse die gracefully. Such extrinsic motivators may effectively carry the patient through an acute illness. Yet, particularly in the home situation, once the goal is achieved (e.g., the grandchild finally graduates or the spouse dies), the patient may once again lose hope and physically decompensate, often to the point of death.

Another way to develop will and decision and responsibility is to suggest a goal for the patient. Ask him to at least temporarily work towards it. After a trial period, the patient evaluates positive and negative effects and decides whether he wishes to continue the plan of care.

Unrealistic Goals

COPD patients exhibiting denial and repression often develop unrealistic goals. For example, the patient may constantly verbalize his intention of flying to a vacation resort as soon as his condition improves, even though the physician counsels against such travel, owing to the adverse effects of high altitude. The patient may insist on signing himself out of the hospital against medical advice because he "feels fine."

Unrealistic goals may appear during acute exacerbations of chest disease and disappear with stabilization. Sometimes they signal the appearance of *conflict motivation,* which occurs when two or more incompatible types of motivated behavior that cannot be pursued simultaneously exist. The inhibitory tendencies of dependency and isolation are in opposition to positive though sometimes unrealistic efforts to improve health. In these cases, the nurse reinforces any health-seeking behavior, such as taking a walk every day. Unrealistic goals are recognized without negation or reinforcement. Attention is directed towards more realistic short-term goals, such as walking a half block rather than a mile per day. Emphasis is placed on symptomatic improvement and the ability to carry out activities of daily living rather than on pulmonary function improvement. Symptomatic improvement may be possible even when objective pulmonary function test (PFT) measurements continue to deteriorate over the years.

Lack of a Mutually Satisfying Goal

Because of the multitude and complexity of problems or the patient's lack of goals, the health care team may tend to establish goals without consulting the patient. Sometimes, unless care is carefully coordinated, the patient, physician, nurse, and respiratory therapist will all have different and incongruent goals. This fragmentation reinforces the patient's lack of motivation.

Ideally, the health care team collaborates with the patient and among themselves to set goals based on the patient's priority of needs (see the next section). All those concerned agree on at least one mutually satisfying goal that is truly acceptable to both staff and patient. A team conference with the patient facilitates this process. For clarity, the patient's goal may be stated in his own words and referred to repeatedly during respiratory care. Staff may set other goals to measure and insure progress, but these goals must never conflict with the patient's goals. Over time, goals are modified according to changing patient needs and reactions to therapy.

In applying the concept of setting a mutually satisfying goal, the nurse must remember that this type of goal does not represent compromise. In compromise, each party settles for something less than what is desired. Value systems do not change. An example of compromise is the nurse who bargains with the difficult patient in the following manner. The nurse insists that the patient practice breathing exercises to strengthen the diaphragm and promote optimal alveolar ventilation. The patient obstinately refuses to do so, explaining that he would rather sit in a chair for 10 minutes. Out of frustration, the nurse reluctantly agrees to this plan, thinking that the sitting position would provide at least some increase in alveolar ventilation. The agreement represents compromise, because the nurse still believes in the more optimal value of breathing exercises for this patient and would not consider the possibility that the act of sitting in a chair may be more acceptable and ultimately more beneficial than infrequently practiced breathing exercises. Sitting in a chair becomes a mutually satisfying goal when value systems change and both nurse and patient truly believe that sitting in a chair is best in the given circumstance.

DOMINANCE OF PHYSIOLOGIC NEEDS

Maslow (1970) relates motivation to basic needs. These needs form a hierarchy or pyramid of relative *potency* or priority, with basic physiologic needs at the bottom and nonphysiologic needs, such as self-actualization and aesthetic needs, at the top, as shown in Figure 16–4. According to Maslow, physiologic needs, such as food and the avoidance of dyspnea, play a dominant role in motivating behavior. Higher level needs do not become primary motivators until lower level needs are met.

The COPD patient with abnormal ABGs is primarily motivated by physiologic needs. Preoccupation with breathing stifles the emergence of behaviors motivated by higher needs. Until dyspnea is relieved and even seemingly minor somatic complaints are addressed, the patient is likely to remain unmotivated to set goals related to higher level needs.

Timing of Assessment and Intervention

When is the patient's physical state stable enough to permit discussion of higher level needs? When should the nurse discuss motivational matters and help the patient become aware of his emotional and physiologic responses to illness? The anxious and tense patient may never appear ready to discuss such matters. Sometimes breathing retraining in conjunction with relaxation therapy, such as progressive relaxation or relaxation with biofeedback techniques, adequately prepares the patient for motivational assessment and intervention. Relaxation helps the patient identify and reduce body tension, thus promoting easier breathing, fuller expression of feelings, and retention of information.

For most patients, the best times for motivational assessment and intervention are as follows:

1. *After a frightening episode of dyspnea* or whenever the patient expresses a desire to discuss his situation.
2. *When ABGs and lung sounds have returned to near normal.* At this time, the patient is more willing and able to discuss old behaviors and learn new ones.
3. *Before weaning from mechanical ventilation.* Since mechanical ventilation permits full emotional expression, the patient may freely express anxieties, concerns, and anger built up from past experiences. This content is a good starting point for further discussions.
4. *After successful weaning and before hospital discharge.* Waiting too long may limit the nurse's capi-

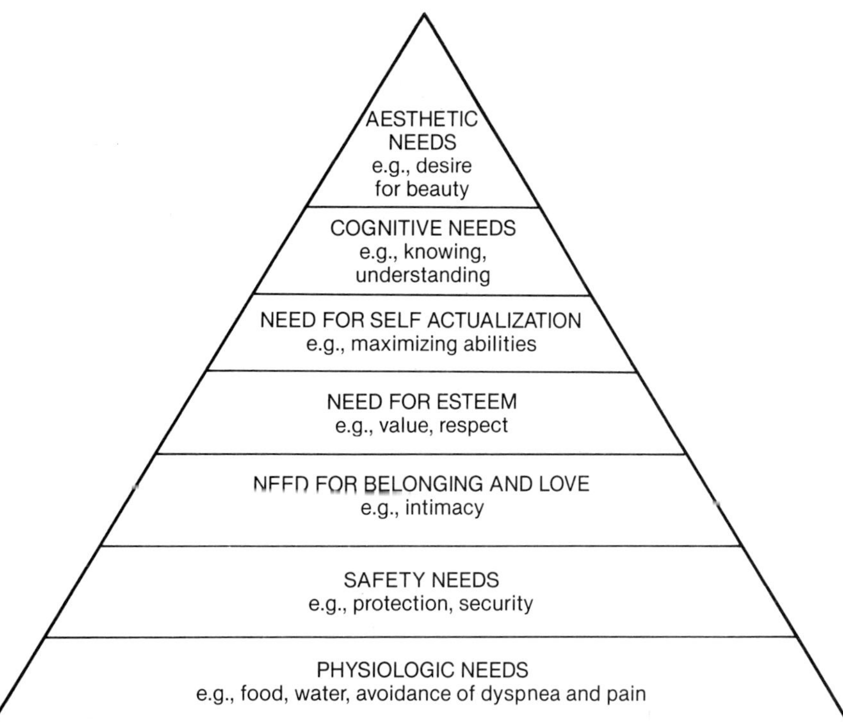

Figure 16–4. Maslow's hierarchy of basic human needs.

talizing on recent experiences and eliminate a deficit motive (described subsequently).

TENSION REDUCTION AND GROWTH THEORIES

Many theories assume that motivation—all excitation, all striving, and all tension—develops from a disturbance of organic equilibrium. Some theories emphasize the negative pole of affect, e.g., avoidance of dyspnea and chest discomfort. Some emphasize the positive pole, e.g., attainment of pleasant feelings. Freud maintained that all instincts make the individual strive for pleasure. For example, the respiratory patient on mechanical ventilation may be motivated either by the desire to avoid dyspnea or the reluctance to give up a sense of well being.

Allport (1955) expanded upon this equilibrium concept to say: yes, the individual strives for stability, but he also wants variety. He described two types of motives: deficit and growth. *Deficit motives* call for the reduction of tension and the restoration of equilibrium. For example, the patient may strive to eliminate dyspnea because it interferes with social interaction. The loss of social interaction is the deficit motive. Once the goal of relief of dyspnea is attained, the patient remains in equilibrium until internal tension creates the desire to set new goals. These *growth motives* generate discrepancies between the present (e.g., feeling good) and possible future (e.g., feeling even better). Though the deficit motive represents a negative approach and the growth motive a positive approach, both types generate discrepancies. Both types motivate behavior by producing a drive toward tension reduction. Hence, this theory is called the *tension reduction theory* of motivation.

In COPD, deficit motives initiate behaviors when disability or acute illness limits opportunities for personal enrichment. Growth motives appear after disease stabilization but may again disappear, when the patient overreacts depressively to minor setbacks.

COMPLEXITY OF THE MOTIVATIONAL PROCESS

Many motivators contribute to the patient's motivational state. Emotional-affective response, need, desire for growth, and tendency towards equilibrium suggest a host of social, psychologic, and physiologic factors, such as interests, sentiments, personality structure, physical state, and family ties. Because no one factor is responsible for altering perception, personal awareness, and subsequent behavior, a holistic approach to the patient is required.

The dynamic nature of the motivational process contributes to its complexity. Depending on the patient's living situation and physical and emotional state, what motivates him one day may have little effect the next day. This is especially true of acutely ill patients as well as ambulatory COPD patients with stable but moderate to severe disease, who normally vacillate between feeling "good" and feeling "bad." With ambulatory COPD patients, good and bad days may not correlate with physical state or any identifiable factor.

Ambulatory care nurses routinely perform *perceptual checks*, i.e., they elicit subjective data to differentiate good and bad days before deciding exactly what nursing interventions are appropriate and how they are best carried out. Some days the COPD patient lacks energy and motivation to cooperate with any activity. If possible, the nurse reserves all energy-consuming, teaching-learning situations for good days.

Long Motivational Process

Because of its complexity, the motivational process takes time. The nurse in the acute care setting may not see any change in the patient's desire and ability to practice self-care strategies. It may take months or years before the patient believes that he must stop smoking. It may take repeated hospitalizations before the patient indicates readiness to take pulmonary medications. Rarely does one intervention have a lasting impact on health behavior. Multiple reinforced interventions over time are required, especially for the multiproblem COPD patient with a complicated treatment regimen. Follow-up care by a visiting nurse trained in psychologic and physiologic aspects of COPD becomes crucial in sustaining patient and family motivation to continue health-seeking behavior after acute hospitalization.

Need for Continuity of Care

Because of the complex and often slowed motivational process in COPD patients in general, it is most advantageous to have one nurse designated as the primary nurse responsible for working with the patient. Once a relationship based on trust is developed, the nurse is more likely to successfully help the patient cope with disease. Few, if any, respiratory patients with the psychologic coping mechanisms of isolation, denial, and repression are willing to reveal life experiences of innermost feelings surrounding illness to more than one or two health professionals. Furthermore, if all disciplines make an effort to avoid changing personnel in the middle of a patient's treatment, then the patient is more likely to receive appropriate and continuous verbal reinforcement, emphasizing the same teaching-learning pointers. Uniform and constant reinforcement, especially during fear-provoking episodes of dyspnea, is key to alteration of awareness enough to motivate the patient to successfully try and repeat desired behavior.

HEALTH BELIEF MODEL (HBM)

This model explains and predicts health behavior. Motivation is defined as ". . . differential emotional arousal in individuals caused by some given class of stimuli (e.g., health matters)" (Becker and Maiman, 1975). It is seen as the "push" factor in compliance. Although the HBM does not fully explain the motivational process, it identifies important variables that hinder or enhance compliance. Based on these variables, Table 16–2 presents the main features of noncompliant patients with examples pertaining to respiratory patients. (Note that Table 16–2 is only a *guide* to understanding noncompliance in respiratory patients; research has yet to validate identified features for respiratory populations.) The presence of one or more of the listed features indicates a possible or potential noncompliance problem.

According to the HBM, patient perceptions of personal vulnerability to disease play key roles in shaping behavior. A patient is more likely to comply with therapy when perceived benefits of preventive action outweigh perceived barriers (see Table 16–2). A stimulus is required to trigger appropriate health behavior; it may be internal (e.g., perceptions of bodily states) or external (e.g., mass media communications, patient education material, advice from others). However, Becker and Maiman (1975) explain that "While it is assumed that diverse demographic, personality, structural, and social factors can, in any given instance, affect an individual's health motivations and perceptions, these variables are not seen as directly causal of compliance."

This model is helpful because it indicates what perceptions are important in motivational assessment and intervention. Once the nurse helps identify perceived benefits and barriers to health behavior, interventions are planned to reinforce benefits and reduce barriers.

Motivational Model for Assessment and Intervention

The model presented subsequently is a modification of one developed by Craig and Craig (1979). It is not meant to help assess all motivational factors in an individual; rather, it is meant as a general theoretic framework for assessment and intervention. In the case of the unmotivated or "difficult" patient, it helps the nurse identify and work with the motivational properties from the patient's awareness context rather than from a medical or nursing context. Because of the large time investment necessary to fully implement the model, it is best used in situations where the nurse has prolonged contact with the patient. Otherwise, it can be utilized to more thoroughly gather subjective data that relate to top priority nursing diagnoses and noncompliance problems. In any case, use of the model almost obligates the nurse to remain involved with the patient. During assessment, misconceptions or lack of knowledge invariably become evident and usually require teaching-learning follow-up. Also, the patient may react emotionally to specific content in the discussion or express feelings of hopelessness and helplessness that require intervention.

Table 16–2. MAIN FEATURES OF NONCOMPLIANT RESPIRATORY PATIENTS*

Feature	Example	Interventions
Denial of personal susceptibility to disease	Patient does not believe in accuracy of diagnosis or has erroneous health beliefs.	Acknowledge and fully explore circumstances. Determine whether beliefs are based on facts or distorted perceptions.
Disbelief of likelihood of recurrence of illness	Patient discontinues medications because he says he feels better already.	Determine whether behavior is due to lack of knowledge or inability to administer proper dosage or whether it represents a psychologic coping mechanism. Point out consequences of behavior and ask patient to reconsider actions.
Low level of perceived severity of disease	Patient claims he is asymptomatic.	Ask family members to comment on presence of symptoms. Check physician's notes, PFTs, and ABGs for objective proof of severity of disease; if discrepancies exist, consult with physician.
Extremely ***high*** level of perceived severity of disease with fear of consequences	Symptomatic patient knows he has a terminal illness and is afraid of becoming a "respiratory cripple."	Encourage verbalization of fears. Ask physician to counsel patient regarding disease process and anticipated levels of subjective and objective improvement. Clarify misunderstandings about disease and treatment. Emphasize positive aspects.
Low level of perceived effectiveness of proposed therapy	Patient discontinues postural drainage at home because he says "it doesn't do any good. A hot shower is more effective."	Acknowledge and fully explore reasons for belief. Monitor physical status, especially lung sounds, to determine level of physical improvement. Assess merits of proposed and alternative therapies. Consult physician.
Presence of perceived barriers to implementation of proposed therapy		
Questionable safety of treatment	Patient refuses to take influenzal or pneumococcal vaccine for fear of adverse side effects.	Clarify any misconceptions regarding vaccine. Respect patient's decision and consult physician.
Excessive costs	For hospital care, home care follow-up, and respiratory equipment	Consult physician and involve social worker to assess financial problems and respiratory therapist to order appropriate cost-effective respiratory equipment for home use.
Fear of discomfort or pain	Patient refuses to walk outside for fear of uncontrollable dyspnea.	Encourage verbalization of feelings. Help patient set a mutually agreed upon, realistic, and easily attainable goal. Repeat activity *with* patient until mastered.
Nature of therapy		
Complex regimen	QID and BID medications with TID respiratory treatments	Consult physician and encourage prescription of as few pills and treatments as possible with use of long-acting (sustained-release) theophylline drugs. Whenever possible, group medications and treatments together to simplify administration schedules.
Long duration	Long, involved program of bronchial hygiene overtires the patient.	Call health team conference to reassess need for and effects of therapy. Encourage the scheduling of activities to allow for longer rest periods between treatments.
Presence of undesirable side effects	Pulmonary medications cause GI upset.	Advise patient to take oral medications with a few crackers or a snack. Consult physician regarding any new appearance of side effects.
Presence of work, family, or other social problems	Family conflict hinders self-care strategies.	Encourage open discussion with patient and family members; help them identify specific actions necessary to support self-care strategies. For multiproblem patients, involve social worker to listen to and counsel family.
Breakdown in patient-physician-nurse communication	Patient views health professional as formal, rejecting, and insensitive to his needs. Professionals never communicate an explanation for diagnosis, purposes of therapies, or sincere willingness to explore emotional as well as physical complaints.	Encourage patient to verbalize feelings. Assign one nurse to coordinate care. Call a health team conference to facilitate problem solving and expression of staff's feelings towards the patient.
Forgetfulness	Because of old age, past episodes of brain hypoxia (cerebrovascular accident or high altitude), presence of abnormal ABGs, or learning disability.	Check ABG results for low Pa_{O_2} or high Pa_{CO_2}. Teach the patient ways to remember important information and activities, e.g., schedule pills with meals, color code pill vials; if necessary, teach a family member to administer medications and treatments.

*Based on the Health Belief Model of Health Behavior.

The motivational model describes a person's subjective motivational state. All four elements of the model represent only what the patient is aware of; they do not represent unconscious processes or objective realities of the situation.

Basic assumptions of the model include, but are not limited to, the following:

1. Subjective experience is critical to any behavioral outcome.

2. The patient rather than the health professional must develop motivation to engage in health-seeking behavior; professionals are health catalysts.

3. Motivation depends on the development of personal awareness of present and imagined future conditions.

4. Since health is a state of complete physical, mental, and social well being, these factors all contribute to the motivational process.

FOUR COMPONENTS OF THE MODEL

The four components of the model are described subsequently and illustrated in Figure 16–5.

1. *Present awareness context.* This element represents the person's conception of "things as they are," i.e., how he sees them. (See element 1 in Figure 16–5.) There are two aspects of this element. The circle (a) represents the person's *raw experiences*—his bodily sensations, feelings, and urges.

The dashed triangle (b) represents the person's interpretation and identification of these experiences or sensations. The triangle is outlined with a dashed line rather than a solid line because interpretations tend to be even more subjective than underlying experiences. Interpretations may have no objective validity. For example, a patient might interpret chest tightness (i.e., raw experience) as a sign of an asthmatic attack, a heart attack, or of no consequence. The present awareness context depends upon how the patient identifies and interprets needs and desires.

2. *Future awareness context.* This element represents a person's conception of "things as they might be," i.e., his conception of alternative futures. (See element 2 in Figure 16–5.) The circle (a) represents *potential experiences of satisfaction or dissatisfaction* (e.g., breathing without chest discomfort) or potential satisfiers (e.g., being reattached to a ventilator and taking an aerosol bronchodilator). A patient can aim for a potentially satisfying experience without thinking of a potential satisfier and vice versa.

The dashed triangle (b) represents the patient's interpretation of the potential satisfiers, satisfying experiences, or both. For example, the patient whose goal is to take the bronchodilator regularly might believe that taking the drug is the only way to control his breathing and eliminate his sense of helplessness.

3. *Strategy bridge.* This element represents the person's conception of alternative strategies he might use to bridge the gap between "things as they are" and "things as they might be." (See element 3 in Figure 16–5.) For example, the patient with chest tightness might contemplate several alternatives that might help him to achieve his goal of breathing without discomfort, including avoidance of exercise or emotionally charged conversations that might precipitate bronchospasm; administration of two puffs of metered cartridge bronchodilator at the first sign of chest discomfort; agreement to let the nurse perform a home assessment of potential allergens; and decision to ignore the symptom.

In Figure 16–5, alternatives are represented by the four lines of the strategy bridge between present and future awareness contexts.

4. *Personal behavior.* This element, which often blends into the third element, represents the person's

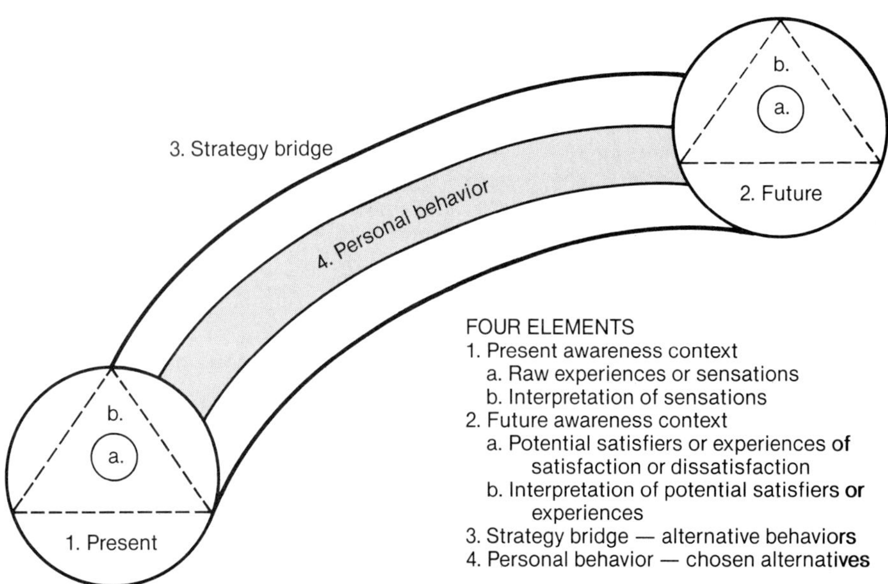

Figure 16–5. Model of a patient's subjective motivational state.

conception of actions he feels he should take. (See element 4 in Figure 16–5.) These actions must be acceptable to him and within his capacity. In the previous example, the patient with chest tightness may decide on the second and third alternatives, the bronchodilator aerosol and the home allergen assessment. These personal behaviors are represented by the shaded lines in Figure 16–5.

DEVELOPING A MOTIVATING GAP

When all four elements in the model are in tune, i.e., developed to the same degree, the *discrepancy* or difference between the present and future becomes a *motivating gap*. The generated tension to eliminate the discrepancy is very intense and energizing. If one or more elements of the model are missing or fail to fit in with the others, a motivating gap is not generated. Assessment strives to determine the presence and relative strengths of the four elements. Intervention strives to strengthen the four elements so that the patient develops an obvious discrepancy or motivating gap between the present and future; he has a goal, sees alternatives, and can choose the action best for him. The development of elements 1 and 2 is key. If the patient cannot conceive of elements 3 and 4, he must at least be confident that a feasible way exists or can be devised for closing the gap, and he must be willing and able to implement the ultimate alternatives once he has identified them with the nurse's help.

IMPLEMENTATION OF THE MODEL

Perhaps the easiest way to implement the motivational model is to integrate the key questions listed in the box into clinical decision-making situations.

KEY QUESTIONS FOR MOTIVATIONAL ASSESSMENT AND INTERVENTION

1. **Present awareness context:**
   What is your respiratory problem?
   Over the past year, has your condition been getting better or worse, or has it remained about the same? Explain your answer.
2. **Future awareness context:**
   Do you have any personal goals that are important to you?
   How would you *like* to feel?
   What would you *like* to be able to do?
3. **Strategy bridge:**
   How do you think you can reach your goal?
4. **Personal behavior:**
   If we help you set realistic goals, would you be willing to try some alternatives to reach the goals we set with you?

CASE STUDY

The following case study illustrates how the model and related motivational theory can be used to deliver respiratory nursing care to a patient with a noncompliance problem. Physiologic aspects have been omitted to stress psychologic aspects of care.

Mr. T. is a 65-year-old white male with severe COPD living with his wife in a small house in a large city. He was forced to retire from his job as a grocer 3 years ago owing to respiratory problems and is now receiving financial assistance from his son, Social Security, and private medical insurance.

While in the hopsital for respiratory insufficiency, rehabilitation was started without using the motivational model framework. Members of the health care team set up the following goals:

1. To promote a maximum activity level within Mr. T.'s physical limitations through a program of breathing and muscle reconditioning exercises.
2. To promote adequate bronchial drainage through bronchodilator aerosol treatments and postural drainage twice a day with coughing and deep breathing.
3. To promote early recognition of complications.
4. To promote an understanding of Mr. T.'s disease, medications, and respiratory equipment.

After discharge, in spite of regular follow-ups by a visiting nurse and the patient's verbal compliance with his program, Mr. T. demonstrated a lack of motivation to follow his treatment program. Although he took his medications, he continued to smoke occasionally, remained in bed most of the day, and frequently skipped respiratory treatments. When his chest assessment findings indicated a deterioration in respiratory status, a respiratory nurse specialist began to visit him once or twice weekly for 6 weeks in lieu of the regular visiting nurse specifically to implement the motivational model. The main goals of therapy were to help Mr. T.:

1. To identify a discrepancy between "things as they are" and "things as they might be."
2. To develop the other elements of the model.
3. To generate a strong motivating gap and desire to follow through with some form of therapy to improve his condition.

PRESENT AWARENESS CONTEXT

To facilitate exploration of his present awareness context, the nurse used several approaches.

First, while performing cardiopulmonary assessments weekly and listening attentively to somatic complaints, she gradually steered conversation towards the patient's emotional response to lung disease and physical disability.

Second, the nurse and patient explored the course of his disease up to the present along with related feelings, concerns, and hopes. It became apparent that Mr. T. was unaware of his feelings, actual behavior, and attitudes in certain circumstances and how they affected his physical condition. The nurse involved Mr. T. in teaching-learning situations to clarify misinterpretations about his disease and to teach new health-seeking behavior.

Third, "things as they are" were discussed from week to week as well as what he thought made the difference. This approach stimulated consideration of a new perspective on therapy. The nurse avoided discussions about his failure to adhere to prescribed treatments.

Finally, the nurse helped Mr. T. become aware of his feelings and how he related to his environment when in a poor respiratory state as opposed to when he is feeling relatively well.

Progress was slow on "bad days" when Mr. T. was doing poorly physically. He blocked stimuli by his mood, abrupt remarks, jokes, and body tension. The nurse respected these defense mechanisms to avoid possible physical decompensation. Instead, she focused on helping Mr. T. verbalize his feelings and actions as they occurred, e.g., "I'm angry, so I'm going to bed." When Mr. T. was feeling better, the nurse explored the incidents and possible reasons for the anger and avoidance behavior.

On "bad days," the nurse spent more time listening to the concerns of the patient's wife and providing her with health education, advice, and emotional support as needed. She seemed to be coping well under the circumstances but was relatively unaware of the facts about COPD, including reasons for her husband's exaggerated emotional responses.

After 3 weeks, Mr. T. became more aware and finally verbalized his present situation and conflict of motivation. Overall, he saw himself as a sick person with little control over his disease process. He described himself as "worthless" because of his inability to maintain the role of provider in the family. He identified different behavior patterns on "good days" and "bad days." On "good days" he was more active, related more to people, had fewer gastrointestinal upsets, experienced less dyspnea, and usually felt no need for respiratory treatments (he skipped them). On "bad days" he felt miserable and expressed feelings of low self esteem. He stayed in bed all day; attempted to block out all noise and people from his room, including his wife; experienced headaches, possibly from a high $Paco_2$; and dyspnea, possibly from a low Pao_2. The nurse reinforced the patient's more positively motivating tendencies and encouraged him to participate in family and community activities as much as possible. Also, the nurse explained how inactivity might precipitate alveolar hypoventilation and hypoxemia and thus contribute to an unstable chest condition and vacillating emotional responses.

FUTURE AWARENESS CONTEXT

Mr. T. could not fully form or verbalize a future awareness context. He only went as far as to wish he were in a stable respiratory state, breathing with minimal difficulty. However, with help, he was able to develop goals or future awareness contexts from week to week, e.g., run one family errand each day and try one aerosol treatment each day for a week.

STRATEGY BRIDGE AND PERSONAL BEHAVIOR

After five weeks, although the future awareness context seemed weakly developed, Mr. T. was able to distinguish between "things as they are" and "things as they might be." The alternatives of the strategy bridge and the personal behavior evolved from further conversation centered around the first two components of the model. After initially choosing to increase activity level in his own way, he physically improved. By taking responsibility for himself and achieving success, Mr. T. felt he had more control over his disease. He started to use his compressor nebulizer, help his wife with family responsibilities, see his doctor, and go on more outings.

In the seventh week, the respiratory nurse specialist terminated services because the patient appeared to be doing well. She would have liked to extend follow-up care and help Mr. T. learn breathing and muscle reconditioning exercises, but his medical insurance would not cover additional home visits. Also, other patients in her case load were more physically unstable and demanded her time.

A few days later, Mr. T. was hospitalized for acute respiratory distress, but no physical reasons were found for the exacerbation of pulmonary symptoms.

DISCUSSION

When Mr. T.'s condition drastically improved, his case was considered a "success" story by the nurses in the home health agency. Then, his rehospitalization caused them to wonder about the appropriateness and effectiveness of the nursing care delivered. Several lessons can be learned from this case.

First, when motivational aspects are emphasized, the patient may learn to depend on the nurse for psychologic support and eventually relinquish responsibility for himself. Nurses with prolonged or intense contact with patients frequently experience this situation. Hence, it is essential to emphasize self-care strategies and the development of family and outside support persons *early* in the rehabilitative process. In Mr. T.'s case, perhaps identification of *mutually satisfying goals* by all concerned, including the visiting nurse, might have facilitated the motivational process before hospital discharge. Also, ideally, to foster patient confidence in self care and to avoid anxiety upon termination, the nurse might have scheduled additional visits and telephone calls and tapered them gradually from once a week to once every 2 weeks and finally once a month. Sometimes, telephone calls can substitute for home visits.

Second, rehospitalization is likely unless the nurse is reasonably confident that the patient and family can cope adaptively to acute dyspnea, especially episodes triggered by emotional response. In Mr. T.'s case, the respiratory nurse specialist had few opportune moments for teaching Mr. T. to control dyspnea because of his defense mechanisms. At the time, he was more depressed than angry. He was not willing to expose himself to increasing amounts of physical activity under direct supervision of the nurse. Never once did he express interest in the prescribed program of breathing exercises and muscle reconditioning. Therefore, although he practiced some self care, he never learned to confidently control acute dyspnea or emotional states of action, in particular. Perhaps working more intensively with the family on coaching Mr. T. to control dyspnea and related emotional upsets might have helped.

Third, the focus on short-term goals, such as running one family errand each day, was crucial to the motivational process. It allowed Mr. T. to at least temporarily achieve his more distant goal, a stable respiratory state, in short manageable steps.

Last, and most important, one wonders whether physical instability was largely responsible for Mr. T.'s inability to fully explore all elements of the motivational model. Unless he decides to stop smoking cigarettes, his physical condition may remain labile, his perceptions altered, and his participation in self-care strategies limited. Moreover, if abnormal ABGs were responsible for his headaches and labile condition, then, as a patient advocate, the nurse should have focused on encouraging medical reevaluation, including possible use of oxygen in the home. Additional information (e.g., recent PFT, ABG, and medical evaluation) would have helped to determine more precisely the severity of Mr. T.'s physical state, his capacity to discuss motivational matters, and the degree of emphasis on physical versus psychologic intervention. At this point, if Mr. T. is not receptive to professional health services, the nurse can only objectively and calmly point out the consequences of his chosen behavior and close the case.

In conclusion, this case study demonstrates an application of the motivational model. Although the patient never fully developed all four elements to generate a strong and long-lasting motivating gap, present and future awareness contexts gradually developed. This development represents a major step for the COPD patient, a step that leads to further development of elements 3 and 4, as the patient passes through the health care continuum.

As a model for continuing care, this approach is time consuming and sometimes difficult to reinforce given the restraints of existing health care delivery systems. However, as a conceptual model for everyday practice, this approach prevents the mistake of the nurse's skipping directly to the patient's personal behavior without allowing the patient to work through his problems and identify mutually satisfying solutions.

Integration of Motivational Concepts into Psychologic Evaluation Tools

The previous case study shows how the motivational model may be directly applied to guide motivational assessment and intervention.

This section of the chapter presents how concepts of the model may be integrated as psychologic evaluation tools and then used as guides to the motivational process. The example is the Self-Concept Evaluation tool (Kersten, 1980), adapted for use with pulmonary patients from the Semantic Differential Scale (Osgood et al, 1957; Tyerman and Humphrey, 1984). Though this tool was developed for an inpatient pulmonary rehabilitation setting, it is appropriate for any situation where the nurse has prolonged contact with patient and family.

At the beginning of pulmonary rehabilitation, the patient is asked to assess his past, present, and future self for each of the 20 concepts or sets of adjectives shown in the box. The *past self* is defined as how the patient thinks he was in good health, i.e., about 6 months before the signs and symptoms of lung disease. Thinking about the past helps the patient rate his present self. The *present self* is analogous to the motivational model's present awareness context. For the patient, it is defined as how he thinks he is now. The *future self*, analogous to the motivational model's future awareness context, is how the patient thinks he will be 6 months into the future.

To assess these concepts, the patient is asked to fill out horizontal rating scales for each concept, as shown for the inactive-active concept in Table 16–3. Note that each scale is relative, with spaces to the far left and far right for extremely inactive and extremely active responses, respectively. (Note there are three scales used for each concept.)

> ***CONCEPTS IN A SELF-CONCEPT EVALUATION TOOL****
>
> unhappy—happy
> bored—interested
> helpless—in control
> worried—relaxed
> dissatisfied—satisfied
> unattractive—attractive
> despondent—hopeful
> lacking confidence—self-confident
> emotional—stable
> worthless—valuable
> forgetful—mindful
> irritable—calm
> unfeeling—caring
> clumsy—skillful
> dependent—independent
> inactive—active
> difficult—cooperative
> withdrawn—talkative
> unfriendly—friendly
> stupid—clever
>
> *From Tyerman, A. and Humphrey, M.: Changes in self-concept following severe head injury. *International journal of rehabilitation research*, 7(1):11–23, 1984.

After pulmonary rehabilitation, the patient is again asked to assess his past, present, and future self concept without consulting the prerehabilitation ratings.

In Mr. M.'s case (see Table 16–3), his postrehabilitation ratings were higher (i.e., marked further to the right on the scale) than his prerehabilitation ratings in 17 of the 20 concepts. Results for the inactive-active concept reflect this improvement. Such improvement indicates a more positive self concept and is an expected outcome of the rehabilitation process, as pointed out in this book. A positive correlation exists between increased activity level and positive self concept (Ben-Shlomo and Short, 1983; Eide, 1982). If expected improvement is not seen in a patient's activity rating, the nurse further assesses the situation by determining whether the health team's assessment of activity correlates with the patient's perceptions.

Besides providing health team members with a measure of perceived changes in self concept, the Self-Concept Evaluation tool provides the patient with visual feedback of his progress from a motivational perspective.

The patient and, if possible, the family are actively involved in the interpretation of results during conferences with the nurse, social worker, or psychologist. At each conference, the nurse might first make a basic interpretation, as shown in Table 16–3. Then, the nurse asks the patient to explain his ratings, concentrating on those that are either extreme or inconsistent with the clinical history. In Mr. M.'s case, during the last conference, the nurse asked him specifically how he was going to implement an exercise program to stay active.

Table 16–3. MR. M.'s RATINGS FOR THE INACTIVE—ACTIVE SELF-CONCEPT

Patient's Ratings								Nurse's Interpretation
Pre Rehabilitation	*Inactive*						*Active*	
Past							X	In good health (i.e., 6 months before lung disease), Mr. M. saw himself as being extremely active.
Present		X						Just before pulmonary rehabilitation, he saw himself as quite, but not extremely, inactive.
Future							X	Six months into the future, he thinks he will be as active as he was in the past.
Post Rehabilitation	*Inactive*						*Active*	
Past							X	Mr. M. still perceives himself as being extremely active in the past (i.e., before lung disease).
Present				X				Now he perceives himself as being equally active and inactive. He has improved his self concept in relation to activity compared with the preprogram rating.
Future						X		Six months into the future, he sees himself as being quite active. The rating is about the same or slightly lower than the preprogram rating. The lower rating is realistic given the severity of his lung disease. The nurse did not consider this rating too high because health team members expected Mr. M.'s activity tolerance to further increase postprogram, as this grossly obese patient gradually lost weight.

Table 16–4. WAYS TO PREVENT BURN-OUT IN PULMONARY NURSES

Focus	Specific Interventions	Rationale
Education	Give classes on pulmonary psychophysiology and the psychologic coping mechanisms of COPD patients.	Once the physiologic basis of behavior is understood, the nurse is more able and willing to cope with difficult clinical situations.
	Introduce a motivational approach to patient care, with emphasis on the patient and not the nurse as motivator. Apply the motivational model described in this chapter to a patient in your clinical setting.	The motivational approach emphasizes self care. Placement of responsibility for health on the patient relieves the nurse of the necessity of experiencing feelings of failure every time the patient's condition deteriorates.
	Familiarize staff with common nursing and patient needs and problems encountered as the patient passes through the health care continuum. Educate acute-care nurses in rehabilitative aspects of care and vice versa (see Chapter 18).	This knowledge helps staff understand the patient and how nursing interventions in specific settings might be modified to promote the motivational process. Separation of nursing needs (e.g., lunch relief) from patient needs (e.g., continual verbal reassurance) prevents staff from projecting their needs onto the patient. Also, it is the first step in resolving the real problem.
Group therapy and team building	Hold periodic conferences with a trained facilitator, such as a psychologist or other mental health specialist, to help nurses express and analyze personal reactions to specific situations, e.g., personal fear of death, anger at patients for smoking.	These sessions encourage verbalization of negative feelings that have built up over days, weeks, and months. Once verbalized, conflicts surrounding the feelings can be dealt with constructively with the help of the facilitator. Also, these sessions encourage verbalization of positive remarks and group decision-making, all factors in team building.
	Hold regular staff meetings to promote communication, address operational tasks, and solve problems.	Comments during staff meetings may indicate a need for a team conference surrounding a particular issue or patient. Also, a smoothly functioning unit is a less stressful workplace.
	Encourage informal meetings and social gatherings, e.g., fun get-togethers at a pizza parlor.	Such gatherings are a pleasant interruption of the daily work routine. Simultaneously, they provide another opportunity to receive the advice, comfort, and positive feedback necessary to cope with the demands of respiratory care.
	Encourage nurse attendance at local, state, and national meetings on respiratory care topics.	Input from these meetings will increase expertise, interest, and motivation to work together to provide the best care possible. Also, outside input and time away from the clinical setting facilitate team evaluation.
Administration and organization of care	Identify and counsel nurses who exhibit signs of burnout. Signs may include apathy, negativism, low tolerance for the difficult patients, reluctance to participate in psychosocial intervention, disrespect for patients.	Ready identification and treatment of burned-out nurses buffers the rest of the staff from constant exposure to negative remarks and apathy. Counseling may result in a change in patient assignment or vacation time, simple solutions that might renew enthusiasm and increase coping ability.
	Provide varied case loads, i.e., mixture of mild, moderate, and severe pulmonary disease, including "time out" from pulmonary patients. Consider integration of acute-care staffs with staffs of intermediate care units.	A case load of patients with severe COPD or acute illness may be overwhelming. Integration of staffs provides varied case loads and facilitates continuity of care.
	Promote hiring policies that favor nurses with an interest in respiratory care and an ability to readily adapt to high demand levels.	Such policies lead to less mismatch between demand and coping ability (Clarke, 1984), a low employee turnover rate, and more opportunity to build a supportive team.
	Encourage use of a primary nurse to coordinate care. Whenever possible, involve the visiting nurse in motivational assessment and intervention.	The COPD patient is more likely to participate in the motivational process when he has one primary nurse whom he knows and trusts.
	Provide staff access to a respiratory clinical nurse specialist for bedside rounds and problem solving.	Ready access to expertise reduces stress associated with the uncertainty and unpredictability of acute or difficult situations.
Ethics and the dying patient	Encourage patient, family, and physicians to address ethical and moral issues, as the terminal patient approaches death. Team conferences (described previously) may be helpful.	The nurse may feel stressed when the suffering patient with irreversible disease repeatedly asks for the discontinuation of life-support systems while medical interventions continue indefinitely.
	Provide medical-legal counseling so that all concerned understand such implications for the withdrawal of life-support systems.	Physicians and nurses may be reluctant to discontinue life-support systems for fear of possible malpractice suits.
	Encourage the family to reach a consensus about their wishes for the patient and then discuss specifics with the physician, e.g., resuscitate versus do not resuscitate.	Family may remain uninvolved in decisions because they do not realize their desires are important, they do not reach a consensus on an approach, or staff does not involve them in decision making.
	Provide PRN pain medication and psychologic support. Encourage use of a social worker and supportive significant others to help family and patient with the grieving process and to work out other problems, e.g., finances, temporary housing close to the hospital.	Coping abilities of both patient and nurse are increased when physical and psychologic support are readily available.

Information gained during discussion is as important as changes in the ratings themselves. It facilitates exploration of present and future awareness contexts, of goal setting, and of alternatives related to developing a more positive self concept. In addition, the information helps the patient verbalize sensitive areas in the history that he neglected to mention during the admitting interview, and it helps him to solve problems under the guidance of a trusted health team member.

When a spouse or significant other is asked to fill out a Self-Concept Evaluation on the patient, a discussion of differences in ratings between spouse and patient may provide insight into communication problems or other problems in the home. Moreover, when patient and spouse recognize great improvement in pre- and postprogram ratings, it serves as incentive motivation for setting more goals for the future.

Burnout in Nurses—A Barrier to the Development of Patient Motivation

Facilitation of the motivational process is emotionally and physically draining for nurses and others who constantly work with respiratory patients. As the patient approaches end-stage disease, motivational states constantly change with vacillating physical and emotional conditions. The nurse cannot rely on any set nursing care plan because of the need to constantly reassess each situation and alter interventions accordingly. When progress becomes evident, the patient may suffer a major setback. When the patient appears to be a candidate for a hospice, his condition may drastically improve. As a health professional responsible for total patient care, the nurse is the major support person for patient and family and usually has the added responsibility of coordinating care with other health professionals. In patients with defense mechanisms and perceptual problems, constant repetition of educational content may be necessary before patient and family finally understand the relevance of various preventive measures and the need to follow specified procedures for respiratory care. Furthermore, not only must nurses cope with patients' psychologic coping mechanisms, but they also must perform or supervise time-consuming intensive respiratory care procedures within a limited time period. The acuteness and unpredictable nature of clinical circumstances may place demands on a nurse beyond the ability to cope. Emotional stress results (Clarke, 1984). It reaches unbearable levels when the patient is angry, anxious, and overtly unappreciative.

Because of unrelieved stress, pulmonary nurses may begin to experience burnout, defined as ". . . emotional exhaustion in which the professional person no longer has any positive feelings, sympathy, or respect for patients or clients" (Maslach, 1979). The process of burnout becomes a major barrier to the development of motivation because of the central role of the nurse in rehabilitative care.

Burnout may be combatted by focusing on education, group therapy, and team building administration and organization of care, and ethics (Table 16–4). Most of the interventions in Table 16–4 contribute either directly or indirectly to the development of personal-professional support systems, a prerequisite for effective team building. On the one hand, when an effective health care team is in operation, nurses and others can collaborate with administrators to plan changes and eliminate sources of burnout. On the other hand, when the health team is fragmented and expertise limited, administrators must take the lead and actively help staff organize care and implement those interventions summarized in Table 16–4.

Conclusion

This chapter has reviewed motivational states of respiratory patients, motivational theory, motivational models for clinical practice, and ways to reduce burnout, a potential barrier to the motivational process. The motivational model serves as a guide for continuing and comprehensive care or as a new way to approach selected noncompliance or other problems. The model's implementation helps patients change from within and take responsibility for the change. Though in most cases use of the model or selected aspects facilitates respiratory care, patient and nurse may encounter barriers to the development of motivation, e.g., physical instability, fears, self doubts, and lack of skills. Some of these barriers are insurmountable. Others may be reduced over time with exploration of the patient's subjective motivational state. Whatever the case, the patient's chosen personal behavior is respected. Not only does this approach promote self care, but it also is more cost effective for both patient and society over time.

REFERENCES

Allport, G.: Becoming. New Haven, Yale University Press, 1955.

Becker, M. and Maiman, L.: Sociobehavioral determinants of compliance with health and medical care recommendations. *Medical care*, 13(1):10–24, 1975.

Ben-Shlomo, L. and Short, M.: The effects of physical exercise on self-attitudes. *Occupational therapy in mental health*, 3(4):11–28, 1983.

Clarke, M.: Stress and coping: constructs for nursing. *Journal of advanced nursing*, 9(1):3–13, 1984.

Craig, J. and Craig, M.: Synergic Power: Beyond Domination, Beyond Permissiveness, 2nd ed. Berkeley, Proactive Press, 1979.

Devereux, G.: Some criteria for the timing of confrontation and interpretations. *International journal of psychoanalysis*, 32(Part I):19–24, 1951.

Dudley, D., Sitzman, J., and Rugg, M.: Psychiatric aspects of patients with COPD. *Advances in psychosomatic medicine*, 14:64–77, 1985.

Dudley, D. L., Wermuth, C., and Hague, W.: Psychosocial aspects of care in the chronic obstructive pulmonary disease patient. *Heart and lung*, 2(3):389–393, 1973.

Dudley, D., et al: Psychosocial concomitants to rehabilitation in chronic obstructive pulmonary disease. Part I. Psychosocial and psychological considerations. *Chest*, 77(3):413–420, 1980.

Eide, R.: The relationship between body image, self-image and physical activity. *Scandinavian journal of social medicine*, 29:109–112, 1982.

Habenger, T. L., et al: The Nebraska Chronic Obstructive Pulmonary Disease Rehabilitation Project. (Project #RD-2517-M). Omaha, Social and Rehabilitation Service, Department of Health, Education and Welfare, 1971.

Johnson, D.: Reaching Out: Interpersonal Effectiveness and Self Actualization, 2nd ed. Englewood Cliffs, New Jersey, Prentice-Hall, 1981.

Joseph, L. S.: Self-care and the nursing process. *Nursing clinics of north america*, 15(1):131–143, 1980.

Kersten, L.: Self Concept Evaluation. A tool used in the Medical Respiratory Care Program. City of Hope National Medical Center, Duarte, California, 1986.

Lazarus, R.: Psychological Stress and Coping Process. San Francisco, McGraw-Hill Book Co., 1966.

Light, R., Merrill, E., Despars, J., et al: Prevalence of depression and anxiety in patients with COPD—relationship to functional capacity. *Chest*, 87(1):35–43, 1985.

Lindemann, J.: Psychological and Behavioral Aspects of Physical Disability—A Manual for Health Practitioners. New York, Plenum Press, 1981.

Maslach, C.: The burn-out syndrome and patient care. In Stress and Survival: The Emotional Realities of Life (C. Garfield, ed.). St. Louis, C. V. Mosby Co., 1979.

Maslow, A. H.: Motivation and Personality, 2nd ed. New York, Harper and Row, 1970.

May, R.: Love and Will. New York, W. W. Norton, 1969.

Osgood, C., Suci, G., and Tannenbaum, P.: The Measurement of Meaning. Urbana, University of Illinois Press, 1957.

Rosillo, R., Fogel, M., and Freedman, K.: Affect levels and improvement in physical rehabilitation. *Journal of chronic diseases*, 24(10):651–660, 1971.

Strain, J.: Psychological reactions to acute medical illness and critical care. *Critical care medicine*, 6(1):39–44, 1978.

Tyerman, A. and Humphrey, M.: Changes in self-concept following severe head injury. *International journal of rehabilitation research*, 7(1):11–23, 1984.

Vernon, M. D.: Human Motivation. Cambridge, Great Britain, Cambridge University Press, 1969.

Windsor, R., Green, L., and Roseman, J.: Health promotion and maintenance for patients with chronic obstructive pulmonary disease: A review. *Journal of chronic diseases*, 33(1):5–12, 1980.

Self-Care Education

17

Main Objectives

1. **Compare the focuses and assumptions of self-care education with those of patient education.**
2. **Name five barriers to the use of self-care education in the clinical setting.**
3. **List the basic educational content for respiratory patients.**
4. **Identify the six steps of the teaching-learning process.**
5. **Give an example of a learning need in each of the four learning areas described in this chapter.**
6. **Describe how to identify teaching-learning needs and maintain a self-care orientation in your clinical setting.**
7. **Define readiness to learn.**
8. **Develop a teaching-learning plan for a respiratory patient in your clinical setting:**
   a. **Identify a need and appropriate respiratory intervention.**
   b. **Write the main objective.**
   c. **Write subobjectives with evaluation criteria.**
   d. **Rank needs and objectives.**
   e. **Identify appropriate teaching methods.**
9. **Describe the importance, purpose, and process of ongoing evaluation and reteaching and relearning of educational content.**

This chapter discusses self-care, teaching-learning needs of respiratory patients. The assessment parameter is called "self-care education" rather than "patient education" because, except in special circumstances, the patient rather than the health professional is assumed responsible for the knowledge and skills necessary for disease treatment and health promotion.

Content focuses on the six steps of the teaching-learning process, with emphases on needs and problems associated with respiratory clinical applications. Specific educational content delivered during teaching-learning sessions is presented in Chapters 18 through 23.

Definition of Self-Care Education

Self-care education is defined by Levin (1976) as "a process whereby a lay person functions on his/her own behalf in health promotion and prevention in disease detection and treatment . . . ." Orem (1980), a nursing theorist who stresses the use of self-care concepts within the framework of the nursing process, defines self-care as "the practice of activities that individuals personally initiate and perform on their own behalf in maintaining life, health and well being." In the self-care approach, the learner is assumed responsible for his own health. Hence, he takes an active role in the teaching-learning process and clinical decision-making.

In contrast, patient education has the same goals of health promotion and prevention and disease detection and treatment, but the health professional rather than the patient plays a dominant role.

The two types of educational approaches are compared and contrasted in Table 17–1. Note that the two approaches represent two poles on a continuum. Health professionals strive to promote self-care because an active, participating patient is essential for informed consent and health maintenance from hospital to community setting. Yet, the nurse may need to revert to patient education to accommodate acute illness or special teaching-learning needs that limit self sufficiency.

Barriers to Self-Care Education

Major barriers to self-care education relate to overemphasis of the medical model for care, restraints of the current health care delivery system, nursing's task orientation, confusion over professional roles in the clinical setting, and overemphasis of the acute-chronic care dichotomy.

FOCUS ON THE MEDICAL MODEL

Interdisciplinary focus on the medical model for health care delivery has reinforced the nurse's view of the patient as a passive, dependent learner. Nurses and other health professionals have come to view themselves as extensions of physicians rather than extensions of patients (Steckel, 1982). Interventions have focused on following the physician's orders, resolving the acute exacerbation, and discharging the patient after disease stabilization without addressing self-care needs that, if met, might have prevented the acute exacerbation in the first place.

For self-care education to work, all concerned must perceive their complementary roles as extensions of the patient, and a more holistic, motivational approach to the patient must be implemented to help the patient through each step of the teaching-learning process.

In addition, focus on the medical model has reinforced the patient's view of himself as a passive learner. Hence, before implementation of self-care education, the nurse may need to educate the patient and family of the need for and the purpose of the self-care approach to respiratory care.

RESTRAINTS OF THE HEALTH CARE DELIVERY SYSTEM

Financial reimbursement policies focus primarily on relief of acute signs and symptoms and secondarily on preventive therapies that arrest or slow chronic disease progression or improve quality of life. Hence, many patients do not receive needed health education, particularly when distance, transportation, family circumstances, insurance policy limitations, and other factors limit access to health care.

Perhaps the most effective way to facilitate reimbursement for services is to carefully document contin-

Table 17–1. FOCUSES AND ASSUMPTIONS OF SELF-CARE VERSUS PATIENT EDUCATION

Variables	Self-Care Education	Patient Education
Goals	Set by patient in anticipation of risk for disease	Set by professional in response to patient's illness
Role of learner	Primary role for learner Staff encourages self-sufficiency	Dependent role for learner Staff encourages compliance and cooperation
Regulation of teaching-learning process, e.g., content, methods, etc.	Patient regulates processes	Professional regulates processes
Patient motivation	Focus on internal motivation Patient develops his own skills and resources	Focus on external motivation Patient depends on professional skills and services
Health care system	Health care system adapts to patient needs and preferences	Patient adapts to health care system
Patient's health status	Determined by forces in the environment that shape behavior	Determined by personal behavior and health activities

ued need for nursing care, including health education and follow-up. Documentation should include any change in pulmonary function tests (PFTs), arterial blood gases (ABGs), chest x-rays, pulmonary symptoms, or chest assessment findings that might indicate an unstable condition and a need for monitoring. Though self-care education may be a major patient need, the unstable condition may be the only acceptable basis for follow-up care reimbursed by third party payers in our current health care delivery system.

NURSING'S TASK ORIENTATION

Though most nurses endorse self-care education and preventive interventions, many do not practice them owing to those previously mentioned or other restraints, such as inadequate staffing, educational resources, administrative support, or teaching skills. Moreover, the orientation of many medical-surgical departments gives highest priority to tasks related to medical orders and physical care, e.g., bedmaking and bathing, and lowest priority to tasks related to teaching-learning needs (Mullin, 1980). Inattention to these needs, however, may relate to the nurse's inability to adapt teaching-learning theories to individual patient situations rather than to inadequate knowledge of the theories themselves.

Redirection of nursing's task orientation to include self-care education requires professional commitment to consider teaching-learning needs along with other physiologic and psychosocial problems. This commitment must be strong, since new prospective financial reimbursement systems have built-in incentives for the reduction of patient services, early hospital discharge or case closure, and treatment of low-risk, single-problem patients rather than multiproblem respiratory patients with major teaching-learning needs.

One way to redirect a nursing department's task orientation is to hold discussions with staff nurses, nurse administrators, and nurse educators regarding ways to incorporate teaching-learning needs into nursing care. Possible interventions might include new guidelines for staff patient assignments that include teaching-learning tasks, appointment of a teaching-learning resource person, modification of a system to include self-care education charges, initiation of problem-oriented charting, and additional budgeting for teaching materials.

CONFUSION OVER PROFESSIONAL ROLES

Confusion may arise in the clinical setting as to *who* shall do the teaching and specifically *what* shall be taught. Miller (1976) suggests that confusion among health professionals over roles and responsibilities is a major barrier to the actualization of self-care education. For example, the physician, nurse, and respiratory therapist may identify different, conflicting learning needs when they do not meet together to agree on overall treatment goals or when a patient coordinator is lacking to facilitate collaboration and coordination. As a result, the patient may become noncompliant owing to confusion and exasperation related to too much conflicting information or too little information at the wrong time.

Generally, the physician is responsible for initially informing and teaching the patient regarding diagnosis, prognosis, and treatment plan. Nurses, respiratory therapists, social workers, pharmacists, physical and occupational therapists, and others complement the physician's role, meeting patient needs related to their respective areas of expertise.

The role of the nurse is to help the patient verbalize learning needs, identify additional information needs implied in observed behavior, and then plan and implement teaching activities to meet individual teaching-learning needs (Pender, 1974). Most important, the nurse is the best person to coordinate teaching-learning activities or any other type of rehabilitative care among health team members. The reasons supporting the nurse as coordinator are listed hereafter.

1. Along with the physician, the nurse is already responsible and accountable for total patient care.
2. The nurse is already a coordinator of patient services by virtue of her central role in direct patient care.
3. Severely disabled individuals often lack the desire and energy to develop trusting relationships with more than one or two persons, usually the nurse and physician. The quality of the nurse-patient relationship is a crucial feature affecting motivation to follow through with all steps in the teaching-learning process.
4. The role of the nurse spans all health care settings. She can participate in evaluation and reteaching of the chronically ill patient as well as health promotion for others at high risk to develop pulmonary disease.
5. The nurse is prepared in basic teaching-learning theory, though in-service education is usually necessary to facilitate applications to respiratory populations. In many settings, a respiratory clinical nurse specialist or nurse educator with a pulmonary background coordinates care or acts as a resource to a primary staff nurse in charge of a patient's care.
6. The nurse's broad pharmacology and medical-surgical background enables her to integrate respiratory self-care teaching with teaching related to coexisting nonrespiratory problems.

Whatever the situation, important prerequisites for self-care education include the identification of a coordinator and assembly of a health care team with clearly delineated roles and a highly developed communication network. These prerequisites are crucial, since in many cases the teaching-learning process becomes integrated with a long treatment plan involving many disciplines.

ACUTE-CHRONIC CARE DICHOTOMY

The dichotomy between acute and chronic care has prompted acute care nurses to concentrate on acute interventions, leaving self-care education and health promotion activities to ambulatory or home care nurses in the community. This dichotomy is very slowly disappearing as acute care units become involved in health promotion (Flynn and Giffin, 1984) and as acute technologies move into ambulatory and home settings. Yet, owing to shorter hospital stays, more emphasis is needed on *early* teaching-learning needs assessment in acute care settings. For example, the critical care patient may be too ill to learn cognitive or psychomotor skills. Nevertheless, the critical care nurse can begin the teaching-learning process by interviewing the family, assessing basic teaching-learning needs, and intervening in the area of health beliefs and attitudes. Together health team members can formulate a tentative teaching plan for more aggressive self-care education once the patient is transferred to the medical floor.

Educational Content for Self-Care

Basic educational content for patients with acute or chronic respiratory problems includes the items listed in the following box.

BASIC EDUCATIONAL CONTENT

Respiratory anatomy and physiology
Pathophysiology of chest disease
Preventive measures
  e.g., pulmonary medications, diet, fluid intake, environmental control, signs of chest infection
Chest therapy
  e.g., relaxation, controlled coughing, breathing retraining, postural drainage
Progressive exercise conditioning
  e.g., walking programs, treadmill or bicycle exercise training, arm or leg range of motion exercises
Respiratory equipment
  e.g., hand-held nebulizer, mechanical ventilation, mist therapy, oxygen therapy

---

This content is adapted to individual situations. On the one hand, for example, the patient with severe chronic obstructive pulmonary disease (COPD) may need all of the content delivered over days, weeks, or months. (See Part Four.) On the other hand, the preoperative thoracotomy patient may need only one or two teaching sessions for content pertinent to surgery, including normal lung anatomy; explanation of the surgical procedure; and postoperative interventions to prevent complications, e.g., analgesics, controlled coughing, and arm range of motion (ROM) exercises.

Content may be delivered in many different ways, such as one-to-one or nurse-to-patient teaching sessions, group sessions, or formal or informal pulmonary rehabilitation programs. A *formal* pulmonary rehabilitation program refers to an organized self-care education program for groups of patients with respiratory problems. In contrast, an *informal* pulmonary rehabilitation program is comprised of individual teaching learning sessions, given as indicated by the situation.

Whatever the teaching method, the nurse evaluates patient progress in each step of the teaching-learning process.

The Teaching-Learning Process

The goal of self-care education is to help the patient through the teaching-learning process, thus helping him to maintain life, health, and well being.

The teaching-learning process is divided into six steps.

STEPS OF THE TEACHING-LEARNING PROCESS

1. Identify need to learn.
2. Identify readiness to learn.
3. Set learning goals.
4. Implement teaching-learning interventions.
5. Evaluate outcomes.
6. Reteach and relearn.

These steps are diagrammed conceptually in Figure 17–1. Note that this conceptualization closely parallels the motivational model presented in the previous chapter (see Fig. 16–5). In fact, the teaching-learning model is actually an extension of the motivational model. Hence, the content of Chapter 16, such as the motivational states of respiratory patients, the goals, the timing of interventions, and the complexity of the motivational process, applies to the teaching-learning situation as well as to the overall care of the patient. Recognizing the parallelism between motivational and teaching-learning models, educators agree that the adult learner is motivated when he recognizes a *motivating gap* between what he knows and what he wants to know, formally called the teaching-learning goal (Rankin and Duffy, 1983).

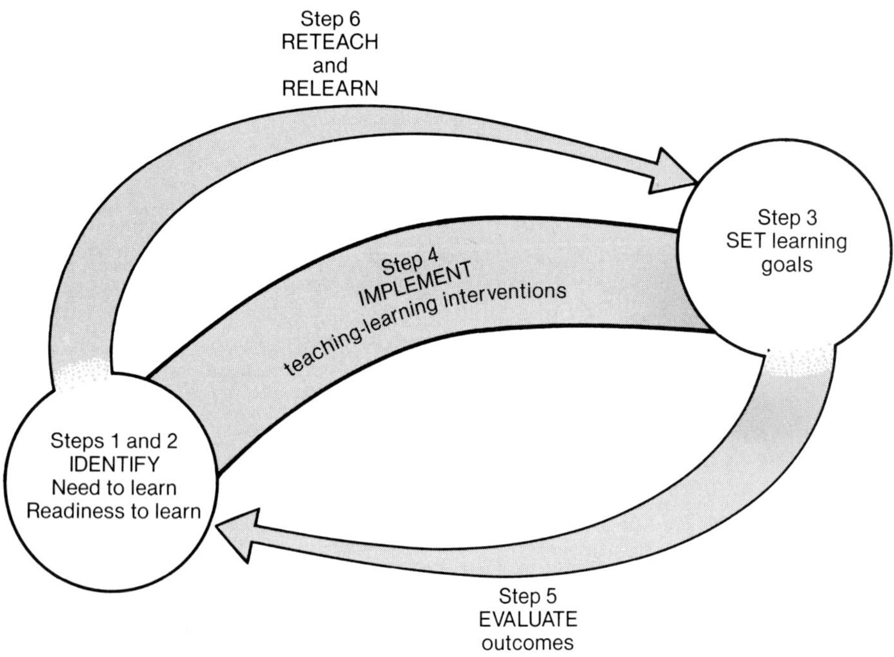

Figure 17–1. Conceptual model of the teaching-learning process.

STEP 1: IDENTIFY NEED TO LEARN

First, patient and health professional must identify a learning need. A *learning need* is defined as a *lack of knowledge, skill, competence, desirable behavior, or attitude.*

Learning Areas. Teaching-learning needs fall within four learning areas (Table 17–2). All learning areas require varying degrees of attention, depending on the acuity and disability of the disease and the individual situation. The intubated patient may need emphasis on knowledge and attitudes, e.g., knowledge that aphonia is temporary and expected during intubation and a hopeful attitude to sustain energy during the recovery period. In comparison, a clinic patient may need emphasis on skills and practices, e.g., using an inhaler correctly and regularly over time.

Assessment Tools. Teaching-learning needs become evident as the clinician implements other assessment parameters as presented in this book. If an initial nursing assessment is unavailable, the nurse may formulate a patient profile that summarizes personal information, physical and psychologic conditions, home living situations, medications and treatments, and patient desires, goals, hobbies, and interests. An example of an interview form is shown in Table 17–3. Answers to the questions at the bottom of this form will help assess need and readiness to learn and help plan interventions. For example, if the patient does not speak English, the nurse finds an English-speaking family member or translator to facilitate assessment and intervention. If a patient indicates no previous teaching about his disease process, the nurse may plan for provision of supplementary educational materials, simple diagrams, and brief explanations.

When special or complex teaching-learning needs are present, the clinician may interview from a check list, such as the list for COPD patients (see Table 17–4) or the list for ventilator-dependent patients (see Chapter 28). These assessment tools may be used during the teaching-learning process to evaluate progress, plan for hospital discharge, and summarize needs for the visiting nurse who is following the patient in the home setting.

Approach to the Patient. Unless staff actively look for teaching-learning needs in respiratory patients, these needs will go unrecognized. They do not become evident until a frightening experience or a complication—accumulation of mucus, increase in wheezing, or pneumonia—prompts the patient to seek care. The nurse approaches the patient with this perspective and the following points in mind.

Assume the patient has teaching-learning needs until

Table 17–2. FOUR LEARNING AREAS*

Learning Area	Example
Knowledge (cognitive)	Knowing the name, dosage, therapeutic effects, and side effects of pulmonary medications
Skills (psychomotor)	Using an inhaler with correct hand coordination and breathing technique
Attitudes (affective)	Believing that bronchodilators will help control pulmonary symptoms and facilitate return to a normal or near-normal life style
Practices (behavior patterns)	Taking pulmonary medications and aerosol treatments at regularly scheduled times

*Adapted from Chatham, M. A. and Knapp, B. L.: Patient Education Handbook. Bowie, Maryland, Robert J. Brady Co., 1982.

proved otherwise. Many, if not most, respiratory patients fall into one or more of the categories listed in the next box, indicating the likely presence of a teaching-learning need.

FACTORS ASSOCIATED WITH TEACHING-LEARNING NEEDS

Surgery
Theophylline level less than 5 mcg/ml
History of noncompliance
Child or adolescent
Elderly person
Recurrent acute exacerbations of chronic disease
Critical or terminal illness
Complex treatment regimen
Limited ability to communicate; e.g., language barrier, endotracheal intubation
Psychologic coping mechanisms of denial, depression, repression, social isolation

The very young patient and very old patient are included in this list because Becker (1979) indicates that noncompliance is associated with extremes of age rather than with factors such as sex, ethnic group, race, education, occupation, income, marital status, intelligence, and religion. Many respiratory patients fall into these two age groups, e.g., young asthmatic and older persons who develop COPD signs and symptoms in the 50s and 60s.

The chronic COPD patient with psychologic coping mechanisms of denial, repression, and isolation typically is unaware of teaching-learning needs. Sometimes, adaptation to chronic dyspnea is accompanied by an unquestioned acceptance of physical limitations that could be at least partially eliminated by pulmonary rehabilitation. In other cases, intense concentration on frequently scheduled medications and treatments leaves the patient little energy or perspective to identify teaching-learning needs.

Similarly, the acutely ill patient with hypoxemia or fluid, electrolyte, or acid-base disorders relies on staff to identify needs until his condition and mental functioning improve. The terminally ill patient and his family will need knowledge of the normal grieving process. In the critical care unit, both patient and family typically require knowledge of the disease process, medications, treatments, and supportive measures throughout the crisis. In addition, they require a basic orientation to the bedside setup, ventilator, cardiac monitor, intravenous lines, and other technologic equipment that may elicit anxiety reactions in persons unfamiliar with their purposes and normal functions.

Self-care education will probably still be necessary, even if the patient does not fall into one of the categories listed in the previous box. According to Eraker and coworkers (1984), noncompliance is estimated at 50% for patients with chronic diseases. Knowledge can significantly reduce this rate, particularly in the case of reversible diseases, such as asthma and congestive heart failure. Moreover, patients tend to have persistent need for reteaching and relearning, since they forget almost immediately as much as one half of what the physician has told them.

Look for affective or attitudinal needs. Though not always readily apparent, affective needs are almost always present in persons with underlying chronic disease, owing to the long motivational process (see Chapter 16). Moreover, acute illness serves as a crisis, forcing the patient to reexamine and modify his attitudes and beliefs. In many cases, unless the acute care nurse recognizes verbal or nonverbal willingness to discuss the illness and acts on these cues, the patient is transferred to the ward, and he quickly reverts to old attitudes and habits.

To foster the identification of affective needs, the nurse (1) encourages verbalization of feelings and beliefs about respiratory disease and health enhancement and (2) explores factors that might have prevented health enhancement and precipitated acute illness, e.g., smoking, refusal to take bronchodilator medications. The goal of intervention is to determine (1) whether the individual has developed an attitude of acceptance versus denial of his disease and (2) whether he takes responsibility for caring for himself.

Use good interviewing skills (see Chapter 10 for history taking skills) as follows:

(1) Use open-ended questions such as "What concerns you now?" to identify needs, unanswered questions, and concerns.

(2) Give the patient plenty of time to explain past experiences. Remember, many patients are reluctant to reveal teaching-learning needs for fear of being labelled "clumsy," "mentally slow," or "problem patient."

(3) Always maintain a positive attitude and reinforcing manner towards the patient. Patients are more likely to listen and comply with therapy when they have a *positive reflexive self concept* (Currie, 1978). A positive reflexive self concept is present when the patient or the family member caring for the patient thinks the nurse has a positive image of him.

Maintain a self-care orientation. The nurse may revert temporarily to patient education to orient the patient and family to agency rules and regulations, visiting hours, meal times, and so forth. She may then present a self-care orientation for matters pertaining more directly to care of the patient. In other situations, total self care is impossible, owing to a disabling or critical illness. Nevertheless, the nurse strives to maintain a self-care orientation to help the patient and family move away from learned helplessness and towards disease acceptance and self-care activities. For example, the nurse may ask the intubated patient to indicate "yes" or "no" to simple choices about the arrangement of bedside objects and treatment schedules. While delivering patient care, the nurse may freely share information, such as temperature, amount

Text continued on page 482

Table 17–3. SAMPLE PROFILE FORM FOR COPD PATIENTS*

Personal Information

Name: ______
Age: ______ Sex: ______ Marital Status: ______
Occupation: ______
Socio-economic status/financial limitations: ______

Description of Condition

Type of COPD: ______
Suspected duration: ______
When diagnosed: ______
Smoker? ______ If yes, what? ______
Light or heavy? ______ How long? ______
Degree of concern/anxiety about condition: ______
Any specific concerns? ______
______
Comments: ______
Current activity level: ______
Desired activity level: ______
Other medical conditions: ______

Living Situation

Special dietary habits affecting treatment (likes to use salt; enjoys fish; hates vegetables; not a dessert eater; enjoys smoked foods): ______
______
Persons living w/patient: ______
Type of residence: ______
Does patient have to use stairs? ______
Characteristics of neighborhood: ______
Is it safe for walking? ______
Household responsibilities; Current: ______
Desired: ______
Persons available to help patient: ______
Consulted? ______ yes ______ no ______ not available ______

Desires, Goals, Hobbies, Interests

Goals expressed by patient: ______
______
Special interests pertaining to teatment: ______
______
Hobbies patient wishes to continue or to learn: ______
Recreational abilities; current level: ______
Desired level: ______
Typical daily activities: ______
______
______
______
______

*Reproduced by permission form Freedman. C.: Teaching Patients. San Diego: Courseware, Inc., 1978, 52.

Table continued on opposite page

Table 17–3. SAMPLE PROFILE FORM FOR COPD PATIENTS* *Continued*

Treatment		***In Hospital Only***	***To Be Continued At Home***
Medications			
(Include name,			
dosage, and			
frequency)			
Special equipment			
(Linde walkers,			
IPPB, oxygen,			
nebulizer or			
vaporizer, ultrasonic			
nebulizer)			
Bronchial hygiene			
General physical			
Reconditioning			
exercises			
Dietary regulations			

Readiness and Ability to Learn

Educational background: ______

Language level (as seen by conversation, books read, etc.): ______

Language limitations: ______

Learning limitations (hearing, sight, exhaustion, pain, senility, arthritis): ______

Level of interest in learning about treatment: ______

Knowledge of disease and treatment: ______

______

Outside affiliations: ______

Anyone else consulted about patient (relatives): ______

Major areas of resistance to learning or to treatment compliance: ______

______

Willingness to take responsibility for condition: ______ High

______ Moderate

______ Low

Table 17–4. ASSESSMENT TOOL FOR TEACHING-LEARNING NEEDS

Directions

For initial assessment: Rate the patient using the scale below. Write the score in the first column. Fill in other information as indicated by the situation.

0 = Unable to perform; no understanding
1 = Poor coordination and technique; minimal understanding
2 = Barely passable technique; basic understanding
3 = Good technique with intermittent coaching; good understanding
4 = Good to excellent technique without supervision; excellent understanding

For discharge planning: Check appropriate columns and fill in information as indicated. Comment about patient progress in the space provided.

Date and initial all evaluations.

Patient's Name	*Initial Assessment Score*	*Demonstration (Verbal Explanation)*	*Return Demonstration*	*Written Instructions Provided*	*Care-giver(s):*
Educational Content					**Comments**
I. General understanding or recognition of disease process					
II. Preventive measures A. Knowledge and recognition of: 1. Medications Name/dosage Schedule Purpose Side effects Refill information					
2. Signs of overexertion					
3. Signs of infection					
4. Signs of fluid retention					
5. Importance of flu shot/ Pneumovax					
B. Adequate diet and fluid intake					
C. Environmental control 1. Avoidance of persons with URI*					
2. Abstinence from smoking					
3. Avoidance of irritants					
D. Has been advised: 1. What to do when ill					
2. Whom to call for advice					
3. What to do in case of a smog alert					

Table continued on opposite page

Table 17–4. ASSESSMENT TOOL FOR TEACHING-LEARNING NEEDS *Continued*

Patient's Name	*Initial Assessment Score*	*Demonstration (Verbal Explanation)*	*Return Demonstration*	*Written Instructions Provided*	*Care-giver(s):*
Educational Content					**Comments**
III. Chest therapy A. Relaxation and posture					
B. Deep breathing and coughing					
C. Breathing retraining 1. Pursed lip breathing					
2. Diaphragmatic breathing a. With resp. treatments, e.g., compressor/nebulizer, MDD† b. At rest c. While walking					
3. Breathing while walking miles, city blocks, or yards: Goal:					
4. Breathing while stair climbing: No. of stairs or flights:					
5. Controlling dyspneic episodes					
D. Activities of daily living (ADLs) that aggravate pulmonary symptoms					
E. Muscle reconditioning exercises: 1. Passive/active (ROM)‡ 2. Arm exercises 3. Leg exercises					
F. Postural drainage 1. With percussion and vibration (P and V) 2. With mechanical percussion 3. Without P and V					
G. Other					
IV. Use of equipment Type: Brand/model				Last gas sterilized	
A. Measuring and storing medications					
B. Cleaning and storing equipment					
C. Assembly and disassembly					
D. Proper technique in taking treatment					
E. Proper use of O_2					
F. Has been advised: 1. Whom to contact for O_2 refill or equipment problems					
2. What to do in case of bronchodilator side effects					
V. Other					

*Upper respiratory infection.
†Metered dose device.
‡Range of motion.

and color of sputum, goals of respiratory treatments, and anticipated outcomes if therapy is not followed. The ongoing flow of small amounts of information throughout the day or week is easier for the patient to ponder and assimilate compared with the delivery of large amounts of information given without sufficient time for reflection, discussion, and integration. Simultaneously, the nurse may ask a patient's friend or willing and able family member to participate in care, e.g., hold a patient's hand during endotracheal suctioning, help turn the patient, give the patient a bath, or supervise the patient's range of motion exercises.

Insistence on patient involvement in at least some aspects of self-care sends an important message, i.e., *the patient is responsible for his own health.* Insistence on at least some family member's or friend's involvement reminds all that their support is desired and needed for health enhancement and maintenance.

Use direct observation of respiratory techniques rather than reliance on historical data to identify needs. For example, direct observation of pursed-lip breathing while the patient is walking is better than reliance on verbal reports, because COPD patients commonly deny breathing difficulties when obviously dyspneic. Chronically ill persons may unknowingly practice faulty techniques for months or years due to lack of knowledge, e.g., no one told them to keep their nebulizer solution in the refrigerator at home or to relax their upper chest muscles during abdominal-diaphragmatic breathing.

Sometimes lack of awareness, carelessness, or poor eyesight is responsible for the patient's failure to identify teaching-learning needs. For example, the home patient may know that respiratory equipment should be completely dry before use. Nevertheless, he may miss detection of small water droplets in nebulizer reservoirs or breathing tubes, owing to poor eyesight, preoccupation with personal problems, or dyspnea.

STEP 2: IDENTIFY READINESS TO LEARN

Readiness to learn is present when the patient

1. *Identifies a learning need,* e.g., need to stop smoking.
2. *Sets or agrees to a learning goal,* e.g., smoking cessation within 2 months.
3. *Understands how to achieve the goal,* e.g., sudden cessation or gradual reduction in cigarettes smoked per day.

Similar to motivational assessment and intervention, prerequisites 1 and 2 are mandatory. Prerequisite 3 may be incompletely developed as long as the patient is willing to try an agreed upon plan. However, when annoyance, resistance, or inconsistent verbal or nonverbal behavior appears, the nurse must take more time with the patient, using open-ended questions and long pauses to elicit suppressed feelings, questions, fears, and misconceptions about anticipated interventions. The nurse does not proceed to steps 3 and 4 until the patient meets the listed three prerequisites and shows an eagerness to proceed with the teaching-learning process.

Common barriers blocking readiness to learn are listed in Table 17–5, along with goals and interventions for reducing these barriers.

The establishment of an effective communication system is a vital component of readiness to learn as well as respiratory care in general (see Table 17–5 and Fig. 17–2). Though many respiratory patients can identify appropriate teaching-learning needs, they cannot communicate them owing to shortness of breath, intubation, or head and neck surgery. The chronically ill patient may not consider vocalization of needs worth the resulting increase in dyspnea, cough, and sputum production. Unless a communication system is established well before the need for teaching arises, both patient and staff become frustrated by the limitations of lip reading and by futile attempts at sign language. The patient becomes more and more agitated and discouraged. Limited in time and resources, the nurse never fully answers all the patient's questions. Hence, the patient either gives up all effort to communicate (an overt sign of depression and helplessness), or he goes through the motions of the teaching-learning process without actually learning the self-care content.

In addition to an effective communication system, three other factors help establish readiness to learn as follows: (1) an interpersonal relationship of trust, caring, and mutual respect; (2) an optimum physical environment; and (3) the presence of a family member or friend. Ideally, the primary nurse caring for the patient implements all teaching-learning sessions. The physical environment should be pleasant, comfortable, and well lit for careful observation of demonstrations. Distractions should be kept to a minimum by limiting telephone calls, visitors, unnecessary alarms, and unrelated nursing care during teaching-learning sessions. Whenever possible, teaching-learning should not begin until a family member or friend is present, since this person is crucial for support and reinforcement of self-care activities at home and in the hospital.

STEP 3: SET LEARNING GOALS

The nurse sets goals with the patient on a daily, weekly, or monthly basis as indicated by the situation. The process is basically the same as that described for the motivational process in Chapter 16.

Use of a Contingency Contract

Before or during implementation of teaching-learning interventions, the nurse may negotiate a contingency contract between herself and the patient or the patient and a family member or friend. A *contingency contract* is a written agreement outlining desired behavior in measurable terms that are acceptable to all persons involved. An example is provided in the box on page 485.

Table 17–5. COMMON BARRIERS TO READINESS TO LEARN

Barrier	Clinical Manifestations	Goals for Intervention	Inverventions
Poor nutrition	Depression Confusion Headaches Fatigue Irritability Poor dietary intake Signs of malnutrition, e.g., poor skin turgor, alopecia	Optimize nutritional status	Obtain a nutritional assessment, with attention to nutrient and caloric analysis, fluid intake and output, and psychosocial variables, including income, food habits, cultural influences, impaired taste, smell, and chewing ability Provide appropriate dietary instruction to patient and family
Dementia, cognitive-affective disorders	Memory impairment Mental confusion Apathy Depression Helplessness	Optimize mental functioning	Utilize experts in psychology and gerontology to determine precise cause of signs and symptoms, e.g., boredom versus true senility Help alter external and internal variables to promote normal mental functioning, e.g., environment, self-confidence level, support system, other medications affecting sensorium Maintain self-care orientation and avoid interventions that reinforce learned helplessness Direct family in self-care activities to reorient patient and help him develop sense of worth, self esteem, accomplishment
Hypoxemia, acid-base and electrolyte disorders	Pa_{O_2} less than 60 mmHg Pa_{CO_2} less than 35 or greater than 45 mmHg pH greater than 7.45 or less than 7.35 Signs of electrolyte imbalance Signs of delirium	Attain a normal sensorium and normal Pa_{O_2} and pH Optimize fluid and electrolyte status	Provide oxygen to normalize Pa_{O_2} at the lowest possible O_2 concentration. Correct fluid and electrolyte disorders. Normalize pH (see Table 13–3) Monitor for signs of hypoxemia, ventilatory failure, change in sensorium, fluid and electrolyte imbalance
Inadequate communication system	Limited patient-nurse communication Signs of frustration, hopelessness, and helplessness Endotracheal or tracheal intubation Laryngectomy or other head and neck surgery	Establish effective and efficient communication system between patient and nurse	Establish communication system before intubation, whenever possible, i.e., preoperatively Use lip reading; encourage patient to clearly form vowels and consonants without vocalization (vocalization may damage vocal cords of intubated patients) Use sign language, e.g., one hand squeeze for "yes" and two squeezes for "no" Provide a magic slate or pad and pencil for longer messages or thoughts Keep communication tools ready at bedside, e.g., an alphabet with large block letters for spelling words, and a table of common needs for the patient to point to (Fig. 17–2). Place the intubated patient in Fowler's position, suction endotracheally and oropharyngeally, and deflate cuff partially or fully for speech; whenever possible, use a cuffless or talking tracheostomy tube (described in Chapter 26) Encourage the use of speaking devices, e.g., Passy-Muir tracheostomy speaking valve; Venti-Voice communication aid (Bear Medical Systems, Inc.) for ventilation dependent patients; Blom-Singer amplifier for laryngectomy patients.
Hearing impairment	Complaints of difficulty hearing Little to no response when spoken to Limited comprehension of simple messages Limited number of social interactions Dead batteries in hearing aid Refusal to wear a hearing aid	Increase verbal comprehension, nurse-patient communications, and social interactions with others	Encourage patient to verbalize feelings about his hearing aid, wear the device, and keep an extra battery readily available Speak directly to the patient, clearly enunciating words if necessary For group teaching sessions, provide front row seating or an amplification device Encourage periodic medical and audiology evaluations Remind the patient that it is his responsibility to indicate when he has difficulty hearing; stress the benefits of hearing, e.g., increased social interaction, and so forth
Pain	Complaints of pain Tachycardia Hypertension Tachypnea Splinting respirations Diaphoresis Inability to concentrate	Increase pain threshold to enhance mental and physical functioning	Give appropriate pain medication before teaching-learning sessions Maintain proper body alignment and good posture Promote use of guided imagery, yoga exercises, or biofeedback techniques to help reduce stress and anxiety related to pain
Fatigue	Complaints of fatigue Somnolence Signs of sleep deprivation Signs of hypercarbia	Minimize fatigue associated with illness	Group patient care activities to provide for uninterrupted sleep Plan interventions when the respiratory patient is least tired and most comfortable, e.g., afternoons, before or after weaning from mechanical ventilation, after bronchodilator medications Check Pa_{CO_2} when signs of hypercarbia are present

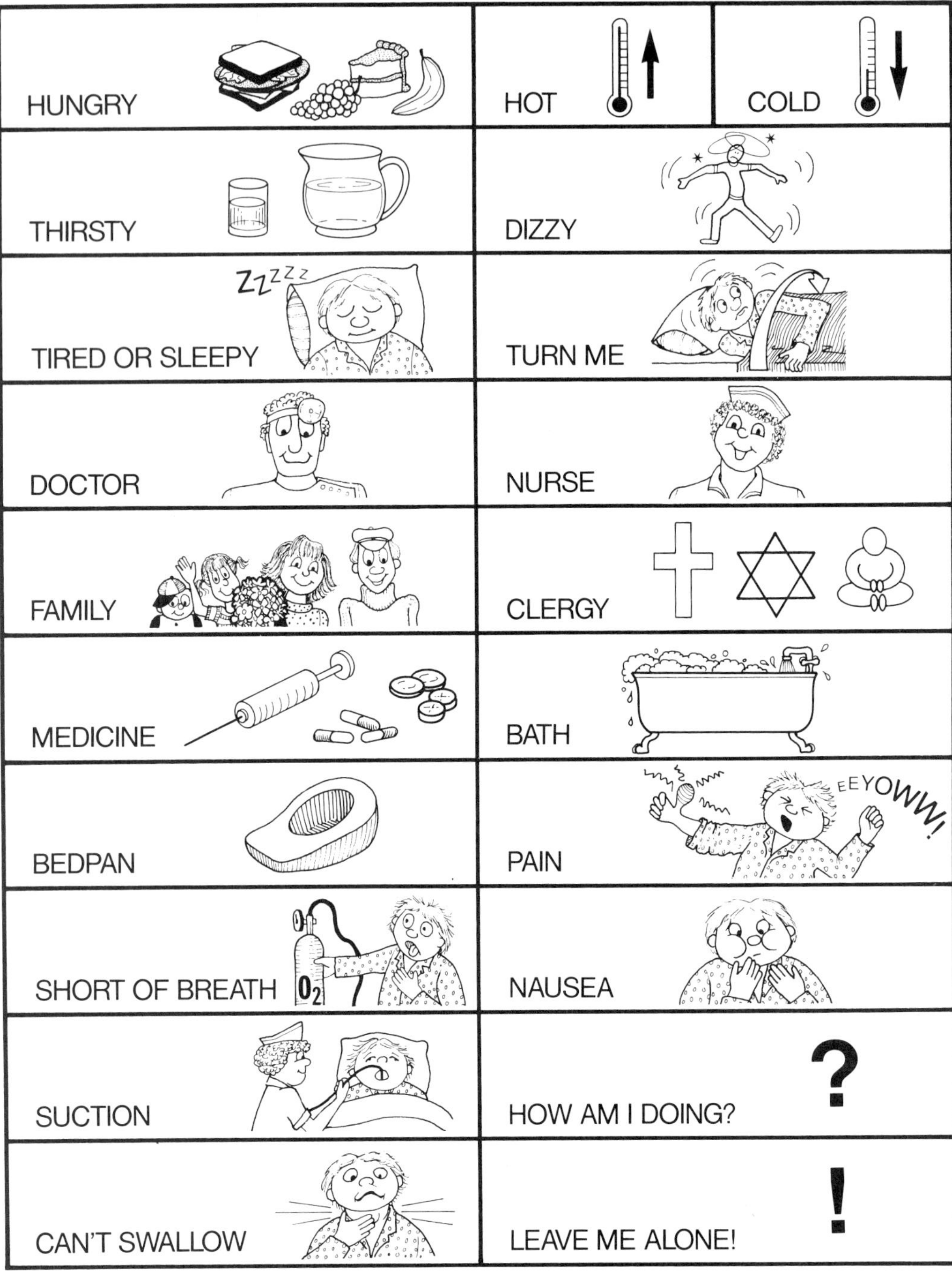

Figure 17–2. Example of a communication chart for a respiratory patient who cannot speak because of intubation, surgery, or trauma. The patient is instructed to point to the appropriate problem or need represented on the chart. (Adapted and reproduced by permission from a chart drawn by Terry Lewis and Susan Oshiro, Los Angeles, California.)

A CONTINGENCY CONTRACT

I, Joe Smith, will take an aerosol treatment before bed and upon arising in the morning.

In return, you, Mary Smith, will arrange for oxygen cylinder changes once a week on Mondays.

Signed:________________
Signed:________________
Date:________________

In this example, Mary's agreement to arrange for oxygen cylinder changes is Joe's reward for keeping the contract. If Joe did not keep the contract (i.e., did not take his aerosol treatments), Mary would not order the oxygen. Joe would have to order the oxygen himself.

Examples of patients likely to benefit the most from this approach include (1) the anxious patient who reluctantly discontinues tranquilizers during a pulmonary rehabilitation program, (2) the obese patient who needs or wants a reward for weight loss, and (3) the patient with a new tracheostomy who is reluctant to try cleaning his respiratory equipment.

A contingency contract may be offensive to some patients because of its legal nature. However, standard inclusion of a reward, called a *reinforcer*, provides many patients with a needed incentive for the practice of health-seeking behavior. Also, once the advantage of having a built-in reinforcer is explained, use of such a contract may be placed in higher regard by persons who were initially offended by its legal nature.

Reinforcers vary, depending on the situation. They may be intangible, such as words of encouragement or departure from strict agency visiting rules; or they may be tangible, such as filling out insurance forms, changing a bed or room assignment, or supervising the first three attempts to clean respiratory equipment. In all cases, the patient is asked to identify a reward that is truly reinforcing to him, regardless of its relation to health and illness (Steckel, 1982). Sometimes merely asking. "How can I help you achieve your goal?" helps the patient identify a meaningful reinforcer.

Patient and nurse or family member sign the contract, date it, and keep a copy for evaluation purposes.

Learning Objectives and Evaluation Criteria

The nurse translates the patient's goal into specific learning objectives. A *learning objective* states what the patient is to learn in behavioral objective form. A *subobjective* is a specific learning objective used to further delineate behaviors for accomplishment of the main objective. In a teaching-learning plan, several subobjectives may be listed under one main objective.

Robert Mager's text, *Preparing Instructional Objectives* (1984), clearly explains how to write a behavioral objective. Essentially, an objective includes a simple statement of a single task. It is learner- rather than teacher-oriented. In addition, it is written with an action verb that has, ideally, only one interpretation. Examples of acceptable verbs follow.

ACTION VERBS FOR OBJECTIVE WRITING

administer	describe	prepare
apply	differentiate	read
auscultate	drain	repeat
call	examine	report
clean	explain	set up
collect	identify	state
compare	implement	store
contrast	list	suction
cough	measure	use
deep breathe	oxygenate	walk
define	perform	write
demonstrate		

Verbs with many interpretations are avoided. Examples of unacceptable ambiguous verbs include to know (meaning to recall, relate, understand, or identify?), to be familiar with, to realize, to appreciate, to believe, and to think.

Most important, the behavioral objective must be stated in measurable terms. For example, *calling* an equipment company can be measured or evaluated by checking with the spouse or equipment company. *Thinking* of three side effects of a medication is not measurable because of the impossibility of determining thought content.

When a teaching-learning need is identified, an overall objective is written with specification of conditions under which the behavior is expected to occur. For example, patient and nurse might agree on a main objective of administration of an effective aerosol treatment without assistance, as shown in Table 17–6. Next, patient and nurse agree on specific criteria that, when met, indicate successful attainment of the goal or objective (see Table 17–6). Evaluation criteria vary, depending on individual situations. They may contain a patient component for self evaluation at home and a professional component for more objective evaluation. In the latter case, changes in lung sounds, PFTs, ABGs, or other physical findings are used.

For complex techniques, the nurse writes subobjectives with corresponding evaluation criteria, as shown in Table 17–6.

To identify appropriate subobjectives, the nurse might ask the following key question:

> What changes in this patient's knowledge, skills, attitudes, and practices are needed to attain the main objective?

In Table 17–6, subobjectives are categorized into four learning areas, but since content areas often overlap, this delineation is not mandatory.

To help write specific evaluation criteria, the nurse may use the evaluation criteria in Part Four of this book as a guide. Then, the nurse may further define the criterion in terms of the following:

> *How much*: e.g., list *three out of five* side effects for metaprotereno (Alupent).
> *How well* (percentage of accuracy): e.g., perform pursed-lip breathing *with 80% accuracy*.
> *How long* (time): e.g., administer daily medications as scheduled *for 4 weeks*.

Ranking Needs and Objectives

Respiratory patients typically have more than one learning need. Once identified, needs and corresponding objectives are categorized into acute, preventive, and maintenance categories. Next, they are ranked from highest priority to lowest priority, considering the patient's personal goals and the clinical circumstances surrounding the illness. Acute needs are ranked as highest priority. The nurse initially focuses intervention on these needs and later addresses lower priority preventive and maintenance needs, described in Table 17–7. These three categories are extremely fluid and not necessarily, mutually exclusive. For example, the need to learn the correct use of an inhaler is an acute one for an unstable asthmatic at home. It becomes of lower priority when a hand-held nebulizer is substituted for the inhaler in the hospital's emergency room. Once the acute asthmatic attack subsides, preventive and maintenance needs (i.e., objectives) are given higher priority, because their fulfillment is crucial to health enhancement and prevention of another acute exacerbation.

STEP 4: IMPLEMENT TEACHING-LEARNING INTERVENTIONS

Step 4 of the teaching-learning process is planning and implementating teaching-learning interventions. This step blends into step 3 (set learning goals), since planning actually begins once goal identification prompts the formation and ranking of objectives based on needs. In other cases, step 4 blends into step 5 (evaluate outcomes), and teaching the patient and evaluating reactions add new information to the data base and alter initial impressions and the teaching-learning plan.

Table 17–6. EXAMPLE OF RESPIRATORY LEARNING OBJECTIVES AND EVALUATION CRITERIA

Main Objective	Main Evaluation Criteria
To administer an effective bronchodilator aerosol treatment without assistance.	In 3 days (1) the patient reports minimal to no wheezing and no difficulty taking scheduled aerosol treatments, (2) the nurse observes correct technique, and (3) the nurse auscultates good ventilation over all lung lobes with minimal to absent wheezing.
Subobjectives by Learning Areas	**Subjectives are Met When the Patient Meets These Following Corresponding Criteria**
Knowledge	
1. To state the name, dosage, therapeutic effects and side effects, of the bronchodilator medication.	1. Repeats the name, correct dosage, one therapeutic effect, and three side effects of metaproterenol (Alupent) when asked by the nurse.
2. To state the purpose of the hand-held nebulizer used to deliver aerosol.	2. Explains how the nebulizer's aerosol transports bronchodilator deep into the lungs when asked by family members.
3. To state what to do when the nebulizer does not work properly.	3. Looks up the equipment vendor's name and telephone number in the telephone book when asked to do so.
Skills	
4. To demonstrate correct technique for addition of medication to the nebulizer.	4. a. Uses a dropper to measure the correct amount of medication. b. Adds the medication to the nebulizer correctly. c. Holds the nebulizer so that the medication lies by the nebulizer's capillary.
5. To demonstrate correct technique during aerosol delivery.	5. Demonstrates a comfortable deep breathing pattern with (a) finger occlusion of the activator valve coordinated with inspiration, (b) 1- to 3-second end-inspiratory pause, and (c) a treatment lasting no longer than 10–20 minutes.
Attitudes	
6. To take responsibility for learning and refining treatments.	6. Remembers and takes his own treatments at home as reported by the spouse.
Practices	
7. To administer own treatments at bedtime and upon arising without assistance.	7. Takes treatment at scheduled times for 1 month without fail and without assistance as reported by patient and spouse.
8. To call spouse or equipment vendor whenever equipment problems arise.	8. Successfully calls the equipment vendor within 12 hours when an equipment problem arises at home.

Table 17–7. PRIORITY SYSTEM FOR TEACHING-LEARNING NEEDS AND OBJECTIVES

Type of Teaching-Learning Need	Characteristic Features	Example	Related Objective
Acute need—top priority	Causes psychosocial anguish, physical deterioration, or both Requires immediate attention	Need to learn correct use of inhaler	Use inhaler at scheduled times with 80% accuracy
Preventive need	Patient exhibits risk factors for disease (e.g., stress, smoking), or environmental factors increase risk for disease (e.g., smog, unkempt and dusty living quarters) Need may cause mild to moderate chronic disease Need likely to become acute when unmet	Need to ingest 2 to 3 qt liquid daily to keep mucus thin	Ingest 2 to 3 qt liquid daily as evidenced by spouse
Maintenance need—lowest priority	Present when patient exhibits learning disability or low psychosocial assets that make periodic reteaching and relearning necessary When met, compliance and avoidance of pulmonary complications results When neglected, acute needs eventually develop Common in elderly chronically ill respiratory patients (they usually need long-term follow-up teaching every 6–12 mo.)	Need to understand the appropriate scheduling of daily bronchodilators to achieve 24-hr bronchodilatation	State an optimal schedule with rationale for administation of bronchodilators

Teaching Methods

One or more teaching methods may be used to attain the overall teaching-learning objective (Table 17–8).

Several factors are considered before selection of a method, including the type of learning objective; the teacher's knowledge and expertise; the time available; the teaching resources; and the learner's comprehension level, motivation, and prior knowledge.

The nurse can use Table 17–9 as a guide to choosing an appropriate teaching method. All methods have advantages and disadvantages that affect their appropriateness for specific patients and settings. For example, audiovisual aids are ideal for sparking patient interest in subjects related to lung diseases. However, they can be quite expensive. Also, they require a quiet space for viewing, adequate time for presentation, and a previewing session to assess the appropriateness of content, educational level, and cultural bias. When audiovisuals are inappropriate or unavailable, printed materials and discussions serve to deliver the same educational content.

Demonstration is a common teaching method of choice because of the numerous skills required for use of inhalers, nebulizers, intermittent positive pressure breathing (IPPB) devices, incentive spirometers, suctioning devices, and other respiratory interventions. To teach by demonstration, the nurse follows the steps in the next box for an effective teaching-learning session (see Steps for an Effective Learning Session).

Demonstrations and other methods require reinforcement with printed materials. The most effective printed materials have most of the desirable characteristics (see the box entitled Characteristics of Effective Printed Materials).

An example of an effective teaching poster is shown in Figure 17–3. Note that it is clearly labelled, with use of arrows and enlarged diagrams for illustrating key information.

Individualizing Interventions

The following points guide the nurse in individualizing teaching-learning interventions.

1. *Use printed material specific to the patient's disease, comprehension level, and interest.* An avid reader may wish to read a whole book on COPD. Others may wish to read only enough information to resolve their immediate problems. To avoid information overload, health professionals may develop education material specific to their particular patient population. Then, the nurse presents only one instruction sheet per teaching-learning session. This approach provides for gradual introduction of material as the patient's condition stabilizes. Also, it helps maintain congruence between printed materials and verbal instructions (Fig. 17–4).

2. *Whenever possible, use short informal discussions, supported by handwritten comments and diagrams.* Patients may not understand formally delivered educational content until subsequent informal conversations make key concepts more relevant and meaningful.

3. *Keep family and friends involved in teaching-learning interventions.* They provide emotional support and sometimes necessary skills, such as percussion and vibration (P and V) during postural drainage or cleaning nebulizers at home. Their ability and willingness to reinforce content influences the patient's ability and willingness to transfer content from the hospital to the home setting (Fig. 17–5).

STEPS FOR AN EFFECTIVE LEARNING SESSION*

1. Set up respiratory equipment (if applicable).
2. Confirm readiness to learn. Postpone the session if the patient is overly drowsy, anxious, or in pain.
3. Tell the patient what you would like to demonstrate and why.
4. Explain the objective of the teaching-learning session.
5. Confirm prerequisite information by asking the patient what he has already learned about the subject, e.g., during the last teaching-learning session.
6. Give a printed handout listing steps or key information you plan to cover.
7. Slowly and simply explain the steps or information, demonstrating skills or giving examples as you go along.
8. Point out common mistakes or misconceptions, ask and answer questions, and use diagrams and models when necessary.
9. Ask the patient to return the demonstration or repeat key concepts or essential instructions. Supervise each step, until performed correctly, giving plenty of positive feedback for small as well as large accomplishments.
10. Document the session in the patient's chart. State the information covered, the problems encountered, and the plan for the next teaching-learning session.
11. Arrange for a repeat demonstration on another day to assure retention of the learned skill.

*After Freedman, C.: Teaching Patients. San Diego: Courseware, Inc., 1978.

CHARACTERISTICS OF EFFECTIVE PRINTED MATERIALS

Simple language
- Layman's terms, 8th grade level of comprehension
- Action verbs

Appropriate title
- Reflects purpose of material

Clear diagrams

Clear labelling

Key information is emphasized
- Bold-faced print

Optimal size
- Narrow pamphlets are best. Comprehension is increased when reading narrow-column material

Aesthetic
- Good spacial arrangement, clear print, no smudges, colorful

Interesting
- Pleasing cover or title, funny diagrams

4. *Conduct demonstrations using the patient's own equipment.* Ask equipment companies to deliver to the patient's hospital room. This policy facilitates learning and permits trouble-shooting for equipment problems before the patient goes home.

5. *Concentrate on only a few interventions at a time.* Choose one or two major interventions aimed at accomplishing top priority objectives. When these interventions are mastered, be sure to integrate them with the patient's overall activity and treatment schedule, e.g., write them down and list times on the patient's schedule.

6. *For each intervention, break complex skills down into small steps and proceed only as the patient masters each step.* For example, consider the head and neck surgery patient with a fresh tracheostomy who must learn to suction himself before leaving the intensive care unit. The nurse teaches from a list of subobjectives, each corresponding to a key step in the procedure. As soon as the patient accomplishes the first subobjective (i.e., learning the anatomy of the tracheobronchial tree), the nurse checks it off on the teaching-learning plan and proceeds to the next subobjective (i.e., learning the purpose of and indications for suctioning).

7. *Adapt standard objectives to the patient's situation.* Some patients are fast learners. They may accomplish the main objective within 15 minutes, using an acceptable variation of the standard technique. The nurse modifies subobjectives accordingly. Other patients are slow learners. They may become extremely anxious and need continual reassurance just to get the suction catheter tip to the tracheostomy opening during the suctioning procedure. For learners with special needs, the nurse adds subobjectives to the teaching-learning plan. For the anxious patient, the nurse might add "Call son to bedside before suctioning" or "Use bedside mirror to help locate tracheostomy opening."

8. *Place the teaching-learning plan in the chart.* The plan should include a check list or record including: learning objectives and subobjectives, teaching methods, evaluation criteria, dates for objective accomplishment, and comments or special problems.

9. *Encourage nurses and other caregivers to teach from the same teaching-learning plan to maintain consistency among teachers.* Emphasize technique details that relate to evaluation criteria listed in the care plan. For example, if holding one's breath for 3 seconds is the evaluation criterion for effective aerosol delivery, then the nurse and all involved must tell the patient 3 seconds, not 5 or 10 seconds. If the patient can easily hold his breath for a longer period of time, breath

Table 17–8. TEACHING METHODS AND TECHNIQUES*

Methods/Techniques	Examples	Advantages	Disadvantages
Audiovisuals	Films, slide-tape shows, and video cassettes available through the American Lung Association, American Thoracic Society, American Cancer Society, and other organizations.	Provide in-depth, clear presentations of specific topics, e.g., lung disease, learning to breathe better. Short 15 to 20 minute audiovisual aids are best. Are very effective as long as the nurse is present in room to encourage attention and reinforce learning afterward. May facilitate discussion of sensitive topics, such as sexuality. Serve to vary the stimuli for learning, providing a welcome change of pace in pulmonary rehabilitation programs.	May be oriented to a high comprehension level, move too fast through content, or be too long in duration for a person with breathing problems. The nurse may tend to think the patient understood the content if he watched the program. A knowledgeable nurse must be available to answer questions. Expense or logistics may limit use.
Behavioral contracting	Contingency contracting with options to renegotiate conditions at any time. Informal verbal agreement.	Holds patient and nurse accountable for mutually agreed upon conditions. Good for patients with compliance problem or who need a reinforcer to shape health-seeking behavior.	The legal nature of the contract is offensive to some persons. May be initially time-consuming to negotiate conditions.
Case example	Introducing the patient to another person who has already learned to live comfortably within the limitations of lung disease.	Helps patients to personally relate to content and express feelings about their condition. May facilitate learning when the patient appears disinterested in teaching or states that the nurse "doesn't understand what he is going through." May help patient understand and accept his medical diagnosis.	Unless the nurse knows what the case patient is going to say, this method may not work. May be time-consuming for the nurse to find an appropriate case example, i.e., one with similar personality, disability, and level of disease acceptance and who can communicate well.
Demonstration	Taking an aerosol treatment Using an inhaler Cleaning respiratory equipment	Provides an opportunity for observation and practice of needed skills. Is time efficient in the long run for the teaching and follow-up of complex skills.	Best for skills, not for cognitive domain of learning. Return demonstrations may be initially time-consuming, although in the long run they may prevent acute exacerbations of lung disease.
Drills	Assembly and disassembly of breathing circuits Taking pulmonary medications	Repetition of learned skills and information facilitates quick implementation of content. Good for learning practices or skills that can be broken down into small steps. Good for slow learners.	Patient may learn skills/practices without rationale and require further teaching later.
Discussions: individual/group (often supplemented with lecture or other methods)			
Individual	Discussion on asthma triggers and how to avoid them Discussion on recognition of signs and symptoms of bronchospasm and chest infection.	Promotes adaptation of content to individual learning needs and maximal learning within a short period of time.	Is cost and labor intensive.

Table continued on following page

Table 17–8. TEACHING METHODS AND TECHNIQUES* *Continued*

Methods/Techniques	Examples	Advantages	Disadvantages
Small group (2 to 8 persons)	Lecture and discussion on sexuality and lung disease, how to make a decision, or how to cope with thoracic surgery or lung disease at home. Informal "rap" sessions organized by a community service organization.	Excellent for affective or cognitive learning areas and process-oriented classes (e.g., decision-making). More cost effective for staff compared with individual teaching. Provides emotional support. Best used in stable ongoing groups.	Some persons still require individual teaching for adaptation of content to specific needs.
Medium group (8 to 30 persons)	Lecture or discussion on lung disease, oxygen delivery devices, or community resources available to persons with lung diseae.	Excellent for cognitive learning area. Cost effective for the initial introduction of material. Facilitates support groups.	Still must provide for the individualization of content. Content may not be applicable in some cases.
Large group (over 30 persons)	A Better Breather's patient club may organize a lecture on Traveling With Oxygen, followed by discussion or question-and-answer period.	Cost effective for cognitive learning. Facilitates support groups and promotes sense of community. May facilitate recruitment of patients for health enhancement or pulmonary rehabilitation programs.	Structure is relatively inflexible. Not optimal for psychomotor or affective learning domains. Planning and implementation are time-consuming.
Lectures	Teaching facts, concepts, and generalizations related to the diagnosis and treatment of lung disease.	Allows delivery of extensive amounts of information in a relatively short period of time. Best used with audiovisuals, demonstrations, case studies, printed materials, or anecdotes to maintain audience interest.	Same as for medium to large group discussions.
Printed materials	Books, pamphlets, brochures, and others available through professional and volunteer organizations, libraries, book stores, schools, hospitals, public health departments, pharmaceutical companies, and respiratory equipment vendors.	Excellent for reinforcement of demonstrations and verbal communications. Used for waiting rooms, examining rooms, schools, homes, and other places where access to other media is limited.	Verbal instruction or reinforcement is still needed. Materials may not be appropriate for the reading level of the patient and family. See Redman (1984) for reading level tests.
Problem solving and decision making techniques	Use of motivational model (see Chap. 16) to help the patient learn how to best adapt to lung disease. Use of decision making techniques for selection of an alternative solution for control of dyspnea.	Process orientation facilitates long-term behavior changes. Individual or small group discussions with family present are best. Cost effective; patient/family learn to correct mistakes in mental information processing that have led to ineffective coping patterns.	Family or significant other may not be available to participate. Requires intense or time-consuming nurse involvement in patient and family dynamics. Staffing patterns may not permit this degree of involvement. Patient's learning disability, hypoxemia, or denial of disease may prevent or limit use.
Question-and-answer sessions	Interviews Asking open-ended questions, e.g., "What might have you done differently to avoid the wheezing episode?" Question categories include: *who, what, when, where, how,* and *why.*	Used to collect additional data, stimulate new thought, and evaluate past behavior.	Open-ended questions may provide opportunity for patient to concentrate on peripherally related topics.

Table continued on opposite page

Table 17–8. TEACHING METHODS AND TECHNIQUES* *Continued*

Methods/Techniques	Examples	Advantages	Disadvantages
Role playing	Asking a friend to enact the role of a patient waking up in the middle of the night with wheezing and dyspnea. The role play should be short (5 minutes), with time allotted afterward to discuss feeling, outcomes, and what are learned.	Best for teaching attitudes, feelings, and problem solving. Reverse role playing allows the patient to evaluate alternative behaviors and feelings.	Time-consuming. Some patients refuse to participate or cannot owing to disability.
Self-instructional materials	Printed material presented in a step-by-step format with use of audiovisuals, demonstrations, programmed text, or other teaching methods. Built-in reinforcers may include drills or short question-and-answer segments to promote learning.	Allows the motivated patient to learn complex concepts at his own pace. Sources include publishers, audiovisual manufacturers, universities, libraries, health insurance companies, pharmaceutical companies, or health supply companies. A valuable supplement in the absence of adequate staff for teaching. An alternative for homebound or geographically isolated patients.	Patient still needs individualized teaching or reinforcement of material relevant to his situation. Equipment and materials may be unavailable or too costly. Some patients lack mental concentration, motivation, or ability to use material or pace themselves.

Adapted from Chatham, M. A., and Knapp, B. L.: Patient Education Handbook. Bowie, Maryland, Robert J. Brady Co., 1982.

holding may be lengthened to 10 seconds on the care plan. In any case, teaching is based on the care plan, so that the patient *always* receives consistent and individualized instructions (Fig. 17–6).

This approach facilitates continuity of care among the respiratory therapist, nurse, physician, and other health professionals. Also, when health team members collectively and consistently refer to the patient's teaching-learning plan and emphasize the same evaluation criteria, the clinical research is facilitated, and evaluation of specific respiratory techniques becomes more reliable and valid.

Table 17–9. GUIDE TO CHOOSING A TEACHING METHOD*

Learning Area	Teaching Method
Knowledge	Audiovisuals Printed materials Discussions and dialogues Lectures Question-and-answer sessions Self-instructional materials
Skills	Audiovisuals Demonstration Supervised practice (return demonstration) Self-instructional materials Drills Problem solving
Attitudes	Group discussions and sharing experiences Role playing Dramatizations and simulations Case examples Counseling (listening and feedback)
Practices	Behavioral contracting Behavioral modification Brainstorming Problem solving Counseling (listening and feedback)

*Adapted from Chatham, M. A., and Knapp, B. L.: Patient Education Handbook. Bowie, Maryland, Robert J. Brady Co., 1982.

STEP 5: EVALUATE OUTCOMES

Evaluation of outcomes is ongoing, beginning with implementation of teaching-learning interventions and ending with discontinuation of respiratory care services. It is a relatively simple process, if team members have written clear evaluation criteria before proceeding to interventions.

To evaluate outcomes, the nurse observes and documents the knowledge, skill, attitude, or practice specified as the outcome in the objective. For example, for subobjective 1 in Table 17–6, if the patient repeats the name, correct dosage, one therapeutic effect, and three side effects for metaproterenol (Alupent), the evaluation criteria for that subobjective are met. If all the listed criteria in the table are met, the desired outcome, administration of an effective bronchodilator treatment, is achieved.

If evaluation criteria are *not* met, the outcome is not achieved. In this case, the nurse investigates question categories likely to clarify exactly why the patient did not learn the educational content. Key questions are shown in Table 17–10.

If the patient meets the main objective—administration of an effective aerosol treatment in this case—without meeting all the subobjectives, then the subobjectives were not properly adapted to the patient's situation. This mistake occurs when standard care plans are not adapted to individual needs. The inclusion of objective indicators in the main objective facilitates the ready identification of this mistake.

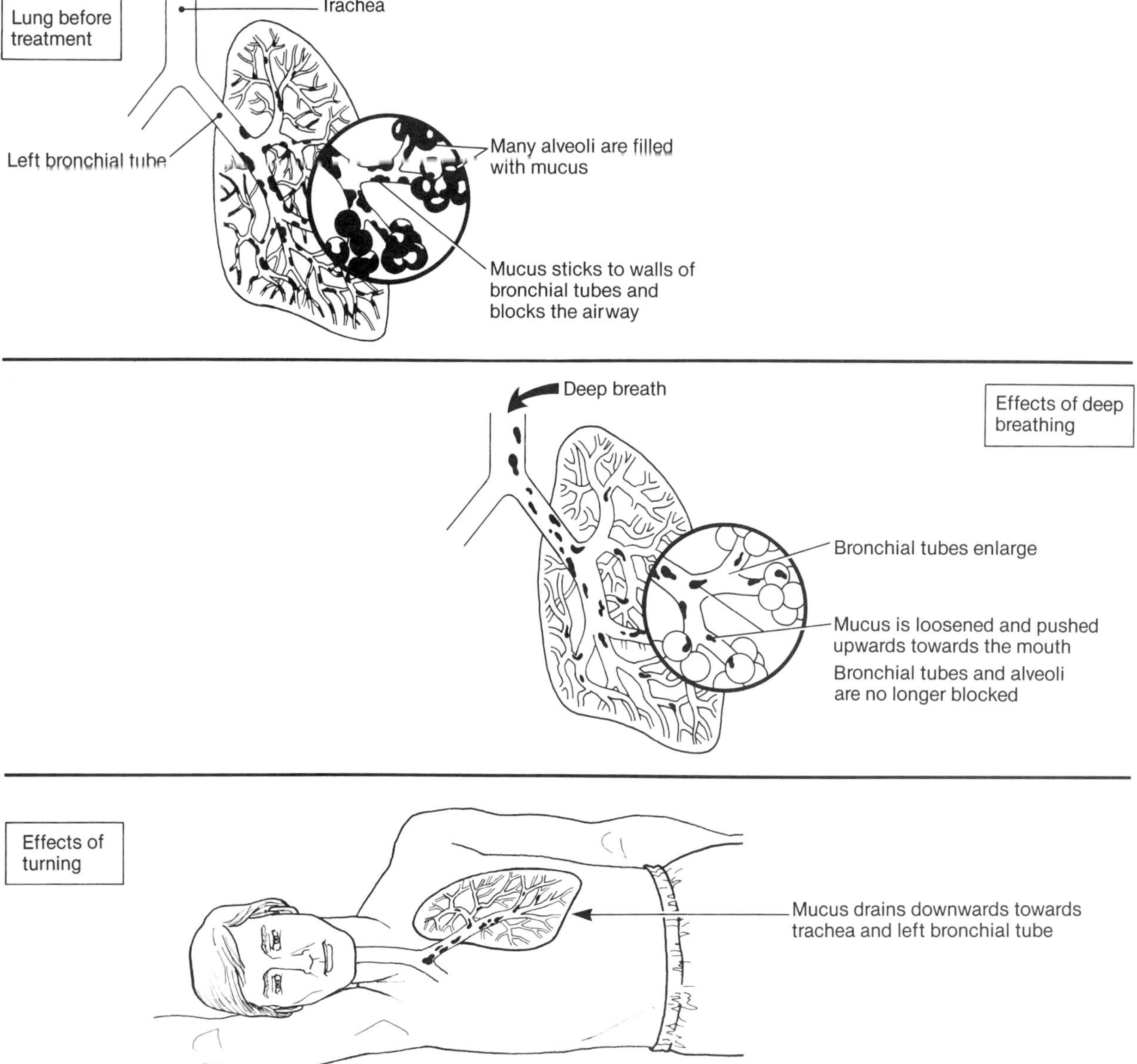

Figure 17–3. Example of an effective poster for self-care education. The poster is appropriately titled and clearly labelled, with "before" and "after" treatment sections. Arrows and exploded diagrams emphasize key information—lung expansion, mucus mobilization, and drainage out of the lungs. (Redrawn from Freedman, C.: Teaching Patients. San Diego, Courseware, Inc., 1978.)

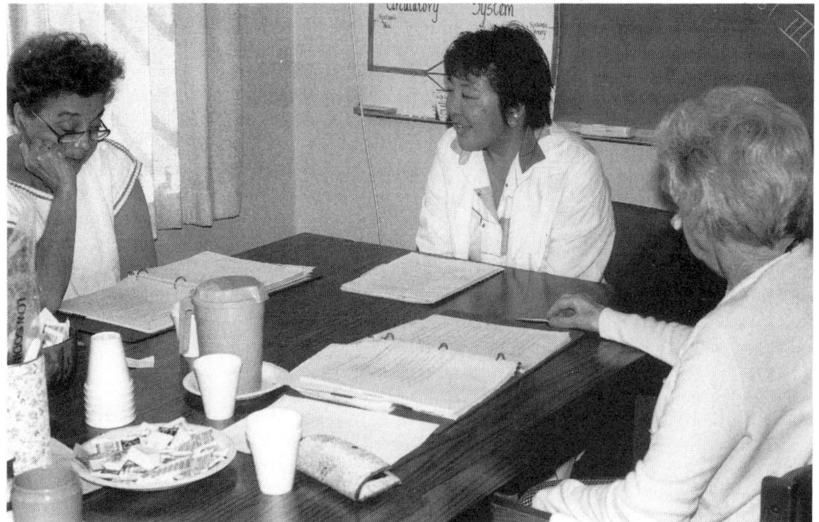

Figure 17–4. A small group of respiratory patients discuss self-care content with an educator. Verbal advice is reinforced with appropriate printed material in each patient's respiratory handbook.

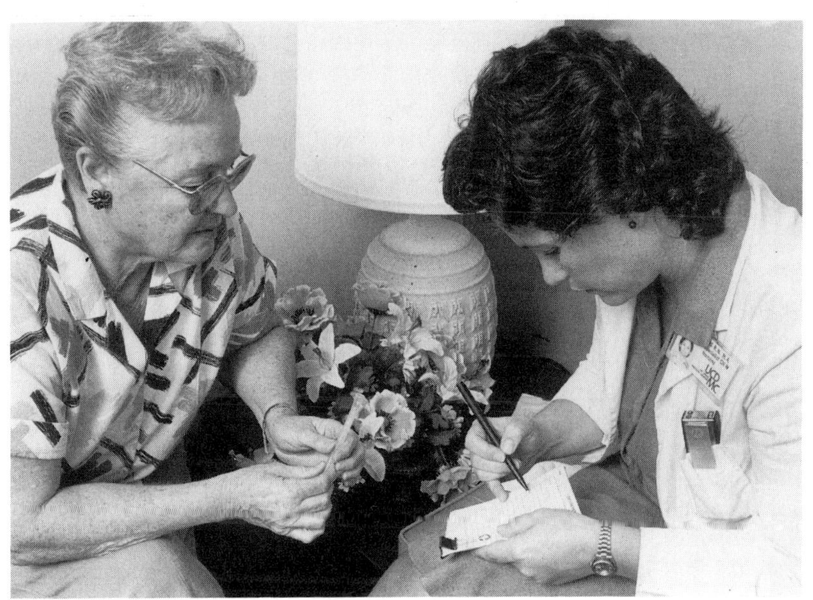

Figure 17–5. A clinical nurse specialist keeps the wife of a patient who has undergone head-and-neck surgery involved in the teaching-learning process through an informal discussion on tracheostomy care at home.

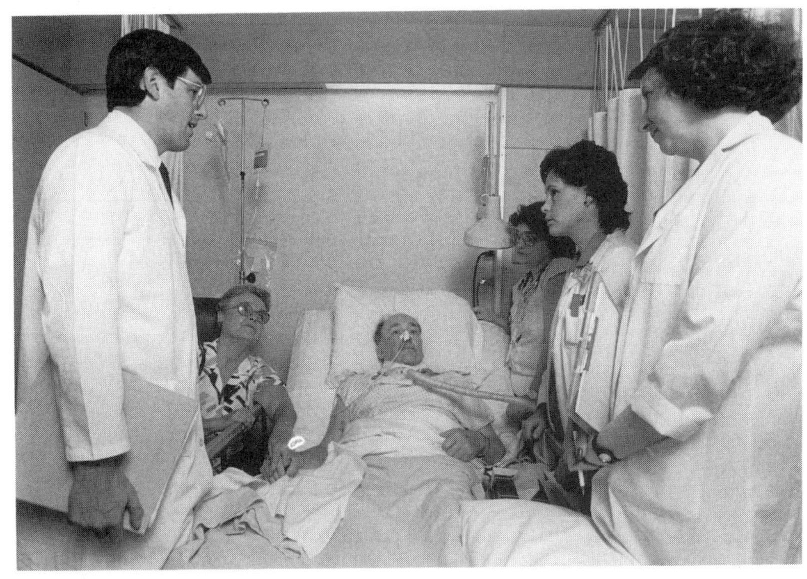

Figure 17–6. During rounds, health team members collaborate to discuss the general progress of the patient and to agree on the specifics of a comprehensive teaching-learning plan for the duration of the hospitalization.

Table 17–10. KEY QUESTIONS TO ASK IF TEACHING-LEARNING GOALS ARE NOT MET

Question Category	Questions
Patient needs	Does the intervention still relate to the patient's most pressing health need?
	Is it relieving pulmonary signs and symptoms?
Readiness to learn	Was the patient ready to learn?
Goals	Were goals (objectives) appropriate? Realistic?
	Agreed upon and understood by both teacher and patient?
	Written clearly in behavioral objective form?
	Broken down into small, easily attainable steps?
Teaching methods	Were teaching methods appropriate for the patient's setting, needs, and interest level?
Reinforcement	Was enough reinforcement available to sustain the new behavior?

Evaluation Methods

Evaluation methods for teaching-learning situations include the following:

1. *Interviews, question-and-answer method*: e.g., "Do you believe you are benefiting from this treatment?" In the case of lack of subjective benefit, ask the patient to at least try the intervention for a mutually agreed upon period of time.

2. *Direct observation*: e.g., watching the patient clean the tracheostomy.

3. *Informal conversations*: plan informal encounters with patients and their families, e.g., a telephone call or brief visit. Frequent contact provides an opportunity to evaluate progress, reinforce content, and reteach specifics if necessary.

4. *Paper and pencil methods*: e.g., questionnaire, true and false, multiple-choice, fill-in-the-blank tests.

5. *Problem solving and simulation*: e.g., "What would you do if you ran out of oxygen on the weekend?"

6. *Record reviews*: e.g., medical, nursing, respiratory therapy, and physical therapy records, health histories, patient health diaries. This method provides the most objective data for evaluation purposes. The nurse searches for ABGs, PFTs, pulmonary symptoms, chest assessment findings, theophylline levels, and pill counts for evidence of patient compliance and benefit from therapy. The absence of benefits suggests noncompliance, poor technique, or inappropriate respiratory intervention.

Program Evaluation

Previous content has focused on evaluation of individual teaching-learning sessions. When educational content is given in a group or within a well-established self-care education program, the nurse evaluates individual sessions as well as the program as a whole. Program evaluation is beyond the scope of this text. However, Table 17–11 may be used to begin the assessment of program inputs, processes, and outcomes in the systems model. Reference to Billie (1981) will clarify how to develop a protocol for evaluation of an educational program.

STEP 6: RETEACH AND RELEARN EDUCATIONAL CONTENT

The last step in the teaching-learning process is reteaching and relearning educational content previously presented. Reteaching and relearning occur once evaluation indicates a need to improve, modify, or reinforce technique, learn new information, or modify goals and objectives.

Health professionals may tend to skip this final step of the teaching-learning process. They assume that once a teaching-learning plan is implemented, the patient will learn the information, and his condition will improve by the next evaluation session.

Unfortunately, few respiratory patients learn under ideal circumstances. Many need the same verbal message repeated several times, with assurance that the situation is under control. Others cannot apply infor-

Table 17–11. SYSTEMS APPROACH FOR EVALUATION OF RESPIRATORY TEACHING PROGRAMS*

Inputs	Processes	Outcomes
Educational content	Teaching activity	Patient
Teachers	Teaching methods	Incidence of acute exacerbations
Nurse/physician team	Program format	Number of hospital days per year
Multidisciplinary team	Patient contact	Sense of well-being
Patients	Teacher attitude	Staff attitudes
Age, sex, lung disease, severity of illness, socioeconomic level	Patient's status	Family's or friends' attitudes
Facilities/setting	Wellness	Cost of program per patient
Inpatient, outpatient	Anxiety level	
Hospital, home	Pain level	
Individual, group	Degree of dyspnea	
Classroom, equipment available	Time spent with patient	

*Adapted from Billie, D.: Practical Approaches to Patient Teaching. Boston, Little, Brown & Co., 1981.

mation because of forgetfulness or transient hypoxemia, or they cannot apply hospital-learned knowledge to the home setting. Moreover, owing to denial and the previously described emotional straightjacket, the chronically ill patient commonly nods his head in agreement during teaching in the absence of understanding. In other cases, readiness to learn is present, but shortness of breath and fatigue cause the patients to concentrate on the basic information, e.g., exactly how many pills to take and when to take them. They then "tune out" during discussions that require more mental concentration, e.g., the purpose and side effects of the medication. In any case, incomprehension may not become evident until the patients fail the evaluation test.

Sometimes the need to reteach educational content arises from the family's ineffective coping behavior. Family members may deny the severity of the patient's illness and fail to reinforce the patient's efforts to follow his teaching-learning plan. This situation is best dealt with by teaching the patient in the absence of unsupportive family members and eventually recruiting another supportive person for the patient.

In other cases, the family is overprotective and insists on doing everything for the patient once he returns home. This situation illustrates the importance of constantly educating both family and patient about the need and purposes of self care. Once overprotective family members observe the patient practicing self care without physical deterioration, they often become convinced of the merits of the self-care approach. At this point, the nurse may withdraw from the teaching-learning situation, as family members actively and appropriately reinfore the patient's teaching-learning plan on their own. In other cases, overprotective family members may be unable to relinquish care duties to the patient without psychologic problems themselves. Patients and families in a long-standing mutual dependency pattern are referred to a family counselor, psychologist, or psychiatrist for counseling or treatment.

The need to reteach educational content is related to other factors in addition to the nature of the respiratory patient and ineffective family coping behaviors. Other contributing factors include inadequate financial reimbursement, inadequate time allotted for teaching, and the nature of respiratory interventions (described next).

Unpredictability of Respiratory Interventions

In respiratory care, reteaching and relearning are mandatory and inevitable because outcomes for common physical therapy and respiratory therapy techniques are largely unpredictable. Because of the lack of controlled studies, research conclusions about pursed-lip breathing, IPPB, deep breathing and coughing, incentive spirometry, and other techniques are conflicting or they do not apply to all phases of illness, all types of lung disease, or all clinical circumstances. For example, some patients do not benefit from pursed-lip breathing. Others may benefit but only when performed with a technique unique to the patient. Consider another example, the patient with lobar atelectasis benefits from a "standard" regimen of chest physical therapy (Marini et al, 1979); however, the patient with uncomplicated pneumonia does not benefit from the same therapy (Graham and Bradley, 1978). Numerous other examples may be found in the respiratory literature.

Therefore, until variables relating to respiratory techniques are more clearly understood, the nurse emphasizes ongoing, thorough evaluation early in the teaching-learning process. When complex skills are broken down into several short teaching-learning sessions, evaluation at the end of each session reduces the amount of reteaching and relearning needed at the end of the teaching-learning process.

Conclusion

This chapter discusses self-care education and the teaching-learning process. The content prepares the nurse to assess patient progress in each of the six teaching-learning steps presented and then to intervene, as the patient moves through the health care continuum. Adherence to these six steps may lead to the reversal or remission of pulmonary disease within a relatively short period of time. At other times, the patient becomes unable to move from step 1 or step 2, and health professionals must implement the motivational model (see Chapter 16) over weeks, months, or years before the patient decides to set a teaching-learning goal. Whatever the case, maintenance of a self-care orientation in the teaching-learning process will always foster a sense of reponsibility, dignity, and power, qualities essential for wholeness, health, and optimum learning.

REFERENCES

American Health Association: Staff Manual for Teaching Patients About COPD. Chicago: American Hospital Association, 1982.

Becker, M.: Understanding patient compliance: The contributions of attitudes and other psychosocial factors. In: New Directions in Patient Compliance (S. Cohen, ed.). Lexington, Massachusetts, Lexington Books, 1979.

Bell, W., Blodgett, D., et al: Home Care and Rehabilitation in Respiratory Medicine. Philadelphia, J. B. Lippincott Co., 1984.

Billie, D.: Practical Approaches to Patient Teaching. Boston, Little, Brown & Co., 1981.

Bloom, B. (ed.): Taxonomy of Educational Objectives: The Classification of Educational Goals. New York, David McKay Co., 1956.

Chatham, M. A. and Knapp, B. L.: Patient Education Handbook. Bowie, Maryland, Robert J. Brady Co., 1982.

Currie, B. (ed.): Patient Education in the Primary Care Setting. Madison, Wisconsin: University of Wisconsin-Madison Center for Health Sciences, 1978.

Czerwinski, B. S.: Manual of Patient Education for Cardiopulmonary Dysfunctions. St. Louis, C. V. Mosby Co., 1980.

Eraker, S. Kirscht, J., and Becker, M.: Understanding and improving patient compliance. *Annals of internal medicine*, 100(2):258–268, 1984.
Flynn, J. B., and Giffin, P. A.: Health promotion in acute care settings. *Nursing clinics of north america*, 19(2):239–250, 1984.
Freedman, C.: Teaching Patients. San Diego, Courseware, Inc., 1978.
Graham, W., and Bradley, D.: Efficacy of chest physiotherapy and IPPB in the resolution of pneumonia. *New england journal of medicine*, 299(12):624–627, 1978.
Hindi-Alexander, M.: Decision making in asthma self-management. *Chest*, 87(1):100S–104S, 1985.
Joseph, L. S.: Self-care and the nursing process. *Nursing clinics of north america*, 15(1):131–143, 1980.
Kee, C. C.: A case for health promotion with the elderly. *Nursing clinics of north america*, 19(2):251–262, 1984.
Levin, L.: Patient education and self-care: How do they differ? *Nursing outlook*, 26(3):170–175, 1978.
Levin, L., Katz, A. and Holst, E.: Self-care: Lay Initiatives in Health. New York, Prodist, 1976.
Mager, R.: Preparing Instructional Objectives, 2nd ed. Belmont, California, Pitman Management and Training, 1984.
Marini, J. Pierson, D., and Hudson, L.: Acute lobar atelectasis: a prospective comparison of fiberoptic bronchoscopy and respiratory therapy. *American review of respiratory disease*, 119(6):971–978, 1979.
Miller, M.: Patient Education—A Growing Concern of Many. Patient Education. New York, National League for Nursing, 1976.
Mullin, V.: Implementing the self-care concept in the acute setting. *Nursing clinics of north america*, 15(1):177–190, 1980.
Orem, E.: Nursing: concepts of practice, 2nd ed. New York, McGraw-Hill Book Co., 1980.
Pender, J. N.: Patient identification of health information received during hospitalization. *Nursing research*, 23(3):262–267, 1974.
Rankin, S. and Duffy, K.: Patient Education: Issues, Principles and Guidelines. Philadelphia, J. B. Lippincott, Co., 1983.
Redman, B.: Patient education—fad or reflection of changed standard of care? *Archives of internal medicine*, 141(2):163, 1981.
Redman, B. K.: The Process of Patient Education, 5th ed. St. Louis, C. V. Mosby Co., 1984.
Steckel, S. B.: Patient Contracting. Norwalk, Connecticut, Appleton-Century-Crofts, 1982.

BASIC INTERVENTIONS

Part Four

This part describes basic respiratory interventions. Though it is written for the nurse who implements self-care educational content in chronic settings, content has been adapted for use in acute-care clinical settings as well.

Basic respiratory interventions are implemented after assessment of teaching-learning needs (see Table 17–4). Chapter 18 presents *pulmonary rehabilitation and basic self care.* The content on pulmonary rehabilitation explains how basic concepts, whether taught in the form of individual or group sessions, apply to nursing practice in all settings, including the critical care unit. The content on basic self care presents concepts that help patients understand their lung diseases and practice preventive measures, such as the cessation of smoking and the taking of pulmonary medications on time.

Chapter 19 and Chapter 20 focus on *chest physiotherapy, energy conservation*, and *exercise conditioning.* Interventions provided in these chapters help patients eliminate or control problems, such as mucus retention, respiratory panic, exercise intolerance, and respiratory muscle deconditioning.

The last three chapters in this part help the nurse implement basic interventions involving respiratory equipment. Chapter 21 discusses the *use of respiratory equipment in the home.* Chapter 22 and Chapter 23 discuss *aerosol therapy*, intermittent positive pressure breathing (IPPB), and *oxygen therapy* in home and hospital settings. These chapters prepare the nurse as follows:

1. To monitor patients receiving any form of respiratory therapy.
2. To collaborate with the respiratory therapist.
3. To solve equipment-related problems that arise when a respiratory therapist is unavailable.

The format for this part of the book differs from other parts of the book in two ways. First, sample self-care educational content, labelled *patient information*, is interspersed throughout the section to help with content implementation. More specifically, the sample content explains exactly what to tell the patient and the family during teaching-learning sessions.*

Second, *indications, goals, practice schedule*, and *evaluation criteria* for each main intervention are written in outline form for quick reference in the clinical setting. Then, at the end of each intervention, the *implementation* discussion explains how the nurse teaches self-care content to patient and family.

Evaluation criteria are divided into two parts; criteria *for correct technique* and criteria *for overall improvement in condition.* These criteria help the nurse plan and modify basic respiratory interventions and overall teaching-learning plan. The list of criteria for each intervention is tailored to meet the needs of each patient, as explained in the chapters Self-care Education and Nursing Diagnosis and Intervention.

To implement basic interventions, the nurse is encouraged to utilize the knowledge and special skills of other health team members, such as the respiratory nurse specialist, chest physiotherapist, and respiratory therapist. Their expertise is invaluable for learning skills, such as chest percussion and vibration, that are best perfected through guided practice. In addition, consultation with other team members usually facilitates the efficiency and effectiveness of techniques, particularly in the case of the multiproblem patient with special teaching-learning needs.

Terms commonly used to describe chest physiotherapy, aerosol and oxygen therapy, and other basic interventions are listed next.

Glossary of Commonly Used Terms in Basic Interventions

aerosol—liquid or solid particles suspended in a gas.

aerosol therapy—delivery of bland or bronchodilator aerosol to the respiratory mucosa.

air entrainment—the movement of room air into a respiratory device caused by a pressure drop in the device.

Bernouilli's principle—the lateral pressure of a gas decreases as its velocity of flow increases. This principle is utilized to produce aerosol in most respiratory therapy devices.

breathing circuit—gas delivery system between patient and ventilator or other device, consisting of breathing tubes, manifold, and mouthpiece.

breathing retraining—use of pursed-lip breathing, diaphragmatic breathing, and other techniques to control shortness of breath and establish a normal or near normal breathing pattern.

---

*Sample educational content was originally developed in collaboration with Oscar Scherer, M.D. and subsequently modifed for use in a variety of hospital, clinic, and home settings. Original adaptations are reproduced by permission from L. Kersten: *Your respiratory home care program* (patient booklet). Berkeley, CA, 1978, Herrick Hospital and Health Center of the East Bay.

bronchial hygiene—condition of the airways. A general term for respiratory interventions that prevent mucus retention, atelectasis, and hypoventilation.
chest percussion—rhythmic clapping on the chest to loosen mucus and facilitate expectoration.
chest physiotherapy—use of breathing exercises, controlled coughing, postural drainage, and other techniques to promote optimal bronchial hygiene and muscle conditioning.
chest vibration—shaking or vibrating the chest to loosen mucus and facilitate expectoration.
controlled coughing—use of maximal inspiration, followed by two to three forceful, low-pitched coughs.
cool or cold aerosol—aerosol delivered at room temperature.
deep breathing—use of sustained maximal inspirations.
diaphragmatic breathing—"belly" breathing to improve lung ventilation and help control dyspnea.
durable medical equipment (DME)—equipment designed for home use.
E cylinder—small green tank used for portable oxygen.
energy conservation techniques—work simplification techniques that help decrease dyspnea and fatigue associated with activities of daily living.
equipment vendor—company that sells or rents equipment.
exercise conditioning—use of a regular exercise program to decrease tissue oxygen extraction during exercise, improve neuromuscular coordination, and thereby increase exercise tolerance.
exercise prescription—physician's guidelines for mode of exercise, along with intensity, duration, and frequency of practice.
exercise stress test—a treadmill or bicycle ergometer test to determine exercise and oxygen prescription.
forced exhalation techniques—a "huffing" technique used instead of coughing to avoid uncontrollable coughing and bronchospasm.
glossopharyngeal breathing (GPB)—"frog" breathing, a technique used by paralyzed neuromuscular patients to sigh and cough unassisted.
H cylinder—large green or yellow tank used for oxygen or compressed air at home.
heated aerosol—aerosol heated to body temperature.
high-flow system—gas administration whereby inspiratory gas flow is provided totally by the administration device, e.g., Venturi's mask.
humidifier—device that provides humidification for oxygen delivery systems and other forms of respiratory therapy.
incentive spirometry—use of a deep breathing device that provides immediate visual feedback upon achievement of a preset goal (e.g., inspired volume).
inhaler extension device (spacer)—device that attaches to the mouthpiece of an inhaler and helps to minimize the oropharyngeal deposition of aerosol.
intermittent positive pressure breathing (IPPB)—10- to 15-minute respirator treatment to deliver medication, inflate the lungs, or both.
long-term oxygen—oxygen administration for more than 30 days.
low-flow system—gas administration system whereby inspiratory gas flow is provided partially by the gas administration device and partially by room air, e.g., nasal cannula.
mainstream smoke—smoke inhaled by a smoker.
manifold—connector in a breathing circuit that provides attachment for a nebulizer, exhalation valve, and supporting arm.
mist therapy—obsolete term for bland aerosol therapy.
nasal cannula—low-flow oxygen delivery via two plastic prongs in the nose.
nebulizer—device that delivers aerosol.
Nicorette—brand of nicotine chewing gum that may help the addicted smoker gradually reduce smoking.
oxygen concentrator—electrically powered device that converts room air to near 100% oxygen.
oxygen-conserving device—oxygen administration device with reduced oxygen utilization compared with standard nasal cannula.
oxygen prescription—physician's guidelines for oxygen use during rest, exercise, and sleep.
Oxymizer—a brand of oxygen-conserving nasal cannula.
passive smoking—indirect inhalation of cigarette, cigar, or pipe smoke, e.g., breathing air in a smoke-filled room.
postural drainage—positioning of the body for gravity drainage of mucus.
pulmonary rehabilitation—an informal or formal, multidisciplinary program that aims to stabilize or reverse pulmonary disease and maximize functional capacity.
pursed-lip breathing—a breathing technique used to increase tidal volume (V_T), decrease respiratory rate, and control dyspnea.
respiratory muscle training—exercising respiratory muscles to reduce or avoid respiratory muscle fatigue.
sexuality—sexual adaptation to lung disease and all somatic, emotional, intellectual, social, and ethical dimensions of the pulmonary patient's life.
sidestream smoke—smoke released directly into the air from a burning cigarette tip.
short-term oxygen—oxygen administration for a duration of 30 days or less.
sustained maximal inspiration—full inspiration followed by a 3-second breath hold.
transtracheal oxygen—an oxygen-conserving device that provides oxygen via a small catheter inserted surgically into the trachea above the suprasternal notch.
turboinhaler—special inhaler for administration of cromolyn antiasthma medication.
ultrasonic aerosol—aerosol produced by an ultrasonic nebulizer; aerosol particles are smaller than those produced by jet nebulization.
Venturi mask—a special oxygen mask that provides a stable preset inspired flow of oxygen (FIO_2) between 0.24 and 0.50.

Pulmonary Rehabilitation and Basic Self Care

18

Main Objectives

1. **Define pulmonary rehabilitation and describe its relevance to self-care education in both acute and chronic settings.**
2. **Describe the general sequence of events for a pulmonary rehabilitation program; specify goals, subgoals, and criteria for referral and entry.**
3. **State at least four criteria for home respiratory care. Name six advantages to implementation of self-care education in the home setting.**
4. **An emphysema patient asks you to explain what is wrong with him. Describe the pathophysiology of emphysema, using simple terminology and a simple drawing of the respiratory system.**
5. **A patient insists he is addicted to nicotine and cannot stop smoking. Describe how you would counsel the patient.**
6. **Explain how to help the patient schedule pulmonary medications to achieve maximal bronchodilatation with minimal side effects at the lowest cost possible.**
7. **Name at least five evaluation criteria for correct inhaler technique.**
8. **Describe how to teach a patient to use a metered dose device (MDD) inhaler.**
9. **Name three advantages and three disadvantages for use of extension devices (i.e., spacers) on inhalers.**
10. **For chest infection or bronchospasm, name three classic signs and symptoms and describe how to determine *early* signs and symptoms.**

11. State basic advice for a chronic obstructive pulmonary disease (COPD) patient who complains of dyspnea during activities of daily living.
12. Describe how to counsel the pulmonary patient on nutrition and appropriate body weight.
13. Explain the rationale for encouraging intake of 2 to 3 quarts of fluids per day.
14. State basic information appropriate for pulmonary patients continually exposed to allergens or lung irritants, such as dust, paint, and smog.
15. An asthmatic patient states that wheezing and fear of suffocation prevent him from continuing sexual activity; describe how you would counsel the patient.

Self-care education is the main structural component of pulmonary rehabilitation.

The first section of this chapter introduces pulmonary rehabilitation as a broad concept that applies to patients in all clinical situations, including critical care units, in-patient and out-patient pulmonary rehabilitation programs, and home settings. This all inclusive approach facilitates the application of self-care concepts and the teaching-learning process across the health care continuum.

The remainder of this chapter discusses basic self care appropriate for the majority of patients with chronic pulmonary diseases. Three content areas are covered. First, *understanding the respiratory system and lung disease* helps the patient understand his particular disease process. Second, *preventive measures* serve to enhance health and prevent acute exacerbations of lung disease. Third, *sexual adaptation to lung disease* helps the patient maintain sexual relations and strengthen existing support systems.

Overview of Pulmonary Rehabilitation

Self-care education is such an integral part of *rehabilitation* that the two terms are considered synonymous in this text.

DEFINITIONS

The term *rehabilitation* was defined in the 1942 statement by the Council on Rehabilitation (Inter-Society Commission for Heart Disease Resources, 1974), as follows:

> "Restoration of the individual to the fullest physical, medical, mental, emotional, economic, social and vocational potential of which he is capable, taking into consideration his totality."

The term *pulmonary rehabilitation* was defined by the American College of Chest Physicians, Committee on Pulmonary Rehabilitation, at its annual meeting in 1974. The definition reads as follows:

> "Pulmonary rehabilitation may be defined as an art of medical practice wherein an individually tailored, multidisciplinary program is formulated which through accurate diagnosis, therapy, emotional support, and education stabilizes or reverses both the physiopathology and psychopathology of pulmonary diseases and attempts to return the patient to the highest possible functional capacity allowed by his pulmonary handicap and overall life situation."

PULMONARY REHABILITATION SPANNING THE HEALTH CARE CONTINUUM

Because of the previously described acute-chronic care dichotomy (see Chapter 17), pulmonary rehabilitation, similar to self-care education, is commonly associated with chronic care. Though currently most pulmonary rehabilitation activity takes place in chronic care settings, the process of health restoration is seen here as a process spanning the entire health care continuum. Restoration begins in whatever clinical setting the patient first finds himself. It continues, taking on different forms, as the patient becomes better or worse and seeks care in various settings. For example, in critical care, the nurse's self-care orientation begins pulmonary rehabilitation and prepares the patient for more structured rehabilitative measures in chronic settings. At the other end of the continuum, the visiting nurse might initiate informal pulmonary rehabilitation for a homebound patient who lacks the desire or means to participate in a hospital based, formal, pulmonary rehabilitation program.

GOALS

The main goal of rehabilitation is to return the individual to the highest level of functional activity that he is capable of achieving. Subgoals based on benefits include the following (California Thoracic Society, 1979):

1. Improve self-care ability
2. Improve exercise tolerance
3. Decrease rate of progression of disability
4. Reduce frequency and duration of hospitalization. Rehabilitation reduces hospitalizations by 50% compared with the year prior to a rehabilitation program (Moser, 1980), or by 55% compared with the following year (Johnson et al, 1980).
5. Improve effectiveness and efficiency of patient-physician interaction
6. Reduce overall medical costs
7. Maintain or reestablish employment
8. Reduce time lost from work

In simple terms, pulmonary rehabilitation is the provision of high quality, comprehensive care for patients with pulmonary disease (American Thoracic Society, 1981).

Individual goals depend on the patient's health status. The overall goal for a young asthmatic might be to play tennis without wheezing and dyspnea. In contrast, the goal for a severely disabled person might be to perform activities of daily living, such as taking a shower, combing hair, or walking to the grocery store, without assistance from others.

Note that improvement in pulmonary function is not included in the list of subgoals. Though patients may receive considerable symptomatic improvement from therapy, pulmonary rehabilitation does *not* alter the rate of pulmonary function deterioration in COPD, i.e., 80 cc/year decline in forced expiratory volume in 1 second (FEV_1), nor does it alter the natural disease course of COPD (Petty, 1977). This lack of objective improvement sometimes causes medical insurance coverage problems. (Pulmonary rehabilitation is not reimbursed when an insurance company limits financial coverage to the treatment of acute diseases and conditions with objective proof of patient progress.)

PULMONARY REHABILITATION PROGRAMS

The need to reduce the respiratory patient's repeated admission into expensive intensive care units brought about the proliferation of formal in-patient and out-patient pulmonary rehabilitation programs in the United States. The target population for these programs has been that of the severely disabled COPD or restrictive disease patients, who require a broad range of comprehensive services to keep them clinically stable and out of the hospital for long periods of time (Table 18–1).

Table 18–1. SERVICES REQUIRED FOR COMPREHENSIVE CARE OF COPD PATIENTS*

Comprehensive assessment and ongoing evaluation
Medical and nursing services
Pulmonary function tests
X-rays
General laboratory services
Electrocardiogram
Immunization
Emergency services
Acute respiratory care
Drugs, medical supplies, respiratory, and other equipment
Other supportive services
Provision for meals (Meals-on-Wheels)
Homemaking or housekeeping services
Psychosocial, vocational, and financial counseling
Patient-sitting services
Transportation and communication services
Self-care education
Bronchial hygiene
Breathing instruction
Physical conditioning
Energy conservation training
Dietary instruction
Environmental control
Patient clubs and visitation groups
Education of family, friends, and work associates
Consultation services for health professionals
Community referral networks for patients and the public
Staff in-service education
Education of the public

*Adapted from the American Lung Association—American Thoracic Society: Report on comprehensive care for patients with chronic lung disease, 1975, and American Thoracic Society: Skills of the health team involved in out-of-hospital care for patients with COPD. *American review of respiratory disease,* 133(5): 948–949, 1986.

Formal programs are usually associated with large, university medical centers, community hospitals, or regional centers in rural areas (Braun et al, 1981). They are few in number because of the time, expertise, and money necessary to initiate, develop, and maintain programs that are truly comprehensive.

The length of a typical rehabilitation program varies, but it usually lasts 2 to 3 weeks for in-patient programs and 4 to 6 weeks for out-patient programs. During this time, the patient learns and practices self-care skills under close supervision of health team members. The team is composed of physicians, nurses, respiratory therapists, and others specially trained in pulmonary care and rehabilitative measures, including physical therapists, occupational therapists, nutritionists, psychiatrists, vocational counselors, and pharmacists.

Though most nurses are not associated with a formal program, general knowledge of such programs is useful for two reasons. First, this knowledge may help the clinician form similar informal programs that span acute care, out-patient, and home settings. Second, most pulmonary rehabilitation programs are grossly underutilized. Clinicians in the community are either unaware of the existence and purpose of local programs, or they refer only patients with overt needs, e.g., severely disabled COPD patients. Those with severe lung disease, however, are the group with the least expected improvement after rehabilitation. Improvement is greater in patients with less impairment.

Hence, to better integrate pulmonary rehabilitation with all aspects of care—prevention, treatment, and health enhancement—clinicians are encouraged to follow these suggestions:

1. Become familiar with local pulmonary rehabilitation programs.
2. Refer appropriate patients with all levels of respiratory impairment, not only the severely disabled.
3. Become familiar with the general sequence of events for most pulmonary rehabilitation programs (described next).

Sequence of Events

Patient Referral. Referral by a physician is required for consideration of a patient for rehabilitation. This requirement increases the likelihood of follow-up treatment, after the conclusion of the program. Nurses may facilitate referral by alerting physicians to patients who might benefit from a program or by encouraging patients to talk to their physician about a referral. Criteria for referral are listed in the box.

CRITERIA FOR REFERRAL TO A PULMONARY REHABILITATION PROGRAM

HISTORICAL FEATURES

Dyspnea on exertion
Inability to carry out selected activities of daily living
Repeated hospitalizations or need for home care services
Time lost from work or school
Desire for disability retirement from work
Desire for educational update of self-care techniques

LABORATORY FEATURES

Reduced vital capacity in restrictive disease
Reduced expiratory flow rates
Increased $Paco_2$
Hypoxemia, at rest or during exercise

Patient Selection. The pulmonary rehabilitation staff screens all referred applicants and selects only those likely to benefit from their programs. Selection criteria vary, depending on the target patient population, the services offered, and the medical director's preferences. Common selection criteria used as a guide for selection are summarized in Table 18–2.

To show how selection criteria are considered guides rather than rules, consider the FEV_1 data. An FEV_1 equal to or greater than 1.0 L is a favorable criteria because the patient's pulmonary function is good enough to permit full participation in rehabilitation activities. Also, improvement after rehabilitation is greater in patients who are less impaired (Moser, 1980). Nevertheless, many severely disabled but highly motivated patients with FEV_1s well below one L (e.g., 500 cc range) prove to be excellent candidates for rehabilitation. Though level of dyspnea may not change significantly after rehabilitation, they may drastically improve their exercise tolerance, self-care ability, and quality of life at home.

Table 18–2. COMMON SELECTION CRITERIA FOR ENTRY INTO A PULMONARY REHABILITATION PROGRAM

Favorable Criteria (present in excellent candidates)	Unfavorable Criteria (present in poor candidates)
Stable asthma; COPD; restrictive disease, particularly neuromuscular disorders.	*Unstable* or rapidly progressive chest disorders, incomplete recovery from acute ventilatory failure.
FEV_1 equal to or greater than 1.0 Liter; class III or better on the Dyspnea-Disability Scale (see Chapter 10).	FEV_1 less than 1.0 Liter, severe pulmonary signs and symptoms, Class IV to V on the Dyspnea-Disability Scale (see Chapter 10).
Other medical disability is stable or well controlled.	Other medical disability is unstable.
Many psychosocial assets—high level of motivation, strong support system, history of personal achievement.	Few psychosocial assets—low level of motivation, lack of support system, history of noncompliance.
Patient does not smoke or agrees to stop smoking *before* entry into program.	Patient continues to smoke or expresses intent to quit *after* entry into program.
Referral by a physician with interest or expertise in ongoing management of chronic respiratory disease.	Lack of a referring physician with interest or expertise in management of chronic respiratory disease.
	Senility, personality disorders

Initial Comprehensive Assessment. If baseline information is not provided by a referring physician, the pulmonary rehabilitation team comprehensively assesses the patient using the following parameters:

ASSESSMENT PARAMETERS FOR COMPREHENSIVE ASSESSMENT

History and physical examination
Basic laboratory tests, e.g., complete blood count, hemoglobin and hematocrit values
Pulmonary function tests, with resting arterial blood gases
Chest x-ray
Psychologic screening, with motivational assessment
Exercise testing to measure level of functional disability, e.g., treadmill, ergometer, distance walking, and stair climbing

The team then makes a decision regarding admission into the program, if it has not already been made, and formulates a plan for program delivery.

Program Delivery. The team teaches self-care educational content and implements a program of bronchial hygiene and physical conditioning, based on needs identified during the initial assessment. Group and individual instruction and counseling are provided by a variety of personnel, e.g., medical director, nurse, respiratory therapist, physical therapist, occupational therapist, dietician, social worker, pharmacist, vocational counselor, and psychiatrist.

Ongoing Evaluation. Patient progress is evaluated utilizing respiratory assessment parameters and teaching-learning tools already discussed in this chapter.

Final Evaluation. A final evaluation with recommendations for long-range treatment is forwarded to the referring physician.

Long-term Follow-up. Reinforcement and updating of individualized plans are accomplished via telephone calls, out-patient visits, patient clubs, and home care in cooperation with a home health agency and respiratory equipment vendor (see Chapter 21).

HOME CARE

Patients with severe lung disease require home care follow-up when discharged from the hospital with new or complicated treatment plans. Specific criteria for referral to home care are listed in the box (McDonald, 1981; American Thoracic Society, 1987).

CRITERIA FOR REFERRAL FOR HOME CARE

Unstable cardiopulmonary status or complex treatment program
Patients who require only periodic medical supervision
"Revolving door" syndrome, i.e., frequent hospitalizations
Confused, highly anxious, or depressed patients
Patients whose behavior or care places an unusual burden on the family
Patients who do not have the support of family or significant others
Patients with new equipment who are discharged from the hospital

---

Elderly pulmonary patients are the most likely ones in need of home care follow-up. The three Medicare eligibility requirements for financial reimbursement are (1) homebound status, (2) medical instability, and (3) need for skilled nursing care rather than custodial care. Though the trend in the United States is towards resolution of acute illness without rehabilitation, some rehabilitation may be covered under Medicare eligibility requirements, depending on interpretation of the words "homebound" and "medical instability." The fiscal intermediaries used by home care agencies often interpret these words differently in different regions of the United States.

Rehabilitative care in the home has advantages not always present in other settings; some of these advantages are summarized as follows:

1. Patients may feel more relaxed and willing to practice new skills in the home. Individuals who respond poorly to formal pulmonary rehabilitation programs in the hospital, as inpatients or outpatients, may respond more favorably to informal programs in the home (Shenkman, 1985).
2. Observation of the family's dynamics and the home environment adds new information to the initial data base. It provides an opportunity to help families and friends support patients in a way that fosters rather than hinders self care. Also, a home environmental assessment may lead to the identification of allergens responsible for wheezing episodes in patients with extrinsic asthma.
3. Observation of bronchial hygiene measures leads to the identification of misconceptions and mistakes in technique not identified in the controlled hospital setting.
4. When the visiting nurse cares for the patient over a relatively long period of time, the relationship of trust is a bond that strengthens communication and cooperation between patient and all care givers. In addition, the relationship of trust facilitates counseling of anxious and depressed patients who automatically avoid potentially, emotionally charged topics or activities associated with dyspnea.
5. Data from the home setting are crucial to comprehensive respiratory assessment. When shared with staff members in the hospital, formulation of a teaching-learning plan becomes more efficient and effective.
6. The nurse is in a central position to coordinate other health professionals in the home (e.g., physical therapist and occupational therapist) as well as other supportive services (e.g., Meals-on-Wheels, transportation, home delivery of groceries and medications, and financial aid).
7. Home health agencies may enlist the services of homemakers for routine household tasks, e.g., cleaning, laundry, shopping, and meal preparations. Also, a home health aide is frequently employed to help with the patient's personal care, leaving the registered nurse more time to coordinate overall care of the patient. Both the homemaker and health aide are major support persons who greatly relieve spouses and other family members of the sometimes overwhelming burden of total patient care at home.
8. Home services may include hospice care for terminally ill respiratory patients.

Thus far, pulmonary rehabilitation has been presented as a concept that applies to acute care settings, pulmonary rehabilitation programs, and home settings. Application depends on knowledge of basic, self-care strategies introduced here and discussed further in subsequent chapters of this book. During the initiation of self-care education, the nurse begins with what is wrong with the patient.

Understanding the Respiratory System and Lung Disease

The *Patient's Bill of Rights* states: "The patient has the right to obtain from his physician complete current information concerning his diagnosis, treatment and prognosis in terms the patient can be reasonably expected to understand" (American Hospital Association, 1972). Although the primary physician bears responsibility for the disclosure of information and informed consent, patients often ask the nurse questions about the respiratory system in general and the particular disease process in particular. Use of a simple drawing, such as the one presented here, may be necessary to facilitate the teaching-learning process.

PATIENT INFORMATION

The purpose of breathing is to provide oxygen for the needs of the body's tissues and to remove carbon dioxide, the body's respiratory waste product.

As you breathe in, air moves through the nose and mouth, past the larynx (voice box), the trachea (windpipe), and to the lungs via the two main bronchi or airways. Past the main bronchi, air moves through *many* airways of different sizes until it reaches tiny air sacs called alveoli. Oxygen leaves the alveoli here and enters the blood stream, while carbon dioxide leaves the blood stream and enters the alveoli to be exhaled.

The pleurae cover the lungs and allow for easy movement of the lungs in the chest cavity.

The diaphragm and the rib muscles are the two main respiratory muscles that help you breathe. The diaphragm is the dome-shaped muscle between the lungs and abdomen.

You can have a breathing problem if any of the aforementioned parts of the respiratory system are not working properly.

THE RESPIRATORY SYSTEM

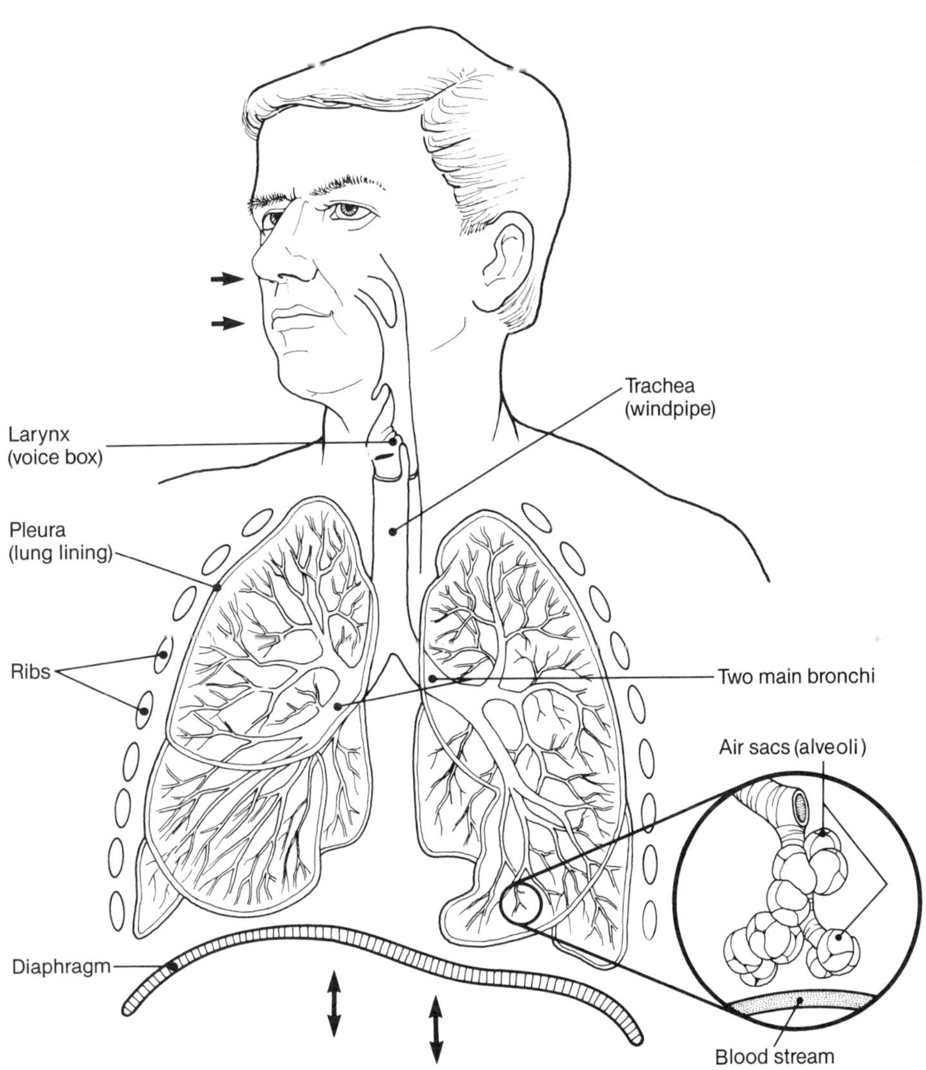

For the majority of COPD patients with mixed chest pathology, the nurse may use Table 18–1 as a guide for presenting the main obstructive diseases, i.e., bronchial asthma, chronic bronchitis, and emphysema. This knowledge base provides the patient with the vocabulary and conceptual framework necessary for asking appropriate questions about his own disease and medical treatment. As the result of exposure to this content, the COPD patient may better understand the components of his disease and ask for appropriate treatment, e.g., bronchodilator, when the asthmatic component, for example, is out of control.

Note that Table 18–3 reduces content on pathology to a bare minimum. The goal of teaching is to facilitate comparison of the three obstructive diseases, emphasizing the relationships among pathology, signs and

Table 18–3. BASIC EDUCATIONAL CONTENT ON CHRONIC OBSTRUCTIVE PULMONARY DISEASE (COPD)

Lung Disease	Definition and Pathology	Main Signs and Symptoms	Main Treatment	Points to Emphasize
COPD	A general term for chronic diseases with obstruction to air flow due to asthma, bronchitis, emphysema, or other disease. Specific pathology varies, depending on the diseases involved.	Shortness of breath due to trouble breathing air out of the lungs	Treatment of underlying obstructive diseases	The patient often complains of difficulty breathing air in. Inability to get fresh air in is actually due to inability to get all the old air out. Obstructive disease is a type of lung disease. It is different from restrictive lung disease.
Bronchial asthma	Muscle spasm causing airway narrowing	Wheeze from air passing through narrowed airways	Bronchodilators to reverse muscle spasm	Asthma cannot be cured, but symptoms can be controlled.
	"Twitchy" lungs	Cough from airway irritability and muscle spasm	Identification and reduction or elimination, if possible, of asthma triggers	It is considered a reversible airway disease because bronchodilators significantly reduce airway obstruction on the breathing test. Both emotional and physical factors may be asthma triggers.
Chronic bronchitis	Mucus secreted into airway, causing airway obstruction	Cough and mucus production	Smoking cessation to decrease mucus secretion and stop damage to the airway	Signs and symptoms may be eliminated or drastically reduced with smoking cessation.
			Bronchodilators to reduce airway obstruction Bronchial hygiene program, e.g., drink fluids, deep breathe, and cough	Acute signs and symptoms may occur, as in acute bronchitis. Obstruction of airway by secretions predisposes the patient to oxygenation problems (V/Q mismatching); hence, optimal bronchial hygiene is crucial for treatment.
Emphysema	Destruction of air sacs (alveoli) Loss of lung elasticity	Barrel chest and lung hyperinflation—air sacs do not recoil (spring back) to resting position on expiration. Shortness of breath as old air is trapped in diseased air sacs; little fresh air can get in for gas exchange.	Smoking cessation to end tissue destruction Bronchodilators to reduce airway obstruction detected on breathing test	Emphysema is an *irreversible* disease. Destroyed lung tissue cannot be replaced, but medications, oxygen breathing retraining, and exercise may decrease shortness of breath. Though the patient typically does not respond to bronchodilators on the pulmonary function test (PFT), bronchodilators may still improve signs and symptoms over an extended period of time. The disease usually occurs with acute or chronic bronchitis.

symptoms, and treatment. Emphasis of these relationships clarifies each disease process and makes subsequent information more meaningful to the patient.

During teaching, comprehension is enhanced by frequently referring to vivid illustrations of bronchospasm (asthma), obstructive secretions in the airway (bronchitis), and tissue destruction and air sac enlargement (emphysema). Learning is also enhanced by showing the patient pertinent pathologic features of his own chest x-ray. Content is modified to emphasize disease components relevant to the patient and to allow enough time for the patient to ask questions about his own case.

Preventive Measures

Once the patient knows the name, basic pathology, and related signs and symptoms of his lung disease, the nurse explains basic preventive measures, as described in the patient information section to follow. These measures will alleviate current pulmonary symptoms and reduce their incidence and severity in the future.

PATIENT INFORMATION

How well you feel largely depends upon how well you protect yourself from conditions that might aggravate your breathing problem. Take these following preventive measures:

1. First and foremost, *stop smoking*:
   a. To help prevent further lung destruction and disability.
   b. To get the maximum benefit from your treatment program. Cigarette smoking is a physical and

psychological addiction that develops from a habit. It is never too late to achieve benefits from stopping the habit. Research indicates that the "cold turkey" approach works the best. So decide on the best time to stop in the near future and develop a positive attitude towards becoming a nonsmoker.

2. *Become familiar with your medications*: Take only the prescribed dosages and do not stop a medication without your doctor's approval. Avoid over-the-counter cold remedies—these drugs may dry up your tissues or interact with your other medications. Avoid sedatives and sleeping pills—they tend to slow down your breathing too much. If you have special needs regarding medications, talk to your doctor.
3. *Recognize possible signs of overexertion in yourself*, such as the following:
   a. Increased breathing rate during or after taking a walk; it's easy to go too fast.
   b. General feeling of tiredness or shortness of breath—slow down, pace yourself, and get plenty of rest.
4. *Recognize signs of a cold or infection*:
   a. An increase in the amount of sputum, thick sputum, or yellow, green, red, or brownish sputum; use white tissues to be more aware of color changes.
   b. A temperature elevated above 100°F or 38°C (not always present).
   c. Other symptoms include increased coughing, chest tightness, or shortness of breath.

   For these signs, make sure you are following the other preventive measures. Call your doctor or start antibiotic medication, as prescribed by your doctor.
5. *Recognize the following signs of bronchospasm*:
   a. Wheezing
   b. Increased coughing
   c. Tightness in the chest

   For these signs, take an extra dose of bronchodilator medication, as prescribed by your doctor Call your doctor if the bronchospasm does not go away.
6. *Watch your diet.*
   a. Eat a well-balanced diet. Good nutrition will help you avoid respiratory infections and build up muscle strength. Each day you should eat food from the four main food groups, with emphasis on the *poultry, meat, and fish* and *fruits and vegetables* groups. The four main groups are poultry, meat, and fish; dairy products; cereals; and fruits and vegetables.
   b. Watch your weight—if you need to gain weight, exercise to develop an appetite, and eat more concentrated foods. If you are overweight, lose weight to lessen the work of your heart and lungs.
   c. Avoid foods that stimulate mucus production or are irritating to you, e.g., milk products.
   d. If too much food causes discomfort or shortness of breath, eat smaller meals with snacks in between.
7. *Drink plenty of fluids*, unless your doctor has restricted them because of a heart condition.
   a. Drink at least 2 to 3 quarts of water or other fluids each day to keep your body well hydrated. If your sputum becomes thick, drink more fluids.
   b. Avoid excessive alcohol intake. Alcohol de-
   c. Call your doctor if you notice the following signs of fluid retention or heart failure:
      (1.) Puffy extremities or ankle swelling
      (2.) Sudden weight gain (e.g., 3 to 5 lbs overnight)
      (3.) Increased shortness of breath and fatigue
8. *Control your environment.*
   a. Avoid contagious sick people, especially those with the flu, the sniffles, a chest cold, or a sore throat. You cannot afford to get sick.
   b. Talk to your doctor about having a *pneumonia shot* and yearly flu shot.
   c. Beware of irritants. Avoid freshly painted rooms; crowded, smoky rooms; humid laundromats; aerosol sprays, such as oven cleaners, hair sprays, deodorants, and insecticides; fireside or barbecue smoke; and other irritants you know you react to.
   d. Avoid dusty environments. If possible, arrange to have someone else do the heavy dusting and vacuuming. Dusting should be done regularly with a damp cloth. Be sure to keep furnace vents dust free and change air filters once a month for better filtration. Keep your bed away from the main air vent. Consult your doctor if you think you need better protection, i.e., central air conditioning with filtration and humidification. Last, avoid house furnishings that collect dust, such as high pile or shag carpets, ornate furniture, and open bookshelves.
   e. In case of a "pollution" alert or "smog advisory":
      (1.) Stay inside. Keep the doors and windows closed. Use your air conditioner, if you have one.
      (2.) Take it easy—no strenuous physical activity.
      (3.) Avoid any irritants, especially smoking. You are much more susceptible to serious respiratory problems at this time. If you must drive, avoid rush-hour traffic and congested areas. Keep your windows up, and vents closed as much as possible. If you have air conditioning, use it most of the time.
      (4.) Call your doctor if you develop respiratory problems.
9. *Seek support from family and friends* to help you to live within your limitations. Emotional, physical, personal, and family adjustments to a chronic respiratory problem are easier if all involved express feelings and concerns and work together on changing personal or family responsibilities and roles. Also, family and close friends can make it easier for you to regularly follow your treatment program and achieve a better sense of well being, if they understand you, your problems, and your disease.
10. *Call or visit your local American Lung Association* to learn about community resources for respiratory patients. Resources may include nonsmoking clinics, Better Breathers' Clubs, equipment loan programs, patient education clubs, and other support groups associated with pulmonary rehabilitation programs.

SMOKING CESSATION

The nurse may be the only person available to actively listen to the patient's concerns and fears related to smoking and smoking cessation, particularly when family and friends have become disgusted with the patient's smoking habit. Pamphlets and other educational materials, available through the American Lung Association and National Cancer Institute, prepare the nurse to counsel patients on how to stop smoking. Counseling involves these basic steps.

Understanding

Understand the patient's smoking habit, including motivation for its continuance.

As the patient begins to talk about contemplation of smoking cessation, the nurse must remember that the nicotine in cigarettes produces physical as well as psychologic addictive behavior. Dependence becomes apparent when elimination of the nicotine produces one or more of the following withdrawal symptoms: craving for tobacco; increased anxiety, irritability, and restlessness; difficulty concentrating; headache; drowsiness; and gastrointestinal disturbances (Sachs, 1985).

Though patients may intellectually recognize the benefits of smoking cessation, they may not be able to give up certain benefits of smoking continuation, including the avoidance of nicotine withdrawal symptoms. Other benefits of smoking under current investigation include improved short-term memory and improved performance under stress, which are related to increased blood arginine vasopressin levels and increased blood β-endorphin levels.

While recognizing the minor benefits of smoking, the nurse encourages careful consideration of the advantages of smoking versus the disadvantages of smoking. This approach provides an opportunity to emphasize the overwhelming advantages of smoking cessation, i.e., the development of greater self control, a positive self image, and improved present and future health.

In emphasizing the positive aspects of not smoking rather than the "taking away" of this valued habit, the nurse reminds the patient that it is never too late to stop smoking (Fig. 18–1). The benefits of smoking cessation are immediately apparent and accumulate the longer one discontinues the habit.

Disadvantages of smoking continuation include progression of lung disease, further disabling illness in the future, and involuntary smoking by household members and associates who breathe the same air. As mentioned in the chapter, Pulmonary History, cigarette smoke is a toxic irritant to others in the same room. Approximately two thirds of all smoke produced from one cigarette ends up in the atmosphere. Also, sidestream smoke (i.e., smoke released directly into the air from a burning cigarette tip) contains 2½ times the nicotine and carbon monoxide and over 100 times

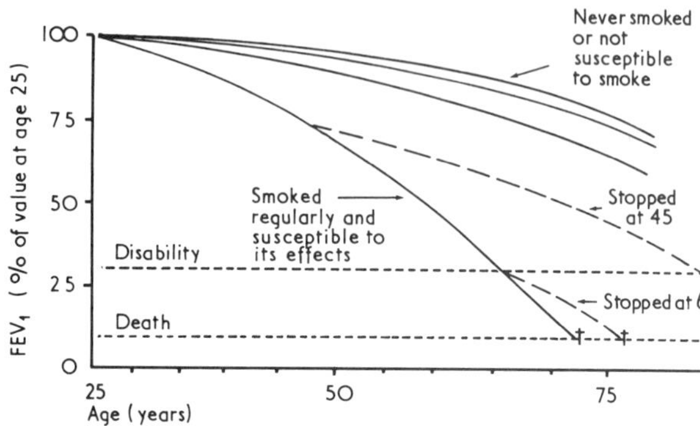

Figure 18–1. Decline in FEV_1 with age for a person who smoked regularly (bottom curve) compared with a person who never smoked or who is not susceptible to smoke (top curves). Smoking cessation slows the decline in FEV_1 (dotted curves), regardless of age at the time of cessation. The underlying cause of death (†) was COPD for the male subjects represented by this display of data. (Reproduced by permission from Fletcher, C. and Peto, R.: The natural history of chronic airflow obstruction. *British medical journal,* 1(6077):1646, 1977.)

the ammonia found in mainstream smoke (e.g., smoke inhaled by the smoker) (Splitter, 1976).

The nurse helps the patient examine his smoking habit, specifically, the time of day cigarettes are smoked; the activity or occasion engaged in; and the mood or feeling achieved. Use of a logbook or diary may facilitate accurate data collection.

Smoking often meets a need that can be met in another way. Identification of the need is the first step to finding an acceptable substitute activity. For example, if the patient states that smoking occurs to promote relaxation after meals, the cigarette might be replaced with a leisurely walk outdoors, a visit with a friendly neighbor, or a cup of decaffeinated coffee.

Encouragement

Encourage the patient to strive for an unequivocal decision to stop smoking. Determination must be strong enough to sustain the patient through withdrawal symptoms, should they arise, and other pressures to smoke a cigarette. The decision may be impossible without support from a nonsmoking friend or family member, a "buddy" to quit smoking with, a contingency contract, or a smoking cessation clinic. In some cases, the patient may give nonsmoking a try for a specified period of time, to better evaluate the benefits of smoking cessation.

Whenever possible, the nurse encourages an unequivocal decision to stop smoking. This "cold turkey" approach forces the patient to rely on inner-directed processes of change. An inner-directed decision process results in more successful attempts at smoking cessation than reliance on environmental change processes, e.g., hiding ashtrays to remove the urge to smoke (Prochaska et al, 1982). In addition, it prompts the patient to deal with quality of life issues. Moreover, if the patient contemplates switching to cigar or pipe smoking, the nurse informs the patient that pipe and cigar smokers have lower mortality rates than cigarette smokers, but higher rates than those of nonsmokers.

During counseling, the nurse uses a straightforward, factual approach to the patient, avoiding moralistic overtones. Advice is best given when the patient is suffering from acute symptoms or illnesses, so that it is seen as highly relevant to the situation. Nevertheless, advice on smoking cessation is routinely given to any smoker, regardless of the presence and severity of symptoms. At unexpected times, this advice serves as a catalyst for those contemplating smoking cessation in the near future.

When the patient verbalizes concern with possible weight gain, the nurse states that most smokers who stop smoking do not gain weight afterwards. Statistics indicate that only one third of patients gain weight; one third have no change in weight at all; and one third lose weight because of an accompanying exercise program (Petty, 1985).

Techniques

Help the patient choose and implement a technique. Techniques include sudden and complete smoking cessation after a certain date and gradual abstention over a specified period of time. In the latter case, the patient sets daily and weekly limits for the number of cigarettes allowed. The number is gradually reduced to zero, ideally over 1 to 3 months. Longer periods of time may be necessary for addicted patients but do not always result in success.

The patient may use other techniques to support smoking cessation and prevent relapse (Fischer et al, 1988). The nurse can call the local American Lung Association or Cancer Society for a list of local resources for nonsmoking clinics, individual and group counseling, and aversive conditioning therapy (i.e., rapid smoking therapy). The last technique is associated with a 2-year cure rate of 50% in patients with histories of smoking relapses (Hall et al, 1984). There are no well-controlled research studies with follow-ups that prove the efficacy of hypnosis and acupuncture for smoking cessation (Sachs, 1985).

Once the patient chooses a technique, the nurse may make one or more of the following suggestions:

1. Change your daily routine to break habit patterns. You may get up earlier or later, eat at different times, or change your evening activity to reading a book instead of watching television. Remember, *smoking is habit related.*
2. Do not carry matches or a lighter.
3. Take fewer draws on the cigarette and avoid deep inhalations.
4. Buy packs, not cartons, of cigarettes.
5. Try cigarette filters that gradually reduce the amount of inhaled tar and nicotine.
6. Plan to suck on mints, chew on gum, or utilize another diversion to reduce the urge to smoke.
7. Talk to the physician about prescription of nicotine-containing chewing gum, when addiction appears severe.

The aforementioned smoking cessation techniques are facilitated by drinking plenty of fluids (2 to 3 quarts per day) to enhance nicotine clearance from the body. To control nervousness, the patient is encouraged to schedule frequent relaxation periods, e.g., daily warm baths or hot showers, entertainment, guided imagery, and other relaxation techniques. Stimulants, such as coffee, tea, and cola beverages, are best avoided to reduce craving for tobacco. A simple, well-balanced diet is planned to optimize health and reduce intake of heavy, richly spiced foods that might precipitate a craving for tobacco (American Hospital Association, 1982).

Nicotine Chewing Gum. In a minority of patients, nicotine addiction plays a major role in foiling attempts to stop smoking (Hudson, 1984). In such cases, nicotine chewing gum (i.e., nicotine polyacrilex or Nicorette) provides an alternate source of nicotine, as the patient gradually reduces smoking. By alleviating withdrawal symptoms, it helps many patients concentrate on psychologic and social factors that reinforce the smoking habit. Chewing a single 2 mg piece of nicotine gum produces blood nicotine levels equivalent to the smoking of half a cigarette per hour. Though nicotine is known to induce cardiac spasm and arrhythmias, adverse reactions to the gum have been minor. Most frequent side effects are mouth, throat, and jaw soreness. Other reactions include nausea, vomiting, nonspecific gastrointestinal distress, hiccups, and rare severe systemic symptoms of nicotine intoxication (Mensch and Holden, 1984).

Most adverse reactions are avoided by proper chewing technique. *Nicotine chewing gum is not to be chewed in the same manner as ordinary chewing gum.* The patient is instructed to chew *very slowly* until he feels slight tingling in the mouth—usually after 15 chews. Each piece of gum lasts about 30 minutes, when most of the nicotine is released. Though 10 to 12 pieces of gum per day are usually enough to control the urge to smoke, some patients require up to 30 pieces per day. Most important, the gum is used on a temporary basis—about 3 to 6 months. It is gradually tapered, as the patient deals with psychologic aspects of his addictive behavior.

Reinforcement

Plan reinforcement of the nonsmoking habit. Maintenance of a nonsmoking environment is key to successful smoking cessation. The nurse encourages the patient to

1. Remove all ashtrays, cigarettes, pipes, tobacco, pipe cleaners, racks, and matches from the home or work place.

2. Seek the company of nonsmoking friends who can understand and support the patient's effort to stop smoking.

3. Clean rugs, draperies, other furnishings, and clothes that are saturated with tobacco smoke.

4. Designate at least one smoke-free room in the house for relaxation, when living with a smoker.

5. Sit in nonsmoking designated areas in public places. When necessary, tactfully ask smokers to extinguish their cigarettes or to move to smoking areas.

In addition, nonsmoking behavior may be reinforced by written reminders of progress, e.g., a chart or wallet calendar scorecard of the number of nonsmoking days achieved. Rewards provide incentive to continue nonsmoking, e.g., contribution to a piggy bank after successfully resisting the urge to smoke and using this piggy bank money for a shopping spree or party, celebrating 6 months of nonsmoking.

Regular Checkups

Encourage the patient to continue regular checkups with his physician. Referral to the physician is important because it facilitates the physician's reinforcement of nonsmoking behavior and the monitoring of signs of tobacco withdrawal and nicotine side effects, when nicotine-containing gum is used.

All patients are encouraged to accept the fact that tobacco withdrawal symptoms are likely, but they will disappear as the urge to smoke passes. Symptoms are usually limited to the signs of tobacco withdrawal mentioned. They may be accompanied by cough and sputum production for several weeks, which are normal reactions of healing airways. In rare cases, severe symptoms occur, including dyspnea, vertigo, chest tightness, visual disturbances, sweats, severe headache, and gastrointestinal disturbances.

MEDICATIONS

Teaching patients about medications has top priority because failure to take prescribed dosages at appropriate times can precipitate acute dyspnea and rehospitalization. At least initially, emphasis is placed on knowing the medication's name; dosage; general purpose, in simple terms; and administration times. Side effects and more detailed information may be presented later, after a medication schedule is established.

Scheduling of pulmonary medications is a joint activity between patient and nurse. To assure optimal therapy and compliance, both should agree upon definite times that

1. *Promote 24-hour bronchodilatation*—as discussed in Chapter 11, bronchodilator administrations should be appropriately timed during waking hours.

2. *Promote aerosol deposition in the lungs*—inhaled steroids or cromolyn are taken after, not before, aerosol bronchodilators.

3. *Minimize side effects*—administration with food or crackers may help minimize gastrointestinal side effects. Also, consistently taking pills with a whole glass of water may increase absorption, while providing the side benefit of hydration of retained secretions.

4. *Fit in with preset activities of daily living*—meals, breaks at work, household duties, and so forth. Compliance is higher when medications are grouped around the existing lifestyle.

5. *Coincide with other treatments*—aerosol treatments, breathing exercises, and so forth.

Cost is a major factor in the patient's willingness and ability to comply with a proposed medication schedule. When cost is a concern, the nurse encourages the patient to locate a pharmacy with reasonable prices; prices may vary dramatically among pharmacies. Patients are reminded that many inhaler prescriptions may be refilled without the plastic adaptor, an extra expense. Repeated complaints about expensive medication are indications for medical evaluation and a less expensive medication regimen. In general, the cost of oral theophylline is relatively low. A beta-adrenergic aerosol is slightly higher in cost, and cromolyn is most expensive. In some cases, prednisone, a relatively inexpensive drug, may be more practical than bronchodilator aerosols that cost more and are improperly administered. Unit dose vials of bronchodilator nebulizer solution (e.g., metaproterenol) are convenient but cost more than bottled nebulizer solution.

In addition to helping the patient reduce cost, the nurse helps the patient devise ways to remember the names and administration times of pulmonary medications. Many individuals require a written list of medications with special instructions, such as the one in Figure 18–2. Such a list might be kept in the patient's purse, wallet, and at home next to the patient's vials of pills for frequent reference. Individuals who do not rely on medication lists may prefer to place medications in a readily visible or accessible place at home, such as a bedside table, bathroom medicine cabinet, or kitchen counter, and link administration times to routine activities, such as getting up in the morning, shaving, and putting children to bed. Sometimes the nurse must use creativity and foresight to help the individual find an administration system that works. The COPD patient in Figure 18–3 took so many daily medications, he and his visiting nurse decided to set up an egg carton system. Each morning, the patient allocated pills in one or more of four slots clearly labelled *8:00*, *12:00*, *5:00*, and *9:00*. The advantage of this system is its use of an egg carton, a common household item. Use of a special medication administration set, such as Mediset, may serve the same purpose. Ideally, such self-medication programs are started before hospital discharge so that individuals have a chance to practice medication administrations with close supervision.

Once a medication schedule is established, the nurse introduces more detailed information on medication actions and side effects. To prevent information over-

DAILY MEDICATION SCHEDULE

RESPIRATORY MEDICATIONS	7am	12 noon	6 pm	10^{30} pm	
Theo-Dur 200 mg (1 pill)	X		X		Take pills just
Prednisone 10mg (2 pills)	X				before meals
Proventil inhaler 2 puffs	X	X	X	X	wait at least 1 min. between puffs
Vanceril inhaler 2 puffs (steroid)	X	X	X	X	Take 15 min. after Proventil
*For wheezing at night:	Take	1-2 pu	ffs of	your	Proventil inhaler

Figure 18–2. A daily medication schedule made in collaboration with an ambulatory care patient.

load, several short teaching sessions may be necessary. Learning may be reinforced with a handout or card listing the medication's name, purpose, and side effects, and advice or cautions for use at home.

Inhaler Technique

The two types of inhalers are the *metered dose device* (MDD) and *turboinhaler* (see Fig. 11–8). The MDD is a cartridge-type inhaler containing an autonomic active, steroid, or cromolyn medication. The turboinhaler is a special inhaler specifically designed for delivery of the powder in cromolyn capsules.

Note in the subsequent patient information that techniques for the MDD and turboinhaler are different. Technique for the autonomic active MDD and steroid MDD is basically the same, though monitoring instructions to the patient are different.

Optimum Technique. Since inhalers are frequently prescribed for both acute and chronic pulmonary disease, working with the patient to perfect technique has become an important nursing duty. Research indicates that optimum bronchopulmonary aerosol delivery occurs when the MDD is activated 4 cm from the wide-open mouth, inhaling the dose over 5 or 6 seconds from functional reserve capacity (FRC) and holding the breath for 10 seconds at total lung capacity (TLC) (Dolovich et al, 1981).

The problem remains, however, of application of optimum technique in the clinical setting. For example, some patients cannot spray into the mouth, unless the MDD is between the lips. Dyspneic individuals can hold their breath for only 1 to 3 seconds not the optimum 10 seconds. Others modify standard technique and still achieve significant improvement in pulmonary function tests and breath sounds (Epstein, 1983).

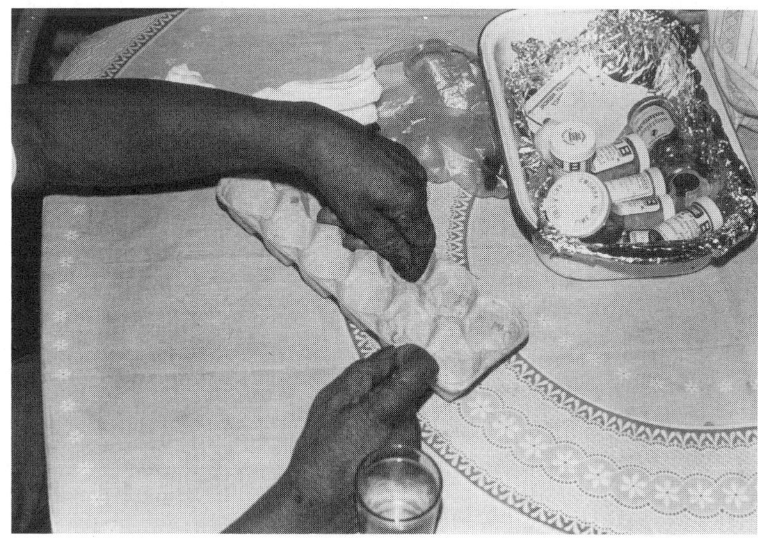

Figure 18–3. The egg-carton system for self medication at home is inexpensive and easy to implement when needed. The patient labels receptacles with daily administration times.

PATIENT INFORMATION

Use of Your Inhaler

Use this procedure to get the maximal effect from your inhaler.

To Prepare

1. Follow the manufacturer's instructions and shake medication before use.
2. Place medication cartridge in the plastic oral adapter and take the cap off the mouthpiece.

Then

1. Breathe all your air out through pursed lips without straining.
2. Place mouthpiece between lips or about 1½ inches away.
3. Keeping your mouth wide open (do not seal lips around mouthpiece), take a *slow deep* breath in. At the same time, firmly press down on the metal vial to give one puff of medication.
    a. Concentrate on the slow deep breath *in* to deposit the medication deep into the lungs.
    b. Keep your tongue down and out of the way.
4. Remove mouthpiece from mouth. Hold your breath for 10 seconds or as tolerated (i.e., minimum of 1 to 3 seconds).
5. Breathe your air out slowly and completely through pursed lips without straining. If two puffs are prescribed, take the second puff 2 to 5 minutes after the first puff.
6. Rinse mouth with tap water (optional). This precaution may reduce the incidence of side effects.

Tips

1. Wash the plastic oral adapter once a day with liquid soap and water. Rinse and dry completely. Store in a clean plastic bag or container.
2. Use only as directed by your doctor. Do not overuse your inhaler. You may develop side effects, such as dizziness, headache, fast beating heart with skipped beats, or resistance to the drug.
3. Call your doctor if you find yourself using your inhaler frequently.

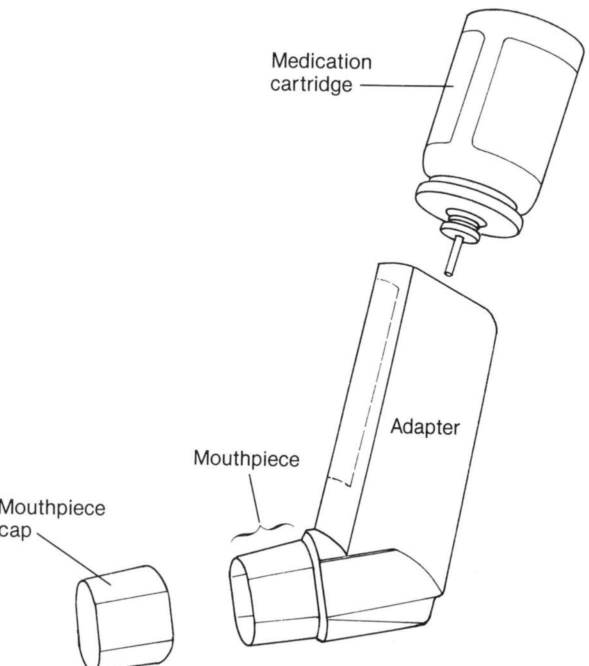

Use of Your Steroid Inhaler

Your doctor has prescribed a steroid inhaler, e.g., Vanceril or Beclovent (beclomethasone), because other drugs have not successfully controlled your respiratory symptoms, or you wish to discontinue your oral steroids (pills). If you are now on steroid pills, the steroid inhaler will be added. Then your steroid pills will be gradually reduced and eventually discontinued, if possible. Carefully follow your doctor's orders and these instructions to keep the right amount of steroids in your body.

1. If ordered, first inhale a bronchodilator to open your airways. Use your inhaler or compressor with nebulizer.
2. Then, use your steroid inhaler as follows:
    a. Shake inhaler well.
    b. Place medication cartridge in the plastic oral adapter and take the cap off the mouthpiece.

To Inhale

1. Breathe all your air out through pursed lips without straining.
2. Place mouthpiece between lips or about 1½ inches away.
3. Keeping your mouth wide open (do not seal lips around mouthpiece), take a *slow deep* breath in. At the same time, firmly press down on the metal vial to give one dose of medication.
    a. Concentrate on the slow deep breath *in* to deposit the medication deep into the lungs.
    b. Keep your tongue down and out of the way.
4. Remove mouthpiece from mouth. Hold your breath for 10 seconds or as tolerated (i.e., minimum of 1 to 3 seconds).
5. Breathe your air out slowly and completely through pursed lips without straining. Wait 1 minute before taking a second puff if 2 puffs are prescribed.
6. If at home, rinse mouth with water or mouthwash (e.g., Listerine and Cepacol) to avoid a mouth infection.

Cleaning

1. Remove medication cartridge and wash plastic oral adapter once a day with liquid soap and water.
2. Rinse and dry completely.
3. Reassemble and store in a cool place.

Tips

1. Do not use your steroid inhaler for episodes of shortness of breath. The inhaled steroid *prevents* breathing problems; it does not relieve shortness of breath once it happens.
2. The inhaled steroid takes time to work. If you are on a reduced number of steroid pills, you may experience symptoms of steroid withdrawal for a few weeks or months until your body adjusts.
   Main signs of steroid withdrawal are joint and muscular pain, depression, and nasal stuffiness.
3. Report any new signs and symptoms, e.g., signs of steroid withdrawal, increased wheezing, shortness of breath, mouth sores, sore throat, difficulty swallowing to your doctor.

Use of the Turboinhaler (SPINHALER)

A

The **Body** consists of a white tube with a gray sleeve which slides up and down.

B

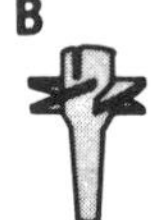

The **Propeller** rests on the steel spindle and holds the capsule.

C

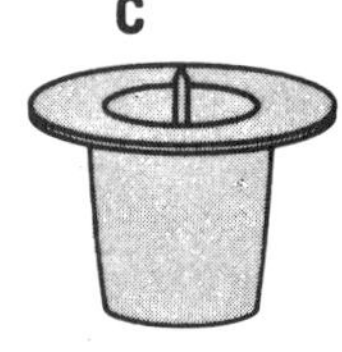

White **Mouthpiece** with flange and stainless steel spindle.

1

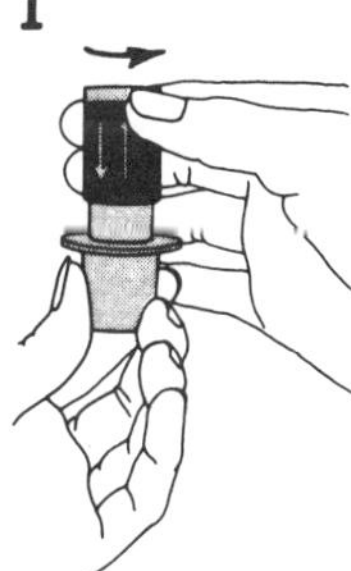

Make sure your hands are clean and dry.

Loading the SPINHALER

Hold SPINHALER vertical with white mouthpiece held downwards. Unscrew body of inhaler counter-clockwise.

2

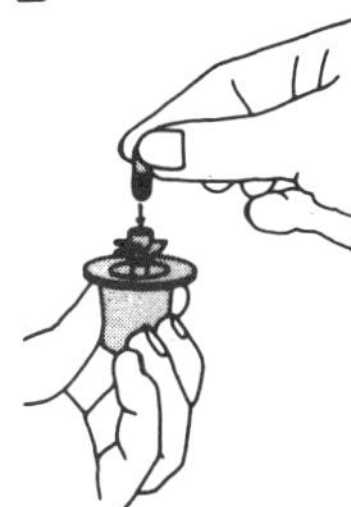

Keep mouthpiece downwards and propeller on spindle. Insert **colored** end of capsule **firmly** into propeller cup. Excessive handling of the capsule causes it to soften.

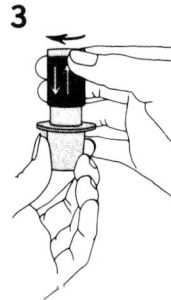

3

Screw body back into mouthpiece, making certain it is securely fastened.

4a

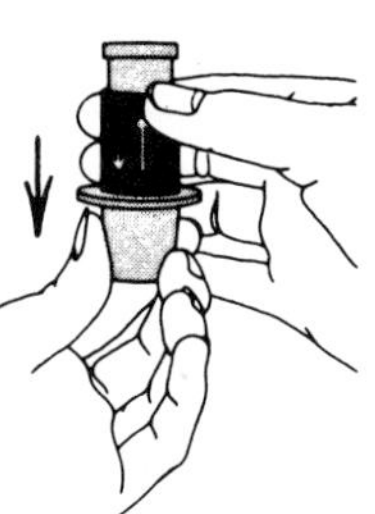

Keep SPINHALER vertical and mouthpiece downwards...slide the gray sleeve down firmly until it stops (to pierce the capsule)...then slide the gray sleeve up as far as it will go.

Do this only once. Do not repeat.

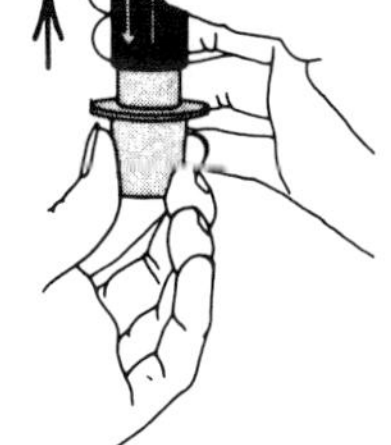

4b

5

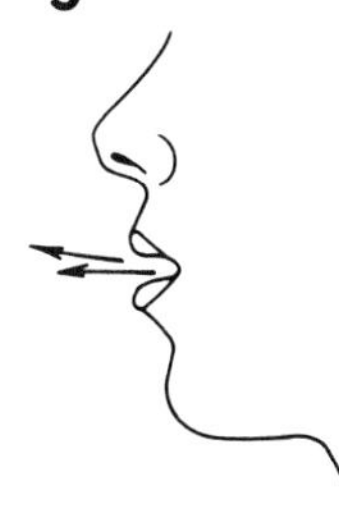

Use of SPINHALER

Check again to make sure that the mouthpiece is securely attached to the body. Holding SPINHALER well away from mouth breathe out fully emptying air from lungs as much as possible.

6

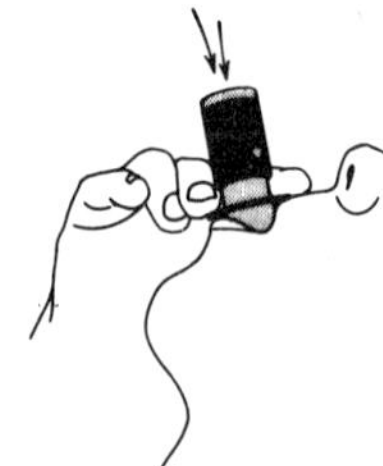

With head tilted backwards and teeth apart, close lips and teeth around the mouthpiece.

Inhale a deep and rapid breath.
DO NOT BREATHE OUT THROUGH SPINHALER ®

7

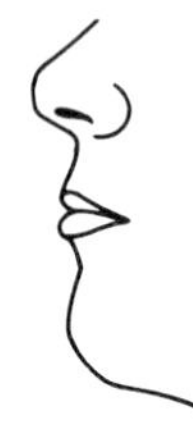

Remove SPINHALER from your mouth and hold your breath for a few seconds.

8

Holding SPINHALER well away from mouth breathe out completely.

Repeat steps 5, 6, 7, and 8 several times until the powder is inhaled.

A light dusting of powder remaining behind in the capsule is normal and is not an indication that the SPINHALER or capsule is faulty.

Caution: Breathing out through the SPINHALER causes moisture to deposit and interferes with proper functioning.

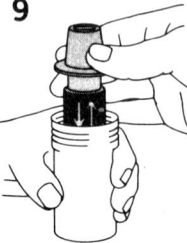

9

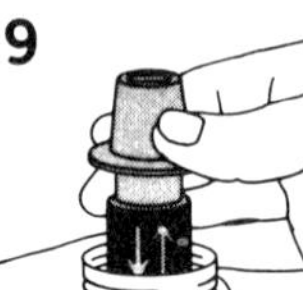

Discard empty capsule, return SPINHALER to container and screw lid on securely.

10

Cleaning SPINHALER

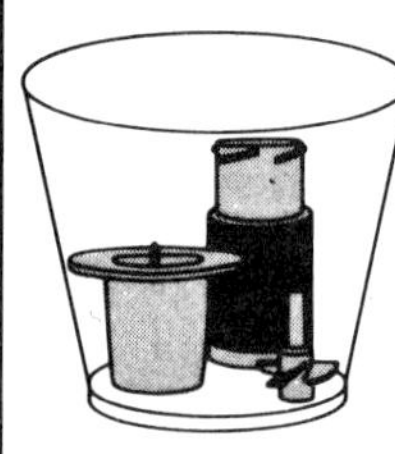

At least once a week, dismantle parts A, B, and C and wash them in clean, warm water. Pay particular attention to washing the inside of the propeller shaft, by moving the propeller on and off the steel spindle under water. Shake out excess water and allow all parts to dry before re-assembly.

How to care for the capsules

1. Do not remove capsules from foil except for immediate use.

2. Do not handle capsules excessively. Moisture from hands may make capsules soft.

3. Protect from extremes of temperature.

Note: In case of difficulty, consult your physician or pharmacist.

With care the SPINHALER should provide useful service for up to 6 months. The SPINHALER should be replaced after 6 months.

Courtesy of Fisons Corporation.

The following evaluation criteria presented in the box below and Figure 18–4 serve as guides to helping the patient perfect technique. As suggested, however, the nurse may need to greatly modify criteria, depending on clinical circumstances and the inhaler-delivery system prescribed (Newman, 1983).

EVALUATION CRITERIA FOR CORRECT INHALER TECHNIQUE

Shaking the canister before use
- To maximize drug delivery during each actuation

Holding the canister upright
- The metering chamber will not refill unless the canister is upright.

A slow steady, full inspiration with head tilted backwards
- To minimize impaction losses in the oropharynx and to facilitate distal penetration

Ten-second breath holding
- To allow particles to settle on airways before exhalation

Inhaler held between the lips or 4 cm away from the mouth (see Fig. 18–4)
- Aerosol particles travel at a slower rate when actuation occurs away from the mouth. Hence, they are more likely to enter distal bronchi.

Synchronization of inhalation with "firing" of the MDD at one third the way into inhalation.
- A steady air stream is necessary to carry particles to the lungs

A 5 to 10 minute wait between consecutive puffs
- The first puff opens airways so that aerosol from the second puff travels deeper into the lungs.

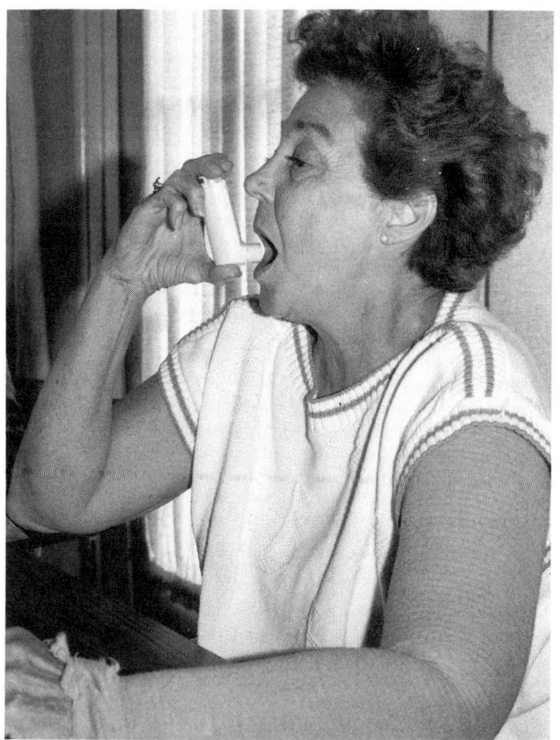

Figure 18–4. An asthmatic patient improvises and uses a one-hand instead of a two-hand technique for aerosol delivery via a metered dose device.

Use of a Mirror and Placebo Inhaler. Patients who exhibit coordination difficulties may benefit from practicing correct inhaler technique before a mirror. A mirror provides a different visual and spatial orientation. The patient sits or stands sideways to the mirror (left side to the mirror for a right-handed person). The head is turned slightly towards the mirror to permit viewing of details, such as the position of the mouthpiece to the lips and timing of actuation during inspiration. If the canister is pushed too early or late during inspiration or during inadequate airflow, the patient can actually see the aerosol "bounce back out" of the oral cavity (Brashear, 1983). This type of visual feedback may decrease learning time and provide a way for the patient to check for correct technique at home.

Use of a placebo inhaler (i.e., propellant without medication) allows repeated practice in front of a mirror without risk of side effects from overdose. Placebo inhalers are available through many pharmaceutic companies that manufacture inhalers.

Use of Arthritic Aids. An aid may be used for arthritic patients, elderly patients, and others who cannot coordinate hand movements for actuation of a MDD. In Figure 18–5, the patient merely squeezes the device between fingers and thumb to produce aerosol. Otherwise, the technique is basically the same as that described for patients without hand coordination problems.

Use of Extension Devices (Spacers). An *extension device* attached to the mouthpiece of the inhaler is

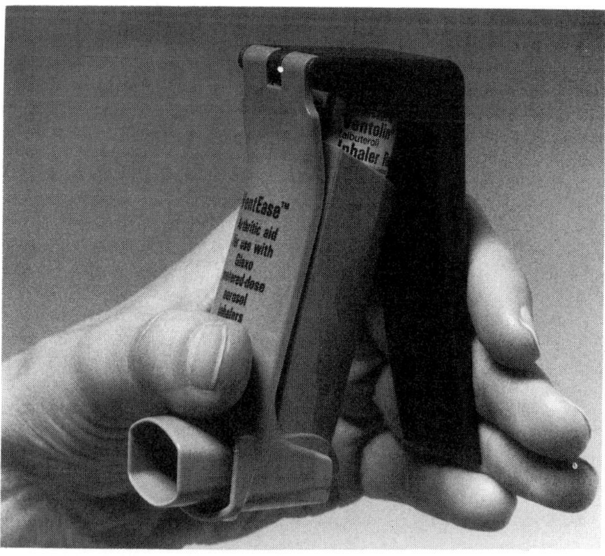

Figure 18–5. The VentEase arthritic aid (Glaxo) for use with a medication cartridge from a metered dose device.

sometimes referred to as a *spacer*. Different types of extension devices are available, as shown by the examples in Figure 18–6. The extra distance between the inhaler and the patient's mouth allows large propellant droplets to condense on the sides of the spacer rather than in the patient's oropharynx. Because air resistance slows down aerosol movement, the remaining cloud of small aerosol particles travels slowly to the back of the mouth, with reduced oropharyngeal impaction (Newman, 1981).

The three main clinical advantages of an extension device are described, as follows. First, technique is simpler, since the patient places his lips completely around the mouthpiece. In some cases, e.g., *InspirEase* in Figure 18–6, rebreathing through a reservoir bag provides longer aerosol contact time for sedimentation on airways. This technique eliminates the need to worry about synchrony between MDD actuation and inhalation.

Second, extension devices decrease the incidence of side effects—candidiasis from steroid inhalers and arrhythmias from sympathomimetics with beta 1 action—owing to excessive oropharyngeal absorption into the systemic circulation.

Third, extension devices increase aerosol delivery to the airways. Hence, they are more likely to maximize bronchodilatation compared with inhalers without extension devices. Whereas only 10% of each MDD puff is normally delivered to the lungs, use of a reservoir bag delivery system may increase this amount up to 53% (Tobin et al, 1982). The InspirEase in Figure 18–6 has a sound monitoring device warning the patient when inspiratory flow rates exceed 0.3 L/sec. This warning assures a slow flow rate to maximize peripheral aerosol deposition.

The nurse may be asked to evaluate a need for an extension device or spacer. The advantages and disadvantages of extension devices may be used to guide evaluation of individual situations (Table 18–4). Different devices in the clinical setting are described in Table 18–5.

Table 18–4. ADVANTAGES AND DISADVANTAGES OF EXTENSION DEVICES

Advantages	Disadvantages
Increases lung deposition of medication.	Added cost to patient.
Simplifies technique and may provide for synchronization of actuation with inhalation and solve hand-lung coordination problems.	Bulky and obtrusive design may cause some patients to avoid use outside the home.
Decreases the incidence of side effects, e.g., oral candidiasis.	May complicate treatment plan, e.g., another technique to learn; spacer may be more difficult to clean and maintain than MDD adapter.
Prevents cold Freon in MDD* cartridge from hitting back of throat and stopping inhalation.	
Decreases irritant receptor stimulation and associated coughing.	May not adapt to all MDDs.
May help control inspiratory flow rate.	Requires staff time for teaching of correct use.
Reduces bad taste of medication in mouth.	

*Metered dose device.

CONTROLLING DYSPNEA: BASIC APPROACHES

Basic self care includes the learning of basic approaches for the control of dyspnea. Dyspnea is a pulmonary symptom that may cause considerable anxiety and panic reaction for a pulmonary patient. The anxiety and panic increase, as past unsuccessful coping patterns cause the patient to immediately associate loss of control with any sensation of dyspnea. Thereafter, the patient projects a negative attitude towards the possibility of learning new techniques that might help him.

To help the patient understand how to control dyspnea and develop a more positive self concept, the nurse implements relaxation and breathing retraining techniques (see Chapter 19) and energy conservation

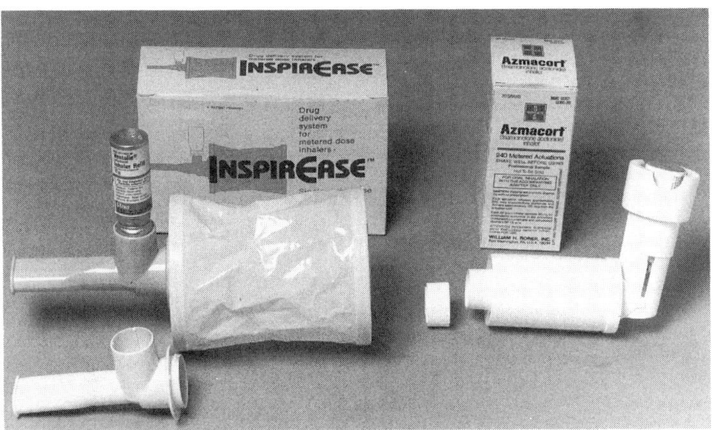

Figure 18–6. Extension devices (spacers) for inhaler aerosol delivery. *Left*, Switching mouthpieces allows the patient to use this InspirEase device with more than one brand of inhaler. The reservoir bag is disposable and collapsible for increased portability. *Right*, Some extension devices, such as this one for Azmacort, come with the medication cartridge.

Table 18–5. CHARACTERISTICS OF EXTENSION DEVICES*

Device	Description	Requires Synchronization of Actuation and Inhalation	Aerosol Deposition in Oropharynx	Adapts to Different MDDs†	Regulates Inspiratory Flow
Brethancer	Straight tube spacer	Yes	Moderately reduced	Adapts to terbutaline	No
Azmacort	Straight tube spacer	Yes	Moderately reduced	Only adapts to triamcinalone	No
Inhal-Aid	700 ml rigid plastic reservoir with one-way valves designed for children	No	Markedly reduced	Adapts to all available MDDs	Yes (visual feedback)
InspirEase	700 ml collapsible plastic reservoir bag	No	Markedly reduced	Adapts to many but not all MDDs	Yes
Aerochamber	145 ml rigid holding chamber with a one-way valve	No	Markedly reduced	Adapts to all available MDDs	No

*Reproduced by permission from Salzman, G: Spacer devices for aerosol therapy. *Clinical challenge in cardiopulmonary medicine*, 3(6):3, 1985.

†Metered dose device.

techniques (see Chapter 20). As adaptive behavior is rewarded with words of encouragement, the patient gains enough self confidence to begin practicing techniques along with daily living activities.

Besides implementing special techniques, perhaps the easiest and most effective way to help the patient is to tell him to "*slow down!*" Because of worry over whether or not he will "make it" to his destination, a patient may walk at a fast pace that nearly guarantees severe uncontrollable dyspnea. Similarly, the patient may race through morning chores and become too dyspneic and tired to participate in other activities in the afternoon.

To counteract this tendency, the nurse encourages the patient: (1) to slow his walking pace, (2) to periodically use basic resting positions to avoid fatigue (Fig. 18–7), and (3) to space daily chores throughout the day, preferably at times when he usually feels good. Moreover, because concerned family members tend to quickly complete unfinished chores for the patient, the nurse counsels them to resist this tendency. Periodic help is appropriate, but too much help reinforces the patient's feelings of dependence and helplessness.

In addition, family and staff are encouraged to remain calm, whenever the patient with chronic pulmonary disease develops dyspnea. Composure sends the nonverbal message that dyspnea is an expected symptom that can be controlled with appropriate techniques. It does not signal a life-threatening emergency. If oxygenation is a concern, family can be taught to check for cyanosis of the lips, an early physical sign of hypoxemia.

RECOGNITION OF SIGNS OF COMPLICATIONS

The patient information relating to preventive measures contains the three following complications that pulmonary patients must learn to recognize: chest infection, bronchospasm, and fluid retention or heart failure.

Counseling focuses on recognition of *early* signs of complications. Because these signs are slightly different for each patient, the nurse asks a COPD patient to recall how the chest infection started—whether the first sign was change in sputum, postnasal drip into the lungs at night, or some other sign. The patient with cor pulmonale may not recognize that he has puffy feet, the sign routinely given in patient education material; but he may acknowledge that he has difficulty putting his shoes on. Similarly, the asthmatic may verbally deny early symptoms of bronchospasm, but on further questioning, he may realize that increased coughing was present the day of an asthmatic attack.

Because little correlation may exist between symptoms and deteriorating lung functions, on the pulmonary function tests, asthmatics may be instructed to keep symptom and activity diaries and record daily peak flow meter results (Fig. 18–8). This type of self monitoring at home allows patients and staff to discover reliable early signs of bronchospasm for the patient. In addition, it allows for the identification and further assessment of asthma triggers that precipitate bronchospasm in the first place.

To emphasize the importance and cost effectiveness of self-monitoring techniques for the patient, consider a relatively asymptomatic asthmatic who notices a significant drop in peak flow values at home. The patient telephones the physician and obtains a bronchodilator medication adjustment, without an extra clinic visit. Moreover, when cough is identified as an early sign of bronchospasm, the same type of medication adjustment may result from the information provided in the symptom (e.g., cough) diary.

NUTRITION

The incidence and severity of nutritional depletion in nonhospitalized respiratory patients are less than

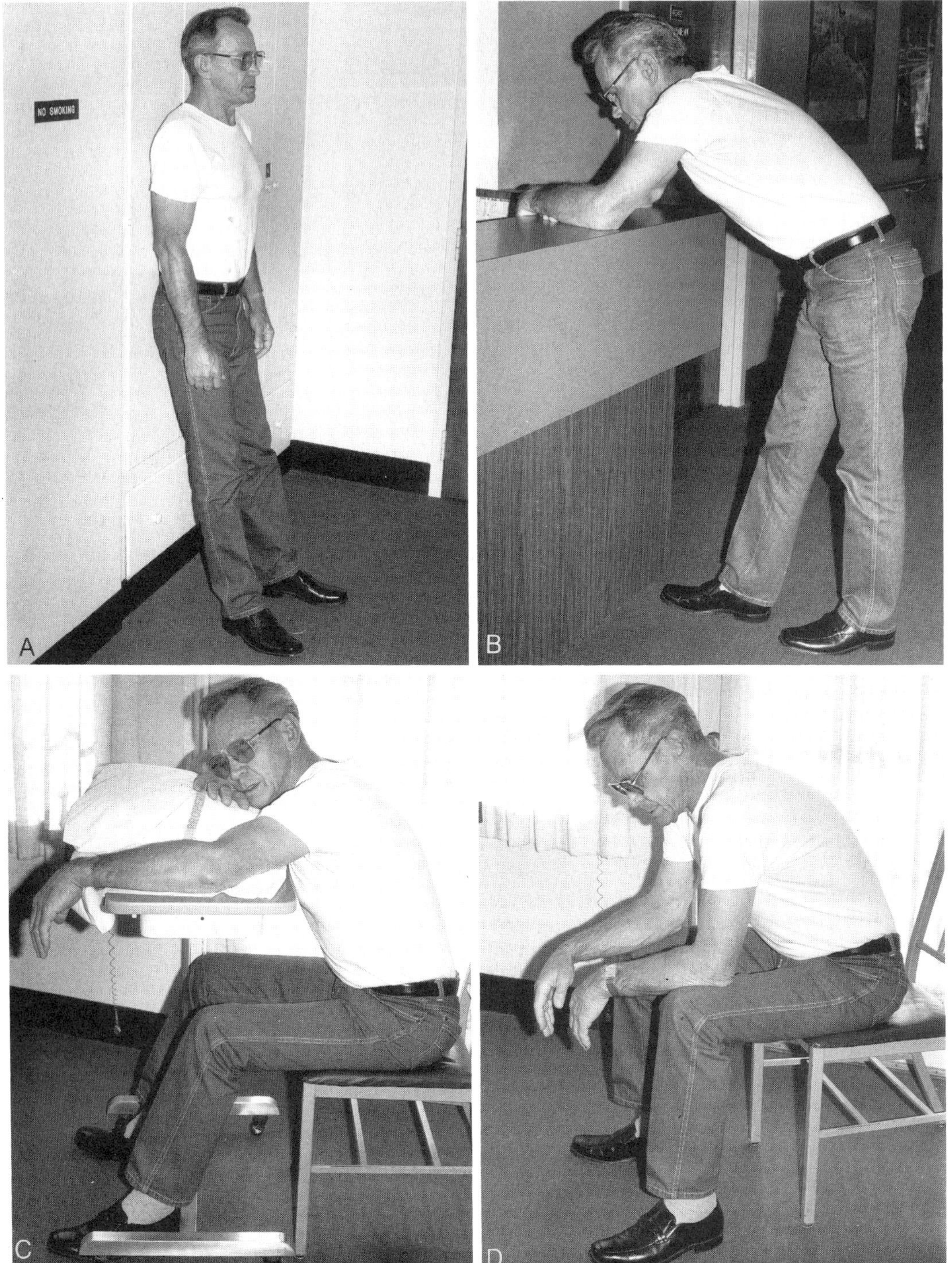

Figure 18–7. Basic resting positions to avoid fatigue and dyspnea.

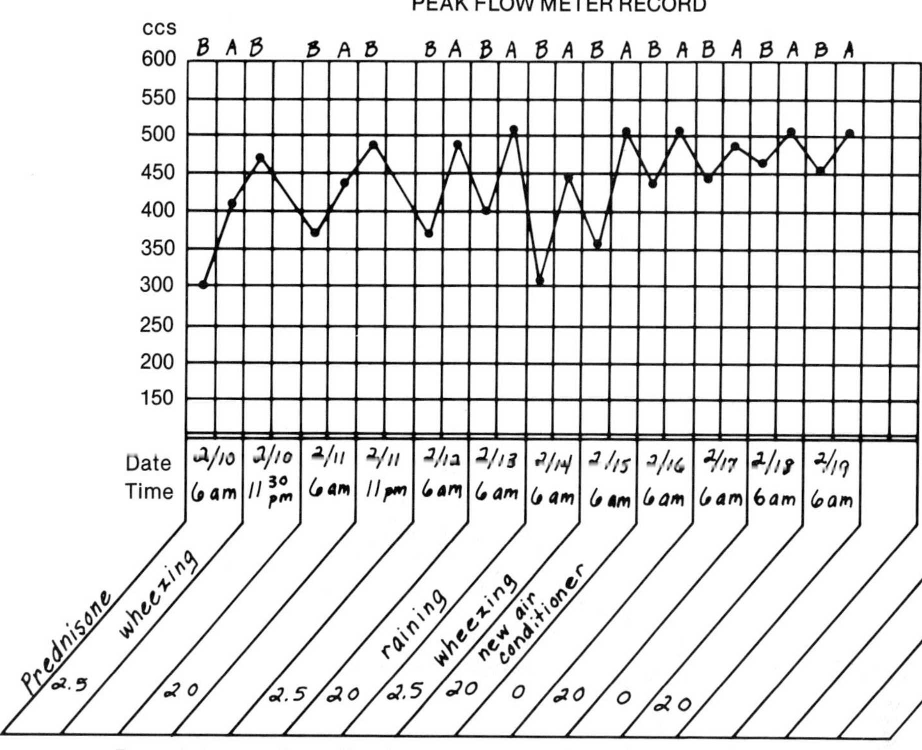

Figure 18–8. Symptom and activity diary to record daily peak flow meter results, allowing identification of early signs of bronchospasm and asthma triggers that precipitate bronchospasm. (B = before aerosol bronchodilator; A = after aerosol bronchodilator.)

those found in hospitalized patients. Nevertheless, nutritional problems are common in the home setting. When untreated, malnutrition develops (see Table 28–5 for clinical manifestations), increasing the likelihood of respiratory failure.

Nutritional deficiency manifested by weight loss may arise due to decreased caloric intake. A variety of factors may be involved, including depression, anorexia, stomach discomfort from air swallowing or medication side effects, fatigue, economic factors, cultural factors, dental problems, inability to prepare meals, and lack of knowledge of community resources.

Nursing interventions focus on three aspects as follows: (1) assessing the patient's daily dietary intake and consulting nutritional specialists and other sources, as needed (Bell et al, 1984; O'Ryan and Burns, 1984); (2) helping the patient identify and solve specific problems affecting dietary intake, e.g., ordering a new pair of dentures and arranging for Meals-on-Wheels or a homemaker to prepare meals; and (3) planning an increased intake to 2700 calories for men and 2000 calories for women. Simple caloric guides are available in grocery stores, discount stores, and hospital dietary departments for patient use.

From another perspective, Braun et al (1984) conclude that increased caloric utilization rather than decreased caloric intake is largely responsible for weight loss and nutritional depletions in ambulatory patients. In their group of patients, weight loss occurred in 26%, despite a normal caloric intake. The *tricep skinfold measurement*, an estimate of the body's fat reserves, was less than 60% of standard in 33% of patients. The *midarm circumference* was mildly reduced, indicating a mild reduction in the body's protein stores.

The exact mechanism for the respiratory patient's increased demand for calories is unknown. It is assumed that it is related to increased work of breathing, increased dead space ventilation (V_D/V_T), inefficient gas exchange, and increased oxygen consumption.

Monitoring Body Weight

Perhaps the easiest and most reliable way to monitor nutritional status is to teach the patient to weigh himself at home once or twice a week and record the weight on a chart for trend analysis. The patient's weight should be maintained as close to ideal as possible. A method to estimate ideal weight is presented in the box (O'Ryan and Burns, 1984).

ESTIMATION OF IDEAL BODY WEIGHT

(Actual height in inches − 60) (5) = x
x + 100 = ideal weight for women
x + 110 = ideal weight for men

Weight is difficult to assess when the patient is affected by right heart failure. Fluid from edema often replaces lean body mass, resulting in a stable or increased weight, when in fact lean body mass is decreased. This situation requires two approaches. First, the patient needs diuretics to eliminate excess fluid; potassium supplement to replace potassium lost in the urine; and a no added salt (NAS) diet to reduce sodium retention, occurring with use of diuretics and steroids.

In addition, the patient needs to increase muscle mass. Specific interventions include eating high protein foods (e.g., meat, fish, poultry, and dairy products), protein additives (e.g., nonfat dry milk), and a well-balanced diet to assure intake of vitamins and trace elements.

As edema is eliminated and nutritional status improves, lean body mass and inspiratory muscle strength both increase, making breathing and muscle strengthening exercises easier to perform.

Sexual Adaptation to Lung Disease

Sexual adaptation to lung disease involves sexuality, a concept that extends beyond sex to include all somatic, emotional, intellectual, social, and ethical dimensions of life. The motivational model in Chapter 16 may be used to help the patient change how he thinks and feels about himself and how he relates to family, friends, and sexual partners. Discussion focuses specifically on the counseling of patients whose sexual activities are restricted by lung disease. When sexual partners do not know how to appropriately modify sexual activities, lung disease may disrupt satisfying sexual relations and precipitate family maladaptation and social isolation at a time when such support systems need to be at their maximum.

SEXUAL NEEDS OF PULMONARY PATIENTS

Both health professionals and patients tend to overlook sexual needs. Health team members may not discuss sexual matters because of knowledge or training deficits, time limitations, social taboos, or uncomfortableness with their own sexuality. Patients, particularly the elderly, also hesitate to bring up the topic. Social norms suppress sexual expression and adjustments in the elderly, and since most disabled respiratory patients are elderly, many have few opportunities to fully explore sexuality and the problems related to maintaining sexual activity, as pulmonary disease progresses.

Whether imagined or real, sexual needs are almost always present in respiratory patients. At least 50% of patients with COPD indicate that their illness negatively affects physical sexual expression (Hanson, 1982). Dyspneic patients may abstain from any form of sexual expression because of past frightful and uncomfortable experiences associated with sexual intercourse. Abstention in turn may prompt both sexual partners to retreat into their own separate worlds. They may share the same living space, but lack the physical, spiritual, and emotional closeness that might help them talk about their frustrations, seek help, or experiment with other forms of sexual expression besides intercourse. Both partners may experience a sense of failure as a man or woman or guilt for not meeting the other partner's sexual needs.

This pattern of isolation and repression is reinforced by changes in lifestyle that accompany the steady downhill disease course of COPD. Rather than returning to work and resuming normal activities of daily living, the emphysematous patient often loses his job and becomes severely disabled. These losses compound the loss of sexual satisfaction. In addition, they reinforce low self esteem, helplessness, and depression and exacerbate the original sexual adjustment problem.

Because of these many losses, the pulmonary patient has a greater need for sexual satisfaction than the cardiac patient or any other patient who is fortunate enough to resume fairly normal work, family life, and outside activities.

COUNSELING THE PATIENT

To determine whether a sexual need exists, the nurse may integrate the sexual assessment questions (see the box) with history, physical, or motivational assessment questions (Tibbals, 1982).

SEXUAL ASSESSMENT QUESTIONS

1. Are you currently active sexually? If so, what is the approximate frequency of sexual activity?
2. Are you satisfied with your sex life? If not, please explain.
3. (*Men*): Do you have difficulty obtaining or maintaining an erection?
   Do you have any difficulty with control of ejaculation?
4. (*Women*): Do you have any difficulty becoming sexually aroused?
   Do you ever experience pain during intercourse?
   Do you have difficulty reaching orgasm?
5. Do you have questions or problems related to sex that you would like to discuss?

Broad, open-ended questions may be followed by specific questions, such as "Has your breathing problem affected your sex life?" Introduction of the possibility of sexual problems gives the patient permission to talk about this private matter more comfortably.

Some patients do not want to talk about sexual activities, even when the nurse implies acceptance and gently encourages discussion; their wishes are respected.

Other patients deny such problems but subsequently send cues, indicating a need or desire to talk about sex. Cues range from a subtle joke about sexual inadequacies to an overt comment such as "I can't even make love with my wife." The nurse asks the patient to explain indirect or vague comments. Subsequent conversations focus on two aspects. First, the nurse tries to discover the patient's sexual attitudes, fears, preferences, and possible difficulties associated with sexual activities and relationships both before and after the onset of pulmonary disease. Second, as questions arise, the nurse discredits myths about sex and pulmonary disease.

Discrediting Myths about Sex and Pulmonary Disease

Seven common myths about sex and pulmonary disease are listed. Information is provided to discredit each of these myths.

Myth 1—Disabled Persons are Asexual. On the contrary, disabled persons have sexual needs. Though sexual activity may be absent or infrequent during acute exacerbations of pulmonary disease, thoughts, fantasies, and feelings about sex do not disappear. Sex is an activity of daily living that affects the patient's self concept and ability to cope with pulmonary disease.

Myth 2—The Elderly are Asexual. On the contrary, older persons have sexual needs. Moreover, aging is not a primary cause of sexual dysfunction. In older men, erections are less frequent, and ejaculations less forceful and frequent. However, satisfying sexual activity and, in some cases, procreation may occur into the seventh and eighth decades of life. Older women require increased time in the first and second phases of intercourse (the excitement and plateau phases). Once at orgasmic levels, older women have the same potential for multiple orgasms as younger women (Shomaker, 1980).

Myth 3—Sexual Problems are due to Pulmonary Disease. On the contrary, most problems are due to the person's adaptation to pulmonary disease rather than the disease itself. The four most common problems or situations associated with sexual dysfunction are explained as follows:

1. Increasing dyspnea and fear of suffocation turn sexual activity into a nightmare experience, causing the patient to abstain completely, as previously described.
2. Aesthetically unpleasing pulmonary symptoms—wheezing, coughing, and sputum production—interrupt sexual activities, interfering with sexual arousal, orgasm, and satisfaction for both partners. Though pulmonary symptoms may be minor, the patient is unwilling to resume sexual activity for fear of uncontrollable dyspnea.
3. An altered body image causes the patient to develop excessive body preoccupation, sometimes leading to impotence or lack of sexual desire. Unaesthetic physical clinical manifestations of pulmonary disease cause the patient to feel unattractive. At least half of all single adults with cystic fibrosis see themselves as physically unattractive, due to their thin or short stature, clubbed fingers, or stained teeth (Coffman et al, 1984). Similarly, the emphysematous patient with a cachectic body and barrel chest may feel unattractive and unworthy of sexual attention. The patient may become depressed, irritable, and blame sexual dysfunction on his pulmonary disease, his spouse, or effects of aging.
4. Other psychologic problems cause the following sexual dysfunctions:
   a. Boredom or anger with sexual partner
   b. Preoccupation with career or work
   c. Mental or physical fatigue
   d. Overindulgence in food or drink
   e. Fear of failure, i.e., the most common cause of erectile problems (Davis, 1981).

A minority of pulmonary patients may have a physical reason for sexual dysfunction, though exact incidence is unknown because of sparse research on the topic. Some COPD patients claim sexual dysfunction, ranging from decreased libido to complete impotence, generally coinciding with the progression of advanced pulmonary signs and symptoms (Fletcher and Martin, 1982). At least some of this decline in sexual function may be related to hypoxemia. Petty (1986) states that correction of hypoxemia improves neurotransmitter and hormonal function, thus allowing otherwise impotent patients to become sexually active again. In other cases, sexual dysfunction is associated with an accompanying disease, such as diabetes, cerebrovascular disease, postmyocardial infarction, paraplegia, and multiple sclerosis. In cystic fibrosis, a disease associated with sexual dysfunction, a relatively small number of patients (5 out of 30 married patients in one study) have sexual problems directly from cystic fibrosis (Levine and Stern, 1982). The majority of adult cystic fibrosis patients have a reasonable chance for normal sexual functioning.

Myth 4—Sexual Problems are due to Pulmonary Medications. On the contrary, pulmonary medications—autonomic active agents, theophylline derivatives, and steroids—generally do not cause sexual dysfunction in pulmonary patients. Tremulousness, a side effect of autonomic active drugs, may interfere with erection. However, it may be avoided by appropriate medication adjustment.

The patient may be on other drugs that affect sexual functioning. For example, antidepressants, sedatives, and antihypertensives decrease libido in both sexes and interfere with potency in males.

Myth 5—Sexual Activity will Precipitate Respiratory Distress. On the contrary, shortness of breath during sexual intercourse is a natural response that can almost always be tolerated by patients with severe lung disease, provided they are on appropriate pulmonary medications. Sexual intercourse itself requires expenditure of few calories and is relatively unstressful. It is the associated anxiety and fear that precipitates respiratory distress. Documented evidence of death during sexual intercourse is rare (Petty and Nett, 1984).

Myth 6—Dyspneic Disabled Persons are Fragile and Need to be Protected. On the contrary, dyspneic disabled persons are not fragile. They can learn how to control their symptoms and lead relatively normal social and sexual lives.

In cystic fibrosis, families tend to overprotect female patients. Overprotectiveness impedes the young woman's sense of autonomy, self worth, and socialization as a sexual being. These patients have far more developmental sexual problems than physically healthy females the same age (Levine and Stern, 1982).

PATIENT INFORMATION

Guidelines for Sexual Activity

These guidelines will help you control pulmonary symptoms and maintain satisfying sexual relations.

1. Talk to your partner about your "likes" and "dislikes" in your sexual relationship. *Open communication is essential!*
   a. Explore factors that are associated with increasing pulmonary symptoms.
   b. Plan changes to overcome barriers to a satisfying sexual experience.
2. Plan sex at a time when pulmonary symptoms are minimal.
   a. Always 20 minutes after an aerosol bronchodilator.
   b. In the afternoon or anytime you are relatively free of symptoms.
3. Avoid sex when you are fatigued, during a chest infection, after a large meal, and after a large amount of alcohol ingestion.
4. Make sex a total body response.
   a. Use a slow deliberate approach to intercourse—*Do not rush!*
   b. Use relaxation techniques to reduce anxiety before sex (e.g., sauna, bath, glass of wine) or during sex (e.g., frequent rest periods).
   c. *Be flexible!* Try different body positions to reduce physical work. Examples of positions are shown. Note that the partner with breathing problems is tinted gray.
      1. Some couples prefer the side-by-side position. Others experiment with different sitting and standing positions.
      2. The partner with lung disease may conserve energy by using a secure stationary position, such as the supine. The other partner may be positioned superiorly and should be free to perform most of the body movement.
   d. Try a water bed to facilitate body movement with minimal energy expenditure.
   e. Develop a broad range of ways to express yourself, such as handholding, hugging, caressing, stroking, total body massage, oral-genital sex, or any other techniques pleasurable to both of you.
5. Use oxygen and breathing retraining techniques, described subsequently, to control shortness of breath during sex.
6. Avoid kissing when it interferes with your breathing.
7. Talk to your doctor if pulmonary symptoms continue to interrupt sexual activity. You may need a medication adjustment.

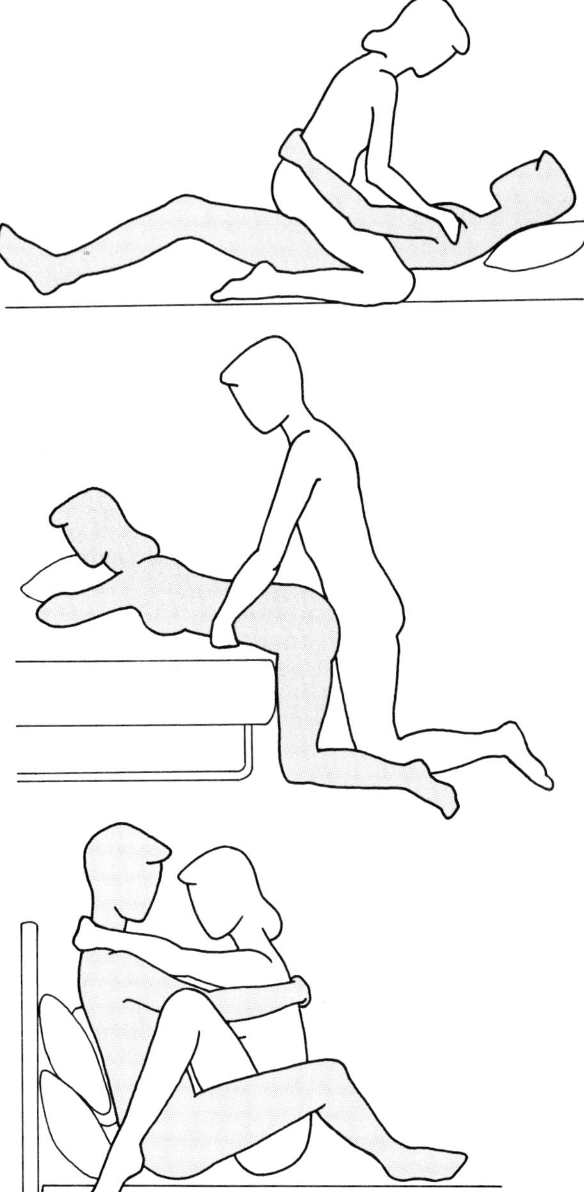

8. See a marriage counselor or psychologist if interpersonal relations interfere with your ability to have satisfying sex.

Myth 7—A Spontaneous and Active Role in Lovemaking is Essential. On the contrary, any type of mutually satisfying sexual behavior is acceptable. To adapt to lung disease, partners will need to communicate needs and experiment with new sexual patterns that emphasize planned rather than spontaneous sex and a passive rather than an active lovemaking role for the partner with lung disease.

Guidelines for Sexual Activity

While discrediting myths about sex and pulmonary disease, the nurse shares the guidelines on page 522 with interested patients.

The nurse may use a variety of ways to communicate sexual guidelines, such as individual conferences, pamphlets, audiovisual materials (Kravetz, et al, 1981) and discussions with other disabled persons and their sexual partners. While most patients with adequate sex education will understand and appreciate advice offered, younger patients or those with limited sex education may need an explanation of normal anatomy and physiology before other information is provided. Patients with a longstanding sexual dysfunction are referred to a specially trained therapist for treatment.

Conclusion

This chapter provides an overview of pulmonary rehabilitation. In addition, it introduces basic self-care educational content, including understanding the respiratory system and lung disease, preventive measures, and sexual adaptation to lung disease.

Emphasis must be placed on the applicability of self-care content to respiratory nursing care in both acute and chronic settings. For example, though smoking produces emphysema, a chronic lung disease, counseling on smoking cessation is best initiated in the acute rather than chronic setting, immediately after recovery from acute ventilatory failure. Counseling may have little influence on the relatively asymptomatic patient at home. Though dyspnea control during sexual activity may not be a concern in the hospital, providing the patient and significant other with the opportunity to discuss the topic before discharge may allay anxiety and eliminate fear of suffocation or heart attack during sexual activity at home.

REFERENCES

American College of Chest Physicians—Committee on Pulmonary Rehabilitation. Statement at the annual Scientific Assembly, 1974.

American Hospital Association: A Patient's Bill of Rights. Chicago, American Hospital Association, 1972.

American Hospital Association: Staff Manual for Teaching Patients about COPD. Chicago, American Hospital Association, 1982.

American Lung Association—American Thoracic Society: Report on Comprehensive Care for Patients with Chronic Lung Disease, 1975.

American Thoracic Society: Pulmonary rehabilitation. *American review of respiratory disease*, 124(5):663–666, 1981.

American Thoracic Society: Skills of the health team involved in out-of-hospital care for patients with COPD. *American review of respiratory disease*, 133(5):948–949, 1986.

American Thoracic Society: Standards for the diagnosis and care of patients with chronic obstructive pulmonary disease (COPD) and asthma. *American review of respiratory disease*, 136(1):225–244, 1987.

Bell, C., et al: Home Care and Rehabilitation in Respiratory Medicine. Philadelphia, J.B. Lippincott Co., 1984.

Brashear, R.: Pressurized aerosol bronchodilator instruction. *Chest*, 84(1):117, 1983.

Braun, S., et al: A decentralized rehabilitation program for chronic airway obstruction disease patients in small urban and rural areas of Wisconsin: a preliminary report. *Public health reports*, 96(4):315–318, 1981.

Braun, S., Dixon, R., and Anderegg, A.: The prevalence and determinants of nutritional changes in COPD. *Chest*, 86(4):558–563, 1984.

California Thoracic Society: CTS Guidelines for Pulmonary Rehabilitation. *Statement of the respiratory care assembly*, May 11, 1979.

Coffman, C., et al: Sexual adaptation among single young adults with cystic fibrosis. *Chest*, 86(3):412–418, 1984.

Cooper, D.: Sexual counseling of the patient with chronic lung disease. *Focus on critical care*, 13(3):18–20, 1986.

Davis, K.: Sexual counseling for the patient with chronic lung disease. *Sexual medicine today*, 5:10–15, 1981.

Dolovich, M., Ruffin, R., Roberts, R., and Newhouse, M.: Optimal delivery of aerosols from metered dose inhalers. *Chest*, 80(6):911–915, 1981.

Epstein, S.: A comparison of three means of pressurized aerosol inhaler use. *American review of respiratory disease*, 128(2):253–255, 1983.

Fischer, D. A.: Patient Selection Criteria for Pulmonary Rehabilitation Programs. Downey, California, Rancho Los Amigos Hospital (unpublished).

Fischer, E., Bishop, D., et al: Implications for the practicing physician of the psychosocial dimensions of smoking. *Chest*, 93(2):69S–78S, 1988.

Fisons Corporation: Instructions for Use of the Spinhaler Turbo-inhaler. Bedford, Massachusetts, Fisons Corporation, 1978.

Fletcher, C. and Peto, R.: The natural history of chronic airflow obstruction. *British medical journal*, 1(6077):1645–1648, 1977.

Fletcher, E. and Martin, R.: Sexual dysfunction and erectile impotence in COPD. *Chest*, 81(4):413–421, 1982.

Haas, A., et al: Sexual aspects of the COPD patient. In Pulmonary Therapy and Rehabilitation: Principles and Practice. Baltimore, Williams & Wilkins, 1979.

Hall, R., et al: Two-year efficacy and safety of rapid smoking therapy in patients with cardiac and pulmonary disease. *Journal of consulting and clinical psychology*, 52(4):574–581, 1984.

Hanson, E.: Effects of chronic lung disease on life in general and on sexuality: perceptions of adult patients. *Heart and lung*, 11(5):435–441, 1982.

Hodgkin, J., Zorn, E., and Connors, G.: Pulmonary Rehabilitation—Guidelines to Success. Boston, Butterworth Publishers, 1984.

Hogan, R.: Human Sexuality—A Nursing Perspective, 2nd ed. Norwalk, Connecticut, Appleton-Century-Crofts, 1985.

Hudson, L.: Management of COPD—state of the art. *Chest*, 84(6):76S–81S, 1984.

Inter-Society Commission For Heart Disease Resources: Report on community resources for rehabilitation of patients with COPD and cor pulmonale. *Circulation*, 49(5):A–1, 1974.

Johnson, N. R., et al: Inpatient comprehensive pulmonary rehabilitation in severe COLD: Barlow Hospital study. *Respiratory therapy*, 10(3):15–19, 1980.

Kravetz, H., Weiss, L., and Meadows, R.: "A Visit with Harry" (Slide and Tape Presentation). Phoenix, Arizona, Howard M. Kravetz, 1981.

Kravetz, H., Garland, A., and Harner, D.: "A Visit with Helen" (Slide and Tape Presentation). Phoenix, Arizona, Howard M. Kravetz, 1982.

Levine, S. and Stern, R.: Sexual function in cystic fibrosis. *Chest*, 81(4):422–428, 1982.

McDonald, G.: A home care program for patients with chronic lung disease. *Nursing clinics of north america*, 16(2):259–273, 1981.

McDonald, G. and Hudson, L.: Important aspects of pulmonary rehabilitation. *Geriatrics*, 37(3):127–134, 1982.

Mensch, A. and Holden, M.: Nicotine overdose after a single piece of nicotine gum. *Chest*, 86(5):801–802, 1984.

Merrell Dow Pharmaceuticals: *Nicorette (Nicotine Resin Complex)*. Cincinnati, Merrell Dow Pharmaceuticals, Inc., 1984.

Moser, K.: Rehabilitation for COPD patients: Why, who, when, what, and how? *The journal of respiratory diseases*, 2(10):42–55, 1980.

Moser, K., et al: Results of a comprehensive rehabilitation program—physiologic and functional effects on patients with COPD. *Archives of internal medicine*, 140(12):1596–1601, 1980.

Mullin, V.: Implementing the self-care concept in the acute care setting. *Nursing clinics of north america*, 154(1):177–190, 1980.

Newman, S.: Factors influencing the efficacy of inhaled bronchodilators. *Respiratory therapy*, 13(4):37–45, 1983.

Newman, S., et al: Deposition of pressurized suspension aerosols inhaled through extension devices. *American review of respiratory disease*, 124(3):317–320, 1981.

O'Ryan, J. and Burns, D.: Pulmonary Rehabilitation: From Hospital to Home. Chicago, Year Book Medical Publishers, Inc., 1984.

Petty, T.: Pulmonary rehabilitation. *Respiratory care*, 22(1):68–79, 1977.

Petty, T.: Comprehensive care of COPD. *Clinical notes on respiratory diseases*, 20(3):3–12, 1981.

Petty, T.: Chronic Obstructive Pulmonary Disease, 2nd ed. New York, Marcel Dekker, Inc., 1985.

Petty, T.: Health, sex, and better quality of life for your COPD patient. *Medical aspects of human sexuality*, 20(8):70–85, 1986.

Petty, T. and Nett, L.: Enjoying Life with Emphysema. Philadelphia, Lea & Febiger, 1984. (For patients.)

Prochaska, J., et al: Self-change processes, self-efficacy and self-concept in relapse and maintenance of cessation of smoking. *Psychological reports*, 51(3):983–990, 1982.

Sachs, D.: Assisting the patient in smoking cessation: a clinical science. *Clinical challenge in cardiopulmonary medicine*, 1(6):1–8:1–7, 1985.

Salzman, G.: Spacer devices for aerosol therapy. *Clinical challenge in cardiopulmonary medicine*, 3(6):(entire issue), 1986.

Shenkman, B.: Factors contributing to attrition rates in a pulmonary rehabilitation program. *Heart and lung*, 14(1):53–58, 1985.

Shomaker, D.: Integration of physiological and sociocultural factors as a basis for sex education to the elderly. *Journal of gerontological nursing*, 6(6):311–318, 1980.

Splitter, S.: Non-smokers (involuntary smokers): the silent majority. *Heart briefs*, Winter: 4–6, 1976.

Tibbals, S.: Symposium on Sexual Counseling in the Patient with Chronic Lung Disease. American Thoracic Society, Section on Nursing, Annual Meeting, 1982.

Tobin, M., et al: Response to bronchodilator drug administration by a new reservoir aerosol delivery system and a review of other auxiliary delivery systems. *American review of respiratory disease*, 126(4):670–675, 1982.

19

Chest Physiotherapy

Main Objectives

1. **Define the following terms: sustained maximal inspiration, manual cough, glossopharyngeal breathing, forced exhalation technique or huffing, and lower costal breathing.**
2. **Describe indications for use: list at least two evaluation criteria for correct technique, overall improvement in condition, or both, and describe**

implementation in the clinical setting for the following techniques:
- **a. General relaxation**
- **b. Deep breathing**
- **c. Controlled coughing**
- **d. Pursed-lip breathing at rest and while walking**
- **e. Diaphragmatic breathing**
- **f. Postural drainage**
- **g. Chest percussion**
- **h. Chest vibration**

3. **Discuss deep breathing and coughing in acute and chronic settings, with attention to optimal technique, physiologic goals, the role of respiratory devices for hyperinflation, and alternatives to standard technique.**
4. **Describe how to teach the patient to use an incentive spirometer to obtain a sustained maximum inspiration.**
5. **Explain the physiologic reason why experts discourage the use of devices such as the blow bottles and the blow glove in respiratory care.**
6. **Explain the physiologic reason why some patients with severe COPD never master diaphragmatic breathing.**
7. **Describe how to help the asthmatic control acute dyspnea.**
8. **Discuss alternatives to manual chest percussion and vibration.**
9. **Name six complications of postural drainage with percussion and vibration.**
10. **Name and explain optimal lateral positioning for a patient with a unilateral chest infiltrate observed on the chest x-ray.**

This chapter presents chest physiotherapy, a form of respiratory intervention that traditionally includes breathing exercises, controlled coughing, forced expiration techniques, postural drainage, percussion, and vibration. Discussion extends beyond these basic techniques to include various associated interventions, such as general relaxation and incentive spirometry, because the effectiveness of chest physiotherapy largely depends on the proper integration of related techniques towards the goals of optimal bronchial hygiene and normal mechanics of breathing.

General Relaxation

GOALS

1. To decrease sympathetic nervous system stimulation and signs of stress
2. To promote general muscle relaxation, bronchodilatation, and alveolar ventilation
3. To increase the effectiveness of chest physiotherapy techniques

INDICATIONS

1. Moderate to severe chronic pulmonary disease
2. Physical or emotional stress
3. Postsurgical incisional pain

Chest physiotherapy is more effective when the patient is relaxed and ready to learn a new technique. Some patients are unaware of the need for relaxation until the nurse massages tense shoulder muscles or guides the patient through a simple relaxation exercise, such as the following.

PATIENT INFORMATION

General Relaxation

Make it a point to rest and relax your mind and body a few times each day. Relaxing regularly relieves muscle tightness and mental and physical discomfort. In this way, it promotes easier breathing.

To Completely Relax

1. In a quiet environment, sit down in a comfortable chair or lie down on a comforrtable cot or bed.
2. Rest your head against the back of the chair and close your eyes.
3. Relax your mind by assuming a passive attitude; do not think about anything.
4. Let your shoulders and arms become limp.
5. Relax the rest of your body and use quiet, easy pursed-lip breathing (PLB).
6. As you breathe out, feel the tenseness in your shoulders, chest, and rest of your body disappear.
7. Maintain this relaxed state for 10 to 15 minutes or until your tenseness disappears.

When Relaxing Your Mind is Difficult

1. Try focusing mental energy on a single word or phrase, such as "breathe in and relax out" or "p-e-a-c-e."
2. Imagine yourself in a peaceful location—walking on a deserted beach or sailing on a quiet lake.
3. Listen to soft music or use another distraction to promote relaxation.

To Promote Relaxation Throughout the Day

1. Use good posture at all times to ease the strain on your body.
2. Wear comfortable clothes.
3. When sitting, choose a straight-backed chair for more support. You may wish to roll up a small towel and place it in the small of the back for added support.
4. Stretch your arms, legs, and back frequently during the day.
5. Have a friend or relative give you a neck, upper back, and shoulder massage.
6. Avoid emotional stress. Try to work out your personal problems in the least stressful way. Stress causes more muscle tension and will aggravate your breathing problem.

PRACTICE SCHEDULE

Once or twice a day at home or at work.

EVALUATION CRITERIA

For Correct Technique

1. Good body alignment (i.e., no slumping)
2. Relaxed facial muscles
3. Shoulders completely dropped and relaxed
4. Quiet controlled breathing

For Overall Improvement in Condition

1. Decrease in signs of stress, e.g., nervous gestures, tense or rigid posture, irregular breathing, increased heart rate and respirations, diaphoresis, headaches, indigestion, emotional lability, and so forth.

2. Decrease in number of dyspneic or wheezing episodes.

IMPLEMENTATION

With this general exercise, relaxation of the shoulder muscles is most difficult for the patient with chronic obstructive pulmonary disease (COPD). Obstructive disease, notably emphysema, produces abnormal mechanics of breathing manifested by en bloc movement of the chest during respiration, as previously described in Chapter 12. Another person, such as the nurse, friend, or spouse, may have to gently press down on the patient's shoulders during expiration. Gentle pressure prompts the patient to relax the shoulders and chest and to expire more completely to minimize air trapping in the lungs.

General relaxation with pursed-lip breathing may promote sufficient relaxation for the patient. However, when muscle tension is severe, implementation of a few arm exercises may be necessary before full chest relaxation is achieved.

Patients with restrictive disease may use the previously described relaxation exercise, but pursed-lip breathing is not essential.

Other Relaxation Techniques

General relaxation may be supplemented by other techniques, including guided imagery, hypnosis (Ben-Zvi et al, 1982), relaxation response (Benson and Klipper, 1976), progressive muscle relaxation, yoga exercises, transcendental meditation (Blodgett, 1984), and biofeedback training (Holliday, 1984).

Of these methods, progressive muscle relaxation is commonly used for pulmonary patients. One method involves placing the supine patient in a quiet, semidark room. The patient is instructed to systematically tense and relax specific muscle groups, starting with the arms and working down the body as follows: head and neck, shoulders, back, chest, abdomen, legs, and feet. After the patient masters tension release, he is instructed to relax without first tensing his muscles (Walsh, 1986). After successful relaxation with supervision, the patient is given a cassette tape of training sessions to practice on his own. He is instructed to practice two to three times weekly and as needed to assist with sleeping, stress reduction, and panic control.

Though most progressive relaxation protocols are satisfactory for most pulmonary patients, staff may need to make adaptations for severely disabled individuals. For example, when patients are more dyspneic and uncomfortable in the supine position, they may relax better in a semireclined or sitting position (Fig. 19–1). When muscle tensing reinforces accessory respiratory muscle use in severely dyspneic patients, staff may focus on relaxation without initial muscle tensing.

General relaxation and similar techniques represent one way to help the pulmonary patient cope with the often phenomenal amounts of muscle tension he experiences in association with anxiety, stress, and abnormal mechanics of breathing. Physical therapy techniques help the patient adapt to abnormal mechanics of breathing. They are marginally effective, however, unless the patient learns to cope with anxiety and stress, the psychologic factors that contribute to the

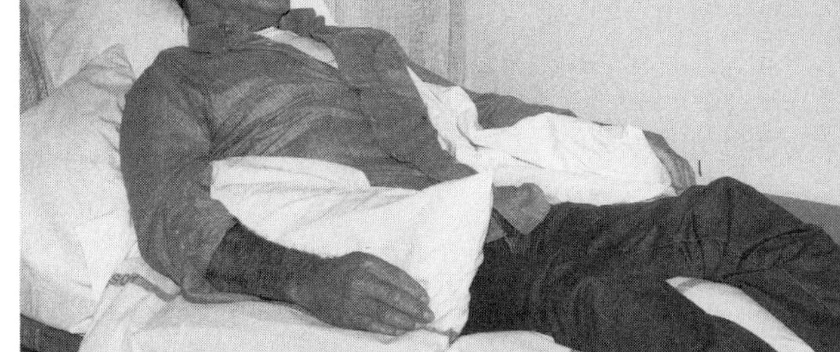

Figure 19–1. General relaxation in a semireclined position for the dyspneic respiratory patient.

muscle tension. The nursing interventions in Chapter 16 serve as a guideline for anxiety and stress reduction in the pulmonary patient. They may be supplemented by assertiveness training. The assertive patient is one who knows what he wants and makes it clear to others in an open, direct, and nonthreatening way. To reduce dyspneic episodes and the need for general relaxation, the assertive patient may, for example, ask a friend not to smoke or not to wear a certain perfume.

Because of the integral relationship between general relaxation and stress reduction, the nurse should focus more on psychosocial intervention, assertiveness training, and decision-making processes that affect coping behavior whenever general relaxation techniques do not work.

Deep Breathing—Foundation for Learning Breathing Retraining

Though deep breathing is presented before the section on breathing retraining, it is not typically considered a breathing retraining technique. Rather, it is a bronchial hygiene technique most commonly associated with coughing and the treatment and prevention of mucus retention problems. Moreover, as a bronchial hygiene technique, deep breathing emphasizes the inspiratory phase of respiration and lung inflation. In contrast, breathing retraining in COPD typically emphasizes the expiratory phase and the reduction of expiratory air trapping in the lungs.

Nevertheless, certain aspects of deep breathing, such as relaxation and the reduction in respiratory rate, apply to pursed-lip breathing and other breathing retraining techniques. In some cases, when the patient cannot perform breathing retraining techniques, owing to a lack of mental concentration or other problems, deep breathing with more emphasis on expiration may be a viable substitute. Also, it may be easier for the nurse to teach a breathing retraining technique in relation to deep breathing, a technique most patients are already familiar with.

For all of these reasons, the nurse is encouraged to keep in mind the basic deep breathing techniques, which involve the three following steps: (1) taking a slow deep breath in, (2) pausing slightly, and (3) breathing out in a relaxed manner. Technique details are thoroughly discussed in subsequent sections of this chapter.

Breathing Retraining

Breathing retraining for individuals with chronic disease begins after establishment of a program of bronchial hygiene and stabilization of acute chest disease. However, some of the techniques, such as diaphragmatic breathing, are also taught to postoperative patients and other acutely ill patients who are alert and able to cooperate.

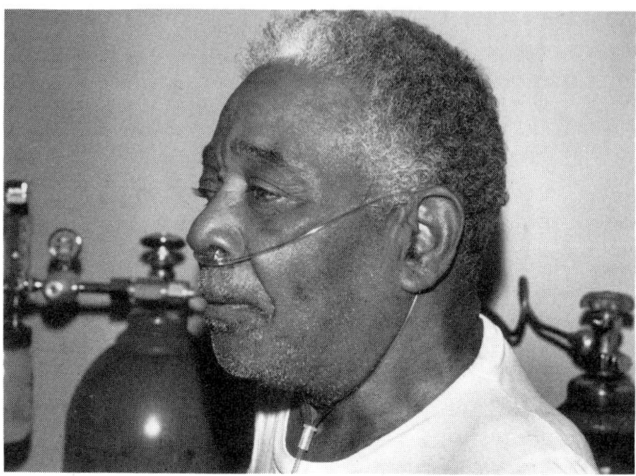

Figure 19–2. Pursed-lip breathing with supplementary oxygen and full dentures in place. Without dentures, this individual was unable to properly purse the lips for control of dyspnea.

GOALS

1. To improve alveolar ventilation and oxygenation
2. To increase strength, coordination, and efficiency of respiratory muscles
3. To mobilize or maintain mobility of the chest wall
4. To promote a relaxed and controlled breathing pattern at rest and during exercise
5. To decrease the work of breathing
6. To promote general well being

PURSED-LIP BREATHING

Indications

1. Chronic obstructive disease
2. Dyspnea

PLB is taught to help the patient control acute dyspnea as well as exertional dyspnea associated with moderate to severe chronic pulmonary disease. If the patient wears dentures, they must be in place to provide adequate support for the pursing of the lips (Fig. 19–2).

As a guideline, when the nurse initiates breathing retraining with the COPD patient, teaching begins with PLB, with reference to deep breathing (described previously) only as needed to clarify technique.

PATIENT INFORMATION

Breathing Retraining

Breathing retraining is necessary to retrain your respiratory muscles and to establish a new breathing pattern that is less tiring and more efficient.

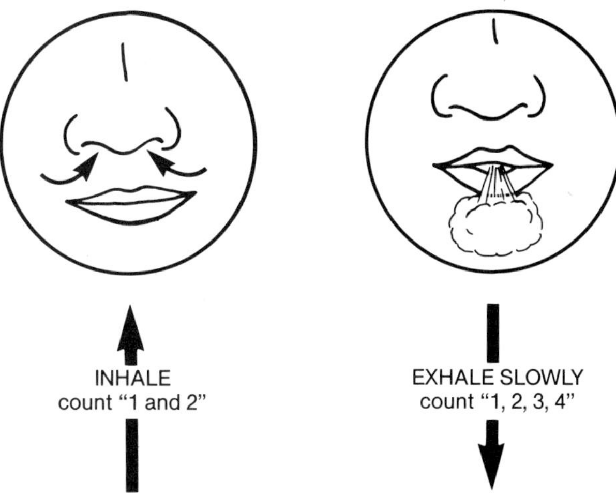

Pursed-Lip Breathing

Pursed-lip breathing will help you to do the following:

1. Slow your respiratory rate.
2. Increase the amount of air moving in and out of your lungs with each breath.
3. Keep your smaller airways open when you breathe out.
4. Control your shortness of breath.

To Pursed-Lip Breathe

1. Take a normal-sized breath in through your nose, as illustrated above.
2. Breathe out *slowly* through pursed lips. Make breathing out at least twice as long as breathing in.

Occasionally, hold your hand up to your mouth and feel the air you are blowing out through your pursed lips. The air flow should be constant and even throughout expiration. If you are breathing out through pursed lips in this slow, relaxed manner, the back pressure in your lungs will help keep your airways open. You will be able to empty the lungs more completely and take in more fresh air with each breath. With practice you can make pursed-lip breathing your natural breathing pattern, control your shortness of breath, and reduce muscle fatigue.

Practice Schedule

Once or twice a day with general relaxation.

Evaluation Criteria

For Correct Technique

1. Decrease in respiratory rate to 8 to 16 per minute. Symptomatic relief appears to be related to the slowed respiratory rate and increases in V_T that pursed lip-breathing achieves (Mueller et al, 1970).
2. A *normal* inspiration through the nose. COPD patients tend to exaggerate inspiration, using accessory muscles of respiration rather than concentrating on exhalation.
3. A relaxed, prolonged expiration through pursed lips. Use of pursed lips causes a rise in intra-airway pressure. The back pressure keeps airways open during expiration, thus preventing airway collapse and air trapping in the lungs.
   a. Expiration (E) is at least twice as long as inspiration (I) (I:E ratio of 1:2).
   b. Expiration is not strained in any way. The patient should not force air out through pursed lips.
   c. A constant, even air flow throughout most of expiration. Hold your hand a few inches from the patient's mouth and feel for this air flow.
4. Lack of frequent sighs, fatigue, or discomfort during breathing. When these signs of improper technique occur, the patient may not be pursed-lip breathing enough air out in a relaxed manner; or he may be breathing too much air out, collapsing airways and increasing the work of breathing. Work on relaxation and adjustment of pursed lips to achieve proper air flow and the right length of expiration.
5. At least a 3 to 4% increase in Sa_{O_2} above the Sa_{O_2} achieved without use of PLB (Tiep et al, 1986). Use portable ear or finger oximetry (described in Chapter 23) for noninvasive measurement of Sa_{O_2} with and without PLB. Help the patient adjust his technique to achieve the highest possible Sa_{O_2}.

For Overall Improvement in Condition

1. Patient states that the breathing pattern feels comfortable and that it helps to control dyspnea.
2. Improvement in level of perceived dyspnea as measured by the Borg scale (see Chapter 10).
3. At least a 3 to 4% increase in Sa_{O_2}.

Implementation

Two facts guide the nurse in implementing PLB in the clinical setting. First, breathing exercises do not alter the course of respiratory disease, although many patients claim significant subjective relief from PLB or other breathing techniques. Second, some patients receive symptomatic benefit from PLB, and others do not. One research study found PLB increases Pa_{O_2} and decreases Pa_{CO_2} at rest but not during exercise. This finding was true for persons receiving symptomatic relief from PLB as well as for those without symptomatic relief. Relief was not associated with improvement in arterial blood gases (ABGs) (Mueller et al, 1970).

More recent research verifies that many patients improve Sa_{O_2} by at least 3 to 4% by use of PLB (Tiep et al, 1986). The mechanism responsible for the improvement is incompletely understood. In COPD it is not always related to increased intra-airway pressure preventing airway collapse during expiration, as originally thought. The mechanism may be related to the slowing of early expiratory flow rates during PLB. Slow flow rates reduce the pressure drop across small airways, which in turn prevents airway collapse due to Bernouilli's effect.

Moreover, in the majority of patients, improvement in Sa_{O_2} may relate more to the decrease in respiratory rate and increase in tidal volume associated with the

PLB technique. Patients are able to expire more CO_2-rich gas with each breath. Minute ventilation stays the same. Also, oxygen demand is less because a lower respiratory rate decreases airway resistance, dead space ventilation, and work of breathing. This explanation is the theoretic basis for dyspneic patients trying PLB, even though the primary diagnosis may be a restrictive lung disease.

Since PLB training methods vary and may affect the level of improvement in Sao_2, clinicians may use oximetry to monitor Sao_2 at rest and during exercise. If Sao_2 remains the same or decreases, the nurse coaches the patient to alter his technique—breathe out more steadily, purse the lips more to prolong expiration, or whatever else is necessary to improve Sao_2. If Sao_2 increases, the nurse coaches the patient to continue his technique. In this way, oximetry serves as a biofeedback device for teaching the patient PLB or similar forms of breathing retraining.

Because of conflicting research on the benefit of PLB, the most practical approach to the patient is to divide teaching into small steps, constantly monitor symptomatic improvement, and whenever possible monitor Sao_2 as the most reliable objective sign of benefit.

The following are the progressive steps for the teaching-learning situation:

1. Teach PLB while the patient is at rest (Fig. 19–3).
2. Teach PLB while the patient is walking, as described in Patient Information.
3. Teach PLB while the patient is stair climbing and during activities of daily living.

For panic control during acute dyspnea, PLB is described subsequently. The nurse discontinues therapy if the patient demonstrates lack of improvement in level of dyspnea and oxygen saturation.

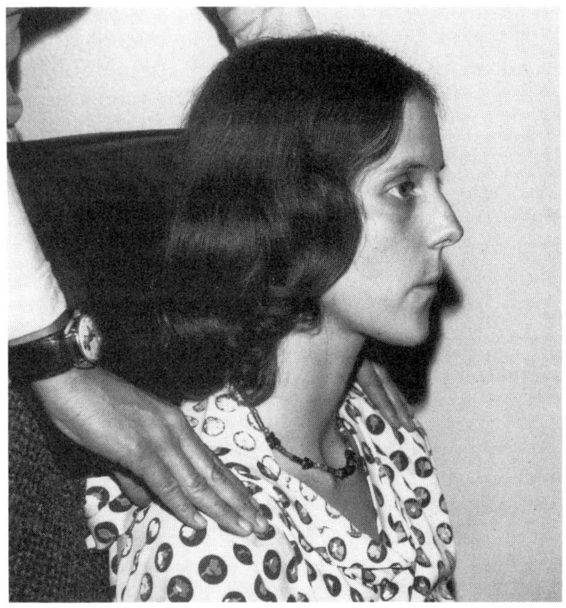

Figure 19–3. Pursed-lip breathing at rest. Gentle pressure on the shoulders prompts the patient to relax the shoulders and expire completely.

PATIENT INFORMATION

Pursed-Lip Breathing While Walking

Your best position for walking is slightly bent forward with your shoulders relaxed and your arms hanging loosely at your sides.

1. Breathe in through your nose at rest or while you are pausing.
2. Slowly blow out through pursed lips as you walk one or two steps.
3. Repeat. Always take *at least* twice as many steps with breathing out as you took with breathing in. For example, with faster walking, take two steps as you breathe in and four to six steps as you breathe out.

Tips

1. Always breathe slowly and concentrate on pursed-lip breathing all your air out.
2. TAKE YOUR TIME. A little shortness of breath every now and then will not hurt you; it increases your exercise ability. But *never overdo it!* To reduce shortness of breath, walk with a slow but steady pace, slow enough so that you reach your destination without having to stop and rest. Stopping and starting are tiring. Start with short walks and set goals for yourself to increase your walking distance.
3. If you do become short of breath, stop and rest.

Walking Up or Down Stairs

Keep the previous walking tips in mind as you walk up or down stairs.

Walking Downstairs

1. *Pause* on the top level and *breathe in* through your nose.
2. *Walk* down one or two stairs as you pursed-lip *breathe out*. Hold onto the handrail.
3. Repeat. Always walk down at least twice as many steps while breathing out as you walked down while breathing in. Walk downhill or down an incline in the same way.

Walking Upstairs

1. *Pause* and *breathe in* through your nose.
2. As you pursed-lip breathe out, step up one or two stairs. Hold onto the handrail and place your whole foot *flat* on each stair as you climb.
3. Repeat. Practice this technique while climbing one flight of stairs.

Tips

1. Think in ratios. Use 1:2 for a slow walking pace and 2:4 for a faster pace.

   1:2 = *1 stair* (while breathing in) to *2 stairs* (while breathing out).

   2:4 = *2 stairs* (while breathing in) to *4 stairs* (while breathing out).
2. Especially if stairs are difficult for you, always pause slightly while breathing in. The pause slows your pace and helps you conserve energy. Later, you may not need to pause.
3. If necessary, stop briefly to rest.

Evaluation Criteria

For Correct Technique

1. Correct body position: patient bent forward

slightly, shoulders relaxed, and arms hanging loosely at sides.

2. Slow but steady pace while walking.
3. I:E ratio of 1:2.
4. Coordinated breathing pattern during stair climbing; the patient exhales while stepping up or down. Initially, the patient may need to start exhalation a little ahead of time (e.g., just before stepping up) to learn proper coordination.
5. Absence of adverse signs and symptoms: obstructed breathing pattern, excessive rest stops, excessive fatigue lasting 1 to 2 hours after exercise, gasping respirations, chest pain, dizziness or nausea, marked tachycardia (over 120 beats per minute) or irregular pulse, signs of hypoxemia.
6. At least a 3 to 4% increase in Sa_{O_2}.

DIAPHRAGMATIC BREATHING

Indications

1. Chronic obstructive disease
2. Postoperative chest
3. Impaired ventilation of nasal lung segments
4. Dyspnea
5. Augmentation of deep breathing maneuvers

PATIENT INFORMATION

Diaphragmatic Breathing With Pursed Lips

The two major muscle groups used in normal breathing are the diaphragm and the rib muscles. Because of a weakened diaphragm, patients with lung problems usually develop a breathing pattern using the neck, shoulder, and rib muscles, i.e., the upper chest. Diaphragmatic breathing will correct this habit and strengthen the diaphragm as well as the abdominal muscles that help it move. More air will move in and out of the lungs without tiring the chest muscles.

When used with pursed-lip breathing and practiced regularly with a few simple breathing exercises, diaphragmatic breathing will increase your exercise tolerance and help you feel better.

Preparation

1. Lie with your knees bent or sit up with your head and back supported.
2. Place your hand on your abdomen.
3. *Relax.*

Procedure

1. Breathe *in* through your nose and gently push your abdomen or belly *out,* as shown in the illustration (top, right). With your belly out, the diaphragm can drop down further to make more room in the lungs for air.
2. Gently push *inward and upward* with your hand as you slowly pursed-lip breathe your air *out.* Breathing out in this manner will empty your lungs more completely.
3. Repeat. Practice this technique in sitting and standing positions.

Tips

1. Remove your hand from your belly. Try placing a small book on the belly for visual reinforcement of correct belly movement during breathing.

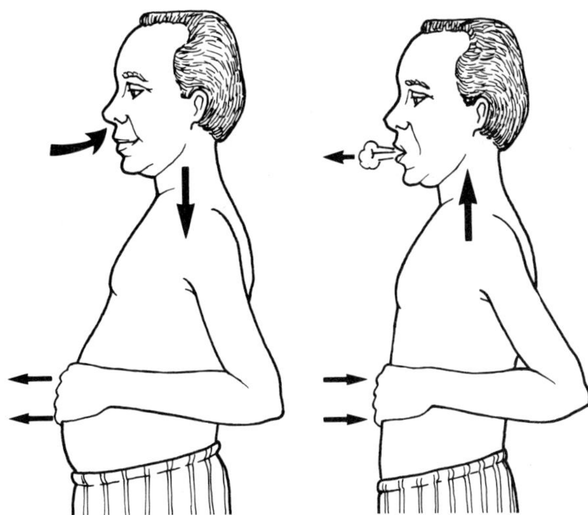

2. As you improve your coordination, concentrate on relaxation and *letting* your belly go out or rise as you breathe in.
3. Remember to breathe slowly.
4. Keep your upper chest and shoulders still while your diaphragm and abdominal (belly) muscles do the work. Do not strain. If necessary, place a hand on your upper chest to be sure it is still or moving very little.

Remember this pattern:

Belly goes out as you *breathe in*

Belly goes in as you *breathe out*

Lower Costal Breathing

After you have mastered diaphragmatic breathing, move your hand from your abdomen up to your lower ribs. Now, upon inspiration your lower ribs as well as your waist and upper belly will swell as your diaphragm drops down. You will get even better lower chest expansion with this modification. Try this lower costal (rib) breathing while sitting, standing, and walking.

Practice Schedule

1. During deep breathing and coughing, relaxation with pursed lips.
2. During aerosol or intermittent positive pressure breathing (IPPB) treatments; a side benefit is the promotion of aerosol deposition to more peripheral areas of the lungs.

Evaluation Criteria

For Correct Technique

1. Proper body alignment with head of bed at 30 to 45 degrees. A semireclined position promotes maximal diaphragmatic excursions and relaxation.
2. An active but gentle push (rise) of the belly or abdomen *out* on inspiration. Until a pattern is estab-

lished, the patient must concentrate and think about "spot" breathing with the belly.

3. Inward and upward movement of the abdomen on exhalation. Until the diaphragm is strengthened, which takes weeks of practice, and to avoid a strained exhalation, the patient or nurse should use one or two hands to slowly push the abdomen upward and inward. Muscle strengthening occurs owing to improved muscle contractility and endurance (Sharp, 1985).

4. Relaxed shoulders and upper chest with little to no movement during respiration. Overuse of the upper chest is a common problem. Instruct the patient or significant other to place a hand on the shoulder or upper chest to make the patient aware of excessive movement.

5. I:E ratio of 1:2 or more.

6. Absence of abdominal "bloating" or back hyperextension; these serve to push the abdomen out but do not increase diaphragmatic excursion.

7. Absence of frequent sighs, fatigue, or discomfort during breathing.

Implementation

Diaphragmatic breathing is a normal breathing pattern. Nevertheless, many healthy and disabled persons are unable to coordinate appropriate chest and abdominal movements with respiration in spite of continuous encouragement from concerned staff. Moreover, some patients with severe hyperinflation, neuromuscular dysfunction, and excessive fatigue will never learn the technique because of limiting mechanics of breathing or neurologic functioning or low motivation. Others who might benefit from diaphragmatic breathing are reluctant to spend additional time and energy learning it when they already receive significant relief of dyspnea from PLB alone. For these reasons, introduction of diaphragmatic breathing requires optimal learning conditions.

Optimal Learning Conditions. Correction of dehydration and fluid-electrolyte imbalances will facilitate muscle coordination. Initial concentration on general relaxation and various reconditioning exercises, such as arm exercises or inspiratory muscle training (see Chapter 20) may save time in the long run because the resultant muscle reconditioning facilitates upper chest stabilization and smooth coordination of diaphragmatic movement.

If the patient is already taking aerosol, IPPB, or incentive spirometry treatments, staff can help the patient perfect relaxation of the upper chest and shoulder muscles during these treatments before concentrating on correct chest and abdominal movements.

IPPB is a particularly useful learning tool, though the clinician's chance to practice it is becoming limited to selected acute situations. Aerosol treatment with a compressed gas source is now preferred over IPPB for aerosol delivery. With IPPB, the patient can concentrate on relaxation and chest and abdominal movements, since he only has to trigger inspiration to receive a relatively large inspired volume. Comparison of the diaphragmatic breath with the patient's normal breath is facilitated. The patient can actually feel extra air ventilate lung bases during the diaphragmatic breath. Convinced of the benefit of the new breathing pattern, he becomes motivated to perfect the technique for home use.

Initially, the patient may have to sacrifice some relaxation to learn how to coordinate respiratory movements at rest and with activity. Ultimately, however, *diaphragmatic breathing should feel comfortable to the patient.* If the previous evaluation criteria are not met after several practice sessions, discontinue therapy and try again at a later date when the patient demonstrates more physiologic or psychologic readiness to learn. If most of the evaluation criteria are met, instruct the patient to practice the technique during the following increasingly difficult activities: sitting upright in a chair or on the edge of the bed; standing; walking; and, finally, climbing stairs. This sequential approach is essential for success.

"Belly" Versus Lower Costal Breathing. Note in the previous patient information section that diaphragmatic breathing is first performed with the hand on the upper abdomen. Hence, it is frequently referred to as *abdominal*-diaphragmatic breathing. Once the technique is mastered, the hand is moved up to the costophrenic angle and edge of the lower ribs (Fig. 19–4). Spot breathing from this location enhances lower chest expansion.

This lower costal breathing is most appropriate for patients *without* severe lung hyperinflation. To understand this point and summarize the rationale for use of other breathing retraining techniques in COPD, consider the effects of severe lung inflation on mechanics of breathing and breathing pattern, summarized in Figure 19–5.

Lung hyperinflation puts the COPD patient at a

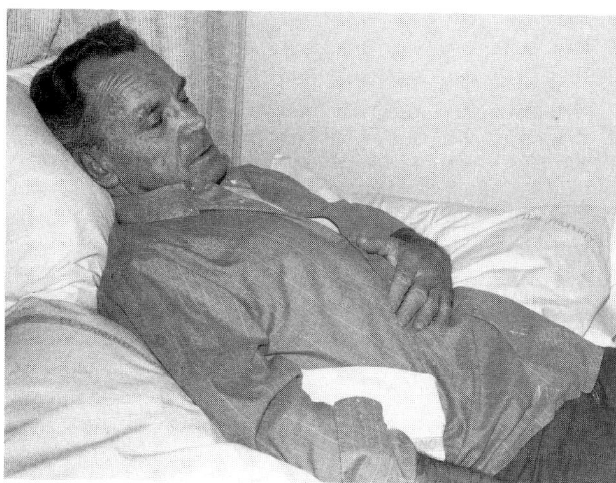

Figure 19–4. The patient practices diaphragmatic breathing during general relaxation. The hand is placed over the costophrenic angle and lower ribs for the lower costal type of diaphragmatic breathing.

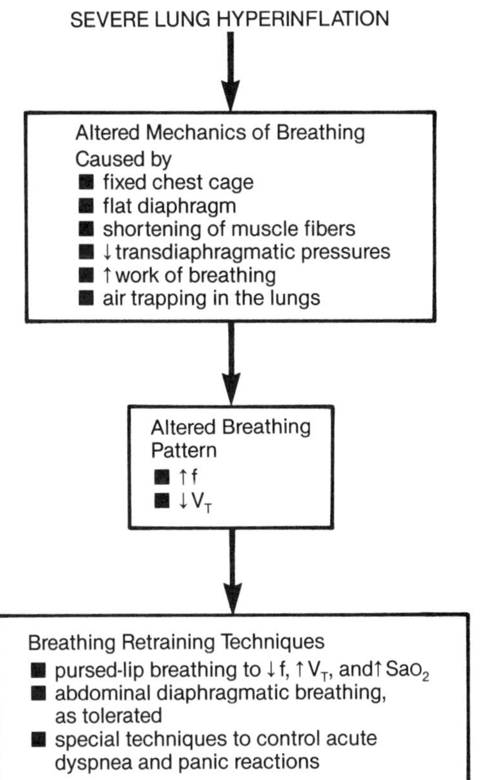

Figure 19–5. Effects of severe lung hyperinflation in chronic obstructive pulmonary disease (COPD). Altered mechanics of breathing explain the altered breathing pattern and rationale for breathing retraining techniques. (f = respiratory rate; V_T = tidal volume; Sao_2 = % saturation of hemoglobin with oxygen in arterial blood.)

mechanical disadvantage and causes a deterioration in inspiratory muscle function. The altered mechanics of breathing is due to a relatively fixed chest cage. Mobilization of the chest wall and stretching of the costophrenic angle are difficult, if not impossible, for the patient to achieve on inspiration. This explains why staff may allow the COPD patient to resort to abdominal or "belly" breathing rather than lower costal breathing. Also, it explains why some patients with severe emphysema may not benefit from any form of abdominal-diaphragmatic breathing.

Deterioration in inspiratory muscle function is related to the flat shape of the diaphragm in lung hyperinflation and the associated shortening of individual muscle fibers. These changes reduce the transdiaphragmatic pressures necessary for normal breathing. To compensate for reduced pressures, the patient resorts to a rapid, shallow breathing pattern (Sharp, 1985). However, this breathing pattern is maladaptive because it increases air trapping and ultimately worsens the effects of lung hyperinflation in addition to increasing the work of breathing. As shown in Figure 19–5, the nurse may use a variety of breathing retraining techniques mentioned in this chapter to help the COPD patient compensate for the effects of lung hyperinflation.

CONTROLLING DYSPNEA

Indications

1. Acute and chronic pulmonary disease
2. Dyspnea
3. Anxiety or fear of suffocation
4. Panic reaction

Controlling dyspnea is an important component of breathing retraining. (Basic approaches to the patient are introduced in Chapter 18.) This section focuses on special techniques to control acute dyspnea and avoid panic reactions. The topic is referred to as "controlling your shortness of breath" instead of the often referred to phrase "panic control" because intervention focuses on the dyspnea, not the panic. The panic will disappear with control of dyspnea.

Controlling dyspnea is basic to coping successfully with the limitations of pulmonary disease. Disabled patients who live alone may become acutely dyspneic while carrying out simple household tasks. In acute asthmatics, the first signs of dyspnea may trigger a vicious circle of anxiety leading to more bronchospasm and dyspnea, similar to the circle illustrated in Figure 16–1. A panic reaction may occur in spite of previous counseling on energy conservation techniques and use of bronchodilators for control of symptoms.

PATIENT INFORMATION

Controlling Your Shortness of Breath

Generally, you should be able to slow and control your shortness of breath by positioning yourself in one of the following ways and pursed-lip breathing (see Fig. 18–7):

1. Sit in a chair with arms supported, head resting against the back of the chair, and feet apart and flat on the floor. If you are not comfortable, try leaning forward with your back straight, elbows on your knees, and hands hanging loosely. You can also use this position while leaning forward and resting your head on a pillow on a table. Hug the pillow with your arms.
2. Stand with one foot in front of the other. Lean forward with a straight back. Rest your forearms on a fence, railing, chair, or some other available object until you catch your breath.
3. If no chair or object is available to sit on or lean against, just lean back against a wall. Your feet should be about 1 ft from the wall. Bend your knees slightly. Relax your arms and shoulders and let your head fall forward slightly.

Panic Control

If you lose control of your breathing, do not panic. Instead, follow these basic steps to gain control of your breathing:

1. Take appropriate medication, if prescribed by your physician.
2. Sit down.
3. Then concentrate all your attention on breathing your air out through very slightly pursed lips.
4. Gradually slow your respiratory rate by breathing out a little slower or longer every 5 to 10 breaths.
5. When you have gained control over your breathing, think about relaxation. Relax your upper chest. Drop your shoulders.

Do not get up until your respiratory rate is near normal. If your respiratory rate does not return to normal, seek medical attention immediately.

Implementation

The previous breathing technique applies to both the restrictive and the obstructive pulmonary disease patient. The only difference is that the restrictive patient may not use PLB unless underlying obstructive disease is present.

The technique is introduced to the patient when he is clinically stable or able to discuss his feelings and past experiences with acute dyspnea. Thereafter, however, it is best taught as acute situations naturally arise in the clinical situation. By this time, the patient has already mastered relaxation and PLB, the basic maneuvers used in controlling dyspnea. The patient's main problem is controlling his mind—thinking about reducing respiratory rate and relaxing rather than fearing suffocation and helplessness. Unless the patient reorients his mind and concentrates fully on technique, he will never develop confidence in his ability to control dyspnea. His attempts to control dyspnea will fail.

For these reasons, and particularly in the case of irrational or completely helpless patients, establishing an effective coping pattern is difficult, if not impossible, to achieve without coaching and reinforcement from another person during a dyspneic episode. At the first sign of dyspnea, anxiety, or wheezing, the nurse instructs the patient in the previously described technique. Other points for the nurse follow:

1. Respond promptly to early complaints of dyspnea.
2. Insist that the patient stop all activity and sit down or lie down in a high Fowler's position.
3. Use touch. Place your hands on the patient's shoulders to encourage relaxation, as already shown in Figure 19–3.
4. Use a calm and reassuring voice. Use relaxation techniques for distraction and mind control during the gradual reduction in respiratory rate.
5. Give positive feedback regarding progress.
6. Do not leave the patient until the dyspnea is controlled.
7. Teach a family member or friend to coach the patient and call the doctor if dyspnea is not controlled within 20 to 30 minutes.

Once dyspnea is controlled, the nurse investigates possible precipitating events, such as an argument with a spouse, increased mucus retention, inability to pace activities, or exposure to an allergen.

As mentioned in Chapter 18, use of a symptom diary over several days to weeks may help the uncomplaining patient recognize pulmonary symptoms before acute dyspnea develops. In addition, discussion of early precipitating events helps patients who complain too much learn other ways to reduce the frequency and intensity of pulmonary symptoms.

Sometimes the patient never has an acute dyspneic episode in the presence of the nurse or other health professional and therefore does not receive coaching for dyspnea control. The patient continues to avoid physical activity for fear of dyspnea. In this case, distance walking, stair climbing, or treadmill walking is used to produce the sensation of dyspnea under controlled conditions and close monitoring. Once the patient learns to control dyspnea, he is less likely to restrict his activity to avoid symptoms.

Deep Breathing and Coughing

GOALS

1. To promote full lung expansion and adequate oxygenation.
2. To mobilize secretions.
3. To prevent atelectasis, mucus retention, and pneumonia.

INDICATIONS

1. Presurgery and postsurgery. Intensify instruction to individuals with risk factors for postoperative pulmonary complications (see Table 4–2).
2. Chronic lung disease.
3. Signs of fluid or mucus retention in the lungs, e.g., abnormal breath sounds, crackles and rhonchi, mucus production.
4. Complete bed rest, shallow breathing, and alveolar hypoventilation (deep breathing only).

Deep breathing and coughing are bronchial hygiene techniques traditionally considered together. Whereas

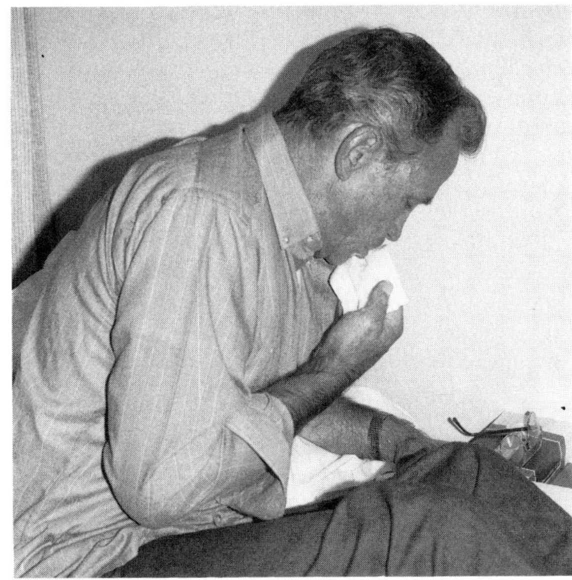

Figure 19–6. The patient leans forward to cough up mucus into a white tissue for inspection.

deep breathing may be used regardless of the presence of mucus in the lungs, coughing is used only when mucus is present (Fig. 19–6). When these techniques do not successfully relieve a mucus retention problem, they are used with more aggressive forms of chest physiotherapy, such as postural drainage, discussed in Chapter 20.

PATIENT INFORMATION

How To Deep Breathe

Deep breathing will help keep your lungs expanded and your airways clear of mucus.

1. Sit up straight or lean forward slightly while sitting on the edge of a chair.
2. Take a slow, deep breath in.
3. Pause slightly or hold your breath for at least 3 seconds, if possible. Holding your breath allows for better distribution of air to all areas of the lungs.
4. Breathe your air out in a relaxed manner. Exhale through pursed lips if you have COPD.
5. Practice this type of sustained deep breath 10 times. Rest or breathe less deeply between sustained breaths to avoid fatigue.

Controlled Coughing

Use an occasional controlled cough during deep breathing when you feel mucus in your chest and you need to cough it up.

1. First, deep breathe as previously directed.
2. While breathing out, cough two to three times in succession, using your abdomen and not your throat. Place your hands on your abdomen and feel your abdominal muscles contract with an effective cough.
3. Repeat as needed to expectorate mucus.

Tips

1. Keep your head forward when you cough.
2. Keep your mouth open to avoid the buildup of pressure in your lungs.
3. *Rest* between coughs with slow, deep breathing. Do not tire or strain yourself.
4. Avoid the continual, hacking cough; it only irritates your airways and causes more nonproductive coughing. If hacking continues, concentrate on deep breathing and cough *only* when absolutely necessary to raise mucus. Try soothing your throat with a few sips of warm liquid.
5. *Remember: Control your cough!* Don't let it control you.

PRACTICE SCHEDULE

Hospital Setting

1. As ordered and PRN.
2. At least ten sustained maximal inspirations every hour in the immediate postoperative period (Bartlett, 1984).
3. After respiratory treatments to mobilize secretions.

Home Setting

1. PRN and after respiratory treatments.
2. Immediately after rising in the morning for COPD patients with sputum production.

EVALUATION CRITERIA

For Correct Technique

Deep Breathing

1. Slow inspiratory phase; promotes recruitment of alveoli instead of overinflation of already patent alveoli.
2. At least a 1- to 3-second pause after maximal inspiration.
3. Respiratory rate no greater than 12/min.

Controlled Coughing

1. Head in neutral or flexed position.
2. Tense abdominal muscles during cough.
3. Cough has a low-pitched deep sound rather than a short high-pitched sound.
4. Cough is *controlled*: forceful but not strained or hacking.

For Overall Improvement in Condition

1. Production of mucus in the case of mucus retention.
2. Decrease in the production of mucus, resolving mucus retention problem.
3. Normal or improved breath sounds.
4. Decrease in adventitious sounds.
5. Decrease in temperature to normal level.
6. Decrease in respiratory rate.
7. Improved vital capacity and forced expiratory volume in one second (FEV_1).
8. Return to normal breathing pattern: normal tidal volumes (400 to 500 ml) interrupted every 5 to 10 minutes by sighs, yawns, or deep breaths to total lung capacity (see Fig. 8–12).
9. Restoration of $Pa{O_2}$ and $Pa{CO_2}$ to normal levels.
10. Absence of atelectasis and pneumonia on the chest x-ray.

FORCED EXHALATION TECHNIQUE (HUFFING)

The *forced exhalation technique* (FET) is informally referred to as "huffing." Similar to the cough, it is indicated for mucus production and retention problems. Recently, it has been suggested as a substitute for voluntary coughing (Sutton et al, 1982).

Huffing consists of one to two forced expiratory efforts or "huffs" made with an open glottis (i.e., compressive phase of a normal cough) at mid to low lung volume, followed by a period of relaxation and diaphragmatic breathing (described subsequently). The technique is described in more detail here.

PATIENT INFORMATION

Huffing Technique

The huffing technique is used in place of coughing to expectorate mucus. When performed properly, it helps to avoid the nonproductive or uncontrollable hacking cough.

To Perform Huffing

1. Learn forward slightly while sitting up in bed or in a chair.
2. Take a deep breath in.
3. Breathe out (exhale) forcefully with your mouth and throat open and with firm contraction of your abdominal muscles. The expulsion of air will make a huffing noise.
4. Relax immediately after the huff.
   a. Drop your shoulders. Let your arms fall limp in your lap.
   b. Continue slow diaphragmatic breathing between each forced exhalation.
5. Repeat the technique two or three times or until you expectorate all the mucus in your chest.

Tips

1. *Remember*: The sequence is *breathe in, huff out,* and *relax.*
2. Try two or three huffs instead of one huff on each forced exhalation. Successive huffs will clear progressively deeper portions of airways.
3. Concentrate on *full* relaxation after each forced exhalation to avoid uncontrollable coughing.
4. Use huffing during your postural drainage treatment. It will increase the amount of sputum produced.

Implementation

With the FET, the nurse stresses the importance of the huff at mid to low lung volumes as well as the relaxation period before reaching residual volume. Relaxation avoids precipitating uncontrolled coughing and worsening bronchospasm, problems associated with other forced expiratory maneuvers, such as coughing or blowing into a glove or blow bottles. The huff causes less airway compression than a cough because transpulmonary pressure is less during the huff, as compared with the cough. Airways remain more patent, thus facilitating mucus drainage and expectoration. In fact, research indicates that huffing is more effective than vigorous coughing in cases of severe obstruction with copious sputum production (Sutton et al., 1983). Huffing increases the efficiency and effectiveness of postural drainage in patients with sputum production (Pryor et al., 1979). In addition, the technique of two or three huffs per forced expiration may be used in postoperative patients whose splinting respirations prevent deep breathing and coughing.

MANUAL COUGH

The *manual cough* is also referred to as the *diaphragmatic push* or the augmented cough. It is used for quadriplegics and other neuromuscular disease patients with impaired diaphragmatic functioning and insufficient expiratory muscular force for coughing.

For the manual cough, the patient is instructed to inspire maximally either spontaneously or from an IPPB device. While the patient sustains the inspiration for 3 seconds, the nurse places one or two hands across the upper abdomen and then *quickly* and *forcefully* pushes inward and upward as the patient coughs. The push helps increase air flow necessary for an effective cough.

COUGHING WITH GLOSSOPHARYNGEAL BREATHING

Neuromuscular patients with little to no respiratory muscle function may use *glossopharyngeal breathing* (GPB), also called *frog breathing,* to double or triple their vital capacities and cough themselves. As with manual cough, it is not used for COPD patients. The technique involves using mouth, tongue, and throat muscles to force small quantities of air into the lungs in quick gulps (Fig. 19–7), until a vital capacity of up to 1000 ml is achieved (Dail et al., 1979). Then the

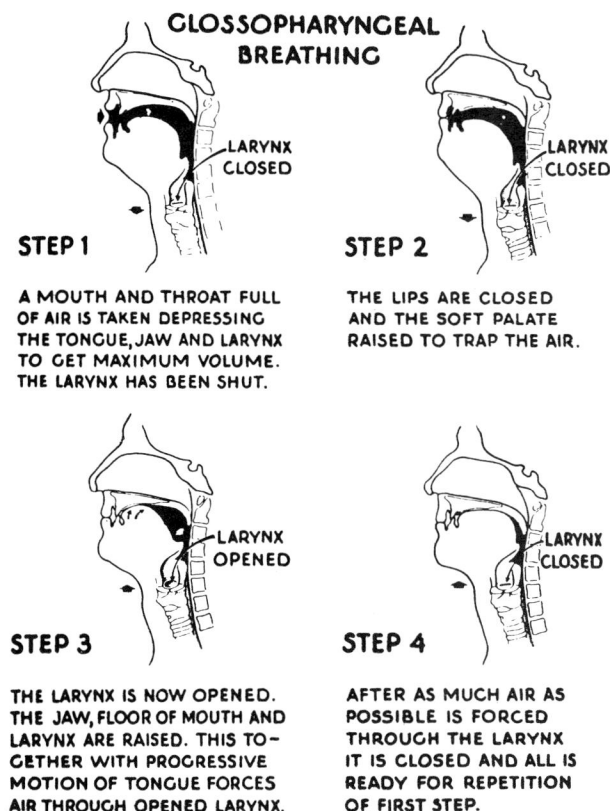

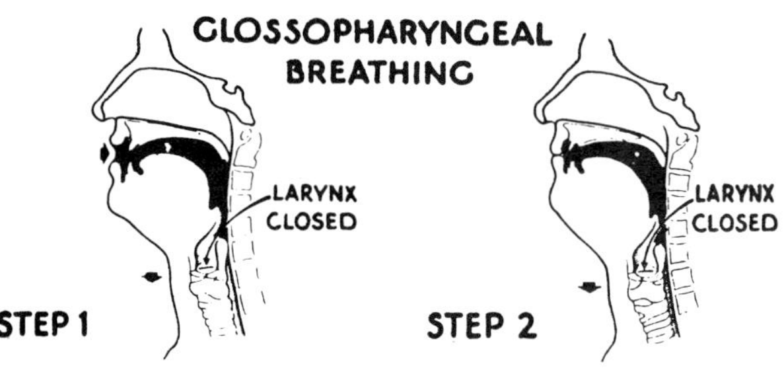
GLOSSOPHARYNGEAL BREATHING
LARYNX CLOSED
STEP 1
A MOUTH AND THROAT FULL OF AIR IS TAKEN DEPRESSING THE TONGUE, JAW AND LARYNX TO GET MAXIMUM VOLUME. THE LARYNX HAS BEEN SHUT.
LARYNX CLOSED
STEP 2
THE LIPS ARE CLOSED AND THE SOFT PALATE RAISED TO TRAP THE AIR.

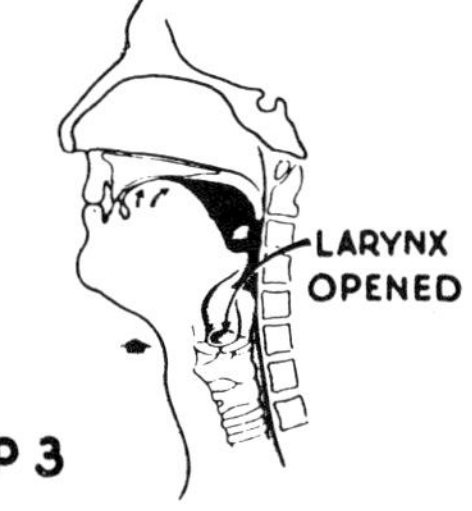
LARYNX OPENED
STEP 3
THE LARYNX IS NOW OPENED. THE JAW, FLOOR OF MOUTH AND LARYNX ARE RAISED. THIS TOGETHER WITH PROGRESSIVE MOTION OF TONGUE FORCES AIR THROUGH OPENED LARYNX.

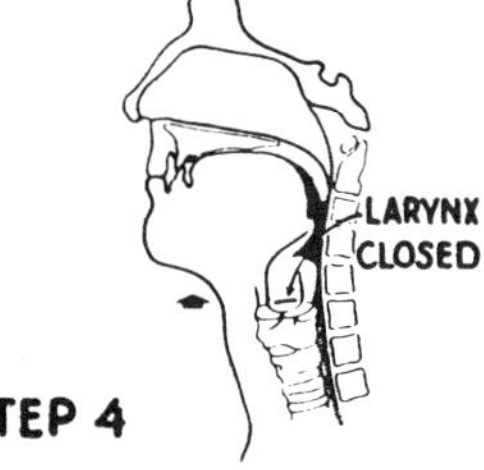
LARYNX CLOSED
STEP 4
AFTER AS MUCH AIR AS POSSIBLE IS FORCED THROUGH THE LARYNX IT IS CLOSED AND ALL IS READY FOR REPETITION OF FIRST STEP.

Figure 19–7. Glossopharyngeal breathing. The taking in of a small quick gulp of air is illustrated in Steps 1 through 4. Repetitive gulping in this manner is necessary to fill the lungs completely. (Reproduced by permission from Hirschberg, G., Lewis, L., and Vaughan, P. Rehabilitation—A Manual for the Care of the Disabled and Elderly, 2nd ed. Philadelphia, J. B. Lippincott Co., 1976.)

patient exhales to residual volume to cough himself, or the nurse uses a diaphragmatic push to improve cough force and facilitate mucus expectoration.

GPB offers other advantages besides improved cough force. Patients at home may perform the technique prophylactically for up to 10 minutes once or twice a day to help prevent mucus retention and atelectasis. Patients may breathe by themselves for several hours during ventilator failure. Many others use it to sing or converse for prolonged periods (Hodgkin et al, 1984).

Although GPB may improve bronchial hygiene and quality of life, not all patients are candidates for the technique. It is difficult to learn, requiring good control of mouth, tongue, and throat muscles as well as an instructor who can demonstrate the technique for the patient to imitate. Patients who might benefit from GPB should be evaluated at a health center that specializes in care of ventilator-dependent neuromuscular patients.

DEEP BREATHING WITH INCENTIVE SPIROMETRY

Incentive spirometry is a method of encouraging deep breathing by giving immediate visual feedback regarding achievement of preset goals (i.e., inspired volumes). Goals start out low and are gradually increased until maximal inspired volumes are achieved. The patient may be asked to cough or huff on expiration after maximal inspiration to facilitate mucus expectoration.

Indications for use of incentive spirometry are basically the same as those for deep breathing and controlled coughing. In addition, the patient must demonstrate either a reduced vital capacity or inability to deep breathe with standard deep breathing techniques (California Thoracic Society, 1981). About 95% of hospitals in the United States routinely order incentive spirometry for the prevention of postoperative atelectasis associated with thoracic and abdominal surgery (O'Donohue, 1985). Moreover, relatively inexpensive disposable spirometry units are available to help the home patient monitor his ability to take a maximal inspiration.

The hazards of incentive spirometry are few. They include hyperventilation and transmission of infection. Hyperventilation is avoided with use of proper technique. Infection is a concern but remains undocumented in the literature. Patients with nondisposable units use disposable circuits to avoid cross contamination. Patients with disposable units at home are advised to wash the mouthpiece daily, cover the unit between treatments, and replace the unit after recovery from each acute exacerbation of pulmonary disease.

Two types of incentive spirometers are used in the clinical setting; flow and volume spirometers.

Flow Incentive Spirometers

Flow incentive spirometers are flow dependent. They consist of one or more plastic chambers containing a freely movable pingpong–type ball, as shown in Figure 19–8. The patient is asked to inhale briskly to elevate the balls and keep them floating in air as long as possible to achieve a sustained maximal inspiration.

Flow spirometers have several limitations. First, maximal inspiration cannot be accurately or practically measured, though it may be grossly estimated by multiplying flow rate by the length of time the ball is suspended in air.

Second, the patient must learn to produce an optimal inspiratory flow rate and sustain it. These two feats are difficult to achieve owing to the device's design. On the one hand, a very brisk flow rate will snap the balls to the top of the chamber on a relatively low volume breath. On the other hand, an excessively slow flow rate may achieve a total lung capacity (TLC) breath without moving the balls. The ideal flow rate lies somewhere between these two extremes. Once it is achieved, the patient may find it difficult, if not impossible, to sustain inspiration longer than 2 seconds without the balls dropping to the bottom of the chamber.

Last, flow incentive spirometers are disposable and for single patient use. Maintenance may be a problem. Patients must be cautioned not to obstruct the air port during use. Obstruction decreases flow rate and the inhaled volume required to reach the preset goal.

Nurses are encouraged to check all disposable spirometers periodically to assure proper working order. Items to check include an unobstructed air port (i.e., flow type), freely moving goal indicator (i.e., volume type), intact plastic body, and unobstructed mouthpiece.

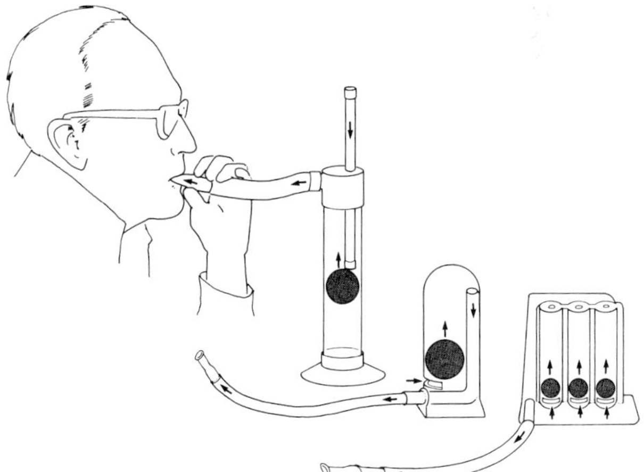

Figure 19–8. Flow incentive spirometers. Patients are instructed to inhale briskly to elevate the ball(s) and to keep them floating for as long as possible. The volume inhaled is unknown. (Reproduced by permission from Luce, J., Tyler, M., and Pierson, D. Intensive Respiratory Care. Philadelphia, W. B. Saunders Co., 1984.)

Although flow spirometers have many limitations, they are cheaper and more portable than many volume incentive spirometers. Also, as Bartlett (1984) points out, using some kind of incentive device as a reminder to deep breathe is clearly better than none for acutely ill patients.

Volume Incentive Spirometers

A volume incentive spirometer is better than a flow spirometer because its operation includes selection of a preset volume and visual feedback of the actual volume achieved. Also, the design permits slower, more sustained inspirations, with breath holds for up to 10 seconds.

The nondisposable type of volume spirometer functions as a pneumotachometer. It uses a spinning turbine that relates rate of rotation to volume inhaled. Lights are used to register preset goal and volume achieved.

In the less expensive type of volume spirometer, a bellow or piston is used to register volume (Fig. 19–9). The nurse slides an indicator or pointer to a desired goal.

Setting Goals for Maximal Inspiration

Clinical judgment is required to determine a realistic inspiratory goal for the patient. Ideally, the patient should achieve an inspiratory capacity (IC) equal to that recorded on a baseline pulmonary function test result. However, since most patients using incentive spirometers are weak or debilitated or in pain, a value about ½ to ¾ the normal value serves as a realistic goal (Luce et al, 1984). Without access to a complete PFT report, the nurse starts at half the patient's vital capacity and gradually increases the preset goal by 100 to 250 ml as tolerated. For anxious patients and those with drastically reduced tidal volumes at rest, the nurse starts at a low volume—200 to 300 ml, if necessary—to insure success with each breathing attempt, thus maintaining incentive motivation to continue therapy. With this approach, three to five sustained inspirations may be required to find a maximal preset goal for each practice session. Once it is established, the nurse stays with the patient, encouraging him to reach the goal ten times and rest between attempts to avoid fatigue and hyperventilation. Specific patient instructions are explained hereafter.

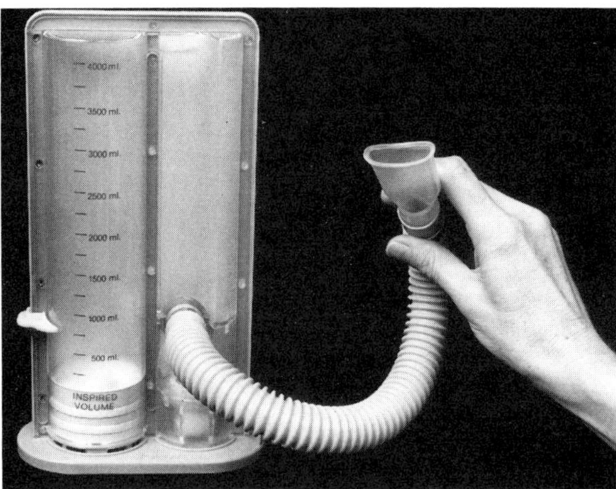

Figure 19–9. A disposable volume incentive spirometer. During inhalation, the bellow at the bottom of the spirometer is raised to the level of the adjustable goal indicator on the left side.

PATIENT INFORMATION

Using Your Deep Breathing Exerciser

Your doctor has prescribed a deep breathing exerciser to make it easier for you to deep breathe and cough up mucus.

Preparation

1. Sit up straight or lean forward slightly while sitting on the edge of a chair.
2. Hold or place the exerciser on the table in an upright position.
3. Slide the volume pointer to the goal suggested by your nurse, therapist, or doctor.
   Goal ______________________

Deep Breathing Technique

1. Place your lips and teeth firmly around the mouthpiece to keep a seal.
2. Breathe out normally.
3. Breathe in *slowly* to raise the piston or bellows in the chamber.
4. Continue breathing in until you reach your goal.
5. Hold your breath for at least 3 seconds, keeping the piston or bellows suspended.
6. Breathe out normally, letting the piston or bellows fall to the bottom of the chamber.
7. Try increasing your goal (i.e., inspired volume) by 100 to 250 ml on each successive deep breath. When you reach your maximal volume, practice inspiring to this volume 10 times.

Tips

1. If you wear dentures, keep them in and use noseclips when you have difficulty keeping a seal around the mouthpiece.
2. *Take your time!* Rest between breaths to avoid dizziness and fatigue.
3. Cough during exhalation if you feel mucus in your chest.
4. Establish a practice schedule.
   Number of deep breaths ______________________
   Frequency ______________________

Deep Breathing and Coughing in Perspective

Deep breathing and coughing in acute and chronic settings are discussed in detail because of their central importance in all aspects of respiratory care. Research in acute care is emphasized because, thus far, implementation of deep breathing and coughing is based mostly on data gathered in acute care settings.

OPTIMAL TECHNIQUE

Research indicates that the *sustained maximal inspiration* described in the previous patient information section is the best method of preventing and treating pulmonary complications after surgery (Breslin, 1981; Risser, 1980). Maximal inspiration to TLC achieves full lung inflation. Sustaining each breath is important, since Ward and associates (1966) found that use of one deep breath held for 3 seconds increases PaO_2 more than unheld single or multiple deep breaths. To be effective, the sustained maximal inspiration must be practiced regularly *ten times each hour* when awake (Bartlett, 1984).

Though these crucial findings apply to patients in the immediate postoperative period, they have implications for all patients receiving respiratory care in hospital and home settings. They have profound implications for respiratory nursing care because the nurse has primary responsibility for deep breathing and coughing and associated interventions, such as turning, ambulation, and aerosol or IPPB treatments.

ACUTE SETTING

In the preoperative period, the surgical nurse must teach deep breathing measures and supervise practice until techniques are mastered. Mastery is necessary for success. Then, in the first 24 to 48 hours postsurgery, the nurse must work closely with the respiratory and physical therapist to be sure the patient takes at least ten sustained breaths per hour.

This task is no small feat for patient or nurse. In spite of preoperative instruction, the patient may be reluctant to move or deep breathe owing to intense incisional pain or anxiety and restrictions imposed upon him by chest tubes, abdominal drains, and intravenous lines. The nurse has the challenge of providing pain medication and timely reassurance, turning the patient every 1 to 2 hours, and spending up to 10 minutes per hour for supervision of deep breathing maneuvers when a respiratory therapist is unavailable. Particularly when patient case loads are heavy, successful accomplishment of these and other tasks require quick assessment of patient problems and optimal cooperation among health team members for appropriate intervention.

HOME SETTING

The visiting nurse is responsible for teaching deep breathing measures and supervising their implementation during acute disease exacerbations. This task remains a challenge. Patient and family may be overburdened with numerous treatments and remain unable to incorporate extra deep breathing maneuvers into the daily routine. In other cases, the COPD patient may deny the need for breathing exercises in spite of increasing rhonchi and sputum production. The challenge of the nurse is to help patient and family integrate deep breathing maneuvers with other aspects of respiratory care and still remain a welcome visitor in the home. In stressful situations, the patient may ask the nurse to discontinue services if a goal seems unattainable or unrealistic given the patient's perception of his situation.

The nurse may meet the challenge in one of three ways. First, she may perform much of the direct supervision and care herself until the patient or family member is able to participate effectively in care. Then, using motivational and teaching models presented in the previous unit of this book, the nurse can gradually help patient and family participate in self care.

Second, as long as financial reimbursement is available, the nurse may utilize a chest physiotherapist for integration of deep breathing maneuvers with chest physiotherapy. Respiratory therapists involved in home equipment maintenance are also resources for reinforcement of educational content.

Last, for mucus-producing bronchitics, deep breathing maneuvers should be intensified in the morning to clear the chest well before noon, thus permitting a more normal life style. Patients with poor technique or infrequently scheduled maneuvers may find themselves coughing nonproductively all morning. This practice produces unnecessary fatigue and locks the patient into "the sick role" for longer periods of time during the day.

Two key interventions in the home setting include (1) optimizing the technique at a time when the patient feels good and able to concentrate on learning and (2) teaching the patient how to intensify procedures when such production increases and how to decrease the frequency and intensity of procedures when mucus production decreases. As an example of the second intervention, a chronic bronchitic patient may need to deep breathe quite frequently during an acute exacerbation—immediately after his early morning aerosol treatment and q1h for 3 hours. However, in his stable state, the extra q1h morning exercises may be unnecessary. Their prompt discontinuation allows the patient more uninterrupted personal time. Also, it facilitates the move away from the sick role in the family and towards a more healthy body image.

WHICH METHOD IS BEST?

Though the topic remains controversial, the literature supports the following conclusions and recommendations for deep breathing, coughing, and other hyperinflation techniques.

1. The goal of controlled coughing is mucus production.
   a. Routine coughing in the absence of lung congestion has no physiologic rationale and may be detrimental to the patient's pulmonary status (Breslin, 1981).

b. The cough is used to clear large not small airways of mucus. It is only effective to Z-6 or Z-7 in Weibel's model of the lung (review Fig. 2–7) (Sutton et al, 1982). Hence, the nurse emphasizes the cough when rhonchi and coarse crackles are present and discourages its use when the lungs are clear.
c. The nurse discontinues coughing and implements huffing, if a cough becomes uncontrollable or if it produces bronchospasm.

2. The physiologic goals of deep breathing are *maximal alveolar inflation* and *maintenance of a normal functional residual capacity* (FRC).
   a. Forced expiratory maneuvers, such as coughing, use of blow bottles, and induced coughing with a suction catheter have been criticized because they do not always meet these two aforementioned goals. During forced expiration, FRC becomes reduced. Pleural pressure rises above airway pressure, and acinar units collapse, producing atelectasis.
   b. Deep breathing maneuvers ideally start at FRC and end at FRC, as demonstrated in the incentive spirometry patient information.
   c. Routine use of blow gloves, blow bottles, transtracheal irrigation and stimulation, and prophylactic endotracheal suctioning has no role in respiratory care (Bartlett, 1984).
   d. If your health agency still uses blow bottles emphasize the importance of taking a maximal inspiration before blowing the colored fluid from one bottle to the next and again after completion of the forced expiratory maneuver. The last maximal inspiration will insure alveolar reinflation.
3. Deep breathing and coughing, IPPB, and incentive spirometry may be equally effective in preventing atelectasis (Celli et al, 1984; Indihar et al, 1982).
   a. The key factor appears to be the patient's motivation and the nurse's or therapist's ability to frequently stimulate the patient with or without use of a respiratory device (Hiller, et al, 1980; Lederer, et al, 1980; Stock, et al, 1985).
   b. Incentive spirometry is preferred over IPPB because it is cheaper and the device is easier to operate. Also, its use may shorten the length of hospitalization (Celli, et al, 1984).
   c. IPPB is indicated when the patient cannot or will not perform spontaneous deep breathing maneuvers.
4. *There is no one best technique for deep breathing and controlled coughing.*
   a. Each patient presents a different set of clinical circumstances, requiring adaptation of standard technique. Practical alternatives to standard technique are reviewed in Table 19–1.
5. During maximal inspirations, distribution of the inflating volume is as important as the volume delivered.
   a. The nurse encourages frequent position changes and ambulation to ventilate all lung lobes, mobilize secretions, prevent hypoxemia, and increase exercise tolerance.

Postural Drainage and Chest Percussion and Vibration

Postural drainage is therapeutic positioning of the body for mucus drainage. It is used alone with deep breathing and coughing or huffing or in combination with *chest percussion* (i.e., clapping on the chest) and *chest vibration*.

Though frequently underutilized in the United States, this form of chest physiotherapy may be more effective than cough for clearing lung periphery of mucus. In the acute care setting, it is as effective as aspiration through a fiberoptic bronchoscope for removal of mucus causing postoperative atelectasis (Sutton et al, 1982).

GOALS

Postural Drainage (PD)

1. To drain peripheral pulmonary secretions by means of gravity into major airways.
2. To improve respiratory mechanics and gas exchange.
3. To decrease the incidence of respiratory infection.

Percussion and Vibration (PV)

1. To augment postural drainage by dislodging and mobilizing secretions from the lung parenchyma into larger airways where they can be easily expectorated or aspirated with a suction catheter.
2. Note: when PV is used with PD, the procedure is abbreviated PD and PV.

INDICATIONS

1. Lobar pneumonia; not indicated in uncomplicated pneumonia (Graham and Bradley, 1978).
2. Copious sputum production (e.g., greater than 25 to 30 ml/day) (Mazzocco et al, 1984).
3. Bronchiectasis.
4. Chronic bronchitis but controversial.
5. Cystic fibrosis.
6. Draining lung abscess.
7. Atelectasis after cardiac surgery.

PD is used only when indications are clearly present. Moving into the many required body positions is taxing on the patient. PV require skill and cooperation from

Table 19–1. ALTERNATIVES TO STANDARD DEEP BREATHING AND COUGHING TECHNIQUE

Technique	General Description	Clinical Uses
Standard deep breathing and coughing technique	The patient inhales slowly and maximally, holds the breath for at least 3 seconds, and exhales normally. When mucus is present, the patient contracts abdominal muscles and coughs 2 to 3 times on exhalation.	Patients with an actual or potential respiratory problem, such as alveolar hypoventilation, atelectasis, and mucus retention.
Series of three coughs	The patient takes a small breath and produces a small cough, a bigger breath and more forceful cough, and finally a maximal deep breath and a forceful cough.	Patients with excessive pain, fatigue, or anxiety.
Huffing (forced exhalation technique)	The patient inspires maximally, holds the breath, and breathes out sharply with firm contraction of abdominal muscles. The vocal cords and mouth remain open. The expulsion of air makes a huffing noise. Bronchitic and asthmatic patients can try 1 big huff, followed immediately by relaxation. Postoperative patients may prefer to huff 2 to 3 times during 1 exhalation.	Used as a substitute for coughing in patients with thoracotomy or upper abdominal surgery, chest pain, excessive fatigue, bronchospasm, or uncontrollable paroxsysmal coughing.
Deep breathing with incentive spirometry	The patient exhales normally, takes a maximum sustained inspiration (i.e., at least a 3-second hold), and exhales normally. Goals (i.e., inspired volumes) are gradually increased as tolerated.	Preferred over IPPB for patients with reduced vital capacities, chest pain, excessive fatigue, thoracotomy, or upper abdominal surgery.
Coughing with IPPB	The patient takes a deep breath from the IPPB machine, holds it, removes the mouthpiece, and coughs twice.	Patients with reduced vital capacities, excessive fatigue, or unwillingness or inability to use simple respiratory devices or spontaneous deep breathing and coughing techniques.
Manual cough (diaphragmatic push, augmented cough)	The patient takes a deep breath in via IPPB if available or with the use of glossopharyngeal breathing. The nurse places one or two hands on the upper abdomen and quickly and forcefully pushes inward and upward as the patient coughs.	Quadriplegics and other neuromuscular patients with impaired diaphragmatic functioning.
Oral and tracheobronchial suctioning (intubated patients)	See Chapter 27 for technique. Teach patients to advance catheter only far enough to stimulate cough or to aspirate secretions already partially raised by coughing. Remember, intermittent suction during catheter withdrawal should last no longer than 10 to 15 seconds. For nasopharyngeal secretions, patients can be taught to use a suction catheter (or Yankauer suction tip) continuously hooked up to suction and readily available at the bedside.	Patients with permanent tracheostomy or those on long-term mechanical ventilation with: History of mucus production Audible secretions or coarse rhonchi that persist in spite of efforts to cough Pooled oropharyngeal secretions Stable mental and physical status Good hand coordination Willingness to learn
Cough simulation (intubated patients)	Staff follow this procedure: 1. Make sure tube cuff is inflated. 2. Give a large, rapid inspiration by manual resuscitation bag. 3. Hold inspiration 3 seconds. 4. Release bag and allow expiration to ensue. 5. Ask another person to vibrate or compress chest during expiration and release pressure on inspiration (sometimes called chest springing). 6. Suction as needed.	Intubated patients with ineffective or absent cough and mucus retention. Though staff perform this procedure, the patient needs to know the purpose and general procedure before it is implemented.

a willing and able family member or friend. Also, though complications are infrequently reported, when they do occur they are usually severe.

Perhaps the most reliable indication for use of postural drainage is sputum production of over 25 to 30 ml per day. Postural drainage is not generally recommended as a prophylactic measure in patients with minimal sputum production (i.e., less than 25 to 30 ml/day). Connors and coworkers (1980) demonstrated that in acutely ill medical patients with minimal to small amounts of sputum production, mean PaO_2 dropped 16.8 mmHg immediately after PD and PV. It dropped another 5.3 mmHg 30 minutes after return to pretreatment body position.

CONTRAINDICATIONS

The nurse withholds therapy and checks with the physician whenever any of the contraindications listed in Table 19–2 are present. In addition, the doctor is consulted whenever the exertion, position changes, or

Table 19–2. CONTRAINDICATIONS FOR POSTURAL DRAINAGE (PD) WITH CHEST PERCUSSION AND VIBRATION (PV)

Contraindication	Rationale for Withholding Therapy
Acute myocardial infarction	Low head position and PV will worsen myocardial ischemia and extend the infarct.
Hemorrhage	Low head position, frequent position changes, and PV promote bleeding and possibly exsanguination if the bleeding is in the respiratory system.
Acute pulmonary embolism	PD and PV are not needed because consolidation is due to pulmonary embolism, not mucus retention.
Pulmonary edema	Fluid retention, not mucus retention, is the basic problem in the lungs.
Bronchopulmonary fistula	PD and PV may make the fistula bigger.
Frank hemoptysis	Pulmonary hemorrhage may occur.
Increased intracranial pressure (ICP)	Low head position and physical stimulation will further increase ICP to a dangerous level.
Pneumonectomy with open pericardium	The heart may fall out of the pericardium. In some cases, PV may weaken suture lines and cause a bronchial or vascular leak.
Acute chest trauma with severe parenchymal involvement or flail chest	Physical stimulation, particularly PV, promotes bleeding and further injury by the already traumatized tissue. PV are never done over or near a healing flail chest area because they will cause chest wall instability and worsen the flailing.
Conditions that allow gastric reflux or a recent meal or nasogastric feeding within the past hour	The head down position may cause aspiration of stomach contents into the lungs. PV may predispose to nausea and vomiting.
Extreme agitation or nervousness	The patient may panic during the procedure and develop severe dyspnea and hypoxemia.

percussion involved in therapy might adversely affect other medical-surgical conditions. For example, aggressive therapy might cause (1) myocardial ischemia in the patient at risk for angina, (2) eye injury in an immobilized postoptic surgery patient, (3) suture strain in the patient with postsurgical anastamoses of major blood vessels, and (4) hypertension in the cardiac patient.

In some cases, however, even though PD and PV is contraindicated, the physician may order it for a limited period when benefits are anticipated to outweigh possible complications. For example, the benefit of improved bronchial hygiene may significantly reduce the risk of pneumonia and outweigh the risk of increased intracranial pressure, a complication of PD and PV in the neurologic patient.

PATIENT INFORMATION

Postural Drainage with Percussion and Vibration

Postural drainage is a way of draining mucus from your lungs by means of gravity and changes in body position.

Percussion and vibration help loosen mucus so that it can drain out of the lungs better. You will need a friend or relative to do all or most of the percussion and vibration while you are in difficult drainage positions.

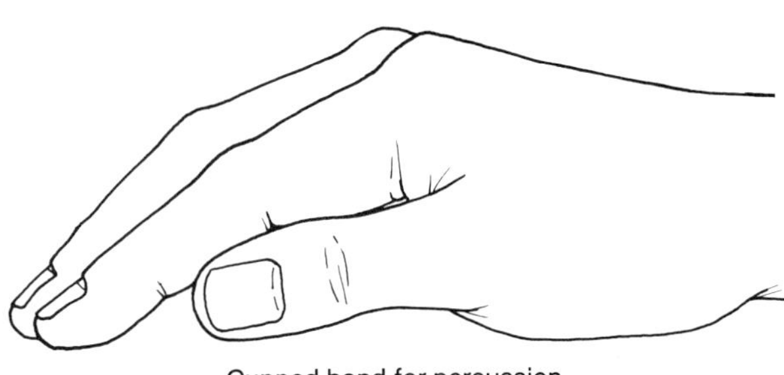

Cupped hand for percussion

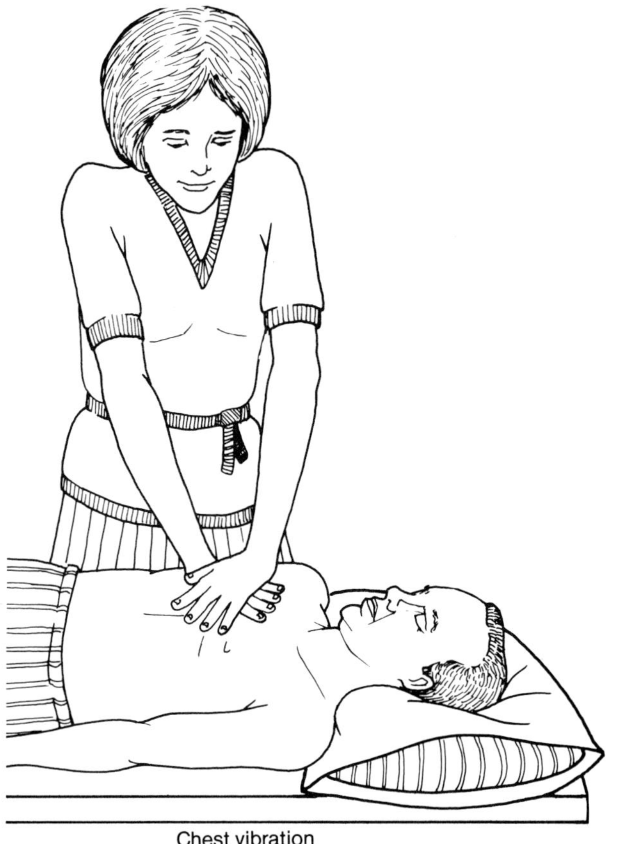

Chest vibration

To Prepare

Wear comfortable clothes, including a light shirt or blouse to protect the skin during percussion.

To Percuss

With hands cupped to trap air, strike the chest with firm pressure. Alternate hands (first one, then the other) in a rhythmic pattern similar to trotting horses. Percuss 20 to 30 seconds. Then vibrate.

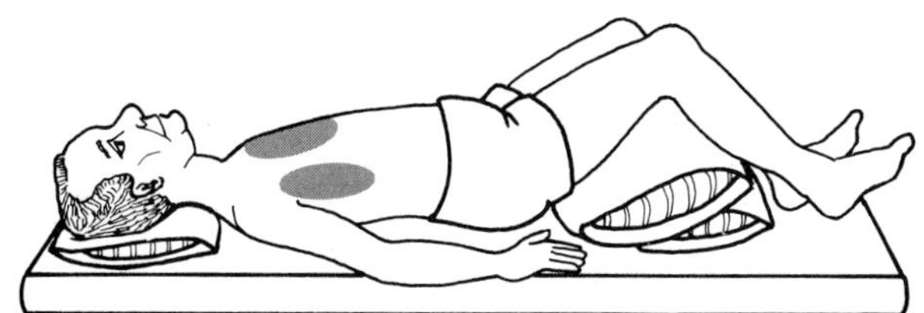

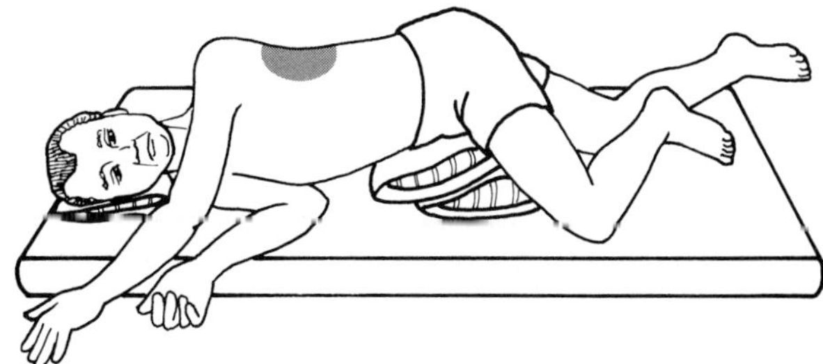

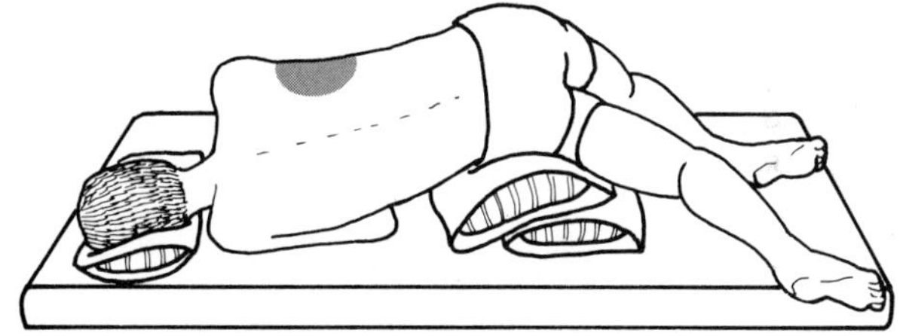

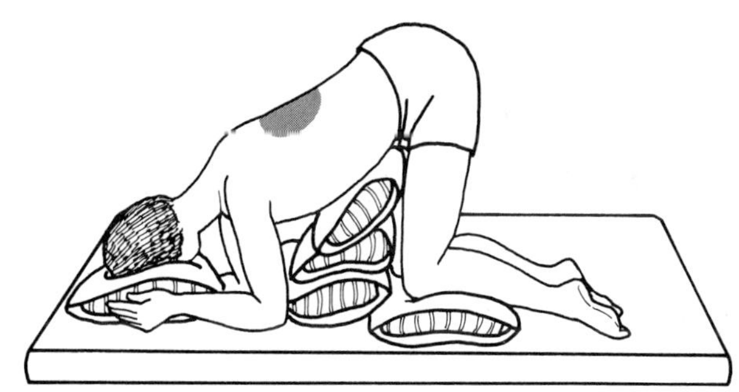

To Vibrate

Place one hand firmly on the chest; place the other hand on top. When the patient breathes out, move the palms of your hands up and down to shake the chest. Stop the shaking or vibration as the patient starts to breathe in again. Vibrate only when he breathes out, three or four breaths in a row. Then percuss again.

Basic Drainage Positions in Sequential Order

Try these positions on your bed at home. You may place a small pillow under your head for all positions. Percussion areas are marked in the illustrations to the right.

1. *Lie flat on your back.*
   Pillow under hips and knees. Percuss on each side of chest from just below the collar bone down to the lower ribs.
2. *Lie on your right side.*
   One or two pillows under hips so that the head is in a downward position. Bend left knee forward.
3. *Lie on your left side.*
   Pillows under hips so that the head is in a downward position. Bend right knee forward.
4. *On arms and knees.*
   Head in a downward position. Pillow under knees to elevate hips. May use a pillow in the space under the hips for increased comfort. *Alternative*: Head down position with hips on the edge of the bed and forearms on a pillow on the floor. Percuss on each side of the spinal cord.

With the help of a friend or relative, follow this sequence for each drainage position:

1. Percuss and vibrate for 2 to 3 minutes.
2. Cough or huff to expectorate mucus.
3. Drain for up to 10 minutes, with use of slow deep breathing.

Tips

1. If short on time, spend most of your time in position 4.
2. Slowly deep breathe throughout the whole procedure.
3. Use plenty of pillows for support and relaxation. If necessary, fold up blankets or tie up a 6-inch stack of newspapers, place in a pillow case, and use for a bottom pillow.
4. Do not sit up between positions. The mucus will slip back down. Keep tissues handy.
5. Keep your mouth and throat open while breathing out during vibrations. Let all your air out without straining.

Your Orders

PRACTICE SCHEDULE

1. Schedule *after* respiratory treatments and bronchodilator medications and *before* meals.
2. Acute disease: 10- to 30-minute sessions every 2 to 6 hours with modified positions to avoid adverse effects and excessive fatigue.
3. Chronic disease: 20- to 40-minute sessions as ordered or PRN.
4. QD: upon rising in the morning.
5. BID: upon rising in the morning and 1 hour before bedtime.
6. TID: early AM, before lunch, and 1 hour before bedtime.
7. QID: add a treatment before dinner.

EVALUATION CRITERIA

For Correct Technique

Postural Drainage

1. The draining segment is *uppermost,* with its bronchus in a vertical or near vertical position to maximize gravity drainage.
2. The lungs are drained from top to bottom, starting with the upper lobes first and ending with the posterior basal segments of the lower lobes.
3. Pathologic segments, posterior basal segments, or both are always drained for at least 5 to 10 minutes.
4. *The patient looks comfortable.* Knees and hips are flexed in all positions. At least two pillows are used to provide support and promote full muscle relaxation.

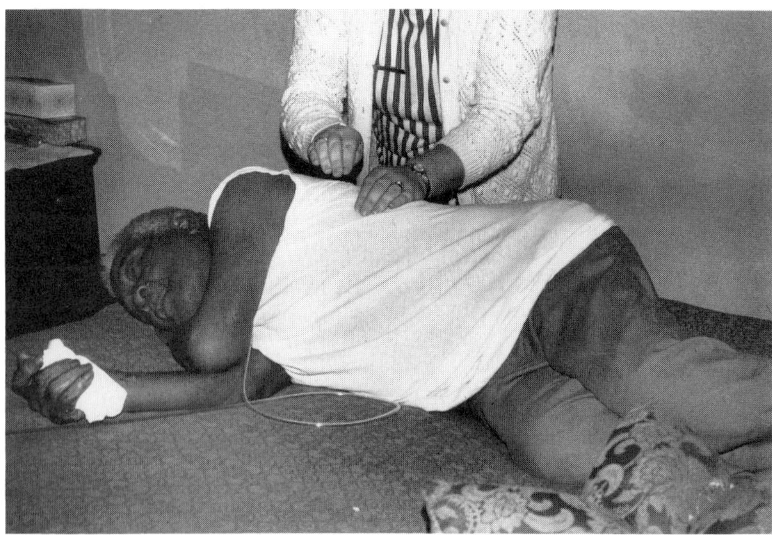

Figure 19–10. Percussion over the lateral chest area with the patient on supplementary oxygen.

If the patient looks tense and uncomfortable, modify drainage position if necessary.

5. Slow controlled breathing throughout the procedure with avoidance of forced expiratory maneuvers except for coughing to remove secretions.

Percussion (**Fig. 19–10**)

1. Peripheral edges of cupped hand exert equal and firm pressure on chest wall upon contact.

2. A loud low-pitched "cupping" sound is produced, likened to the sound of a horse trotting, when the trapping of air within the palm produces suction on the chest's surface. Adjust the cup of the hand when the patient reports feeling thumbs pressing into the chest wall or "stinging" skin from slapping movements.

3. Slow, *rhythmic* percussion rate.

Vibration (**Fig. 19–11**)

1. Vibration results in shaking of the chest wall as opposed to chest wall compression. Compression during vibration may result in rib fractures.

2. Vibration is done *only* during expiration with the patient's mouth and throat open (i.e., no PLB).

Criteria for Overall Improvement in Condition

These are generally the same as those for deep breathing and coughing in addition to the following:

1. Moderate to large amounts of mucus produced. Wait 1 to 2 hours after treatment to see if patient expectorates secretions. Small amounts of *thick* mucus suggest dehydration and a need to push fluids before PD & PV can be effective. Thick mucus does not drain well.

2. Absence of damage to skin, soft tissues, bony structures, and internal organs. Percussion is never done over bare skin, but over a single layer of light clothing. This precaution and avoidance of nearby organs (Fig. 19–12) during PV help meet this criterion.

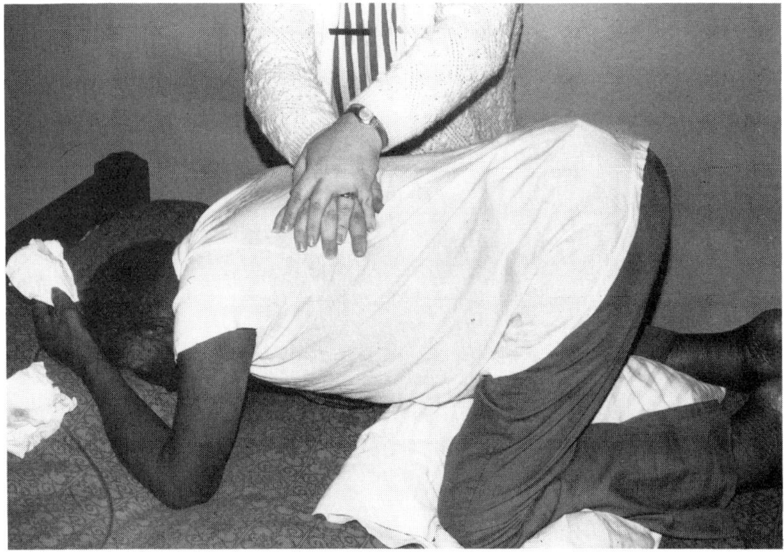

Figure 19–11. Vibration over the left lower lobe with the patient in a head-down position, on arms and knees.

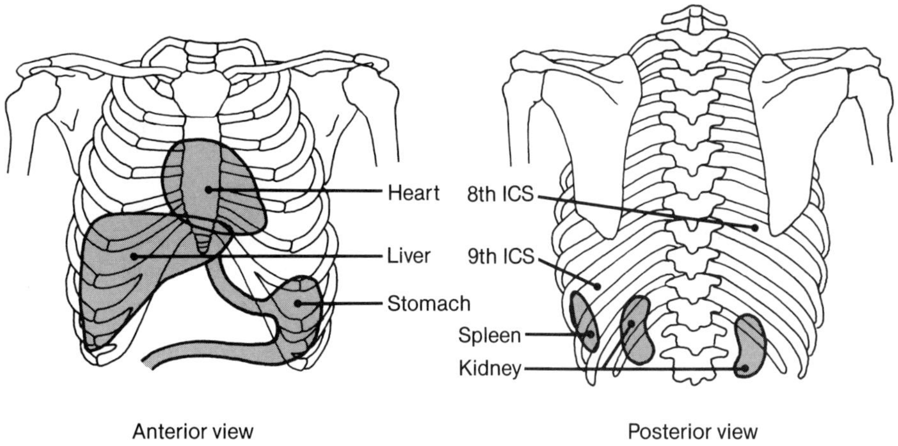

Figure 19–12. Relationship of internal organs (shaded gray) to the bony thorax. These organs are avoided during percussion of the chest wall. (ICS = intercostal spaces.)

3. Absence of signs of hypoxemia, bronchoconstriction, increased dyspnea, increased airway obstruction, drastic changes in blood pressure, and increased arrhythmias.

If necessary, elevate the head of the bed to avoid adverse effects, check with the physician regarding additional supplementary oxygen, or do both.

IMPLEMENTATION

Staff use this general procedure for a PD & PV treatment:

GENERAL PROCEDURE FOR STAFF

1. Check the chart or referral form for orders and possible contraindications.
2. Within prescribed orders, plan a treatment that takes into consideration physical findings, x-ray findings, and physical tolerance.
3. Give the treatment. In each PD position
   a. Percuss 20 to 30 seconds and vibrate 3 to 4 times, as tolerated.
   b. Ask the patient to cough or huff.
   c. Drain 5 to 10 minutes or until clear.
4. Chart the effects of therapy, including changes in breath sounds, adventitious sounds, quantity and quality of sputum.

Once the home patient experiences an effective treatment and the family observes at least one treatment, the nurse teaches one or more family members to perform PV.

Partial Versus Complete Postural Drainage

The physician may leave the decision regarding partial or complete postural drainage to the nurse and therapist caring for the patient. Partial drainage, consisting of the four positions or similar positions illustrated in the previous patient information section, is quite sufficient for most COPD patients. Position 4 is preferred by many disabled persons over other methods of draining the lower lobes because it requires no position aids. Compliance is increased because implementation is simple. The patient can easily position himself on the floor or bed, as shown in Figure 19–11. Many patients claim increased security and relaxation in this position, as opposed to a head down position over the edge of a bed or on a slanted board.

In contrast, patients with cystic fibrosis and bronchiectasis and others who produce well over 30 ml of sputum daily may require complete PD with implementation of all or most of the body positions presented in Figure 19–13.

SEQUENCE FOR REMEMBERING BODY POSITIONS FOR COMPLETE POSTURAL DRAINAGE

Head of bed up 60 to 75 degrees
- Apical segments of upper lobes
- Left posterior segments

Bed flat
- Right posterior segments of upper lobe
- Superior segments of lower lobes
- Anterior segments of upper lobes

Foot of bed 12 inches in Trendelenburg's position
- Lateral and medial segments of right middle lobe
- Lingular segments of left upper lobe

Foot of bed up 14 to 18 inches in Trendelenburg's position for lower lobe segments
- Anterior (medial) basal
- Lateral basal
- Posterior basal

Text continued on page 551

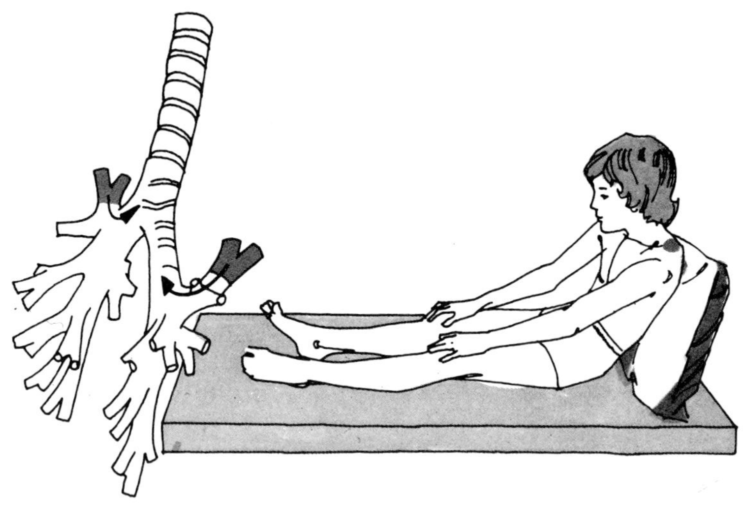

Figure 19–13. Positions for complete postural drainage (in sequence). Percussion areas are shaded gray, when visible in the illustrations. (Adapted and reproduced by permission from Hilman, B. The "How" and "Why" of Bronchial Drainage—A Guide for Your Home Care Program. New York, Breon Laboratories (Winthrop-Breon Company), 1978. Copyright, Sterling Drug, Inc.)

Apical segments, UPPER LOBES
Bed flat. Patient leans back on pillow at 30-degree angle, or elevate head of bed 60 to 75 degrees. Arms forward. Percuss over area between clavicle and top of scapula on each side.

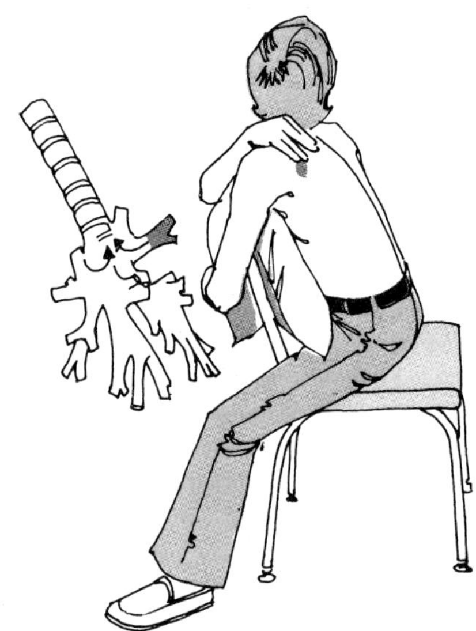

Posterior segments, UPPER LOBES
Choose upright or reclining position.

Upright position for left and right posterior segments
Patient sits in chair and leans over folded pillow at a 30-degree angle (left posterior segment) or at a 45-degree angle (right posterior segment). Arms forward. Percuss over back.

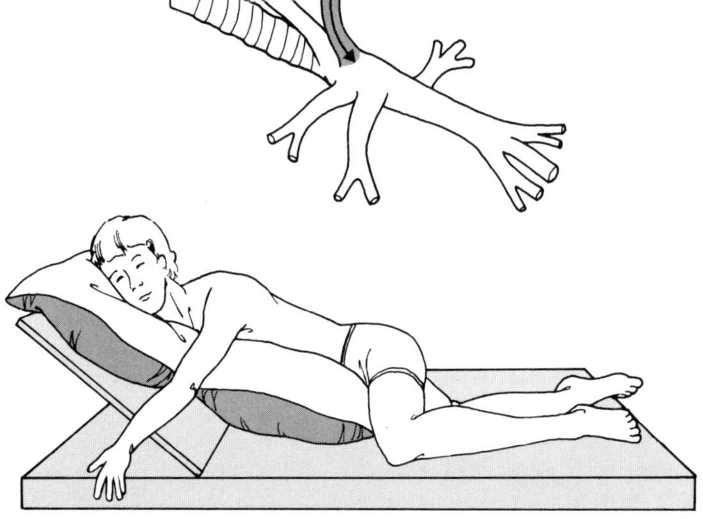

Reclining position for left posterior segment
Head of bed elevated 45 degrees. Patient lies 45 degrees from prone position. Right arm outstretched behind. Left arm extended forward or hanging over edge of bed. Left knee and hip flexed. Percuss upper back.

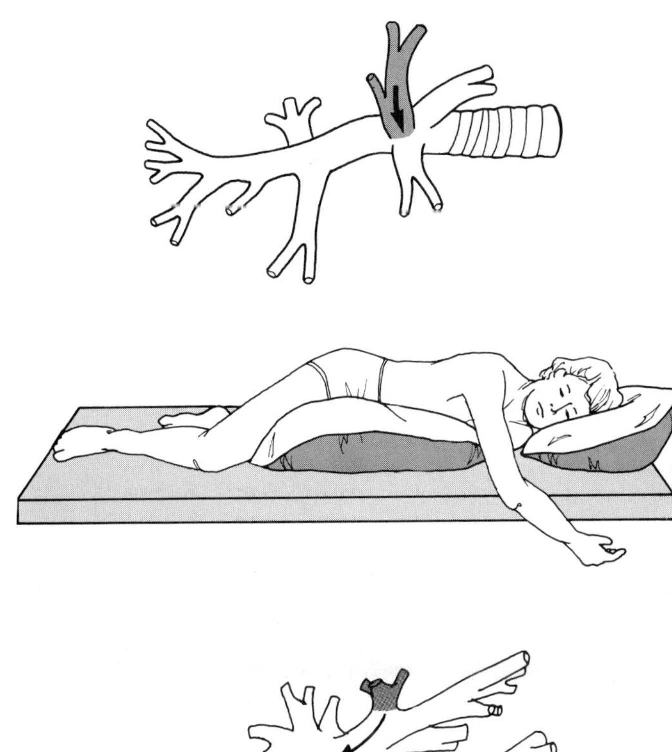

Figure 19–13 *Continued*
Reclining position for right posterior segment
Bed flat. Patient lies 45 degrees from prone position. Left arm outstretched behind. Right arm extended forward or hanging over edge of bed. Right knee and hip flexed. Percuss upper back.

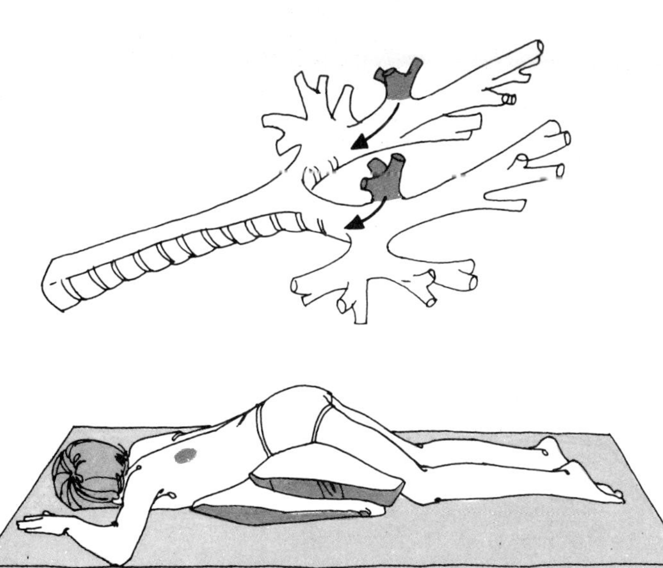

Superior segments, LOWER LOBES
Bed flat. Patient lies on abdomen with pillows under hips. Arms forward. Percuss area between T4 or below tip of scapula on either side of spine.

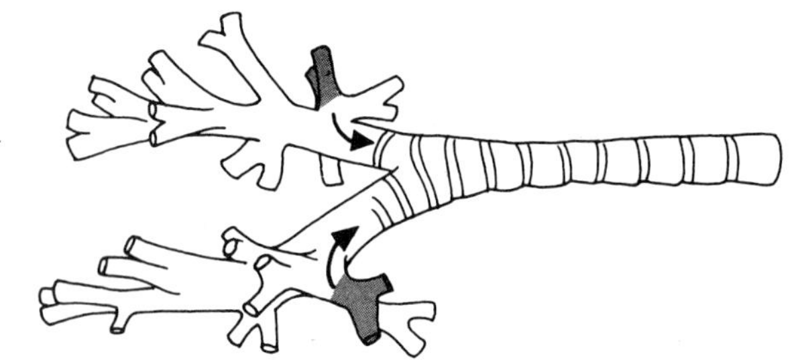

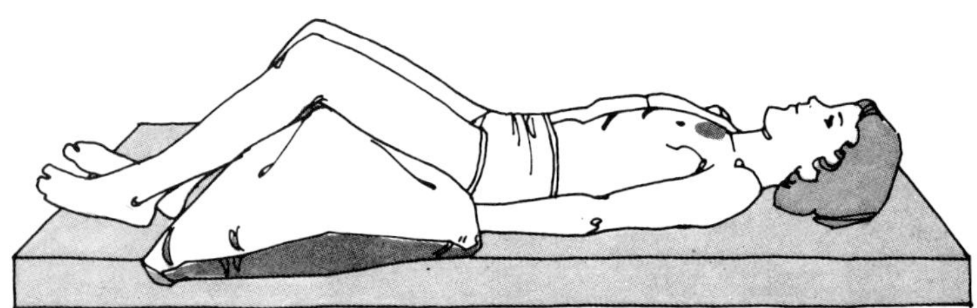

Figure 19–13 *Continued*
Anterior segments, UPPER LOBES
Bed flat. Patient lies supine with pillow under knees. Percuss between clavicle and 4th rib or nipple on each side of chest.

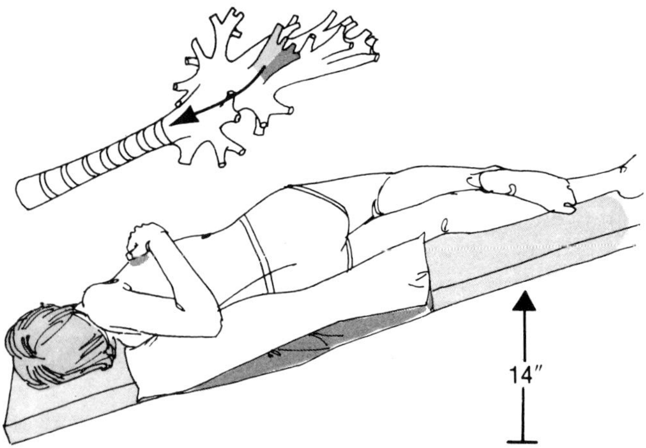

Lateral and medial segments, RIGHT MIDDLE LOBE
Foot of bed elevated 12 to 14 inches (15 degrees). Patient lies supine and turns 45 degrees to the left. Place pillow behind patient to support shoulder, back, and hip. Knees flexed. Percuss anterior chest just below 4th rib or nipple.

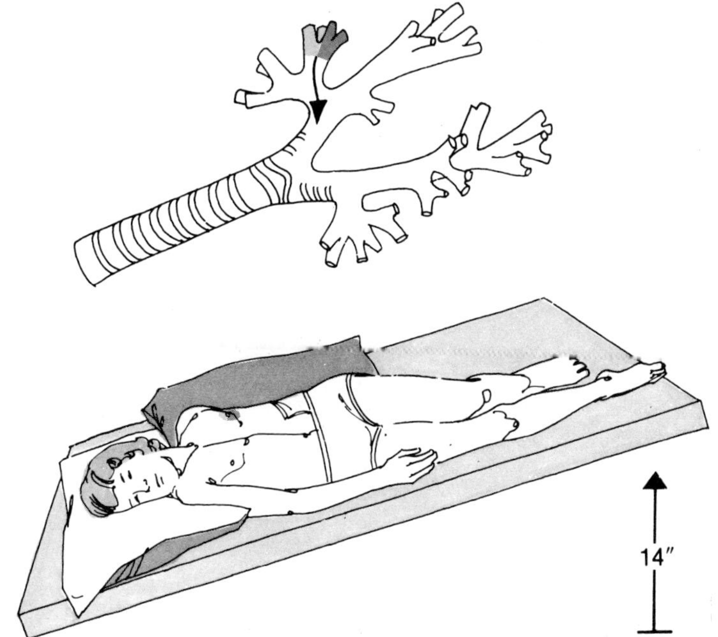

Figure 19–13 *Continued*
Lingular segments, LEFT UPPER LOBE
Foot of bed elevated 12 to 14 inches (15 degrees). Patient lies supine and turned 45 degrees to the right. Place pillow behind back for support. Knees flexed. Percuss over left nipple area.

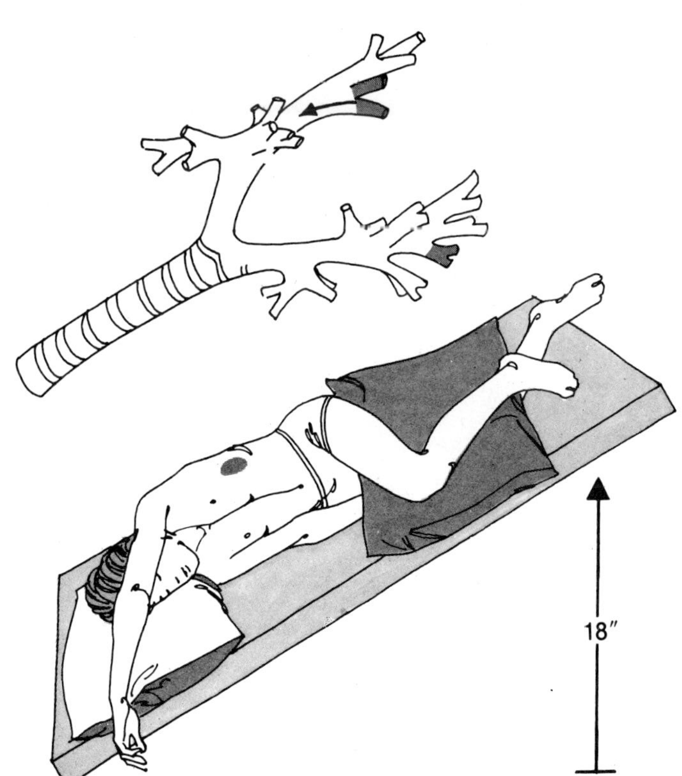

Anterior (medial) basal segments, LOWER LOBES
Foot of bed up 14 to 18 inches (30 degrees). Patient lies on side with upper leg flexed over a pillow for support. Supine position is also acceptable. Percuss over lower ribs, anterior axillary line.

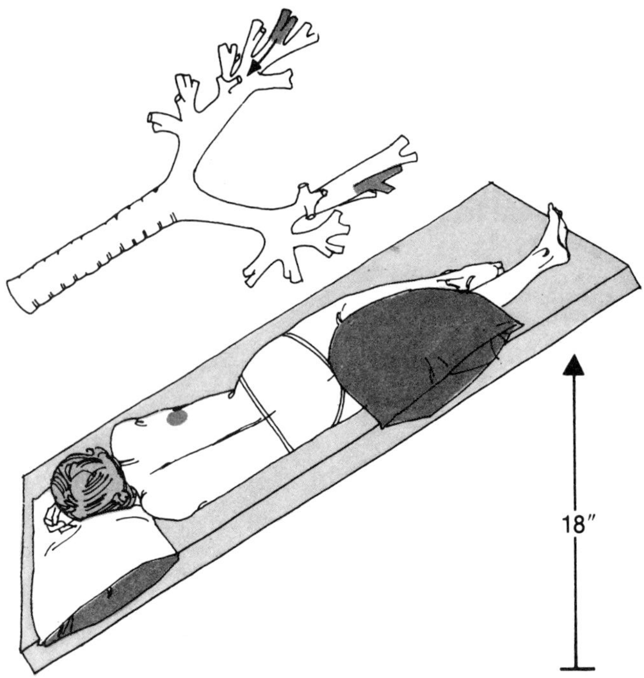

Figure 19–13 *Continued*
Lateral basal segments, LOWER LOBES
Foot of bed elevated 14 to 18 inches (30 degrees). Patient turns to far right or left side. Upper leg flexed over a pillow for support. Percuss over uppermost portion of lower ribs.

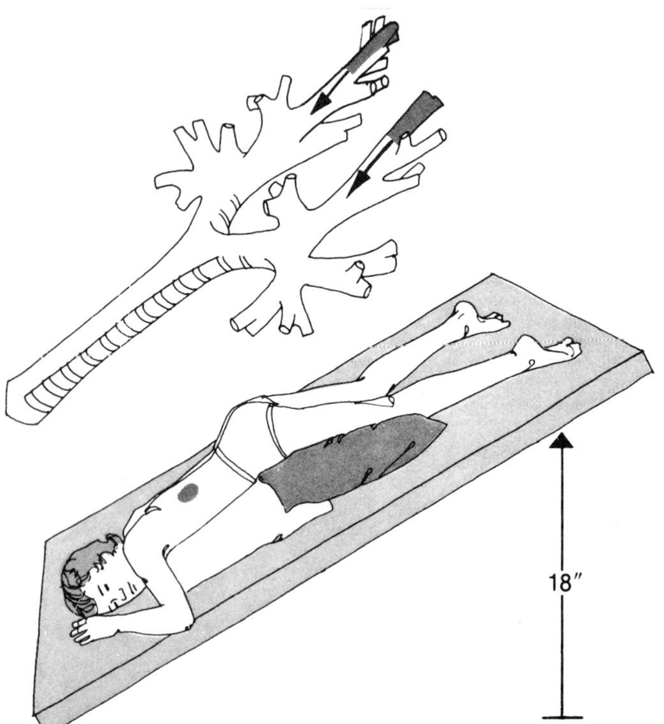

Posterior basal segments, LOWER LOBES
Foot of bed elevated 14 to 18 inches. Patient lies on abdomen, with pillow under hips and thighs. Spine should be straight. Percuss over lower ribs close to spine on each side of chest.

The practice schedule and evaluation criteria for complete PD and PV are the same as those already listed for partial drainage. However, frequency of treatments may be reduced to QD or BID, with supplementary partial drainage during treatment intervals as needed.

As for partial drainage, the lungs are drained from top to bottom; other positions are added between upper lobe and posterior basal positions to accommodate all lung segments. Additions and deletions are made without altering the proper drainage sequence. For complete PD and PV, the head of the bed always moves from high Fowler's position to Trendelenburg's position as shown in the last box on page 545.

Not all patients tolerate complete PD and PV. However, many young patients with chronic bronchitis or cystic fibrosis require aggressive chest physiotherapy and are able to comfortably perform complete PD and PV with use of a hospital bed, portable postural drainage positioner, or other aid for positioning, such as a slant board, magazines or newspapers tied in a stack, or a bean bag chair. Moreover, older, more disabled patients may tolerate complete PD and PV during an acute exacerbation with use of appropriate positioning aids and supplementary oxygen to prevent hypoxemia.

Modifying Standard Procedure

The effectiveness of PD and PV largely depends on two factors: (1) the nurse's assessment skills, i.e., the ability to recognize mucus-filled lung regions, which invariably change from day to day or week to week; and (2) the nurse's ability to modify drainage positions and duration and intensity of PV, according to changing chest assessment findings and physical tolerance. As with other respiratory treatments, modification of standard procedure is the rule rather than the exception.

The following are suggestions to help patient and nurse modify therapy appropriately:

1. Keep a copy of positions for partial and complete PD in the clinical setting for quick reference.
2. Auscultate the chest to identify pathologic segments, i.e., segments with abnormal breath sounds, rhonchi, and crackles. Look at the chest x-ray if available.
3. Check with the patient to see if he is aware of rhonchal fremitus over pathologic segments or other signs of mucus retention. Eventually the patient must learn to modify positions without outside help.
4. Plan therapy to concentrate on pathologic segments. These segments are top priority.
   a. Use the four basic drainage positions. Use Figure 19–13 as a guide for adapting and adding extra positions to accommodate pathologic segments not reached by these basic positions.
   b. Prolong PV and drainage times over pathologic segments.
5. Plan positions appropriate to the patient's acuity level and exercise tolerance.
   a. For dyspneic patients, drain posterior segments in the supine rather than Trendelenburg's position. If necessary, raise the head of the bed slightly.
   b. For exhausted patients, restrict drainage to pathologic and posterior segment positions.
   c. Eliminate less crucial drainage positions.
   d. Encourage use of oxygen during and 30 minutes after therapy to prevent hypoxemia.
6. Keep patient and family actively involved in the planning and implementation of therapy.
   a. Show pictures of ideal drainage positions so that patient and family understand the necessary positioning for effective treatment.
   b. Encourage patient and family to think of creative, convenient, and economic ways to achieve optimal positioning at home when means are limited. Unless staff try the patient's ideas, the patient may discontinue or alter therapy on his own, sometimes to his disadvantage.
   c. Advise the patient to report trends toward decreased or increased sputum production. These signs indicate a need for reassessment and either discontinuation or modification of therapy.

Alternatives to Manual Percussion and Vibration

Two problems commonly arise in the implementation of PV. First, percussion and vibration are difficult techniques to master. In spite of intensive instruction, some persons never perform them well enough to effectively and consistently drain retained secretions from the lungs. Second, no one may be available to perform PV at scheduled times.

To work around these problems, the nurse may train two persons instead of just one in the home, one serving as an alternate. A neighbor or other volunteer may be recruited to implement therapy during a family member's working hours.

In addition, other alternatives to standard PV may be appropriate. The nurse may teach the patient to drain himself by combining huffing with selected drainage positions. As alluded to earlier, the forced exhalation technique (FET) clears more sputum in less time than conventional chest physiotherapy (Pryor et al, 1979).

The patient may percuss anterior and lateral chest areas himself, provided he can do so without sacrificing relaxation.

The family member who complains of general fatigue, arthritis of the hands, or poor muscle strength in the wrists and arms may use a manual cup (Fig. 19–14) or a mechanical percussor (Fig. 19–15 and Fig. 19–16). A mechanical percussor with a speed selector is as effective as hand percussion (Maxwell and Redmond, 1979). Many individuals with cystic fibrosis routinely use mechanical percussion because, compared with hand percussion, it allows them to reach more chest surface with less exertion. Since they can perform most of the treatment themselves, this method

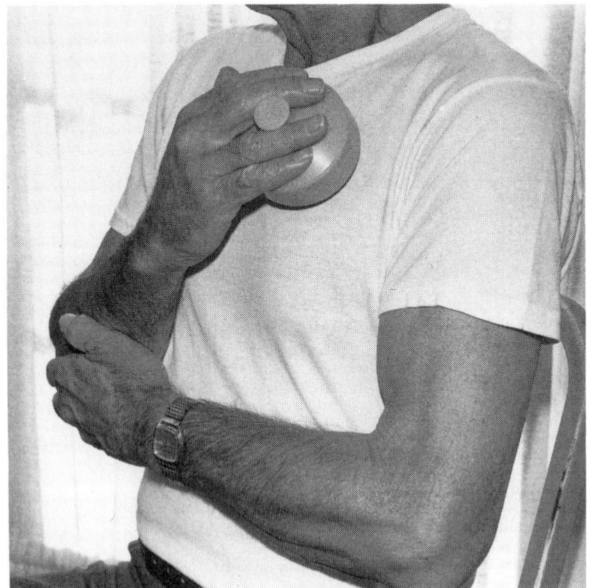

Figure 19–14. Use of a manual (palm) cup for self percussion over the left upper lobe. (Manual percussor 240, DHD Medical Products, Canastota, New York.)

allows them more independence, more control over their daily schedules, and more positive self concepts.

Some patients may use an automatic mechanical percussor that straps onto the chest for independent percussion of posterior lung segments (Fig. 19–17). In these cases, the nurse should caution the patient to securely position the percussor. If it becomes loose and slides off the chest, trauma may occur to kidneys and soft tissues in the vicinity.

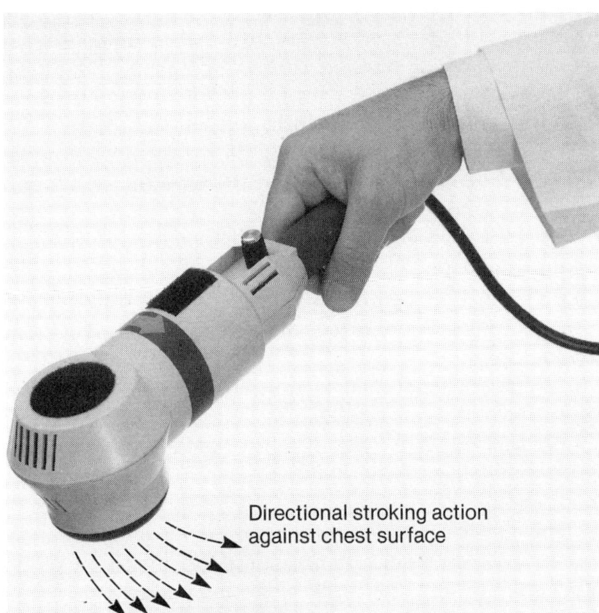

Figure 19–15. Vibracare mechanical percussor. The percussor's directional stroking action has two force components as follows: (1) an up-and-down movement against the chest to loosen mucus (incorporated into most mechanical percussors) and (2) an additional stroking movement parallel to the chest to promote drainage towards the mouth. (Courtesy of General Physiotherapy, Inc., St. Louis, Missouri.)

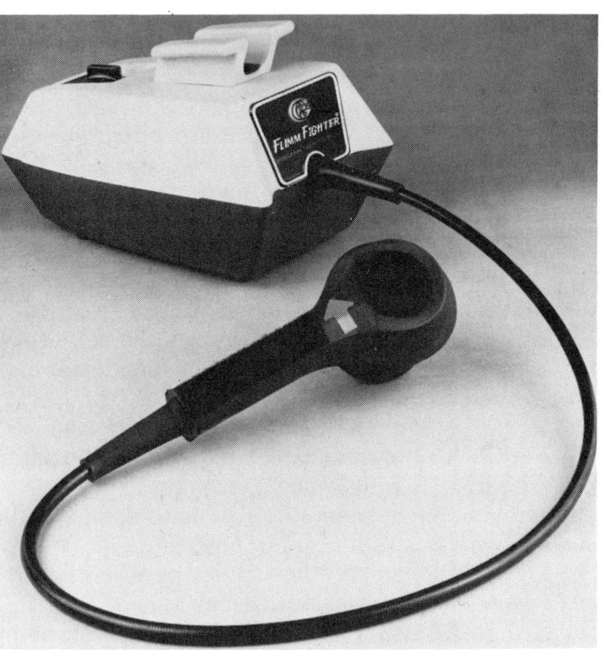

Figure 19–16. Flimm Fighter mechanical percussor with directional stroking feature for home use. (Courtesy of General Physiotherapy, Inc., St. Louis, Missouri.)

Some patients who agree to try a mechanical percussor revert to a small commercial hand vibrator. Though not intended for PD and PV, this relatively inexpensive drugstore item sends fine vibrations through the chest, thus helping the patient raise secretions in a less expensive and obtrusive way. Though clinical experience with commercial vibrators appears favorable, research applicable to adults is lacking. Such a device may be useful in adults who tolerate manual percussion poorly or who are prone to rib fractures. In a study involving neonates, vibration with a mechanical toothbrush resulted in a higher PaO_2 compared with vibrations with a padded nipple or no vibrations (Curran and Kachoyeanos, 1978).

Monitoring for Complications

During PD and PV, the nurse monitors the patient for signs of complications. Primary complications in acute and chronic care settings with interventions aimed at reducing their incidence are listed in Table 19–3. Otherwise, the best method of preventing complications is careful consideration of indications and contraindications before therapy is ordered.

The Acute Setting

Basic principles for PD and PV in the acute care setting are the same as those for the home setting. Methodology is also the same, since in both the nurse must modify drainage positions to accommodate the

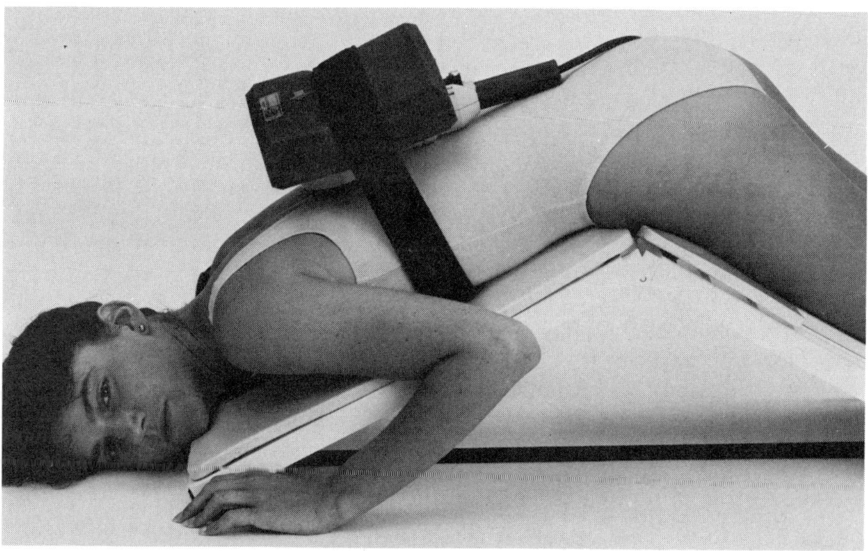

Figure 19–17. Velcro belt system for self application of mechanical percussion to the posterior segments of the lungs. The individual is lying on a portable tilt table to promote bronchial drainage during percussion. (Courtesy of General Physiotherapy, Inc., St. Louis, Missouri.)

Table 19–3. COMPLICATIONS OF POSTURAL DRAINAGE WITH PERCUSSION AND VIBRATION

Complications	Interventions to Decrease Incidence
Increased intracranial pressure From Trendelenburg's position, coughing, and physical stimulation	Use PD & PV with caution in neurologic patients and only as instructed by the physician. Emphasize huffing instead of coughing. Modify drainage positions, e.g., keep head of bed up 20 to 30 degrees; concentrate on lateral positions; use gentle PV or omit it. Use intracranial pressure (ICP) monitoring (critical care). Apply therapy only as long as ICP remains within normal range.
Hypoxemia Most common in these situations: Low resting Pa_{O_2} before therapy Cardiovascular instability Minimal sputum production (Connors et al, 1980) Copious sputum production (Gormenzano and Branthwaite, 1972) Unilateral chest infiltrate with "bad" side down	Provide O_2, as ordered by physician, to patients with low resting Pa_{O_2}, Pa_{O_2} below 60 mmHg, or copious sputum production. Withhold or discontinue therapy if sputum production falls below 25 to 30 ml per day. Withhold therapy if cardiovascular status becomes unstable or patient complains of increasing dyspnea. Drain unilateral chest infiltrate with "bad" side up, good side down.
Wheezing or decreased expiratory flow rate From bronchospasm, airway hyperirritability, or incomplete clearance of mucus from large airways	Schedule bronchodilator aerosol 20 minutes before therapy to decrease bronchospasm, open airways, and facilitate drainage. Allow adequate drainage time in last PD position. Encourage use of sustained maximum inspiration during therapy. Suction prn inability to deep breathe and expectorate mucus.
Decreased cardiac output and tissue oxygen delivery From increased O_2 consumption during therapy, decreased venous return (from increased intrathoracic pressure), low intravascular volume, failure of compensatory mechanisms in unconscious or acutely ill patients, or any combination thereof	Monitor pulse, heart rhythm, respirations, and blood pressure during treatment of acutely ill patients. Withhold treatment if tachycardia (over 120 beats/min), other arrhythmias, tachypnea, hypertension, hypotension, or signs of hypoxemia develop. Measure Pa_{O_2}, $P\bar{v}_{O_2}$, and cardiac output after therapy to assess possible hypoxemia and alteration in cardiac output. Use modified PD positions and gentle PV, as tolerated, in patients with cardiac conditions or potential hemodynamic instability.
Rib fractures From PV Most likely in elderly patients with osteoporosis and steroid dependency	Emphasize PD and huffing (without PV) for high risk patients. Use gentle PV for the elderly.
Pulmonary hemorrhage From tissue trauma, necrosis, or pulmonary vessel rupture into an adjacent bronchus Most likely with coagulopathy and when "bad" lung is in dependent position	Do not use PV in any bleeding state of the lung. Use PD with extreme caution in patients with a coagulopathy, lung contusion, or lung abscess. Discontinue therapy immediately if hemoptysis occurs. Ready suction and intubation equipment in case of sudden vessel rupture and impending exsanguination.
Tissue trauma to Soft tissues of skin Skeletal muscle Kidneys and other vital organs	Do not use PV near vital organs. Avoid use of automatic mechanical percussors or securely strap to chest to avoid slippage. Encourage correct cupping technique. Discourage pounding on the chest. Discontinue therapy if signs of tissue trauma appear: skin discoloration, muscle ache, pain.

needs of dyspneic or disabled patients with borderline low Pao_2 levels.

In critical care, however, the patient's limited mobility in bed and unstable general condition may restrict drainage to positions 1, 2, and 3 (see the previous patient information section), except no pillow is placed under the hips in the lateral positions. The head of the bed may be flat or slightly raised at all times to prevent dyspnea, extreme discomfort, increased intracranial pressure, gastric reflux, or hemodynamic changes.

In addition, other modifications are usually necessary. PV are performed around surgical tubes and dressings and only as tolerated. Patients with thoracoabdominal incisions are given pain medication before therapy to maximize relaxation and, hence, drainage. Several lateral segments may be percussed simultaneously to reduce treatment length to 15 to 20 minutes or as tolerated. The posterior basal segments are reached by turning the patient more laterally towards the prone position. Neurologic patients on CircOlectric beds or Stryker frames are always turned prone, whenever possible, to expand and drain posterior lung segments, those dependent segments that collect the most mucus. (See Mackenzie, 1981, for other modifications of PD and PV and mobilization methods in acute care settings.)

Which Lateral Position Is Best? For patients who need chest physiotherapy but do not tolerate it, the nurse regularly turns the patient every 1 to 2 hours. This routine aspect of nursing care is actually a form of PD. The following points help the nurse decide which side-lying position to place the patient in or which lateral position to utilize during PD and PV.

Patients with bilateral or absent lung infiltrates on the chest x-ray are turned laterally without a predilection for right or left side. Favoring one side promotes mucus retention in dependent lung segments.

Patients with unilateral disease are best drained with the "bad" side up. This approach permits mucus drainage into major bronchi by gravity. Also, local increased transpulmonary pressures facilitate reexpansion of collapsed alveoli and stabilization of other alveoli at a larger alveolar volume. The increased alveolar volume promotes drainage and helps prevent atelectasis.

Drainage of a unilateral chest infiltrate in the opposite lateral position, i.e., with the "bad" side down, is more likely to cause hypoxemia due to V/Q mismatch and intrapulmonary shunting. Remember that both ventilation and perfusion are normally increased in dependent lung regions (see Chapter 5). Placing the "bad" side down produces the following V/Q relationship in diseased, dependent lung regions:

"Bad" Lung Down

$$\frac{V\downarrow}{Q\uparrow} = \downarrow\downarrow\frac{V}{Q}\text{ ratio}$$

Venous admixture or capillary shunt occurs as pulmonary blood flows past partially or totally unventilated alveoli (see Chapter 13).

In spite of possible adverse effects of placing the "bad" side down, some patients with unilateral disease are treated in both lateral positions. The nonaffected lung is placed up to drain any secretions that might have drained into it during treatment of the affected lung. When both lateral positions are used, the nurse or therapist carefully monitors for signs of hypoxemia, particularly in patients with low baseline Pao_2 before therapy. Some investigators have found Pao_2 differences of as great as 100 mmHg between right and left lateral positions in critically ill patients (Tyler et al, 1980).

Conclusion

This chapter discusses basic chest physiotherapy techniques and associated interventions, including general relaxation, breathing retraining, deep breathing and coughing, and postural drainage.

It is hoped that this body of knowledge has prepared both the acute care and visiting nurse for use of chest physiotherapy whenever its indication arises in the clinical setting. It prepares the visiting nurse for implementation of techniques in the home setting. Once the patient integrates basic techniques with other aspects of respiratory care, he is ready for their integration with activities of daily living. Chapter 20 discusses breathing retraining during activities of daily living and various other forms of energy conservation, exercise, and muscle reconditioning.

REFERENCES

Bartlett, R.: Respiratory therapy to prevent pulmonary complications of surgery. *Respiratory care*, 29(6):667–677, 1984.

Benson, H. and Klipper, M.: Relaxation Response. New York, Avon Books, 1976.

Ben-Zvi, Z., Spohn, W., Young, S., and Kattan, M.: Hypnosis for exercise-induced asthma. *American review of respiratory disease*, 125(4):392–395, 1982.

Blegen, M.: Controlled breathing pattern in COPD. *Rehabilitation nursing*, 6(2):10–14, 1981.

Blodgett, D.: Relaxation techniques. In Home Care and Rehabilitation in Respiratory Medicine. Bell, C., Blodgett, D., et al–eds.). Philadelphia, J. B. Lippincott Co., 1984.

Breslin, E.: Prevention and treatment of pulmonary complications in patients after surgery of the upper abdomen. *Heart and Lung*, 10(3):511–519, 1981.

California Thoracic Society, Respiratory Care Assembly. *Criteria for the review of respiratory care services.* Oakland, California Thoracic Society, 1981.

Campbell, A., O'Connell, J., and Wilson, F.: The effect of chest physiotherapy upon the FEV_1 in chronic bronchitis. *Medical Journal of Australia*, 1(2):33–35, 1975.

Casciari, R., et al: Effects of breathing retraining in patients with COPD. *Chest*, 79(4):393–398, 1981.

Celli, B., Rodriguez, K., and Snider, G.: A controlled trial of IPPB, incentive spirometry, and deep breathing exercises in preventing pulmonary complications after abdominal surgery. *American review of respiratory disease*, 130(1):12–15, 1984.

Connors, A., Hammon, W., Martin, R., and Rogers, R.: Chest physiotherapy: the immediate effect on oxygenation in acutely ill patients. *Chest,* 78(4):559–564, 1980.

Curran, C. and Kachoyeanos, A.: A comparison of the effects of two methods of chest physical therapy on the oxygenation of neonates with respiratory distress syndrome. *American review of respiratory disease,* 117(4):201, 1978.

Dail, C., Rogers, M., Guess, V., et al: Glossopharyngeal Breathing Manual. Downey, California, Professional Staff Association, Rancho Los Amigos Hospital, 1979.

Frownfelter, D.: Chest Physical Therapy and Pulmonary Rehabilitation, 2nd ed. Chicago, Year Book Medical Publishers, Inc.

Gaskell, D., and Webber, B.: The Brompton Hospital Guide to Chest Physical Therapy, 4th ed. St. Louis, C. V. Mosby Co., 1981.

Gormenzano, J. and Branthwaite, M.: Pulmonary physiotherapy with assisted ventilation: arterial blood gas tension changes following pulmonary physiotherapy with IPPB. *Anaesthesia,* 27(3):249–257, 1972.

Graham, W. and Bradley, D.: Efficacy of chest physiotherapy and IPPB in the resolution of pneumonia. *New England Journal of Medicine,* 299(12):624–627, 1978.

Gramse, C.: Chest physiotherapy: make the most of this hands-on technique. *Nursing 85,* 15(1):32C–32G, 1985.

Hiller, F., Bone, R., and Wilson, F.: Prevention of postoperative respiratory complications. *Respiratory therapy,* 10(6):87–96, 1980.

Hillman, B.: The "How" and "Why" of Bronchial Drainage—A Guide for Your Home Care Program. New York, Breon Laboratories (Winthrop-Breon Company), 1978.

Hirschberg, G., Lewis, L., and Vaughan, P.: Rehabilitation—A Manual for the Care of the Disabled and Elderly, 2nd ed. Philadelphia, J. B. Lippincott Co., 1976.

Hodgkin, J., and Zorn, E., and Connors, G.: Pulmonary Rehabilitation—Guidelines to Success. Boston, Butterworth Publishers, 1984.

Holliday, J.: Biofeedback. In Pulmonary Rehabilitation From Hospital to Home (O'Ryan, J. and Burns, D.–eds.). Chicago, Year Book Medical Publishers, Inc., 1984.

Hughes, R.: Do no harm—cheaply. *Chest,* 77(5):582–583, 1980.

Indihar, F., Forsberg, D., and Adams, A.: A prospective comparison of three procedures used in attempts to prevent postoperative pulmonary complications. *Respiratory care,* 27(5):564–568, 1982.

Jones, N.: Physical therapy—Present state of the art. *American review of respiratory disease,* 110(6):132–136, 1974.

Jung, R., et al: Comparison of three methods of respiratory care following upper abdominal surgery. *Chest,* 78(1):31–35, 1980.

Kersten, L.: Your respiratory Home Care Program. (Patient booklet.) Berkeley, California, Herrick Hospital and Health Center of the East Bay, 1978.

Kirilloff, L., Rogers, R., and Mazzocco, M.: Does chest physical therapy work? *Chest,* 88(3):436–444, 1985.

Lederer, D., Van de Water, J., and Indech, R.: Which deep breathing device should the postoperative patient use? *Chest,* 77(5):610–613, 1980.

Luce, J., Tyler, M., and Pierson, D.: Intensive Respiratory Care. Philadelphia, W. B. Saunders Co., 1984.

Mackenzie, C. (ed.): Chest physiotherapy in the Intensive Care Unit. Baltimore, Williams & Wilkins, 1981.

Marini, J., Pierson, D., and Hudson, L.: Acute lobar atelectasis: a prospective comparison of fiberoptic bronchoscopy and respiratory therapy. *American review of respiratory disease,* 119(6):971–978, 1979.

Maxwell, M., and Redmond, A.: Comparative trial of manual and mechanical percussion technique with gravity assisted bronchial drainage in patients with cystic fibrosis. *Archives of disease in childhood,* 54(7):542–544, 1979.

Mazzocco, M., Owens, G., Kirilloff, L., and Rogers, R.: Chest percussion and postural drainage in patients with bronchiectasis. *Chest,* 88(3):360–363, 1985.

Mueller, R., Petty, T., and Filley, G.: Ventilation and arterial blood gas changes induced by pursed lips breathing. *Journal of applied physiology,* 28(6):784–789, 1970.

Murray, J.: The ketchup-bottle method. *New england journal of medicine,* 300(20):1155–1156, 1979.

O'Donohue, W.: National survey of the usage of lung expansion modalities for the prevention and treatment of postoperative atelectasis following abdominal and thoracic surgery. *Chest,* 87(1):76–80, 1985.

Petty, T. and Guthrie, A.: The effects of augmented breathing maneuvers on ventilation in severe chronic airway obstruction. *Respiratory care,* 16(3):104–111, 1971.

Pryor, J., Webber, B., Hudson, M., and Batten, J.: Evaluation of the forced expiration technique as an adjunct to postural drainage in treatment of cystic fibrosis. *British medical journal,* 2(6187):417–418, 1979.

Risser, N.: Preoperative and postoperative care to prevent pulmonary complication. *Heart and lung,* 9(1):57–67, 1980.

Shapiro, B., Peterson, J., and Cane, R.: Complications of mechanical aids to intermittent lung inflation. *Respiratory care,* 27(4):467–470, 1982.

Sharp, J.: Therapeutic considerations in respiratory muscle function. *Chest,* 88(2):118S–123S, 1985.

Stock, M., Downs, J., et al: Prevention of postoperative pulmonary complications with CPAP, incentive spirometry, and conservative therapy. *Chest,* 87(2):151–157, 1985.

Sutton, P., Parker, R., et al: Assessment of the forced expiration technique, postural drainage, and directed coughing in chest physiotherapy. *European journal of respiratory disease,* 64(1):62–68, 1983.

Sutton, P., Pavia, D., Bateman, J., and Clarke, S.: Chest physiotherapy: a review. *European journal of respiratory disease,* 63(3):188–201, 1982.

Tiep, B., Burns, M., et al: Pursed lips breathing training using ear oximetry. *Chest,* 90(2):218–221, 1986.

Tyler, M.: Complications of positioning and chest physiotherapy. *Respiratory care,* 27(4):458–466, 1982.

Tyler, M., Hudson, L., Grose, B., and Huseby, J.: Prediction of oxygenation during chest physiotherapy in critically ill patients. (Abstract). *American review of respiratory disease,* 121 (Part 2) (4):218, 1980.

Walsh, R.: Occupational therapy as part of a pulmonary rehabilitation program. *Occupational therapy for the energy deficient patient,* 3(1):65–77, 1986.

Ward, R., Danziger, F., et al: An evaluation of postoperative respiratory maneuvers. *Surgery, gynecology and obstetrics,* 123:51–54, 1966.

Energy Conservation and Exercise Conditioning

20

Main Objectives

1. **State the goals of energy conservation techniques, exercise conditioning, and respiratory muscle training.**
2. **Describe at least six ways to simplify work in the home.**
3. **Name the five indications for an exercise stress test.**
4. **Define the following terms: exercise prescription, oxygen prescription, training threshold, anaerobic threshold, inspiratory resistance training, hyperpnea training, maximum sustained ventilatory capacity.**
5. **Describe the pulmonary patient's physiologic and clinical responses to exercise.**
6. **State three indications and three evaluation criteria for arm exercises.**
7. **Explain how to help a patient implement a home walking program.**
8. **Describe the current role of respiratory muscle training in pulmonary rehabilitation.**

This chapter discusses energy conservation and exercise conditioning. Techniques presented are restricted to a few basic exercises because of the complexity of the pulmonary patient's overall intervention plan. Encouraging the regular practice of a few basic exercises is more realistic than encouraging several exercises that may be quickly and completely omitted when the patient is not feeling well.

Energy Conservation Techniques

GOALS

1. To decrease dyspnea and fatigue associated with activities of daily living.
2. To increase self confidence and independence.

INDICATIONS

1. Inability to perform activities of daily living (ADL).
2. Helplessness or anxiety associated with inability to perform ADL.

Energy conservation techniques are indicated for pulmonary patients who are unable to comfortably perform ADL, due to dyspnea, fatigue, inappropriate work and rest rhythms, poor body mechanics, poor organization of home resources, or other factors. Sometimes the need for intervention does not become evident until the nurse assesses dyspnea using a questionnaire, such as the one in Table 10–3. Use of this questionnaire helps the nurse decide which ADL the patient needs help with. In other cases, the patient denies dyspnea but complains of fatigue and helplessness in performing basic tasks. When the exact sources of fatigue are ambiguous, sharing basic energy conservation techniques (described hereafter) and visiting the home, if possible, facilitate discussion of possible problems and identification of specific ways to conserve energy.

PATIENT INFORMATION

Energy Conservation Techniques

Exercises and ADL will be easier and you will still have energy left over for pleasurable activities if you remember these points:

1. *Take your time.* Space activities over wide intervals of time to conserve energy and avoid fatigue.
   a. Allow for rest breaks.
   b. Do more activities while sitting, such as ironing, cooking, shaving, combing your hair, and washing dishes.
2. *Choose or arrange your physical surroundings* to enable you to perform routine activities with less energy.
   a. If getting up in the morning is difficult, lay out your clothing the night before. Use a footstool or long-handled shoe horn to put your shoes on.
   b. Avoid carrying groceries or using shoulder bags that may restrict chest expansion. Use grocery carts or bags with handles.
   c. Keep commonly used personal or household items within easy reach. You may have to rearrange your kitchen and use space savers, such as peg boards.
   d. Shop in a convenient, uncrowded grocery store. Make a grocery list and shop from one end of the store to the other.
3. *Remember to use pursed-lip breathing (PLB).* It helps prevent airway collapse, a problem for persons with chronic obstructive pulmonary disease (COPD). Also, it slows your breathing rate. PLB allows more old air to empty from the lungs and increases the amount of fresh air that reaches the lung's air sacs for gas exchange.
4. *When you are exerting the most effort, pursed-lip breathe out.* The lips are pursed during exhalation and always during exertional motions because these are the times when your airways are most likely to narrow or collapse. Airway collapse causes air trapping in the lungs and impairs gas exchange.
   a. When you *bend* over to tie your shoes, when you *lift* something up, or when you *push* open a swinging door, pursed-lip breathe out.
   b. Reaching is a little different. As you reach up to a cupboard, take a breath in. Chest expansion is easier when the arms go up. Breathe out as your arms return to your side.
   c. Changing position: when you change position (e.g., from lying to sitting or from sitting to standing), pursed-lip breathe out.

IMPLEMENTATION

Energy conservation techniques are best presented after the patient has implemented general relaxation and PLB while walking. However, when patients see no need for breathing retraining, utilization of principles of work simplification may still significantly reduce the energy required for basic tasks.

In addition to these interventions, the nurse may emphasize the work simplification suggestions in the next box, as indicated by the situation.

When energy conservation is a major patient concern, an occupational therapist (OT) is indicated for evaluation of self-care ability and implementation of energy conservation techniques for special needs. The OT is particularly useful in the home setting when the nurse is limited in time and resources for appropriate intervention.

Exercise Conditioning

GOALS

1. Increased exercise tolerance
2. Increased sense of well being
3. Decreased dyspnea and fear of exercise
4. Improved appetite and sleeping pattern
5. Increased ability to perform ADL

INDICATIONS

All respiratory patients without a medical contraindication to exercise. Conditioning in the form of a regular exercise program is the key to increasing exercise tolerance and improving the patient's ability to perform ADL. The physiologic mechanism is related

SUGGESTIONS FOR WORK SIMPLIFICATION

WORK ORGANIZATION

1. Organize equipment and supplies by grouping related items together, e.g., can opener by canned goods, laundry soap by the washing machine.
2. Group similar tasks together, e.g., washing hair during a bath or shower.
3. Eliminate unnecessary tasks, e.g., let dishes dry in the rack rather than drying them with a towel.
4. Alternate and spread out light and heavy household tasks over the day and week.
5. Use labor-saving devices, e.g., portable mixer, electric can opener, storage organizers in the kitchen.
6. Use easy work heights, e.g., table at elbow or waist height. If necessary, put wooden blocks under table or chair legs or buy leg extenders to achieve an appropriate work height.
7. Use long-handled items, such as dust pans, shoe horns, or sponges, to extend your arm reach with ease.
8. Equip the bath or shower with a chair, handrail, back scrubber, and rubber mat to avoid foot slippage.
9. Plan to work in a cool place. Plan stressful activities, such as gardening, in the cool of the morning, late afternoon, or early evening. Work will be easier to perform if you are comfortable.

WORK PERFORMANCES

10. Perform activities at an even pace, with slow, smooth movements. Avoid fast, jerky movements. Use slow, relaxed breathing.
11. Whenever possible, sit down to conserve energy and prevent pooling of blood in the legs.
12. Allow for 10- to 15-minute work breaks between activities.
13. Use both hands during work to increase efficiency.
14. Use the assembly line approach, e.g., assemble all supplies, sit down, and work from right to left or vice versa for tasks such as washing dishes and stuffing a turkey.
15. Use oxygen, if ordered, to help decrease dyspnea and facilitate work simplification.

to the decrease in tissue oxygen extraction during exercise from increased muscular efficiency, improved neuromuscular coordination, or both (Alpert et al, 1974).

OVERVIEW OF EXERCISE AND THE PULMONARY PATIENT

A brief overview of exercise and the pulmonary patient, including the exercise stress test, exercise prescription, and response to exercise, serves as a theoretic basis for exercise conditioning in the clinical setting.

The Exercise Stress Test

An exercise stress test is ordered for one or more of the reasons listed in the following box.

INDICATIONS FOR THE EXERCISE STRESS TEST

1. To aid in the evaluation of exercise intolerance.
2. To evaluate exercise capacity.
3. To monitor the electrocardiogram during exercise for the presence of ischemic heart disease or dangerous arrhythmias.
4. To assess the amount of oxygen needed during exercise, called the *oxygen prescription.*
5. To establish an exercise prescription for implementation of an exercise program.

The patient may be tested by treadmill walking, by ergometry (leg) on a stationary bicycle, or by a 6- to 12-minute walk. One of these tests may be supplemented by a bicycle-arm ergometer test to assess arm and upper shoulder mobility and muscle endurance (Fig. 20–1).

The treadmill stress test is usually the incremental type, as opposed to the single-stage submaximal test. It may involve sophisticated gas exchange studies in a pulmonary function laboratory, particularly during the initial assessment of the patient (Fig. 20–2A). The headgear attachments worn by the patient in Figure 20–2B allow measurement of oxygen consumption ($\dot{V}CO_2$), anaerobic threshold (AT), and numerous other parameters. In other rehabilitation settings, the treadmill test is simplified. The patient walks on a treadmill without the cumbersome headgear, nose plug, and breathing tube apparatus. Only a few parameters are monitored, such as blood pressure, to detect hypotension and hypertension; heart rate and rhythm, to detect cardiac arrhythmias; and arterial blood gases (ABGs), to detect hypoxemia, alveolar hypoventilation, and acidosis during exercise. In both acute care hospitals and rehabilitation settings, noninvasive continuous monitoring, such as ear or finger oximetry to estimate SaO_2, is used to assess hypoxemia and need for supplemental oxygen at various stages of work. Oxygen is applied during testing and training when PaO_2 is less than 55 mmHg or SaO_2 is less than 85% before or during exercise.

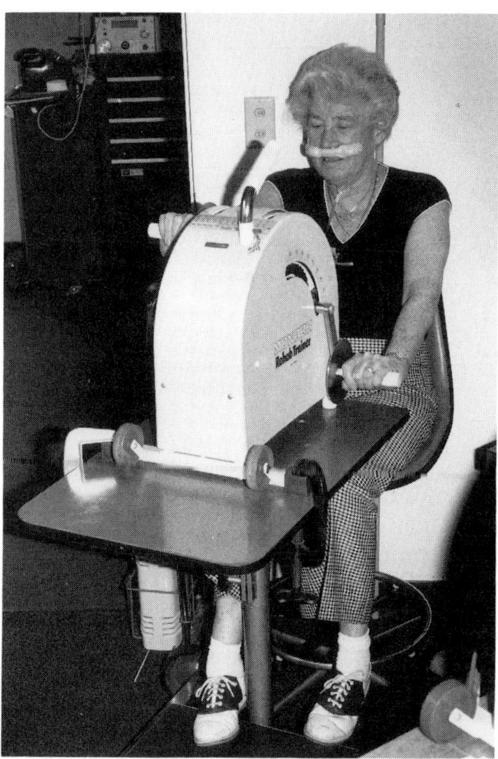

Figure 20–1. Bicycle-arm ergometry. A patient in a pulmonary rehabilitation program tests and trains on a bicycle-arm ergometer, while receiving supplementary oxygen via a reservoir nasal cannula (Oxymizer).

Exercise Prescription

Exercise stress test results interpreted in light of other clinical findings determine the patient's exercise prescription. In essence, the patient's *exercise prescription* is the physician's guidelines for *mode of exercise, intensity, duration,* and *frequency.* These factors are important in the determination of the patient's *training threshold,* the activity level associated with the physiologic effects of muscle conditioning. A recommended exercise prescription for the pulmonary patient is shown in Table 20–1.

Though the exercise prescription in Table 20–1 provides a helpful guideline for implementation of an exercise program for many pulmonary patients, experts do not agree on its usefulness for all pulmonary patients. In addition, they do not agree on the best method for outlining exercise prescription components, especially in the case of severe or disabling disease. The source of this controversy stems from a number of factors, including the pulmonary patient's unique response to exercise and the current incomplete understanding of the training effect after exercise in different lung disorders.

The Patient's Response to Exercise

The normal person is exercised in the laboratory until he achieves his maximum predicted target heart rate, as long as adverse ECG changes or cardiopul-

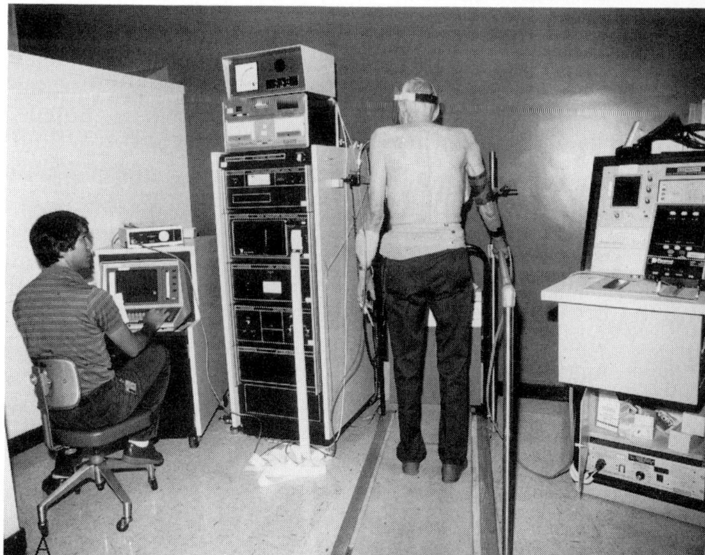

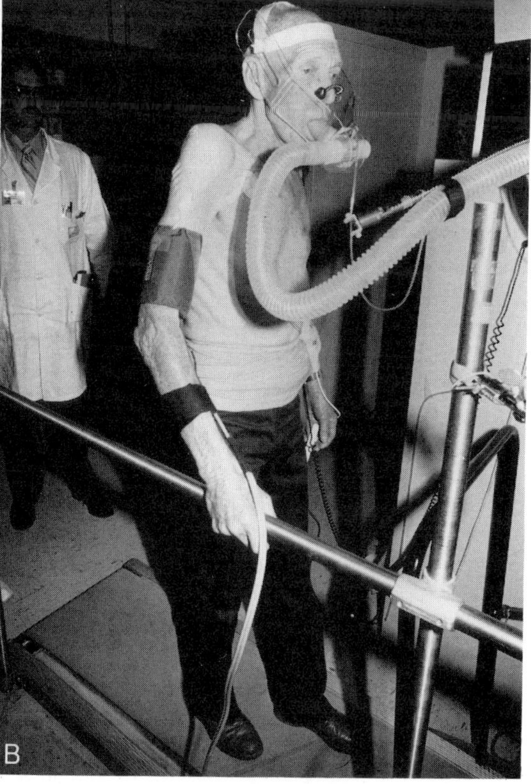

Figure 20–2. The exercise stress test in a pulmonary function laboratory. *A,* The respiratory patient walks on a treadmill, while staff continuously monitor blood pressure (cuff on right arm), heart rate, and rhythm (electrocardiogram electrodes on anterior chest area), Sa_{O_2} (finger oximeter sensor attached to left finger), and other parameters. *B,* The headgear, nose clip, and breathing tube apparatus allow sophisticated gas exchange studies to be done. (Courtesy of Allan Siefkin, M.D.)

Table 20–1. EXERCISE PRESCRIPTION FOR THE PULMONARY PATIENT

Components	Recommendations
Mode of exercise	Treadmill walking Stationary bicycle 6- or 12-minute walk
Intensity	Exercise to target heart rate of 60 to 70% of maximum heart rate (predicted on exercise stress test or calculated as follows: 220 − patient's age). or Exercise to at least 50% of maximal $\dot{V}O_2$ (oxygen consumption) or Exercise to tolerance
Duration	20 to 30 minutes per training session
Frequency	3 to 4 sessions per week for at least 4 weeks

(After Belman, M. and Wasserman, K.: Exercise training and testing in patients with COPD. *Basics of Respiratory Disease*, 10(2):1–6, 1981.)

monary symptoms do not develop. Normal sedentary subjects respond to this stress by increasing maximum oxygen consumption ($\dot{V}O_2$ max), cardiac output, and arteriovenous oxygen difference. Most patients are able to reach their target heart rate and AT without difficulty. *AT or anaerobic threshold*, a common term in exercise physiology, is defined as *the highest $\dot{V}O_2$ during exercise above which a sustained lactic acidosis occurs*. Exercise training results in a decreased heart rate and an increased stroke volume at any given level of exercise. In addition, AT significantly rises on a subsequent exercise stress test. This increase means that the patient is able to perform more work without the accumulation of blood lactate and significant change in blood pH. The patient's work capacity increases.

Unlike the normal person, the COPD patient's expected rise in $\dot{V}O_2$ with exercise is limited by dyspnea secondary to impaired ventilatory mechanics. Though maximum $\dot{V}O_2$ is a reliable guide to increased work capacity in a normal person, in a patient with COPD it is symptom linked at a level below the true $\dot{V}O_2$ max.

Similarly, heart rate is not a reliable indicator of work intensity in a pulmonary patient. Unlike the normal or cardiovascular patient, the dyspneic pulmonary patient typically stops exercising before reaching his target heart rate. The dyspnea is due to increased dead space ventilation (V_D/V_T), increased air trapping, and worsening V/Q ratios with progressive exercise. In other cases, the patient achieves a target heart rate of 110 to 130 beats per minute, but without a corresponding increase in cardiac output or workload. A training effect does not occur at the target heart rate. The physiologic reason for the lack of correlation between heart rate and workload is incompletely understood but is believed to be related to the pulmonary patient's more rapid increase in heart rate compared with normal due to a reduced stroke volume response (Belman and Wasserman, 1981). In spite of its limitations, heart rate is used in the clinical setting because it one of the few objective monitoring parameters readily available to patient and nurse.

For these reasons, the pulmonary patient often does not reach his AT on the exercise stress test. This and other parameters normally monitored for normal and cardiovascular patients may have limited clinical usefulness for pulmonary patients.

Though vigorous exercise is not tolerated by most patients with chronic pulmonary disease, submaximal exercise results in a training effect. In walking programs, progress is assumed as long as the distance walked gradually increases, and baseline heart rate remains unchanged or decreases. Modest progress is not always manifested in exercise test results, but it may significantly improve the patient's sense of well being and ability to perform ADL.

Since improvement in exercise endurance is usually greater when the patient is supervised by experienced personnel, all nurses are encouraged to become familiar with the basic exercises described in the next section. Moreover, keep in mind that the patient may continue to improve exercise endurance up to about 30 to 40 weeks after initiation of an exercise program. Then, exercise endurance tends to plateau (Belman, 1986).

BASIC EXERCISES

Basic reconditioning exercises are integrated with breathing retraining, as indicated by the clinical situation. The exercises described here are samples any nurse can implement. They will achieve a training effect when practiced regularly. In addition, the patient may practice other passive-active range of motion (ROM) exercises to meet special needs. A patient in a formal pulmonary rehabilitation program receives a more intensive program of muscle reconditioning.

PATIENT INFORMATION

Reconditioning Exercises

Persons with respiratory problems tend to limit exercise to avoid the discomfort of becoming short of breath. Hence, the body's muscles become "out of condition." Poor exercise tolerance develops. Reconditioning exercises with the correct breathing pattern will strengthen your muscles and increase your exercise tolerance. If you practice the exercises regularly, you will develop an increased sense of well being and will be able to do more for yourself. Breathing at rest or with activity will become easier.

Walking

Start a home walking program (described on next page) and *walk every day*. A daily walk helps your heart, circulation, and lungs.

Arm Exercises

Arm exercises will recondition and strengthen your arm and shoulder muscles so that you can relax your upper chest better during normal breathing and carry or lift objects more easily.

Exercise 1

1. Sit comfortably with your back supported and your feet flat on the floor.
2. Breathe in through your nose as you raise your arms in front of you to shoulder height. Keep your arms straight.
3. Breathe out slowly as you lower your arms to your sides. Take at least twice as long to pursed-lip breathe out and lower your arms.
4. Repeat, only this time raise your arms in front of you as high as you can without straining.

Exercise 2

1. Start with your arms at your sides.
2. Breathe in through your nose as you extend your arms outward along your sides and upward as far as possible. Keep your arms straight.
3. Breathe out through pursed lips as you *slowly* lower your arms.

Exercise 3

This exercise will help you strengthen the muscles used for activities such as combing your hair.

1. Stand up or sit on the edge of a chair with your feet flat on the floor.
2. Breathe in through your nose as you reach up and touch the back of your neck with your fingertips. Keep your elbows up.
3. Pursed lip breathe out as you slowly bring your arms down and touch the back of your waist with the backs of your hands.

Leg Exercises

Exercise 1

1. Lie down in bed on your back with a pillow under your head.
2. *Relax.*
3. Breathe in through your nose.
4. Blow out gently through pursed lips as you slowly raise your knee to your chest.
5. Breathe in as you lower your leg to the bed.

Repeat this exercise a number of times, alternating legs and developing your own rhythm.

Tips

1. Ask your nurse which exercises are best for you and how to set up a practice schedule.
2. Whenever possible, do the arm exercises standing up so that you increase your tolerance to standing.
3. If you become dizzy, stop exercising, sit down, and rest.
4. Be careful to coordinate your breathing with the correct arm or leg movements. Do not hold your breath.
5. Do not stop between exercises. If absolutely necessary, stop between exercises for 30 to 90 seconds but no longer. If you stop for 2 minutes or more, you will lose the training effect.
6. After exercising, sit in a chair and rest for at least 5 minutes to cool down. *Do not lie down!* This is not good for your heart.

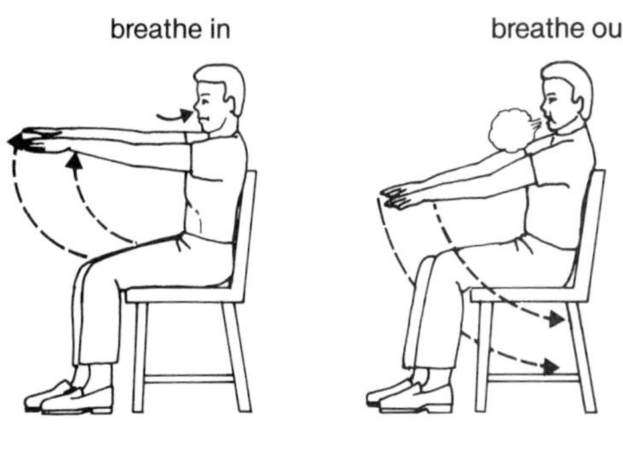

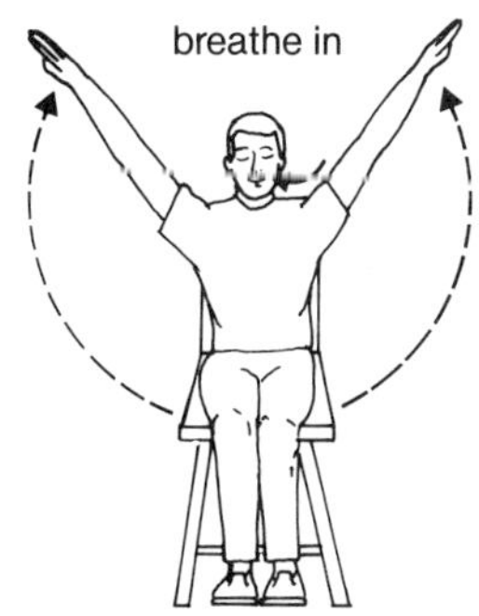

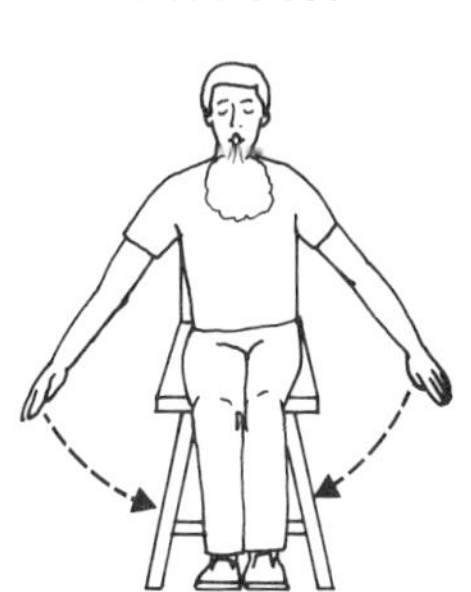

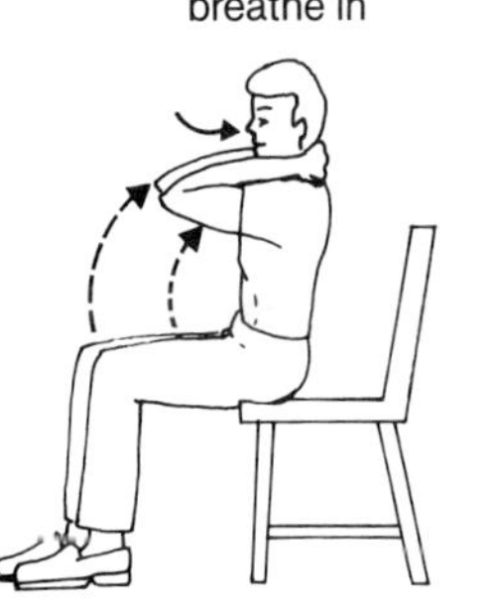

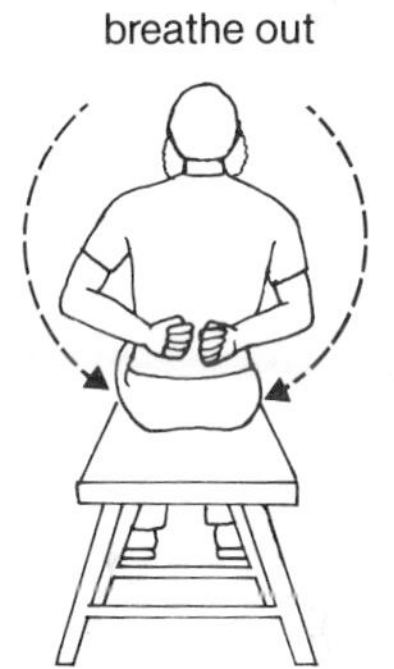

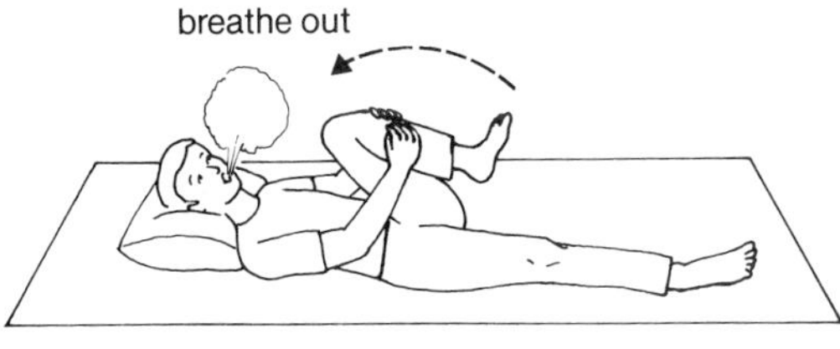

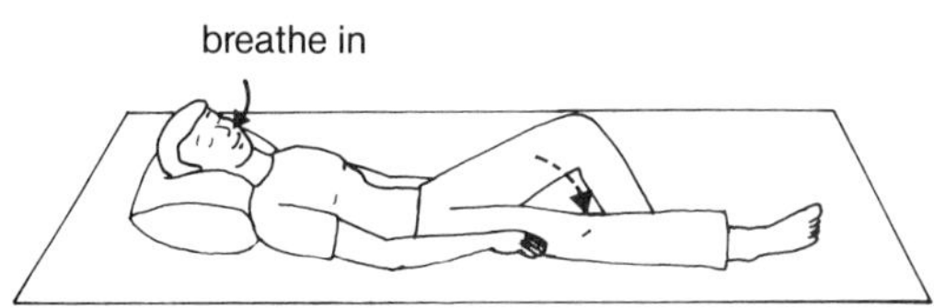

Arm Exercises

Indications

1. Tense patients with difficulties relaxing shoulders and upper chest muscles.
2. Patients with restricted mobility of the upper chest, shoulders, and arms.
3. Highly motivated patients who desire to further increase arm and shoulder strength and exercise tolerance.
4. Patients with mucus retention. Exercises help to loosen pulmonary secretions.

Practice Schedule

1. To begin, do exercises 1 and 2, 5 to 10 times each (referred to as 5 to 10 repetitions), 2 times a day. Schedule exercises after bronchodilator aerosol if prescribed. Arms and shoulders may be slightly sore at first, but patients usually report increased relaxation after 3 to 7 days.
2. Add Exercise 3. Gradually intensify schedule to 10 to 20 repetitions of each exercise a day as tolerated.
3. Add other exercises as advised by physical or occupational therapist.

Evaluation Criteria

1. Correct positioning: standing up straight or sitting up straight in a chair without arm rests.
2. Correct PLB pattern for COPD patients with no breath holding. Patients who know how to do abdominal-diaphragmatic breathing may use this technique as well.
3. End-expiratory position looks relaxed *with shoulders completely dropped.*
4. Absence of excessive fatigue, gasping respirations, chest pain, marked tachycardia or irregular pulse, dizziness, signs of hypoxemia.

Leg Exercises

Indications

1. Patients unable to increase or maintain exercise tolerance by walking (e.g., those on bedrest or those with restricted activity inside due to inclement weather).
2. Patients who request or are ready for leg exercises to further increase exercise tolerance as well as perfusion and ventilation to the lung bases.

Practice Schedule

1. Initially, for 5 minutes twice a day, using one leg at a time with brief 30- to 90-second rest periods in between if necessary.

Evaluation Criteria

1. Slow, well-coordinated leg movements.
2. Correct use of PLB.
3. Absence of excessive fatigue, gasping respirations, chest pain, marked tachycardia or irregular pulse, dizziness, signs of hypoxemia.

WALKING

Most COPD patients prefer walking over any other form of physical exercise (Fig. 20–3). Patient information for a home walking program is described hereafter.

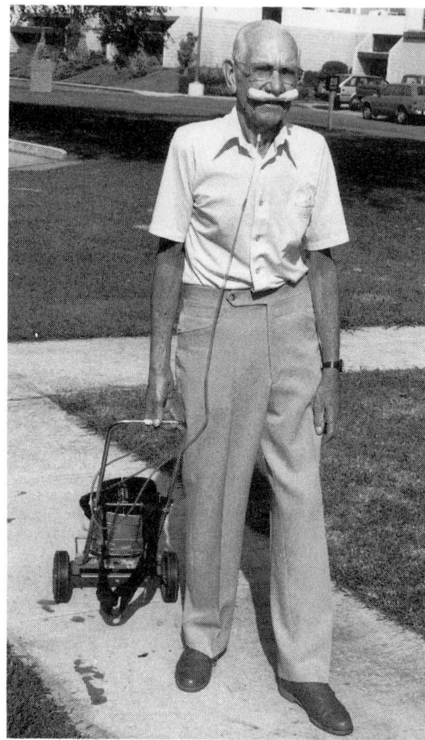

Figure 20–3. Patient walks with a portable liquid oxygen system and oxygen conserving device. The reservoir nasal cannula (Oxymizer) allows the patient to exercise and carry out activities of daily living away from home for extended periods of time. (See Chapter 23.)

PATIENT INFORMATION

Starting A Home Walking Program

Walking is one of the best forms of regular exercise. To get started on a home walking program, decide to take a walk today. The answers to the questions that follow will help you determine an appropriate walking time, walking pace, and weekly frequency so that your body will benefit from the exercise.

For how long should I walk? How far should I go?

Your walking duration is based on time not on distance. To get started, walk as far as you can without stopping and without becoming extremely short of breath. Use a watch to determine the time in minutes that it took you to walk this distance. Gradually increase this walking time over several days or weeks as directed by your nurse. Use the following chart as a guide.

Day or week	1	2	3	4	5	6	7	8	9	10
Walking time (minutes per day)	5	7	9	11	13	15	17	19	21	23

1. You may increase walking time more rapidly and walk up to at least 60 minutes each day.
2. Some people find it more convenient to divide their walking time in half and walk twice a day.

3. If you are extremely short of breath, try walking in intervals. For example, walk 5 minutes, rest 1 to 2 minutes, walk 5 more minutes. The next week, try 10 minutes of continuous walking.

What should be my walking pace?

Your walking pace must be slow enough to avoid severe shortness of breath and respiratory panic. At the same time, it must be fast enough to challenge your leg, heart, and respiratory muscles. Otherwise, you will not train your muscles.

1. Remember that mild to moderate shortness of breath is a normal response to exercise. Instead of being afraid of it, recognize it and use your breathing retraining techniques to control it.
2. Your nurse will teach you how to take your pulse and assign you a heart rate to aim for at the peak of exercise. Walk fast enough to increase your heart rate to your assigned heart rate of ___ beats per minute.
3. To monitor your pulse, take it:
   a. Before exercise to determine your baseline heart rate.
   b. *Immediately* after you stop walking to determine your peak exercise heart rate.
   c. Five minutes after exercise if you feel excessively tired or notice an excessively high heart rate or skipped heart beats.

How often should I walk?

Try to walk every day or at least 3 times a week. The following occurs when you change your walking frequency to

1. *Less than three times a week:* you decondition your muscles and lose the benefits of exercise. You may become frustrated because you cannot improve your walking time.
2. *Three to four times a week:* you maintain or slightly improve your exercise tolerance and develop a more positive self image.
3. *Five to seven times a week:* you greatly improve your exercise tolerance, sense of well being, and ability to cope with lung disease.

Where should I walk?

Walk outside on the level ground.

1. If hills are unavoidable, slow your pace while walking uphill and return to normal pace afterward.
2. Treat walking as an enjoyable recreational activity. For maximal enjoyment, walk in the park, in a safe neighborhood, or any place outdoors with pleasant surroundings.
3. During inclement or smoggy weather, walk indoors—at a local shopping mall or inside your house, room to room. Whatever the case, make a personal commitment to *stick to your exercise schedule!*

What are the danger signs of too much exercise?

Most people with lung disease do not have to worry about doing too much exercise because shortness of breath limits their exercise capacity. However, you should be aware of the following danger signs; they are most likely to occur if you have a heart problem in addition to lung disease.

1. Excessive fatigue lasting 1 to 2 hours after exercise
2. Chest pain
3. Gasping for air or feelings of suffocation
4. Dizziness or nausea
5. Heart rate noticeably faster than your assigned heart rate; your peak heart rate does not come down to your baseline heart rate after exercise
6. Skipped heart beats of no more than 5 to 10 beats per minute, if you have a history of skipped heart beats

Call your nurse or physician if any of these danger signs appear.

Should I stop walking if I'm having a "bad" day?

No! Reduce your walking time or slow your pace but continue to walk as tolerated. Stop walking only when you notice the previously mentioned danger signs.

1. Do not become discouraged. "Bad" days are a normal part of life with lung disease. Be flexible and learn to work around them.
2. When you feel better, gradually work up to your normal pace and walking time.
3. For moral support, plan to walk with your spouse or a friend. Do all you can to keep walking enjoyable!

Implementation

Patient and nurse set walking goals for each day or week in terms of distance in feet or city blocks or, preferably, walking time in minutes per day.

Alternative forms of exercise that achieve a similar training effect include swimming, bicycling on a stationary bicycle, and use of an exercise rebounder. The rebounder is a small trampoline that allows the patient to walk, bounce, or jog to the beat of a metronome, music, or other pace-setting method. The rebounder is indicated for young persons or those with a good sense of balance and coordination.

Implementation of a walking program is facilitated when the patient has had a recent exercise stress test. The nurse can more assuredly emphasize the benefits and safety of exercise. Limits for peak pulse, distance walked, exercise time, and amount of supplementary oxygen are set based on the patient's known response to exercise. When test results are available, the nurse obtains the exercise prescription from the physician, teaches the patient to take his own pulse, and encourages exercise congruent with the prescription (Fig. 20–4). During implementation, the nurse stresses the patient objectives in the box on the next page.

Monitoring during exercise is an important nursing duty, particularly when the patient has not had an exercise stress test to help determine a safe exercise prescription. In some cases, the patient's resting PaO_2 is normal, but the exercise PaO_2 is substantially reduced. Yet, since routine blood gases are always obtained at rest, hypoxemia during exercise may go undiagnosed for years because the patient exercises in the home, away from medical and ECG monitoring. Furthermore, if the patient has coexisting coronary artery disease, he is at risk for arrhythmias that appear only during exercise, when the body is stressed and the patient becomes increasingly hypoxemic. In this case, the physician may order 24-hour Holter ECG monitoring and a daily diary of patient activities to help determine the association of arrhythmias with ADL on the ward or at home.

PATIENT WALKING OBJECTIVES

1. To walk fast enough to achieve the assigned pulse rate (same as target heart rate in Table 20–1).
2. To gradually increase walking distance or time in minutes per day.
3. To increase supplementary oxygen to the prescribed level just before exercising and turn it back down within 5 minutes after exercising. If the patient complains of the extra cost of using more oxygen during exercise, encourage him to obtain an oxygen-conserving administration device (described in Chapter 23).
4. To consider oxygen as a tool rather than as a crutch. Liter flow may be increased to 2 to 5 L/min, depending on each patient's drop in oxygen saturation, to eliminate hypoxemia during exercise. The resultant relief of dyspnea, decreased minute ventilation, decreased pulse rate, and muscle reconditioning occur to a degree not obtainable when room air alone is used (Barach and Petty, 1975).
5. To consider oxygen as a training device. In some pulmonary rehabilitation programs, oxygen may be prescribed during rehabilitation, whether or not the patient demonstrates exercise-induced hypoxemia. The oxygen enables the patient to exercise at a higher workload than that possible without the supplementary oxygen. It is discontinued upon home discharge. Zack and Palange (1985) report that patients who breathe oxygen during training subsequently improve their performance while breathing room air at home.
6. To reduce the exercise goal if resting pulse rate is greater than 120 or postexercise pulse is greater than 145.
7. To use diaphragmatic breathing with PLB whenever possible. In severe COPD, the lungs are more effectively and efficiently ventilated with use of this technique at rest when compared with use of voluntary deep breathing (Petty and Guthrie, 1971). Casciari and associates (1981) showed that COPD patients receiving breathing retraining during exercise demonstrate greater increments in exercise performance, as evidenced by decreased respiratory rate, increased V_T, and increased Pa_{O_2}, compared with control subjects receiving no breathing retraining during exercise.
8. To stop exercising and consult the physician in case of adverse effects.

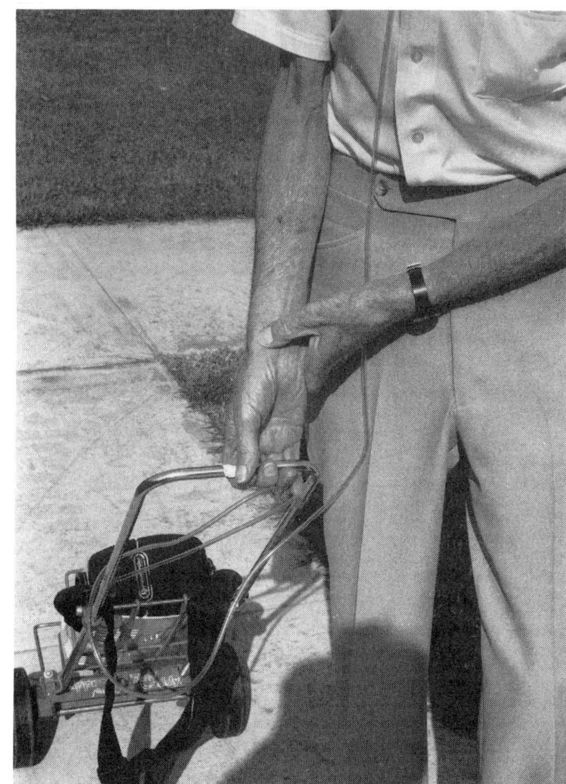

Figure 20–4. Self palpation of the radial pulse is performed to determine heart rate during exercise. (This individual with portable oxygen found it easier to use the thumb rather than forefingers to palpate his strong radial pulse.)

During walking, the nurse routinely monitors the following parameters:

1. Before walk
   a. Baseline pulse: palpate radial artery.
   b. Baseline respiratory rate.
2. At end of walk: while stopping to rest
   a. Peak pulse: instruct patient to lean against a chair, walker, or wall to take pulse.
   b. Peak respiratory rate.
3. After walk: pulse recovery time: measured from peak pulse to when pulse returns to baseline.

In addition, the nurse may monitor other parameters, such as blood pressure, level of dyspnea, and level of leg fatigue (i.e., cramps). The last two parameters are measured by Borg scale discussed in Chapter 10. A portable oximetry device may be used in the hospital, clinic, or home setting to noninvasively monitor Sa_{O_2} before, during, and after exercise (see Chapter 23). In some cases it replaces the ABGs during routine treadmill testing. In the home or ward setting, periodic oximetry monitoring helps the nurse make decisions about the safe implementation of a walking program in hypoxemic or borderline hypoxemic individuals.

After working with a patient, the nurse charts the following information: *distance walked; walking time; liter flow of oxygen;* Sa_{O_2} (if monitored); *baseline and peak pulses; recovery time; subjective response; adverse effects,* if present; and *reason for cessation of exercise,* e.g., leg cramps from lactic acidosis, anaerobic metabolism, or respiratory alkalosis.

During exercise conditioning, the patient's supplementary oxygen may be gradually reduced by 1 L/min. More specifically, a reduction in oxygen is ordered when (1) Sa_{O_2} improves and still remains over 85% and (2) when pulse recovery time improves and is less than 5 minutes. An ABG on room air is always taken before oxygen discontinuation. Many patients who do well on 1 to 3 L/min of oxygen exercise poorly on room air.

Evaluation Criteria

1. Pulse increase (i.e., peak pulse minus baseline pulse) no greater than 20 to 30% of baseline pulse (Frownfelter, 1978).
2. Pulse recovery period no greater than 5 to 10 minutes. The pulse should return to within 10% of baseline pulse within 5 to 7 minutes (Frownfelter, 1978).
3. Absence of signs of hypoxemia. Sa_{O_2} greater than 85%.
4. Absence of excessive fatigue; gasping respirations, but some fatigue and dyspnea are expected; irregular pulse; pulse deficit; chest pain; dizziness; leg cramps; mental confusion.
5. Absence of drastic change in blood pressure (B/P). *Guidelines:* systolic B/P not exceeding 250 mmHg, diastolic B/P not exceeding 150 mmHg, and no more than 10-mmHg drop in systolic B/P.

RESPIRATORY MUSCLE TRAINING

Goals

1. To improve respiratory muscle strength and endurance.
2. To increase exercise capacity.
3. To avoid ventilatory failure.

Indications

1. Respiratory muscle fatigue, particularly in COPD, neuromuscular disease, weaning from mechanical ventilation, postextubation period.
2. Potential ventilatory failure.

Respiratory muscle training is a method of exercising to reduce or avoid respiratory muscle fatigue. It is usually combined with rest and pharmacologic measures when the patient's own compensatory mechanism of alternating work of breathing between primary and accessory respiratory muscle groups becomes increasingly more ineffective. Because it is a relatively new and incompletely developed technique, the discussion here focuses on a general description rather than specific patient information for implementation.

The two respiratory muscle training techniques used in the clinical setting are *inspiratory resistance training* and *hyperpnea training.*

Inspiratory Resistance Training

Inspiratory resistance training is defined as *normal ventilation with added external loading.* The external loading is usually inspiratory loading. The patient breathes at his own rate through the mouthpiece of a trainer, such as the hand-held trainer in Figure 20–5. Inspiratory resistance is added by reducing the size of the inspiratory orifice. Resistance is increased to a predetermined mouth or transdiaphragmatic pressure (Sobush et al, 1985). The pressure is just below the patient's fatigue threshold. When clinical signs are the primary monitoring parameters, the inspiratory resistance is gradually increased until signs of respiratory muscle fatigue appear. Signs include tachypnea, asynchronous breathing, paradoxical chest and abdominal wall movements, and other signs of increased work of breathing. The patient exercises at home at the set inspiratory resistance for 15 to 30 minutes each day, 5 days a week, for 6 to 10 weeks.

Hyperpnea Training

Hyperpnea training is defined as *high ventilation with low external loading.* Methods vary, but they usually require sustained periods of hyperpnea lasting 15 to 30 minutes daily for several weeks. This form of training has been used for COPD patients as well as for acute patients being weaned from mechanical ventilation.

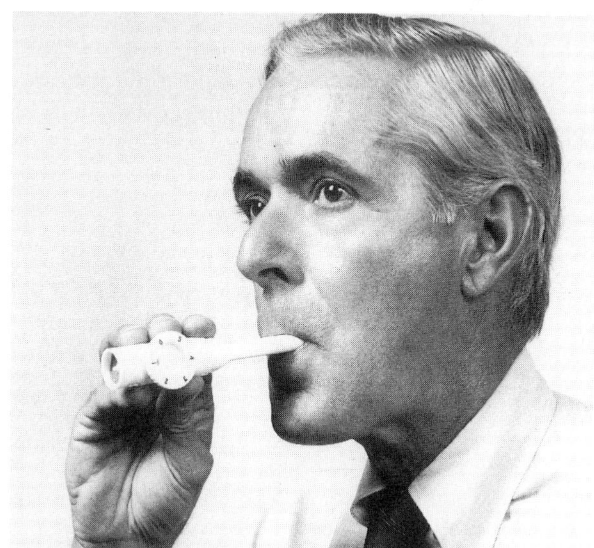

Figure 20–5. Use of the PFLEX inspiratory muscle trainer. (Courtesy of HealthScan Products Inc., New Jersey.)

Training Effects

Training effects appear within 4 to 6 weeks of therapy. Specific effects depend on the particular mode of therapy, because different muscle fiber types are affected by different modes of training. Modes or training devices that increase muscle strength will cause hypertrophy of muscle fibers and increase V_T as well as maximum inspiratory and expiratory pressures.

Modes that increase muscle endurance cause many physiologic changes in muscle fibers, including an increase in vascularity, myoglobin content, aerobic enzymes, and number of fatigue-resistant fibers (Sobush et al, 1985). Though endurance does not increase V_T, it increases *maximum sustained ventilatory capacity*. This measure of endurance is defined as *that level of minute ventilation that can be maintained for 15 minutes* (Pardy and Leith, 1984).

Once a patient achieves a training effect, regular practice is required to prevent deconditioning. However, the intensity or frequency of training may be reduced without decreasing respiratory muscle performance.

Evaluation Criteria

These evaluation criteria serve as a general guideline. Specific criteria will depend on the type of training device, specificity of training, and clinical setting.

1. Normal breathing pattern sustained for 4 weeks.
2. Improvement in inspiratory and expiratory pressures by 40 to 50%.
3. Decreased respiratory rate, increased V_T, increased maximum voluntary ventilation.
4. Absence of intolerable dyspnea, excessive fatigue, shallow and rapid breathing, asynchronous breathing, paradoxical chest and abdominal wall movements, and other signs of inspiratory muscle fatigue described in Table 28–5.
5. Absence of decreased total lung capacity (TLC), increased residual volume (RV), decreased vital capacity (VC) on the complete pulmonary function test (PFT).

Role of Respiratory Muscle Training In Rehabilitation

Though many clinicians employ some form of respiratory muscle training, its role in pulmonary rehabilitation remains largely undefined. Some patients never achieve an increase in muscle strength or endurance. The minority of patients who do respond to therapy may show no change in pulmonary function, exercise performance, or ability to perform ADL (Chen et al, 1985). Belman and Sieck (1982) conclude that ventilatory muscle endurance may not be essential to increase exercise performance, since exercise (e.g., walking) alone achieves similar benefits. Yet, it may increase the patient's resistance to respiratory failure.

One major implementation problem is that COPD patients may not be able to tolerate respiratory muscle training for long enough periods of time to result in a training effect. They may discontinue therapy because they perceive no improvement in their condition. In resistance training, they learn to breathe through higher resistances by changing their breathing strategy. Because breathing strategy can reduce the intensity of the training stimulus and result in no change in respiratory muscle endurance, Belman and coworkers (1986) conclude that some kind of biofeedback signal is needed to be sure that the patient reaches his specified resistive load.

It is hoped that further research will clarify key questions and solve many of the implementation problems related to respiratory muscle training. Current research areas include the specific indications for training; the efficacy of inspiratory loading versus hyperpnea techniques; the regulation of training intensity; and the role of training in relation to other interventions aimed at reducing muscle fatigue, such as nutrition, theophylline administration, and rest.

Conclusion

This chapter has discussed energy conservation techniques and exercise conditioning, including walking, arm and leg exercises, and respiratory muscle training.

Though commonly overlooked, basic exercises are best implemented early, after stabilization of acute chest disease. They are continued indefinitely after hospital discharge to achieve and maintain a training effect. The benefits of exercise, in turn, provide motivation for the patient to achieve other personal goals that make life more comfortable and pleasurable.

REFERENCES

Alpert, J. et al.: Effects of physical training on hemodynamics and pulmonary function at rest and during exercise in patients with COPD. *Chest*, 66(6):647–651, 1974.

American Hospital Association: Staff Manual for Teaching Patients About COPD. Chicago, American Hospital Association, 1982.

Anderson, S.: Exercise and the asthmatic patient. *Respiratory therapy*, 10(3):68–75, 1980.

Barach, A. and Petty, T.: Is COLD improved by physical exercise? *Journal of american medical association*, 234(8):854–855, 1975.

Bell, C., Kass, I., and Hodgkin, J.: Exercise conditioning. In Pulmonary Rehabilitation—Guidelines to Success. (J. Hodgkin et al,—eds.). Boston, Butterworth Publishers, 1984.

Belman, M.: Exercise in chronic obstructive pulmonary disease. *Clinics in chest medicine*, 7(4):585–597, 1986.

Belman, M. and Sieck, G.: The ventilatory muscles—fatigue, endurance and training. *Chest*, 82(6):761–766, 1982.

Belman, M., Thomas, S., and Lewis, M.: Resistive breathing training in patients with COPD. *Chest*, 90(5):662–669, 1986.

Belman, M. and Wasserman, K.: Exercise training and testing in patients with COPD. *Basics of respiratory disease*, 10(2):1–6, 1981.

Berman, L. and Sutton, J.: Exercise for the pulmonary patient. *Journal of cardiopulmonary rehabilitation*, 6(2):52–61, 1986.

Casciari, R. et al: Effects of breathing retraining in patients with COPD. *Chest,* 79(4):393–398, 1981.
Chen, H., Dukes, R., and Martin, B.: Inspiratory muscle training in patients with COPD. *American review of respiratory disease,* 131(2):251–255, 1985.
Frownfelter, D.: Chest Physical Therapy and Pulmonary Rehabilitation. Chicago, Year Book Medical Publishers, Inc., 1978.
Hodgkin, J.: Exercise in the pulmonary patient. *Respiratory care,* 27(6):671–672, 1982.
Kersten, L.: Your Respiratory Home Care Program. (Patient booklet). Berkeley, California, Herrick Hospital and Health Center of the East Bay, 1978.
McGavin, C., Gupta, S., and McHardy, G.: Twelve-minute walking tests for assessing disability in chronic bronchitis. *British medical journal,* 1(6013):822–823, 1976.
Medical Respiratory Care Program Patient Handbook. Duarte, California, City of Hope National Medical Center, 1985.
Pardy, R. and Leith, D.: Ventilatory muscle training. *Respiratory care,* 29(3):278–284, 1984.
Pardy, R., Rivington, R., Despas, P., and Macklem, P.: The effect of inspiratory muscle training on exercise performance in chronic airflow limitation. *American review of respiratory disease,* 123(4):426–433, 1981.
Petty, T. and Guthrie, A.: The effects of augmented breathing maneuvers on ventilation in severe chronic airway obstruction. *Respiratory care,* 16(3):104–111, 1971.
Rochester, D.: The respiratory muscles in COPD—state of the art. *Chest,* 85(6):47S–49S, 1984.
Sobush, D., Dunning, M., and McDonald, K.: Exercise prescription components for respiratory muscle training: Past, present, and future. *Respiratory care,* 30(1):34–42, 1985.
Unger, K., Moser, K., and Hansen, P.: Selection of an exercise program for patients with COPD. *Heart and lung,* 9(1):68–76, 1980.
Zack, M. and Palange, A.: Oxygen supplemented exercise of ventilatory and nonventilatory muscles in pulmonary rehabilitation. *Chest,* 88(5):669–675, 1985.

Use of Home Respiratory Equipment

21

Main Objectives

1. Name five factors to consider before suggesting the use of respiratory equipment in the home.
2. Name nine variables to consider in the selection of a durable medical equipment (DME) vendor.
3. Describe six desirable characteristics of respiratory DME.
4. Explain how to order respiratory DME for a patient.
5. Discuss how to teach a patient to measure and store medications for an aerosol device and to clean and disinfect respiratory equipment.
6. Identify the two most important aspects of equipment cleaning; explain the rationale for emphasizing these aspects in the teaching-learning situation.

This chapter discusses general information related to the use of respiratory equipment in the home. Content is organized according to the steps the nurse must take before the patient can begin aerosol, oxygen, or other forms of respiratory therapy at home.

When home respiratory therapy is contemplated, the hospital nurse or visiting nurse consults with the patient, family, physician, and respiratory therapist in the decision to order equipment. If health team members and patient determine that the benefits of therapy at home outweigh cost and risks, the nurse may be involved in the choosing of an equipment vendor or supplier and the ordering of specific devices. Before the patient initiates therapy, the nurse initiates the teaching of crucial self-care educational content, specifically, the measuring and storing of medications and the cleaning and storing of equipment. Unless patient or family demonstrates competence in these areas, respiratory therapy may be contraindicated, and a different and simpler approach to the patient's problem may be best.

The Decision to Use Home Respiratory Equipment

After recovery from an acute exacerbation, the patient with chronic pulmonary disease may benefit from respiratory treatments at home. In spite of an obvious need, however, the decision to implement therapy may be a difficult one. The patient's existing care plan may already be complex, involving diet restrictions, multiple daily medication administrations, and continuous psychologic support. The addition of another therapy, such as aerosol therapy via hand held nebulizer, introduces other demands on the patient, including the need to learn a new technique, to adjust to an overall daily routine, to find an equipment vendor, and to maintain the device required. Unless demands are anticipated and details worked out before equipment is ordered, the patient may become overwhelmed and frustrated.

The role of the nurse is to provide information that will help in the decision to order respiratory treatments at home. Factors to consider include cost of equipment, maintenance requirements of equipment, adequacy of patient's breathing technique, availability of appropriate equipment vendor, and availability of supervision. Information is best gathered in collaboration with other members of the health care team, including the respiratory therapist, social worker, and local equipment personnel.

COST

The patient's medical insurance or financial reimbursement policy is checked to determine whether it covers rental and purchase costs of the desired equipment. When respiratory equipment is ordered, the patient is encouraged to rent it for a month rather than buy it. During this time, patient and staff evaluate the effects of therapy and determine the need for therapy in the future. When cost is a main concern, the nurse, social service worker, or other knowledgable person carefully checks the details of financial coverage, including amount of copayments (percent of the total bill paid by the patient), billing procedure, time lapse between billing and reimbursement, and equipment service coverage. In addition, staff help the patient evaluate the benefits of renting versus buying equipment in the future. In some cases, for example, buying equipment may be less expensive over time, but patient and family may decide to rent because they have full financial reimbursement, and they do not want to lose the service agreement associated with renting. Since wide variation exists in reimbursement policies, vendor fees and services, and individual needs and preferences, the nurse and other staff must be careful to evaluate costs within the context of each patient's unique set of circumstances.

EQUIPMENT MAINTENANCE

Respiratory equipment is not ordered unless patient, family member, or another person is able to maintain the equipment. Disinfection of tubings, nebulizers, and humidifiers is of prime concern. Unless the equipment is disinfected properly and regularly, the patient is at increased risk for respiratory infection from microorganisms growing in mist droplets and water reservoirs.

PATIENT'S BREATHING TECHNIQUE

The patient must be able to safely and knowledgeably administer medications for nebulization. In addition, the patient must be able to coordinate the required breathing technique. Ideally, the patient demonstrates this competency in the clinic or hospital using equipment that is identical to anticipated home equipment. Home equipment is ordered if the patient meets most of the evaluation criteria for correct technique (see Chapter 22 and Chapter 23). In the home, the visiting nurse uses clinical judgment to determine whether the patient will be able to meet most of the evaluation criteria for the proposed therapy. In equivocal cases, treatments may be ordered for a trial period.

EQUIPMENT VENDOR

A vendor must be available to provide and service the desired respiratory equipment.

Follow-up Supervision. As explained in the self-care education (see Chapter 17), the respiratory patient almost always requires follow-up supervision for reteaching and perfection of technique. In addition, a primary physician is required for periodic medical evaluation and direction of health team members. Home health care nurses are excellent resources, but financial coverage for such skilled nursing care in the home is usually limited. A periodic telephone call is becoming more of a necessity to facilitate monitoring and trouble shooting for equipment-related problems. Moreover, in ambulatory care, the patient may be asked to bring the equipment, or at least the nebulizer or breathing circuit, to the clinic or physician's office for inspection and follow-up supervision during treatment.

REQUIREMENTS FOR OPTIMAL RESPIRATORY DURABLE MEDICAL EQUIPMENT

SAFE

Easy to operate to avoid errors.

Easy to disassemble, to allow for thorough disinfection and drying, and easy to reassemble.

Heating devices for humidifiers and nebulizers do not overheat and cause burns.

Ventilators have controls that cannot be tampered with by children and have appropriate alarm systems.

RELIABLE

Few and infrequent equipment problems.

Nondisposable rather than disposable parts for nebulizers and ventilator circuits because they are more dependable and easier to disinfect and dry.

EASY TO OPERATE

Simple and lightweight design.

Settings are clearly labelled, calibrated, and few in number.

Absence of unnecessary alarms and controls that may be confusing and disturbing to patient and family.

Easy to trouble shoot, e.g., intermittent positive pressure breathing (IPPB) device should have pressure gauge for visual confirmation of hyperinflation during treatment.

VERSATILE

Portable, e.g., fits on a walker or wheelchair and in a car or airplane.

Provision for changing ventilatory support and comfort requirements, e.g., ventilator with more than one mode of ventilation and internal battery as a reserve power source.

Aesthetic, i.e., fits in with work or home environment.

COST EFFECTIVE

Calculate cost including the price of the main piece of equipment; accessories (e.g., holding devices, extension tubing, oxygen tank regulator); additional monitoring equipment (e.g., alarms); electricity for powered devices, as estimated by vendor; and service charges, e.g., oxygen tank refills.

Compare cost of alternative equipment.

ACCEPTABLE TO PATIENT AND FAMILY

Patient and family agree to use equipment model recommended by health care team.

Choosing an Equipment Vendor

Choosing an appropriate equipment vendor is just as important as deciding whether or not to order therapy. Variables to consider in selection of a DME vendor are presented in Table 21–1. DME refers to equipment that is designed to withstand repeated use in the home. Some hospital equipment may qualify as DME, but usually modifications are made to prolong longevity and facilitate home disinfection procedures.

Choosing Respiratory Equipment

The nurse recommends equipment that is safe, reliable, easy to operate, versatile, cost effective, and acceptable to patient and family. These desirable characteristics are outlined in the box to the left.

Patient and family acceptance of equipment recommendations is sometimes overlooked when discharge planning is complex, and the patient is still recuperating from acute illness. Yet, acceptance is mandatory to assure use of equipment in the home. Problems may arise when the chronic respiratory patient becomes emotionally and intellectually attached to old equipment, even though it is out of date and stained with medication. Switching to new equipment is done only after careful consideration of the patient's feelings and beliefs about existing and recommended equipment. Unless the patient agrees to at least try new equipment, he is likely to revert to old equipment after hospital discharge or discontinuation of home care services.

ORDERING EQUIPMENT

After patient and health team members choose appropriate equipment, the physician writes medical orders in the chart for therapy. Orders should state all of the components listed in the box below.

ORDERS FOR RESPIRATORY TREATMENTS

Type of therapy—e.g., aerosol therapy, IPPB, incentive spirometry, and mechanical ventilation.

Frequency—e.g., QD, BID, TID, or QID.

Duration of treatment—e.g., 5 to 10 minutes, 15 to 20 minutes.

Medications—concentration, dosage, dilution ratio, and diluent.

Settings—e.g., L/min, peak inspiratory pressure, FIO_2, V_T, and inspiratory to expiratory ratio.

Table 21–1. VARIABLES TO CONSIDER IN SELECTION OF A DURABLE MEDICAL EQUIPMENT VENDOR

Variables	Recommendations
Geographic location	Patient resides within the vendor's service area and within 1 hour's travel time of the vendor's office.
Hours of coverage	24 hours a day, 7 days a week coverage for routine and emergency service.
Charges	Reasonable patient charges for equipment and services. Compare charges between vendors in your area.
Staffing	Vendor employs courteous and knowledgeable office personnel, trained delivery personnel, and a registered or certified respiratory therapist or a respiratory nurse specialist for consultation and teaching.
Self-care education	Vendor provides self-care instruction, reinforced with educational materials. Shows a willingness to coordinate instruction with content already given by other members of the health care team.
Equipment	Full line of respiratory and nonrespiratory equipment so that the patient does not have to use several vendors. Equipment is approved for third party reimbursement.
Quality assurance	Vendor periodically evaluates patient needs and vendor services via questionnaires, surveys, verbal communications, equipment checks, and so forth.
Finances	Minimal patient involvement in finances. Vendor bills fiscal intermediary and accepts payment directly from intermediary. Option to rent or purchase, with rental fee applied to purchase price. Reduced charges to patients of physicians or agencies who regularly refer patients.
Reputation	Efficient patient referral system, prompt equipment delivery, regular billing, prompt follow-up on equipment problems or complaints, favorable public relations.

Team members implement therapy using hospital equipment, until home equipment can be ordered. They chart actual dates and times of respiratory treatments during practice, therapeutic effects, any adverse effects, self-care education presented, and patient and family response to instruction. If patient response is favorable, the physician writes a prescription for appropriate DME. If time permits, the vendor is instructed to deliver equipment directly to the patient's hospital room to facilitate familiarity with it and to practice under close supervision before hospital discharge. In other cases, pulmonary departments provide home equipment for use in the hospital, and the vendor delivers the same equipment model to the home immediately after hospital discharge. In any case, communication must flow freely among hospital personnel, visiting nurse, and equipment vendor to assure prompt and timely delivery of equipment and presentation of self-care instruction that does not conflict with that previously provided by other health team members.

The prescription for DME usually includes the items as listed in this box.

DATA FOR THE DME PRESCRIPTION

Date
Patient's name and address
Type of equipment
Diagnosis and prognosis
Duration and frequency of prescription
Medication—dosage and dilution ratio
Pertinent PFT and ABG results
Physician's signature and registration number

Some equipment vendors have special forms or check lists that include other details, such as FIO_2, peak inspiratory pressure, and liters per minute.

The nurse may be asked to provide the equipment vendor with more detailed information to document the need for specific therapy, such as oxygen. Though Medicare guidelines in the United States are changing, the information in the box below may be used as a

DOCUMENTATION REQUIREMENTS FOR HOME OXYGEN THERAPY

MEDICAL DIAGNOSIS

Primary lung disease, e.g., COPD, interstitial fibrosis
Hypoxia-related symptoms, e.g., polycythemia, cor pulmonale
Other conditions, e.g., angina pectoris

OXYGEN FLOW RATE (L/MIN) AND CONCENTRATION (%)

FREQUENCY

Hours per day
Minutes per hour, if applicable
PRN is unacceptable

DURATION OF NEED

Number of months
"Lifetime" is unacceptable

LABORATORY EVIDENCE OF HYPOXEMIA

$PaO_2 \leq 55$ mmHg on room air (ABG)
or
$SaO_2 \leq 85\%$ on room air (ABG or oximetry)
"Borderline" cases may be acceptable with medical explanation of need

ADDITIONAL MEDICAL DOCUMENTATION

Statement indicating that other treatments for hypoxemia or hypoxia-related symptoms were unsuccessful.

guide for obtaining documentation requirements for patients who need oxygen therapy. Later, the equipment vendor contacts the physician for documentation of continued need for therapy. Unless such verification is obtained, the patient may not receive financial reimbursement.

A recent PaO_2 or SaO_2 is used to document continued need for an oxygen setup in the home. If ABGs are unavailable, some vendors and Visiting Nurses's Associations provide the extra service of measuring SaO_2 noninvasively by oximetry during a home visit. When the patient's condition improves (i.e., SaO_2 increases above 85% on room air), the nurse notifies the physician, who may in turn discontinue oxygen therapy.

Return once more to the hypothetical case in this chapter of a patient who has just received a prescription for home respiratory equipment. After the ordering of appropriate equipment and the documenting of medical need from information in the chart, the nurse may begin instruction on two crucial topics as follows: (1) measuring and storing medications and (2) cleaning and storing equipment.

Measuring and Storing Medications

The following sample education material instructs the patient in measuring and storing medications utilized in aerosol devices.

PATIENT INFORMATION

Measuring and Storing Medications

Order

1. Drop ______drops or ______ml of ____________________ into the nebulizer cup of your setup.
2. Pour a small amount of ________________________into a small measuring cup, and draw up ________________________ into a small syringe. Add to the nebulizer cup.

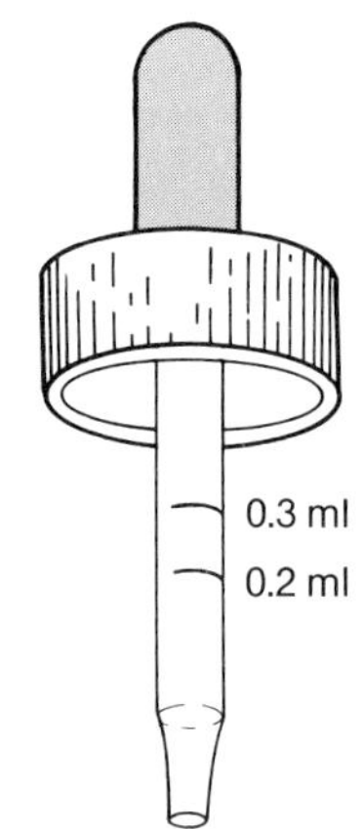

Dropper used for Alupent
Mark prescribed dose

3. Keep opened medication bottle in refrigerator. Store unopened bottles in a cool place.

Tips

1. Do not dip dropper from one medication to another without rinsing under water.
2. Always keep medication tightly capped.
3. If your eye dropper is not attached to the cap of your medicine bottle and you must use a separate dropper, always rinse after use; shake dry; and store in a clean, covered, but unsealed container with your measuring cup.
4. Wash measuring utensils (e.g., any separate droppers, measuring cups, and plastic syringes taken apart) daily, along with other equipment. Disinfect twice a week, as directed.

EVALUATION CRITERIA

1. Medication is correctly measured and diluted according to instructions.
2. Nebulizer solution is stored in the refrigerator between uses.
3. Measuring utensils are cleaned and disinfected regularly with other respiratory equipment.

IMPLEMENTATION

The following points help the nurse decide how to help the patient develop a system for measuring medications.

1. The patient may prefer to use a teaspoon or some other household device to measure the diluent.
2. Avoid teaching the patient to use a needle attached to a syringe to draw up diluent. Needles are dangerous and difficult to clean and dry thoroughly.
3. Many elderly persons or persons with poor eyesight prefer to learn to measure correct dosage by counting drops. Always check the dropper for correct dosage. Some patients may substitute a larger dropper (e.g., Mucomyst dropper) for a smaller one (e.g., Bronkosol dropper) and, hence, receive drug overdosage.
4. Medication and diluent are added to any *empty* nebulizer cup. Instruct the patient to discard any residual solution after each treatment. Able individuals may be encouraged to rinse the nebulizer cup under tap water and let drip dry between treatments.

Which Diluent Is Best?

The prescribed diluent may be sterile water or normal saline, commonly used in hospitals, distilled water, or tap water. Hodgkin (1979) recommends water over saline solution for aerosol bronchodilators because water dilution results in maximal decrease in solute concentration. As aerosol particles are inhaled into airways, they tend to become smaller and deposit more peripherally when compared with the more hypertonic saline particles that tend to grow rapidly in aerosol form. Many clinicians prefer distilled water for home use. Though over-the-counter distilled water is not entirely bacteria free, it is cheaply and readily available in grocery stores. It can also be utilized for mist therapy (bland aerosol) and avoids the needle and syringe system utilized for vials of sterile normal saline or water.

If distilled water is the diluent, patients must be cautioned not to confuse distilled water for mineral or drinking water—both types may be shelved next to each other in the store and in identical containers with nearly identical labels. Mineral water is undesirable because it contains solutes that readily clog up nebulizer capillaries and prevent adequate aerosol formation.

In addition, the nurse should be aware that as a hypo-osmolar solution, distilled water has the potential of precipitating airway irritability or bronchospasm in asthmatics. Since bronchospasm is most likely to occur in patients with pure asthma rather than in the majority of patients with COPD, who may have a small asthmatic component, the nurse tends not to encounter this problem in the clinical situation. Nevertheless, whenever a patient complains of hacking cough and increased wheezing during an aerosol treatment, distilled water may be replaced with a saline solution for the diluent. Normal saline is available in unit dose form.

The American Association for Respiratory Therapy (1982) notes that some workers prefer tap water over sterile water for reservoir solutions of respiratory therapy devices because tap water dispensed from a non-aerated tap is less likely to become contaminated by poor handling techniques. Yet, water systems in some geographic regions are grossly contaminated. Therefore, unless a surveillance program has demonstrated the absence of pathologic organisms in tap water, distilled water is preferred over tap water as a diluent for any type of aerosol treatment. This rule of thumb applies provided the distilled water is stored properly, e.g., covered, refrigerated, and not stored for long periods of time after the seal is broken.

Premixed Medication

Use of premixed medication in small plastic, easy to administer vials eliminates the need to measure bronchodilator medication and diluent (see Fig. 11–3 and Fig. 11–8). This unit dosage system is more expensive, but it may solve all the patient's measuring problems.

To reduce cost, McLean and associates (1984) recommend sending the patient home with a pint of premixed bronchodilator solution in 1:8, 1:10, or 1:12 strengths that has been prepared by the pharmacy. Measuring medication is simple because it only involves pouring out 3 ml of the premixed medication. A smaller, 120-ml colored dropper bottle and 1-ml dropper are also sent home. The patient is encouraged to measure from the smaller bottle, keeping the larger pint bottle separate as a stock supply.

Cleaning and Storing Equipment

Within 24 to 48 hours after delivery, the patient will have to clean and disinfect the home respiratory equipment. Unless equipment is cleaned and disinfected regularly, infectious agents, such as *Pseudomonas, Proteus, Alkaligenes, Herellea, Flavobacterium,* and others, may grow in nebulizer solutions and water droplets along the sides of tubings, eventually infecting the patient and precipitating hospital readmission.

The following patient information explains a basic procedure for cleaning and storing equipment. (See Chapter 22 and Chapter 23 for description of specific equipment.)

PATIENT INFORMATION

Cleaning and Storing Equipment

Clean your equipment once a day. Failure to use the cleaning procedure *daily* (every 24 hours) makes you a prime candidate for a respiratory infection from germs multiplying in your setup. Keep two setups so that you *always* start the day with a clean setup.

Clean Daily

1. *Take apart your equipment.* For a ventilator or IPPB circuit, separate the three tubes and take apart the manifold. Plug the opening to the exhalation valve, if you do not take the valve apart.
2. *Wash in a clean sink or dish pan* that is used *only* for cleaning your equipment. Use a nonresidue liquid detergent, such as Joy.

   Scrub with a soft brush to remove medications, secretions, and particles from small crevices and the sides of tubing.

   If you are cleaning a nebulizer, pull the nebulizer jet off and wash the insides with a stylet or pipe cleaner.
3. *Rinse completely* with warm tap water.
4. *Dry completely.* Shake excess water off small pieces. Do not towel dry. Place these pieces on a lint-free or clean towel on the bottom of your dish pan to dry. Cover the dish pan, allowing air to circulate underneath.

   Shake or swing excess water out of tubing and hand to drip dry.
5. When all the equipment is *completely* dry, assemble and store in a clean, unsealed plastic bag. A covered container is okay.
6. If you are ready to use the setup and it is not completely dry, assemble, hook up to the machine, and run the machine until tubes are dry.

Disinfect at Least Twice a Week

1. Wash with liquid detergent as described. Rinse thoroughly.
2. In your dish pan, mix 1 part of white vinegar and 2 parts tap water. Make sure you get the proportions right. If the solution is too dilute, the procedure is not effective.
3. Soak for 30 minutes with parts and tubing completely covered with the mixed solution.
4. Rinse completely with warm tap water and follow steps 4, 5, and 6 under *Clean Daily* for drying.

Alternative

You may buy a special disinfection solution to substitute for the vinegar solution. Check with your nurse or respiratory equipment company.

EVALUATION CRITERIA

1. Equipment is cleaned every 24 hours and disinfected at least twice a week.
2. After the procedure, equipment demonstrates the absence of medication stains, mucus, and water droplets within tubings, nebulizers, and other parts of breathing circuits. Carefully inspect crevices and tubing corrugations.
3. New warm soapy water is used with each cleaning. Old water is discarded after each use.
4. White vinegar solution approximates a 1:1 to 1:2 concentration.
5. White vinegar solution is saved in a covered container and preferably refrigerated for no longer than four days.
6. Surfaces of machine are free of dust and dirt. Encourage the patient to wipe it down with a clean damp cloth, cover it between treatments, and store it in a safe place.
7. Scrub brush and basin is used for equipment cleaning.
8. Hair dryers or blowers are *not* used for drying equipment. They introduce lint and may damage parts.
9. The patient has two complete sets of washable equipment, so a clean, dry setup is always available for the following day.

IMPLEMENTATION

The above self-care education material presents only one system for cleaning and storing equipment. Because of the paucity of reliable and valid research on the topic, numerous systems exist. Moser and colleagues (1980) recommend daily cleaning followed immediately by disinfection in a 1:1 vinegar to water solution. The American Hospital Association (1982) recommends a similar procedure. In addition, the patient is encouraged to add one tablespoon of vinegar solution to the IPPB nebulizer and run the machine for 10 minutes before cleaning and disinfecting the IPPB circuit. The same procedure is recommended for ultrasonic nebulizers, only on a weekly basis. The Pennsylvania Society for Respiratory Therapy (1983) recommends rinsing all parts under water after each treatment. Routine equipment is cleaned and disinfected daily with a 2:3 vinegar to water solution. Circuits for continuous mechanical ventilation are cleaned and disinfected every 48 hours, and the vinegar solution is discarded weekly. In contrast, for continuous ventilators, Lucas (1984) recommends a 1:3 vinegar to water solution and the decontamination of ventilator circuitry, aerosol tubing, nebulizers, and humidifiers every 3 days.

Until research further identifies appropriate cleaning and disinfection procedures for different pieces of home equipment and for different types of patients, health team members must be flexible in helping patient and family work out a practical procedure for their unique set of circumstances (Fig. 20–1 and Fig. 20–2). As a general rule, the visiting nurse reinforces the system already presented to the patient in the hospital or pulmonary rehabilitation program. Ideally, but not always, cleaning policies are based on results of local surveillance programs. When patients are forgetful or demonstrate difficulty implementing a system, the nurse attempts to adjust or simplify the system. For example, a 2:3 vinegar to water solution may be simplified to a 1:1. The stronger 1:1 solution is easier to measure and allows for the mistake of adding too much water. In addition, the patient with a busy schedule may agree to buy several extra nebulizer or IPPB circuits to eliminate daily cleaning tasks. Patients who are reluctant to soak equipment in vinegar solution twice a week may agree to do it once a week.

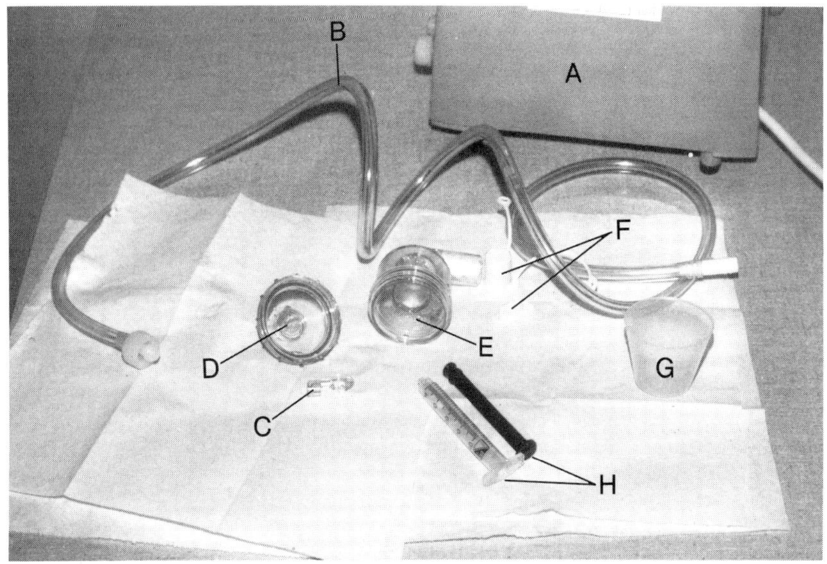

Figure 21–1. Nebulizer and medication administration equipment for compressor-nebulizer treatments may be dried on towels on a tabletop (above) rather than on the bottom of a clean dishpan (described in the patient information section). A, Compressor; B, Tube that connects nebulizer to compressor; C, Capillary that fits into bottom of nebulizer; D, Bottom of nebulizer; E, Top of nebulizer; F, Nebulizer plugs; G, Medication (measuring) cup; and H, Dismantled syringe for measuring diluent.

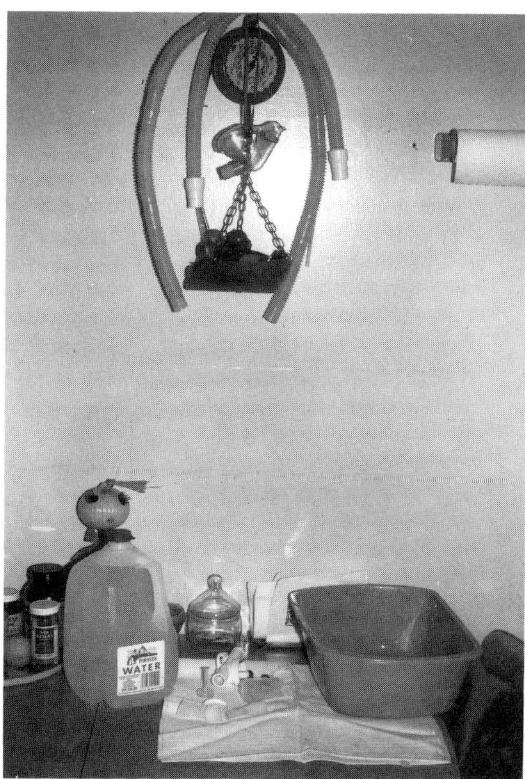

Figure 21–2. Breathing tubes for respiratory equipment may be hung in any available dry place in the home that allows water to drain completely from tubing corrugations. The dyspneic owner of this equipment preferred to hang the tubes above the kitchen table, where they were readily accessible to him.

In working out a reasonable system with the patient, the nurse keeps in mind these seven summary points

1. *Be flexible!* Tradeoffs between practicality and recommended procedures are inevitable. In difficult situations, a minimum cleaning procedure is better than no cleaning procedure at all. As a general guideline, reinforce a strict daily cleaning procedure for nebulizer devices and a more lenient procedure for humidifier devices (e.g., every 2 to 3 days). Contaminated aerosol particles inhaled to distal airways increase risk for pulmonary infection.
2. Encourage patient and family to commit themselves to specific and realistic times for cleaning and disinfection. Then establish a regular schedule, posting a chart or checkoff list, if necessary.
3. Cleaning should be meticulous whenever it occurs. Equipment must be thoroughly cleaned and thoroughly dried.
4. Some patients may wish to use other solutions for disinfection, e.g., glutaraldehyde or quaternary ammonium compounds. The popular disinfectant, Control III, is a double quaternary ammonium chloride. These solutions are obtained through equipment companies and vendors and diluted according to the manufacturer's instructions. Lucas (1984) reports that double- and triple quaternary ammonium compounds are cheaper than vinegar and more effective against gram-negative and gram-positive organisms. However, these compounds have the disadvantage of limited availability, since, unlike vinegar, they are not common household items.
5. Gas sterilization with ethylene oxide is recommended once a year for major pieces of equipment, such as ventilators. Many equipment companies and local hospitals agree to perform this service.
6. A strict cleaning and disinfection system is stressed for individuals most likely to develop infection. These include patients with tracheal tubes, dermatitis or skin lesions (potential for cross contamination during cleaning), diagnosed respiratory infection, and history of repeated infections. Other patients at risk are those receiving immunosuppressive cytotoxic therapy, high dose oral steroids, or broad-spectrum antimicrobial drugs. Most patients with end-stage pulmonary disease fall into this high risk group.
7. A relatively lenient cleaning and disinfection system may be acceptable for some patients with uncomplicated medical courses. A study by Witek and associates (1986) suggests that colonization of nebulizers is minimal during the first 72 hours of use by postoperative patients with uncomplicated clinical courses.
8. Research has yet to identify the best cleaning and disinfection procedure. Results from one research study suggest that use of Control III or vinegar and water solutions may not be any more effective than soap and water (Dettenmeier et al, 1985). With this perspective in mind, the nurse should emphasize the following two aspects during instruction: (a) thorough and daily soap and water cleaning to remove saliva and medication stains and (b) thorough drying between cleanings to eliminate bacterial growth in moisture.

CONCLUSION

This chapter discusses general information related to use of respiratory equipment in the home. This information helps the hospital or clinic nurse coordinate discharge planning; it helps the visiting nurse supervise the acquisition, use, and care of respiratory DME in the home. Once the patient obtains appropriate equipment and understands the obligation to clean and disinfect it regularly, the nurse helps the patient learn specific administration techniques discussed in Chapter 22 and Chapter 23.

REFERENCES

American Association for Respiratory Therapy: Recommendations for Respiratory Therapy Equipment Processing, Handling, and Surveillance. In Staff Manual for Teaching Patients about COPD, 2nd ed. Chicago, American Hospital Association, 1982.

American Hospital Association: Staff Manual for Teaching Patients about COPD, 2nd ed. Chicago, American Hospital Association, 1982.

American Thoracic Society: Home use of equipment for patients with respiratory disease. *American Association of Respiratory Disease,* 115(5):893–895, 1977.

Bell, C., Blodgett, D., et al: Home Care and Rehabilitation in Respiratory Medicine. Philadelphia, J. B. Lippincott Co., 1984.

Dettenmeier, P., Vogt-Yanta, M., et al: Comparison of home nebulizer cleaning/disinfecting techniques reported to decrease bacterial growth. *American Association of Respiratory Disease,* 131(4):A166, 1985.

Foster Medical Home Health Care: Understanding the New Oxygen Coverage Guidelines. Conshohocken, Pennsylvania, Foster Medical Corp., 1985.

Hodgkin, J.: COPD—Current Concepts in Diagnosis and Comprehensive Care. Park Ridge, Illinois, American College of Chest Physicians, 1979.

Kersten, L.: Your Respiratory Home Care Program. Berkeley, California, Herrick Hospital and Health Center of the East Bay, 1978.

Lucas, J.: Home Ventilator Care. In Pulmonary Rehabilitation: From Hospital to Home. (O'Ryan, J. and Burns, D.—eds.). Chicago, Year Book Medical Publishers, 1984.

McLean, D., et al: Respiratory Therapy Techniques. In Pulmonary Rehabilitation—Guidelines to Success. (Hodgkin, J., Zorn, E., and Connors, G.—eds.). Boston, Butterworth Publishers, 1984.

Moser, K., Archibald, C., et al: Better Living and Breathing, 2nd ed. St. Louis, C. V. Mosby Co., 1980.

Pennsylvania Society for Respiratory Therapy, Patient and Home Care Committee: Pennsylvania Society For Respiratory Therapy, Inc., 1983.

Pierce, A., Sanford, J., et al: Long-term evaluation of decontamination of inhalation therapy equipment and the occurrence of necrotizing pneumonia. *New England Journal of Medicine,* 282(10):528–531, 1970.

Walton, J.: A new controversy in respiratory equipment management: reusables versus disposed disposables versus reused disposables. *Respiratory Care,* 31(3):213–217, 1986.

Witek, T., York, R., et al: Bacterial colonization of ultrasonic nebulizers: Implications for frequency of circuit changing. *Respiratory Care,* 31(12):1207–1210, 1986.

Aerosol Therapy and Intermittent Positive Pressure Breathing (IPPB)

22

Main Objectives

1. Define the following terms: aerosol, bland aerosol, medication aerosol, Bernouilli's principle, baffle, air-entrainment port, cool aerosol, heated aerosol, ultrasonic aerosol.
2. Discuss how aerosol is produced by jet nebulization.
3. Name at least five factors that affect aerosol deposition in the lungs.
4. Name goals and indications for use; name six evaluation criteria for correct technique and two for overall improvement in condition; describe implementation in the clinical setting, including a typical daily treatment schedule; and explain how treatments in the hospital differ from those in the home for the following:
    a. bland aerosol treatment
    b. bronchodilator aerosol treatment
    c. IPPB treatment
5. Name three aerosol delivery devices.
6. Describe a procedure for making sterile water or normal saline at home.
7. Identify one compressor-driven nebulizer and

one respirator used for IPPB treatments in the home.
8. Describe how the role of IPPB in respiratory care has changed in recent years.
9. Describe the flow of gas in a respirator's breathing circuit.
10. A patient receiving aerosol therapy complains that his nebulizer is not making "mist." A patient on IPPB treatments states that the needle on the pressure gauge rarely reaches the preset peak pressure. Describe how to troubleshoot these two common problems.

This chapter presents aerosol therapy and IPPB. *Aerosol therapy* is the practice of delivering aerosol to the respiratory mucosa; an *IPPB treatment* is the practice of delivering positive pressure to the lungs for aerosol deposition or lung hyperinflation.

The first part of this chapter presents an overview of aerosol therapy to clarify the respiratory terminology and to explain the basic principles related to the generation of aerosol particles and their deposition in the respiratory tract. The remainder of the chapter explains how to give aerosol and IPPB treatments and to monitor their effects in the clinical setting.

The patient information in this chapter and Chapter 23 includes a few specific details on how to care for respiratory equipment at home. These details complement the more general information on the cleaning and disinfection of home equipment presented in Chapter 21.

Overview of Aerosol Therapy

The main purpose of aerosol therapy is to deliver medication or large quantities of liquid to help liquefy and mobilize respiratory secretions.

DEFINITIONS

The term aerosol is defined as *liquid or solid particles suspended in a gas.* It is delivered by a *nebulizer*, a device sometimes confused with a *humidifier.* Though both devices may be similar in appearance, a nebulizer produces aerosol mist. A humidifier produces humidified gas (water vapor) or warm moist air when a heater is in place (Fig. 22–1). Table 22–1 clarifies the basic differences between aerosol and humidification and between a nebulizer and a humidifier. (Humidification is discussed more thoroughly in Chapter 23.)

Though a nebulizer is intended to deliver aerosol, certain nebulizers (e.g., heated and ultrasonic) can provide up to 100% relative humidity as well.

TYPES OF AEROSOL

When aerosol therapy is initiated, the physician specifies the type of aerosol. The two main types of aerosol are *bland aerosol* and *medication aerosol.*

Bland aerosol contains water or isotonic, hypertonic, or hypotonic saline solution nebulized from a reservoir container. Nebulization of large quantities of bland aerosol is sometimes referred to as *mist therapy* because of the dense mist or fog produced (Fig. 22–2). This type of aerosol is most likely to benefit patients with inflammation or edema or the upper airway. Mist therapy is sometimes used to treat mucus retention problems, though little data support its use over conventional bronchial hygiene measures for secretion liquefaction and mobilization.

Medication aerosol is aerosol with medication added. It is delivered in small quantities via an inhaler, e.g., metered dose device (MDD); hand-held nebulizer, usually powered by a compressed gas source; and/or IPPB device. The medication is usually a bronchodi-

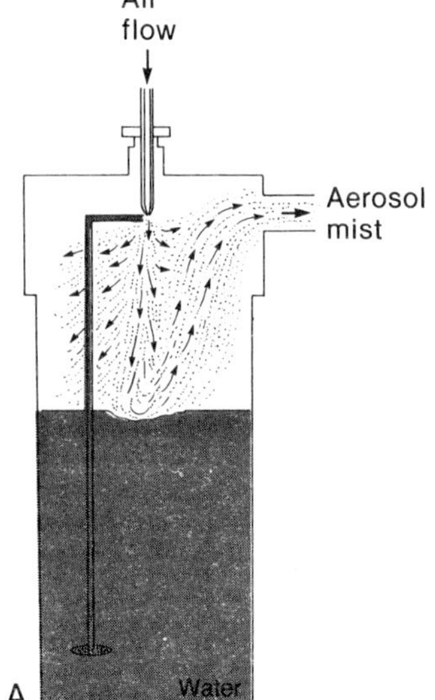

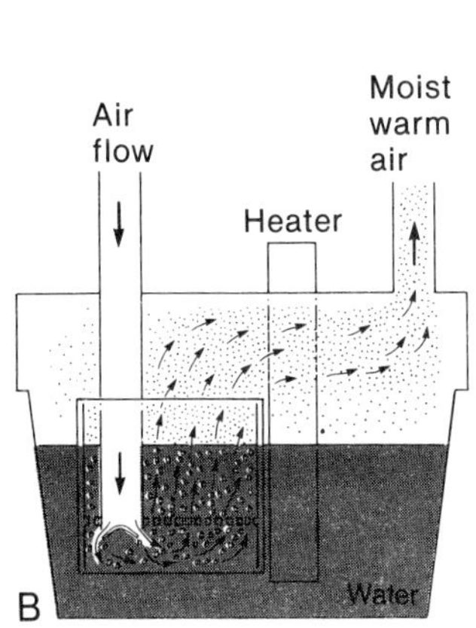

Figure 22–1. Nebulizer compared with a humidifier. *A*, A jet nebulizer produces aerosol particles that are incorporated into the carrier gas. The amount and size of the particles determine the water content of the gas. *B*, A Cascade type of heated humidifier produces warm moist air (water vapor) by bubbling the gas mixture through a heated water bath. (Reproduced and adapted by permission from Luce, J., Tyler, M., and Pierson, D. *Intensive Respiratory Care.* Philadelphia, W.B. Saunders Co., 1984.)

Table 22–1. AEROSOL COMPARED WITH HUMIDIFICATION

	Definition	Example	Respiratory Device
Aerosol	Liquid or solid particles suspended in a gas	Water or medication droplets suspended in air	Nebulizer delivers aerosol to respiratory tract; humidifies inspired gas
Humidification	Water in gaseous form	Water vapor	Humidifier humidifies inspired gas; a heater in the humidifier warms the moist air

lator, but others, such as a mucolytic agent, steroid, antibiotic, or alpha-adrenergic sympathomimetic, may be used as discussed in Chapter 11 on pulmonary medications.

AEROSOL PRODUCTION—PRINCIPLES OF JET NEBULIZATION

Most types of aerosol are produced in a *jet nebulizer* by a process called *jet nebulization.* Basic principles of jet nebulization are discussed in detail here because they provide an important theory base for understanding many respiratory techniques discussed elsewhere in this book. Moreover, these details will help the nurse better understand and remember the function of the main parts of any jet nebulizer.

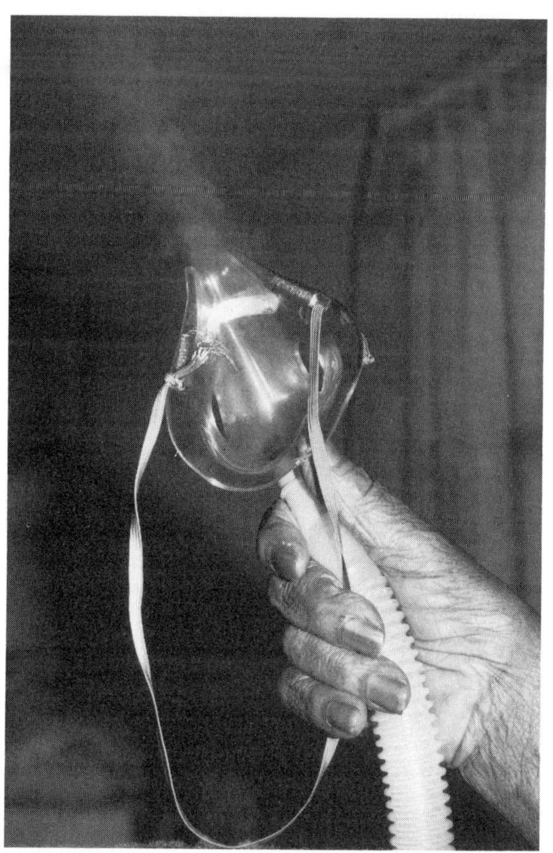

Figure 22–2. Dense fog or mist produced by nebulization of bland aerosol.

Jet Flow and Bernouilli's Principle

In a jet nebulizer, a high-velocity gas (i.e., jet flow) enters the nebulizer through a long tube (Fig. 22–3). The jet passes through a restricted orifice and across the end of a long capillary tube immersed in a liquid. The pressure drop at the end of the restricted orifice (Bernouilli's effect) draws liquid up the long capillary tube. When liquid reaches the jet flow, it is drawn into it and shattered into small aerosol particles.

Bernouilli's effect is explained by the principle of the same name. Bernouilli's principle is important to understand not only because of its role in respiratory therapy but also because of its role in the creation of adventitious lung sounds. This effect is responsible for the pressure drop in the postulated wheeze mechanism (review Fig. 12–52) as well as airway narrowing associated with inspiratory stridor (review Table 14–3). Bernouilli's principle is defined as follows:

> ***BERNOUILLI'S PRINCIPLE***
>
> The lateral pressure of a gas decreases as its velocity of flow increases.

For further explanation, consider a gas molecule moving down a relatively wide tube (Fig. 22–4A). It changes direction and hits the sides of the tube more frequently than a gas molecule moving down a much narrower tube (Fig. 22–4B). In the second case, the reduced number of impacts against the tube's wall is responsible for a *lateral pressure drop.* As lateral pressure decreases, gas flow through the center of the tube increases proportionally. Hence, whenever a tube becomes twice as narrow, molecules must travel twice as fast to maintain the same output within a given time period. Simultaneously, lateral pressure drops by half.

In a jet nebulizer, the lateral pressure drop occurs around the jet flow. The pressure drop at the end of the restricted orifice draws liquid up a small capillary tube as in a hand-held nebulizer or an IPPB device or up a longer capillary tube as in a large volume reservoir nebulizer.

When mist exits from the nebulizer uninhibited, as shown in Figure 22–3A, the nebulizer is more specifically called an *atomizer.* Hand-held atomizers are commonly used in otolaryngology and endoscopy procedures for application of local anesthetic.

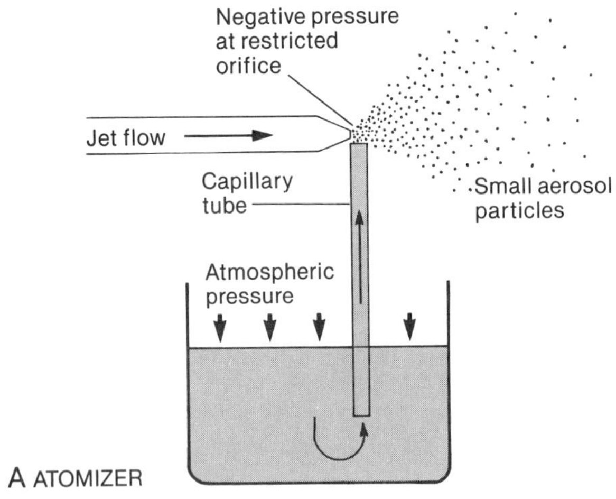

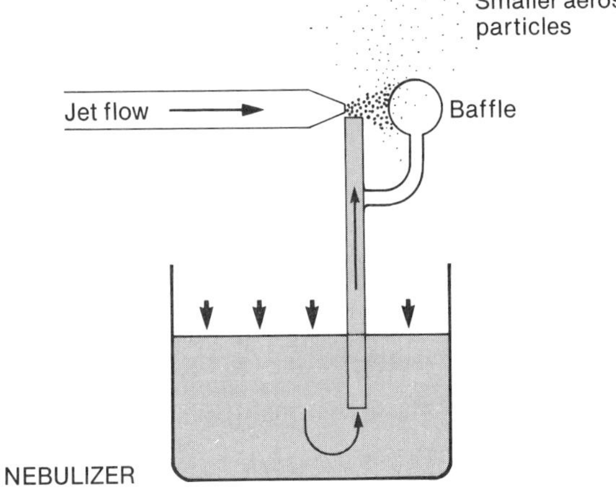

Figure 22–3. Atomizer without a baffle *(A)* compared with a nebulizer with a baffle *(B)*. Both aerosol devices use Bernouilli's principle to generate negative pressure at the restricted orifice.

Most jet nebulizers, however, have at least one *baffle* located by the jet flow. A *baffle* is any barrier—rod, sphere, plate, sides of a container, or surface of a liquid in a container—that helps reduce the average size of aerosol particles. In Figure 22–3B aerosol particles are further fragmented as they are blown against the baffle located directly in front of the jet flow.

Once aerosol is produced, small particles leave the nebulizer to be inhaled, whereas others coalesce into masses too large for transport. These masses return to the nebulizer's reservoir, or they "rain out" (i.e. condensation) in the breathing tube on the way to the patient.

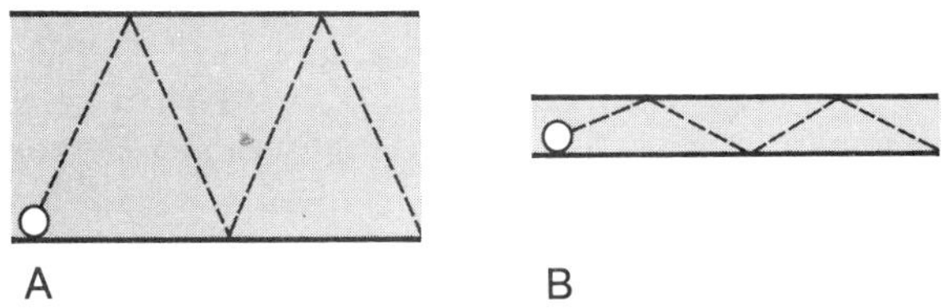

Figure 22–4. Movement of a gas molecule through a wide tube *(A)* compared with movement through a narrow tube *(B)*.

Air Entrainment and the FIO_2 Dial

Nebulizers have adjustable air entrainment ports that vary in size with the FIO_2 setting. When Bernouilli's effect occurs, the pressure drop *sucks in* room air through this *air entrainment* port (Figure 22–5). When the port is wide open (e.g., 0.35 FIO_2 in disposable units and 0.40 FIO_2 in some nondisposable units), aerosol output may increase by 50% and gas flow may increase fourfold compared with aerosol output and gas flow at the 1.0 FIO_2 setting (McPherson, 1985). The air-entrainment port is always kept wide open in the home setting, since compressed air rather than oxygen is the typical gas source and since occlusion may adversely decrease flow rate below the patient's inspiratory flow rate.

In the hospital setting, the nebulizer is attached to an air mix or oxygen source. This permits treatment of hypoxemia by adjustment of the nebulizer's FIO_2 setting. Increasing the FIO_2 setting gradually closes the air-entrainment port and decreases the dilution of pure oxygen from the gas source. In addition, a flow meter is attached to regulate gas flow. Liter flow is increased to at least 10 to 12 L/min or to a level that exceeds the patient's inspiratory flow rate.

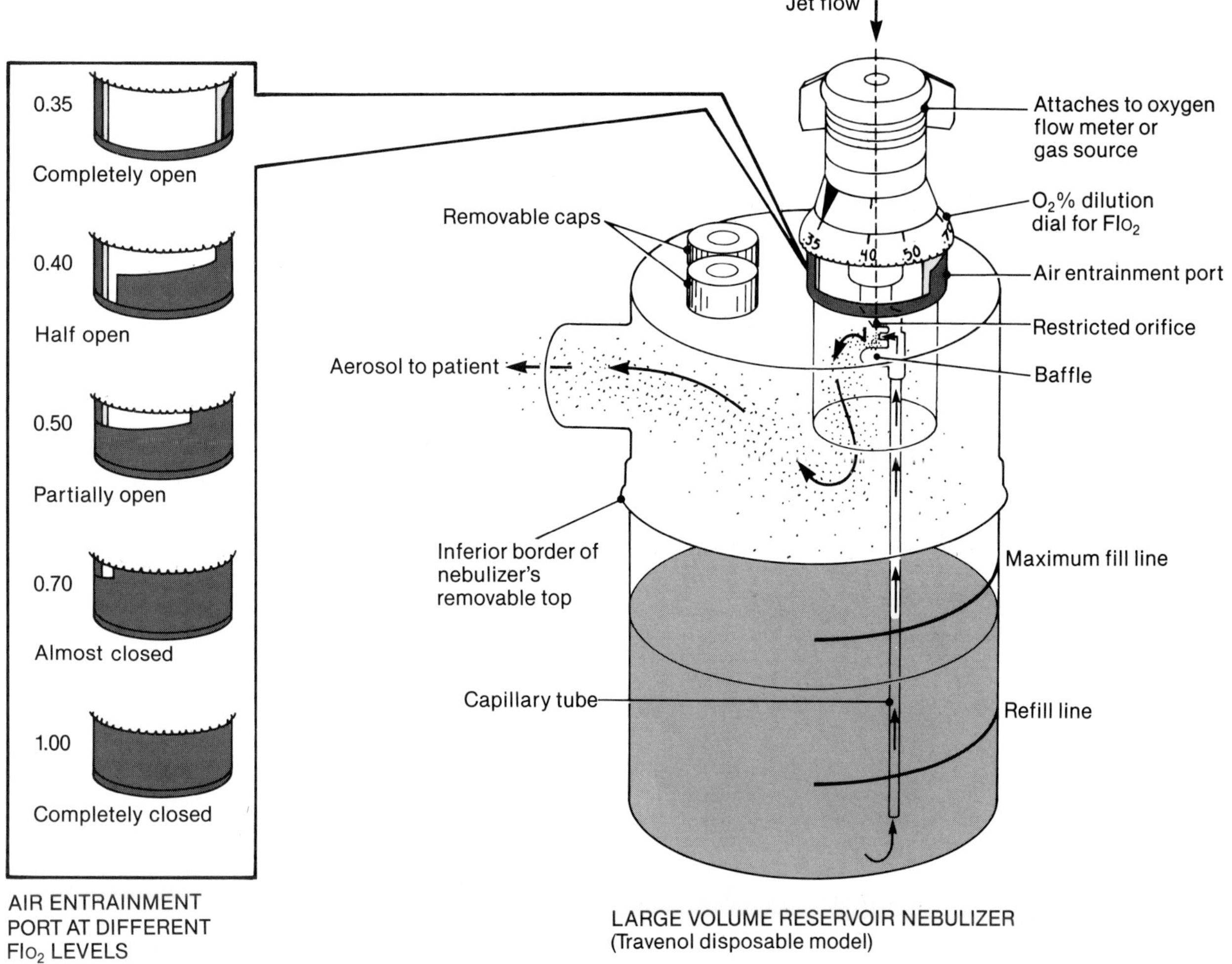

Figure 22–5. Large volume reservoir nebulizer (bottom) with air entrainment port at different FIO_2 levels (top).

When the patient's inspiratory flow rate is low, the respiratory therapist may dial in an FIO_2 of 1.0 to totally occlude the air entrainment port; he or she then uses an oxygen blender to dial in a more precise oxygen concentration. When the patient's inspiratory flow rate is normal to high, the air entrainment port may be kept wide open to increase the flow of gas through the system. A flow meter without a blender attached may be placed *in-line* between the gas source and nebulizer and patient, as shown in Figure 22–6. Whenever oxygen is used, oxygen concentration is checked by measuring actual FIO_2 with a probe attached to an oxygen analyzer and inserted near the patient's mouth.

AEROSOL DEPOSITION IN THE LUNGS

The effectiveness of medication or bland aerosol largely depends on the depth of aerosol deposition in the lungs. Several factors affect the depth of aerosol deposition, including particle size, particle density, gas viscosity, kinetic activity of gas molecules, particle inertia, patient's breathing pattern, and other factors mentioned in Pulmonary Pharmacology (see Chapter 11).

Particle size is a major factor. Generally, the smaller the particle, the deeper the penetration into the respiratory tract, as shown in Figure 22–7.

For bronchodilator aerosol delivery, nebulizers should produce a particle size in the range of 1 to 5μ (micron) for maximal deposition in small conducting airways and alveoli and for minimal systemic effects. Because less drug impacts in the mouth and upper respiratory tract, locations where rapid absorption into the blood stream normally occurs, minimal side effects are observed.

In contrast, a particle size in the 5- to 10-μ range produces maximal deposition in large conducting airways. The large particle size is appropriate when the goal of therapy is to deliver large volumes of bland solution to the respiratory tract, as in tracheitis, and when side effects are not concerns (e.g., no medication is in the solution).

As particle size increases, the probability of oropharyngeal deposition also increases. The probability of deposition in the oropharynx may exceed 50% for a

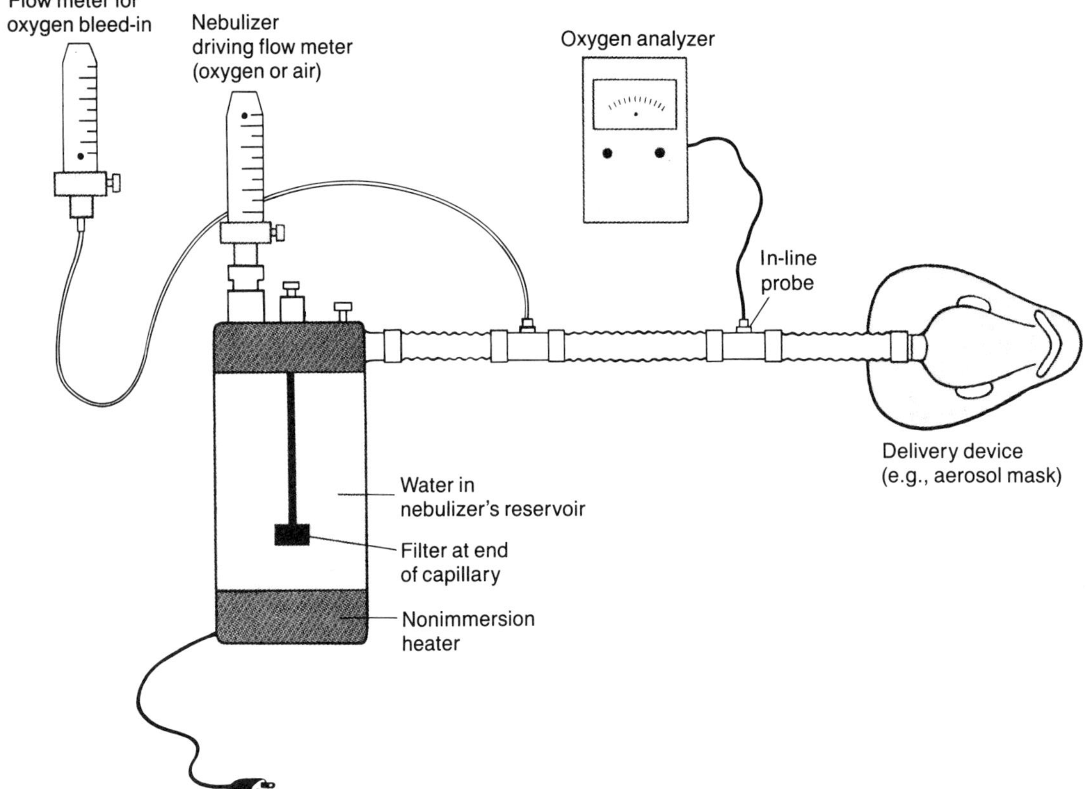

Figure 22–6. Controlled oxygen delivery via nebulizer. For oxygen above 35%, or lowest setting on nebulizer, both flow meters are oxygen powered. For oxygen less than 35%, air is used for driving the nebulizer. The air-entrainment port is left wide open in both cases to establish high total flow. (Reproduced and adapted by permission from McPherson, S.: Respiratory therapy equipment. St. Louis, C.V. Mosby Co., 1985.)

particle 8μ in diameter and is about 100% for a particle 16μ in diameter (Newman, 1985).

Bland Aerosol Treatment

GOALS

1. To add humidification to the respiratory mucosa.
2. To liquefy and mobilize secretions.
3. To improve alveolar ventilation.
4. To obtain sputum for diagnostic purposes.

INDICATIONS

1. Bypassed upper airway, e.g., tracheostomy.
2. Difficulty raising thick or tenacious secretions.
3. Mucus retention problem, unresponsiveness to conventional bronchial hygiene measures, e.g., hydration, coughing, deep breathing, and so forth.
4. Sputum induction for cytologic or bacteriologic studies.
5. Postextubation or postbronchoscopy.
6. Laryngotracheobronchitis.
7. Laryngeal edema.
8. Chronic obstructive pulmonary disease (COPD); atelectasis; and pneumonia, which is controversial.

TYPES OF BLAND AEROSOL

The physician may order a treatment with cool aerosol, heated aerosol, or ultrasonic aerosol.

Cool aerosol is aerosol delivered at room temperature.

Heated aerosol is aerosol heated to body temperature before delivery. Heat increases the moisture-carrying capabilities of delivered aerosol. The increase in humidity facilitates delivery of larger amounts of liquid to the respiratory tract.

Heated aerosol is not recommended for medication aerosol; when aerosol is heated, it impacts relatively high in the upper respiratory tract. The extra humidity coalesces on heated particles as they cool on the way to the patient. This coalescence increases particle size, thus causing early impaction on airways.

Ultrasonic aerosol is produced by a special type of nebulizer called an *ultrasonic nebulizer*. Unlike a jet nebulizer, an ultrasonic nebulizer produces sound waves that travel through a liquid, producing ultrasonic vibrations that break up water into small aerosol particles. Particle sizes range from 1 to 10μ. Most particles

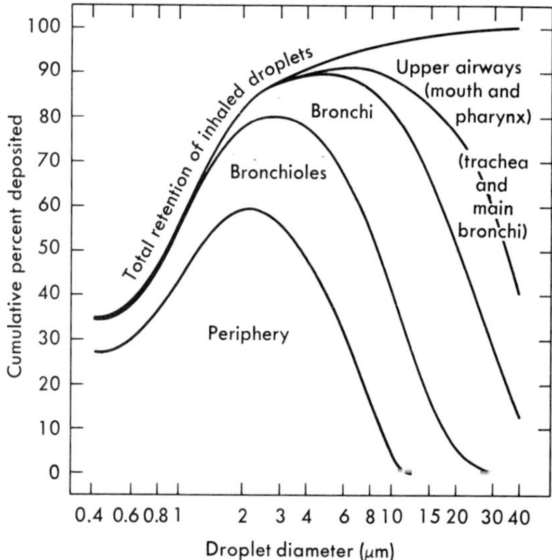

Figure 22–7. Particle deposition in the respiratory tract. The smaller the particle, the deeper into the respiratory tract the particle will potentially deposit. (Reproduced by permission from Cushing, I. and Miller, W. Nebulization Therapy. In *Respiratory Therapy*. (Safar, P.—ed.) Philadelphia, F. A. Davis Co., 1965.)

produced by ultrasonic nebulization are smaller than those produced by jet nebulization.

Important Points

These important points help keep the use of different types of bland aerosol in perspective. First, many clinicians do not use bland aerosol therapy because its efficacy is questionable. No research study supports its routine use in respiratory care. However, bland aerosol may benefit selected patients, such as those with mucus retention problems unresponsive to conventional bronchial hygiene measures.

Generally, cool aerosol is attempted first, followed by heated or ultrasonic aerosol if therapy ineffectively liquefies secretions. Ultrasonic aerosol is reserved for sputum inductions and for retention of thick secretions in peripheral lung regions.

There are exceptions to these guidelines. For example, some clinicians routinely avoid cool aerosol as a first choice. Because cool aerosol particles land more distally in the lung compared with heated particles, cool aerosol may increase the risk for infection, particularly in patients likely to have contaminated equipment or bland solutions.

Moreover, the nurse must keep in mind that response to therapy can be highly variable among patients. Asthmatic patients and others with hyperirritable airways may wheeze with the addition of bland aerosol to respiratory intervention. Bland aerosol is not appropriate for these patients. Other persons tolerate cool and ultrasonic aerosol but not heated aerosol. Some who tolerate cool and heated aerosols develop bronchospasm from the small particles delivered by ultrasonic nebulizers. Most important, aerosol therapy is likely to be ineffective unless conventional bronchial hygiene measures are implemented simultaneously. Since the efficacy of bland aerosol therapy is questionable, it may be the accompanying cough and deep breathing rather than the aerosol that is responsible for improvement in the patient's condition. Also, when therapy produces scattered rhonchi throughout the lungs, expectoration is mandatory to relieve airway obstruction.

HOME RESPIRATORY EQUIPMENT

Nebulizers

Cool aerosol is delivered via a durable, nondisposable unit, such as the *Puritan nebulizer* (Fig. 22–8A) or the *Ohio Deluxe nebulizer*. Numerous disposable nebulizers are available, but they are best reserved for hospital use (Fig. 22–8B).

Heated aerosol is delivered with the same nebulizer as that used for cool aerosol, except the water in the reservoir is heated with a *nonimmersion* or an immersion heater. The best type of heater for the home setting is the *plate* nonimmersion heater, a device placed underneath the nebulizer reservoir (Fig. 22–8C, left). Alternatively, the water can be heated by placing an *immersion-type heating probe* or heating rod through one of the ports on top of the nebulizer jar and into the solution to be aerosolized, as shown in Figure 22–8A. Though used in many hospitals, the heating probe is not recommended for home use because it increases the risk of airway burns from aerosol overheating and bacterial contamination from heating rod contact with solution. The *doughnut* heater is another alternative (Fig. 22–8C, right). However, similar to the heating rod, it is designed for hospital use.

Bland aerosol is occasionally delivered by ultrasonic nebulizer in the home setting.

Delivery Devices

Aerosol is delivered from a nebulizer to the patient via one of three devices as follows: an *aerosol mask; face tent*, also called a *face shield*; and a *tracheostomy collar* if a tracheostomy is present (Fig. 22–9). Persons who do not tolerate the aerosol mask owing to a feeling of suffocation can switch to the less occlusive face tent.

TEACHING THE PATIENT

The following self-care education material is appropriate for cool aerosol using a Puritan nebulizer in the home. However, the instructions for use of any type of large reservoir nebulizer are similar.

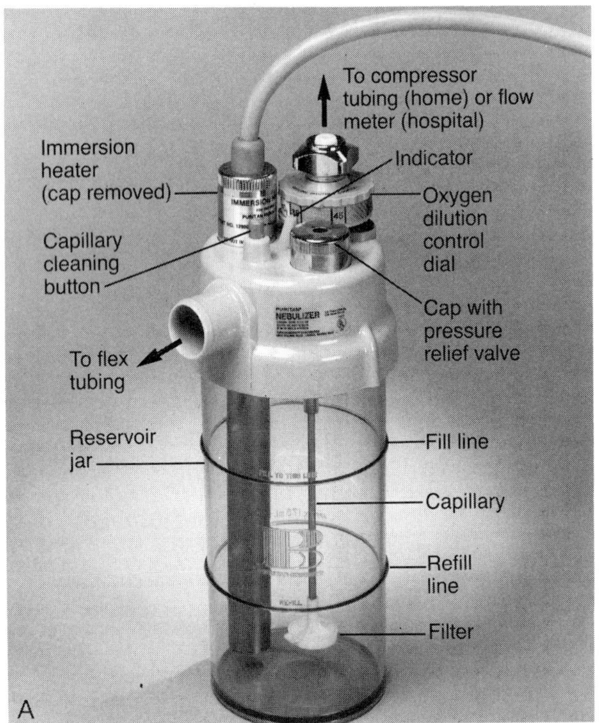

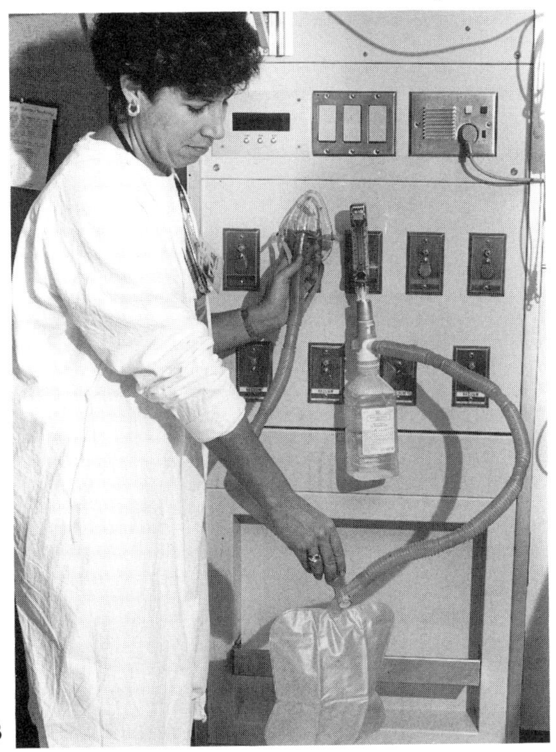

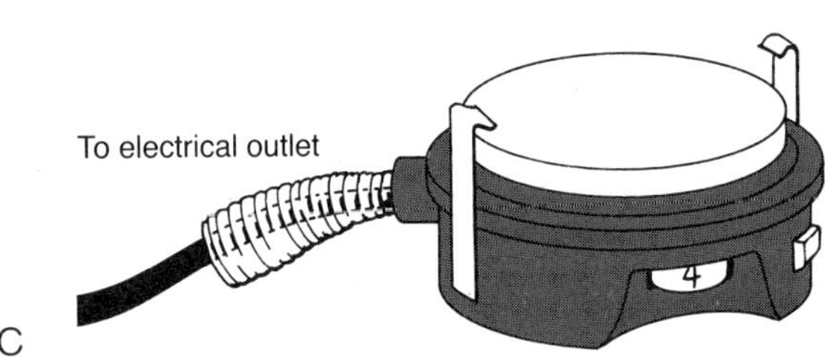

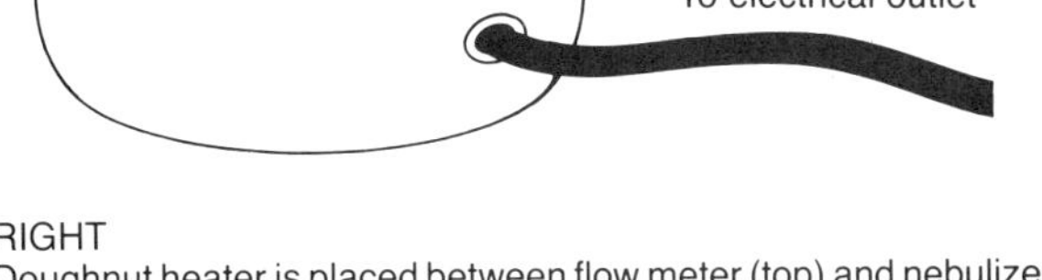

LEFT
Plate heater mounts on bottom of nebulizer jar and has a temperature control dial.

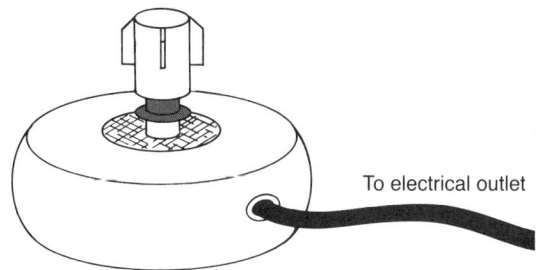

RIGHT
Doughnut heater is placed between flow meter (top) and nebulizer (bottom) and heats to a fixed temperature.

Figure 22–8. Nebulizer equipment for the delivery of bland aerosol. *A*, Non-disposable Puritan nebulizer with immersion heater. (Courtesy of Puritan-Bennett Corporation, Lenexa, KS.) *B*, Disposable nebulizer attached to flex tubing and delivery device. The plastic bag is a water trap used to prevent condensation from draining backwards into the nebulizer reservoir. The trap is rarely used in the home setting because it is difficult to clean, disinfect, and dry completely. *C*, Plate and doughnut types of nonimmersion heaters.

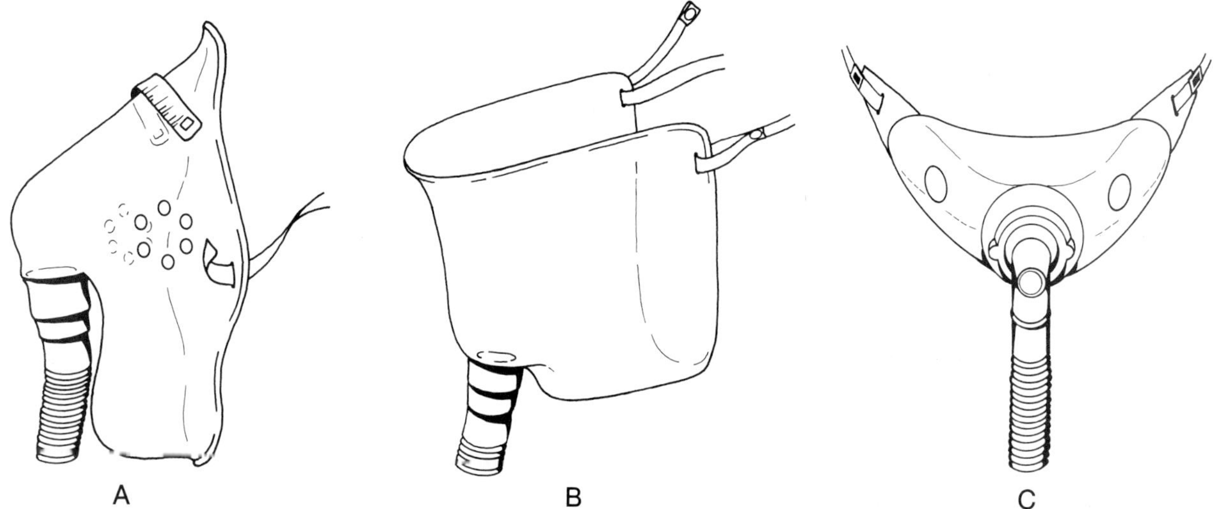

Figure 22–9. Aerosol delivery devices. *A*, Aerosol mask. *B*, Face tent. *C*, Tracheostomy collar.

PATIENT INFORMATION

Bland Aerosol Treatment

Your doctor has ordered bland aerosol to humidify the air you breathe and to liquefy any mucus in your lungs. Thin, liquefied mucus is much easier to cough up than thick mucus that sticks to your lung tissues.

Treatment Times

Preparation

1. Place the nebulizer jar in the stand.
2. Fill jar to "fill" line with ____________. (Refill when fluid level reaches "refill" line.)
3. Screw top on and make sure the oxygen dilution control dial is always on 35 or the lowest number. Turn the dial either way until the big indicator points to 35.
4. Connect the mask to the large flextubing and the other end of the flextubing to the nebulizer.
5. One end of the compressor tubing should already be screwed onto the compressor; screw the other end onto the top of the nebulizer.
6. Plug the compressor's electrical cord into the wall outlet.

Treatment

1. Relax in a comfortable chair.
2. Turn on the compressor, and make sure mist is coming out of the mask. If you are not getting enough mist, try pressing the cleaning button on the nebulizer top.
3. Secure mask to your face with elastic strap.
4. Breathe the mist in through your *mouth*; droplets are carried deeper in the lungs if they are inhaled through the mouth and not through the nose.
5. Halfway through and after your treatment, deep breathe and try to cough up any loose mucus.
6. Wipe face mask dry and place in clean plastic bag until next treatment.

Tips

1. If your shortness of breath, wheezing, or both become worse during aerosol therapy, stop your treatments and call your physician.
2. Regularly empty flextubing of accumulated fluid.
3. If you are using your mist unit as instructed and are still not getting enough mist output, call your visiting nurse or service company for further advice.

Cleaning

Daily

1. Discard leftover fluid.
2. Wash nebulizer jar with its top, mask, and flextubing with liquid detergent and water. Note, caps on the nebulizer top may be removed by turning them counterclockwise and lifting up.
3. Rinse well with warm tap water
4. Drip dry all parts and reassemble.

At Least Twice a Week

1. After washing with liquid detergent, rinse equipment.
2. Disinfect as directed.

Schedule

1. 20- to 30-minute treatments BID, TID, or QID.
2. Always schedule before postural drainage.
3. Bronchodilator aerosol may be given before or after bland aerosol, depending on clinical response. Many clinicians give the bronchodilator before bland aerosol to open airways and facilitate deeper penetration into the lungs. Others give bland aerosol first to clear airways of mucus before bronchodilator administration.
4. Continuous therapy for upper airway edema and swelling in acute care setting.
5. Continuous or nocturnal therapy for new tracheostomy patients to prevent dried mucus plugs.

Evaluation Criteria

For Correct Technique

1. The patient is sitting or lying comfortably with good posture and body alignment. Correct positioning promotes maximal lung expansion, deeper breaths, and more peripheral deposition of aerosol in the lungs.

2. The patient slowly *deep breathes* with his *mouth open* for at least half the duration of the treatment. Breathing through the nose results in increased aerosol deposition in the nose and pharynx rather than in the lungs.

3. Liter flow is at least 10 to 12 L/min, or mist is observed to *continually* drift out of the aerosol mask's exhalation ports. Note that aerosol density and oxygen concentration drop unless total flow from a mist setup equals or exceeds the patient's inspiratory flow demands. Patients with high minute ventilations have high inspiratory flow demands and may need a liter flow greater than 12 L/min. Hence, evaluation of liter flow is *best* accomplished by watching the amount of mist drifting out of the aerosol mask's exhalation ports.

4. The length of the delivery tube is as *short* as possible. A long flextube promotes the deposition of aerosol along the sides of the tubing, thereby decreasing the amount of aerosol reaching the patient. In heated nebulizers, it promotes excessive cooling of gases, loss of humidification, and "rain out" (i.e., condensation) in the tubing before moisture reaches the patient.

5. Minimal to small amounts of condensation in the unit's flextubing. Accumulation of large amounts of liquid slows air flow through the unit, decreases aerosol delivery, and promotes the drainage of liquid back into the nebulizer jar (a source of contamination). Whenever fluid accumulates in flextubing, the patient or nurse disconnects the tubing *near the nebulizer*; empties the fluid onto a towel or into a container, stretching the tubing if large corrugations are present; and reconnects the tubing to the nebulizer. When condensation is a problem, a small plastic bag or trap container may be inserted in line to catch drainage before it reaches the nebulizer (see Fig. 22–8B).

6. Flextubing is arranged in a downward direction from the face mask. The downward direction prevents rain out accumulation and the accidental flow of water into the patient's mouth.

7. Maintenance of the proper liquid level in the nebulizer jar. When the level is allowed to drop below the lowest limit line, less aerosol is made and delivered to the patient.

8. For heated aerosol units and humidifiers, temperature reading measured at the patient is never greater than 40°C (104°F), or the nebulizer or humidifier is never too hot to touch anywhere on its exposed surfaces (Health Devices, Inc., 1980). Higher temperatures may cause airway burns, manifested by sore throat, pain, edema, or blister. Nebulizers should not be allowed to warm up longer than 15 to 30 minutes before a treatment (check equipment manual for recommended time). Prolonged warm-up periods cause overheating. In the acute care setting, temperatures greater than 40°C (104°F) measured at humidifer or nebulizer outlets should be monitored continuously with a sensor in-line near the patient and an effective alarm system to signal overheating.

9. Adequate bubbling (i.e., water movement) in the nebulizer jar. Reduced bubbling may indicate inadequate liter flow, infrequent changing of water in the jar, or failure to thoroughly clean the capillary tube and attached filter (see Fig. 22–6).

10. Adequate face seal (e.g., aerosol mask) without signs of skin irritation or pressure sores from the elastic headband or edges of the mask. If necessary, pad mask edges or elastic with gauze or tape.

For Overall Improvement in Condition

1. See criteria for deep breathing and coughing, page 535.
2. Mucus is less tenacious and thick.
3. Absence of adverse effects.
   a. Flushing of the face.
   b. Increased airway obstruction, such as feeling of suffocation, dyspnea, chest tightness, coughing, wheezing, stridor, tachypnea, increased or irregular pulse, reduced FEV_1, and reduced PEF rate.
   c. Signs of hypoxemia when airway obstruction is severe.
   d. Increased fluid retention manifested by weight gain, crackles in lungs, and peripheral edema. Patients at risk are infants, children, and adults with histories of heart failure and patients' receiving continuous aerosol therapy, particularly ultrasonic aerosol.

IMPLEMENTATION

When the patient first starts on bland aerosol treatments, the nurse monitors signs and symptoms before, during, and after therapy. Key assessment parameters include history (i.e., chief complaint), pulse, respiratory rate, lung sounds, and skin color.

When adverse effects appear, the nurse stops therapy and notifies the physician. If mild dyspnea or wheezing develops, a bronchodilator aerosol may be given 20 minutes before the bland aerosol to control adverse effects. Aerosol therapy is promptly discontinued when the patient's condition improves, and mucus retention is no longer a problem.

If the patient does not respond, therapy may be ineffective, and a medical evaluation is indicated. More aggressive bronchial hygiene measures may need to be initiated for successful mucus expectoration. In rare cases, aerosol therapy is ineffective because the gas flow from the nebulizer dries retained secretions and causes mucosal swelling.

Using Bland Solutions

In the hospital, sterile water or sometimes normal saline (NS) (0.45 or 0.90) is added to the nebulizer's reservoir. Commercially prepared saline and sterile water are not used in the home setting because of cost and limited availability in the community. Distilled water is the preferred substitute for sterile water because it is practical, relatively inexpensive, and widely available in major grocery stores. If distilled water is unavailable, the patient can boil tap water for 15 to 20 minutes and allow it to cool to a lukewarm temperature before use. The sterilization procedure is summarized here.

PATIENT INFORMATION

Home Preparation of a Distilled Water (Normal Saline) Substitute*

Sterilization of the Storage Container

1. Select a jam jar or juice bottle to serve as a storage container for your aerosol solution.
2. Wash bottle and lid with liquid detergent. Rinse thoroughly.
3. Completely submerge the bottle and lid in a pan of tap water. Cover the pan with a lid and gently boil the contents for 15 to 20 minutes.
4. Use the pan lid to drain water out of the pan. Leave bottle and lid in the pan to cool.
5. Place bottle and lid on a clean counter to air dry. *Do not turn items upside down or touch inside surfaces.*

Sterilization of Tap Water

1. Pour twice the desired amount of tap water into the pan used to boil the bottle and lid.
2. Boil water gently for 15 to 20 minutes.
3. Let the water cool.

To Make Normal Saline Solution

1. Follow the same steps, but use distilled water rather than tap water.
2. Add salt to the water before boiling.
3. The correct proportion is ¼ teaspoon of salt to every 2 cups of water.

Storage

1. Pour sterilized water (saline) into sterilized container. Cover with lid and store in the refrigerator.
2. Discard unused sterile water once or twice a week and prepare a new batch.
3. To avoid contamination:
   a. Pour solution directly from the storage container to the nebulizer jar,
   b. Never pour extra solution back into the storage container,
   c. Never place unsterilized measuring device into the sterilized solution.

*After Moser, K., Archibald, C. et al. Better Living and Breathing, 2nd ed. St. Louis: C.V. Mosby, 1980.

When the patient prepares for an aerosol treatment, the nurse instructs him to allow adequate time for the hot sterile water (saline) to cool before use. Cooling prevents the risk of airway burns. Conversely, when refrigerated solution is used, the nurse instructs the patient to pour the cold solution into the nebulizer 15 to 30 minutes before treatment time to allow warming to room temperature. Though some patients are not sensitive to small changes in temperature, persons with increased bronchomotor tone may experience bronchospasm during inhalation of cold aerosol.

Though normal saline is not practical for home use, sometimes it is prescribed because of the patient's intolerance to distilled water. The procedure for making normal saline is the same as that for sterilizing tap water (described previously), except distilled water is the preferred mixing solution, and salt is added before boiling.

One problem with the making of saline solution is the precipitation of salt out of solution during cooling. Salt and solutes in tap water may clog up the nebulizer's filter, located at the tip of the capillary tube. Use of distilled rather than tap water helps prevent this equipment problem.

Furthermore, patients who use saline for any form of aerosol therapy and who do not meticulously clean the equipment parts more commonly run into problems, such as fused parts and clogged capillaries.

Water Versus Saline. The related literature does not support the use of any one best therapeutic agent for humidification and nebulization. In the past, water has been used for problems of humidity deficit, croup, cystic fibrosis, and sputum deficit, and normal saline mostly for problems of mucosal crusting and thick mucus plugs in small airways. Both agents, however, can produce local and systemic problems. The addition of water to the respiratory tract may cause airway irritation, coughing, wheezing, and overhydration. Excess normal saline can cause fluid overload and electrolyte imbalance with hypernatremia. Findings by Stehlin and Schare (1980) indicate that the inhalation of water aerosol may have more deleterious systemic effects than the inhalation of 0.9 or 0.45 NS aerosol.

Hence, in light of this information and administration problems at home, the best agent is one that is most practical and beneficial based on the patient's circumstances at home and clinical response to therapy.

Monitoring the Patient Receiving Ultrasonic Nebulization. Adverse effects are most likely in patients receiving ultrasonic nebulization. Since ultrasonic nebulizers can deliver large quantities of solution to the respiratory tract in a relatively short period of time, fluid overload is of special concern, particularly in the patient with a history of heart failure. The nurse monitors carefully for signs of fluid retention as well as for signs of bronchospasm. Bronchospasm is most likely because, as mentioned previously, ultrasonic particles are smaller and travel deeper into the lungs than jet nebulization particles. Monitoring for correct cleaning of equipment is given top priority for essentially the same reason. Contaminated ultrasonic aerosol reaches more peripheral lung regions compared with other forms of aerosol. From this perspective, the patient using an ultrasonic nebulizer is at increased risk for infection, unless proper follow-up supervision is provided.

Home Humidification—Alternative to Bland Aerosol Therapy? Some patients may verbalize a preference for using their over-the-counter home humidifier or vaporizer rather than a prescribed aerosol device for mucus retention problems. In most cases, home humidifier therapy is not an acceptable substitute for bland aerosol therapy because evidence is lacking regarding its efficacy. Though it may have a favorable placebo effect, a home humidifier may introduce other problems, such as increased potential for airway burns due to the poor design of the heaters of some heated humidifiers. Also, the patient may be at extremely high risk for infection because many humidifier models do not come apart completely to permit thorough cleaning and drying of parts.

The Hospital Setting. Monitoring in the hospital setting is basically the same as monitoring in the home setting, except for a few differences. First, the routine bland solution is sterile water, (sometimes sterile NS), available in disposable plastic bottles. Second, chest assessment findings of acutely ill patients, particularly those with upper airway problems and those on ultrasonic nebulization, are monitored more frequently, along with other vital signs. Third, patients with an endotracheal or tracheostomy tube may receive aerosol via a T-tube or T-piece delivery device (see Part 5, Specialized Interventions). Last, a water trap, such as a small plastic drainage bag, is usually routinely placed in-line to prevent condensation from accumulating in corrugations and draining back down into the nebulizer reservoir.

Bronchodilator Aerosol Treatment

GOALS

1. To bronchodilate airways and keep airway obstruction or chronic air flow limitation to a minimum.
2. To mobilize secretions.
3. To reduce mucosal edema (California Thoracic Society, 1981).

INDICATIONS

1. Pulmonary function test (PFT) evidence of air flow limitation or difficulty in removing bronchial secretions.
2. Lack of benefit from bronchodilator metered dose device (MDD) inhaler, e.g., no improvement in PFT values in a patient expected to improve.
3. Inability to properly use MDD, e.g., lack of manual dexterity.

HOME RESPIRATORY EQUIPMENT

Bronchodilator medication solution is delivered by either a jet nebulizer or an ultrasonic nebulizer.

Common jet nebulizers include the *Pulmo-Aide nebulizer* and the *Maximyst nebulizer*. These and other nebulizers are powered by small portable compressors, such as the one shown in Figure 22–10. The equipment setup is called a *compressor-driven nebulizer* setup or a *compressor nebulizer*.

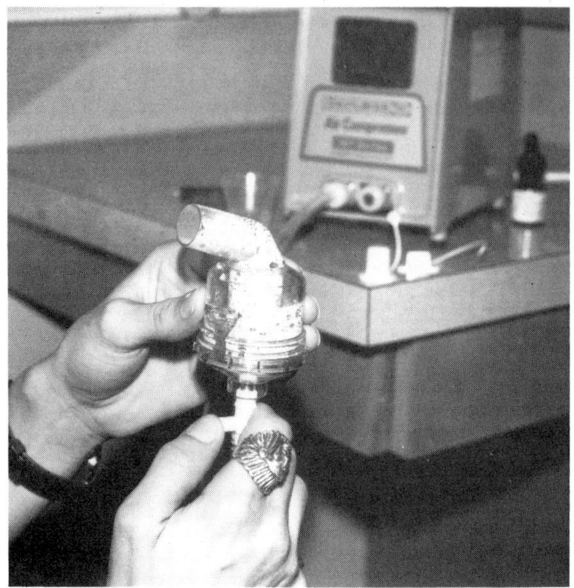

Figure 22–10. A compressor-driven nebulizer setup. The durable DeVilbiss model #645 nebulizer is attached to the small portable Pulmo-Aide compressor in the background. The plugs to the mouthpiece and air entrainment port (located by left thumb) are removed and rest on the table. The right finger is placed over the actuator valve to test for mist output before a treatment. NOTE: Though this nebulizer model is no longer available, many patients continue to use it because it is more durable than the newer DeVilbiss model presented elsewhere.

Ultrasonic nebulizers are sometimes used to deliver medication aerosol because home models are small,

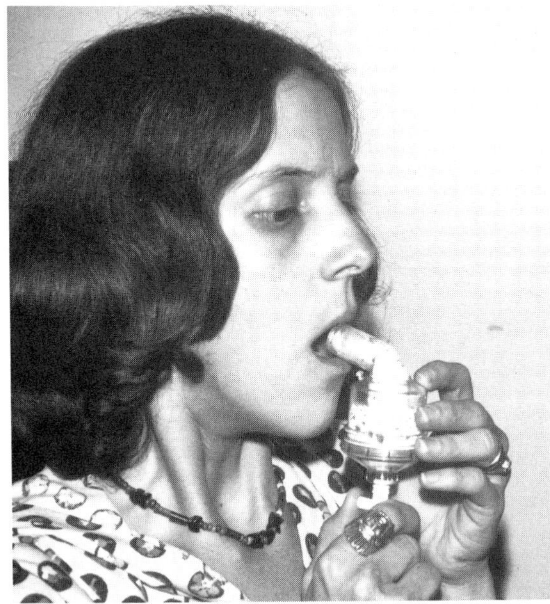

Figure 22–11. The inspiratory phase of respiration during a compressor nebulizer treatment.

portable, and relatively easy to operate. Also, they are easy to clean, since the reservoir lacks a capillary tube.

TEACHING THE PATIENT

The educational material that follows is written for nebulizers with an actuator valve and air-entrainment port, e.g., DeVilbiss Pulmo-Aide (645) compressor-driven nebulizer setup. However, the basic content may be applied to other compressor nebulizers encountered in the clinical setting.

PATIENT INFORMATION

Using Your Compressor-Driven Nebulizer

Scheduled Times

Your morning and evening treatments are especially important to help open your airways and clear your lungs for a more comfortable day and a good night's sleep. Do not miss these important treatments.

A cloud-like mist is made from the medicated fluid in the nebulizer and the constant air flow coming from the motor-driven compressor. If you properly breathe in the mist, the medication will land deeper in the lungs and open up your airways. Additional coughing and deep breathing will help keep your lungs well aerated and clear of mucus.

Preparation

1. Place compressor driven nebulizer setup on a table next to you. Plug in the compressor's power cord to the wall outlet.
2. Assemble unit as instructed in your manual but *do not attach or use white mouthpiece.* Remove cap to the nebulizer's mouthpiece as well as the cap to the side air vent.
3. Add the ordered medication to the nebulizer through the mouthpiece.
4. Sit in a comfortable, straight-backed chair with your feet flat on the floor, with tissues close by.
5. Turn the compressor switch to *ON*.
6. Test to make sure the nebulizer is working; mist should be coming out of the nebulizer when you hold it upright, and put your thumb or finger over the white activator valve beneath the nebulizer.
7. *Relax.* Let your shoulders drop.
8. Get nebulizer ready by placing it up to your mouth.

Proper Breathing Technique

1. Pursed-lip breathe all your air out without straining.
2. Place finger or thumb over activator valve and take a slow, deep breath in. Remember, do not seal your lips around the mouthpiece. The room air you breathe in with the mist increases the air flow into your lungs.
3. Remove thumb or finger from the valve and hold your breath for at least 1 to 3 seconds (10 seconds, if possible).
4. Breathe your air out slowly and completely through pursed lips without straining.

Tips

1. To avoid wasting medication, remember to put your thumb or finger over the activator valve *only* when taking a breath in.
2. Occasionally tap on the side of the nebulizer with your fingers to make droplets fall to the bottom of the cup where the capillary is located.
3. Repeat the relaxed breathing technique until medication is gone. Rest whenever necessary. Deep breathe and cough to aerate lungs and clear airways of mucus.

Cleaning Procedure

Always store nebulizer in a plastic bag or covered container.

Daily

1. Take nebulizer apart. Be sure to pull out capillary.
2. Wash with liquid detergent (e.,g., Joy) and water. Clean small holes with cleaning wire or pipe cleaner.
3. Rinse well; drip dry.
4. Reassemble.

At Least Twice a Week

1. Wash compressor tubing with liquid detergent. Rinse.
2. Disinfect nebulizer and compressor tubing as directed.

Tips

1. Once you have mastered this breathing technique, try abdominal breathing with pursed lips while taking your treatment. With better lung expansion and better air flow, medication will go deeper into the lungs.
2. If the compressor makes an unusual sound during operation, the air filter may need cleaning or changing. Check your equipment manual for instructions.
3. If your machine takes excessively long to nebulize solution, it may need cleaning. Check with your equipment company.

Schedule

1. As ordered:
   QD: upon rising in the morning.
   BID: upon rising in the morning and just before bedtime.
   TID: Early am; before lunch, as chronic obstructive pulmonary disease (COPD) patients have more secretions in the morning; and at bedtime.
   QID: add a treatment before dinner.
2. Never schedule treatment immediately after meals or nasogastric feedings.
3. Before treatment, give PRN sedation or pain medication for tense patients and patients splinting with pain in the acute care setting.
4. Pain relief and relaxation facilitate deep breathing and more peripheral deposition of aerosol in the lungs.

Evaluation Criteria

For Correct Technique

1. A comfortable breathing pattern. See criteria for deep breathing, pursed-lip breathing (PLB), and diaphragmatic breathing.
2. Finger occlusion of activator valve is coordinated with inspiratory phase of respiration (see Fig. 22–11).
3. With finger occlusion, compressed air is directed through the nebulizer's capillary to make mist.
4. If patients cannot use the activator valve owing to coordination problems, remove it from the nebulizer circuit.
5. To compensate for wasted medication during continuous nebulization, check with the physician regarding a medication dosage adjustment; dose may be doubled.

6. At least a 1- to 3-second end-inspiratory pause at total lung capacity (TLC).

7. The longer the pause, the more likely that aerosol will impact in peripheral lung regions.

8. Treatments lasting 8 to 15 minutes for best results with minimal side effects (Helmholz and Burton, 1984).

9. Lengthy treatments may indicate a clogged nebulizer capillary and inadequate nebulization, or the patient may be adding too much diluent to the nebulizer or forgetting to discard leftover medication from a previous treatment.

10. To avoid excessive patient fatigue, the physician usually orders only 1.5 to 3 ml of diluent.

For Overall Improvement in Condition

1. See criteria for deep breathing and coughing.

2. An increase in intensity of normal breath sounds, a decrease in wheezes, crackles, and rhonchi after treatments, or both.

3. Absence of adverse effects, such as dizziness from hyperventilation, excess fatigue, medication side effects.

4. Improved pulmonary symptoms and general sense of well being.

5. Improved PFTs (VC, PEF, FEV_1, and $FEF_{25-75\%}$) after bronchodilator aerosol treatment.

6. On complete PFT, prebronchodilator results are better than results from a previous day. Postbronchodilator results approximate prebronchodilator results.

Implementation

The patient information and evaluation criteria for correct technique apply to aerosol treatments using a certain type of nebulizer. In the clinical setting, however, nebulizers may vary in design. For example, in the Mada model (Fig. 22–12A) and in the newest DeVilbiss Pulmo-Aide model (Fig. 22–12B), the top to the medication cup attaches to a T adapter, also referred to as a T piece (Fig. 22–12). This design requires utilization of a mouthpiece, so that the patient can inspire room air through the other end of the adapter. In the Mada model, neither an actuator valve nor an air entrainment port is used. Though these changes may drastically simplify breathing technique for patients' having problems taking their treatments correctly, the main disadvantage is the potential for increased deposition of medication in the mouth and on the tongue rather than in the lungs. Closure of the mouth around the mouthpiece may impede laminar inspiratory airflow.

When working with patients using the T-piece design, the nurse adapts the aforementioned evaluation criteria, emphasizing the following: upright posture (i.e., not bent over or lying down); slow, deep breathing; 1- to 3-second end-inspiratory pauses; and frequent rests, as needed. The compressor should be turned off during rests to avoid medication wastage.

The monitoring of patients' taking bronchodilator aerosol treatments is similar to the monitoring of patients' taking bland aerosol treatments. The nurse monitors the patient's verbal complaints, pulse, respiratory rate, lung sounds, and skin color before, during, and after the initial aerosol treatment and thereafter during periodic evaluation home visits. Emphasis is placed on assessing ventilation and wheezing to determine whether the patient benefited from the bronchodilator aerosol. (See Chapter 11 for monitoring patients on bronchodilator medications.)

When a compressor or electrical outlet is unavailable, the patient may use a hand-bulb nebulizer for aerosol delivery. The technique is basically the same except that the patient manually squeezes a rubber bulb, instead of occluding an actuator valve, during inhalation to produce mist. Hand-bulb nebulizers are rarely used because many disabled persons have trouble squeezing the bulb at the right time. Also, whenever possible, aerosol bronchodilators are always delivered by inhaler, as described in Chapter 18. Inhalers are similar to hand-bulb nebulizers in that they can be difficult to coordinate manually. Yet, compared with nebulizers in general, inhalers are much easier to care for: the cartridges are disposable, and the plastic oral adapter is easy to wash and disinfect along with the rest of the patient's equipment.

The Hospital Setting. In the hospital setting, the bronchodilator aerosol treatment is commonly referred to as the *hand-held nebulizer* treatment, abbreviated *HHN Tx*. The technique is basically the same as that previously described except the setup is slightly different. A disposable nebulizer is attached directly to an air mix or oxygen flow meter. Flow is set at 4 to 8 L/min. An actuator valve is usually omitted, since many patients are too ill to coordinate inhalation with actuator occlusion. Also, a mouthpiece is added in accordance with the T adapter design of many of the disposable models on the market. Both omission of the actuator valve and use of a mouthpiece facilitate the learning process for acutely ill patients in the hospital.

For patients on mechanical ventilation, a nebulizer is inserted along the inspiratory breathing circuit close to the endotracheal tube for periodic treatments. (See Fig. 28–10.)

Intermittent Positive Pressure Breathing (IPPB) Treatment

IPPB refers to the inhalation of a gas by an intermittent pressure–cycled respirator followed by passive exhalation to atmospheric pressure. The gas is delivered in 15- to 20-minute treatments, with humidity, medication aerosol, or both added, depending on the goals of therapy.

GOALS

1. To improve alveolar ventilation and lung expansion above that achieved with spontaneous deep breathing.

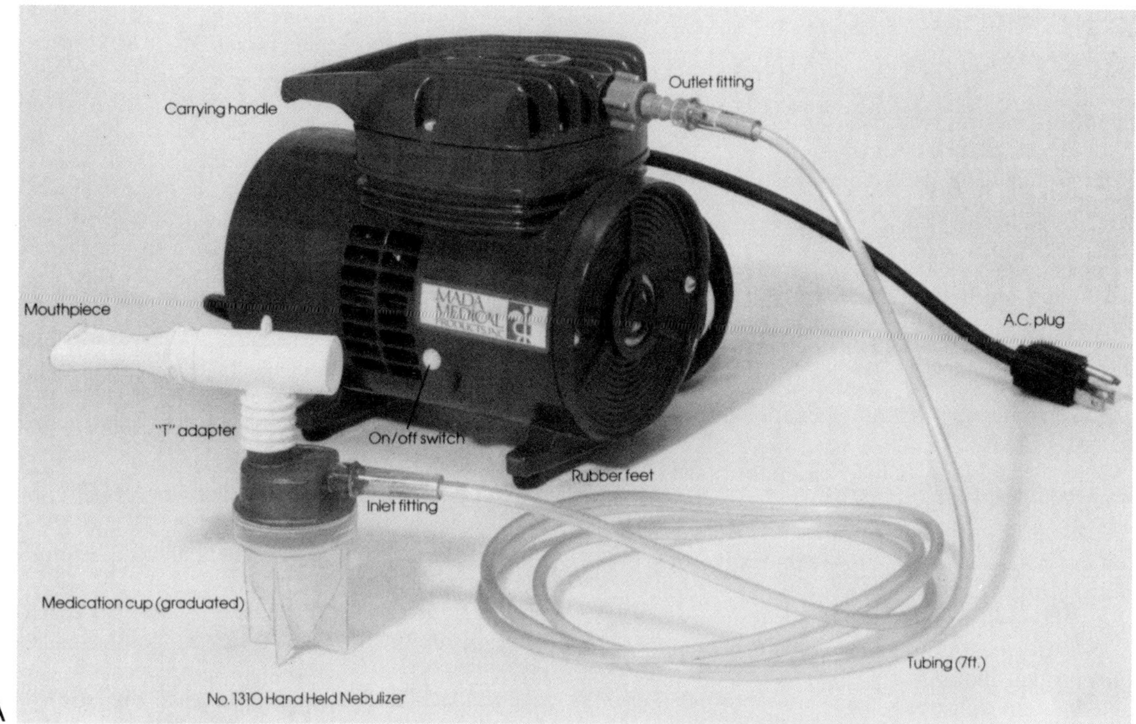

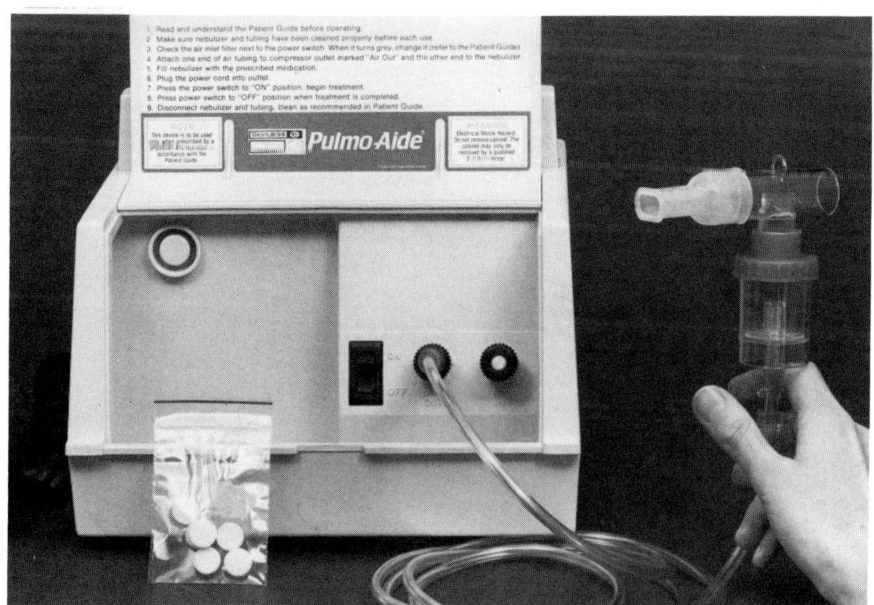

Figure 22–12. Compressor-nebulizer setups with a *T* adapter attached to the nebulizer. *A*, Mada model. (Courtesy of Mada Medical Products, Inc., Carlstadt, New Jersey.) *B*, DeVilbiss Pulmo-Aide model. The plastic bag contains filters for the air-inlet filter located to the right of the nebulizer tubing's compressor connection. (Courtesy of National Medical Homecare, Sacramento, CA.)

2. To prevent atelectasis and pneumonia.
3. To improve delivery of aerosol medications, coughing, and expectoration and thereby help keep airway obstruction or chronic airflow limitation to a minimum.

INDICATIONS

1. Difficulty in raising respiratory secretions.
2. PFT evidence of airflow limitation.
3. Reduced vital capacity (VC) with ineffective deep breathing and coughing.
4. Unsuccessful trial of simpler and cheaper approaches, e.g., inhaler, compressor nebulizer (hand-held nebulizer), voluntary deep breathing, incentive spirometry, hydration, and postural drainage.
5. Special situations
   a. Acute pulmonary edema secondary to left ventricular failure.
   b. Acute respiratory failure in nonintubated patients with COPD.
   c. Weak patients with neuromuscular deficits, e.g., loss of consciousness and degenerative nerve or muscle disorders.
   d. Restrictive disorders that impair lung expansion, e.g., severe kyphoscoliosis, ascites, alveolar or interstitial disease.
   e. Medication delivery.
   f. Sputum induction for diagnostic studies.

The role of IPPB in respiratory care has changed in recent years. Clearly, the trend is toward less reliance on IPPB and more reliance on simpler methods for aerosol deposition, lung expansion, and secretion mobilization. IPPB provides no clear advantages to patients able to inhale breaths of 15 to 20 ml/kg of body weight (Hodgkin and Webster, 1982). Results from a study by the Lung Division of the National Heart, Lung, and Blood Institute indicate that IPPB provides no benefit over a simple compressor-driven nebulizer in stable outpatients with COPD (The IPPB Trial Group, 1983).

In restrictive disease, IPPB may be used to improve lung compliance and decrease the work of breathing rather than to deliver aerosol to the lungs. Yet, even this use is in question for selected patients. A study by McCool and associates (1986) indicates that patients with quadriplegia or muscular dystrophy do not show immediate improvement in mechanics of breathing from IPPB treatments.

CONTRAINDICATIONS

The main contraindications for IPPB are listed in the box. Some contraindications, such as hypotension, hemoptysis, and increased intracranial pressure, are relative rather than absolute depending on the clinical situation.

CONTRAINDICATIONS TO IPPB

1. History of pneumothorax with IPPB.
2. Pneumothorax, untreated with bronchopleural fistula or treated without chest tube.
3. Tracheoesophageal fistula.
4. Bullous emphysema.
5. Subcutaneous or mediastinal emphysema.
6. Cardiovascular insufficiency, e.g., hypotension, hypovolemia, arrhythmias.
7. Subjective deterioration, e.g., treatment causes increased dyspnea or patient distress.
8. Esophageal or gastric surgical procedure.
9. Hemoptysis.
10. Increased intracranial pressure.

HOME IPPB RESPIRATORS

Home IPPB respirators are electrically operated machines, such as the Bennett AP-4 and AP-5 respirators (Fig. 22–13), the Monaghan 515 respirator, and the Portabird respirator.

The Bennett respirator is the most popular because it is durable, easy to operate, flow sensitive, and equipped with a practical nondisposable breathing circuit. It is flow sensitive because this respirator has an internal Bennett valve that automatically adjusts inspiratory flow according to changing airway resistance (Fig. 22–14). This feature facilitates ventilation of COPD patients with turbulent air flow.

Familiarity with the knobs and tubes of a common respirator, such as the Bennett respirator, is essential before the nurse can teach the patient and troubleshoot common equipment-related problems in the home setting.

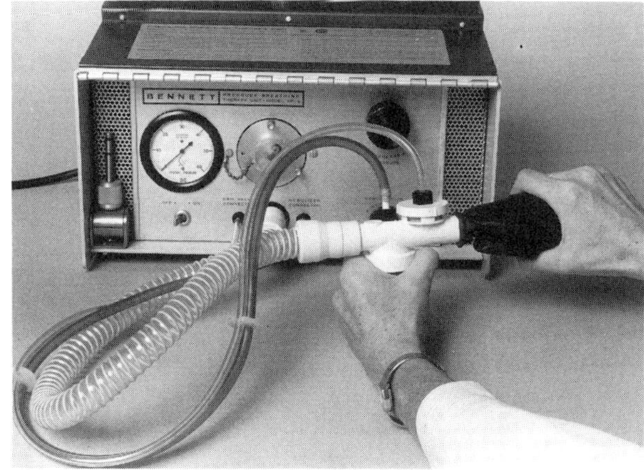

Figure 22–13. The Bennett model AP-4 respirator. The AP-4 and AP-5 models are basically the same except for accessory parts. Here, a test lung is used to check sensitivity and peak inspiratory pressure.

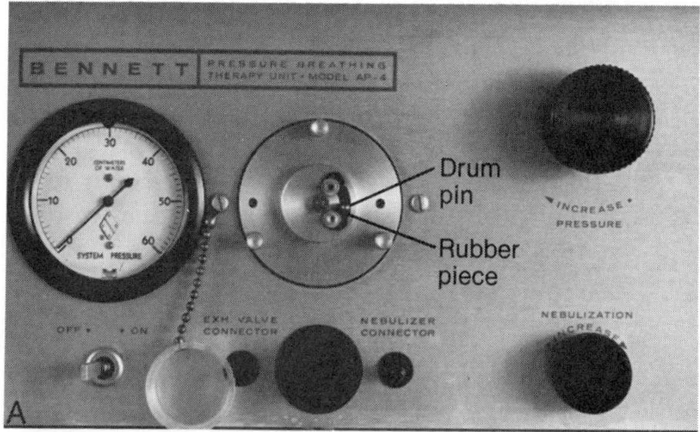

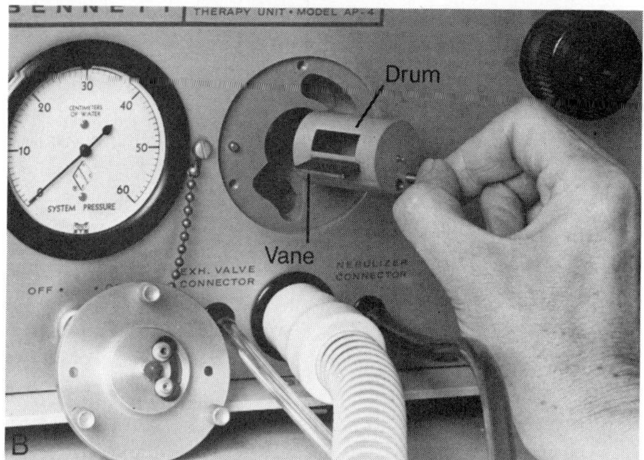

Figure 22–14. The flow-sensitive Bennett valve. *A, Outside view.* Ventilator sensitivity is changed by manually moving the rubber piece up or down. *B, Inside view.* The valve's drum is carefully removed for cleaning by handling the drum pin.

The Flow of Gas in a Breathing Circuit

Most breathing circuits used for IPPB as well as for continuous mechanical ventilation are the same as or similar to the Bennett circuit. Regardless of the model, air moves through the three following tubes: (1) *main breathing tube,* (2) *exhalation valve tube,* and (3) *nebulizer tube* (Fig. 22–15).

Once the patient triggers the respirator, the respirator forces air down the *main breathing tube,* through the *manifold* and *mouthpiece* to the patient. Simultaneously, air flows through the exhalation valve and into or against an internal diaphragm (Fig. 22–16). This pressure against the diaphragm occludes the exhalation valve or port during inspiration.

Inspiration continues until the patient reaches a preset peak inspiratory pressure that is controlled by adjustment of the pressure knob on the respirator. Pressure is displayed visually on a manometer located above the power switch in cm H_2O.

When the manometer's needle reaches the preset pressure, all inspiratory gas flow stops. The patient exhales passively through the exhalation valve port as the needle on the pressure manometer falls to zero (Fig. 22–17).

Nebulization

When the nebulization control is turned on, air flows through the *nebulization tube* and to the nebulizer, producing an aerosol by the previously described Bernouilli's effect.

The patient's breathing circuit has a mainstream or sidestream type of nebulizer. In a *mainstream nebulizer* (Fig. 22–18, left), the nebulizer is located directly in the path of the main gas flow along the main breathing circuit. The Bennett Slip/Stream nebulizer (Fig. 22–19) and the Bird micronebulizer are examples of mainstream nebulizers.

In a *sidestream nebulizer* (Fig. 22–18, right), the nebulizer is located well below the circuit's manifold. Aerosol is injected into the gas stream from the side. The Bennett Twin with two jets and capillary tubes is an example of a sidestream nebulizer.

The mainstream nebulizer has the advantage of a higher aerosol output compared with the sidestream nebulizer. The last delivers less aerosol because of excess rain out or condensation before aerosol drifts into the main gas flow. Though output is reduced, however, the sidestream nebulizer has the advantage of delivering a smaller particle size, a factor favoring more peripheral deposition in the lungs.

TEACHING THE PATIENT

The information that follows is written for the Bennett AP-4 and AP-5 respirators; basic principles of operation may be applied to other IPPB machines as well.

PATIENT INFORMATION

Your Respirator IPPB Treatment (Bennett AP-4, AP-5)

Scheduled Times
Your morning and evening treatments are especially important to help clear your lungs for a more comfortable day and a good night's sleep. Do not miss these treatments.

Your respirator delivers air with moisture, medication, or both to your lungs under positive pressure. If taken correctly, respirator treatments with additional coughing and deep breathing will help keep your lungs well ventilated and clear of mucus.

Preparation
1. Set your respirator on a table in front of you where you can see the dials. Connect the electrical power cord to the wall outlet.
2. To put your setup together, look at the picture in your respirator manual.
   a. Connect the large breathing tube to the black air outlet.
   b. Connect the blue nebulizer tube to the *NEBULIZER CONNECTOR* outlet on the front of the machine. Connect the other end to the opening just above the nebulizer cup.

c. Connect the smaller clear tube to the *EXH. VALVE CONNECTOR* and to the exhalation valve.
d. If you have set up your equipment properly, the exhalation valve will be a little closer to your mouthpiece than your nebulizer cup.
e. Add medication and distilled water to the nebulizer cup. Screw the cup back on. Be sure the little tube or nebulizer jet inside is below the level of the fluid in the cup.

Treatment

1. Sit in a comfortable, straight-backed chair with your feet flat on the floor. Keep tissues close by.
2. Relax. Let your shoulders drop.
3. Flip the power switch to *on*. Turn the *Nebulization* or *Neb* knob on until you can see mist coming out of the mouthpiece.
4. Place your lips firmly around the mouthpiece to keep a seal.
5. Start to take a deep breath in to trigger the machine, relax, and let the machine fill your lungs with air; pause 1 to 3 seconds before breathing out.
6. Breathe out slowly and completely through the mouthpiece without straining. Pause before taking the next breath.
7. Note that with each breath in, your machine is set to automatically stop when the needle on the pressure dial reaches cmH_2O.
8. Stop and cough whenever you feel mucus in your chest.

Tips

1. Try to make the pressure needle go up evenly with each breath by relaxing and breathing slowly.
2. For a more effective treatment, use diaphragmatic breathing while keeping a continual seal around the mouthpiece. If you feel relaxed and comfortable, try to actively inspire throughout inspiration to increase the volume of each respirator breath.
3. End your treatment early if your nebulizer cup runs out of medication or water. You might have to adjust the nebulization knob so that you run out of medication when your treatment is supposed to be over.
4. If you feel your heart beating faster or skipping beats or if you feel dizzy, slow your breathing rate down. If symptoms persist, cut the dose of your medication in half, use the same amount of distilled water or normal saline, and try a treatment. Call your physician if problems persist.

Schedule

1. Same as for aerosol treatments, with treatments lasting 10 to 20 minutes.

2. 5- to 10-minute treatments, TID, QID to ql to 2h in restrictive disorders when lung expansion is a primary goal.

3. 5- to 10-minute treatments qlh to avoid endotracheal intubation in the acute setting (Ziment, 1984).

Evaluation Criteria

For Correct Technique

1. Volume provided by IPPB exceeds the patient's spontaneous inspired volume, preferably by 25%.

2. Initial treatments should be monitored with a bedside spirometer.

3. Patient adherence to preset peak pressure, usually set at 10 to 15 cmH_2O for normal lungs to 15 to 25 cmH_2O for COPD.

Some patients may indiscriminately increase pressure, not realizing the dangers of high pressures over 30 to 35 cmH_2O. Hence, in the home setting it is most practical to stick with *one* present pressure and work on relaxation and other ways to increase volume. To determine optimal pressure, if it has not already been determined, the nurse starts at 12 to 15 cmH_2O and raises pressure 2 to 3 cm at a time *until* adequate inspired volumes are achieved and *as long as* the increased pressure does not cause undue patient discomfort. Remember, *preset pressure never guarantees adequate volume.*

4. Avoidance of premature exhalation or excessive inspiratory effort during inhalation.

After the patient learns the basic technique, he or she can be coached to *actively* inspire to increase volume (Welch et al, 1980). However, inspiratory effort should never be excessive, and the therapist or nurse should monitor volumes or breath sounds during coached breaths to be sure volumes increase along with inspiratory effort.

5. Slow inspiratory flow rate as evidenced by the smooth steady ascent of the pressure needle during inspiration.

A slow flow rate promotes laminar flow, ventilation of lung regions with decreased compliance, and peripheral deposition of aerosol. In contrast, a rapid inspiratory flow rate promotes a rapid respiratory rate, hyperventilation, dizziness, and more proximal deposition of aerosol in the respiratory tract.

6. End-inspiratory pause for at least 1 to 3 seconds. The pause increases aerosol deposition before exhalation and promotes equal distribution of gas to all lung regions.

7. Inspiratory:expiratory (I:E) ratio of 1:3 to 1:4. The long expiratory phase facilitates complete alveolar emptying and decreases the likelihood of air trapping in the lungs and hyperventilation.

8. Treatment lasts no longer than 20 minutes, and the medication in the nebulizer is gone at the end of the treatment.

9. Respiratory rate during IPPB is less than the patient's spontaneous respiratory rate.

10. Sensitivity is set so that the patient initiates each breath with between -0.5 and -1.5 cmH_2O (negative) pressure. The pressure needle moves to the right of 0 this much. A setting closer to 0 causes the respirator to trigger prematurely. A setting below -1.5 increases work of breathing.

For Overall Improvement in Condition

1. See criteria for deep breathing and coughing (page 535) and aerosol treatment (page 590).

2. Absence of adverse effects, e.g., lightheadedness, fatigue, dizziness, anxiety, paresthesias, seizures, ar-

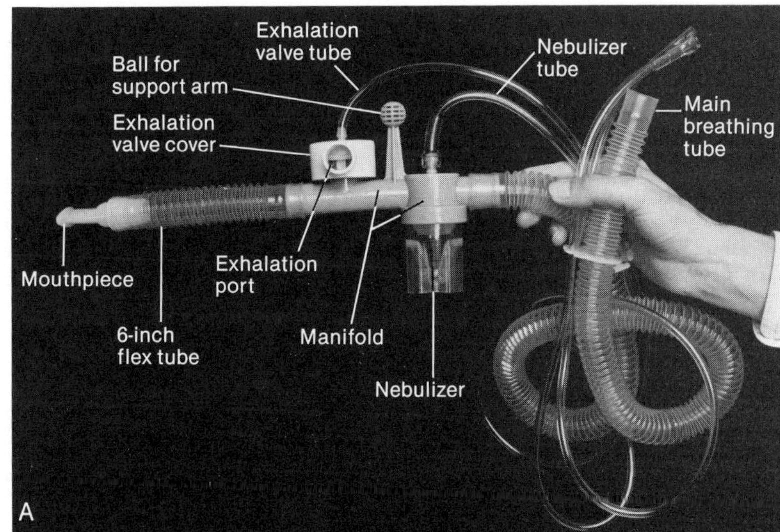

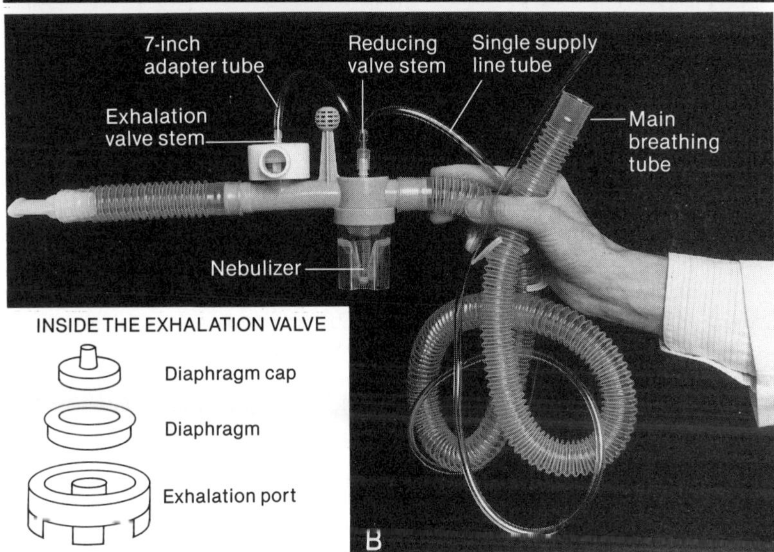

Figure 22–15. A breathing circuit for intermittent positive pressure breathing IPPB. Though setups vary, gas travels through tubes with the same function. *A, Double supply line setup*. The exhalation valve tube and nebulizer tube are separate. *B, Single supply line setup*. A single supply line tube is attached to a reducing valve stem and 7-in adapter tube. Breathing circuits packaged as universal IPPB setups include a reducing valve stem and adapter tube to facilitate the conversion of a double supply line setup into a single supply line setup.

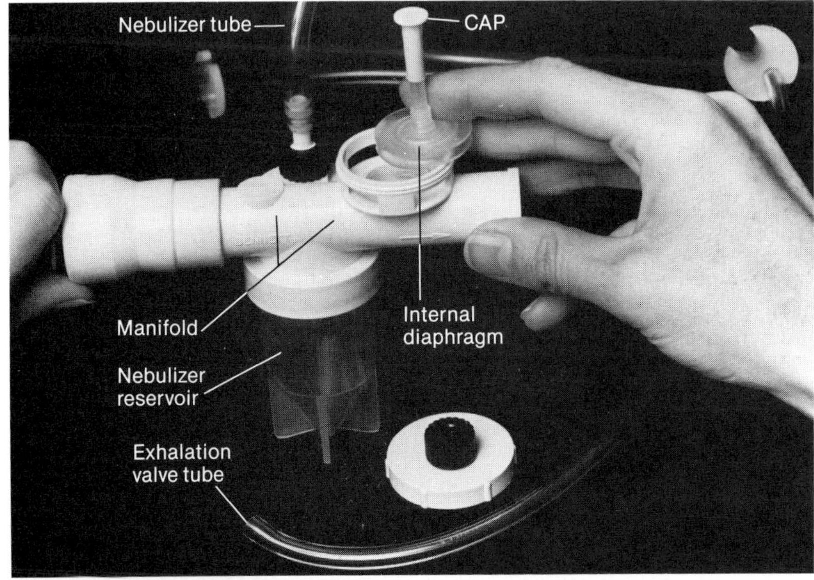

Figure 22–16. The internal diaphragm of a Bennett exhalation valve. The top of the diaphragm may be capped with a plug to simplify the home cleaning procedure (see Chapter 21.)

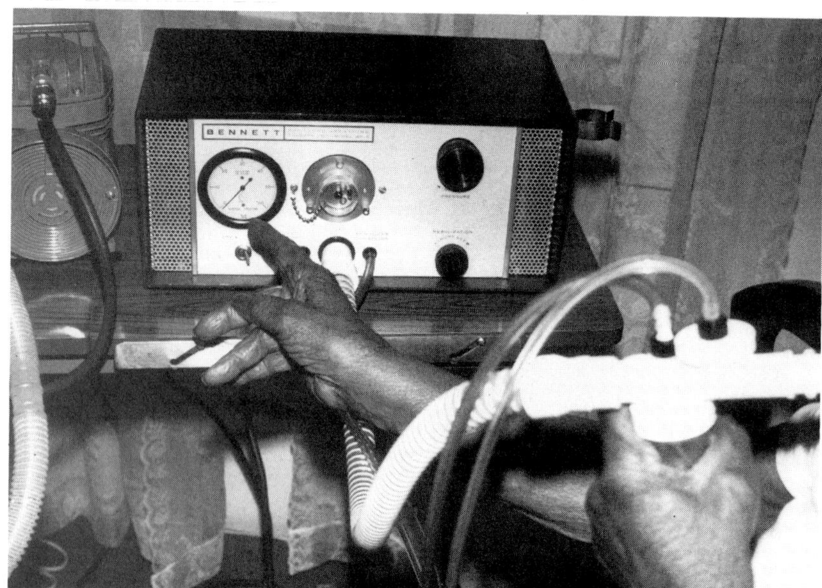

Figure 22–17. A patient watches to be sure the needle on the respirator's pressure manometer rises smoothly to peak pressure and falls to zero with each breath.

rhythmias, headache, hypernatremia, other symptoms in Table 10–2, and development of an air leak in a chest tube drainage system in acute care settings.

Implementation

The nurse may be asked to help assess whether a bronchodilator is best delivered by IPPB or compressor nebulizer. Though Cherniack and Svanhill (1976) point out that the use of IPPB or a compressor nebulizer results in no difference in number of hospital admissions, days spent in the hospital, or mortality, research data on the subject were gathered from stable outpatients. IPPB may be appropriate for unstable or borderline-unstable patients with mucus retention and failure to perform deep breathing.

A successful IPPB treatment largely depends upon the clinician's ability to work with the patient, encouraging relaxation and providing continuous positive feedback and emotional support. Otherwise, the patient may become upset with the machine, mobilize accessory muscles of respiration, and "fight" rather than relax to receive an adequate volume of air.

Monitoring. As with aerosol therapy, the nurse monitors verbal complaints, pulse, respiratory rate, lung sounds, and skin color before, during, and after treatment. Until the patient masters the technique, the nurse monitors inspired volumes to insure delivery of inspired volumes of at least 25% over spontaneous inspired volumes.

The incidence of complications associated with IPPB is low when treatments are properly administered. Of the complications listed in Table 22–2, increased airway resistance, barotrauma, and nosocomial infection are documented in the literature with specific cause-and-effect relationships (Shapiro et al, 1982).

Cleaning IPPB Circuits. The cleaning instructions provided in Chapter 21 instruct the patient to plug the top opening of the exhalation valve before cleaning and disinfecting IPPB circuits (see Fig. 22–16). The equipment vendor provides the cap for plugging the port. Plugging the port is recommended for teaching

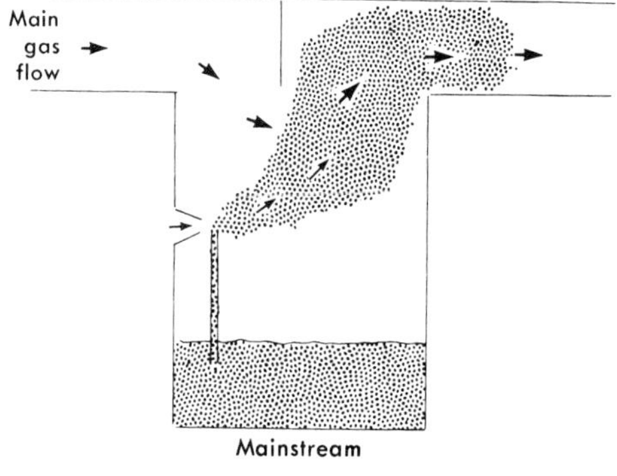

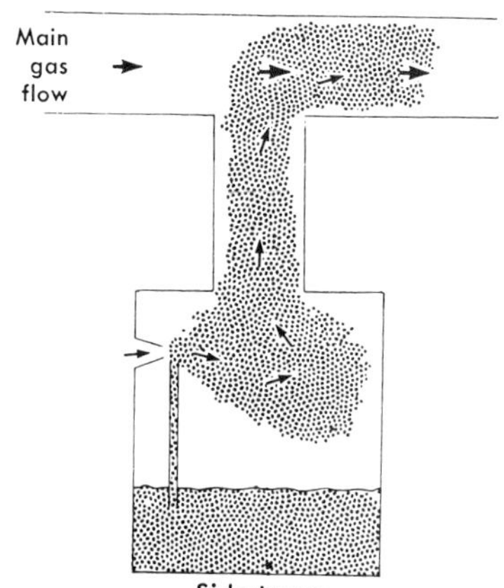

Figure 22–18. Aerosol from mainstream and sidestream nebulizers. *Left,* Main gas flow passes through a mainstream nebulizer, carrying aerosol particles with it. *Right,* Aerosol simply drifts upward and into the main gas flow in a sidestream nebulizer. (Reproduced by permission from McPherson, S. *Respiratory Therapy Equipment.* St. Louis, C.V. Mosby Co., 1985.)

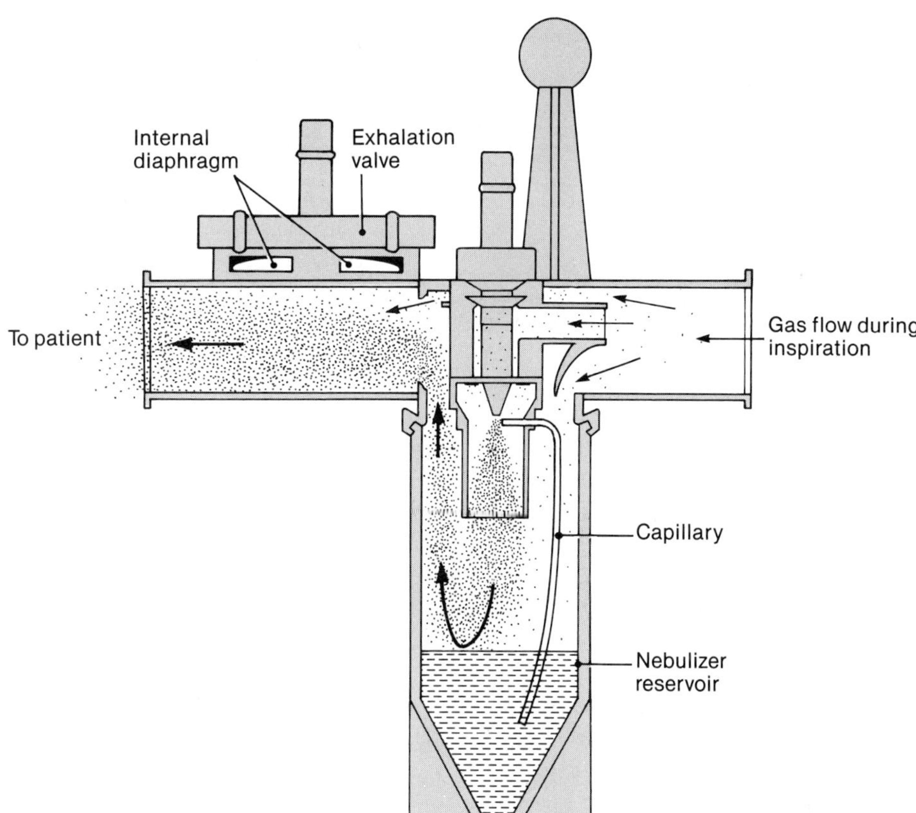

Figure 22–19. The Bennett Slip/Stream nebulizer functions primarily as a mainstream nebulizer. (Redrawn from Puritan-Bennett Corp., Lenexa, Kansas.)

inexperienced or disabled patients who have difficulty disassembling and reassembling IPPB circuits. This technique allows cleaning to be divided into small, easily accomplished steps. Eventually, however, the valve should be fully disassembled to insure removal of medication stains from areas not accessible to a scrub brush.

Durable nondisposable IPPB circuits are recommended for home use (see Chapter 21). Nevertheless, the nurse may encounter patients who prefer to use cheaper disposable circuits, even though the circuits are unreliable for long-term use and more difficult to clean and dry properly. They are difficult to clean because of their large accordion-like corrugations that readily collect water droplets and medication. The nurse stresses the importance of stretching and swinging the main breathing tube to drain out excess water after cleaning and allowing extra time for drying.

The other problem with disposable units pertains to the exhalation valve. Unlike Bennett's exhalation valve, a disposable valve is usually a flat diaphragm. Capping the port above the valve for cleaning has limited usefulness because the diaphragm is not a circular self-contained unit. Water may still reach the inside of the diaphragm and cause valve malfunction. Furthermore, sometimes patients can disassemble valves but have difficulty with reassembly.

Clearly, disposable circuits are not designed for repeated use. When finances are limited, the patient is encouraged to adjust his or her personal budget and buy at least one dependable nondisposable breathing circuit for the respirator.

Troubleshooting. In addition to the problems associated with disposable equipment, the two most common equipment problems in the home setting are failure to reach the preset peak inspiratory pressure and inadequate nebulization.

If the patient does not achieve preset peak pressure, the nurse may take one or more of the following courses of action:

1. Check for adequate mouth seal. Noseclips may be necessary if air leaks out of the nose during inspiration.
2. Check all connections and tubes for leaks.
3. Check proper functioning of the exhalation valve. Water in the diaphragm may be causing a malfunction.
4. If the patient fails to trigger the machine, increase the sensitivity slightly. Sensitivity is increased in the Bennett AP-4 or AP-5 by pushing the rubber stopper piece, as shown in Figure 22–14, upward a few millimeters.
5. If the exhalation tube keeps popping off from the machine, cut ½ off the end and reattach.
6. If the pressure needle fails to rise or rises sluggishly, the internal part of Bennett's valve may be stuck because of dirt or medication stains. Check with the patient or equipment company representative for permission to remove the sensitive and expensive valve and inspect for dirt and stains. Check equipment manual for procedure.

Table 22–2. COMPLICATIONS OF IPPB

Complication	Mechanism	Prevention/Intervention
Barotrauma	Hyperinflation with air trapping may increase the size of a bulla and cause lung rupture and pneumothorax.	Do not use IPPB in high risk patients, e.g., those with bullous emphysema or histories of pneumothorax with IPPB. Avoid use of coached breaths in these patients also.
Decreased venous return	Positive pressure pinches shut alveolar vessels and increases right atrial pressures to produce decreased venous return, decreased cardiac output, and hypotension. Simultaneously, positive pressure reflected superiorly may increase intracranial pressure.	Monitor blood pressure (BP) when adverse circulatory effects are suspected or when peak pressure is greater than 30 cmH_2O. Monitor neurologic signs for indications of increased intracranial pressure.
Excessive oxygenation	Hyperoxia depresses ventilatory drive and causes alveolar hypoventilation. May occur with hyperventilation or when a respirator, with an air dilution knob (Bird), is connected to an oxygen gas source. With this arrangement, the respirator delivers between 40 to 100% O_2, even when the FIO_2 knob is set at air mix. Use electrically driven respirators in the home setting. Instruct patient in correct breathing technique to avoid hyperventilation.	Connect gas-driven respirator to compressed air rather than to compressed O_2 gas source. Use nasal prongs for supplementary O_2, during IPPB treatment.
Gastric distention, vomiting	Air enters stomach, precipitating vomiting and increasing risk for aspiration of stomach contents. Gastric insufflation occurs more often when the patient is restless, tense, and uncooperative.	Check for gastric distention before treatment. Schedule treatment before, not after meals. Encourage relaxation and proper body position during treatment. Withhold treatment when patient is tense, uncooperative, nauseated, or vomiting.
Hyperventilation	Associated with rapid, deep breathing and incorrect use of IPPB. Causes hyperoxia, hypocapnia, and respiratory alkalosis.	Watch for signs of hyperventilation: dizziness, lightheadedness, paresthesias. Slow respiratory rate to 6 to 10 breaths/min with I:E ratio of 1:4. Monitor inspired volumes. Encourage relaxation.
Impaction of secretions	Positive pressure may loosen secretions and push them distally.	Encourage coughing or huffing between respirator breaths. Monitor lung sounds. If ventilation decreases after treatment, consult physician regarding use of bronchodilator aerosol. Consider discontinuation of IPPB, use of a hand-held nebulizer, and more aggressive bronchial hygiene program.
Increased airway resistance	Associated with use of normal saline or distilled water.	Watch for signs of airflow limitation, e.g., wheezing, decreased breath sounds. If they occur, try another diluent.
Increased work of breathing	Associated with "fighting" the respirator.	Encourage relaxation and proper technique during treatment. Withhold treatment if dyspnea or signs of hypoxemia appear.
Nosocomial infection	From contaminated respiratory equipment, diluent, or medication.	Teach proper technique for cleaning equipment and measuring and storing medications. Observe medication bottle for discoloration and sedimentation; discard solution if present. In hospital, use unit dosage system rather than multidose vials of diluent.
Psychologic dependence	Patient believes treatments help, though signs of physiologic benefit are lacking.	Use motivational model (Chapter 16) to help patient evaluate IPPB in light of overall health status. Consult physician regarding patient's need for IPPB versus alternative interventions to achieve same goal.
Side effects related to aerosol drug	See Table 11–5 for medication side effects	Monitor for side effects. Call physician when they occur.

7. Increase flow or decrease preset pressure slightly, as a last resort.

The following actions may correct an inadequate nebulization problem:

1. Check the patient's system and frequency of equipment cleaning, with special attention to the jet or capillary extending into the nebulizer, since it may be clogged.

2. Check whether the jet actually extends into the bottom of the nebulizer where the medication rests. Be sure the tip does not lie flush against the side of the nebulizer cup.

3. Check the position and tilt of the nebulizer during the IPPB. With some nebulizers, e.g., Bird micronebulizer, a slight tilt to the right or left results in a shift of the medication away from the capillary or jet. This shift prevents nebulization.

One important concept to remember in troubleshooting is that most dial settings are relative rather than absolute. Adaptations may need to be made, depending on the physical condition of the patient (e.g., changing lung compliance or airway resistance) and the machine chosen to deliver the treatment. Most important, when equipment problems arise, focus primarily on the patient's response to therapy and only secondarily on the prescribed dial settings. Briefly, *never trust a dial*! Encourage the patient to have his or her respirator serviced if the dial settings seem totally inappropriate.

The Hospital Setting. Most of the previous information on technique also applies to IPPB in the hospital setting, with a few exceptions. First, treatments may be performed with more sophisticated respirators, such as the Bird Mark 7 or Bennett PR-1 and PR-2 series discussed in Chapter 28. Second, the clinician utilizes the coached inspirations to increase volumes up to twice the patient's capacity to re-expand collapsed alveoli (Welch et al, 1980). The coached breath is safer and more practical in the acute care setting because a respiratory therapist is available to appropriately adjust flow and pressure, to monitor for complications, to measure inspired volumes, and to encourage optimum technique. Last, more parameters may be monitored in the hospital setting to assess the effect of treatment and detect possible complications in potentially unstable patients. For example, the high technology available in acute care units permits continuous monitoring of blood pressure and heart rhythm via monitors. When an aerosol bronchodilator is administered, the clinician may measure bedside PFT (e.g., PF and VC) before and after each IPPB or aerosol treatment. Results are recorded on a flow sheet or graph to facilitate the analysis of trends. When the patient has a chest tube, the water seal chamber of the drainage system is monitored for the development of an air leak caused by excessive positive pressure.

Conclusion

This chapter discusses aerosol therapy and IPPB. This knowledge facilitates either nurse or patient initiation of bland or bronchodilator aerosol treatments or IPPB treatments. Specific content on goals, indications, respiratory equipment, and teaching the patient prepares the nurse to make theory-based decisions that ultimately result in quick resolution of common problems, such as bronchoconstriction, mucus retention, and alveolar hypoventilation.

If the patient on aerosol or IPPB treatment shows signs of hypoxemia, oxygen therapy is indicated (see Chapter 23).

REFERENCES

Brain, J. and Valberg, P.: Aerosols: Basic and Clinical Considerations. In Bronchial Asthma—Mechanisms and Therapeutics, 2nd ed. (Weiss, E., Segal, M., and Stein, M.—eds.) Boston, Little, Brown & Co., 1985.

Cherniack, R. and Svanhill, E.: Long-term use of IPPB in COPD. *American review of respiratory disease*, 113(6):721–728, 1976.

Cushing, I. and Miller, W.: Nebulization Therapy. In Safar, P., ed.: Respiratory Therapy. Philadelphia, F. A. Davis Co., 1965.

Health Devices, Inc.: Evaluation—heated humidifiers. *Health devices*, 9(7): 167–176, 1980.

Helmholz, H. and Burton, G.: Applied Humidity and Aerosol Therapy. In Respiratory Care—A Guide to Clinical Practice, 2nd ed. (Burton, G. and Hodgkin, J.—eds.) Philadelphia, J. B. Lippincott Co., 1984.

Hodgkin, J. and Webster, J.: IPPB: worthwhile for which patients? *The journal of respiratory diseases*, 3(3): 97–107, 1982.

The IPPB Trial Group: Intermittent positive pressure breathing therapy of chronic obstructive pulmonary disease: a clinical trial. *Annals of internal medicine*, 99(5): 612–620, 1983.

Kersten, L.: Your Respiratory Home Care Program. Berkeley, Herrick Hospital and Health Center of the East Bay, 1978.

McCool, F., Mayewski, R., et al.: Intermittent positive pressure breathing in patients with respiratory muscle weakness—alterations in total respiratory system compliance. *Chest*, 90(4): 546–552, 1986.

McPherson, S.: Respiratory Therapy Equipment, 3rd ed. St. Louis, C.V. Mosby Co., 1985.

Moser, K., Archibald, C., et al.: Better Living and Breathing, 2nd ed. St. Louis, C.V. Mosby Co., 1980.

Newman, S.: Aerosol deposition considerations in inhalation therapy. *Chest*, 88(2): 152S–159S, 1985.

Shapiro, B., Peterson, J., and Cane, R.: Complications of mechanical aids to intermittent lung inflation. *Respiratory care*, 27(4): 467–470, 1982.

Spearman, C., Sheldon, R., and Egan, D.: Egan's Fundamentals of Respiratory Therapy, 4th ed. St. Louis: C.V. Mosby Co., 1982.

Stehlin, C., and Schare, B.: Systemic and pulmonary changes in rabbits exposed to long-term nebulization of various therapeutic agents. *Heart and lung*, 9(2): 311–315, 1980.

Welch, M., et al.: Methods of IPPB. *Chest*, 78(3): 463–467, 1980.

Ziment, I.: Intermittent Positive Pressure Breathing. In Respiratory Care—A Guide to Clinical Practice, 2nd ed. (Burton, G. and Hodgkin, J.—eds.) Philadelphia, J. B. Lippincott Co., 1984.

Oxygen Therapy

23

Main Objectives

1. Define the following terms: short-term oxygen therapy, long-term oxygen therapy, nocturnal oxygen, H cylinder, E cylinder, flow-meter, regulator, bubble humidifier, and low-flow and high-flow systems of gas administration.
2. For short-term and long-term oxygen therapy, state
   a. Goals.
   b. Indications.
   c. Documentation needed for continued use.
   d. Respiratory equipment for hospital or home use.
3. Discuss the efficacy of long-term oxygen therapy.
4. Compare and contrast use of oxygen tanks or cylinders, liquid oxygen systems, and oxygen concentrators.
5. Discuss the controversial topic of humidification, including goals, indications, and factors affecting water vapor content of bubble humidifiers.
6. Recognize and explain the uses of the following oxygen delivery devices in hospital or home settings: simple face mask, nasal cannula, oxygen-conserving nasal cannula, partial rebreathing mask, nonrebreathing mask, Venturi mask, and transtracheal oxygen device.
7. State the advantages and disadvantages of one oxygen-conserving delivery device.
8. State a typical order for low flow oxygen at rest and during sleep.
9. Name six evaluation criteria to assess correct technique and at least four evaluation criteria to assess overall improvement in condition.
10. Explain how monitoring in the hospital setting differs from monitoring in the home setting.

11. A physician asks you to talk to a patient who expresses reluctance to use nocturnal oxygen at home. Explain how you might use the motivational model in Chapter 16 as well as content in this chapter to assess the clinical situation and intervene appropriately.
12. Explain the indications for and uses of pulse oximetry in the evaluation of oxygen therapy.

This chapter discusses oxygen therapy, with emphasis on home oxygen equipment, patient teaching, and monitoring in the clinical setting. It is designed to complement the content on oxygenation in Chapter 13 (Blood Gases).

Overview of Oxygen Therapy

DEFINITIONS

In this chapter, *oxygen therapy* refers to the administration of increased concentrations of oxygen at one atmosphere.

Short-term oxygen therapy is administered for a duration of 30 days or less. *Long-term oxygen* is administered for longer than 30 days.

Generally, short-term oxygen is for acute disorders, and long-term oxygen for chronic disorders. Knowledge of both types of therapy is essential, regardless of clinical setting. For example, the visiting nurse usually supervises long-term therapy but may implement short-term therapy, when the patient is discharged relatively early from the hospital or when acute signs and symptoms develop in the patient at home. Similarly, the hospital based nurse usually supervises short-term therapy. Yet, pulmonary patients admitted for an unrelated health problem, such as hip fracture or eye injury, may require continuation of long-term therapy for chronic cor pulmonale.

SHORT-TERM OXYGEN THERAPY

Goals

1. To relieve or prevent hypoxemia.
2. To reverse signs, symptoms, and physiologic abnormalities arising from tissue hypoxia.

Indications (California Thoracic Society, 1981)

Documented by invasive or noninvasive analysis of Pa_{O_2} or Sa_{O_2} as follows:

1. Pa_{O_2} less than 60 mmHg or Sa_{O_2} less than 90%.
2. Normal Pa_{O_2} and normal Sa_{O_2} with signs of significant hypoxia.

or

Presence of one of the following diagnoses:

1. Myocardial infarction.
2. Carbon monoxide poisoning.
3. Methemoglobinemia.
4. Acute anemia.

or

Presence of one of the following clinical circumstances in high risk patients:

1. Postanesthesia
2. Postcardiopulmonary arrest
3. Reduced cardiac output, demonstrated by cardiac index less that 1.5 l/min/m^2 and $P\bar{v}_{O_2}$ less than 75% or Pa_{O_2} less than 40 mmHg.
4. Others include hypotension, tachycardia, cyanosis, chest pain, dyspnea, and acute neurologic dysfunction.
5. Stressful procedures and situations, such as endotracheal suctioning, bronchoscopy, thoracentesis, pulmonary artery catheterization, travel at high altitudes, postural drainage in deep Trendelenburg's position.

Documentation of continued need is at least every 24 hours (unstable patients) to every 3 to 4 days (stable patients). All intermittent oxygen orders must state specific circumstances when oxygen therapy is required.

Important Points

Short-term oxygen therapy is provided to relieve hypoxemia without causing an abnormally high Pa_{O_2}. As pointed out in Chapter 13, oxygen is a powerful drug that must be prescribed in appropriate doses to avoid the hazards of hypoventilation, absorption atelectasis, retrolental fibroplasia, and oxygen toxicity.

In addition, oxygen is routinely given when hypoxemia or hypoxia is a potential problem. For example, oxygen is ordered for at least a few hours postoperatively because decreased lung volumes and increased venous admixture are associated with use of the inhaled agents given during general anesthesia. It is ordered for all myocardial infarction patients because oxygen is known to reverse the commonly present mild hypoxemia found in uncomplicated cases. In these conditions, discontinuation of therapy may be based on clinical signs and symptoms at the bedside rather than on analysis of Pa_{O_2} or Sa_{O_2}. However, when the patient develops signs of hypoxemia or when hypoxemia or hypoxia is suspected, blood gas measurement is always obtained to document the need for continuation or discontinuation of therapy.

One further concept about short-term oxygen therapy needs emphasis. In emergency situations, the rule is to *give oxygen—and give it in generous amounts*! Do not worry about alveolar hypoventilation, except in COPD patients with known hypoxic ventilatory drives (see Chapter 13). The need to immediately maximize oxygenation takes precedence over the risk of hypoventilation, at least until a physician becomes available to more thoroughly evaluate the clinical situation.

Oxygen Equipment

Oxygen equipment for short-term oxygen therapy is basically the same as that described next for long-term therapy. However, in the hospital setting, short-term therapy may involve use of delivery devices that deliver a high FIO_2, such as the partial or nonrebreathing mask presented subsequently. Also, most large hospitals have compressed oxygen and compressed air sources piped into devices in the wall. Bedside wall outlets are readily available for attachment to an administration device (Fig. 23–1).

LONG-TERM OXYGEN THERAPY

Goals

1. To relieve hypoxemia.
2. To reverse signs, symptoms, and physiologic abnormalities arising from tissue hypoxia.
3. To provide overall clinical benefit, e.g., improvement in exercise tolerance, self-reliance, and cognitive ability.

Indications

1. Other therapy fails to optimize oxygenation status. *Note*: A 3- to 4-week observation (i.e., stabilization) period is recommended to see if PaO_2 returns to an acceptable level without oxygen therapy at home.
2. Significant hypoxemia (hypoxia) at rest or during sleep documented by invasive or noninvasive analysis of PaO_2 or SaO_2: (a) PaO_2 of 55 mmHg or less or SaO_2 of 85% or less; (b) PaO_2 of 55 to 59 mmHg or SaO_2 of 86 to 89% with evidence of tissue hypoxia, manifested by pulmonary hypertension, cor pulmonale, erythrocytosis, impaired mentation, signs of central nervous system dysfunction, and increasing severity of hypoxemia with exercise.
3. Significant hypoxemia during exercise: (a) PaO_2 of 55 mmHg or less or SaO_2 of 85% or less and (b) improvement in duration, performance, or capacity during exercise with oxygen.

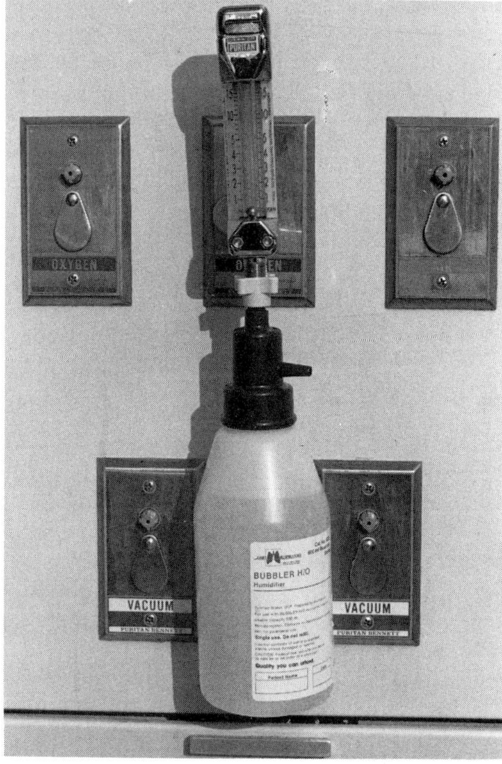

Figure 23–1. A disposable bubble humidifier with a flow meter attached is plugged into a compressed oxygen outlet in the wall not in a similar looking compressed air or vacuum outlet.

Documentation of continued need is 1 month, 6 months, 12 months, and subsequently yearly after initiation of oxygen therapy (see Chapter 21 for documentation requirements for financial reimbursement).

For practical guidelines, long-term oxygen is prescribed when the chronic pulmonary patient is clinically stable and meets one or more of these main criteria as follows:

1. PaO_2 of 55 mmHg or less or SaO_2 of 85% or less on room air while resting, sleeping, or exercising.
2. A hematocrit level greater than 50% for women and 55% for men.
3. Hypoxia suggested by the presence of cor pulmonale with or without right-sided heart failure.

Flenley (1985) adds another criteria, i.e., abstinence from cigarette smoking; cigarette smoking is determined by a blood carboxyhemoglobin level over 3% in two measurements made 3 weeks apart. This recommendation is based on three factors as follows:

1. Increased incidence of burns in patients who smoke while receiving oxygen at home.
2. Evidence that secondary polycythemia is not reversed by 1 year of home oxygen in patients who smoke.
3. Ethical concern over providing scarce resources to patients who will not help themselves by stopping the habit of smoking.

Even though a patient who needs long-term oxygen usually has a PaO_2 below 55 mmHg, no specific level of oxygenation is an absolute indication for home therapy. Each patient under consideration has slightly different pathology and intervening variables.

Two important variables include cost and ability to safely store and use oxygen in the home. The cost of home oxygen is estimated at 200 to 300 dollars per month for 12 hours/day to 400 to 500 dollars per month for 24 hours per day, when liter flow is at 2 L/min (Hodgkin et al, 1984). Portable oxygen ranges from 200 to 1000 dollars per month, with an average of 300 dollars per month, according to Tiep and colleagues (1985d).

Efficacy

The efficacy of long-term oxygen therapy is largely based on results from two important research studies performed in the late 1970s, involving large populations of COPD patients. In the United States, the Nocturnal Oxygen Therapy Trial (NOTT) study (1980) compared the use of nocturnal oxygen with the use of continuous oxygen. The term *nocturnal oxygen* refers to the provision of oxygen at times that include sleeping hours—during the night for most patients. In Britain, a study by the Medical Research Council Working Party (1981) compared nocturnal oxygen with no oxygen prescription. Largely from these studies, experts conclude that low flow oxygen given for 15 hours in the 24-hour day (i.e., nocturnal oxygen) will significantly reduce mortality of COPD patients compared with no oxygen. Continuous oxygen (i.e., 19 to 24 hours per day) further decreases mortality by almost twofold, compared with nocturnal oxygen (Fulmer and Snider, 1984). In addition, continuous oxygen may prevent the progression of pulmonary hypertension, cor pulmonale, and arrhythmias. In patients with sleep apnea or hypoventilation and irregular breathing at night, nocturnal oxygen improves daytime somnolence, morning headache, and nocturnal arrhythmias.

In the clinical setting, oxygen is prescribed for 15 to 18 hours and preferably for 20 to 24 hours per day to increase survival time, overall brain function, and quality of life (Petty, 1985). At least 8 hours per day during sleep is necessary for sustained improvement in polycythemia (Flick and Block, 1977). The physician may vary oxygen prescription, depending on the patient's need and history of adherence to recommended therapy.

Specific clinical effects of long-term oxygen therapy vary. Most, but not all patients, show dramatic improvement in signs and symptoms. Improvement may be evident during the first week of therapy, or it may take 6 weeks or longer. Beneficial effects are increased PaO_2, relief of dyspnea and hypoxia, improved cognition, decreased pulmonary artery pressures, improved right ventricular performance, and other signs mentioned previously. (See Chapter 4 for further discussion.) Ultimately, therapy decreases the number of days spent in the hospital each year and permits return to gainful employment for a few patients. Relief of dyspnea on exertion increases the individual's ability to carry out activities of daily living and improves overall quality of life.

Home Oxygen Equipment

Home oxygen equipment includes an oxygen system (source), an optional humidification device, and an oxygen delivery device connecting the patient to the oxygen source.

OXYGEN SYSTEMS

Oxygen at home is provided three ways as follows: (1) compressed gas in tanks or cylinders, (2) liquid oxygen in reservoirs, and (3) oxygen concentrators or enrichers.

Oxygen Tanks or Cylinders

Compressed oxygen in tanks is one method of delivering oxygen. For nocturnal or continuous therapy, a large *H cylinder* may be ordered, along with stand, regulator, flow meter, and humidifier (Fig. 23–2). The

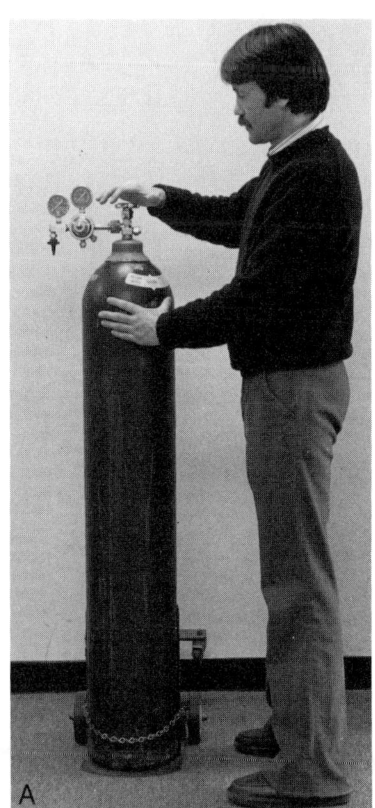

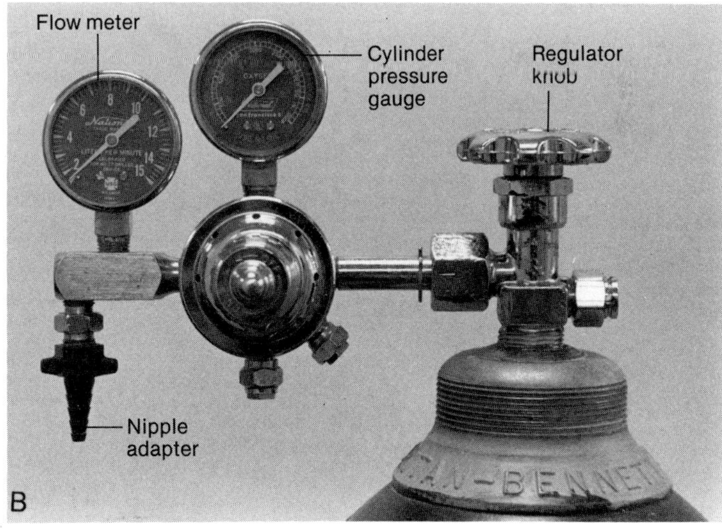

Figure 23–2. Large H cylinder with stand, regulator, and flow meter. *A*, Size of the cylinder compared with the size of an adult. *B*, Close-up view of attachments.

oxygen cylinder is green and stands about 5 ft high. Compressed air cylinders are yellow. The regulator reduces the high tank pressure of 2200 (psi) pounds per square inch to a working pressure of about 50 psi before gas enters the flow meter. The regulator's pressure gauge reads *2200 psi* when the tank is full, and *0 psi* when it is empty. The flow meter controls and measures liter flow of oxygen to the patient. A calibrated flow meter with ¼ L/min gradations is recommended for COPD patients with hypoxic drives who are sensitive to slight changes in oxygen flow (Fig. 23–3). In addition, the flow meter should be the *back-pressure compensated* type, when long extensions of tubing are added to allow ambulation around the house. This type of flow meter compensates for increased back pressure in extension tubing and insures accurate liter flow of oxygen to the patient.

The small *E cylinder* is put into a stroller for patient ambulation or travel in a car (Fig. 23–4). Though the E cylinder is portable, it weighs about 17 lb and may be difficult for the patient to push or lift into a car or bus. Smaller cylinders, such as the D cylinder (10 lb), C cylinder (7 lb), and small Mada cylinders (5 or 7 lb), are available and convenient to the patient during short walks (Fig. 23–5). Most cylinders weighing less than 10 lb may be carried by a shoulder strap and refilled from the larger H cylinder at home, as directed by equipment vendor personnel.

Liquid Oxygen Reservoir and Walker

Liquid oxygen is an alternative to compressed gas in tanks. Oxygen gas is cooled to a liquid at −300°F. In its liquid form, oxygen occupies only 1/860 the

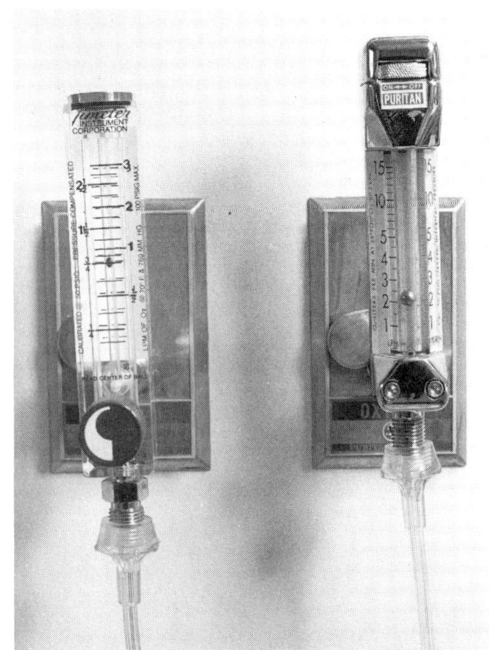

Figure 23–3. A calibrated oxygen flow meter with 1/4 L/min gradations (left) compared with the standard oxygen flow meter (right).

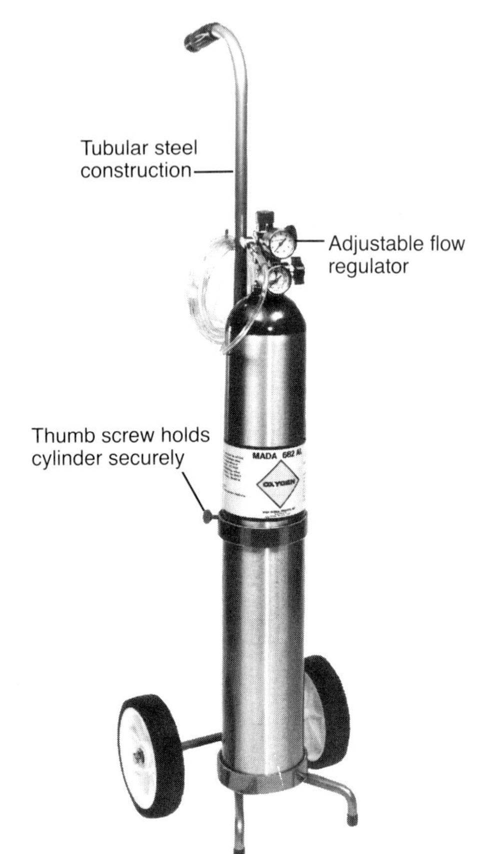

Figure 23–4. An aluminum E cylinder in its portable stand. (Courtesy of Mada Medical Products, Inc., Carlstadt, N.J.)

volume of gas at 1 atmosphere pressure. A nurse or ambulatory patient may fill a portable walker system from the large reservoir (Fig. 23–6). The liquid system is preferred by many patients because it has a portable walker that weighs less than 10 lb and may be carried on the shoulder or in a stroller with enough oxygen for about 8 hours at 2L/min (see Fig. 20–3). Also, portable units are easily refilled from the larger reservoir. (More detailed data comparing commonly used oxygen tanks with a typical liquid oxygen system are provided in Table 23–1.)

Oxygen Concentrators and Enrichers

An *oxygen concentrator* is an electrically powered device that takes in room air, compresses it, and passes it through filters (i.e., molecular sieves) to remove nitrogen, water, and carbon dioxide (Fig. 23–7). The residual gas—oxygen—passes to the patient via a flow meter and humidifier. Most concentrators provide flow rates of 1 to 10 L/min or 1 to 4 L/min. However, unlike tank or liquid systems, oxygen from a concentrator does not provide pure oxygen (FIO_2 of 1.00).

Oxygen concentration depends on flow rate. The higher the flow rate, the lower the FIO_2. Low flow rates of 1 to 4 L/min usually provide an FIO_2 of 0.85 to 0.90 in new concentrator models. Flow rates over

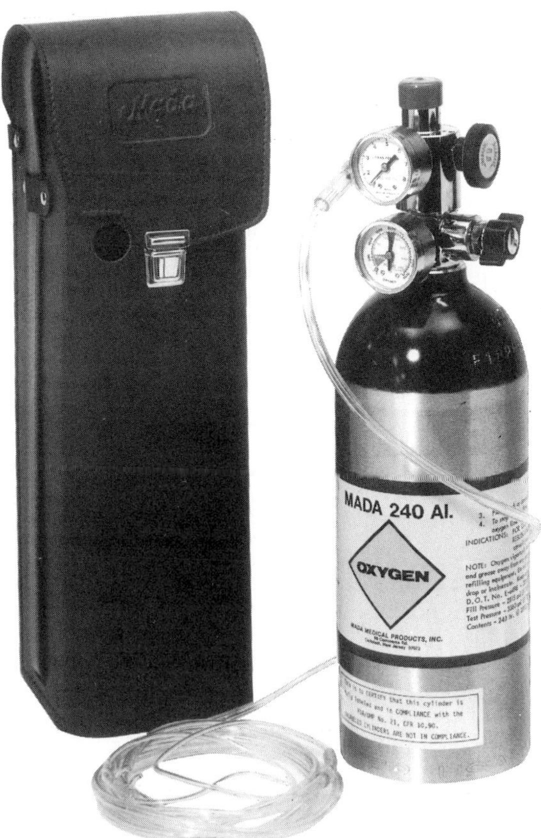

Figure 23–5. Example of a small portable C cylinder with case and shoulder strap. (Courtesy of Mada Medical Products, Inc., Carlstadt, N.J.)

10 L/min provide an FIo_2 of 0.50. From this perspective, the oxygen concentrator is not recommended for the restrictive lung disease patient who requires at least 5 L/min of 100% O_2 and who may be bothered by the nasal and sinus discomfort associated with high flow rates.

Oxygen concentrators are becoming more compact for increased portability within home and work settings. In addition, suitcase models, such as the one in Figure 23–8, are now available to facilitate long distance travel outside the home.

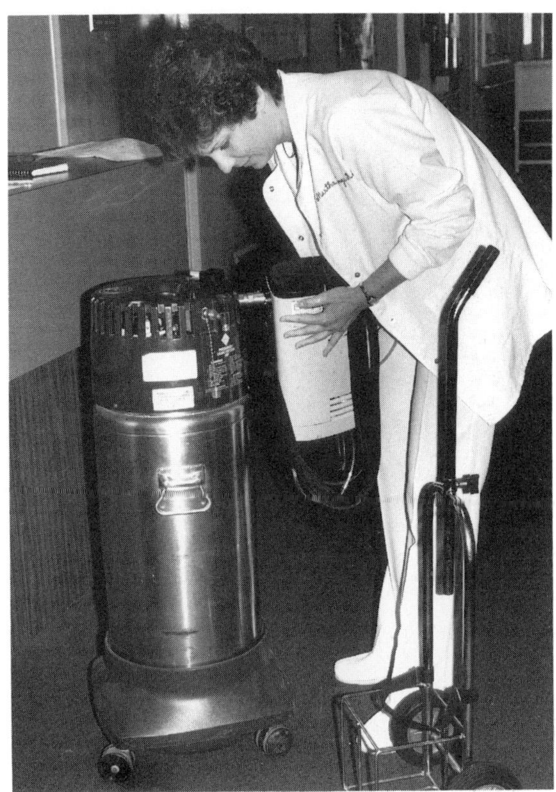

Figure 23–6. A nurse prepares to fill a portable walker unit (Liberator stroller) from the larger 20-L reservoir of liquid oxygen.

An *oxygen enricher* is nearly the same device as an oxygen concentrator, with two exceptions. First, it provides humidified oxygen, since the filter, a polymeric membrane, is permeable to both oxygen and water vapor. Second, it provides a lower FIo_2 (0.30 to 0.40) at flow rates of 1 to 10 L/min. It is not often recommended; compared with an oxygen concentrator, higher flow rates are required to achieve similar Pao_2 values. The high flow rate tends to cause intolerable nasal discomfort. Moreover, patients acclimated to high flow rates may experience "air hunger," when treated with lower flow rates of pure oxygen.

A comparison of the three main home oxygen sys-

Table 23–1. COMPARISON OF COMMON OXYGEN TANKS WITH A LIQUID OXYGEN SYSTEM*

Type of System	Weight (lb)	Volume (gaseous L)	Hours of Continuous O_2 1 L/min	2 L/min	3 L/min	4 L/min	5 L/min
Oxygen Tanks							
H tank	153	6905	115	57	38	28	23
E tank	17	623	10	5	3.5	2.5	2
Liquid Oxygen							
Liberator System† (Cryogenic Associates)							
20 L reservoir	84	17,200	226	126	88	66	55
30 L reservoir	120	25,800	323	188	132	100	82
Stroller	9.6	1058	14	7.8	5.4	4.2	3.4
Stroller sprint	6.9	513	6.6	3.8	2.6	2.0	1.7

*Data based on approximate values, with device full of oxygen.
†Values assume a normal evaporation rate of 1.0 lb (499 cc) per 24 hours.

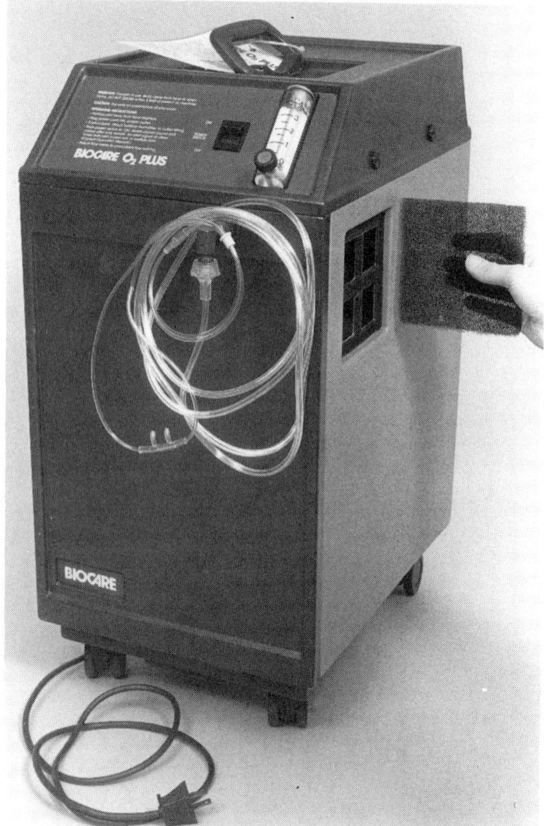

Figure 23–7. Oxygen concentrator with a washable air inlet filter mounted on the side of the device. Here, a humidifier is not attached because the patient is to receive an oxygen flow rate of less than 3 L/min. (Courtesy of National Medical Homecare, Sacramento, CA.)

tems is provided in Table 23–2. When evaluating the cost, keep in mind that differences between systems may vary considerably, depending on geographic areas of the country. Though the generalizations provided in the table apply to most situations, the nurse is encouraged to obtain specific costs from the local durable medical equipment representative and to periodically monitor costs. Monitoring is necessary to note price changes and evaluate changes in the cost effectiveness of individual delivery systems.

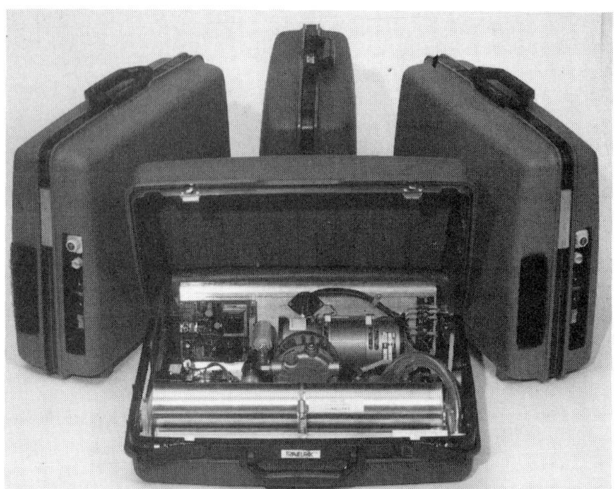

Figure 23–8. The Travelpak suitcase oxygen concentrator. (Courtesy of TravoMed, Inc., Inglewood, Colorado.)

HUMIDIFICATION—A SEPARATE ISSUE

Patients on short-term or long-term oxygen therapy may have *humidifiers* attached to the flow meters. The standard *bubble (diffusor) type humidifier* (Fig. 23–9) produces moisture in the form of water vapor with a relative humidity between 60 and 70%. Some humidifiers produce up to 80 to 100% relative humidity.

The goal of humidification is to prevent the adverse effects associated with breathing dry medically prescribed gas, i.e., decreased mucociliary activity, drying of the respiratory tract mucous membrane, increased body heat loss, and decreased static compliance (Darin et al, 1982).

Indications for humidification are considered separately from indications for oxygen or any other form of respiratory therapy. Moreover, because the topic is controversial, the nurse will find that not all patients with oxygen setups will have humidifiers. Clinicians who omit humidification emphasize the incapacity of bubble humidifiers to deliver clinically significant amounts of moisture to patients receiving low concentrations of oxygen by nasal prongs or masks (Lasky, 1982; Darin, 1982). Currently, humidification is believed beneficial in the following situations (Helmholz and Burton, 1984):

PATIENTS WHO BENEFIT FROM HUMIDIFICATION

Patients with bypassed upper airways
Patients on ventilators
Patients with an O_2 flow rate greater than 2 L/min or O_2 concentration greater than 30%

Patients with croup, bronchiolitis, exercise-induced asthma, and other disorders may benefit from humidification, but research has not identified clear indications.

In the home setting, when benefits are questionable, humidification is best omitted because of the economic and social costs of maintaining equipment. A statement sponsored by the American College of Chest Physicians claims that "...there is no subjective or objective evidence that routine humidification of oxygen is necessary at flow rates of 1 to 4 L/min when environmental humidity is adequate" (Fulmer and Snider, 1984).

Factors Affecting Humidification

For most bubble humidifiers, maintenance of high water vapor content depends on three main factors as

Table 23–2. COMPARISON OF THREE HOME OXYGEN SYSTEMS*

Variable	Tank (Cylinder)	Liquid System	Concentrator
Cost	Cost varies among geographic regions Usually cheaper than concentrator, when used for intermittent or nocturnal therapy at low flow rate	Cost varies between geographic regions. Most expensive system for intermittent therapy. Least expensive system for ambulation when in 24 hour use.	Usually the cheapest system, when used for continuous oxygen therapy or high liter flow rates. Increases monthly electricity bill.
% Oxygen delivered	100% concentration	100% concentration	85 to 90% concentration at flow rates of 1 to 4 L/min Oxygen concentration decreases as flow rate increases. Oxygen prescription may need adjustment to compensate for difference in PaO_2.
Oxygen storage	Oxygen may be stored in aluminum or cast iron tanks for long periods without loss. Two or more H tanks may be joined in series to decrease the number of weekly or monthly tank deliveries. Requires adequate space for storage.	Oxygen cannot be stored for extended periods of time. It must be used within several days because both reservoir and walker types normally vent gaseous oxygen to the atmosphere at a rate of about 1lb/day. Reservoir requires frequent refilling—usually once or twice a week.	Storage is not a major concern. Concentrator provides a limitless supply of oxygen, without tank exchanges or reservoir refills. However, extra service may be required to change filters and check equipment regularly.
Aesthetics	*Low rating*—some patients regard the H tank as an obtrusive sight that reinforces feelings of dependency and helplessness.	*Medium rating*	*High rating*—the console resembles a piece of home furniture. The continuous "hum" during operation is noisy in old models and reasonably quiet in new models. May be undesirable in hot or enclosed environments (e.g., trailer homes), because heat radiating from concentrator may increase environmental temperature to an uncomfortable level.
Portability	*Medium rating*—the H tank is stationary. Smaller tanks are available for ambulation, but they do not provide as much oxygen as liquid walker systems.	*High rating*—light-weight, walker units are "transfilled" from a stationary reservoir. They permit activity outside the home for up to 8 hours (at 2 LPM via standard nasal cannula). Refills are available in most major cities for traveling convenience.	*Low rating*—unit is electricity dependent. Casters facilitate movement within a home or building. Small units may be transported in car trunks for use outside the home, e.g., in motel rooms, offices, and vacation resorts.
Safety	*Average rating*—the high pressure in tanks respresents a potential explosive hazard. Unsafe for weak patients who do not adjust knobs or transfill smaller tanks correctly. Safe at liter flows greater than 4/min.	*Average rating*—frostbite-type injury may result from touching metal tubing or connectors containing liquid oxygen. Unsafe for patients unable to correctly transfill walker. Liter flows greater than 4 to 6/min may cause system to freeze.	*High-rating*—easier to operate and safer than tank or liquid systems. However, a back-up oxygen tank is required in case of electric power failure. Not recommended for patients living in regions with frequent power failures. Liter flows greater than 4/min may endanger the patient, since FIO_2 is reduced at high flow rates, and since patients tend to reduce prescribed flow rates for comfort.
Indications based on safety and cost effectiveness	Continuous or nocturnal oxygen therapy Intermittent use of oxygen Venturi's mask or simple face mask. They require high flow rates.	Best for ambulatory patients' requiring 1 to 4 L/min continuously.	Best for bedridden or homebound patients' requiring 2 to 4 L/min continuously.

*Assumes use of a standard oxygen delivery device, such as the standard nasal cannula.

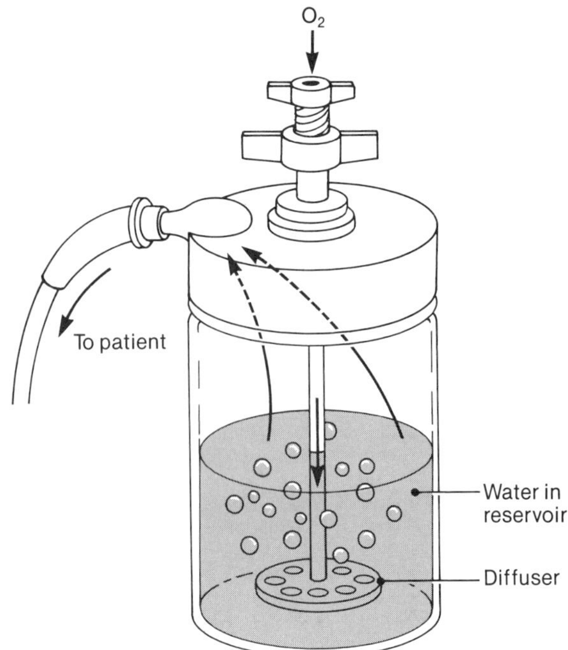

Figure 23–9. A bubble humidifier. The diffuser breaks up the oxygen into smaller bubbles. The bubbling increases the gas/water surface area and promotes evaporation to form humidity (arrows).

follows: (1) water level in the humidifier reservoir, (2) design of the bubble diffusor, and (3) flow rate.

Keeping the reservoir filled to the "fill" line with sterile or distilled water insures adequate gas and water exposure time for humidification.

Diffusor designs that produce small rather than large bubbles are best because the small bubbles increase the surface area for diffusion, which in turn promotes humidification.

High flow rates over 4 L/min cool the water and decrease the water vapor–carrying capacity of a gas. Hence, low flow rates provide more humidification than high flow rates. This fact helps explain why a high flow rate usually requires provision for humidification.

In addition, heat increases water vapor content. It is not added to the standard bubble humidifier because it is unnecessary and impractical. In other situations, however, heat may be added to a Cascade type of humidifier for a patient on mechanical ventilation or for a patient with a bypassed upper airway (see Fig. 22–1B).

STANDARD OXYGEN DELIVERY DEVICES

A standard oxygen delivery device or an oxygen-conserving delivery device (discussed subsequently) is attached between the humidifier or flow meter and the patient.

Main types of standard devices are discussed. Of the main types presented, the nasal cannula and Venturi mask are preferred for long-term therapy. Although the Venturi mask has the advantage of delivering precise low concentrations of oxygen, most clinicians order the nasal cannula for reasons related to tradition, familiarity, preference, comfort, economics, availability, and ease of home cleaning.

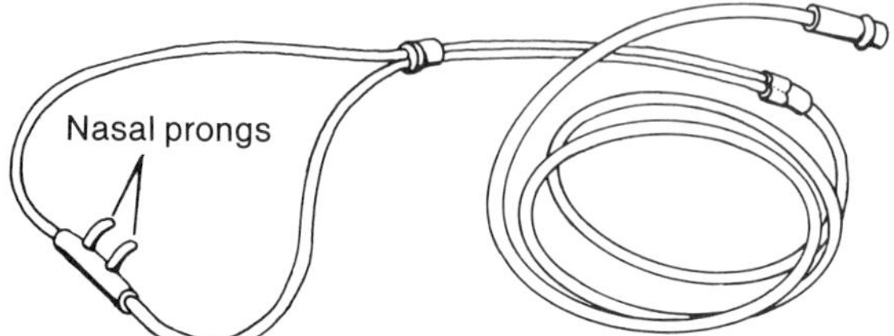

Figure 23–10. Standard nasal cannula (nasal prongs).

Nasal Cannula (Nasal Prongs)

The nasal cannula is a commonly used, relatively comfortable, and inexpensive device for oxygen delivery (Fig. 23–10). The patient inhales oxygen from two plastic prongs inserted 1 cm into each naris. The prongs are held in place by an attached elastic band around the head or by tubing looped behind the ears and under the patient's neck. This device provides an FIO_2 of 0.24 to 0.50, with O_2 flow rates of 1 to 6 L/min. As a rule of thumb, FIO_2 (O_2 concentration) increases by 0.40 (4%) for each 1 L/min increase in flow rate (Table 23–3).

The nasal cannula may be used for short-term or long-term oxygen therapy. It is routinely applied whenever a patient removes the oxygen mask to eat, drink, or perform airway care.

Table 23–3. STANDARD OXYGEN DELIVERY DEVICES WITH FIO_2

Delivery Device	Oxygen flow rate (L/min)	Estimated FIO_2*
Low Flow Systems		
Nasal cannula	1	0.24
	2	0.28
	3	0.32
	4	0.36
	5	0.40
	6	0.44
Simple face mask	5–6	0.40
	6–7	0.50
	7–10	0.60
Partial rebreathing mask	6–10	0.35–0.60
Nonrebreathing mask	6–10	0.60–1.00
High Flow System	**Minimal O_2 Flow Rate**	**FIO_2 Set At**
Venturi mask (Inspiron model)	4	0.24
	4	0.28
	6	0.31
	8	0.35
	8	0.40
	10	0.50

*Assumes normal $\dot{V}_E$.

The following pointers summarize monitoring considerations:

1. For long-term use, order nasal prongs that are soft and pliable; curved rather than straight, to direct flow posteriorly rather than upwards towards the frontal sinuses; and slightly flared at the ends, for smooth gas flow spread over greater surface area (McPherson, 1985).
2. Check for proper position in the nares; malpositioning will decrease FIO_2 and cause hypoxemia.
3. Mouth breathers may still benefit from nasal oxygen, since inspired ambient air flow in the oral pharynx entrains oxygen from the nasopharynx.
4. Flow rates greater than 6 L/min do not significantly increase FIO_2 and are likely to cause adverse effects, such as excessive drying of the mucosa, headaches, sinus pain, skin irritation, and dermatitis.
5. Flow rates greater than 4 L/min indicate the patient may need a more accurate delivery device, owing to a need for a higher FIO_2.

Nasal Catheter

This soft rubber or plastic catheter is inserted into one naris and directed posteriorly until its tip rests in the pharynx behind the uvula (Fig. 23–11). The nasal plus oral pharynx serves as an internal oxygen reservoir. The device provides an FIO_2 of up to 0.50. While it is an alternative to nasal prongs for short-term oxygen therapy, it is not utilized in ambulatory and home settings because it is more invasive and uncomfortable than the nasal cannula.

Monitoring considerations are the same as those mentioned previously for the nasal cannula. The catheter must be changed every 12 to 24 hours to prevent adherence to mucous membranes.

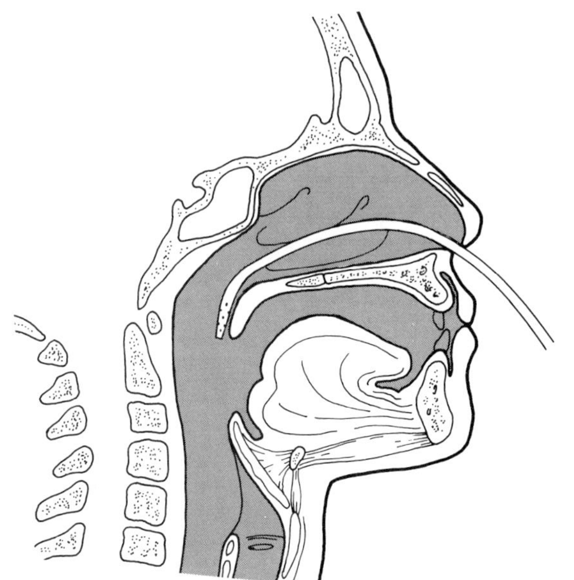

Figure 23–11. Nasal catheter appropriately positioned with its tip behind the uvula.

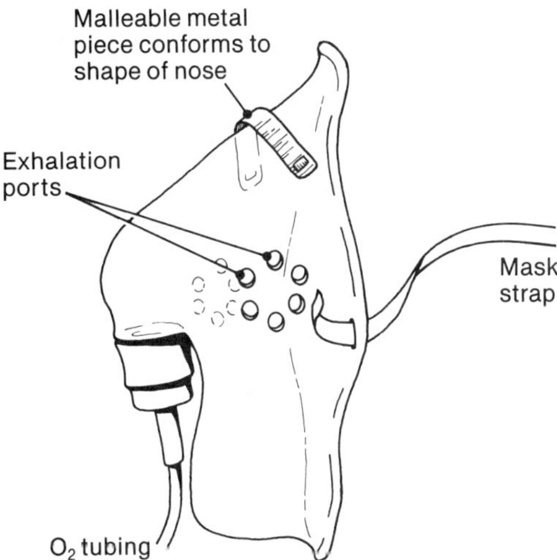

Figure 23–12. Simple face mask.

Simple Face Mask

When a simple face mask is applied, the patient inhales from the mask and exhales through the side exhalation ports (Fig. 23–12). The device provides an FIO_2 of 0.30 to 0.60 with O_2 flow rates of 5 to 10 L/min. The face mask is used for short-term oxygen therapy in patients who do not require low flow oxygen or precise concentrations of oxygen.

Monitoring considerations are as follows:

1. To avoid rebreathing of exhaled CO_2, *never use flow rates less than 5 L/min*!
2. Flow rates greater than 8 to 10 L/min do not significantly increase FIO_2.
3. In choosing a face mask of any kind, remember comfort depends on the shape and dimensions of a patient's face relative to the design, composition, and size of the mask. Small, medium, and large sizes should be available.

Partial Rebreathing Mask

The partial rebreathing mask is similar to a simple face mask, but a reservoir bag is added (Fig. 23–13). The patient inhales oxygen rich air from the reservoir bag (large arrow in A) and then potentially room air from the exhalation ports (small arrows). The first third of exhaled gas (B) goes back into the reservoir bag. This quantity represents oxygen-rich gas in the patient's anatomic dead space. The rest is breathed out the exhalation ports.

The partial rebreathing mask provides an FIO_2 of up to 0.60 with flow rates between 6 and 10 L/min. It is used for acutely ill patients requiring an FIO_2 between 0.40 and 0.60.

During routine monitoring, the nurse checks for a snugly fitted mask and an adequate flow rate. These features are essential to achieve a high FIO_2. Liter flow is increased until the reservoir bag deflates only slightly during inspiration. The bag should *never* de-

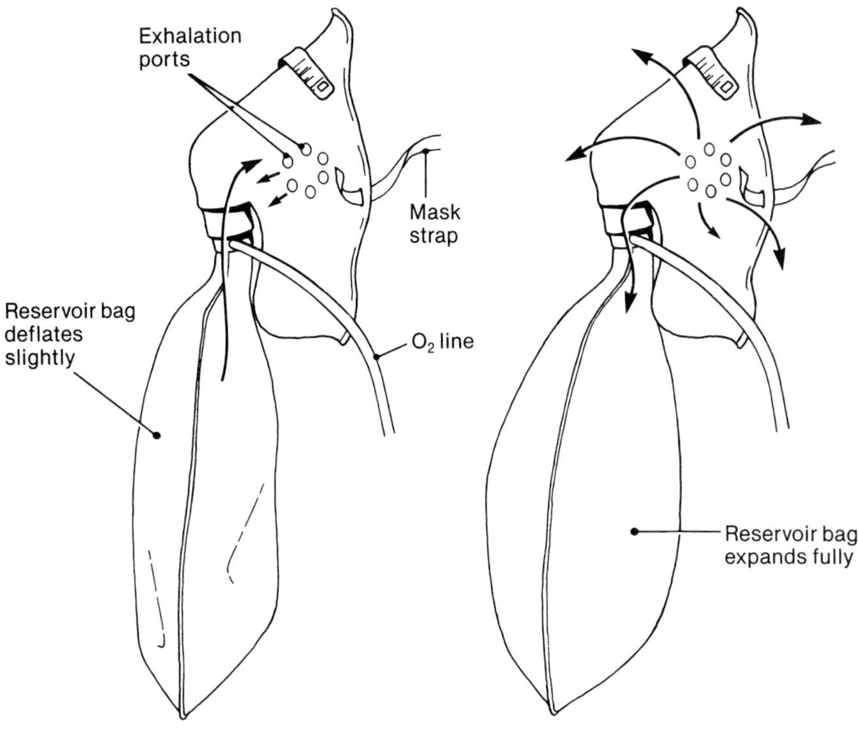

Figure 23–13. The partial rebreathing mask during inhalation (*A*) and exhalation (*B*). The arrows indicate the direction and relative magnitude of gas movement. (See text.)

flate completely. Deflation causes the patient to entrain more room air through the exhalation ports and drastically reduce the FIO_2. In addition, note that FIO_2 can vary greatly when the patient's ventilatory pattern changes. Flow rate may need adjustment as often as every 30 to 60 minutes, as described.

Nonrebreathing Mask

This mask is similar to a partial rebreathing mask, except for two distinguishing features. First, a one-way valve lies between mask and reservoir bag (Fig. 23–14). This valve prevents exhaled gas from entering the bag. Second, one-way valves or rubber flaps on the side-exhalation ports allow gas to leave the mask during exhalation, and they prevent the entrance of room air during inspiration. Hence, the patient inspires pure oxygen from the reservoir bag (A) and exhales completely through the exhalation ports underneath the exhalation valve (B).

The nonrebreathing mask provides an FIO_2 of up to 0.90 to 1.00. Keep in mind that differences in design and resulting FIO_2 may exist among various brands of partial and non-rebreathing masks. When differences are minimal, FIO_2 varies little between the two types of masks.

The nonrebreathing mask is indicated for short-term oxygen therapy for acutely ill patients requiring an FIO_2 between 0.60 and 1.00.

Monitoring considerations are the same as those described for the partial rebreathing mask. The nurse checks for a snug mask fit; a properly inflated reservoir bag—increase flow, if necessary; and properly functioning exhalation port valves. Valves should open during exhalation and close during inhalation. They must be kept free of saliva and mucus to avoid valve failure and drastic reductions in FIO_2. In addition, note that when FIO_2 is greater than 0.50, the patient is at risk for absorption atelectasis and oxygen toxicity (see Chapter 13).

The Venturi Mask (Air-entrainment Mask)

The Venturi mask is the most accurate device for delivering a prescribed dose of oxygen. Pure oxygen and entrained air are inhaled from the flextube in Figure 23–15. Gas is exhaled via side exhalation ports.

Operation is based on Bernouilli's principle. FIO_2 is controlled by changing the size of the narrowed orifice at the base of the flex tube or by changing the size of adjacent air entrainment ports. In the former case, the high velocity jet flow of oxygen enters the larger flex tube. Here, it creates negative pressure, which in turn sucks in room air through one or more air entrainment ports (Fig. 23–15). The size of the narrowed orifice determines the amount of negative pressure, the amount of air entrainment, and hence the FIO_2 inhaled by the patient. In the Inspiron mask, insertion of different color-coded adapters changes FIO_2. FIO_2 settings range from 0.24 to 0.50, as indicated in Table 23–3.

The Venturi mask may be used for short-term or long-term oxygen therapy, though patient acceptance and cost related to the required high flow rates may be prohibitive.

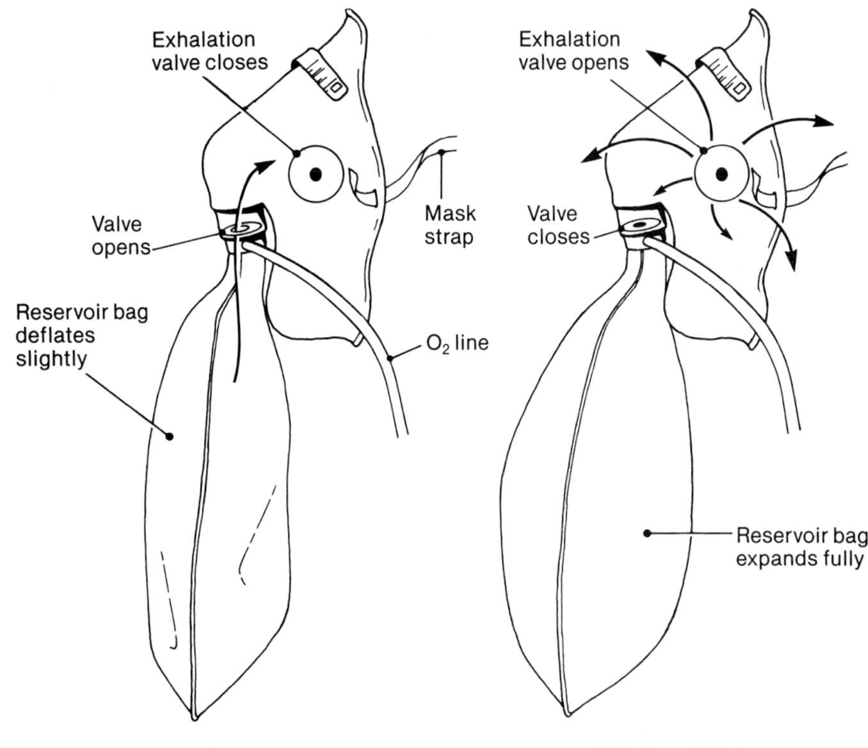

Figure 23–14. The nonrebreathing mask during inhalation *(A)* and exhalation *(B)*. The arrows represent the direction and relative magnitude of gas movement.

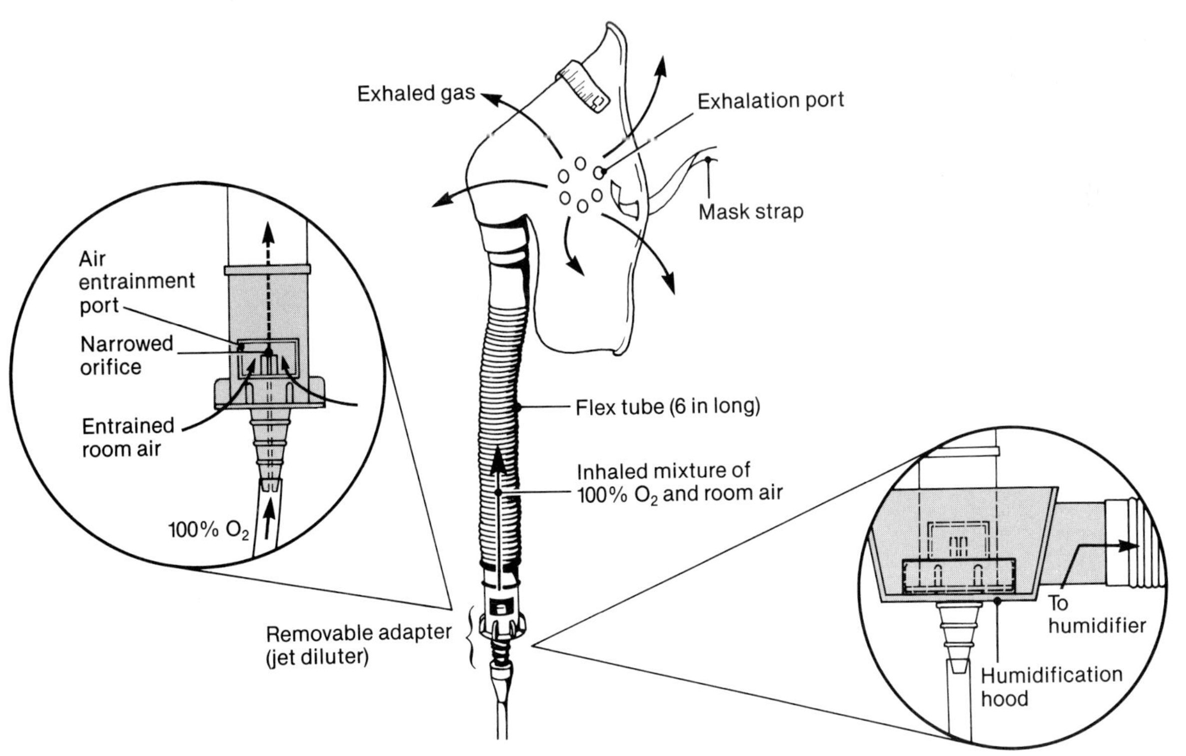

Figure 23–15. Venturi mask. The arrows indicate the movement of gas during respiration. A humidification hood is added to protect air entrainment ports and to provide humidification.

Monitoring considerations are as follows:

1. Prescribed FIO_2 is assured, regardless of ventilatory pattern. Accidental increase in flow rate does not change FIO_2.

2. The mask's air entrainment ports must be kept free and open to prevent a dangerous increase in FIO_2.

3. The mask is not tolerated by some patients because it interferes with eating and talking. It may cause skin irritation, face discomfort, or a feeling of confinement. Some patients are reluctant to wear it because it is cumbersome and obtrusive.

4. It is more expensive than the nasal cannula. Also, it costs more to operate because it requires a higher oxygen flow rate.

Low-flow and High-flow Systems

The aforementioned standard oxygen delivery devices are categorized into *low-flow* and *high-flow systems of gas administration*, as defined in Table 23–4. The nasal cannula is a low-flow system and the Venturi mask is an example of a high flow system. Recognition of low-flow systems is particularly important because, as explained in Table 23–4, *liter flow never guarantees a set FIO_2*. In the assessment of patients on oxygen therapy, monitoring ventilatory pattern is just as important as monitoring flow rate. For adequate oxygenation, oxygen flow rate must meet inspiratory demand.

Changing Delivery Devices

When the patient changes from one oxygen delivery device to another, liter flow may need adjustment to achieve the desired FIO_2. Table 23–3 serves as a guide for estimation of FIO_2 for standard oxygen delivery devices. To understand its usefulness, consider a patient who wishes to remove the 35% Venturi mask and apply nasal prongs for eating dinner. The nurse sets liter flow at 4 L/min because the estimated FIO_2 of 0.36 is closest to the Venturi mask's setting of 35%.

To switch from a standard nasal cannula or Venturi mask to one of the oxygen-conserving devices described subsequently, the nurse follows physician and manufacturer guidelines to adjust liter flow and the oxygen supply system.

OXYGEN-CONSERVING DELIVERY DEVICES

The nurse may find several new oxygen delivery devices in the clinical setting. The main oxygen-conserving delivery devices are the *transtracheal oxygen delivery device* (Fig. 23–16), the *reservoir nasal cannula* (Fig. 23–17), and the *pulse-dose demand valve device* (Fig. 23–18), also called the *demand oxygen delivery device* (Tiep and Lewis, 1987). These devices are described and compared with each other in Table 23–5.

The reservoir nasal cannula and the pulse-dose demand valve device conserve oxygen by restricting flow to the inspiratory phase of respiration, thus eliminating the wasteful flow of oxygen during expiration. A major problem with standard steady-flow devices, such as the standard nasal cannula, is oxygen wastage during expiration, the phase of respiratory cycle that takes the most time.

Oxygen-conserving delivery devices are used mostly for persons on long-term therapy at home. The OXYMIZER is sometimes employed in the hospital setting when the patient in need of oxygen is in an otherwise stable cardiopulmonary condition.

A main advantage is a reduction in oxygen utilization (i.e., flow rate) by at least 50%. This reduction is the

Table 23–4. LOW-FLOW AND HIGH-FLOW SYSTEMS OF GAS ADMINISTRATION

System	Definition	Important Points
Low-flow System Nasal cannula Nasal catheter Simple mask Partial rebreathing mask Nonrebreathing mask	System whereby adequate inspiratory gas flow is provided partially by the gas administration device and partially by room air.	The term "low flow" is not always synonymous with low FIO_2. FIO_2 varies depending on flow rate, ventilatory pattern (e.g., rhythm, respiratory rate, I:E ratio, V_T), and anatomic dead space. In a low-flow system, *high tidal volumes result in a low FIO_2*, because the patient inhales more room air with each breath. *Low tidal volumes result in a high FIO_2*, since less room air is inhaled with pure oxygen from the administration device. Hence, a child or small adult will receive a higher FIO_2 than an adult with the same liter flow of oxygen. For this reason, small persons require reduced oxygen flow rates.
High-flow System Venturi mask Other Venturi devices	System whereby adequate inspiratory gas flow is provided *totally* by the gas administration device.	Venturi devices provide high total gas flow at a fixed FIO_2. FIO_2 does not change with variations in ventilatory pattern. Hence, this system is best for patients with shallow, deep, or irregular ventilatory patterns, or for COPD patients with sensitive hypoxic drives. FIO_2 can be easily measured and adjusted. Since the device provides the entire inspiratory volume, temperature and humidity can be controlled.

Table 23–5. OXYGEN-CONSERVING DEVICES

Type	Oxygen Benefit Ratio*	Examples	Description	Advantages	Disadvantages
Transtracheal oxygen-delivery device	2:1 to 3:1	Trachette catheter (Erie Medical) Scoop catheter (Transtracheal Associates)	Small (one piece) polyethylene catheter that is inserted directly into the trachea above the suprasternal notch. The continuous flow of O_2 enlarges the size of the trachea's reservoir of O_2 at end inspiration.	Patient may use standard O_2 setup with smaller reservoirs for convenience. Humidification is unnecessary. Elimination of nasopharyngeal irritation associated with use of a nasal cannula. High aesthetic value, since the catheter is relatively inconspicuous. Compliance with therapy may be greatly improved. Successful oxygenation may be accomplished in patients refractory to O_2 by standard nasal prongs.	Requires minor surgery for catheter placement. Catheter must be changed every 30 to 90 days by a physician. Requires attachment to retention necklace to guard against accidental dislodgement. Complications may occur, e.g., bleeding, infection, subcutaneous emphysema, increased mucus production, and catheter failure or displacement (Heimlich and Carr, 1985).
Reservoir nasal cannula	2:1 to 4:1	OXYMIZER OXYMIZER pendent (Chad Therapeutics)	An intermittent flow device that looks like standard nasal prongs, except for the addition of a reservoir. The OXYMIZER face-piece model has the reservoir under the nose; the OXYMIZER pendent has it on the upper chest. This passive device stores O_2 during exhalation and delivers it during inspiration. Minimal nasal inspiratory flow triggers operation.	As with the Trachette, the patient may use a standard O_2 setup with smaller portable reservoirs to increase patient mobility. Humidification is unnecessary. Device is noninvasive. The pendent model is a viable option for the patient who wants an O_2-conserving device that is noninvasive and relatively cosmetically appealing. Suitable for hospital use because it is noninvasive, and it easily substitutes for standard nasal cannula with a simple adjustment in flow rate. Used only for patients with a stable cardiopulmonary status.	The OXYMIZER face-piece model has low aesthetic value for patients concerned with the mustache-like appearance. The face piece may become easily dislodged during sleep. Some patients may not benefit from pursed-lip breathing. Current OXYMIZER models require expiration through the nose, not the mouth, for the reservoir to work. Potential problems include lack of acceptance, hypoxemia due to reservoir membrane failure, and O_2 overdosing.
Pulse-dose demand valve device	3:1 to 7:1	OXYMATIC electronic oxygen conserver (Chad Therapeutics) Demand oxygen controller and Pulsair system ($CryO_2$ system)	A standard nasal cannula is connected to a demand-valve system. A fluidics sensor detects the onset of inspiration and causes the release of a preset dose (i.e., volume or pulse) of O_2 through the demand valve. The dose of O_2 varies, according to respiratory rate and desired O_2 flow in L/min marked on the device.	Provides the highest oxygen benefit ratios. Attaches to conventional O_2 tank or liquid O_2 system. Humidification is unnecessary. Eliminates the need to adjust O_2 flow when respiratory rate changes. In case of pulse-mode failure, the patient may conveniently switch to the device's conventional mode. Device is noninvasive.	Clinical experience with the device is limited. High initial cost for the system. Does not adapt to O_2 concentrators. Inspiratory sensor will not work when the cannula becomes clogged or dislodged or when the patient breathes through the mouth. The device is technically complex, expensive, and time consuming to service. When service is needed, the patient may be reluctant to continue future use.

*Standard steady-flow device: O_2 conserving device.

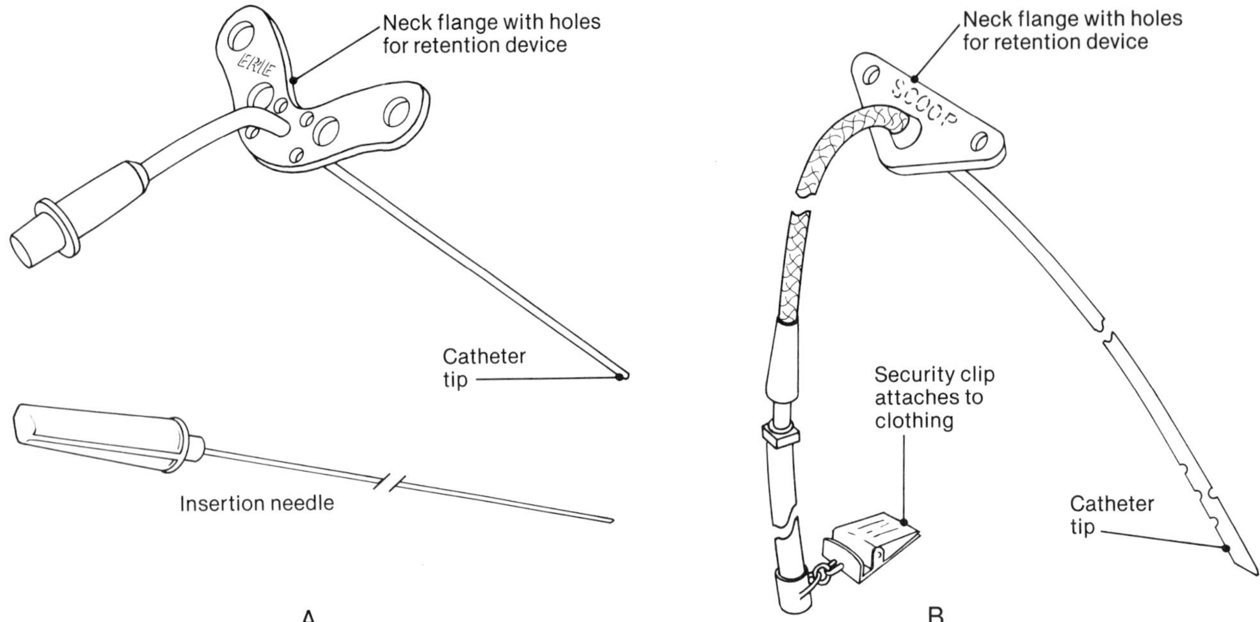

Figure 23–16. Transtracheal oxygen delivery devices. *A*, Erie Medical Trachette with insertion needle. *B*, SCOOP catheter.

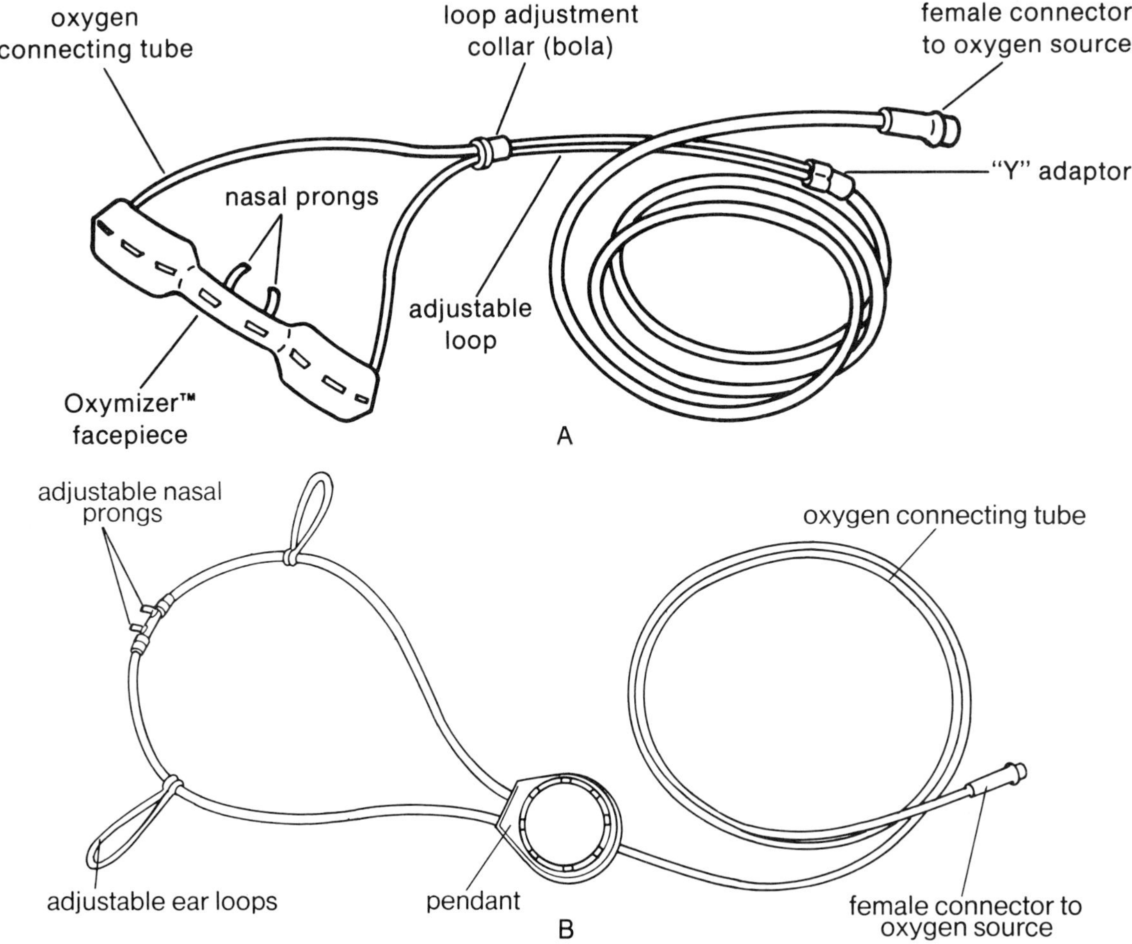

Figure 23–17. Reservoir nasal cannulas. *A*, OXYMIZER oxygen-conserving device with the facepiece reservoir by the nasal prongs. *B*, OXYMIZER Pendant with the reservoir designed to rest on the anterior chest area. (Reproduced by permission from Chad Therapeutics, Inc., Chatsworth, California.)

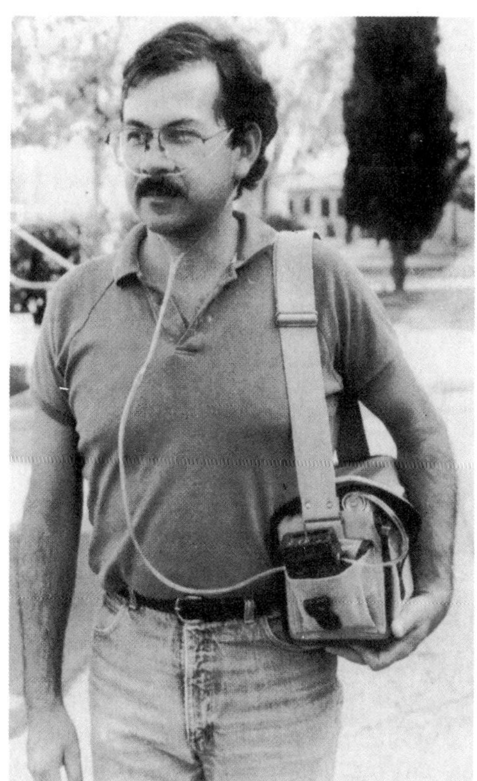

Figure 23–18. A patient receiving oxygen intermittently using an electronic demand delivery system. (Reproduced by permission from Tiep, B., Carter, R., et al. Demand oxygen delivery devices during exercise. *Chest,* 91(1):15–20, 1987.)

same as an oxygen benefit ratio of 2:1. A 2:1 ratio means that the use of standard nasal prongs (i.e., standard steady flow technique) requires twice as much oxygen to achieve a specified Sa_{O_2} as the amount of O_2 required by an oxygen-conserving device, such as the Trachette or OXYMIZER. This saving in oxygen supply amounts to a considerable financial saving to the patient; third-party payers; and, in some cases, taxpayers.

Two other advantages of an oxygen-conserving device are reduced nasal drying and irritation, since flow rates are reduced, and greater patient mobility. Patients tend to extend their time spent out of the home because they do not need as much oxygen and can use smaller, more lightweight, portable reservoir units for ambulation.

Though oxygen utilization is reduced, associated cost savings may be lost, unless the patient uses the device appropriately and keeps the flow rate at the prescribed low level. Patients tend to dial in higher flow rates and become overoxygenated, when they feel poorly or immediately after conversion from standard nasal cannula. Because of this potential problem, an important nursing function is to emphasize the importance of keeping oxygen flow rate at the prescribed low level. When oxygen prescription is the same at rest and during exercise, a flow restrictor sized to a specified liter flow may be inserted in the system to increase compliance.

Oxygen-conserving devices may be supplemented by new cosmetic developments, such as less obtrusive tubing and the mounting of tubing on eyeglasses (Oxyframes, Oxyspects). Intensive research is in progress to refine these and other cosmetic developments and to do so without sacrificing the oxygen-conserving quality of the device. Cosmetic improvements are of prime consideration because they increase patient acceptance of the delivery device and thereby increase patient compliance with oxygen therapy.

Teaching the Patient

The following self-care educational material helps the nurse teach the patient how to use oxygen. Though the material is written for use of oxygen cylinders and the standard nasal cannula, basic information applies to liquid concentrator systems and oxygen-conserving devices.

PATIENT INFORMATION

Use of Oxygen

Your Order

At rest	________	liters per minute
During exercise or any activity	________	liters per minute
During sleep	________	liters per minute
Total hours per day	________	

Your doctor has ordered oxygen at home because you have a low level of oxygen in your blood at rest, during exercise, or during sleep. You may not feel the need for oxygen if you use it only at night. However, if blood is well oxygenated at all times, the heart does not have to work as hard to supply enough oxygenated blood to body tissues. Also, persons with obstructive lung disease tend to have "thicker" blood because of low oxygen levels. Oxygen "thins" blood towards normal.

Preparation and Use

1. If humidification is ordered, fill humidifier bottle to the maximum fill line marked on the bottle (200 to 300 ml level). Use sterile or distilled water.
2. Slowly turn the large regulator knob on top of your cylinder to the open position—counterclockwise two or three full turns. Your service person might have done this already for you.
3. Turn the oxygen flow meter on until the middle of the ball is on your ordered flow rate.
4. Put your nasal prongs in your nose. Stretch the tubing up and around your ears and tighten under your chin.
5. When finished with oxygen, turn off flow meter and store nasal prongs in a clean plastic bag.

Cleaning Procedure

Daily

1. Discard leftover fluid.
2. Wash humidifier bottle and top with liquid soap and water.

3. Rinse well.
4. Air dry and reassemble.

Once or twice a week

1. Wash nasal prongs with liquid soap.
2. Rinse well.
3. Disinfect humidifier bottle and top.

Tips

1. *Oxygen is a powerful drug*! It should be used only as prescribed. Too much or too little may cause medical complications.
2. If you become short of breath during activity, follow the suggestions in the section Controlling Your Shortness of Breath. *Remember*: *do not turn the liter flow up*!
3. Be sure another tank is ordered or is on the way when your oxygen gauge gets down to 500 pounds per square inch. Make sure you have enough oxygen for the weekend.

Fire Prevention

Oxygen is one of the three ingredients of a fire. The others are a combustible or flammable material and a source of ignition. The following rules will help prevent the chance of a fire.

1. *No smoking* in any room where oxygen is being used. Your equipment company or local American Lung Association can provide you with "No Smoking" or "O_2-in-Use" signs to place by your oxygen system.
2. The oxygen system should be at least 10 ft away from any open flame, including pilot lights in stoves, furnaces, and water heaters.
3. Keep the system at least 10 ft away from electric equipment that may spark.
4. Do not use oily lotions, face creams, grease, lip balms, and petroleum jelly around oxygen equipment. These substances are flammable.

Storage and Handling

1. Oxygen should be stored in a well ventilated area, away from direct heat or sun. The corner of a room or other out-of-the-way location is best, to avoid accidental breakage. Do not store in closets.
2. Do not try to repair oxygen equipment or let untrained persons make adjustments. Always call your serviceman, when a problem arises.
3. Oxygen cylinders should be secured by a chain, cord, or stand. Handle small cylinders with extreme care during ambulation.
4. Keep oxygen turned off, when not in use.

Car Travel

1. Transport portable oxygen in the back seat of your car and secure it in an upright position.
2. Open your window about one inch for ventilation.
3. Notify your equipment company of your travel plans.

Airplane Travel

Pressurized cabins of modern jets maintain an altitude of about 5000 to 6000 feet. By law, altitude must be no greater than 8000 feet. People with lung disease who are not short of breath at sea level may become short of breath at these high altitudes. Therefore, always check with your physician regarding the safety of airplane travel for you.

When you plan airplane travel

1. Call the airlines well in advance of departure to arrange for oxygen during travel. Regulations prohibit you from carrying or using your own portable oxygen system on board. However, empty units may be checked with baggage for refill at your destination.
2. Airlines may request an oxygen prescription from your physician, a letter stating diagnosis, and permission to fly with or without an attendant.
3. Postpone your trip if you are not feeling well.

SCHEDULE

1. Continuous—19 to 24 hours per day.
2. Nocturnal—at least 6 to 12 hours per day, depending on the patient's schedule. Schedule during nighttime sleeping hours and daytime naps.
3. Periodic—PRN, as ordered for exercise, cluster or migraine headaches, angina or congestive heart failure, high altitude travel, severe anemia, renal dialysis in patients with history of heart failure, or other conditions.

EVALUATION CRITERIA

For Correct Technique

1. Nasal prongs properly positioned in *both* nares.
2. Flow rate at prescribed L/min rate; FIO_2 on the Venturi mask set at prescribed quantity.
3. Humidifier setup appears clean—distilled water appears clean with absence of sediment on diffusor head and sides of reservoir.
4. Adequate bubbling in the jar for prescribed liter flow. If necessary, experiment with a fresh oxygen setup until you become familiar with bubbling expected for a commonly used flow rate, such as 2L/min.
5. Reduced bubbling may indicate the regulator knob is not all the way to open position; the patient does not change the distilled water daily; the patient inadequately cleans the diffusor head and humidifier jar; or the jar lid is not screwed on tightly.
6. Adequate fluid in the humidifier reservoir.
7. Absence of the following adverse effects: dry or sore skin and nasal mucosa; sores where tubing or elastic rubs side of face or ears, which can be padded with gauze or moleskin, if necessary; and headaches or sinus pain from high flow rates.

For Overall Improvement in Condition

1. Stable or improved PaO_2 or SaO_2.
2. Increased exercise tolerance.
3. Reduced blood hematocrit level.
4. Improved mental functioning and general sense of well being.
5. Improved signs indicating alleviation of cor pulmonale or heart failure.
6. Absence of signs of hypoxemia, tissue hypoxia, and overoxygenation in patients with hypoxic ventilatory drives to breathe.

7. In acute care settings, reduced pulmonary vascular resistance, reduced mean pulmonary artery pressure, increased cardiac output, and increased cardiac index.

IMPLEMENTATION

Before teaching the patient, the nurse clarifies the need for oxygen and the details of the oxygen prescription. "Oxygen PRN dyspnea" is an unacceptable order, because it does not state the disorder that oxygen is intended to treat, nor does it give a PaO_2 or an SaO_2 that documents hypoxemia. As mentioned in Chapter 21, such PRN orders for long-term oxygen therapy are not considered reimbursable by third-party payers.

The order for low flow oxygen is usually for nasal prongs at 1 to 3 L/min at rest. Liter flow is increased by 1 L during sleep. The increase in oxygen may increase $PaCO_2$ but is of little clinical significance at reduced flow rates.

The order for a portable oxygen system should document the need (e.g., to avoid exercise induced hypoxemia and improve exercise tolerance) and conditions for use (e.g., when walking or travelling outside the home). Liter flow is determined by the exercise stress test and response to therapy, as described in Chapter 20.

Clarification of the minimal number of hours per day for nocturnal oxygen is of utmost importance, particularly when noncompliance becomes a problem. Patients tend to reduce total hours per day because of short sleeping hours, dissatisfaction with the appearance of the delivery system, or absence of cardiopulmonary symptoms. To prevent noncompliance, the nurse helps the patient find ways to increase oxygen delivery time. A few simple suggestions, such as oxygen during daytime naps or the addition of a 25- or 50-ft extension tubing to allow ambulation, may solve the patient's problem.

Two other interventions will increase compliance. First, encourage the patient to verbalize feelings about the oxygen system. Feelings of dependency and helplessness are dealt with by using the motivational model presented in Chapter 16. Also, the patient is reminded that oxygen is to be considered a tool to increase activity rather than a crutch. If aesthetics is a problem, the nurse may suggest that the patient consider transtracheal oxygen; or the patient may switch from an oxygen conserving nasal cannula to standard nasal prongs, since the latter is less noticeable. Patients who are embarassed to walk in public with portable oxygen in a stroller may be less embarassed to take shorter walks, carrying a smaller lighter cylinder over their shoulder.

Second, during discussions, the nurse repeatedly emphasizes the benefits of oxygen. As oxygen reduces fatigue and increases exercise tolerance, it moves the patient away from the sick role in the family and towards a more productive life. However, the patient must be warned that benefits may not be fully realized unless oxygen is used for the prescribed amount of time.

Basic Monitoring

The evaluation criteria for oxygen therapy serve as a guide for monitoring patients on oxygen therapy at home. Monitoring for signs of hypoxemia is most important. Key signs include increased dyspnea, tachypnea, increased blood pressure and heart rate, cyanosis, altered mental status, and general fatigue. When these signs occur, the patient may need a medical evaluation, or oxygen equipment may not be working properly.

If the patient is not receiving humidification, check for nasal dryness, an indication for humidification.

Whether a liquid or tank system is in use, always check to be sure the patient knows when to reorder oxygen or refill portable units. A full H tank lasts 57 hours or 2½ days at 2L/min continuous use. A small E tank lasts 5 hours at the same flow rate. The following formula is used to calculate remaining hours of oxygen in tanks.

CALCULATION OF REMAINING HOURS IN OXYGEN TANKS

$$\frac{\text{PSI} \times \text{K}}{\text{flow rate (L/min)}} = \text{minutes}$$

$$\frac{\text{minutes}}{60} = \text{hours}$$

PSI = pounds per square inch (read regulator dial)

K = cylinder constant
3.14 for H tank
2.41 for G tank
0.28 for E tank

This formula helps the nurse advise the patient on when to order more oxygen. Ideally, however, the patient establishes a regular delivery schedule with the equipment vendor usually of once or twice a week, so that he never runs out of oxygen during the night or the weekend. At the time of tank replacement, any oxygen remaining in the used tank is credited to the patient's account.

Monitoring activity level and life situation helps the nurse determine whether the present oxygen delivery system is still appropriate. For example, patients who become homebound and require continuous oxygen may decide to switch to the concentrator system for cost effectiveness and convenience. Patients who feel better and begin to participate in more social activities outside the home may be happier with a liquid system. Study of Table 23–1 will help the nurse identify appropriate changes to discuss with the physician, patient, and equipment vendor.

Hospital Setting

Monitoring the patient in the hospital setting is exactly the same as monitoring in the home setting. The only difference is the increased intensity and frequency and the use of high technology in critical care units. For example, when a pulmonary artery catheter is in place, hypoxemia may be signalled by an increase in pulmonary vascular resistance, increase in mean pulmonary artery pressure, and decrease in cardiac output and cardiac index. Since hospitalized patients are usually sicker and more labile, signs and symptoms may be more severe. They may include late signs of hypoxemia, such as hypotension, or arrhythmias that disappear with an increase in FIO_2. When pneumonia is present, hypoxemia may occur suddenly or intermittently during 1 hour, as shifting mucus plugs alter V/Q relationships in the lungs. Such labile patients require intensive respiratory nursing care and specialized interventions (see the next unit of this book).

MONITORING OXYGEN PERCENT SATURATION (SaO_2) WITH PULSE OXIMETRY

Since clinical signs of hypoxemia may be nonspecific, few in number, or lacking, the nurse periodically monitors PaO_2 or SaO_2 in the evaluation of oxygen therapy. The most practical parameter for routine monitoring in acute and chronic care settings is SaO_2 by pulse oximetry.

Pulse oximetry is a noninvasive method of measuring SaO_2 and evaluating hypoxemia. The oximeter device has a probe that transmits light pulses through highly arterialized capillary beds, such as the ear lobe or finger. Varying degrees of light absorption through tissue are related to arterial hemoglobin oxygen saturation (SaO_2).

Pulse oximetry is considered a supplement rather than a replacement for the ABG. It reduces the time, cost, and invasiveness of taking repeated ABGs to titrate oxygen therapy to an acceptable SaO_2 level. Oximetry is indicated when knowledge of oxygenation alone is adequate for assessment of individual situations and when alveolar ventilation and pH are relatively constant (Petty, 1986).

Besides the evaluation of oxygen therapy, oximetry has numerous other uses, as shown in the next box. Most of these uses are explained in other chapters of this book in relation to specific respiratory interventions, such as mechanical ventilation or pursed-lip breathing.

> ***CLINICAL USES OF PULSE OXIMETRY***
>
> Adjustment of oxygen therapy
> Documentation of continued need for oxygen
> Ventilator adjustments, especially when multiple adjustments are necessary
> Initial emergency room screening
> Treadmill testing
> Evaluation of chest physiotherapy techniques, e.g., breathing retraining
> Evaluation of a patient who becomes dyspneic, lightheaded, or shows other signs of hypoxemia
> Sleep apnea studies
> Bronchoscopy
> Surgical procedure
> Postanesthesia care

Oximetry has two important advantages over ABGs and other methods of assessing oxygenation. First, it allows either continuous monitoring (Fig. 23–19A) or intermittent monitoring (Fig. 23–19B). Second, modern portable oximetry models are small, easy to use, and suitable for monitoring at rest as well as during ambulation. Last, they may be used in the hospital, clinic, or home settings for documentation of Medicare home oxygen reimbursement (Nelson et al, 1986).

The two most commonly used oximeters are the ear oximeter and finger oximeter. Obtaining an ear oximeter SaO_2 measurement involves vigorously rubbing the pinna of the ear for 15 to 30 seconds to increase circulation to the area. As long as a low-perfusion warning is not activated, indicating insufficient signal for accurate readings, a digital read-out is obtained in 30 to 60 seconds. The finger oximeter works the same way except rubbing the finger is unnecessary because it has a greater blood volume than the ear. Compared with an ear sensor, a finger sensor tends to be less cumbersome for the wearer and is less likely to slip off the skin's surface during activity.

Blood SaO_2 and oximetry SaO_2 are interpreted the same way, since a good correlation exists between the two measurements (see A Chapter 13 for interpretation of SaO_2 values). Standard deviation ranges from 1% to 2.6% for most oximetry models in current clinical use. Though both ear and finger oximetry are suitable for monitoring purposes, finger oximetry SaO_2 results correlate with blood SaO_2 to a slightly higher, statistically significant degree (Cecil et al, 1985).

One disadvantage of oximetry is that it is not a reliable indicator of SaO_2 under certain conditions. Erroneous values occur in the presence of poor perfusion states (e.g., low cardiac output, peripheral shunting, hypothermia), elevated bilirubin concentrations, elevated hemoglobin-carboxyhemoglobin levels, and Cardio-Green and other intravascular dyes (Wilkins et al, 1985).

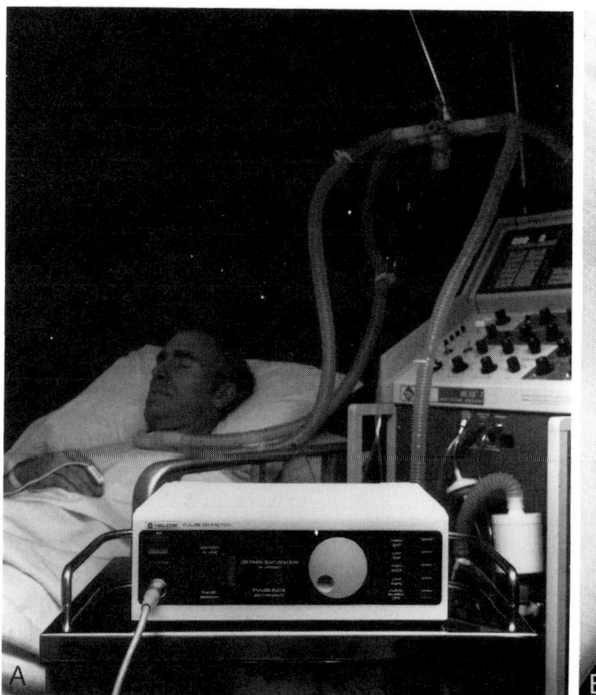

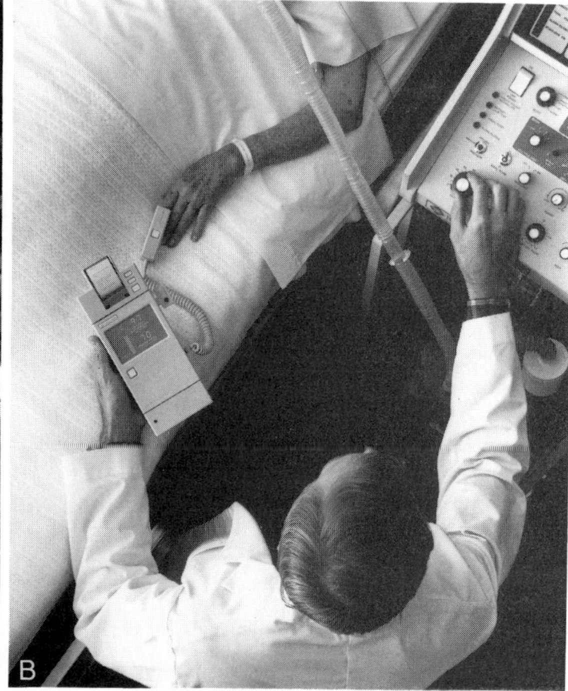

Figure 23–19. Finger pulse oximetry. *A*, The finger oximetry unit may be used at the bedside for continuous monitoring of oxygen saturation (top digital reading) and pulse rate in beats/min (bottom digital reading). *B*, A lightweight portable unit may be carried by the nurse for intermittent, on-the-spot checks in hospital, clinic, or home settings. This Nellcor N-10 model has both a digital display and a printer attachment that provides a copy of patient results for immediate interpretation. (Courtesy of Nellcor Incorporated, Hayward, California.)

When initiated, oximetry Sao_2 is compared with blood Sao_2. If the difference is greater than 4% or if oximetry values vary widely for unknown reasons, measurement error or equipment failure is suspected. Because of the chance of error, oximetry is used for monitoring *trends* in Sao_2 rather than absolute values. Trends provide adequate information to determine, for example, whether a change in liter flow has increased oxygen saturation to above 85% during exercise. If a COPD patient's Sao_2 rises well above 85%, a reduction in oxygen liter flow or a discontinuation of oxygen therapy may be indicated.

Conclusion

This chapter on oxygen therapy prepares the nurse to safely and promptly administer oxygen to relieve hypoxemia and tissue hypoxia.

It also prepares the visiting nurse to make numerous patient- and equipment-related decisions, while delivering home respiratory nursing care. Some decisions will have a major impact on the patient's ability to cope with lung disease, such as the decision to increase oxygen liter flow to relieve signs of hypoxemia or the decision to suggest a liquid oxygen system for the ambulatory patient who begins to socialize outside the home. Other decisions, such as the one to pad oxygen tubing to prevent local skin irritation, may seem to be of low priority at that moment. Yet, these decisions are just as important as seemingly more critical decisions; when a potential problem is not addressed, it may quickly develop into a major problem. In the case of padding, local skin irritation may precipitate patient reluctance to wear the nasal cannula; noncompliance with prescribed oxygen therapy; and, ultimately, acute exacerbation of cardiopulmonary disease.

REFERENCES

American College of Chest Physicians; Continuous or nocturnal oxygen therapy in hypoxemic COLD. *Annals of internal medicine*, 93(3):391–398, 1980.

American Lung Association of California, California Thoracic Society: *Guidelines for the use of home oxygen therapy*. Oakland, California, American Lung Association, 1983.

California Thoracic Society, Respiratory Care Assembly: *Criteria for the review of respiratory care services*. Oakland, California, California Thoracic Society, 1981.

Cecil, W., Morrison, L., and Lamoonpun, S.: Clinical evaluation of the Ohmeda Biox III pulse oximeter: a comparison of finger and ear cuvettes. *Respiratory care*, 30(10):840–845, 1985.

Darin, J.: The need for rational criteria for the use of unheated bubble humidifiers. *Respiratory care*, 27(8):945–947, 1982.

Darin, J., Broadwell, J., and MacDonell, R.: An evaluation of water-vapor output from four brands of unheated, prefilled bubble humidifiers. *Respiratory care*, 27(1):41–50, 1982.

Findley, L., Whelan, D., and Moser, K.: Long-term oxygen therapy in COPD. *Chest*, 83(4):671–674, 1983.

Flenley, D.: Long-term home oxygen therapy. *Chest*, 87(1):99–103, 1985.

Flenley, D.: Long-term oxygen therapy—state of the art. *Respiratory care*, 28(7):876–884, 1983.

Flick, M., and Block, A.: Chronic oxygen therapy. *Medical clinics of north america*, 61(6):1397–1405, 1977.

Fulmer, J., and Snider, G.: American College of Chest Physicians—National Heart, Lung, and Blood Institute (ACCP-NHLBI) National Conference on oxygen therapy. *Chest*, 86(2):234–246, 1984.

Heimlich, H., and Carr, G.: Transtracheal catheter technique for pulmonary rehabilitation. *Annals of otology, rhinology and laryngology*, 94(5):502–504, 1985.

Helmholz, H., and Burton, G.: Applied humidity and aerosol therapy. In Respiratory Care—A Guide to Clinical Practice, 2nd ed. (Burton, G., and Hodgkin, J.—eds.). Philadelphia, J. B. Lippincott Co., 1984.

Hodgkin, J., Zorn, E., and Connors, G.: *Pulmonary Rehabilitation—Guidelines to Success*. Boston, Butterworth Publishers, 1984.

Kersten, L.: Your Respiratory Home Care Program. Berkeley, California, Herrick Hospital and Health Center of the East Bay, 1978.

Kirilloff, J., Dauber, J., et al: Patient response to transtracheal oxygen delivery. *American review of respiratory disease*, 131(4): A162, 1985.

Lasky, M.: Bubble humidifiers are useful—fact or myth? *Respiratory care*, 27(6):735–736, 1982.

McPherson, S.: Respiratory Therapy Equipment, 3rd ed. St. Louis, C.V. Mosby Co., 1985.

McDonald, G.: Long-term oxygen therapy delivery systems. *Respiratory care*, 28(7):898–905, 1983.

Medical Research Council Working Party: Long-term domiciliary oxygen therapy in chronic hypoxic cor pulmonale complicating chronic bronchitis and emphysema. Lancet, 1(8222):681–668, 1981.

Nelson, C., Murphy, E., Bradley, J., and Durie, R.: Clinical use of pulse oximetry to determine oxygen prescriptions for patients with hypoxemia. *Respiratory care*, 31(8):673–680, 1986.

Nocturnal Oxygen Therapy Trial Group: Continuous or nocturnal oxygen therapy in hypoxemic COLD. *Annals of internal medicine*, 93(3):391–398, 1980.

Petty, T.: *Ambulatory oxygen*. New York, Thieme-Stratton Inc., 1983.

Petty, T.: Who needs home oxygen? *American review of respiratory disease*, 131(6):930–931, 1985.

Petty, T.: Clinical Pulse Oximetry. Boulder, Colorado, Ohmeda Life Support, 1986.

Pierson, D., West, G., and McDonald, G. (eds.): Long-term oxygen therapy: a world view. *Respiratory care*, 28(7): entire issue, 1983.

Poundstone, W.: Air travel and supplemental oxygen—friendly skies for respiratory patients. *Respiratory therapy*, 13(1):79–82, 1983.

Rebuck, A. S., Chapman, K. R., and D'Urzo, A.: The accuracy and response characteristics of a simplified ear oximeter. *Chest*, 83(6), 860–864, 1983.

Shigeoka, J., and Bonekat, H.: The current status of oxygen-conserving devices. *Respiratory care*, 30(10):833–836, 1985.

Tiep, B., Belman, M., et al: A new pendant storage oxygen-conserving nasal cannula. *Chest*, 87(3):381–383, 1985a.

Tiep, B., Carter, R., et al: Demand oxygen delivery during exercise. *Chest*, 91(1):15–20, 1987b.

Tiep, B., and Lewis, M. Oxygen conservation and oxygen-conserving devices in chronic lung disease. *Chest*, 92(2):263–272, 1987.

Tiep, B., Nicotra, B., et al: Evaluation of an oxygen-conserving nasal cannula. *Respiratory care*, 30(1):19–25, 1985d.

Tiep, B., Nicotra, M., Carter, R., et al.: Low-concentration oxygen therapy via a demand oxygen delivery system. *Chest*, 87(5):636–638, 1985e.

Wilkins, R., Sheldon, R., and Krider, S.: Clinical Assessment in Respiratory Care. St. Louis, C.V. Mosby Co., 1985.

SPECIALIZED INTERVENTIONS

Part Five

Basic interventions are usually combined with specialized interventions to deliver comprehensive respiratory nursing care. This part of the book describes specialized interventions, i.e., interventions that require special techniques or high technology for implementation. Though it is written for nurses who care for acutely ill respiratory patients in the critical care setting, content on topics such as tracheostomy tubes, care of the intubated patient, and mechanical ventilation, applies to ward, clinic, and home settings as well. Content related to artificial airways and airway care is divided into several chapters to facilitate the retrieval of information for both hospital and home settings.

The first step in respiratory emergencies is *establishing airway patency* (see Chapter 24). When conservative methods of establishing an airway fail, passing an endotracheal tube into the trachea may be necessary. *Endotracheal intubation* is discussed in Chapter 25, along with the complications and consequences of leaving an artificial airway in the trachea for short and long periods of time. When a long intubation period is anticipated, the physician may perform a *tracheotomy* procedure and insert a *tracheostomy tube* (see Chapter 26).

Both endotracheal intubation and tracheostomy require specialized maintenance care. Chapter 27 discusses *care of the intubated patient* and the family.

Patients who require endotracheal intubation almost always require ventilator assistance to maintain normal lung ventilation and oxygenation. Chapter 28 discusses *mechanical ventilation* in considerable detail to prepare the nurse to collaborate with other health team members caring for the patient.

Chapter 29 discusses basic *hemodynamic monitoring* concepts with respiratory applications.

Chapter 30 presents *chest tube drainage systems* in detail, since monitoring these systems is one of the least understood of all respiratory interventions. In addition, this chapter summarizes related *post-thoracotomy care.*

Since this part of the book emphasizes the technology of specialized interventions, it is more procedurally oriented than other parts. The reason for this orientation is threefold. First, mastering technology is a prerequisite for humanizing nursing care. In other words, the knowledgeable and skilled nurse is more efficient and therefore has more time to deliver care in a professional and caring way.

Second, time restraints are crucial in critical care. The nurse moves from assessment to intervention in a matter of seconds and minutes to avoid potentially fatal complications. Reliance on theoretically sound respiratory procedures helps the nurse initiate appropriate interventions, until the assessment process suggests a modified plan of action.

Third, knowledge of current respiratory technologies and monitoring parameters prepares the nurse for more sophisticated technologies that are being developed at major medical centers. Examples of developing technologies are computer-aided ventilator monitoring, high frequency ventilation, differential lung ventilation utilizing two ventilators, and lung and heart-lung transplantation.

In essence, this part of the book prepares the nurse to meet both current and future challenges in respiratory care. What remains for future research is the determination of the cost effectiveness, ethics, and efficacies of new technologies, and the determination of optimal ways to organize critical care nursing services to meet the changing and complex needs of the patient.

Terms commonly used to describe specialized interventions are listed in the glossary.

Glossary of Commonly Used Terms in Specialized Interventions

ABCs of cardiopulmonary resuscitation (CPR)—priorities for emergency intervention: (1) establishment of a patent *airway*, (2) assisted or spontaneous *breathing*, and (3) *circulatory* assistance.

afterload (cardiac)—tension developed by the ventricle during systole or resistance to flow from the ventricle during contraction. Measurements of right ventricular afterload are pulmonary arterial (PA) pressures and pulmonary vascular resistance (PVR). Measurements of left ventricular afterload are arterial systolic blood pressure and systemic vascular resistance (SVR).

artificial airway—any tube that maintains airway patency to the lungs, e.g., oral or nasal airway, endotracheal tube, tracheostomy tube.

assist-control mode—a mode of mechanical ventilation. The patient triggers assisted breaths that are replaced by controlled breaths during hypoventilation.

bagging—use of a manual resuscitator for oxygenation and ventilation.

bronchoscope—flexible or rigid tube passed down the nose or mouth for visualization of the larynx, trachea, and large airways and for tissue biopsy or aspiration of respiratory secretions.

capnography—study and use of capnograms; graphic display of expired Co_2 waveforms.

chest tube—tube inserted into the intrapleural space or mediastinum to drain air, fluid, or both from the chest.

chest tube drainage system—system attached to a chest tube for drainage collection and maintenance of normal pleural and intrathoracic pressures.

chronotropic—relating to heart rate.

continuous positive airway pressure (CPAP)—spontaneous breathing with a fixed amount of positive pressure applied to the airway at all times.

contractility—inotropic state of the myocardium, influenced by many biochemical, neurogenic, and pharmacologic factors.

controlled mode—a mode of mechanical ventilation. The ventilator delivers positive pressure breaths at a fixed time interval.

cuff management—inflation and deflation techniques and pressure monitoring for the cuff of an artificial airway.

cuff pressure monitoring—periodic measurement of artificial airway cuff pressure, using a mercury or aneroid manometer.

decannulation—tracheostomy tube removal.

ejection fraction—proportion of blood ejected from the ventricle per beat compared with end-diastolic volume.

endotracheal tube—tube inserted through the nose or mouth and into the trachea to maintain airway patency and, in some cases, initiate mechanical ventilation.

extubation—endotracheal tube removal.

fenestrated tracheostomy tube—tube with an opening (fenestration) in the outer cannula to increase air flow and decrease airway resistance.

finger sweep—using the index finger to clear the mouth, removing vomitus, mucus, or foreign objects caught against the cheek or in the back of the throat.

fractional inspired oxygen concentration (FIO_2)—oxygen concentration of inspired gas, expressed in decimal form, e.g., FIO_2 of 0.80 = 80% oxygen concentration.

hard cuff—low volume, high pressure cuff on the distal end of an endotracheal or tracheostomy tube.

head tilt/chin lift—method of opening the airway by placing one hand on the patient's forehead and tilting the head backward. The other hand gently lifts the chin so that it is pointing upward.

heart rate—heart beats per minute, a major determinant of cardiac output, coronary blood flow, and oxygen utilization in the body.

hemodynamic monitoring—use of a pulmonary artery catheter to determine pressure relationships in the heart and lungs.

high frequency ventilation—a relatively new mode of mechanical ventilation involving delivery of small tidal volumes at high frequencies.

intermittent mandatory ventilation (IMV)—a mode of mechanical ventilation. The ventilator delivers a preset number of breaths to a spontaneously breathing patient.

inner cannula—the inside shaft of a tracheostomy tube.

inotropic—relating to the force of cardiac muscle contraction.

intubation—insertion of an artificial airway through the nose (nasotracheal intubation), through the mouth (orotracheal intubation), or directly into the trachea (tracheal intubation) to establish airway patency, initiate mechanical ventilation, or both.

jaw thrust—method of opening the airway by first tilting the head back, and then grabbing the corners of the jaw with the fingers and displacing the mandible forward.

Lanz pressure regulating valve—a special valve that is built into the relatively large pilot balloon of some soft cuffed tubes, e.g., original Lanz tube (no longer available) and current Hi-Lo tube.

laryngoscope—a flexible or rigid tube for visualization of the larynx and atraumatic placement of an endotracheal tube into the trachea.

Leuken's trap—sterile specimen container that attaches to a suction catheter for collection of sputum during tracheal suctioning.

long-term mechanical ventilation—mechanical ventilation out of the hospital setting either continuously or for predetermined periods of time during the day or night.

mechanical ventilation—ventilation of the lungs by artificial means, usually by a ventilator.

mixed venous blood—venous blood drawn from the distal port of a pulmonary artery catheter.

mode of ventilation—type of ventilatory pattern provided by a mechanical ventilator, e.g., intermittent mandatory ventilation (IMV) mode.

nasal airway—short rubber tube used to maintain airway patency from naris to hypopharynx.

negative pressure ventilation—lung ventilation by intermittent application of negative pressure to the chest, e.g., iron lung, chest cuirass.

obturator—part of a tracheostomy tube that fits into the outer cannula and is used exclusively to facilitate tube insertion.

oral airway—short rubber or plastic piece that inserts into the mouth and maintains airway patency to the hypopharynx.

overwedging—a falsely high pulmonary capillary wedge pressure tracing caused by overinflation of the pulmonary arterial catheter balloon.

oximeter (ear or digital)—a noninvasive device that attaches to the ear or finger and measures oxygen saturation of hemoglobin in the blood.

peak inspiratory pressure (PIP)—highest pressure (cmH_2O) attained during a tidal volume ventilator breath.

pilot balloon—balloon located along the inflating tube of an endotracheal or tracheostomy tube.

positive end-expiratory pressure (PEEP)—application of positive pressure to the airway at the end of expiration. Used with other modes of mechanical ventilation, such as the assist-control mode.

positive pressure ventilation—lung ventilation by intermittent application of positive pressure to the lungs by mask or artificial airway.

preload (cardiac)—initial stretch of the myocardial fiber at end diastole or volume of blood in the ventricle before contraction. Measurements of right ventricular preload are right atrial pressure and central venous pressure; measurements of left ventricular preload are pulmonary capillary wedge pressure and left atrial pressure.

pressure-cycled (limited) ventilator—ventilator that allows gas flow into the lungs until a present pressure is reached.

psychologic adjustment phases to mechanical ventilation—four phases are (1) preoccupation with survival, (2) denial and fantasy, (3) depression and gradual accommodation to reality, and (4) active participation in rehabilitative care.

pulmonary capillary wedge pressure (PCWP)—pressure measured when the catheter balloon is inflated and the catheter tip is wedged in a branch of the pulmonary artery. The pressure reflects left atrial pressure.

resuscitator, manual—1- to 2-L bag and valve device that self inflates once it has been manually squeezed to provide a positive pressure tidal volume to the patient; sometimes called an air-mask-bag unit (AMBU).

resuscitator, pulmonary—a generic term describing numerous manual and automatic cycling breathing units.

sniffing position—in the supine position, placement of the head slightly above the shoulders to create a straight airway from mouth to glottis.

soft cuff—high volume, low pressure cuff on the distal end of an endotracheal or tracheostomy tube.

speaking tube—special tracheostomy tube that enables the patient to talk with near normal laryngeal speech.

splinting—immobilization of the chest during breathing due to pain, e.g., the post-thoracotomy patient splints by flexing the trunk towards the incision.

stoma—opening.

stripping—manual or mechanical squeezing technique used along the length of a chest tube to insure patency. Utilized only by a physician's order and only as a last resort.

suctioning—passage of a catheter into the upper or lower airway and application of a negative pressure to remove respiratory secretions.

stylet—wire-like instrument used during endotracheal intubation that inserts into the tube to stiffen it.

synchronized intermittent mandatory ventilation (SIMV)—same as the intermittent mandatory ventilation mode of mechanical ventilation, except ventilator breaths are synchronized with patient breaths.

thoracostomy—insertion of a tube through a closed chest.

tidalling—respiratory fluctuation of fluid in the water seal chamber of a chest drainage unit.

time-cycled (limited) ventilator—ventilator that allows gas flow into the lungs until a preset length of time has elapsed.

T-piece or T-tube—a nebulizer adapter or breathing tube apparatus that resembles a T. The base of the T of the breathing tube attaches directly to an artificial airway to permit spontaneous breathing during weaning. This feature may be built into the design of a ventilator, without requiring a separate device.

tracheostomy—opening or stoma made by surgical incision into the trachea.

tracheostomy button—plugged cannula that inserts into a tracheostomy to maintain stoma wall patency during weaning.

tracheotomy—surgical incision into the trachea.

tube stabilization—taping an endotracheal tube, use of a side support for a ventilator circuit, and other interventions that stabilize an artificial airway.

universal adaptor—standard 15 mm adapter, used to connect an artificial airway to a respiratory therapy device.

ventilator check—investigating basic ventilator parameters during the nursing assessment: (1) ventilator mode; (2) FIO_2; (3) respiratory rate f, including ratio of assisted breaths to controlled breaths; (4) preset and exhaled tidal volume (V_T), (5) peak inspiratory pressure; (6) positive end expiratory pressure (PEEP) level; and (7) alarm system.

volume-cycled (limited) ventilator—ventilator that allows gas flow into the lungs until a preset volume is delivered.

water seal—essential chamber of a chest drainage system that prevents air and fluid from being sucked into the chest and maintains normal pleural and thoracic pressures.

weaning—gradual process of reducing FIO_2 to at least 0.40 and withdrawing mechanical ventilatory support.

Yankauer's pharyngeal suction tip—hand-held device attached to a suction source used to quickly clear the upper airway of respiratory secretions and vomitus.

Establishing Airway Patency

24

Main Objectives

1. **Explain why establishing a patent airway comes first in CPR.**
2. **Describe the steps for establishing and maintaining a patent airway for (a) the unconscious patient or patient in respiratory distress and (b) the unconscious choking victim.**
3. **Differentiate between the head-tilt and jaw-thrust methods for opening an airway.**
4. **Describe how to manually bag a patient using a mask and resuscitator.**
5. **Name three factors that determine the actual FIO_2 delivered by a manual resuscitator bag hooked up to a 100% oxygen source.**
6. **In regard to oral and nasal airways**
   a. **Describe basic design.**
   b. **Explain insertion and removal techniques.**
   c. **Explain how to verify patency after airway insertion.**
   d. **Name two complications that may occur during or after insertion.**
   e. **Describe maintenance care.**
7. **Discuss how to modify the standard procedure (see Chapter 27) to suction through the oral or nasal airway of a spontaneously breathing patient.**

This chapter explains (1) how to establish a patent airway during cardiopulmonary emergencies, (2) how to use a manual resuscitator bag, and (3) how to use nasal and oral airways.

This information prepares the hospital-based nurse to collaborate with the respiratory therapist and physician to establish and maintain airway patency. In addition, it prepares nurses in hospital, home, and clinic settings to accomplish the same goal in the absence of other health team members.

The ABCs of Cardiopulmonary Resuscitation (CPR)—The Airway Comes First

The ABCs of CPR include *A*, establishment of a patent *airway*; *B*, assisted or spontaneous *breathing*; and *C*, *circulatory assistance* in the form of external chest compression and appropriate medication (Rosequist, 1987).

In the case of acute respiratory failure of any cause, establishment of a patent airway is always first. Without airway patency, all attempts to ventilate the lungs will fail. Apnea or complete airway obstruction can quickly lead to cyanosis within 1 minute, permanent brain injury within 4 to 5 minutes, and cardiac asystole within 5 to 10 minutes.

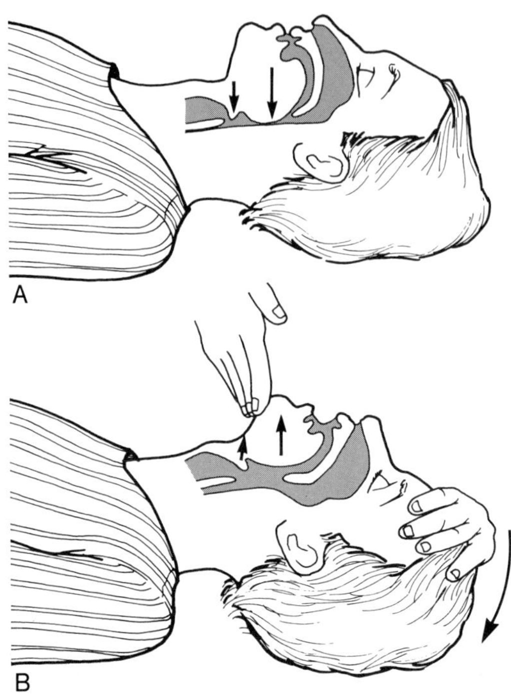

Figure 24–1. Airway obstruction produced by the tongue and epiglottis *(A)* is relieved by the head-tilt/chin-lift method of opening the airway *(B)*.

Steps for Establishing Airway Patency

THE UNCONSCIOUS PATIENT OR PATIENT IN RESPIRATORY DISTRESS

The clinician follows these steps when a patient is found unconscious or in respiratory distress:

Step 1—Evaluate Unresponsiveness. Grab the patient's shoulders and shake him. Call out his name and ask "Are you OK?" For a trauma patient, use a light touch rather than shaking to avoid inappropriate body movements and possible paralysis.

Step 2—Call for Help. If the patient does not respond to verbal or tactile stimulation or if signs of airway obstruction are present (e.g., apnea, use of accessory muscles of respiration), call for help and prepare to establish an airway.

Step 3—Reposition the Patient. Place the patient supine with the arms alongside the body. Remove all pillows from the bed. When possible, ask another person to clear away unnecessary bedside equipment, pull the bed away from the wall, and remove the bed's headboard for better access to the patient.

Step 4—Open the Airway. Tilt the patient's head back and check for breathing, using the head-tilt/chin-lift method for the relief of upper airway obstruction (Fig. 24–1).

Head-tilt/Chin-lift Method. Place the palm of one hand on the patient's forehead and firmly tilt the head backward. To complete the maneuver, place the fingers of the other hand under the bony part of the chin and gently lift, as shown in Figure 24–1 (bottom). These actions will help bring the jaw forward and lift the flaccid tongue away from the posterior oropharynx.

Jaw-thrust Method. This method is sometimes called *jutting the jaw.* It is usually used for patients with neck, back, or facial injuries when opening the airway is desired without neck hyperextension. Neck hyperextension is avoided in these situations because of increased risk for tissue trauma and paralysis. To jut the jaw, grasp the corners of the lower jaw with the fingers. Lift with both hands, while keeping the elbows on the bed for leverage (Fig. 24–2). If ventilation is not possible while lifting the jaw forward in this manner, the patient's head may be tilted back slightly during the lifting motion. In both the head-tilt/chin-lift and jaw-thrust methods, the mouth should not be completely closed. If necessary, use the thumb to retract the lower lip enough to maintain the airway.

Step 5—Check for Breathing. Look for chest movement, listen for air movement, and, if necessary, place the hand over the nostrils and mouth to confirm air

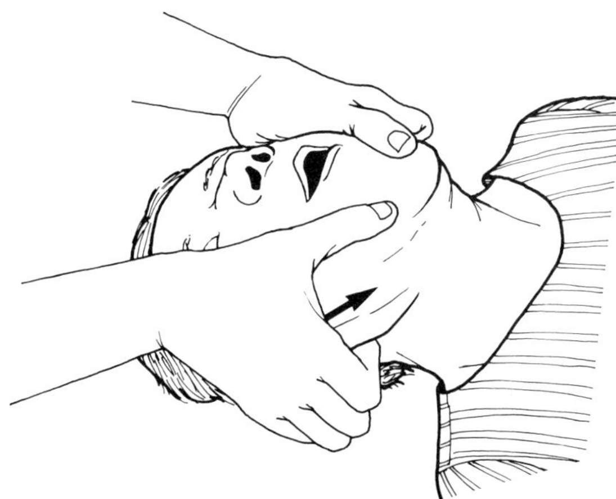

Figure 24–2. A modified jaw-thrust method of opening the airway. Neck hyperextension is avoided.

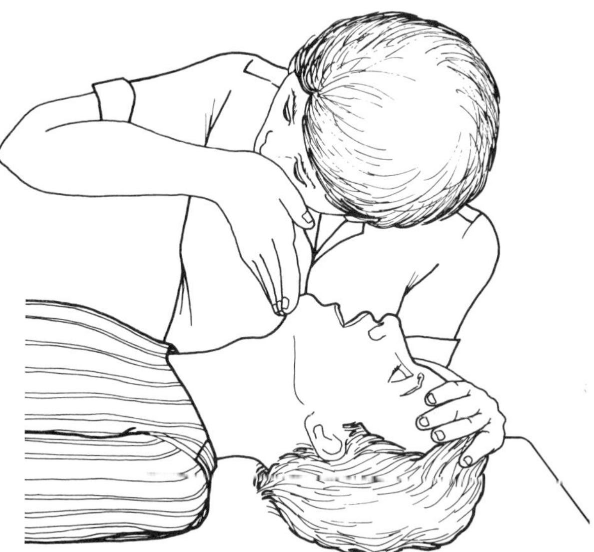

Figure 24–3. Checking for breathing.

movement (Fig. 24–3). If the patient begins to breathe spontaneously, instruct him to take more deep breaths and then apply a face mask for supplementary oxygen. Elevate the head of the bed to facilitate breathing but do not position the head of the patient on a pillow.

Step 6—Positive Pressure Ventilation. If apnea persists, deliver positive pressure ventilation. When resuscitation equipment is not available, the clinician uses the mouth-to-mouth, mouth-to-nose, or mouth-to-stoma technique described by the American Heart Association (1986). Otherwise, a bedside resuscitation device, such as a mouth-to-mask resuscitator (Fig. 24–4) or preferably a manual resuscitator (Fig. 24–5), is used to deliver two slow full breaths in a row (Birdsall and Ruggio, 1987). At this point, do not take time to clear the airway—just concentrate on delivering the initial two breaths. To avoid gastric distention, regurgitation, and pulmonary aspiration, the nurse allows 1 to 1.5 seconds for each inflation. To avoid lung hyperinflation, the nurse allows twice as much time or 2 to 3 seconds for each deflation.

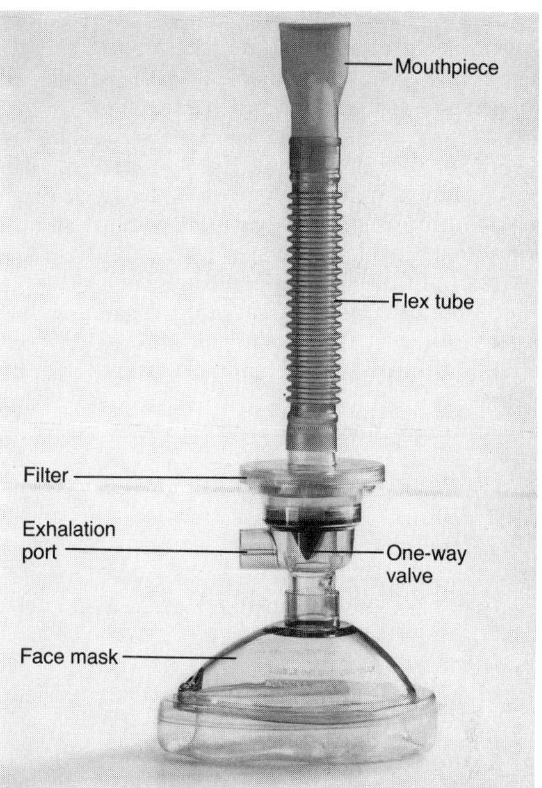

Figure 24–4. A mouth-to-mask resuscitator (Safe-Response model. Courtesy of Intertech Resources Inc., Bannockburn, Illinois.)

Step 7—Relieve Airway Obstruction. Inability to compress the resuscitation bag during positive pressure ventilation indicates increased airway resistance and airway obstruction. In this case, turn the patient's head to the side. Roll him to one side, if possible. Allow pharyngeal secretions to drain out of the mouth,

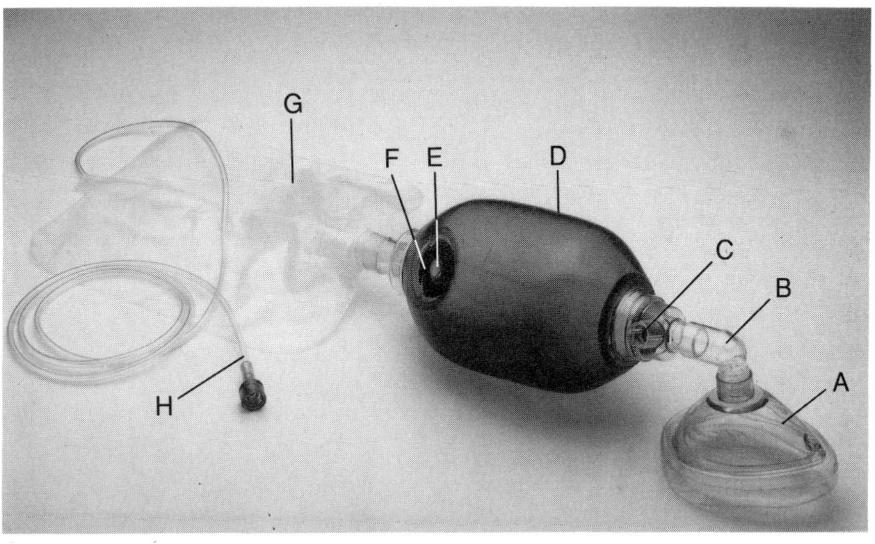

Figure 24–5. A disposable ual resuscitator. A, Face mask (transparent); B, Elbow attachment; C, Exhalation port that may be used for PEEP attachment; D, Self-inflating bag (semitransparent); E, O_2 inlet (inside view); F, Gas inlet consisting of a one-way valve that encircles the O_2 inlet; G, Reservoir bag to ensure 100% O_2 delivery; H, O_2 extension tubing. It attaches to the O_2 flow meter and extends through the reservoir bag to the O_2 inlet. In this 1st Response model, compressing the bag closes the gas inlet valve and allows 100% O_2 to be delivered to the patient. Releasing the bag opens the gas inlet valve and allows O_2 to enter through the O_2 inlet. (Courtesy of Intertech Resources Inc., Bannockburn, Illinois.)

using a finger sweep to loosen and remove vomitus or foreign objects caught in the back of the throat. If available, use a suction catheter or pharyngeal suction tip to aspirate secretions (see Chapter 27).

For the *finger sweep*, grasp the tongue and lower jaw with one hand and pull the jaw up (Fig. 24–6). With the index finger of your other hand, sweep the entire mouth using a hooking motion. Start along the inside of one cheek and sweep across the base of the tongue to the inside of the opposite cheek.

The American Heart Association recommends the steps described in this box for an unconscious victim who does not respond to the initial attempt to ventilate the lungs.

RELIEF OF AIRWAY OBSTRUCTION IN THE UNCONSCIOUS CHOKING VICTIM

1. Reposition the head and try again to give two full, slow breaths.
2. *If ventilation is successful*
   a. Check the pulse and continue artificial ventilations, as needed.
   b. Do not attempt to clear the airway further in the case of partial obstruction. Such attempts may push a foreign object back into the lungs.
   c. Wait for medical assistance or for the patient to spontaneously cough up the object or mucous plugs.
3. *If ventilation is unsuccessful*
   a. Perform 6 to 10 abdominal thrusts with the patient supine (the Heimlich maneuver).

      For an *abdominal thrust*, kneel astride or beside the victim. Place the heel of one hand on the abdomen between the rib cage and waist. Put your other hand on top, as shown in Figure 24–7. With arms straight and shoulders directly over the patient's abdomen, press into the abdomen with a quick upward thrust. To avoid internal injuries, do not press to either side. In the case of gross obesity or advanced pregnancy, use *chest thrusts*, instead of abdominal thrusts. Chest thrusts are delivered with the same body position and hand position as for chest compressions in CPR. The heel of the hand rests over the lower body of the sternum. The chest is compressed 1.5 to 2 in.
   b. Finger sweep the back of the throat to clear the airway.
   c. Reposition the head and attempt to ventilate again.
   d. Repeat the above *thrust, finger sweep,* and *ventilation* steps until medical help arrives or until spontaneous breathing resumes.

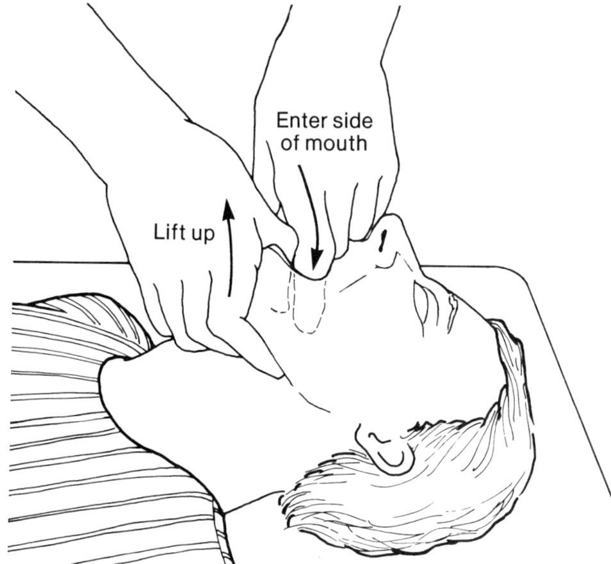

Figure 24–6. Clearing the airway with a finger sweep.

Step 8—Insert an Oral Airway. When an oral airway is readily available, the nurse may insert it (technique described subsequently) before initial ventilation of the lungs in the unconscious or cooperative patient (see step 6—Deliver Positive Pressure Ventilation). In many cases, however, an oral airway is not readily available, and insertion is best performed after initial ventilation and relief of airway obstruction. Moreover, when the patient resists efforts to open the mouth, in spite of words of encouragement, this step is best omitted or delayed until help arrives or an intravenous muscle relaxant is given (e.g., immediately before endotracheal intubation).

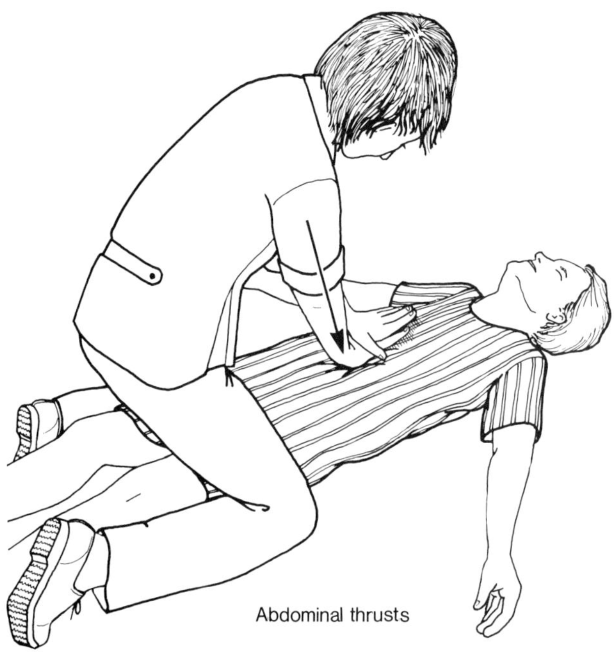

Figure 24–7. Giving six to ten subdiaphragmatic abdominal thrusts (Heimlich maneuver).

Step 9—Check for Spontaneous Breathing and a Carotid Pulse. If no breathing and no pulse are present, begin the CPR procedure with chest compressions. In any case, do not take longer than 5 to 10 seconds to check pulse and breathing.

Step 10—Continue to Ventilate the Lungs. When ventilating the lungs, give one breath (i.e., bag compression) every 5 seconds for adults and one breath every 3 seconds for infants. During a CPR procedure, give one breath for every five chest compressions. Watch for chest expansion with each breath. Ask another person to auscultate the anterior chest area to verify air movement in all anterior lung lobes.

Use of a Manual Resuscitator

Use of a manual resuscitator to ventilate and oxygenate the lungs is commonly referred to as *bagging* the patient. Its use is not restricted to the resuscitation situation, but extends to other clinical situations. Bagging may be used before and after suctioning the trachea to hyperinflate and hyperoxygenate the lungs and to churn up and promote evacuation of secretions. This technique may be used temporarily whenever ventilator malfunction is suspected or respiratory distress becomes worse. In addition, during ventilator circuit changes, bagging is employed to avoid hypoxemia and the anxiety of being off the ventilator for a short period of time.

A resuscitator with mask, oxygen tubing, and attached flow meter should be readily available on each ward's emergency cart and at the bedside of every ventilator dependent patient. Various models are available, e.g., Puritan, Vitalograph, Hope, Air Shields, and Ambu resuscitators.

Perhaps the most important point to remember about resuscitators is that *attachment to a 100% oxygen source does not guarantee delivery of 100% oxygen.* Resuscitators deliver from 30% to 100% oxygen, depending on oxygen flow rate, respiratory pattern, and presence or absence of an oxygen reservoir (i.e., an additional bag or corrugated tubing) at the end of the bag (Barnes and Watson, 1982).

An oxygen reservoir is particularly important. After each bag compression, the bag inflates itself by entraining gas through a one-way valve during expiration. Use of an oxygen reservoir of 400 cc (e.g., Vitalograph) to 2400 cc (e.g., Laerdal), assures self-inflation with mostly oxygen rather than room air. With a reservoir, resuscitators will maintain a high FIO_2, ranging from 0.80 to 1.00 at different ventilatory patterns. Without a reservoir attached, these resuscitators deliver a FIO_2 of about 0.30 to 0.50.

In an emergency situation, the clinician follows these steps to use a resuscitator.

1. Attach the flow meter to an oxygen source. Turn the flow rate to 10 to 15 L/min. A lower flow rate results in a lower FIO_2. A higher flow rate (i.e., flow meter completely open or in "flush" position) is more likely to guarantee a high FIO_2, but in some models, the high flow may cause the resuscitator's valve to chatter and stick in the inspiratory position.
2. Remove the bed's headboard, pull the bed away from the wall, and position yourself at the head of the bed.
3. Hyperextend the patient's neck.
4. Place the mask over the face. The top should seal over the bridge of the nose and the bottom between the lower lip and chin. Your emergency cart should be equipped with different size masks (e.g., infant, child, and small, medium, and large adult), should you need them. Also, all masks should be transparent for visualization of the mouth and possible aspiration.
5. Hook your last three fingers over the jaw, as shown in Figure 24–8. Exert pressure to keep the mask sealed tightly and the neck hyperextended. If both hands are needed to accomplish this, call for another person to compress the bag, while you maintain the airway.
6. Compress the bag slowly but forcefully two times in a row. Each compression should leave the bag at least half empty.
7. Watch for the chest to rise and fall with each breath. In case of no chest excursions, reposition the mask and hands to achieve a better seal and hyperextend the neck a little more.
8. Once ventilation is successful, compress the bag once every 5 seconds for adults (12 breaths/min) and once every 3 seconds for infants (20 breaths/min).

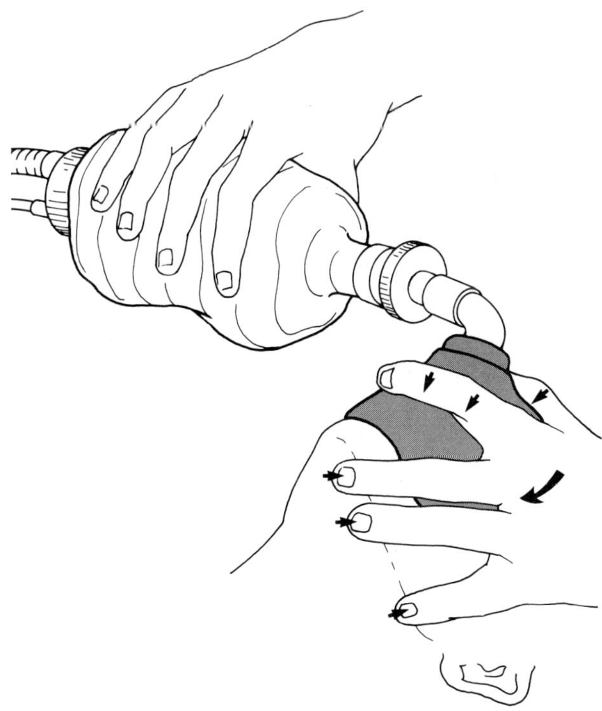

Figure 24–8. Bagging the patient using a mask and manual resuscitator. The nurse holds the mask with one hand, while manually squeezing the resuscitator bag with the other hand. The arrows show the magnitude and direction of pressure to keep the seal.

For a patient with an endotracheal or tracheal tube already in place, the procedure is about the same, except the resuscitator's elbow attachment fits directly onto the tube's 15-mm adapter (Fig. 24–9). If the patient is breathing spontaneously, the clinician carefully watches the chest and compresses the bag just as the patient starts to take a breath. Timing bag compressions to coincide with patient breaths minimizes asynchronous breathing and maximizes alveolar ventilation. If tachypnea persists, the clinician spaces bag compressions to about 12 breaths/min to avoid respiratory alkalosis.

Oral Airways

An oral airway is a rigid curved rubber or plastic tube shaped to follow the natural curvature of the tongue and soft palate (Fig. 24–10A). Inserted in the mouth, it extends past the base of the tongue, holding the tongue away from the back of the throat, maintaining airway patency to the hypopharynx (Fig. 24–10B).

Oral airways are utilized to relieve upper airway obstruction and to provide a route for gas exchange during a variety of situations as follows: cardiopulmonary resuscitation, anesthesia, postoperative care, and maintenance care of unconscious patients. The basic design of these oral airways serves many functions. The outer flange has a flat surface, so that it fits against the lips, permitting placement of the airway under a face mask during bagging or IPPB treatment. Most airways have either a central hollow passageway (e.g., Guedel airway) or two side channels along a center support (e.g., Berman's airway) for insertion of a suction catheter. Suctioning through these channels reduces tissue trauma during catheter advancement and facilitates routine mouth care measures as well as bronchial hygiene measures. Sometimes, an oral airway is positioned next to an oral endotracheal tube to prevent the patient from biting the endotracheal tube and obstructing air flow. Also, during seizures, an oral airway is inserted to prevent the patient from biting the tongue, although its presence may not prevent a powerful jaw spasm from breaking the teeth. Last, the design of the double-ended S tube or Safar airway provides a mouthpiece at one end for artificial ventilation, as shown in Figure 24–10A.

INSERTION OF AN ORAL AIRWAY

The clinician follows these steps to insert an oral airway.

1. Select an appropriate size.
   a. 00 newborn
   b. 0 infant
   c. 1 child, 1 to 3 years old
   d. 2 child, 3 to 8 years old
   e. 3 large child, small adult
   f. 4 medium adult
   g. 5, 6 large adult
2. Explain the purpose of the airway and the procedure to the conscious patient. Position him supine and remove head pillows and dentures, if possible. Apply a water-soluble lubricant to the distal end of the airway, if time permits or if a difficult insertion is anticipated.
3. Hyperextend the neck and allow the mouth to fall open. If necessary, use a crossed-finger technique with finger and thumb to push the teeth apart, as shown in Figure 24–11. If time permits, a topical anesthetic agent, e.g., Cetacaine spray (benzocaine), may be applied to the back of the throat to blunt the patient's pharyngeal (i.e., gag) reflex.
4. With one hand, hold the airway so that its tip points down into the mouth. With your other hand, use a tongue blade to press down on the tongue and at

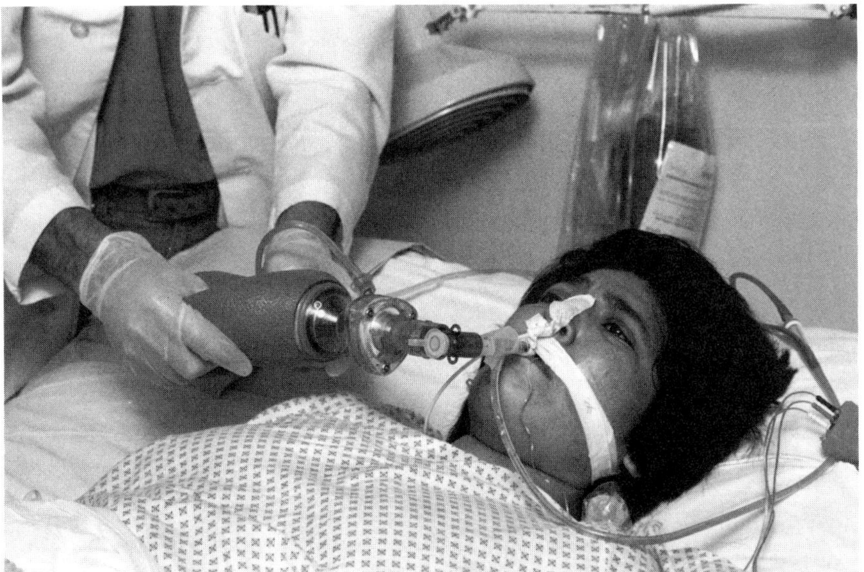

Figure 24–9. Bagging the patient using a Puritan manual resuscitator (PMR) attached to an endotracheal tube.

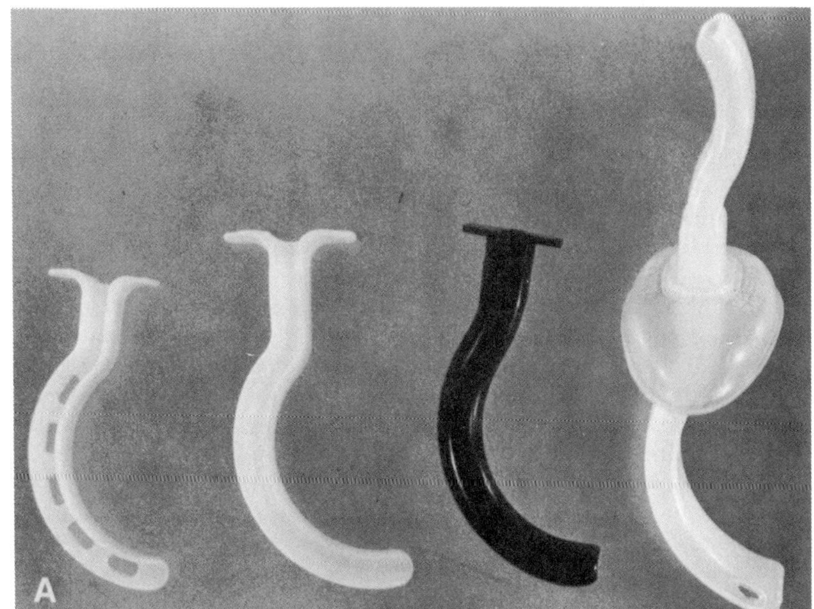

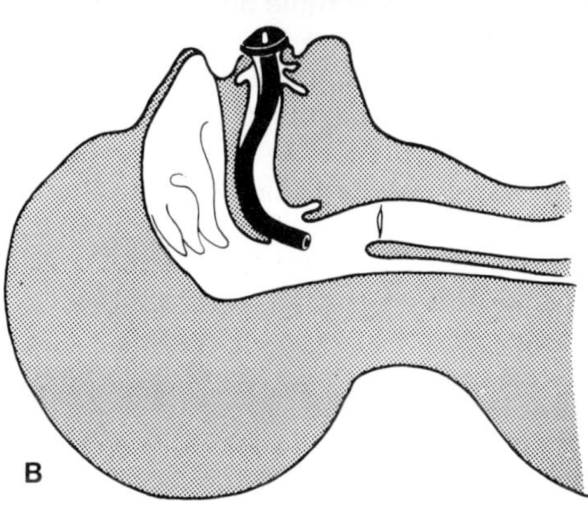

Figure 24–10. Oral airways. *A*, Types from left to right are as follows: (1) Berman with perforations, (2) plain Berman, (3) Guedel, and (4) Safar S tube. *B*, Proper placement of a Guedel oral airway for maintenance of airway patency to the hypopharynx. (Reproduced by permission from Petty, T. Intensive and Rehabilitative Respiratory Care. Philadelphia, Lea & Febiger, 1982.)

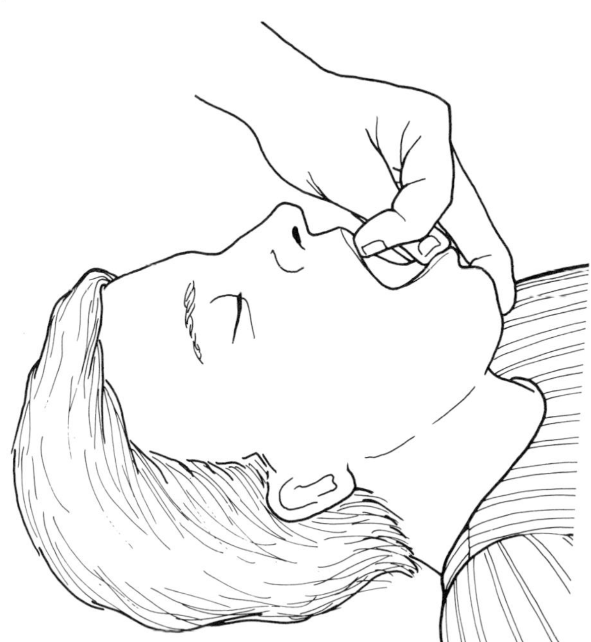

Figure 24–11. Crossed-finger technique for opening the mouth.

the same time displace it forward, away from the back of the throat (Fig. 24–12).

5. Advance the airway along a center curved pathway, until its tip reaches the base of the tongue, as shown in Figure 24–10B. *Alternate procedures* follow:
   a. Place your thumb on the tongue and grab the entire jaw. Lift the jaw upward and outward as you advance the airway with the other hand.
   b. Some clinicians prefer to begin with the airway sideways or with the end curving up toward the roof of the mouth. The airway is rotated into final position when the end reaches the back of the mouth.
6. Verify airway patency by watching chest movement and auscultating breath sounds. Tape the airway in place to prevent dislodgement, being careful not to tape over the air channels. One or two ½-in strips of adhesive tape across the flange and cheek are usually enough.
7. Withdraw the airway slightly, if the patient begins to gag during insertion. Continue airway advancement when he becomes more relaxed, and the gagging reflex disappears. *Important*: Remove the airway immediately if the patient gasps for air, breathes irregularly, continues to gag, or retches. *To remove it*, grasp it by the flange and pull it out toward the patient's feet.

Use of an oral airway is usually temporary. It is removed when the patient regains consciousness and is able to maintain a patent airway without it or when a more permanent airway is inserted for oxygenation and ventilation.

Complications of the oral airway include airway obstruction from inappropriate airway sizes, occlusion of the air channel from secretions, and displacement of the base of the tongue against the oropharynx during insertion (Eubanks and Bone, 1985). Other complications include pulmonary aspiration from gagging or inappropriate patient positioning, laceration of the mouth during insertion, pressure sores, and mouth infection from poor oral hygiene.

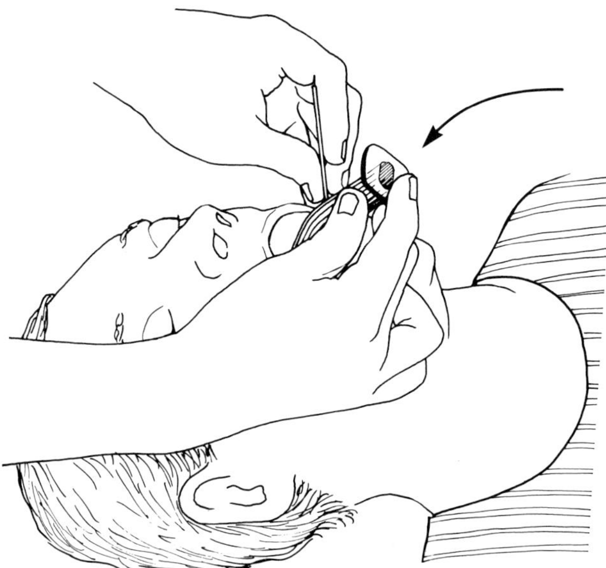

Figure 24–12. Insertion of an oral airway.

When an oral airway is in place for extended periods, it should be changed daily. Meticulous mouth care is given every 4 to 8 hours and PRN to prevent secretion encrustations, mouth infections, and occlusions of airway ports. (See Chapter 27 for mouth care procedure.) Airway repositioning may be needed q1 to 2h to prevent pressure sores and necrosis, particularly where the flange contacts the lips. Application of a cream or of petroleum or water soluble jelly to the lips may be necessary to prevent mucosal drying and cracking. The patient is kept on his side to decrease the possibility of aspiration, and the oropharynx is routinely aspirated to prevent the pooling of secretions.

Nasal Airways

INSERTION OF A NASAL AIRWAY

A *nasal* or *nasopharyngeal airway* is a soft rubber or latex tube (Fig. 24–13A). It is inserted through one of the nares and follows the posterior nasopharyngeal and oropharyngeal walls to the base of the tongue (Fig. 24–13B). Similar to the oral airway, it is used to maintain patency to the hypopharynx. Moreover, it has certain advantages over the oral airway, as described subsequently. First, it is tolerated better for longer periods of time because of its more stable position in the naris and its decreased tendency to stimulate gagging in semicomatose and awake patients. A nasal airway is used whenever a clenched jaw prevents insertion of an oral airway. This type of airway facilitates passage of a fiberoptic bronchoscope, bronchial catheters for suctioning, or bronchography. For any patient who requires repeated tracheal suctioning, the nasal airway decreases tissue trauma in three ways as follows:

1. It eliminates the likelihood of unsuccessful catheter passes to the hypopharynx.
2. Its more direct route to the epiglottis makes it easier to stimulate coughing and expectoration, without actually entering the trachea for aspiration.
3. If deep tracheal aspiration is required, the likelihood of successful catheter passes into the trachea is increased, thus averting poking and subsequent tissue trauma associated with unsuccessful passes.

INSERTION OF A NASAL AIRWAY

The clinician follows these steps to insert a nasal airway.

1. Explain the purpose and procedure to the patient.

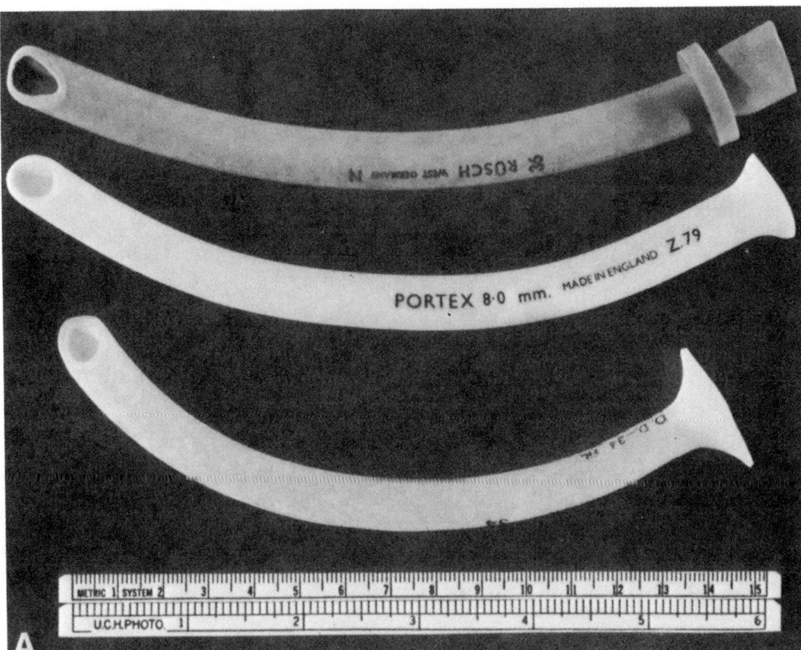

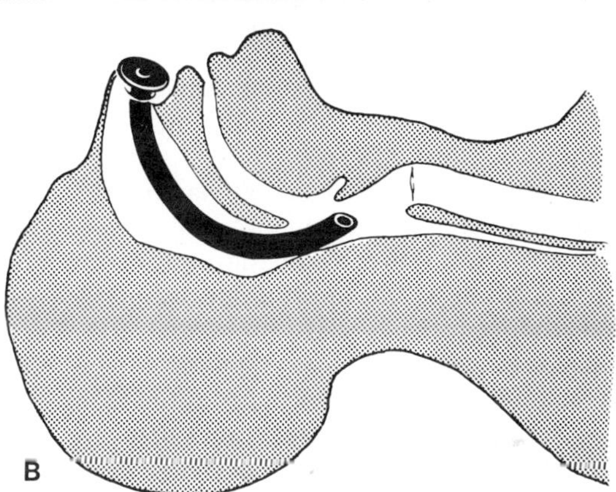

Figure 24–13. Nasal airways. *A*, A variety of different types. *B*, Proper placement of a nasal airway for maintenance of airway patency to the glottis. (Reproduced by permission from Petty, T. Intensive and Rehabilitative Respiratory Care. Philadelphia, Lea & Febiger, 1982.)

2. Select a tube of an appropriate size and length. Airway diameter sizes range from 26 to 36 French (8 to 14 mm). These sizes are available in a variety of different lengths. Some brands are shaped for the right and left nares.

To select a tube, first estimate the size of the patient's external naris opening. The external diameter of the nasal airway should be slightly smaller than this opening. Length is estimated by determining the distance between the naris and tip of the closest ear lobe. This distance plus 1 in is an appropriate length.

3. Choose a patent nasal passageway. Patency is determined by inspecting with a flashlight and feeling for air movement by one nostril, while occluding the other nostril with external finger pressure.

4. Apply a topical anesthetic. Use cotton swabs (Q-tips) to spread cream, jelly, or liquid anesthetics as far as possible into the nasal passageway. When a difficult insertion is anticipated, anesthetics with a vasoconstrictor, such as epinephrine, will help shrink the nasal mucosa and make airway insertion easier and less traumatic.

5. Lubricate the tip and sides of the airway with a water soluble jelly.

6. Gently insert the airway into the naris. Guide it medially and downward with an arcing motion of the hand. If resistance is met, rotate the tube slightly, as the tip moves along the posterior pharyngeal wall (Fig. 24–14).

7. Verify airway patency by feeling for air movement over the tube's flange, watching for chest movement, and auscultating breath sounds. For tubes with a small outer flange, tape the tube to the side of the face to prevent slippage into the nose and larynx. Some clinicians place a large safety pin across the flange's rim for this purpose.

8. Withdraw the airway, if its presence causes shortness of breath, labored breathing, or cessation of air flow through the tube. The tube may be kinked, or its small diameter may be increasing airway resistance and severely limiting airflow.

9. *To remove the nasal airway*, grab it by the flange and pull it out towards the patient's feet. Use one smooth motion, and always withdraw during expiration

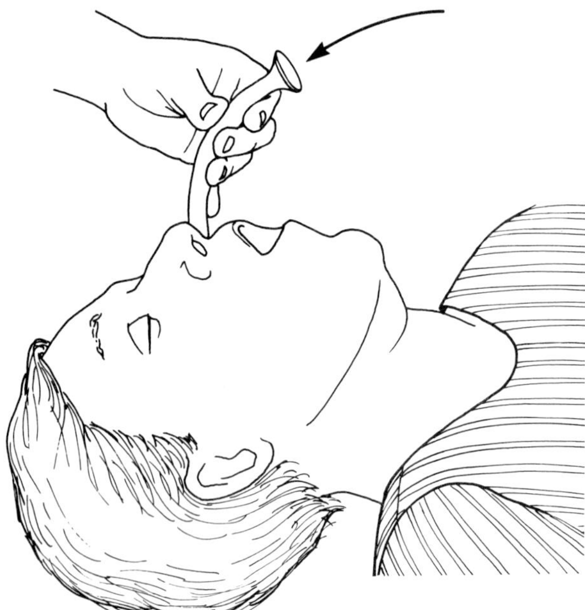

Figure 24–14. Insertion of a nasal airway.

to avoid aspiration. If the tube is stuck, do not use force but lubricate around the tube and nostril and gently rotate the tube until it is free.

Complications of the nasopharyngeal airway include epistaxis, nasal mucosal ulceration, and sinusitis or otitis with long-term use. Most traumatic injuries are prevented by utilization of the appropriate tube size and topical anesthetic, by generous lubrication of the tube before insertion, and by gentle handling during insertion. The airway is changed daily and shifted from one nostril to the other to avoid infection, pressure necrosis, and occlusion of the tip with secretions. With long-term use, humidification via face mask may be necessary to prevent the buildup of secretions along the walls of the tube and the sticking of the tube against the nasal passageway.

Suctioning Through an Oral or Nasal Airway

Immediately after insertion of an oral or nasal airway, suctioning through the airway is often necessary to clear the mouth or oropharynx of secretions and to establish airway patency.

Chapter 27, Care of the Intubated Patient, describes the basic principles and procedures for aspiration of a patient's upper airway. The information applies to suctioning through an oral or a nasal artificial airway as well, with a few adaptations.

First, a second person is advised to hold steady the flange of the airway, while the first person advances the catheter down the inner or side channel of the airway. Complete immobilization of the airway is necessary to prevent pressure on the nose, lips, and mouth, and possible pressure sores with repeated suctioning procedures. This modification reduces trauma as long as the nurse lubricates the suction catheter well to promote smooth advancement, and as long as she chooses an appropriate suction catheter. The catheter should have a standard straight tip not a beaded or curved tip. A catheter with a beaded tip, such as the Aero-flow, may not easily pass down the channel of some oral airways. Ideally, the catheter should be small enough to permit easy advancement and large enough to aspirate thick oral secretions. A size 14 French is standard for adults (see Chapter 27).

In spite of the use of an appropriate catheter, however, airway design may make suctioning through channels difficult. In these cases, the nurse may aspirate along the outside length of the airway to reach oropharyngeal secretions.

Another modification of the suctioning procedure pertains to the distance of catheter advancement. The catheter tip is advanced about 1 in beyond the tip of the airway or until the patient begins to cough. If coughing is unproductive and rhonchi are still auscultated over the chest, the catheter is advanced into the trachea for lower airway suctioning, as directed by standard protocol or a physician's order.

Last, after suctioning the inner channel of an oral airway, the nurse may carefully advance the catheter in one or both sides of the mouth to aspirate pooled secretions. After suctioning the nasal airway, the nurse may ask the patient to spit oral secretions, if present, into a tissue. In the case of the comatose patient, the mouth may be suctioned to aspirate secretions, using gentle motions and a soft, flexible catheter to minimize oral tissue trauma.

Oral care and daily airway replacements are scheduled after rather than before suctioning, a time when the mouth is clear of secretions. For patients with copious secretions, oral airways may be rinsed under tap water to help prevent secretion buildup between suctioning procedures and to promote optimal oral hygiene.

Conclusion

This chapter discusses establishing and maintaining airway patency, with emphasis on the patient who develops signs of respiratory distress or respiratory failure. When these signs develop in the acute care hospital setting, the nurse collaborates with other health team members to implement the ABCs of CPR. After patient positioning to open the airway, the patient is bagged with 100% oxygen, and an oral airway is inserted to maintain patency. Within minutes, the patient may respond to oxygenation, ventilation, and intermittent suctioning to remove obstructive secretions, and he may no longer require further aggressive intervention. If signs of respiratory distress do not disappear or if signs become worse, insertion of an endotracheal tube into the trachea for oxygenation and ventilation may be necessary. Endotracheal intubation is the topic of Chapter 25.

REFERENCES

American National Red Cross: Red Cross CPR Module—Respiratory and Circulatory Emergencies, 2nd ed. Stock No. 321113, 1980.

American Heart Association Standards and Guidelines for Cardiopulmonary Resuscitation (CPR) and Emergency Cardiac Care (ECC). *The journal of the american medical association*, 255(21):2905–2932, 1986.

American Heart Association: Textbook of Advanced Cardiac Life Support (McIntyre, K. and Lewis, A.—eds.). Dallas, Texas, American Heart Association, 1983.

Barnes, T. and Watson, M.: Oxygen delivery performance of four adult resuscitation bags. *Respiratory care*, 27(2), 139–145, 1982.

Birdsall, C. and Ruggio, J. Mouth-to-mouth resuscitation—Is there a safe, effective alternative? *American journal of nursing*, 87(8): 1019, 1987.

Brenner, B.: Comprehensive Management of Respiratory Emergencies. Rockville, Maryland, Aspen Systems Corporation, 1985.

Buschiazzo, L.: What's new in CPR? *Nursing 86*, 16(1):34–37, 1986.

Eubanks, D. and Bone, R.: Comprehensive Respiratory Care—A Learning System. St. Louis, C.V. Mosby Co., 1985.

Petty, T.: Intensive and Rehabilitative Respiratory Care. Philadelphia, Lea & Febiger, 1982.

Rosequist, C. Current standards and guidelines for cardiopulmonary resuscitation and emergency cardiac care. *Heart & lung*, 16(4):408–418, 1987.

Endotracheal Intubation

25

Main Objectives

1. Define the following terms: nasal endotracheal tube, oral endotracheal tube, Murphy style, McGill style, stylet, laryngoscope, Magill forceps, Yankauer pharyngeal suction tip, minimal leak technique for cuff inflation, minimal occluding volume for cuff inflation, lateral tracheal wall pressure, soft cuff, hard cuff, and slope pressure.
2. State four indications for endotracheal intubation.
3. Describe basic features of a modern endotracheal tube, including shaft, depth markings, radiopaque line, pilot balloon, inflating tube, and 15 mm-adaptor (i.e., universal adaptor).
4. Describe how to prepare for endotracheal intubation. In your answer
   a. Explain the importance and role of assisting other health personnel at the bedside.
   b. Name appropriate equipment for an intubation tray.
   c. Explain the use of each piece of equipment during the intubation procedure.
   d. Name an appropriate tube type and size for an average adult male.
   e. Describe how to test a tube's cuff for presence of an air leak.
5. Explain how to mathematically convert a French-sized tube to an internal diameter–sized tube.
6. Explain advantages and disadvantages of orotracheal versus nasotracheal intubation.
7. Discuss how knowledge of technique helps the nurse to assist during intubation and to monitor for complications.
8. Describe appropriate oxygenation and ventilation of the lungs before and during intubation.
9. Name eight complications of endotracheal intubation. Describe interventions to reduce the likelihood of their occurrence.
10. Describe how to check for tube misplacement into the esophagus or right main stem bronchus.

11. **Describe how to stabilize the endotracheal tube after intubation.**
12. **Discuss physiologic events in the pathogenesis of tracheal injury, the most common complication of endotracheal intubation. In your answer**
    a. **Explain in detail how four contributing factors lead to high cuff pressure, high lateral tracheal wall pressure, or mucosal edema.**
    b. **State the safe range for intracuff pressure.**
    c. **Explain how duration of intubation, traction of the tube, self extubation, and presence of a nasogastric tube contribute to tracheolaryngeal injury.**
    d. **Name three clinical circumstances that may cause permanent tracheolaryngeal damage.**
    e. **Discuss a safe length of time for endotracheal intubation in the critical care setting.**

The first part of this chapter discusses endotracheal intubation procedures and postintubation monitoring. Though this content will help the nurse anesthetist and others perform a safe and speedy intubation, it is aimed primarily at the nurse who assists the intubationist and provides nursing care immediately postintubation.

The last part of the chapter presents the pathogenesis of tracheal injury, the theoretic basis for modern airway care practices during the patient's intubation period.

Definitions and Indications

Endotracheal intubation refers to the insertion of an artificial airway called an *endotracheal tube* into the trachea. A *nasal endotracheal (nasotracheal) tube* is inserted via the nose and an *oral endotracheal (orotracheal) tube* via the mouth. Some tubes, such as the one in Figure 25–1A, may be used as either an oral or a nasal endotracheal tube. Indications for endotracheal intubation include the following (Marini, 1981):

1. Upper airway obstruction.
2. Airway protection against aspiration.
3. Clearance of secretions retained in central airways.

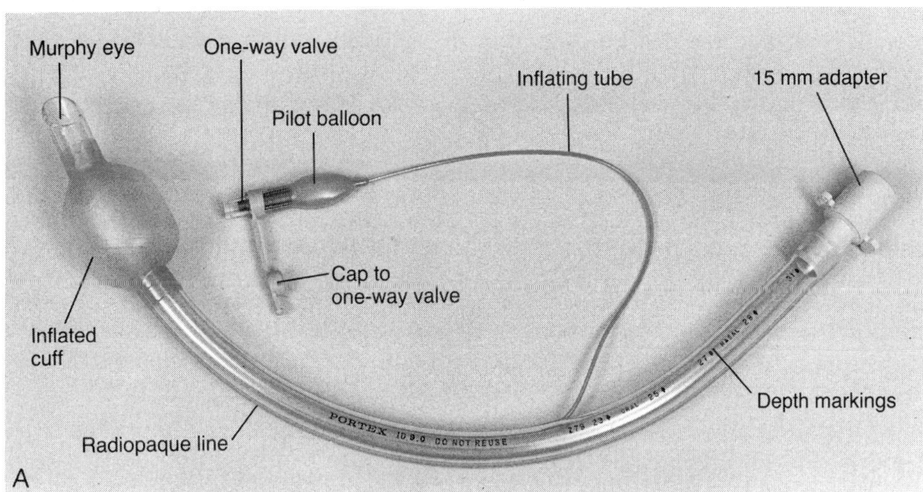

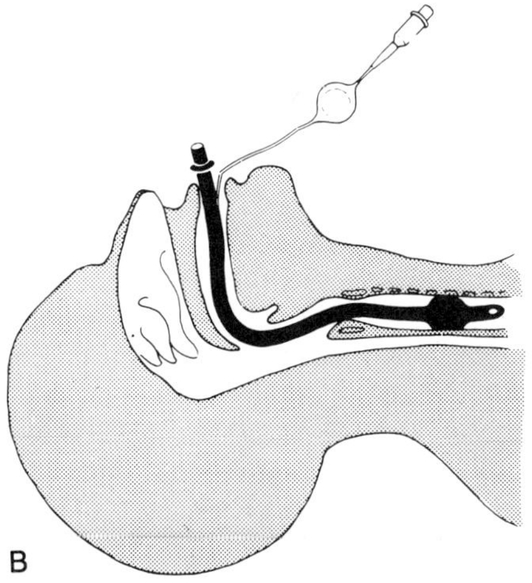

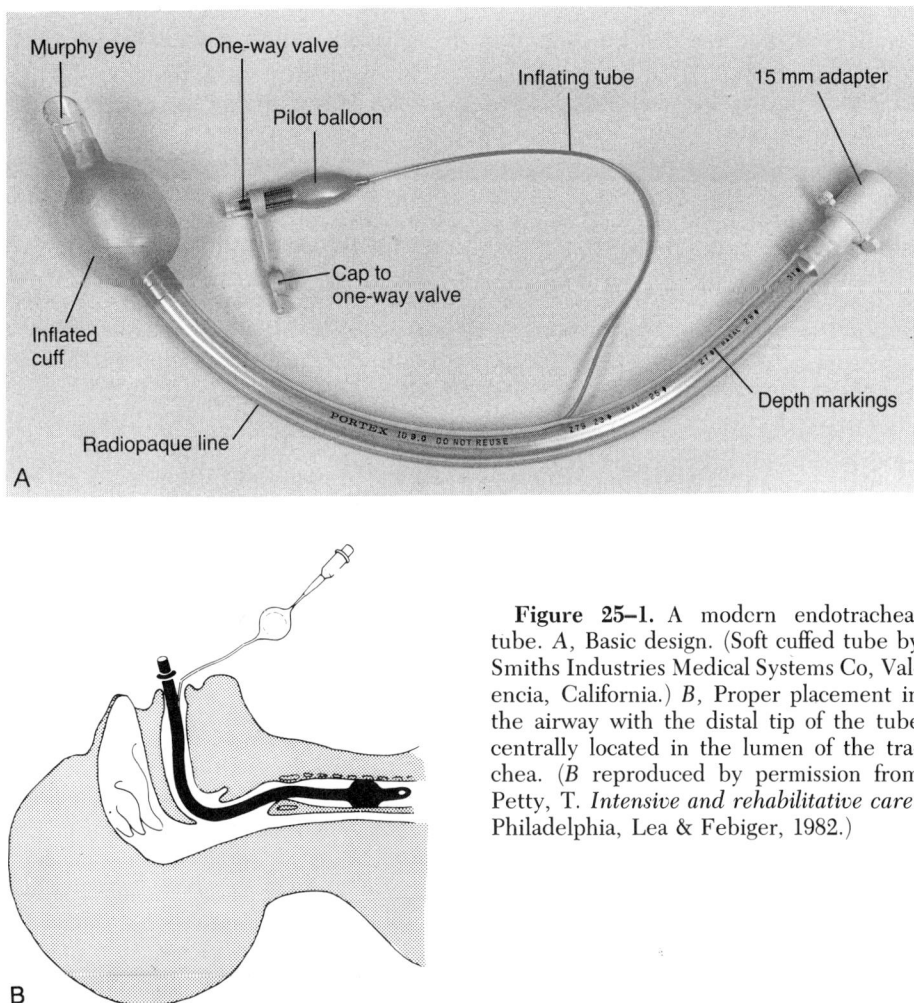

Figure 25–1. A modern endotracheal tube. *A*, Basic design. (Soft cuffed tube by Smiths Industries Medical Systems Co, Valencia, California.) *B*, Proper placement in the airway with the distal tip of the tube centrally located in the lumen of the trachea. (*B* reproduced by permission from Petty, T. *Intensive and rehabilitative care.* Philadelphia, Lea & Febiger, 1982.)

4. Need for positive pressure mechanical ventilation.

The procedure is performed as a last resort when more conservative methods of establishing an airway, normal alveolar ventilation (V_A), and oxygenation have failed or are likely to fail. In the cardiopulmonary arrest situation, bagging by mask and cardiac compressions may be interrupted 10 to 15 seconds, while the patient is intubated.

Basic Design of an Endotracheal Tube

Most modern endotracheal tubes are disposable and made of polyvinyl chloride (PCV) or silicone rubber (Fig. 25–2). Reusable red rubber tubes with latex cuffs are available, but their nonflexible, less malleable quality and relatively high pressure cuff have made them less popular compared with other tubes.

MURPHY STYLE AND McGILL STYLE

Endotracheal tubes are available in a variety of styles, but the most common are the Murphy and McGill. Both have the same features, except the *Murphy tube* has a small port on the side by the distal tip, and the *McGill tube* has no side port. The purpose of a port is to provide another channel for lung ventilation should the distal tip become occluded. In case of accidental intubation of the right main stem bronchus, air can move through the side port and into the left lung, thus avoiding atelectasis of the left lung. In spite of these potential advantages, however, many clinicians believe the Murphy tube offers no proven advantage over the McGill tube. For example, when an endotracheal tube nearly fills the trachea, inadequate space may exist between the trachea and tube for air passage through the side port of the Murphy tube. In case of right bronchial intubation, the side port may lie so close to the tip that it enters the right bronchus and remains occluded by the bronchial wall. Moreover, thick secretions may migrate through the side port to occlude the tip, particularly in a young child.

BASIC FEATURES

Basic features of endotracheal tubes are described as follows (see Fig. 25–1A). The *shaft* of the tube is curved, and the tip is beveled to facilitate insertion through the nasal passageway and past the vocal cords. *Bevel angle* varies from about 30° for nasal tubes to 45° for oral tubes. Tube *length* varies from 12 cm to 38 cm. In addition, the shaft of the tube may have *depth markings* in centimeters to help estimate and maintain tube position during insertion or respositioning in the nose or mouth. Either a *radiopaque line* extends the entire length of the tube, or a small marker lies at the distal tip to aid in its location by x-ray. The shaft is labelled with the *manufacturer's name* (e.g., Portex, Lanz, Shiley, Argyle, and Rusch), *type* (i.e., oral, nasal, or both), and *internal diameter* (ID) in millimeters. Sizes range from an ID of 2.0 mm for a newborn to 11 mm for a large adult. To convert a French size to an ID size, divide the French size by 4. For example, a 32 French tube is the same as an 8 mm ID.

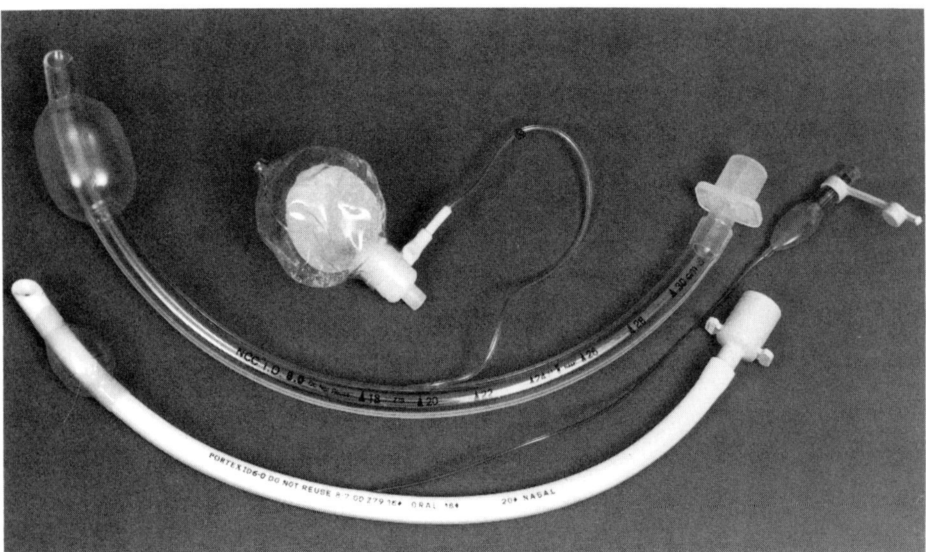

Figure 25–2. Different types of disposable endotracheal tubes. *Top,* Hi-Lo tube with Lanz cuff and pressure regulating valve. (Mallinckrodt, Inc.) (See Chapter 26.) *Bottom,* Portex tube (Smiths Industries Medical Systems Co.)

Adult endotracheal tubes have a 2.0 to 4.0 cm long *cuff* bonded to the distal end of the tube. When inflated with air, the cuff stabilizes the tube in the center of the trachea, and it seals the airway so that all air movement is through the tube; no air escapes around the cuff, past the vocal cords, and up through the nose and mouth.

Neonatal and pediatric endotracheal tubes, however, are used without a cuff. Cuffs are unnecessary because, as mentioned in Table 2–1, the narrowest portion of a child's (i.e., below 5 years of age) upper airway is at the cricoid ring rather than at the vocal cords. Also, cuffs in younger age groups lead to an increased incidence of subglottic stenosis and other complications.

For the adult endotracheal tube, air is injected into the cuff via the *one-way valve* and *inflating tube*. The point where the inflating tube joins the shaft may vary among tubes, depending on tube type. In most cases, this point is relatively close to the 15 mm adaptor in nasal tubes. It is more distal to the 15 mm adaptor in oral tubes and in tubes that may be used for either oral or nasal intubation.

A *pilot balloon* is situated next to the one-way valve. In acute situations, it may be used to quickly determine whether or not the cuff-inflating system is intact. Observation of an inflated pilot balloon suggests that air remains in the distal cuff of the endotracheal tube. Yet, the degree of cuff inflation cannot be determined without completely deflating the cuff with a syringe, as described in Chapter 26.

A standard *15-mm adaptor*, also called a *universal adaptor*, is attached proximally to connect the endotracheal tube to a mechanical ventilator, resuscitation bag, or other respiratory modality.

The Intubation Procedure

GETTING READY

The successful passage of the tube past the vocal cords on the first try largely depends on the presence of optimal patient and environmental conditions. When intubation is anticipated, as in the preoperative or slowly deteriorating patient, the patient is given nothing by mouth (NPO) at least 6 hours before the procedure to avoid aspiration of gastric contents. Similarly, feedings via nasogastric tube are held for at least 6 hours for the same reason. If the patient is conscious, the procedure is explained, and the patient is reassured that discomfort will be brief and sense of well being will become much improved once the tube is in place. In emergency situations, before intubation, metabolic acidosis is corrected, and the patient is bagged with 100% oxygen to correct hypoxia and minimize hypoxemia.

Every effort is made to provide appropriate health care personnel and properly functioning equipment. In critical situations to avoid unnecessary loss of time, intubation attempts must not last longer than 30 seconds. After 30 to 60 seconds, the attempt must be aborted, and oxygen provided to avoid further hypoxemia and cardiopulmonary arrest. Optimal environmental conditions are important because repeated probing of a sensitive larynx during a difficult intubation may result in immediate edema of the vocal cords and abrupt cessation of lung ventilation. Since a higher complication rate is anticipated in emergency intubations, bedside health care personnel must be prepared to deal with any complication that might arise.

Health Care Personnel

At least three persons are needed for endotracheal intubation: (1) a physician, nurse anesthetist, or other person trained in intubation procedure; (2) a respiratory therapist to help manage the airway, provide supplemental oxygen, and set up a ventilator or other respiratory modality for use after intubation; and (3) a nurse to give medications, help with the airway care, and attend to other patient needs.

Intubation Equipment

Equipment for endotracheal intubation is listed in the box.

EQUIPMENT FOR ENDOTRACHEAL INTUBATION

MAIN EQUIPMENT ON INTUBATION TRAY

Soft cuffed endotracheal tubes
Stylet
Topical anesthetic
Laryngoscope handle with blade attached
Magill forceps
Yankauer pharyngeal suction tip
Syringe for cuff inflation

OTHER EQUIPMENT

Portable or wall suction apparatus, ready for use
Self-inflating resuscitation bag with mask connected to 100% oxygen, 15 L min flow
Suction kit with sterile gloves, catheter, and suction cup filled with sterile saline solution
Oropharyngeal airway, tongue blade
Water soluble lubricant without anesthetic
Items for taping the tube: tincture of benzoin or protective dressing swabstick, 1-in adhesive tape, and scissors (or use an endotracheal tube holder).

Main equipment commonly provided on a special intubation tray or basket is shown in Figure 25–3. The intubation tray is stored readily available on top of each unit's or ward's emergency crash cart. Other

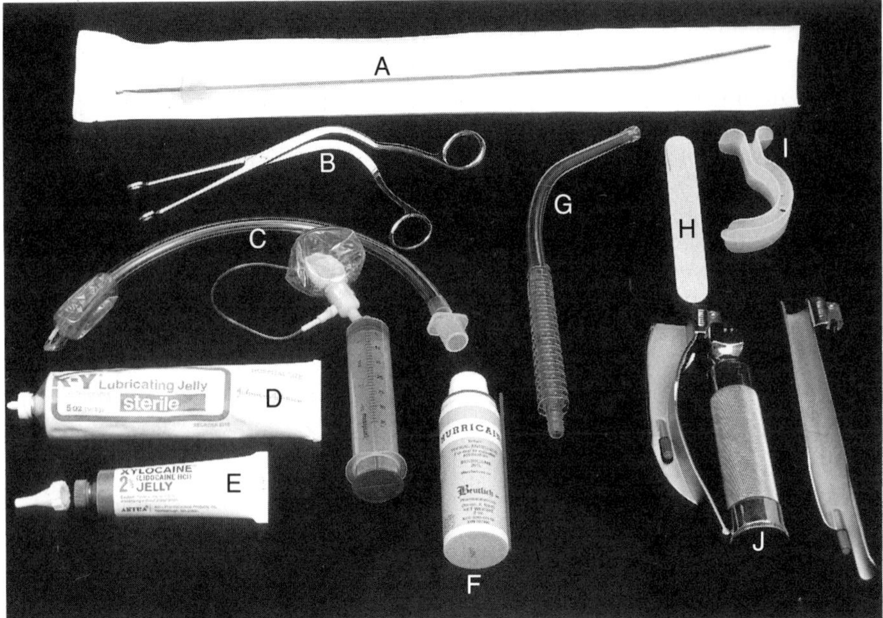

Figure 25–3. Equipment for endotracheal intubation. *A*, Stylet (disposable); *B*, Magill forceps; *C*, Soft cuffed endotracheal tube with syringe for inflation; *D*, Water soluble lubricant; *E*, Anesthetic jelly (optional); *F*, Topical anesthetic with spray stick attached to right side of cannister; *G*, Yankauer pharyngeal suction tip (disposable); *H*, Tongue blade; *I*, Oral airway; *J*, Laryngoscope handle with a curved blade (attached) and straight blade (right).

equipment is stored on the crash cart, at the bedside, or in close proximity to facilitate prompt retrieval. Items on the intubation tray are discussed next.

Soft Cuff Endotracheal Tube (Nasal and Oral). The intubationist will specify the type and size of tube desired. Table 25–1 summarizes the advantages and disadvantages of an oral versus a nasal intubation procedure. Essentially, an oral tube is always used in emergency situations because oral intubation is easier and quicker to perform than nasal intubation. As a general guide, an oral tube is used when intubation is anticipated for up to 5 to 7 days. A nasal tube is preferred when intubation is anticipated for a longer period of time, e.g., 7 to 14 days. After an oral tube

Table 25–1. ADVANTAGES AND DISADVANTAGES OF OROTRACHEAL VERSUS NASOTRACHEAL INTUBATION

	Advantages	Disadvantages
Orotracheal intubation	Easier and quicker to perform, and the patient usually requires less sedation. Avoids nasal and paranasal complications associated with nasal intubation. Permits passage of a larger diameter tube, which in turn decreases turbulent air flow, decreases airway resistance, and increases V_A. Large diameter facilitates secretion management and passage of a fiberoptic bronchoscope. Oral tube permits deeper tracheal suctioning because it usually is shorter than a nasal tube. Oral tubes tend to kink less than nasal tubes.	May not be possible in patients with limited neck mobility. Oral tube is less stable and less comfortable for the patient. More nursing supervision may be necessary to monitor the patient and prevent accidental extubation. Limits access to the mouth for oropharyngeal hygiene. Impairs ability to swallow and communicate. Patients tend to gag more. May stimulate increased salivation, which tends to loosen the tape securing the tube and contribute to pooling of secretions above the cuff.
Nasotracheal intubation	Once in place, the nasal tube causes less discomfort and anxiety than the orotracheal tube. Leaves the mouth more accessible for oropharyngeal hygiene. The patient is likely to demonstrate fewer oral complications and to gag less. Stable position of tube permits increased patient activity with less risk of accidental extubation. Permits swallowing of secretions and small amounts of liquid and communication through use of the lips. May cause less laryngeal injury and fewer posterior glottic ulcers than an oral tube (Stauffer and Silvestri, 1982). Reasons are related to the nasal tube's smaller diameter. Also, with its straighter alignment in the throat, it centers better in the glottis and, hence, exerts less pressure on the posterior glottis.	Nasotracheal intubation is more difficult to perform than orotracheal intubation. May cause nasal hemorrhage during insertion and purulent nasal discharge or sinusitis after several days. Smaller diameter tube may be necessary for passage through the nares. The nares require a smaller diameter than the larynx. Increased airway resistance and decreased V_A may result from the nasal tube's small diameter, its tendency to accumulate encrusted secretions, and its tendency to kink. Longer tube length may limit the depth and extent of tracheal suctioning of secretions. It may also contribute to increased airway resistance.

is in place for a week, it may be replaced with a nasal tube to facilitate the patient's communication, swallowing, and comfort. In this case, the nasal tube chosen should be 1 to 2 mm smaller in ID than the oral tube in place. The narrower diameter is required for passage of the nasal tube through a nares.

A variety of tube sizes should be readily available. An average sized female usually requires a 7.5 to 8.0 mm ID and an average male, 8.5 to 9.0 mm ID.

For pediatric patients, the size of the little finger may be used to estimate the size of the tube. Otherwise the following formula may be used (Penlington, 1974):

$$4.5 + \frac{\text{age in years}}{4} = \text{correct mm ID tube size}$$

For a French size tube, the formula is as follows:

$$18 + \text{age in years} = \text{correct French tube size}$$

Stylet. This flexible instrument inserts into the endotracheal tube to stiffen it and help direct the tip of the tube into the glottic opening. To avoid laryngeal trauma, the stylet tip should never extend beyond the tip of the endotracheal tube.

Topical Anesthetic. If time permits, application of a topical anesthetic, such as Hurricane or Cetacaine spray (benzocaine) or atomized 4% lidocaine, is used to eliminate the pharyngeal gag reflex and to reduce pain and discomfort. For nasal intubation, a topical anesthetic with a vasoconstrictor action, i.e., cocaine 4% or lidocaine with phenylephrine or epinephrine, is used to shrink the nasal mucosa and to reduce the incidence of bleeding. Also, oral and nasal tubes may be lubricated with a water soluble anesthetic jelly (e.g., 2% lidocaine jelly) before insertion.

Laryngoscope. A laryngoscope is introduced into the pharynx to help expose the larynx and to provide light for direct viewing of the vocal cords. It consists of two parts as follows: (1) a handle with batteries enclosed and (2) a blade with a small light bulb. The blade hooks onto a bar located on top of the handle and clicks into place at a right angle, as shown in Figure 25–3J. Before intubation, the nurse makes sure that the light bulb on the blade is tightly screwed in place and briefly locks the blade in place to check bulb and battery function.

The two types of laryngoscope blades are the *curved* (MacIntosh) and *straight* (Miller). The former is used most frequently. The latter may be preferred for better viewing of the vocal cords, particularly in obese patients with stout necks.

Sometimes, the intubationist may use a *flexible bronchoscope* or *flexible intubating laryngoscope* (Fig. 25–4) to facilitate intubation in difficult cases, e.g., elderly patients and patients with cervical arthritis, obesity, short necks, and neck trauma.

Magill Forceps. Once the tip of the endotracheal tube passes into the pharynx, the physician may use the Magill forceps to grasp the tip and guide it into the trachea.

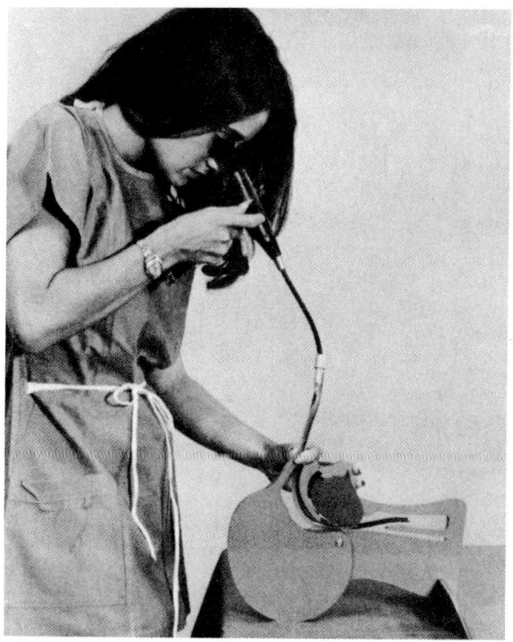

Figure 25–4. Fiberoptic laryngoscope used as an aid to intubation. The intubationist slips the endotracheal tube over the fiberoptic cable; directs the scope's tip into the trachea; and advances the endotracheal tube into the trachea, using the fiberoptic cable as a guide. (Reproduced by permission from Tomie, J. and Birch, A. Anesthesia for the Uninterested, 2nd ed. Rockville, Maryland, Aspen Publications, 1986.)

Yankauer Pharyngeal Suction Tip. This device (disposable or nondisposable) is used to aspirate secretions from the pharynx before, during, and after intubation. Most suction tips aspirate secretions and vomitus more quickly than standard suction catheters utilized for the same purpose.

Syringe for Cuff Inflation. A 30-cc (Lanz cuff) or 12-cc Luer tip syringe is used to inflate the cuff with air after the tube is in place in the trachea. Before intubation, the cuff and pilot balloon are tested for patency and uniform inflation by injection of a volume of air recommended by the manufacturer. Recommended inflation volumes vary greatly among manufacturers and sometimes among different tube sizes from the same manufacturer. If an air leak is suspected, the inflated cuff is immersed in sterile saline and observed more closely. Care is taken to keep the tube sterile during cuff testing.

Other pieces of airway and suctioning equipment used during endotracheal intubation are discussed in Chapter 24 and Chapter 27.

Intubation does not begin until all pieces of equipment are assembled. The tube cuff, laryngoscope, and suction source should already be checked for proper functioning. The tube and stylet should be well lubricated with the water-soluble anesthetic jelly. As the situation permits, the patient should understand what is going to happen and have a chance to verbalize concerns so that appropriate reassurance can be given and full cooperation elicited.

INTUBATION TECHNIQUES

Since endotracheal intubation is rarely a nursing function, most nurses do not need to become familiar with the details of intubation techniques. However, basic knowledge enables the nurse and others to assist the intubationist, anticipate the complications, and help implement suitable interventions that may save the patient's life. Intubation of an adult involves these five interventions:

1. Positioning of the patient.
2. Provision for topical anesthesia and premedication.
3. Airway maintenance.
4. Hyperoxygenation.
5. Visualization of the vocal cords and tube insertion.

Positioning

The patient is placed supine, and the headboard is removed from the bed. A head-tilt/chin-lift technique is used to open the airway. For an orotracheal intubation, a small hard pillow (e.g., folded bath blanket or towel) is placed under the head to achieve the *sniffing position.* Placement of the head above the level of the shoulders, as shown in Figure 25–5, creates a straight airway from the mouth to the glottis, thus increasing the likelihood of intubation on the first try. The head-tilt/chin-lift alone creates an indirect route to the larynx and seldom allows full exposure of the larynx.

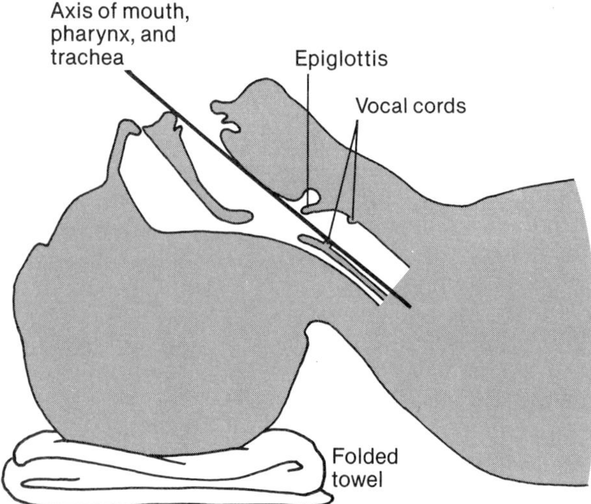

Figure 25–5. Neck hyperextension in the sniffing position aligns the axis of the mouth, pharynx, and trachea before endotracheal intubation.

Topical Anesthesia

As time permits, the nasal mucosa (nasal tube only), the posterior tongue, the pharynx, and the larynx are anesthetized topically. During application of topical anesthetic, a laryngoscope is used for visualization of the last three structures. In some cases, the vocal cords may be partially anesthetized by transcutaneous injection of 4% lidocaine into the larynx through the cricothyroid membrane.

Premedication

For elective intubations, intramuscular (IM) atropine may be given to reduce salivation, bronchial secretions, and potential, vagal-induced bradycardias during the procedure. Agitated or seriously hypoxic patients are quickly sedated with intravenous (IV) morphine sulfate or diazepam (Valium) or, if necessary, temporarily paralyzed with a rapid acting hypnotic, such as thiopental (25 to 100 mg IV), which is optional and used mostly by anesthesiologists, followed by succinylcholine (1 mg/kg), or pancuronium (0.06 to 0.10 mg/kg). Paralysis permits an *apneic intubation.* The apnea shortens time required for intubation as well as time without adequate oxygen. Also, it reduces the likelihood of laryngospasm, insertion trauma, and other hazards associated with intubating agitated, hypoxic patients.

Airway Maintenance and Hyperoxygenation

If worn by the patient, dentures are removed and airway cleared by suctioning the phyarynx, if necessary (see Chapter 27 for oropharyngeal suctioning procedure). If the patient is unconscious, the nurse checks with the family or checks the medical chart to see if the patient wears dentures. In uncertain cases, the nurse inspects the mouth with a flashlight or grips the teeth to remove possible dentures or retainers. The emergency room nurse checks the post-trauma patient for the presence of loose teeth. The intubationist may remove loose teeth beforehand to prevent them from becoming dislodged during the intubation procedure, causing pulmonary aspiration and airway obstruction.

Before intubation, critically ill patients are manually bagged with a mask and 100% oxygen, employing gentle and frequent insufflations rather than forceful and slow ones. Insufflations are gentle rather than forceful to reduce the likelihood of air entering the stomach and causing gastric distention. Also, gentle insufflation decreases airway turbulence and promotes even distribution of ventilation in the lungs. Other patients may be preoxygenated with a high oxygen concentration via a partial or nonrebreathing mask. During intubation, supplementary oxygen is provided by nasal prongs at 6 L min or by holding a tube with dry oxygen at the side of the mouth. Humidification is not used because it may obscure vision.

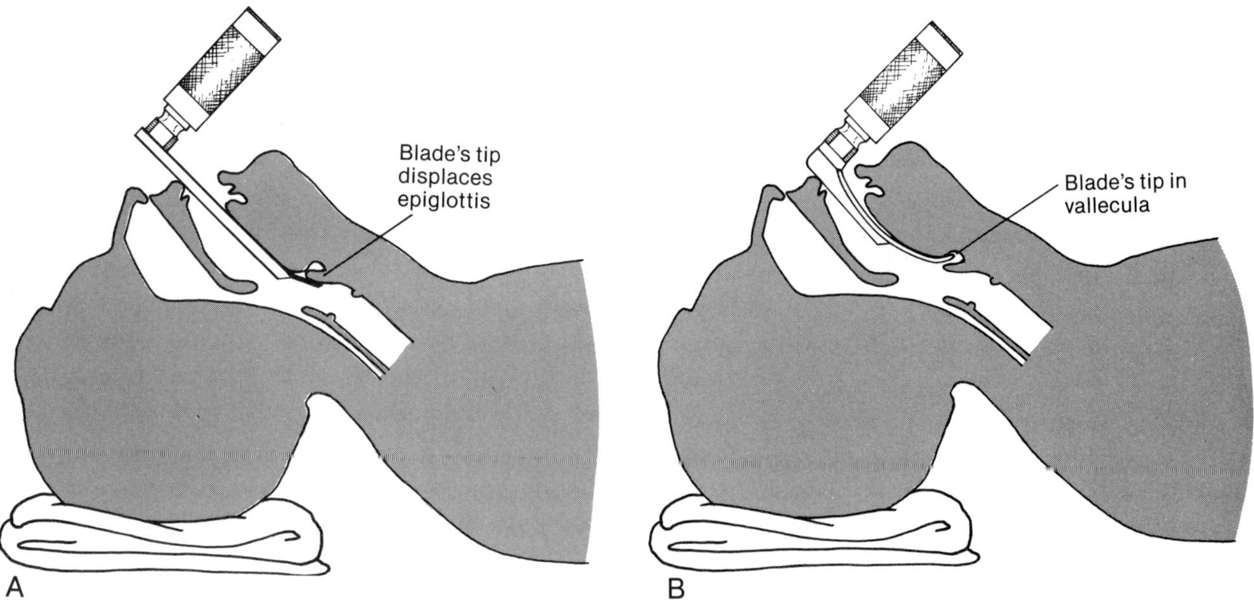

Figure 25–6. Placement of the laryngoscope blade during endotracheal intubation. *A*, The straight blade (Miller). *B*, The curved blade (MacIntosh).

Visualization of the Vocal Cords

For orotracheal intubation, the laryngoscope blade is lubricated with sterile saline, inserted on the right side of the mouth, and pulled to a midline position in the mouth. These actions push the tongue to the left, freeing the right side of the mouth for tube insertion and full visualization of the vocal cords. The straight blade's tip is passed into the hypopharynx and under the epiglottis (Fig. 25–6A). The curved blade's tip is placed into the vallecula between the base of the tongue and epiglottis (Fig. 25–6B). A steady lifting motion of the entire laryngoscope exposes the glottis and prevents the laryngoscope blade from pressing against the teeth.

Tube Insertion

The lubricated oral tube is passed along the right side of the laryngoscope blade and into the glottis during inspiration. Continual visualization of the vocal cords assures tip placement in the trachea and not the esophagus. If necessary, a stylet may be used to direct the tube tip. Gentle external pressure on the larynx may facilitate visualization of the vocal cords and at the same time seal the esophagus from air entry. The tube tip is passed 5 to 6 cm (about 2 in) beyond the vocal cords in adults, the cuff is inflated (described subsequently), and the patient is ventilated with the resuscitator bag.

The nasotracheal tube is inserted with a similar technique, except it is passed through a nostril. Once in the hypopharynx, the tube is passed blindly into the glottis during inspiration. A laryngoscope blade and Magill forceps may be used to pass the tip into the glottis under direct vision.

Other techniques may be tried for difficult intubations, including a fiberoptic bronchoscope or flexible intubation laryngoscope and the threading of an endotracheal tube over an introducer or suction catheter.

COMPLICATIONS

Complications during intubation include insertion trauma (e.g., laryngeal, nasal, pharyngeal, and dental), hypoxia and ischemia, cardiac arrhythmias, gastric aspiration, esophageal intubation, laryngospasm, bronchospasm from stimulation of airway irritant receptors, and right bronchial intubation. Attention to correct technique as described greatly reduces the incidence and severity of most of these complications.

Of all serious complications, pulmonary aspiration and cardiac arrhythmias are most likely. Pulmonary aspiration occurs in about 8 to 19% of intubations in critically ill patients (Stauffer et al, 1981). Ready availability of strong suction at the first sign of gagging helps to prevent aspiration, should the patient vomit. Also, NPO status or stomach decompression before intubation and external laryngeal pressure during intubation may help. If the stomach becomes distended during manual bagging, the tube in the pharynx may stimulate vomiting of gastric contents and aspiration of gasric contents into the lungs.

An important nursing function is the vigilant and continuous monitoring of the patient for hypoxemia and hypoxia and cardiac arrhythmias, while the intubationist concentrates on tube placement. Arrhythmias develop in 32% of oral intubations and 58% of nasal intubations and may result in cardiac arrest (MacKenzie et al, 1980).

Postintubation Monitoring and Tube Stabilization

Immediately following intubation and before taping the tube, the intubationist or nurse verifies correct tube placement during manual bagging by inspecting the chest for bilaterally symmetric chest expansion and by auscultating for equal breath sounds. In addition, the stomach is auscultated to rule out possible esophageal intubation. If breath sounds over the stomach are louder than breath sounds over the anterior chest area, the intubationist *immediately* withdraws the endotracheal tube, oxygenates the patient for several minutes, and prepares for another intubating attempt.

A STAT chest x-ray is ordered to confirm proper tube placement in the trachea and to rule out the relatively common complication of accidental right bronchial intubation. On the x-ray film, the tube tip should rest 5 cm ± 2 above the carina with the head in the neutral position (see Chapter 15). However, if a bronchoscope is used for intubation, visualization of tube position above the carina is easily accomplished during the procedure, and a postintubation chest x-ray is unnecessary.

Two health team members are required for tube stabilization in the mouth. One person holds the tube stable, while the other person tapes the tube to the patient's face or applies a tube holder. The procedure for taping the tube securely to the face is shown in the box. For an oral endotracheal tube, an oral airway may be placed next to the tube to prevent biting the tube and to facilitate pharyngeal suctioning and tube stabilization.

---

*HEAD HALTER TECHNIQUE FOR SECURING AN ENDOTRACHEAL (ET) TUBE**

EQUIPMENT

1-inch wide cloth adhesive tape
Scissors
Benzoin swabstick or protective dressing swabstick (79% isopropyl alcohol, butyl mono ester, dimethyl phthalate)
4 × 4 gauze
Q-tips (cotton applicators)

*This procedure serves only as a guide, since taping methods may vary widely among hospitals and even among clinicians in the same settings.

PROCEDURE FOR A NASAL ET TUBE

One team member holds the tube securely while the other takes the following steps:

1. If the patient is alert, instruct him not to move and to keep his head in the midline position while you tape the tube. Provide reassurance as follows:
   a. State that taping the tube takes about 5 minutes.
   b. Emphasize that the procedure will not interfere with breathing or cause pain.
2. To make a halter, cut two strips of tape, one 26 in long and the other 6 to 8 in long.
3. Lay the 26-in length flat with the adhesive side up. Place the 6-in length sticky side down in the middle of the longer strip, as shown in A on the opposite page. The sticky

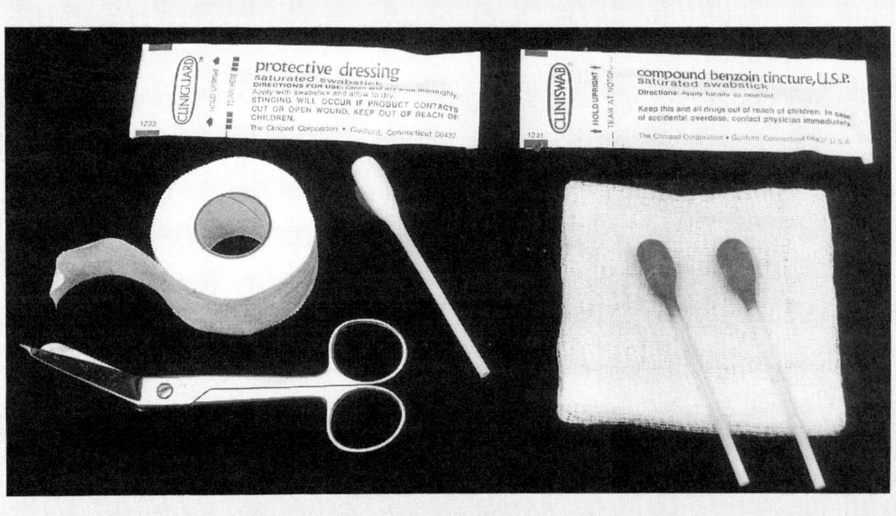

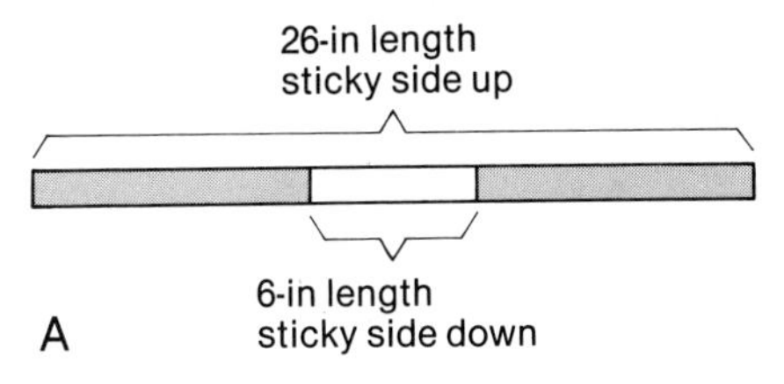

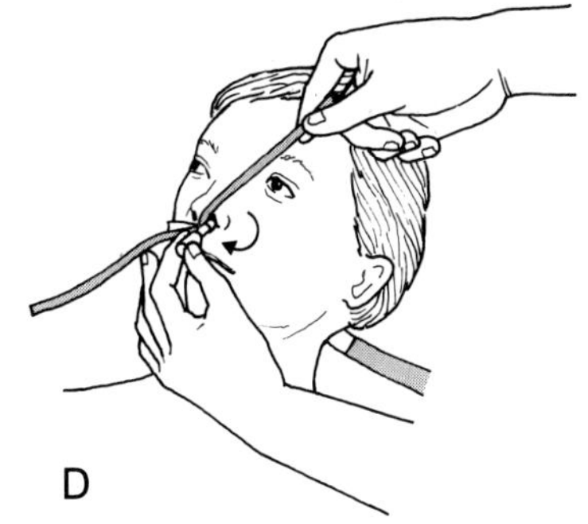

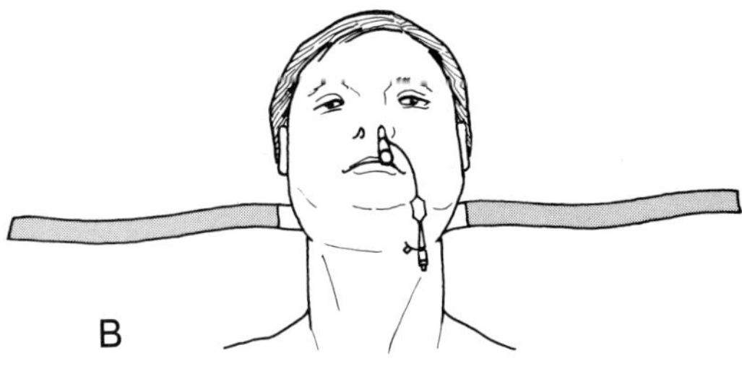

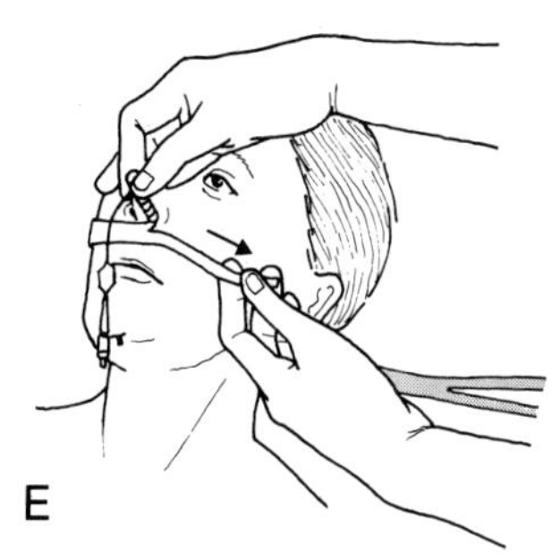

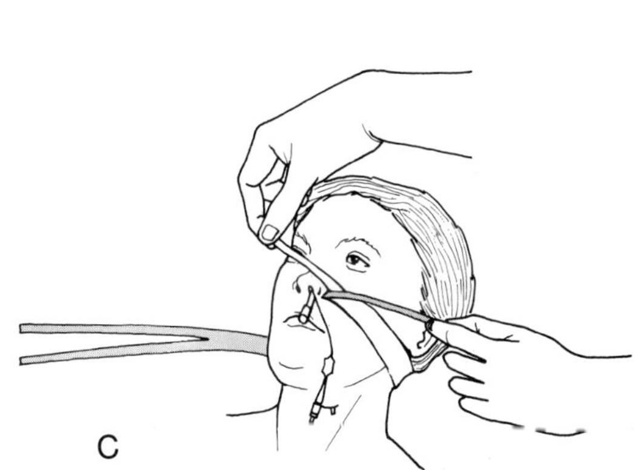

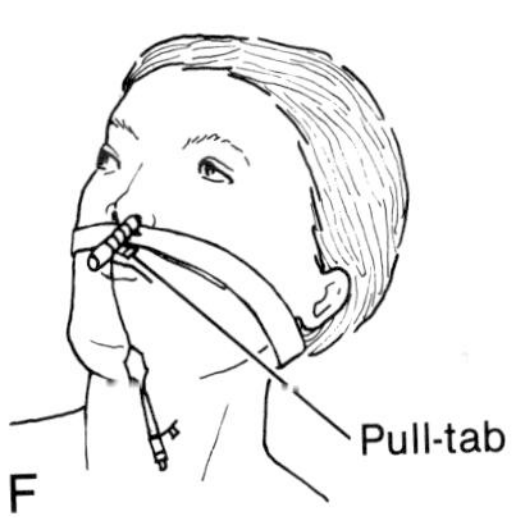

sides of the tape are apposed so that the hair bordering the patient's posterior neck area does not stick to the halter.

4. Place the halter under the patient's neck, as shown in B.
5. Split or tear each tape end lengthwise to the point where the endotracheal tube exits from the nose (C).
   a. Be careful not to tear the tape too far. The halter will not fit if the tape is torn to a point beyond the nostril.
   b. Trim excess tape with scissors, as needed.
6. Prepare the skin by applying benzoin to the face and tube where tape contact is anticipated. Properly prepared skin surfaces are vital for tape adhesion and adequate tube stabilization. Whenever possible
   a. Allow at least 1 min for the benzoin to dry before tape application. Fan the skin with a package of 4 × 4s, if necessary, to reduce drying time.
   b. For diaphoretic skin, wash with soap and water and dry before benzoin application.
7. To tape one side of the face
   a. Apply the tape across the cheek.
   b. Wrap the top split end around the tube in a clockwise fashion (D).

Apply the bottom split end below the nose and towards the opposite cheek for extra tube stabilization (E). (*Note*: Some clinicians prefer to wrap the bottom split end around the tube in a clockwise fashion.)

8. Repeat step #7 with the other end of the tape. When finished wrapping the tube, fold a 1/4-in end of tape back on itself to make a pull-tab (F). This pull-tab facilitates later tape removal.

Box continued on following page

HEAD HALTER TECHNIQUE FOR SECURING AN ENDOTRACHEAL (ET) TUBE Continued

PROCEDURE FOR ORAL ET TUBES

Follow the same steps as described but with the following modifications:

1. One person holds the tube securely at the side of the mouth, while the other person tapes the tube.
2. Reverse the taping of split ends.
   a. The *top* split end is applied beneath the nose and across the opposite cheek.
   b. The *bottom* split end is wrapped around the tube.
3. When an oral (pharyngeal) airway is in place, try to keep it free of tape. The mouth should be left accessible for care, changing of oral airway, and suctioning of secretions.

Various holders are available for stabilization of oral endotracheal tubes (Fig. 25–7). They are used routinely in many intensive care units, particularly when the patient is allergic to adhesive tape, when excessive oral secretions loosen tape by the tube and mouth, or when long-term (4 days or longer) intubation is anticipated. Some patients do not tolerate tube holders because of gagging, pressure necrosis, or inadequate tube stabilization; the head straps slip or the tube slips from the holder in some designs. However, initial research using the design in Figure 25–7 indicates that except in the case of head and neck trauma and short-term postoperative recoveries, tube stabilization with a tube holder may be more efficacious than stabilization with adhesive tape application. A tube holder may significantly decrease internal and external tube movement, decrease skin breakdown, and increase acceptance levels of the nursing staff caring for the patient (Tasota et al, 1987). Patient comfort and acceptance have not been systematically evaluated.

During postintubation monitoring, vital signs are taken q15 to 30 min, until they are stable. The patient is observed for signs of hypoxemia, nasal bleeding, tooth avulsion, and other complications precipitated or caused by the intubation as mentioned subsequently. After the patient is placed on a ventilator or other respiratory modality, an ABG sample is drawn in 10 to 20 minutes to assess oxygenation and ventilation.

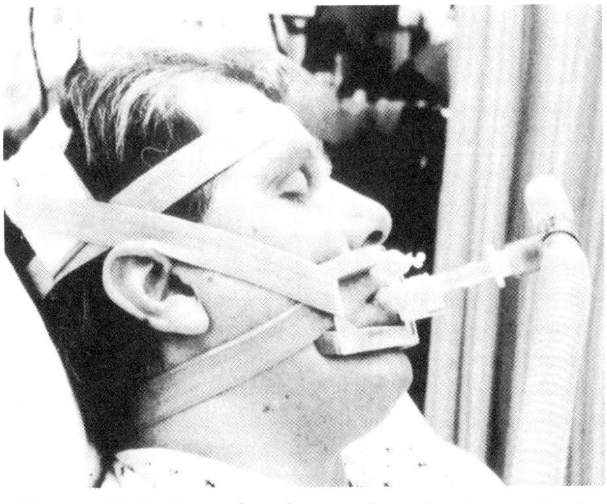

Figure 25–7. Example of an endotracheal tube holder (SecureEasy, Respironics Inc., Monroeville, Pennsylvania.) (Reproduced by permission form Tasota, F., Hoffman, L., et al. Evaluation of two methods used to stabilize oral endotracheal tubes. *Heart & lung*, 16(2):141, 1987.)

Checking for possible incorrect tube placement is a top priority, until chest x-ray results become available, and correct tube position is confirmed. Monitoring involves checking q15 to 30 min for the following signs of right bronchial intubation: *decreased chest expansion* and *decreased breath sounds over the left lung.* Frequent monitoring is especially important in the alert or agitated patient with an orotracheal tube. If the tip of the tube lies at the carina, his neck and mouth movements may advance the tube, causing periodic right bronchial intubations. Conrardy and associates (1976) report an endotracheal tube moves an average of 1.9 cm towards the carina with neck flexion, 1.9 cm away from the carina with neck extension, and 0.7 cm away with lateral head rotation. These measurements may be greater when neck movement is supplemented by mouth manipulations.

If the postintubation chest x-ray film indicates incorrect or suboptimal tube position, tape securing the tube is removed, and the tube is repositioned. Excess tubing is cut so that the 15-mm adaptor is closer to the lip or nostril. The tube is secured again with new tape or the same tube holder.

Complications and Consequences of Endotracheal Intubation

The intubation procedure is the beginning of a short-term or long-term intubation period. During this period, some consequences of intubation such as mild tracheal edema are inevitable, while other such as tracheal stenosis are usually preventable with meticulous airway care. In any case, whenever intubation is anticipated, the clinician and the patient should be aware of adverse effects that may affect the patient's clinical course in the hospital.

The consequences and complications of endotracheal intubation are explained next in relation to the pathogenesis of tracheal injury. Other complications are presented in relation to airway care in Chapter 27.

PATHOGENESIS OF TRACHEAL INJURY

The most common complication of an endotracheal tube is tacheal injury at the tube's tip or at the cuff's site. Most researchers identify excessive cuff pressure as the most frequent problem of endotracheal intubation and the best predictor of tracheolaryngeal injury (Rashkin and Davis, 1986). Although excessive cuff pressure is known to cause tracheal injury, the exact mechanism is complex, usually multifactorial, and incompletely understood.

A current theory of the pathogenesis of cuff pressure–induced tracheal injury is presented in Figure 25–8. This section of the chapter discusses the chain of events presented in this illustration and explains the main contributing factors likely to predispose the patient to laryngotracheal injury. This knowledge serves as a theoretic basis for modern airway care practices discussed in subsequent chapters.

High Cuff Pressure

A cuff is normally inflated until a barely noticeable leak is present (i.e., minimal leak technique) or until the trachea is sealed (i.e., minimal occluding volume), as described in Chapter 27. Minimal air is used to keep intracuff pressure no higher than 20 to 25 mmHg, as measured by a manometer. Too much air results in cuff overinflation and unsafe intracuff pressures over 30 mmHg. When this pressure is transmitted across the cuff and against the tracheal mucosa, the resulting high *lateral tracheal wall pressure* decreases tracheal

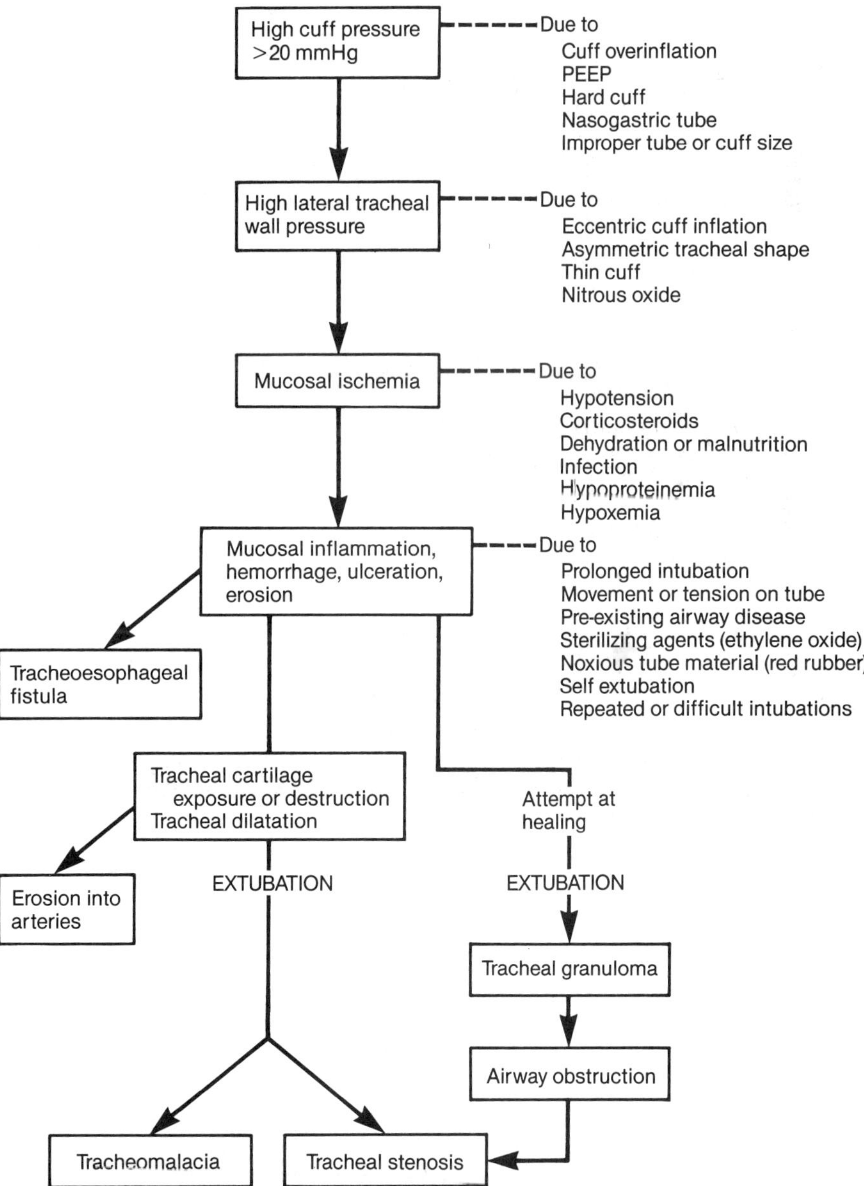

Figure 25–8. Pathogenesis of cuff pressure–induced tracheal injury.

mucosal blood flow and sets the stage for inflammation and destructive changes as summarized in Figure 25–8.

Soft Versus Hard Cuffs. A major contributing factor to high cuff pressure is the use of an endotracheal tube with a hard cuff rather than a soft cuff. Contrasting the two types facilitates understanding of why a soft cuff is optimal and why a hard cuff results in more severe laryngotracheal injury.

A *soft cuff* is a high volume, low pressure cuff (Fig. 25–9, left). Its high volume and high compliance permit the cuff to flatten itself against the tracheal wall, tucking itself into sharp corners, similar to wallpaper (Fig. 25–9, bottom left). In this way, it is able to contact a relatively large surface of the tracheal wall, without exerting much pressure on it.

A *hard cuff* is a low volume, high pressure cuff. Because of its low volume and low compliance, it starts to stretch as it flattens against the tracheal wall. Further cuff inflation dramatically increases intracuff pressure, and the cuff pushes itself into tracheal corners, distorting the cuff and the trachea, until a seal is attained. The high lateral tracheal wall pressure compresses the tracheal mucosa against the stiff tracheal rings.

A soft cuff can maintain a seal without stretching, whereas a hard cuff is likely to do so only when the trachea is perfectly circular. Only 1.8% of adult tracheas are circular, according to MacKenzie (1983). The hard cuff distorts the trachea rather than conforms to individual anatomy, as it *pushes* itself into the corners of the more commonly found C-, U-, and D-shaped tracheas.

Cuff Overinflation. A soft cuff is more likely than a hard cuff to tolerate overinflation without significant increases in cuff pressure. Its *slope pressure* (i.e., cuff-tracheal pressure after the addition of 1 cc of air to a normally inflated cuff) is less than 25 cmH_2O (19 mmHg) during passive exhalation (Emergency Care Research Institute, 1978). The addition of 1 cc or more of air to a hard cuff results in further cuff stretching and a *sharp* increase in cuff-tracheal pressure well over 25 cmH_2O. A low or at least a gradual increase in slope pressure with cuff inflation is crucial in the

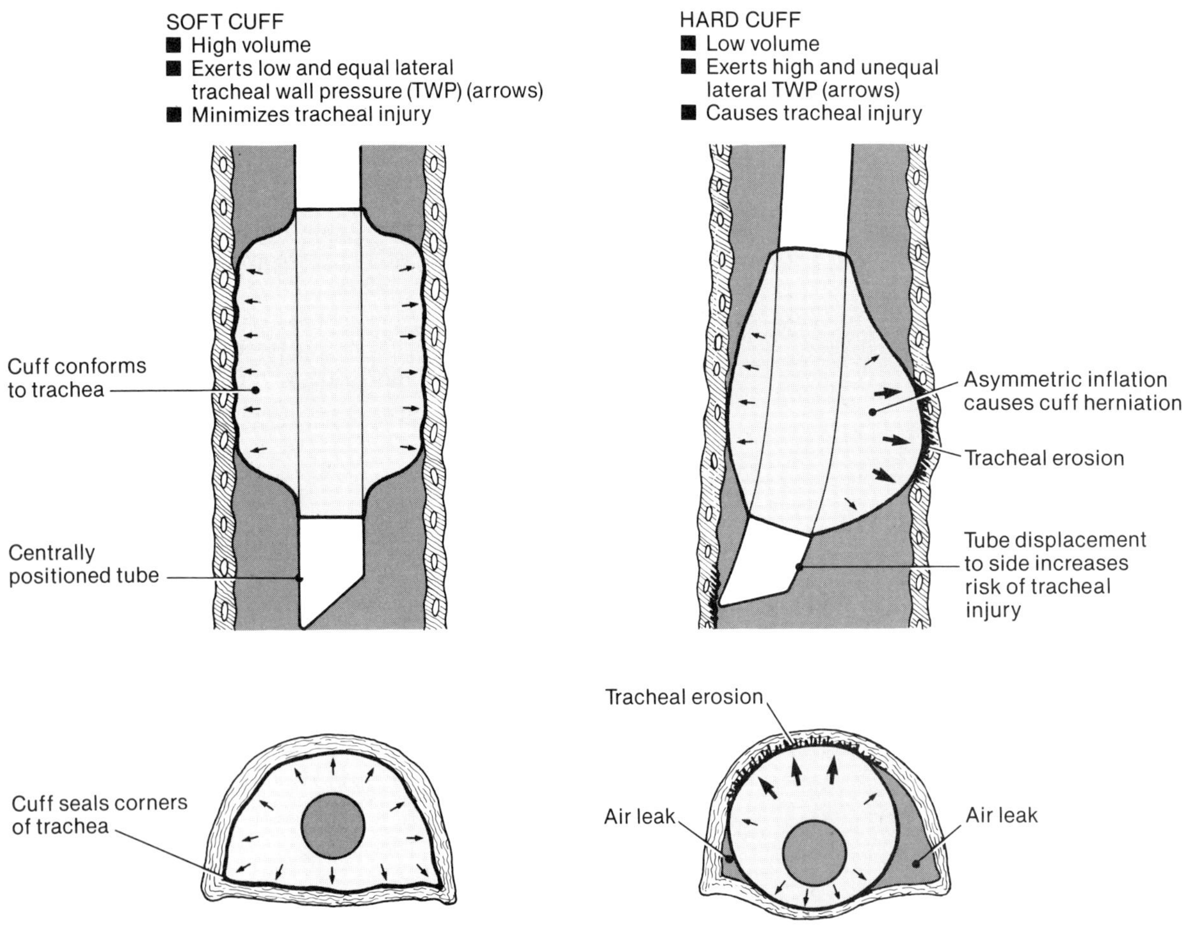

Figure 25–9. Effects of soft and hard cuff inflation on the tracheal wall.

clinical setting because in some circumstances, the addition of only 1 cc of extra air in the cuff will increase cuff pressure considerably, despite use of a soft cuffed tube (MacKenzie, 1983; Crosby and Parsons, 1974). A change of inflation volume of 2 to 3 cc may result in an intracuff pressure change of 30 to 40 mmHg (Lewis et al, 1978).

Overinflation is a major cause of high cuff pressure. It is largely avoidable with the use of soft cuffs; intracuff pressure monitoring; and special devices, such as pressure relief valves on the pilot balloons of tracheal tubes and sideport airway connectors (see Chapter 26). These special devices are particularly useful for reducing cuff overinflation for patients on mechanical ventilation with high levels of positive end expiratory pressure (PEEP). The PEEP is used to keep alveoli open and to increase oxygenation. One disadvantage of PEEP is that high cuff pressure may be necessary to maintain the extra pressure in the lungs at the end of expiration and to prevent air leakage around the cuff.

Tube and Cuff Size. *Improper tube and cuff size* also may contribute to high cuff pressure in the pathogenesis of tracheal injury. For a cuff to seal the trachea at a low intracuff pressure, its diameter must equal or exceed tracheal diameter. The average adult tracheal diameter at breath holding is 24.3 mm for males and 20.5 for females (Bernhard et al, 1982). A large diameter, floppy cuff centers the tube within the cuff, and permits the tube rather than the cuff to move with head flexion and extension. On the one hand, if the tube's ID is too large in relation to the trachea, the underinflated cuff allows eccentric rather than central positioning of the tube within the trachea. The tube's tip may erode into the tracheal mucosa, and secretions may seep along folds in the underinflated cuff and into the lungs, causing pulmonary aspiration. On the other hand, if the tube's ID is too small, cuff overinflation is required to produce a nonleaking seal.

Thick and Thin Cuffs. The *thickness of the cuff material* is also important. Thin-walled cuffs effectively seal the trachea, but they also readily transmit intracuff pressure to the tracheal wall. Although hard cuffs tend to be thick walled and may not transmit all intracuff pressure to the tracheal wall, the comparatively high pressures required for a seal far outweigh this advantage. Furthermore, some thick-walled, low pressure cuffs (e.g., foam or Silastic-aire) may predispose a patient to aspiration when large, lateral, cuff folds form with inflation (Bernhard et al, 1982).

Thin cuffs also are more vulnerable than thick walled cuffs to the inward diffusion of nitrous oxide during general anesthesia and carbon dioxide from surrounding tracheal tissues. The resulting increase in pressure may turn a soft cuff into a hard cuff, thus defeating the purpose of the soft cuff design.

Presence of a Nasogastric Tube. As explained, cuffs made by different manufacturers transmit intracuff pressure to the tracheal wall to varying degrees, depending on design. All cuffs, however, may transmit full intracuff pressure to the tracheal mucosa when a *nasogastric (NG) tube* is in place. An NG tube displaces the posterior tracheal wall and indents the cuff. The indentation destroys the elastic property of the cuff at that point, thus subjecting the mucosa to increased pressure.

MUCOSAL ISCHEMIA AND TISSUE DAMAGE

Mucosal ischemia occurs when lateral tracheal wall pressure (TWP) exceeds capillary perfusion pressure, causing obstruction of mucosal blood flow. Since the venous end of the capillary bed has a perfusing pressure of about 18 mmHg (24 cmH_2O), a pressure greater than 18 mmHg will obstruct venous blood flow. It will also obstruct lymphatic flow, since the lymphatics perfuse at only 5 mmHg (7 cmH_2O). A lateral TWP exceeding 30 mmHg (42 cmH_2O) will obstruct lymphatic, venous, and arterial flow to the tracheal mucosa (Shapiro et al, 1985). A lateral TWP sustained above 50 mmHg (67.5 cmH_2O) for 15 minutes will destroy tracheal columnar epithelium (Bernhard et al, 1985).

The extent of injury to the tracheal mucosa varies from mild mucosal ischemia and inflammation (i.e., tracheitis) occurring within 24 hours postintubation, to mucosal ulceration and eventually frank necrosis of cartilaginous tracheal rings. Tracheitis is practically unavoidable. Progression to ulceration is not uncommon and typically develops without signs and symptoms. Mucosal ulcers at the cuff site are seen in about 15% of patients after 5 days of intubation with a soft cuffed tube (Stauffer et al, 1981).

Tracheal dilatation may occur, becoming more severe as the cuff requires increasingly more air for inflation. These changes may be accompanied by the relatively common complication of laryngeal edema and ulceration where the shaft of the endotracheal tube applies constant pressure to the posterior glottis.

Factors Affecting Tissue Response. Several factors are believed to adversely affect individual tissue response to laryngotracheal injury, including *poor perfusion states, corticosteroids, dehydration, malnutrition, hypoproteinemia, infection,* and *hypoxemia.* Mucosal ischemia occurs more easily when capillary perfusion pressure is reduced by *hypotension,* as during hemodialysis, cardiopulmonary bypass, shock, polyneuritis, and sepsis (MacKenzie, 1983). Corticosteroids are believed to produce qualitatively worse tracheitis and cartilage denudation, but incomplete data exist to support the claim. The other factors mentioned limit the tissue's ability to withstand cuff compression and promote healing.

Duration of Intubation. Duration of intubation seems to be a key factor in estimating extent of injury, even though researchers are still unable to establish undisputed correlations between the two. Clearly, laryngeal damage is greater after several days of intubation than after several hours of intubation for a routine general anesthetic (Stauffer and Silvestri,

1982). Similarly, tube and cuff damage appear to be progressively worse with increasing duration of endotracheal intubation over 1 to 2 weeks.

Traction on the Tube. Traction on the endotracheal tube from unsupported ventilator circuits is conducted along the tube's shaft, placing pressure on the larynx, tracheal wall, and other less well-known sites of pressure-induced injury (Fig. 25–10). Similarly, tachypnea, Kussmaul breathing, or the delivery of large tidal volumes during continuous mechanical ventilation may result in a piston-like motion of the endotracheal tube within the tracheal lumen. The mechanical effects of friction combined with the increased pressures necessary to maintain a seal facilitate the erosion of mucosal tissue. Any kind of patient movement may aggravate these mechanical effects, especially coughing, attempts at speaking, seizure activity, turning, struggling, and breathing out of phase with the ventilator. Patients with chronic obstructive pulmonary disease (COPD) or pneumonia may experience more tube and cuff movement, when secretions are copious and coughing uncontrollable. Since movement significantly contributes to the pathogenesis of laryngotracheal injury, airway care largely focuses on reducing external sources of increased pressure on tube and cuff.

Self Extubation and Other Factors. *Self extubation* is another clinical problem that is common with an incidence of 13%, according to Stauffer and associates (1981), and contributes to injury. As the patient pulls the tube out, the inflated cuff scrapes the tracheal wall and lacerates the laryngeal mucosa as the tube passes through the glottis. Repeated intubations are usually more difficult because of preexisting edema and are more likely to produce additional complications.

Numerous other factors contribute to mucosal damage, including noxious tube material (e.g., red rubber) and resterilization of tubes with ethylene oxide gas.

Healing Versus Permanent Damage. If contributing factors are favorable and cuff pressures are at safe levels, the body attempts to heal itself by forming granulation tissue at the site of the injury. After extubation, the granulation tissue disappears or is expectorated with coughing. In some cases, however, the granulomata may be extensive enough to obstruct air flow and cause tracheal stenosis, requiring surgical resection and anastomosis.

Destructive changes become more severe in the presence of persistently high cuff pressures or multiple adverse contributing factors. The cuff or tube tip may erode the muscle of the posterior trachea and produce a tracheoesophageal (TE) fistula (see Fig. 2–11). This direct access to the stomach permits the constant aspiration of gastric contents. The cuff or tube shaft may erode into a major systemic artery, such as the innominate artery, and cause almost immediate exsanguination.

Severe tracheal ulceration may heal completely, but it sometimes leaves circumferential scarring at the cuff site or at the level of the cricoid cartilage in children, from subglottic ulceration and fibrosis. Accompanying laryngeal lesions may lead to granulomata, synechiae (i.e., webs), and strictures. If mucosal erosion extends to the tracheal cartilaginous rings, tracheomalacia may occur (see Chapter 7). The tracheal portion that loses cartilaginous support becomes dilated, fibrosed, and tends to collapse inward, once the cuff is removed. A permanent stent may be required to maintain airway patency until corrective surgery is performed.

The description of the pathogenesis of tracheal injury clearly points out the need for meticulous respiratory care aimed at reducing cuff and tube related complications. Some patients may tolerate endotracheal intubation for up to 22 days with minimal complications, but other patients experience serious complications within a relatively short period of time, even when they receive the best care possible.

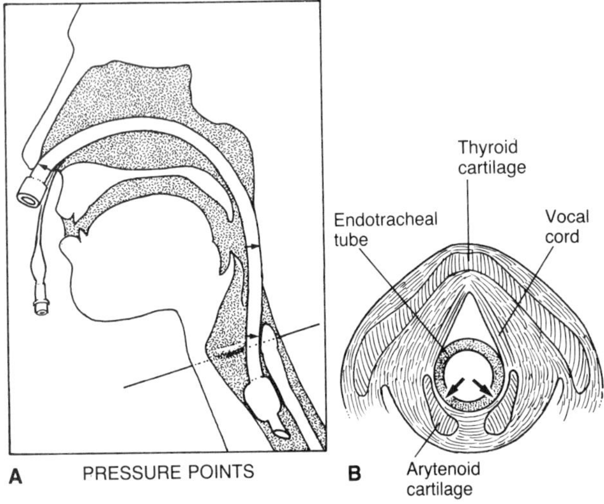

Figure 25–10. Less well-known sites of pressure-induced injury associated with nasal endotracheal tubes. *A*, Main pressure points (arrows). *B*, Cross-sectional view at the level of the larynx (line in *A*). These sites (arrows) are subject to pressure in both nasal and oral endotracheal tubes. (Reproduced by permission form Luce, J., Tyler, M., and Pierson, D. Intensive Respiratory Care. Philadelphia, W. B. Saunders Co., 1984.)

Conclusion

This chapter discusses endotracheal intubation, stressing the crucial role of the nurse in facilitating a safe and speedy intubation and monitoring for postintubation complications. The section on the pathogenesis of tracheal injury provides the rationale for modern airway care practices that serve to reduce the complications associated with intubation.

The discussion of the specifics of airway care is presented in Chapter 27. Chapter 26 introduces another form of intubation, the tracheotomy.

Both endotracheal intubation and tracheotomy procedures mark the beginning rather than the end of intensive respiratory nursing care, particularly for the chronic pulmonary disease patient who requires a long intubation period for clinical stabilization. In this case, the decisions to intubate and then to mechanically ventilate the lungs have far reaching implications for the nurse who has the burden and challenge of providing continuous physical and emotional care to the patient and family experiencing this prolonged crisis situation. Though the challenge is great at times, the nurse can meet the challenge by making decisions based on theory presented in Chapters 26, 27, and 28. Theory-based decisions make the job more efficient, effective, and personally rewarding for patient, family, and nurse.

REFERENCES

Bernhard, W., Yost, L., Turndorf, H., and Danziger, F.: Cuffed tracheal tubes—physical and behavioral characteristics. *Anesthesia and analgesia*, 61(1):36–41, 1982.

Bernhard, W., Yost, L., Joynes, D., Cothalis, S., and Turndorf, H.: Intracuff pressures in endotracheal and tracheostomy tubes—related cuff physical characteristics. *Chest*, 87(6):720–725, 1985.

Conrardy, P., Goodman, L., Lainge, F., and Singer, M.: Alteration of endotracheal tube position. *Critical care medicine*, 4(2):8–12, 1976.

Crosby, L. and Parsons, L.: Measurement of lateral wall pressures exerted by tracheostomy and endotracheal tube cuffs. *Heart and lung*, 3(5):797–803, 1974.

Dripps, R., Eckenhoff, J., and Vandam, L.: Introduction to Anesthesia—The Principles of Safe Practice, 6th ed. Philadephia, W. B. Saunders Co., 1982.

Emergency Care Research Institute: Artificial airways. *Health devices*, 7(3):67–91, 1978.

Lewis, F., Schlobohm, R., and Thomas, A.: Prevention of complications from prolonged tracheal intubation. *American journal of surgery*, 135(3):452–457, 1978.

MacKenzie, C.: Compromises in the choice of orotracheal or nasotracheal intubation and tracheostomy. *Heart and lung*, 12(5):485–492, 1983.

MacKenzie, R., Gould, A., and Bardsley, W.: Cardiac arrhythmias with endotracheal intubation. *Anesthesiology*, 53(35):102, 1980.

Marini, J.: Respiratory Medicine and Intensive Care for the House Officer. Baltimore, Williams & Wilkins, 1981.

Penlington, G.: Endotracheal tube sizes for children. *Anaesthesia*, 29(4):494, 1974.

Petty, T.: Intensive and Rehabilitative Respiratory Care. Philadelphia, Lea & Febiger, 1982.

Rashkin, M. and Davis, T.: Acute complications of endotracheal intubation—relationship to reintubation, route, urgency, and duration. *Chest*, 89(2):165–167, 1986.

Shapiro, B., Harrison, R., Kacmarek, R., and Cane, R.: Clinical Application of Respiratory Care, 3rd ed. Chicago, Year Book Medical Publishers Inc., 1985.

Stauffer, J. and Silvestri, R.: Complications of endotracheal intubation, tracheostomy, and artificial airways. *Respiratory care*, 27(4):417–434, 1982.

Stauffer, J., Olson, D., and Petty, T.: Complications of endotracheal intubation and tracheostomy. *American journal of medicine*, 70(1):65–76, 1981.

Tasota, F., Hoffman, L., Zullo, T., and Jamison, G.: Evaluation of two methods used to stabilize oral endotracheal tubes. *Heart & lung*, 16(2):140–146, 1987.

Via-Reque, E. and Rattenborg, C.: Prolonged oro- or nasotracheal intubation. *Critical care medicine*, 9(9):637–639, 1981.

Tracheotomy and Tracheostomy Tubes

26

Main Objectives

1. Define the following terms: tracheotomy, tracheostomy, stoma, cricothyroidotomy, flange, obturator, inner cannula, outer cannula, decannulation, fenestration, and Tucker valve.
2. State six indications for tracheotomy with tracheostomy intubation.
3. In brief, describe the tracheotomy operation.
4. Name six complications of tracheotomy and the four most common complications of tracheostomy.
5. Describe the basic design of a tracheostomy tube.
6. Describe the special features and uses of the following tracheostomy tubes and attachments: (a) tube with a Lanz pressure-regulating valve, (b) fenestrated tube, (c) foam cuff tube, (d) Olympic tracheostomy button, (e) Kistner button, (f) speaking tube, (g) speaking attachment (i.e., Passy-Muir Tracheostomy Speaking Valve), and (h) metal or nylon cuffless tube.
7. Explain the function and limitations of the Lanz pressure-regulating valve.
8. Explain why the fenestrated tracheostomy tube's cuff is always deflated before insertion of the decannulation cannula.
9. Explain why the foam cuff's inflating tube is never clamped or occluded in any way.
10. Describe the purpose and use of the foam cuff's sideport airway connector.
11. Describe the correct fit and placement of a tracheostomy button.
12. Using a chart, convert a Jackson-sized tracheostomy tube to an outside diameter (OD), internal diameter (ID), or a French-sized tube.

This chapter presents tracheotomy and tracheostomy tubes. Tracheotomy with tracheostomy tube insertion, similar to endotracheal intubation, is another intubation procedure that involves the nurse. It is presented here as a separate chapter for quick reference. The content on tracheostomy tubes explains special features, such as the Lanz cuff and pressure regulating valve, found in many tracheostomy and endotracheal tubes with the same basic design.

Definitions and Indications

The terms tracheostomy and tracheotomy are easily confused. However, many sources use these terms interchangeably. *Tracheotomy* correctly refers to the surgical incision into the trachea during the tracheotomy operation. *Tracheostomy* refers to the opening or *stoma* made during the operation. The *tracheostomy tube* is a short artificial airway inserted into the trachea during a tracheostomy operation (Fig. 26–1).

Tracheotomy with tracheostomy intubation is indicated when a definitive airway cannot be established by oral or nasal endotracheal intubation or when mechanical ventilation is anticipated for at least *3 weeks*. Specific indications are listed subsequently but are not rigidly followed. Each patient presents a different set of circumstances requiring careful consideration to be sure anticipated advantages of tracheostomy (e.g., swallowing, decreased airway resistance, and so forth) are likely to outweigh disadvantages or complications.

1. Prolonged need for an artificial airway, i.e., longer than 3 weeks.
2. Acute upper airway obstruction when passage of an endotracheal tube is impossible or undesirable, e.g., laryngeal or pharyngeal obstructions.
3. Chronic upper airway obstruction, including obstructive sleep apnea.
4. Postcricothyroidotomy (see Chapter 7), to establish a more definitive airway.
5. Intolerance to an endotracheal tube.
6. Retention of bronchopulmonary secretions.
7. Predisposition to pulmonary aspiration, e.g., glottic incompetence.
8. Prophylaxis in anticipation of acute airway management problems, e.g., burns, radical neck surgery, various neurosurgical operations, ventilator management of severe flail chest, and radiation to the larynx.
9. Laryngectomy.
10. Congenital anomalies of the face and neck or severe facial and neck trauma that makes endotracheal intubation impossible.

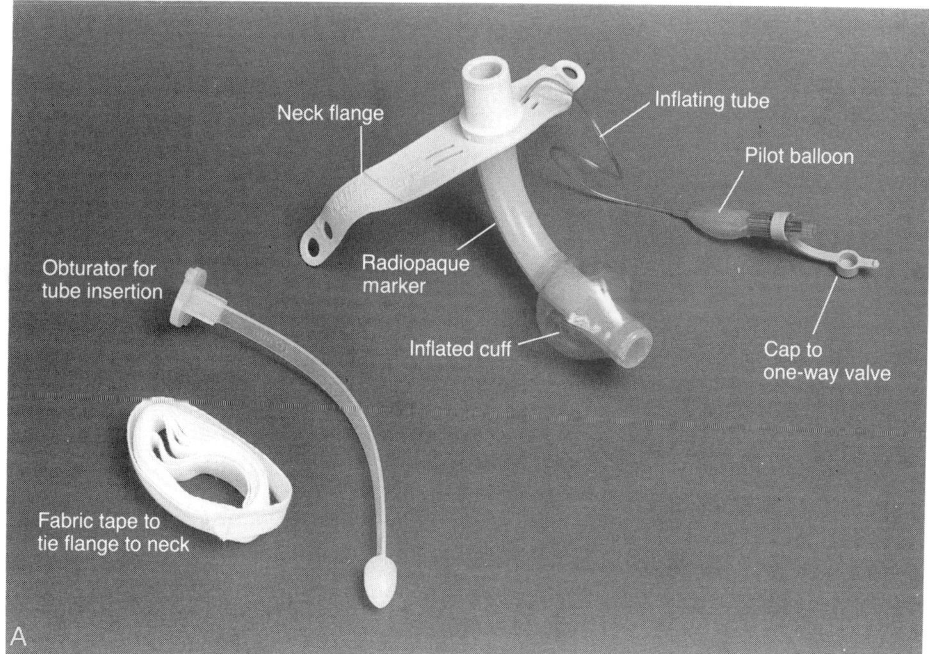

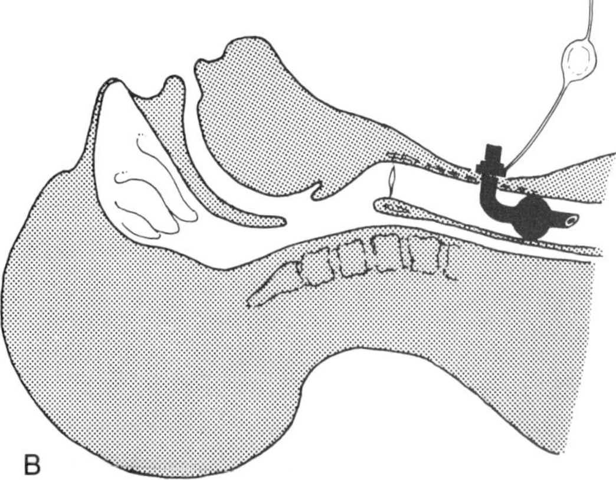

Figure 26–1. The tracheostomy tube. *A*, Basic design (Portex blue line tube from Smiths Industries Medical Systems Co., Valencia, California). *B*, Position in the airway. *B* reproduced by permission from Petty, T. *Intensive and rehabilitative care.* Philadelphia: Lea & Febiger, 1982.

Tracheotomy Procedure

Tracheotomy is considered an emergency procedure best performed in the operating room, where experienced surgeons can work under optimal conditions of controlled asepsis, good lighting, and readily available equipment. Since complications are frequently more severe than those in endotracheal intubation, bedside tracheotomy is performed only on patients too critically ill to be moved.

In brief, the operation is performed utilizing local anesthesia in the intensive care unit or general anesthesia in the operating room, with the neck extended, and the endotracheal tube in place. It involves two incisions. First, a transverse skin incision is made at or slightly below the cricoid cartilage. Second, after the trachea is exposed, a vertical incision is made through the second and third or third and fourth tracheal cartilaginous rings (Fig. 26–2). In other cases, a surgeon may make a horizontal, T-shaped or U-shaped tracheal incision for tube insertion. When a U-shaped incision is made, the window or cartilaginous flap, called a Björk flap, is reflected downward and outward, with the upper border sutured to subcutaneous tissues of the neck. The bridge of tracheal tissue facilitates future tube replacements and avoids creation of a false channel in the case of tube displacement, a major complication of tracheotomy during the first 5 days after surgery. Though critics of this technique claim that tracheal flaps are associated with a higher incidence of severe tracheal stenosis after tube removal, current evidence does not support this claim (Heffner et al, 1986).

The surgeon may omit the tracheal flap but suture the tube's flange (described subsequently) to the skin for extra tube stability. This practice is discouraged by some clinicians because the tight pressure of the tube against the incision may increase the risk of subcutaneous emphysema and infection. Also, it makes cleaning around the stoma more difficult.

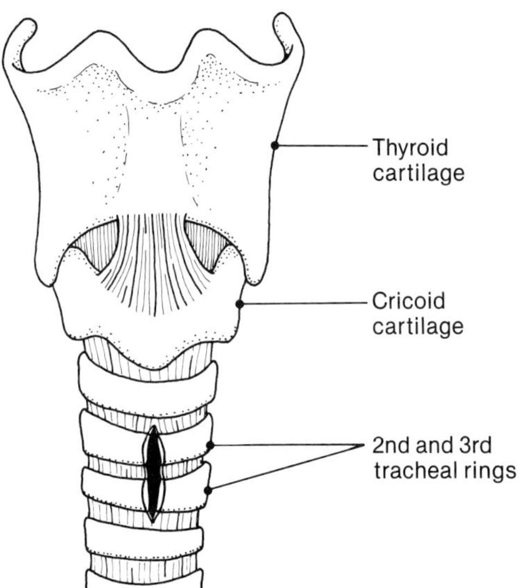

Figure 26–2. Vertical tracheal incision during a tracheotomy procedure.

In a previously intubated patient, the tracheostomy tube is inserted as the endotracheal tube is removed. The tube's cuff is inflated, and the patient is ventilated and oxygenated through the tube. A postoperative chest x-ray film is taken to monitor tube position and detect complications.

Complications

Complications of tracheotomy include hemorrhage, subcutaneous or mediastinal emphysema, pneumothorax, and injury to the thyroid gland, recurrent laryngeal nerve, and other vital structures near the stoma. Cardiac arrest may occur from hemorrhage or from displacement of the tube tip into tracheal tissues. Placement of the stoma too low, i.e., below the second or third cartilaginous ring, increases the chance for erosion of the tube's tip into the tracheal innominate artery.

Cuff- and tube-related complications while the tracheostomy is in place are similar to those described for an endotracheal tube, except laryngeal complications tend to be fewer, since the larynx is bypassed. Also, the stoma introduces other clinical problems, such as mild stomal bleeding, which occurs in the majority of cases. The four most common complications of tracheostomy are *stomal infection*, defined as cellulitus or an unusual degree of purulent exudate at the stomal site (36% of all tracheostomies); *stomal hemorrhage* (36%); *excessive cuff pressure* (23%); and *subcutaneous emphysema* (9%) (Stauffer et al, 1981).

Of these four tracheostomy complications, stomal infection is perhaps the most significant for the nurse to be aware of because of its high incidence and because of its relationship to late complications, such as pulmonary infection and tracheal stenosis at the stoma site (see Chapter 25). Sixty to 100% of patients with long-term tracheostomies experience colonization of tracheobronchial tree with *Pseudomonas* or enteric gram-negative bacillary infections (Heffner et al, 1986). Stomal infection may be associated with this colonization process; inadequate tracheostomy care; and other factors, such as poor nutritional status, that predispose the patient to infection.

Postintubation Monitoring

During the immediate postintubation period, swallowing ability is diminished because of functional glottic incompetence. The head of the bed is elevated at least to 30 degrees. The cuff is kept inflated continuously to prevent aspiration, and the patient is given

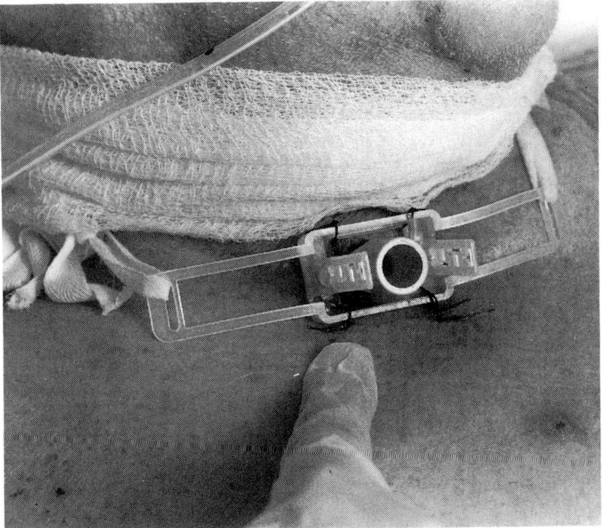

Figure 26–3. Checking the stoma and surrounding skin for signs of inflammation and infection.

nothing by mouth (NPO) for a few days until swallowing ability returns. If, after a few days, dysphagia is suspected, the patient may be asked to swallow a dilute solution of methylene blue prior to a meal to check glottic functioning. If the dye does not appear in tracheal secretions, aspiration is unlikely, and the meal may be given. Blue-tinged secretions indicate aspiration. The patient is fed via a small, pediatric, nasogastric tube until swallowing ability returns. Eventually, when oral feedings begin, many patients find they can swallow semisolid foods, such as Jello, much better than liquids

The stoma is checked q2 to 4h initially, and later it is checked with the routine vital signs for signs of bleeding. A small amount of bleeding over 3 to 4 days is normal. However, a constant ooze may result in significant blood loss and require surgical intervention to ligate a blood vessel. Also, the stoma and neck are checked for signs of subcutaneous emphysema, and the chest is examined for signs of pneumothorax. The tube is palpated for pulsations, suggesting impending erosion of the tube into a major blood vessel. The stoma and surrounding skin are monitored for inflammation and signs of infection, including the oozing of purulent secretions from around the stoma (Fig. 26–3).

Tracheostomy Tubes

The type of tracheostomy tube inserted during intubation largely determines the specifics of respiratory nursing care. To prepare the nurse for care of the patient with a tracheostomy the remainder of this chapter presents the basic and special designs of tracheostomy tubes in the clinical setting.

BASIC DESIGN

A tracheostomy tube is similar to an endotracheal tube, except it is shorter (2 to 6 in long). The adult sized tube does not always have a cuff, and for long-term use it may be made of metal or nylon. As with endotracheal tubes, most tracheostomy tubes are disposable, except for metal tracheostomy tubes and some nylon tracheostomy tubes.

Size may vary among manufacturers—it may be in terms of internal diameter (ID), outside diameter (OD), or a number between the two, called a *Jackson size*. For example, a tube with an ID of 9.0 mm and OD of 13 mm may be listed as a Jackson size 9 tracheostomy tube. As a general guide, the OD of an adult tube is 3 to 4 mm more than its ID. Since many manufacturers carry a limited range of sizes, the clinician must check availability before ordering a specific sized tube.

Unlike the beveled endotracheal tube, the distal tip of a tracheostomy tube ends abruptly, as shown in Figure 26–1A. This design maximizes air flow and prevents occlusion of the tip against the tracheal wall.

Proximally, a neck *flange* stabilizes the tube in the trachea and provides small holes for tying fabric tape to secure the tube to the neck. In other cases, an adjustable tube holder rather than fabric tape is used to secure the tube to the neck (Fig. 26–4).

Each tube comes with an *obturator*. When it is inserted into the tube, its rounded tip extends beyond the tube's tip to facilitate insertion and prevent the tube's tip from scraping against the tracheal wall. After intubation, the obturator is placed in a plastic bag and kept at the bedside for emergency use.

Some tracheostomy tubes consist of an *inner cannula* as well as an *outer cannula* (i.e., main shaft). After the

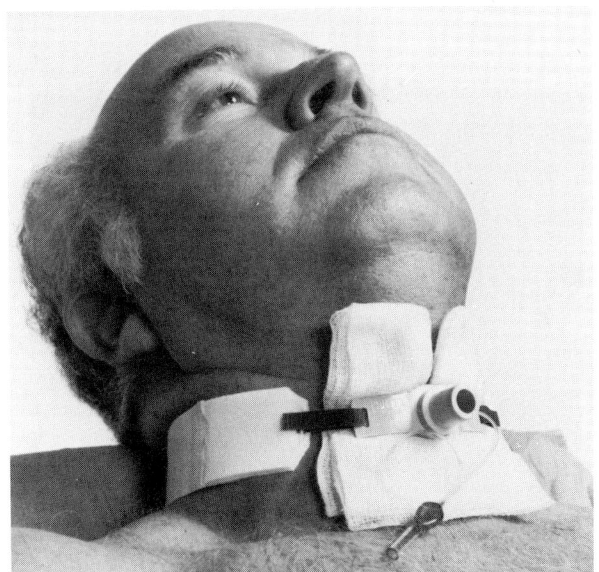

Figure 26–4. Dale tracheostomy tube holder. (Courtesy of Dale Medical Products, Plainville, Massachusetts.)

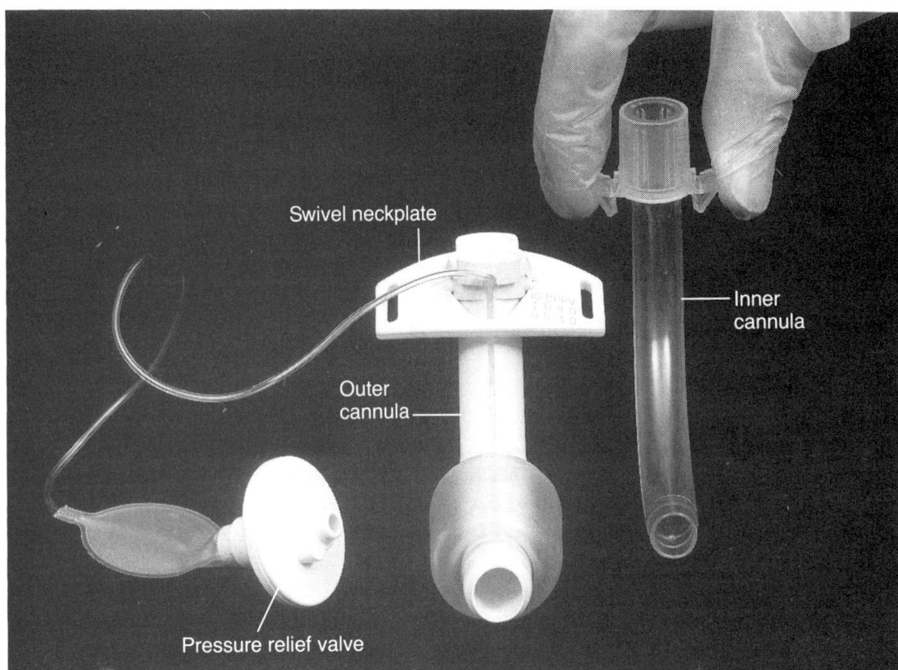

Figure 26–5. Shiley tracheostomy tube with disposable inner cannula and pressure relief valve. Pressure on the sides of the 15-mm, snap-lock connector permits removal and reinsertion of the inner cannula.

obturator is withdrawn, the inner cannula is inserted into the outer cannula. The main advantage of the inner cannula is that it is removable. For tubes with a *nondisposable* inner cannula, this feature permits periodic cleaning and prevents airway obstruction from accumulated secretions along the tube's inner surfaces.

Some tubes, such as the Shiley disposable cannula tracheostomy tube, have a disposable inner cannula to facilitate cleaning (Figs. 26–5 and 26–6). Research is in progress to determine whether tracheostomy care with a disposable cannula is more cost effective than care with a nondisposable cannula that requires the standard cleaning procedure described in Chapter 27.

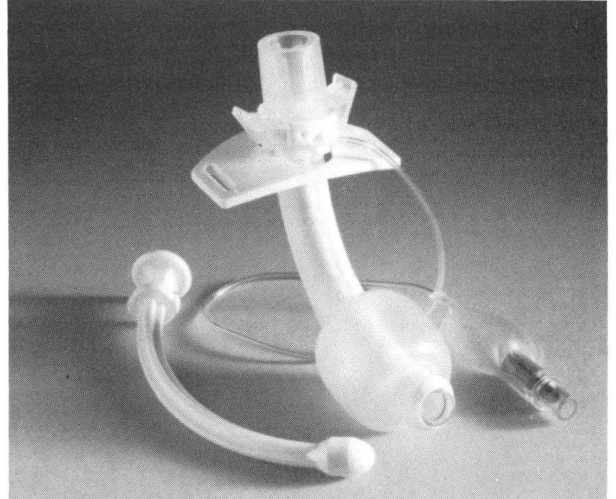

Figure 26–6. Shiley disposable cannula tracheostomy tube with the inner cannula inserted into the outer cannula. (Courtesy of Shiley Inc., Irvine, California.)

SPECIAL DESIGNS

At least ten different types of tracheostomy tubes are available, each with a minor or major alteration in the basic design described. Generally, the cuffed tubes are designed for acute care use (e.g., Lanz, Portex, Shiley, and National); uncuffed tubes are designed for long-term use in patients who have competent glottic functioning (e.g., Dow Corning Silastic, Jackson metal tube, and Martin laryngectomy tube). Some of the tubes have special features designed to facilitate weaning from mechanical ventilation and tube removal (i.e., *decannulation*). Distinguishing features of common tubes are discussed next. Some of these features are also found in endotracheal tubes (e.g., Lanz and foam-cuffed tubes).

Tubes with a Lanz Pressure-Regulating Valve

Tubes with a Lanz pressure-regulating valve are commonly used in acute care settings. The Hi-Lo tracheostomy tube has a high volume, low pressure cuff and a relatively large external pilot balloon encased by a soft clear plastic covering for protection (Fig. 26–7). The cuff usually requires 20 to 30 cc of air for inflation at safe pressures. The flange may be adjusted

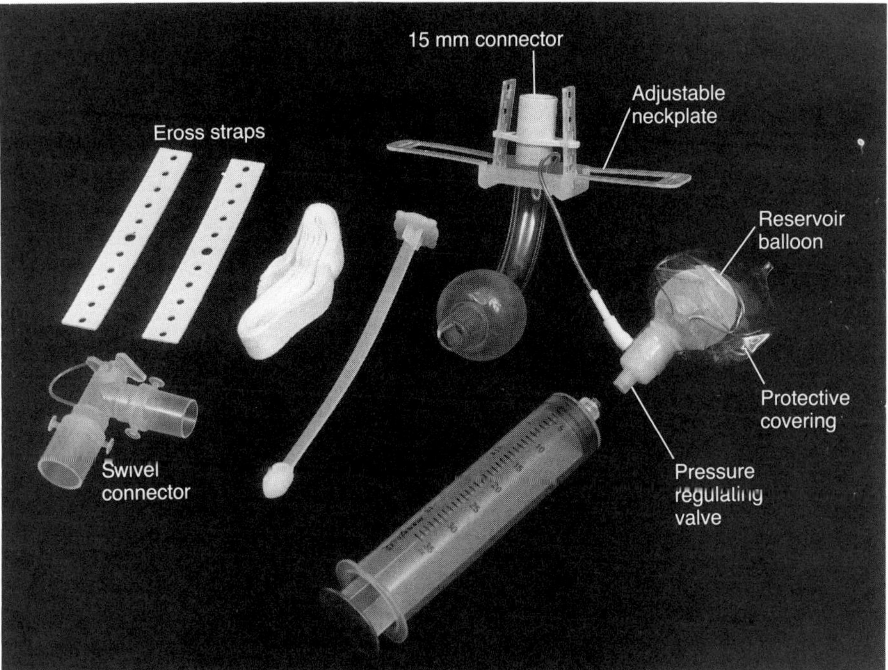

Figure 26–7. Tracheostomy tube with Lanz pressure-regulating valve. (Hi-Lo tube by Mallinckrodt, Inc., Argyle, New York.) An eross strap is used occasionally to secure the swivel connector to the tracheostomy tube's 15-mm connector.

so that its fit against the neck is neither too tight nor too loose. A plastic wedge on both sides of the tube's opening guards against unnecessary tube movement and pressure against the stoma and tracheal wall.

A unique feature of a tube, such as the one in Figure 26–7, is its *pressure-regulating valve* located where the syringe attaches to the pilot balloon. This valve is advertised to maintain a pressure of 20 to 25 mmHg on the tracheal wall during expiration. Although this tube is supposed to prevent cuff overinflation and excess pressure against the tracheal wall, it can do so only when the valve is fully open to allow free communication between the cuff and pilot balloon. Attaching a syringe or stopcock to the pilot balloon opens the valve. Removal of the syringe allows only *one-way* flow from the pilot balloon into the cuff. Hence, a cuff can increase its pressure, but it cannot decrease it. For this reason, external balloons are not manually squeezed to push air into the cuff and eliminate an air leak between the cuff and tracheal wall.

Burns and coworkers (1983) relate three other points to keep in mind about tubes with a Lanz pressure-regulating valve. First, the pilot balloon may not give any indication of increased pressure. Increased pressure is detectable only when the balloon appears obviously overdistended and constrained by the clear plastic protector. Second, because attachment of a manometer immediately decreases pressure, a reading may not reflect high cuff pressure existing before attachment. Most important, a controlled pressure cuff system does not replace the need for frequent monitoring of cuff pressures by standard methods (see Chapter 27).

Fenestrated Tubes

A fenestrated tube has a precut opening *(fenestration)* in the outer cannula. This type of tube is used for weaning patients from mechanical ventilation or for long-term airway management and is available in a variety of cuffed and cuffless designs.

The plastic Shiley fenestrated low pressure cuffed tracheostomy tube has four parts as follows: (1) an *outer cannula*, (2) *inner cannula*, (3) *decannulation cannula* (closed lumen), and (4) *obturator*. The outer cannula has a fenestration above the cuff, as shown in Figure 26–8. The pilot balloon has a one-way valve, and the cuff usually inflates with 3 to 9 cc of air. The flange is a swivel neckplate that conforms to individual neck anatomy, thus reducing unnecessary traction on the tube and facilitating stomal cleaning under the neckplate.

When the inner cannula is inserted into the outer cannula, it obstructs the fenestration. Then, provided the cuff is inflated, the clinician may connect the patient to another device for intermittent positive pressure breathing (IPPB), aerosol treatment, mechanical ventilation, or pulmonary function measurements. The inner cannula will not slip out, as long as it is locked into place by twisting its end connector (i.e., 15-mm adaptor) clockwise, until the blue dots on tube and cannula are aligned.

For the spontaneously breathing patient, the inner cannula is removed, the cuff deflated, and the tube plugged with the short decanulation cannula. Since the fenestration is open, the patient breathes around the cuff as well as through the fenestration, as shown

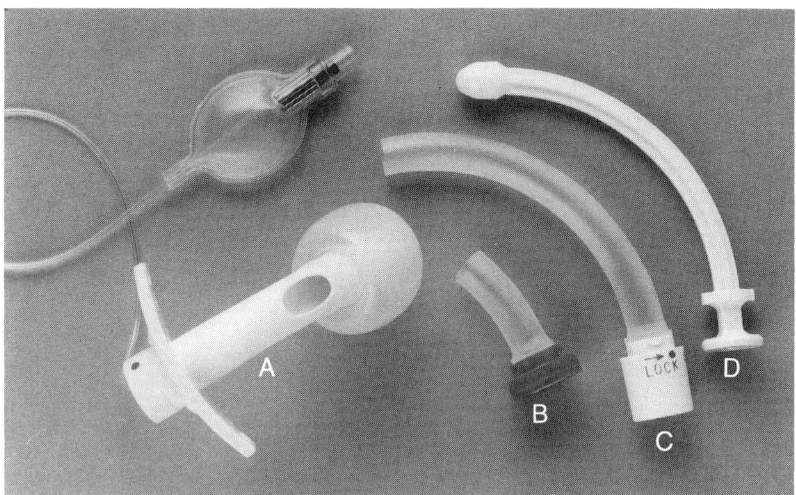

Figure 26–8. Shiley fenestrated low pressure cuffed tracheostomy tube. *A*, Outer cannula with a fenestration above the cuff; *B*, Decannulation cannula used to plug the tracheostomy tube; *C*, Inner cannula; *D*, Obturator. (Courtesy of Shiley, Inc., Irvine, California.)

in Figure 26–9. The increased air flow facilitates breathing and phonation. Unlike other weaning devices (e.g., tracheostomy button) described subsequently, the decannulation cannula is easily removed, permitting access for suctioning or mechanical ventilation.

Perhaps the most important point to remember about fenestrated tubes is that *the cuff must be down before insertion of the decannulation cannula.* The patient cannot breathe with the cuff up and the tube plugged! Also, fenestrated tubes are not for emergency use. When mechanical ventilation is anticipated for longer than 24 hours, the tube is replaced with a nonfenestrated tube. Last, a precut fenestration may be associated with an airway obstruction when the fenestration is not correctly aligned within the trachea. To assure a patent fenestration, many clinicians recommend assessment of the position of the fenestration and, if necessary, enlargement. (Cane and associates in 1982 described a bedside technique.)

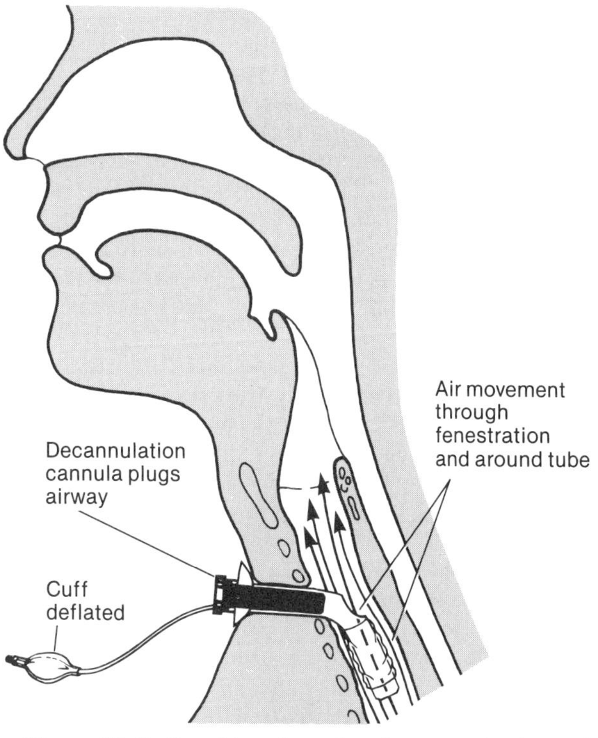

Figure 26–9. Breathing through a fenestrated tube with the decannulation cannula in place and the cuff deflated.

Tubes with a Foam-filled Cuff

A tracheostomy or endotracheal tube with a foam-filled cuff has a silicone rubber shaft and a cuff made of polyurethane foam filling (i.e., Fome-Cuf tube made by Bivona, Inc.). Use of this type of tube permits the maintenance of low cuff pressures in the range of 5 to 15 mmHg.

Before this tube is introduced in the clinical setting, staff must be thoroughly educated about its use, with emphasis on the unconventional functioning of the foam cuff. Unlike air-inflatable cuffs, the foam cuff is deflated by first using a syringe to aspirate air through the inflating tube. Then, the tube is promptly plugged to maintain cuff deflation (Fig. 26–10, left). The cuff is inflated simply by opening the inflating line to air (Fig. 26–10, right). Most important, *cuff inflation is maintained not by clamping the inflating line, as sometimes done with air-inflatable cuffs, but rather by leaving the inflating line open to air.* This practice allows small amounts of air to move in and out of the cuff to keep the low pressure against the tracheal wall relatively stable.

In addition, a manometer is not used to measure the cuff pressure of a foam-filled cuff. Manufacturer guidelines are referred to for measurement of air (cc) in the cuff and estimation of pressure on a Fome-Cuf pressure chart.

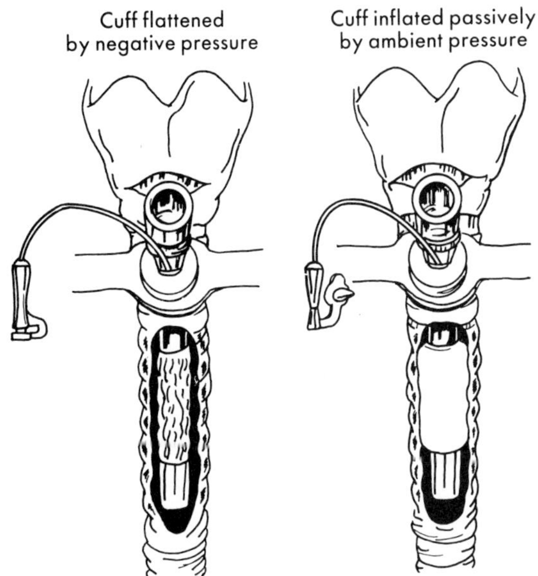

Figure 26–10. The foam-filled cuff positioned in the trachea. Left, Deflated cuff. Right, Inflated cuff. (Reproduced by permission from Bivona Surgical, Hammond, Indiana.)

A relatively new feature of the Fome-Cuf is the sideport airway connector shown in Figure 26–11. The connector is attached proximally to a tube's 15-mm adaptor and distally to the patient's ventilator circuit. When the connector's small stem is attached to the inflating tube, intracuff pressures approach or equal airway pressure during both inspiration and expiration. Furthermore, cuff volume increases and decreases synchronously with increases and decreases in tracheal volume, while continuously ensuring a tracheal seal.

The equalization of pressure throughout the respiratory cycle serves two purposes as follows: (1) it reduces the risk of high cuff-to-tracheal wall pressures during nitrous oxide anesthesia (Greene, 1986) and (2) it minimizes tracheal dilatation associated with greater than 3 days of positive pressure ventilation, particularly in patients on high levels of positive end-expiratory pressure (Cane, 1982).

Tracheostomy Buttons

Besides the fenestrated tracheostomy tube, another type of cannula, called a *tracheostomy button* (Fig. 26–12), is used to provide a step between mechanical ventilation and spontaneous breathing. The tracheostomy button is a preferred means of maintaining a stoma, when the patient needs no assistance clearing bronchial secretions.

Insertion of the Olympic Button. To fit a patient with a tracheostomy button, the clinician utilizes a probe to measure the distance from the anterior tracheal wall to the skin's surface. This measurement is an estimate of the desired button length. A button, such as the Teflon *Olympic tracheostomy button* (Olympic Medical Corporation), of an appropriate out-

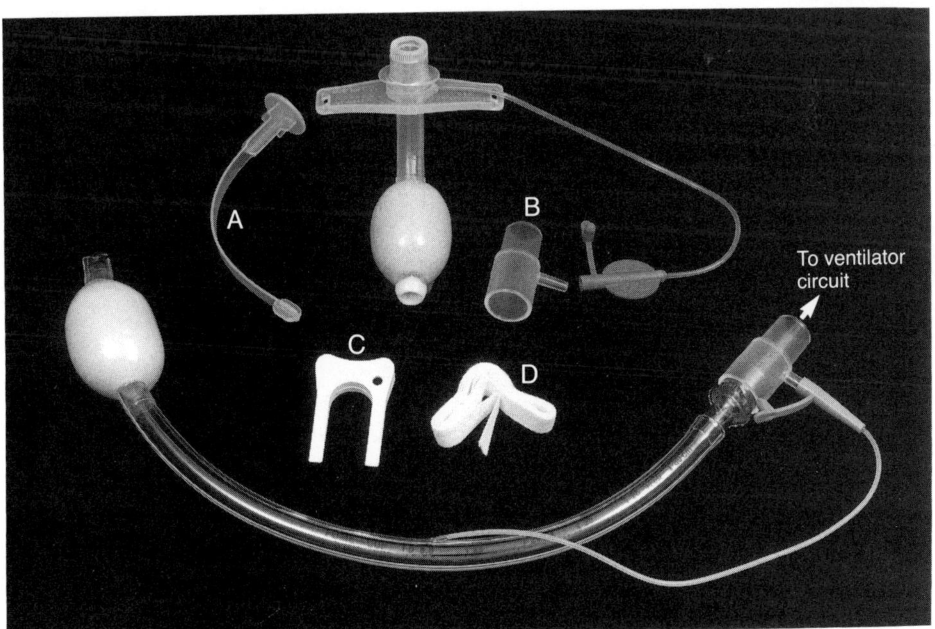

Figure 26–11. Foam-cuffed tubes (Fome-Cuf tubes from Bivona, Inc., Gary, Indiana). *Top*, Tracheostomy tube with obturator (A), sideport airway connector (B), wedge (C) used to facilitate disconnection of sideport airway connector from the tube, and fabric tape (D). *Bottom*, Endotracheal tube. With the sideport airway connector attached, intracuff pressure equals airway pressure.

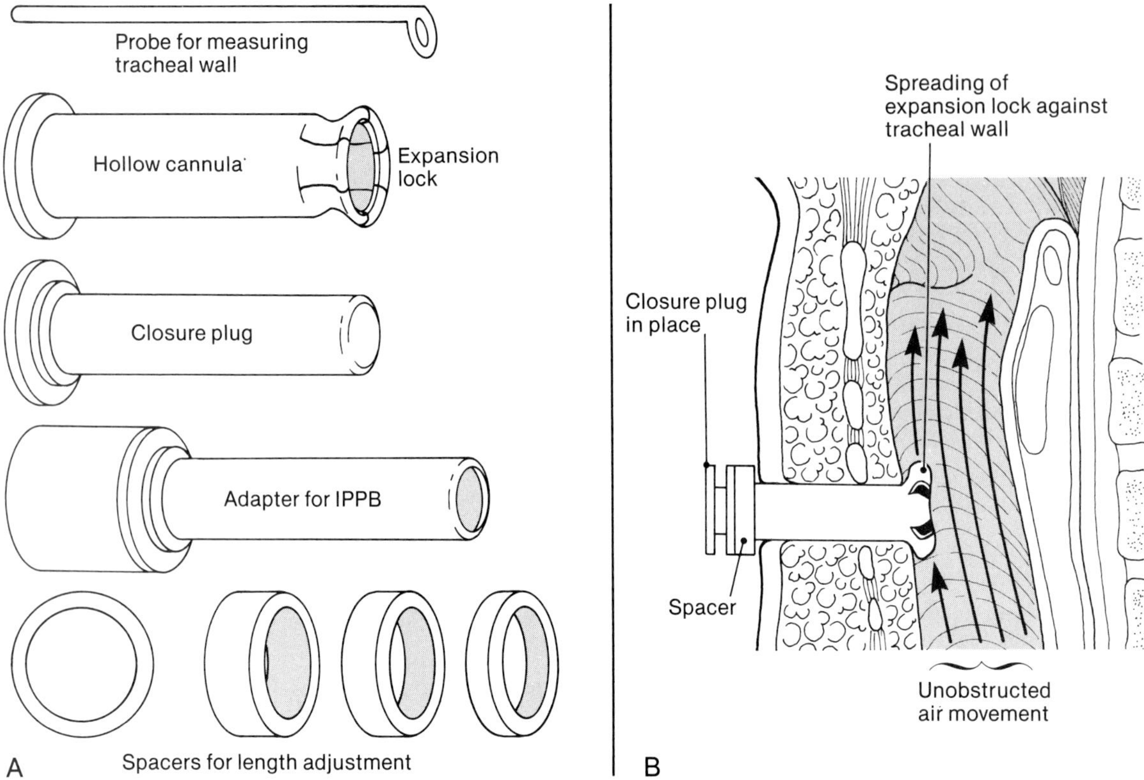

Figure 26–12. Tracheostomy button. *A*, Individual parts. *B*, Breathing with the closure plug in place.

side diameter and length is ordered. The outer cannula is inserted through the stoma. Insertion of the inner closure plug spreads the flanged tip, called the expansion lock of the cannula. This action fixates the cannula to the anterior tracheal wall, as shown in Figure 26–12B.

The clinician keeps in mind three points, when inserting a tracheostomy button. First, to avoid anterior button displacement, the clinician must be sure the flanged tip lies in the tracheal lumen and not in the anterior cervical tissues before inserting the closure plug to spread the flange. Anterior button displacement may cause premature stomal closure. Second, after insertion, the clinician pulls back on the cannula to insure a snug fit. If the button is too long, even after appropriate sizing, it may be removed; rings called *spacers* are added to take up the extra slack between the neck and proximal end of the button. A snug fit is necessary to help prevent dislodgement of the tube and posterior displacement of the button into the tracheal lumen. Third, some button models may have an inner cannula with a 15-mm adaptor for manual bagging or IPPB.

Kistner Tracheostomy Tube. The Kistner tracheostomy tube (Pilling Co.) is sometimes referred to as a tracheostomy button. It has a *one-way valve* that attaches to the outer cannula (Fig. 26–13). The valve allows air to flow in through the tube on inspiration. It closes on expiration, forcing air to exit via the larynx and oral and nasal passages. This arrangement permits speaking, coughing, and PRN suctioning, when the patient cannot clear secretions with only coughing and deep breathing. Then, as the weaning process progresses, the one-way valve is removed, and the closure plug inserted.

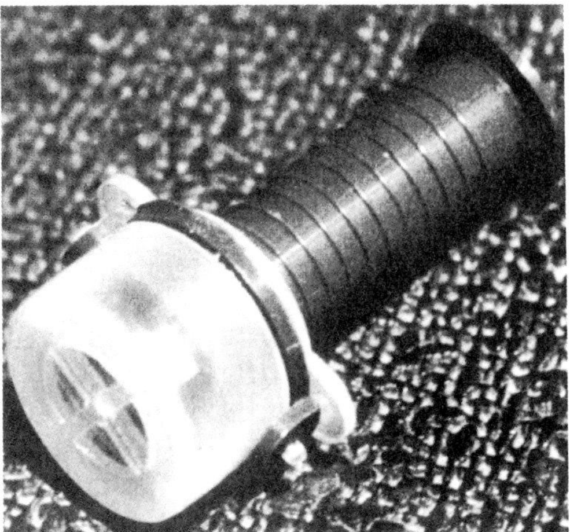

Figure 26–13. Kistner plastic tracheostomy tube. (Reproduced by permission from Caldwell, S. and Sullivan, K. Artificial Airways. In Respiratory Care—A Guide to Clinical Practice, 2nd ed. [Burton, G. and Hodgkin, J.—eds.]. Philadelphia, J. B. Lippincott Co., 1984.)

The Kistner tube is made of flexible inert polyvinyl acetate. The one-way valve is contained in a cap that snaps onto the cannula. A plastic, retaining ring or a cap with valve removed may be added to act as a spacer or to provide external fixation (i.e., the ring is sutured to the skin). The one-way valve may stick owing to water condensation, particularly when oxygen with humidity or mist is provided via the Kistner tube. Wet valves are promptly replaced to prevent breathing room air through the upper airway, and supplementary oxygen via nasal prongs or face mask may be needed if hypoxemia persists.

In addition to valve malfunction, other complications may include local skin irritation, tube dislodgement during forceful coughing, and airway obstruction from protrusion of the tube into the tracheal lumen (Venus, 1980). As with other buttons, the Kistner tube is replaced with a cuffed tracheostomy tube, should a need for mechanical ventilation develop.

Speaking Tubes

Speaking tracheostomy tubes, such as the *Pitt Trach Speaking Tube* (National Catheter Corp.) and *Communitrach* (Implant Technologies, Inc.), are standard cuffed tubes with an extra air (i.e., oxygen or O_2) channel that allows speaking with the cuff inflated. This type of tube provides a means of communication for patients whose aphonia, anxiety, and frustration seem to be hindering the weaning process or the adaptation to long-term illness.

The Pitt Trach Speaking Tube requires continuous air or oxygen to flow through the air (i.e., oxygen or O_2) channel at a rate of 4 to 6 L/min (Fig. 26–14). If a patient wishes to speak, he or she occludes the extra channel's adaptor port with a finger or thumb. This action permits air flow through the small channel, along the curvature of the tracheostomy tube, and out through a port situated under the cuff's flap. As air escapes from under this flap, it exits via the larynx, permitting phonation in a coarse whisper rather than a normal voice.

Some clinicians modify the Pitt Trach Speaking Tube for secretion management in patients with swallowing dysfunction and continual laryngeal aspiration, despite presence of a cuffed tracheostomy tube (Shahvari et al, 1977). The cuff's protective flap is carefully cut off, so that the underlying port is available for secretion aspiration. The external air (i.e., oxygen or O_2) channel is connected to strong intermittent or moderate (60 to 100 mmHg) constant suction to aspirate secretions pooled on top of the cuff. This technique prevents pulmonary aspiration and at the same time provides a means for quantification, since aspirated food and secretions can be inspected and measured.

The Communitrach tube is similar to the Pitt Trach Speaking Tube with three exceptions. First, it has both an inner and outer cannula. Second, the air/O_2 channel is a thin hose that lies between the inner and outer cannulas. Third, air or O_2 moves upward towards the vocal cords after passing through eight small ports in the outer cannula, as opposed to the Pitt Trach Speaking Tube's single port under the cuff's flap.

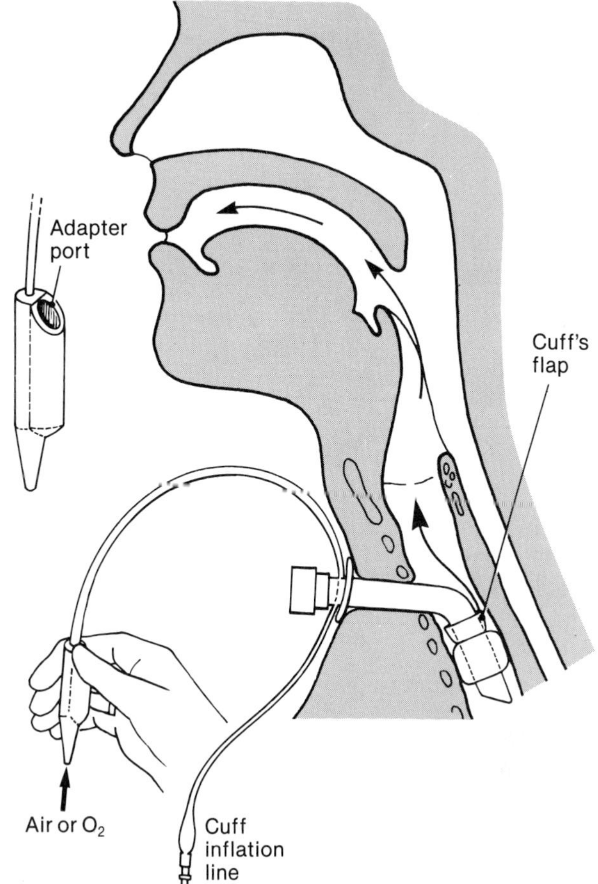

Figure 26–14. Pitt Trach Speaking Tube. Occluding the adapter port with the thumb directs compressed air or oxygen into the trachea above the cuff and underneath the cuff's flap. The gas exits through the vocal cords to produce speech. (Adapted by permission from Luce, J., Tyler, M., and Pierson, D. Intensive Respiratory Care. Philadelphia, W. B. Saunders Co., 1984.)

Speaking Attachments

Some speaking devices, such as the Olympic Trach-talk and Passy-Muir Tracheostomy Speaking Valve, are attachments to the standard tracheostomy tube. The *Olympic Trach-Talk* allows spontaneous breathing and phonation through a T-piece arrangement (Fig. 26–15). It is similar to a Kistner tracheostomy button, and it has a one-way valve that closes during expiration. This closure forces air through the vocal cords and pushes secretions into the oral cavity for expectoration.

The *Passy-Muir Tracheostomy Speaking Valve* is a silastic membrane one-way valve (Fig. 26–16). Unlike other one-way valves that close in response to positive pressure during exhalation, the Passy-Muir valve is a spring-loaded system. It closes *automatically* at the end of exhalation. The automatic closure helps to maintain a closed system and to avoid valve fluttering and malfunctioning, particularly when humidification is added or when secretions are present.

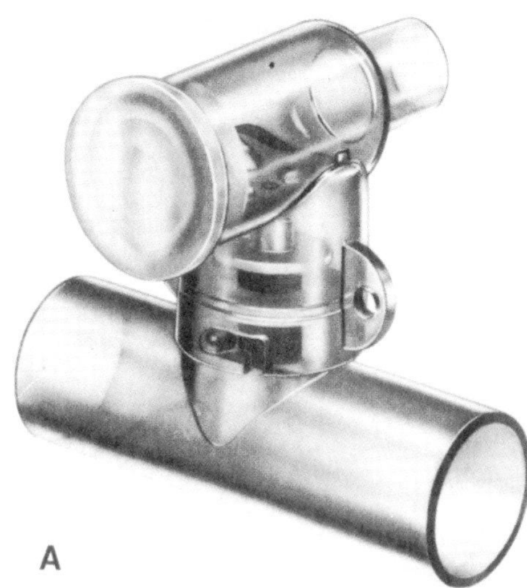

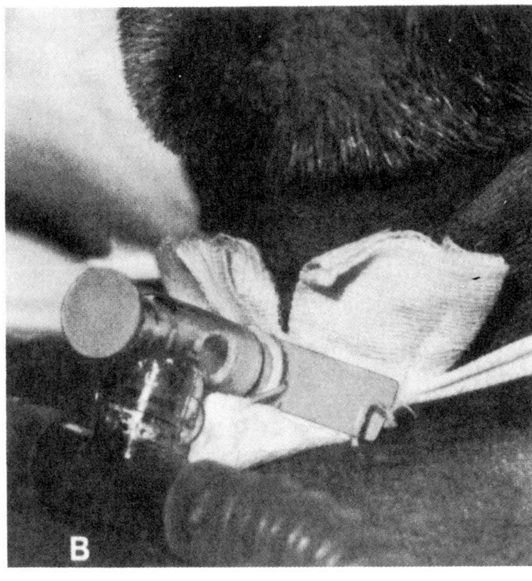

Figure 26–15. An Olympic Trach-Talk. (Reproduced by permission from Caldwell, S. and Sullivan, K.: Artificial Airways. In Respiratory Care—A Guide to Clinical Practice, 2nd ed. [Burton, G. and Hodgkin, J.—eds.]. Philadelphia, J. B. Lippincott Co., 1984.)

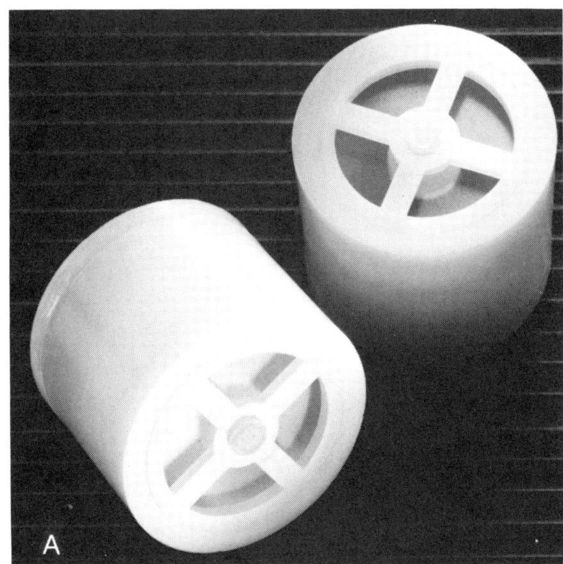

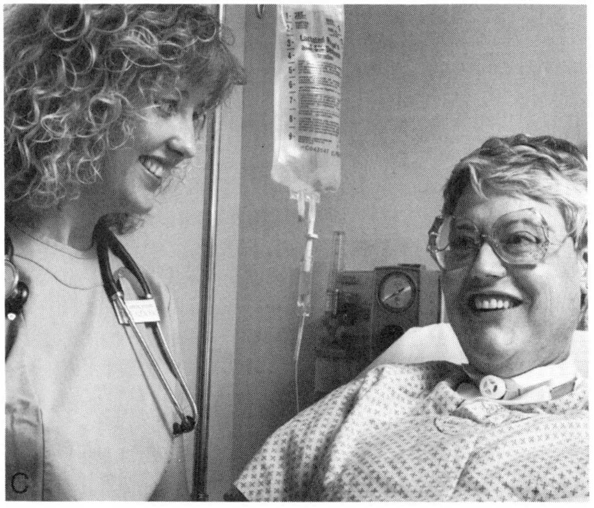

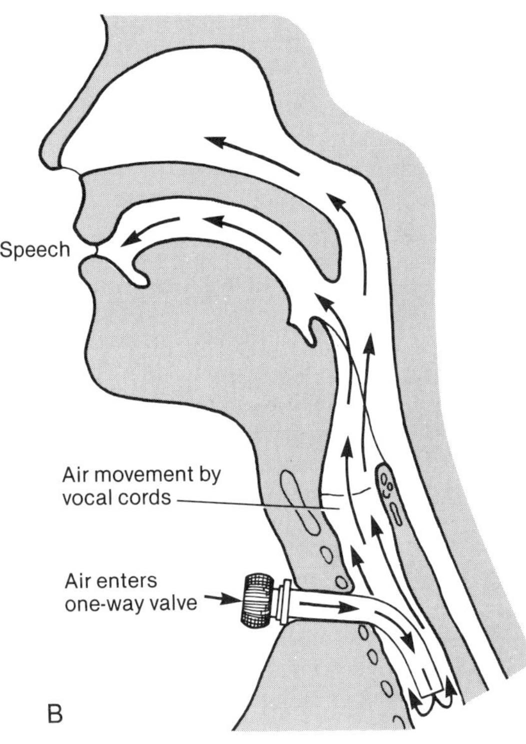

Figure 26–16. Passy-Muir Tracheostomy Speaking Valve. *A*, Basic design. *B*, Air movement through the valve for speech. *C*, Nurse and patient discuss how use of the valve makes speech easier and clearer. (*A* and *C* courtesy of Passy & Passy, Inc., Irvine, California.)

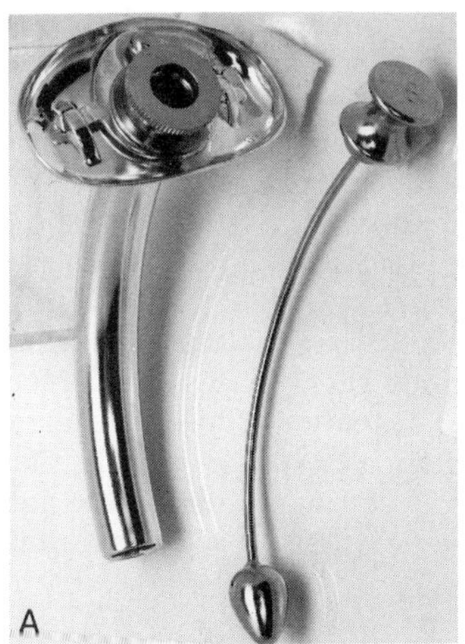

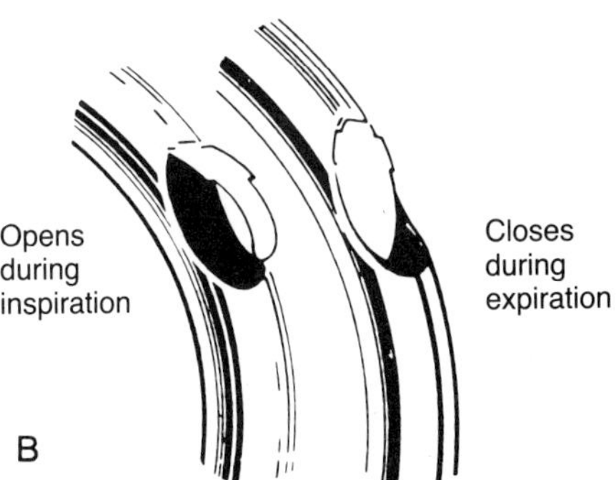

Figure 26–17. Metal tracheostomy tube. *A*, Sterling silver Jackson type with the obturator (right) and the inner cannula locked into the outer cannula (left). *B*, The Tucker valve of an accessory inner cannula (i.e., Tucker valve inner cannula). The valve remains open during inspiration, as the patient inspires through the cannula. On expiration, the valve leaflet closes, forcing air through the trachea and upper passageways. (Courtesy of Pilling Co., Fort Washington, Pennsylvania.)

The Passy-Muir valve facilitates decannulation in patients unable to tolerate tracheostomy plugging and in those with sleep apnea, bilateral vocal cord paralysis, tracheomalacia, neuromuscular disease, head trauma, and COPD. Contraindications are as follows: (1) patients with severe laryngeal or tracheal stenoses; (2) unconscious patients; (3) seriously ill patients; and (4) patients with tracheostomy tubes with inflated cuffs, unless the tube is fenestrated (Passy, 1986). Clinical advantages summarized by Passy include the following:

- Speech (Fig. 26–16B). The patient does not need to use finger occlusion of the tracheostomy tube for phonation. Finger occlusion, a common tendency, is undesirable because it is a source of contamination
- Improved sense of smell associated with the redirection of air high up in the nasal passageways.
- Reduced frustration at not being able to speak, improved sense of well being, and increased involvement in activities of daily living (Fig. 26–16C).
- Maintenance of a more closed tracheobronchial system at all times. This arrangement simulates the normal tracheobronchial tree. Because of this advantage, the Passy-Muir valve may be associated with a reduced risk for pulmonary infection when compared with other valves, according to researchers at the University of California, Irvine. In addition, note that the valve's partial filtration of inspiratory air may help prevent contamination of the tracheobronchial tree.
- Increased ventilation and oxygenation associated with the development of back pressure in the closed pulmonary system.
- Facilitation of mucous expectoration through the oral cavity rather than through the tracheostomy tube.

Metal and Nylon Tubes

Many patients with chronic pulmonary problems have metal or nylon tracheostomy tubes to maintain airway patency and provide a route for aspiration of secretions.

One of the most popular metal tubes is the *Jackson* tracheostomy tube. It is a stainless steel or sterling silver tube with an inner cannula, outer cannula, and obturator (Fig. 26–17A). Although a cuff may be attached, this tube is almost always used cuffless. Detachable cuffs are undesirable because they tend to exert high pressure against the tracheal wall, and they may become damaged or slip off the end of the tube.

A special inner cannula called a *Tucker valve inner cannula* may be used with a sterling silver Jackson or Tucker tube. This cannula has a *Tucker valve* that allows phonation without finger occlusion of the tube (Fig. 26–17B). The cannula works best for patients *without* obstructive disease and clinical problems that commonly impair valve functioning, e.g., increased airway resistance and mucus production.

When ordering a Jackson tracheostomy tube, the clinician must remember that the sizes are different than the OD, ID, and French sizes of other tracheostomy tubes. Table 26–1 may be used as a guide for

Table 26–1. CONVERSION CHART FOR TRACHEOSTOMY TUBE SIZES*

Jackson Size	Outside Diameter (mm)	Internal Diameter (mm)	French Size
00	4.3	2.5	13
0	5.0	3.0	15
1	5.5	3.5	16.5
2	6.0	4.0	18
3	7	4.5–5.0	21
4	8	5.5	24
5	9	6.0–6.5	27
6	10	7.0	30
7	11	7.5–8.0	33
8	12	8.5	36
9	13	9.0–9.5	39
10	14	10.0	42
11	15	10.5–11.0	45
12	16	11.5	48

*Sizes are approximate. (Adapted from Caldwell, S. and Sullivan, K. Artificial Airways. In Respiratory Care—A Guide to Clinical Practice. (Burton, G. and Hodgkin, J.—eds.). Philadelphia, J. B. Lippincott Co., 1984.)

the comparison of sizes. Though the nurse may never care for a patient with a Jackson tracheostomy tube, sizes are important to be aware of because they serve as references for the sizing of other tracheostomy tubes.

Metal and nylon tubes are utilized less frequently in the clinical area because of the following disadvantages. First, metal and nylon tubes are rigid and, hence, are more likely to cause pressure necrosis and increased patient discomfort, compared with soft, thermolabile tubes that conform to the patient's anatomy. Second, metal tubes may cause local skin irritation and stimulate mucus production (Caldwell and Sullivan, 1984). The irritation may be due to the oxidation that normally takes place when the silver of a silver or silver-plated tube is exposed to air. In other cases, irritation may be due to the effect of a silver polish and the failure to clean the tube with an appropriate agent. Last, metal tubes may not have a 15-mm adaptor that facilitates manual bagging with a resuscitator bag in case of emergency.

In spite of these disadvantages, a metal or nylon, cuffless tracheostomy tube is often the one of choice for a patient after laryngectomy. A laryngectomy tube has the same design as a tracheostomy tube, except it is slightly shorter (Fig. 26–18). Similar to other nondisposable tubes, most laryngectomy tubes come in sets that are interchangeable within a size and style.

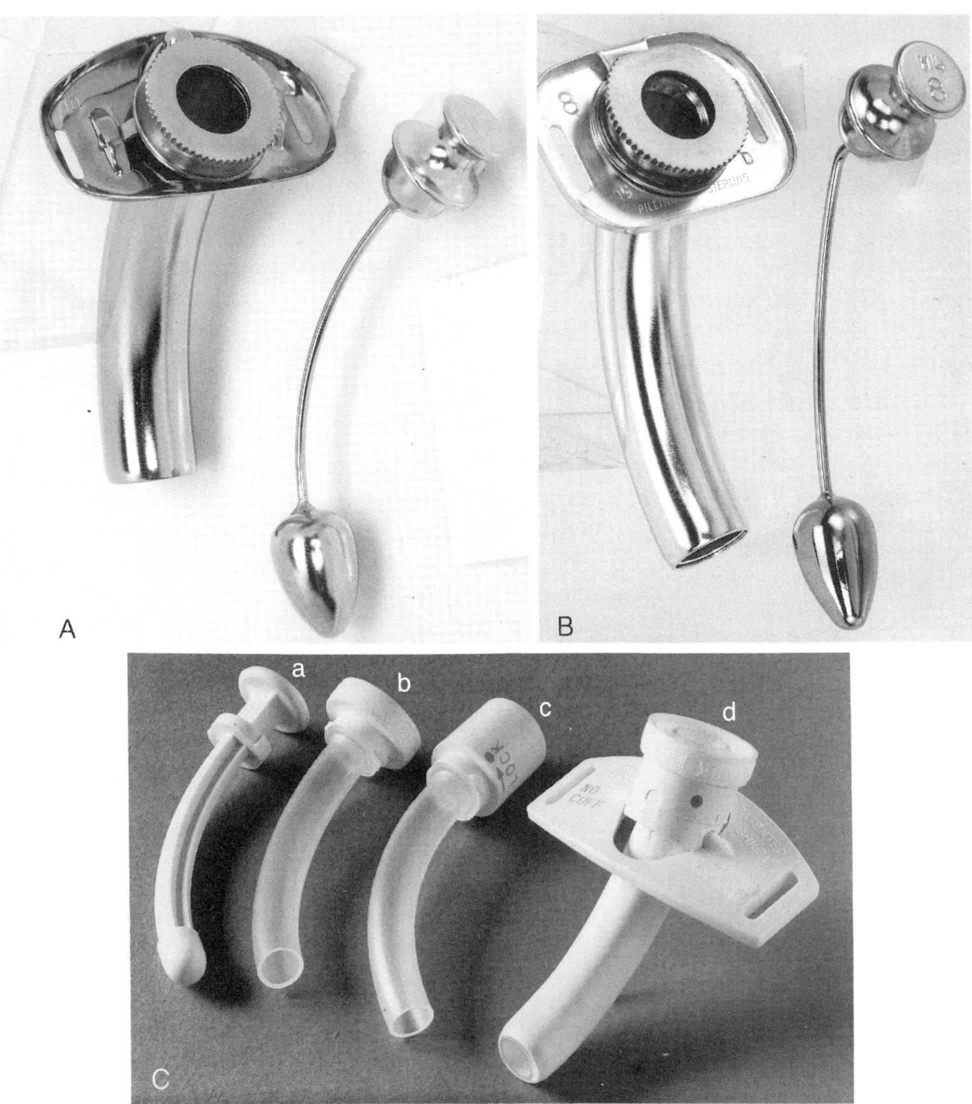

Figure 26–18. Different types of laryngectomy tubes. *A*, The sterling silver Jackson; *B*, The sterling silver Holinger. The tube's outer cannula is the same length (50 mm) as the outer cannula of the Jackson type. Here, the cannula appears longer because the angle of the cannula to the neckplate is only 65 degrees, as opposed to 90 degrees in *A*. *C*, Plastic Shiley. *a*, Obturator; *b*, Inner cannula with low-profile connector to reduce bulk at the stoma; *c*, Inner cannula with integral 15-mm twist-lock connector; *d*, Laryngectomy tube with inner cannula in place. (*A* and *B* courtesy of Pilling Co., Fort Washington, Pennsylvania. *C* courtesy of Shiley Inc., Irvine, California.)

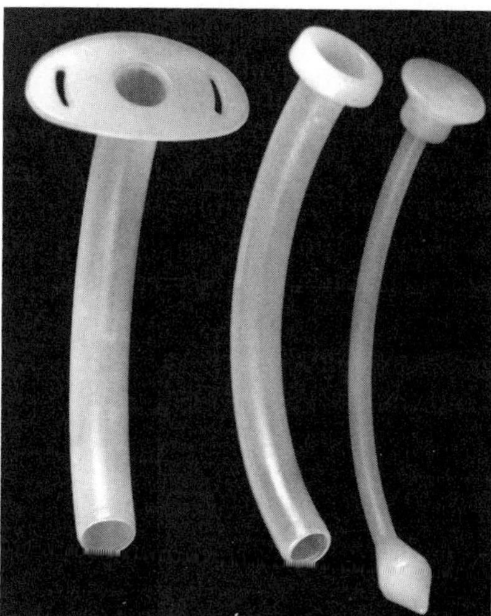

Figure 26–19. Air-Lon tracheostomy tube with inner cannula (center) and obturator (right). This nylon tube is reusable, relatively inexpensive, and nonirritating to the skin. (Courtesy of Pilling Co., Fort Washington, Pennsylvania.)

Though nylon tubes are rigid, they are less rigid than metal and generally more comfortable for the patient. In addition, they have the advantage of being lightweight, easy to clean and change, and nontoxic to tissues (Fig. 26–19).

Conclusion

This chapter discussed tracheotomy with tracheostomy intubation, stressing the complications that the nurse monitors during the postintubation period. The basic design of a tracheostomy tube is reviewed, and common tracheostomy tubes in the clinical setting are introduced. This information complements the information provided in regard to endotracheal intubation in Chapter 25 and provides a firm foundation for the care of the intubated patient, the topic of Chapter 27.

REFERENCES

Burns, S., Shasby, D., and Burke, P.: Controlled pressure cuffed endotracheal tubes may not be controlled. *Chest*, 83(1):158–159, 1983.

Caldwell, S., and Sullivan, K.: Artificial Airways. In Respiratory Care—A Guide to Clinical Practice, 2nd ed. (Burton, G. and Hodgkin, J.—eds.). Philadelphia, J. B. Lippincott Co., 1984.

Cane, R., Shapiro, B., et al: A new technique for minimizing tracheal dilatation in mechanically ventilated patients. Divona, Inc., Gary, Indiana.

Cane, R., Woodward, C., and Shapiro, B.: Customizing fenestrated tracheostomy tubes: a bedside technique. *Critical care medicine*, 10(12):880–881, 1982.

Greene, S., Cane, R., and Shapiro, B.: A foam cuff endotracheal tube T-piece system for use with nitrous oxide anesthesia. *Anesthesia and analgesia*, 65(12):1359–1360, 1986.

Heffner, J., Miller, K., and Sahn, S.: Tracheostomy in the intensive care unit. Part 2. Complications. *Chest*, 90(3):430–436, 1986.

Passy, V.: Passy-Muir tracheostomy speaking valve. *Otolaryngology—head & neck surgery*, 95(2):247–248, 1986.

Shahvari, B., Kicin, C., and Zimmerman, J.: Speaking tube modified for swallowing dysfunction and chronic aspiration. *Anesthesiology*, 46(4):290–291, 1977

Stauffer, J., Olson, D., and Petty, T.: Complications of endotracheal intubation and tracheostomy. *American journal of medicine*, 70(1):65–76, 1981.

Tout, C.: Artificial airways: tubes and trachs. *Respiratory care*, 21(6):513–519, 1976.

Venus, B.: Five year experience with Kistner tracheostomy tube. *Critical care medicine*, 8(2):106–110, 1980.

Care of the Intubated Patient

27

Main Objectives

1. **Define the following terms: ideal intracuff pressure, T-piece or T-tube, high flow cascade, extubation, straight suction catheter, angled (i.e., coudée) suction catheter, preoxygenation—bagging method, preoxygenation—ventilator method, swivel adaptor, self-sealing adaptor, Leuken's trap, and tracheal lavage.**
2. **List the characteristics of the ideal artificial airway that promote optimal airway care, prevent laryngotracheal injury, and maximize patient comfort.**
3. **Explain the following cuff management techniques: minimal leak technique and no-leak technique for cuff inflation, pressure monitoring, and cuff leak assessment.**
4. **Explain why an intubated patient with a nasogastric (NG) tube is likely to have more oropharyngeal secretions than an intubated patient without an NG tube.**
5. **Describe how to tape an endotracheal tube, give daily mouth care, stabilize the ventilator circuit, remove water condensation from tubings, and elicit patient cooperation.**
6. **Explain the rationale and use of humidity for intubated patients.**

7. **Discuss appropriate position changes for intubated patients.**
8. **State signs and symptoms that indicate a complication during intubation. Name at least one nursing intervention for each complication.**
9. **Describe nursing care related to**
   a. **routine tracheostomy care.**
   b. **changing the tracheostomy tube.**
   c. **extubation (i.e., decannulation).**
   d. **postextubation monitoring.**
   e. **psychosocial adjustment.**
10. **State the indications, contraindications, and complications of tracheobronchial suctioning.**
11. **Describe a procedure for nasopharyngeal and tracheobronchial suctioning that minimizes hypoxemia, atelectasis, and tissue trauma.**
12. **Compare and contrast the provision of mouth care to an intubated patient with normal oral mucosa versus one with signs of stomatitis.**
13. **Discuss how to adapt hospital procedures to the home setting for tracheostomy care, tracheal suctioning, and mouth care.**
14. **Explain how to support the patient's family as the patient's intubation or acute exacerbation of chronic pulmonary disease precipitates family disorganization.**

This chapter presents care of the intubated patient, with a focus on airway care. Care related to mechanical ventilation is also relevant (see Chapter 28), since many intubated patients are on mechanical ventilation and since many complications of mechanical ventilation, such as malnutrition and infection, are also complications of prolonged intubation, without application of mechanical ventilation.

As with previous chapters in this part of the book, emphasis is placed on acute care in the hospital setting. However, basic principles of respiratory intervention are applicable to most intubated patients, regardless of setting. Clinical applications unique to the home setting are presented for tracheostomy care, suctioning procedure, and mouth care.

Basic Airway Care

The nurse works closely with the physician and respiratory therapist to provide optimal airway care for the patient with an endotracheal or tracheostomy tube.

TUBE AND CUFF SELECTION

One easy way to promote optimal airway care, prevent laryngotracheal injury, and maximize patient comfort is to make available only soft cuffed tubes in critical care units. More specifically, the tube selected for intubation should come as close as possible to the characteristics of an ideal artificial airway. These characteristics include the following:

1. Soft, flexible, thermolabile tube.
2. Nontoxic, pyrogen free, implant tested material (i.e., labelled Z 79 or IT).
3. Soft cuff (e.g., high volume, low pressure, and low slope pressure).
4. Cuff diameter larger than tracheal diameter.
5. Kink and collapse resistant shaft.
6. Durable inflation valve.
7. Radiopaque line or marker on shaft.
8. Disposable.

Most important, tubes with small diameter, high pressure cuffs should be avoided, e.g., Rusch's latex cuff and Bivona's Silastic "aire cuff" (Bernhard et al, 1985).

CUFF MANAGEMENT

After intubation, the cuff is inflated to an ideal intracuff pressure, defined as the *lowest possible pressure that allows the delivery of adequate tidal volumes and prevents major pulmonary aspiration* (Stauffer and Silvestri, 1982). In most situations, the pressure is maintained below 25 cmH_2O to prevent injury and above 20 cmH_2O to prevent aspiration. However, some ventilated patients require cuff pressures greater than 25 cmH_2O to maintain adequate seals, and other patients are able to maintain seals with pressures less than 20 cmH_2O, depending on tube design, size, and mode of ventilation.

Inflation Techniques

The clinician inflates the cuff with either the minimal leak or no-leak technique. For the *minimal leak technique* (MLT), the clinician places a stethoscope over the larynx and injects 0.5 cc of air into the cuff at a time, until a small inspiratory leak is auscultated. In spontaneously breathing patients, the leak may be barely audible with a stethoscope. In patients on continuous mechanical ventilation, the leak may be readily heard without a stethoscope, as a rush of air moves past the cuff and through the mouth or nose at the peak of inspiration, notably at the peak of a large breath (i.e., sigh). Whatever the case, the MLT should result in no more than a 50-cc to 100-cc loss in tidal volume (V_T); exhaled V_T is less than inhaled V_T by this amount. If a leak is difficult to detect, the cuff may be temporarily inflated with a recommended amount of air and checked later to be sure intracuff pressure is within safe levels.

For the *no-leak technique*, also called *minimal occluding pressure* or *minimal occluding volume*, the same technique is used, except the cuff is inflated just to the point that the air leak ceases, and the trachea becomes sealed.

Both of the aforementioned cuff inflation techniques have special advantages. The MLT decreases mucosal injury because slightly less air and less pressure are required. Also, the intermittent flow of air pushes pharyngeal secretions towards the mouth and prevents the accumulation of secretions above the glottis. Alternatively, the no-leak technique is preferred for recently intubated patients and patients likely to aspirate, e.g., the supine comatose patient with an NG tube in place. It may be used for a patient whose air leak with the MLT changes greatly in size, owing to differences in patient position, tube movement, V_Ts, and peak pressures.

Cuff Deflation

In the era of hard cuffs, hourly 5-minute cuff deflations were advocated to minimize tracheal wall damage. Currently, however, soft cuffs remain inflated continuously and are deflated only when problems arise or periodically (q48 to 72h) to check for cuffs that are overinflated. Researchers have yet to prove that periodic cuff deflation for soft cuffed tubes reduces tracheal damage. Now, the evidence indicates that deflation promotes hypoxemia; overinflation when the cuff is reinflated; and pulmonary aspiration, as pooled secretions drip into the lungs and stimulate coughing (Powaser et al, 1976).

Intracuff Pressure Monitoring

Although intracuff pressure monitoring is a function of the respiratory therapist, the nurse needs this skill when a respiratory therapist is unavailable.

Cuff pressure is measured immediately after cuff inflation and TID thereafter. Precise measurement requires use of a mercury or aneroid manometer, as shown in the box on the opposite page.

When a manometer is unavailable momentarily, the nurse may obtain a rough estimate by feeling the "give" or compliance of the pilot balloon. Though this method is no substitute for precise measurement with a manometer, in acute care situations, it may help troubleshoot and determine whether the cuff is completely deflated (i.e., zero pressure) or obviously overinflated (i.e., high pressure).

The patient usually needs periodic adjustments in cuff pressure. If after cuff inflation, cuff pressure is over 25 cmH_2O, cuff volume is reduced 0.50 cc at a time until a pressure below 25 cmH_2O is achieved, while using a minimal or no-leak technique for sealing the trachea. Pressure may need to be similarly increased or decreased with any dramatic change in sensorium, activity, or position, because corresponding changes in muscle tension, gravitational forces, and breathing pattern will alter pressure relationships within the trachea. Some patients may require a cuff volume adjustment with each position change.

As mentioned previously in relation to the Lanz cuff, currently available self pressure regulating cuffs are not totally reliable in maintaining an ideal pressure. They must be monitored routinely, similar to low-pressure cuffs.

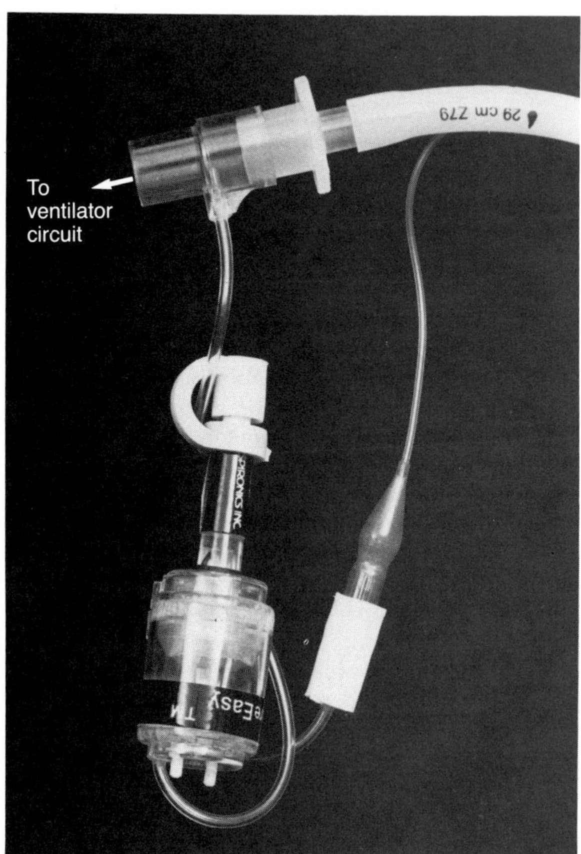

Figure 27–1. PressureEasy cuff pressure controller (Respironics, Inc., Monroeville, Pennsylvania) attached to an endotracheal tube. The T-piece connector (attached to 15 mm adaptor) has the same basic function as the sideport airway connector of the foam cuffed tube in Figure 26–11.

In some cases, a *cuff pressure controller* may be attached to an endotracheal or tracheostomy tube for the automatic and continuous adjustment of pressure. The *PressureEasy* cuff pressure controller in Figure 27–1 controls pressure at 18 to 27 cmH_2O continuously. Though such controllers may effectively reduce the need for frequent pressure measurements and cuff adjustments, similar to any mechanical device with a valve, they may malfunction. They do not eliminate the need for periodic monitoring with a mercury or aneroid manometer.

Other Points

Other points to consider during cuff care follow:

1. Although monitoring of cuff pressure is key, *cuff inflation volume must not be disregarded.* This volume should be recorded in the chart along with cuff pressure. Should cuff problems arise, this knowledge allows the clinician to determine quickly whether further inflation is likely to result in cuff stretching and overinflation, compression of the shaft's lumen, eccentric centering of the tube's shaft within the trachea, and possibly herniation of the cuff over the distal tip of the airway. Recording of cuff inflation volume also helps in identifying the presence of a cuff leak, as described subsequently.

MEASURING CUFF PRESSURE WITH AN ANEROID CUFF PRESSURE MANOMETER (PORTEX)

1. Connect the manometer line, with a three-way stopcock attached to the patient's inflation system. The stopcock to the patient should be turned to off position.
2. Occlude the open port with the thumb or finger. Inject air into the manometer line until the manometer reads between 20 cmH_2O and 25 cmH_2O. This action fills up dead space in the manometer line and helps prevent a falsely low volume for cuff measurement.
3. Turn the stopcock to the open port to off position, so that the manometer communicates with the patient's inflation line. Read the manometer after the needle drifts down a few centimeters and stabilizes.
4. Turn the stopcock to the patient to off position. Disconnect the manometer line from the patient's inflation line. (Portex manometer courtesy of Smiths Industries Medical Systems Co., Valencia, California.)

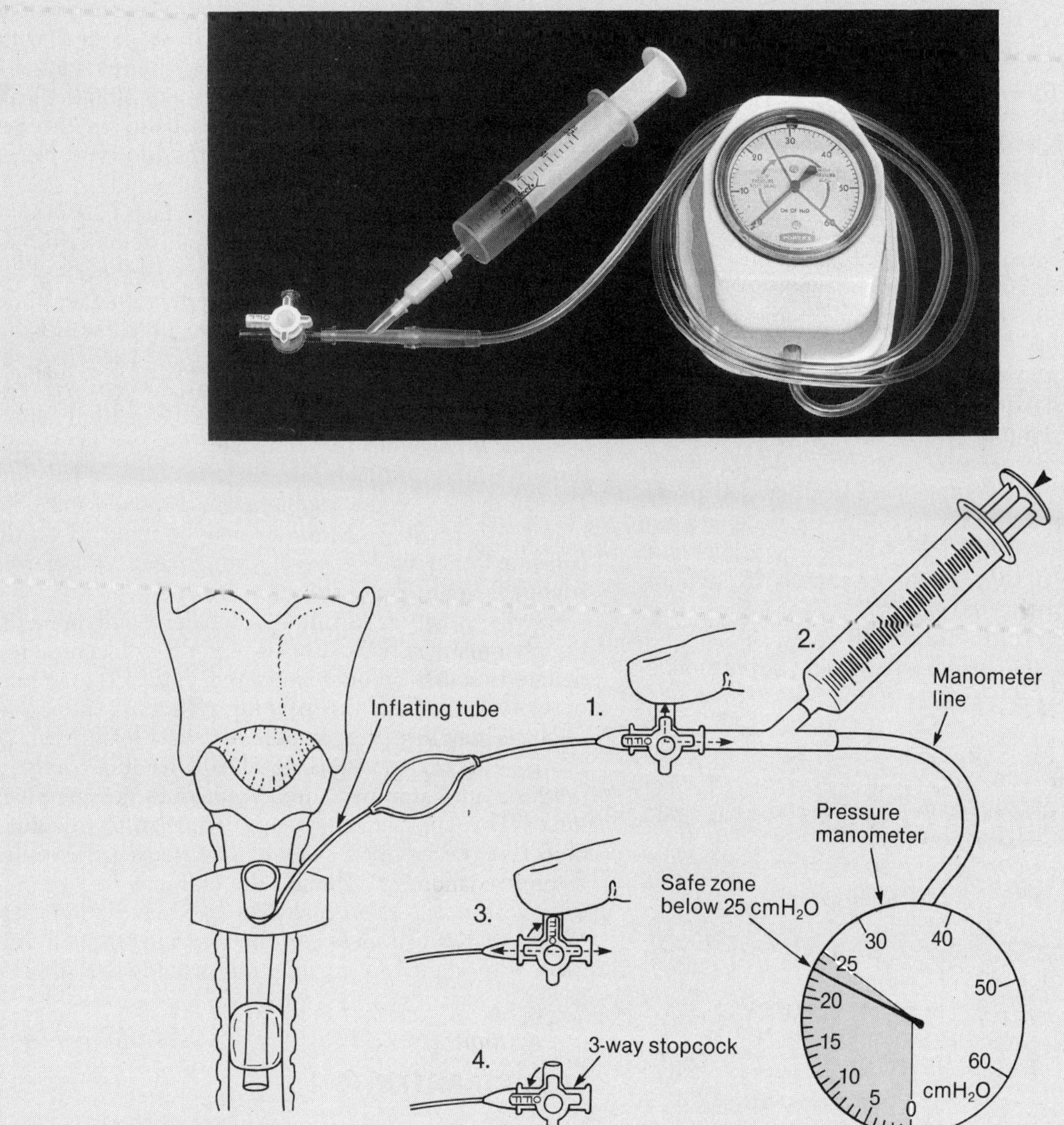

2. Monitor cuff pressure frequently after general anesthesia. As explained previously, nitrous oxide tends to diffuse into thin cuffs and increase pressures.
3. In spontaneously breathing patients, the cuff may be left deflated if aspiration is not a problem. This practice is often incorporated into the weaning process, but the cuff is usually inflated before meals and after meals for 1 hour as precautions.

4. If the inflating valve is absent or malfunctioning, the nurse may insert a three-way stopcock, inflate the cuff, and apply a padded hemostat to clamp the inflating tube distal to the pilot balloon. Turn the stopcock to the patient to off position and remove the hemostat. This measure is a temporary one, until the pilot balloon is replaced (e.g., tube with Lanz cuff) or until the physician is called for medical evaluation and possible reintubation.
5. When the inflating line becomes faulty and the tube needs changing, reintubation may be undesirable because the patient may be at high risk for complications, e.g., mechanical ventilation at high levels of positive end expiratory pressure (PEEP), cervical spine injury, recent upper airway surgery, and recent tracheostomy. In these cases, the nurse may collaborate with the respiratory therapist as follows:
   a. Cut off the faulty end of the inflating line with scissors (Fig. 27–2).
   b. Insert a short 18- to 23-gauge blunt needle.
   c. Attach a three-way stopcock.
   d. Use a 10-ml syringe to inflate the cuff with air, as shown in Figure 27–2.
   e. Turn the stopcock to the patient to off position. The assembled device may be taped to a tongue depressor for stabilization and protection (Sills, 1986).
6. Always note the type of nasogastric (NG) tube in the intubated patient. Change a large NG tube (e.g., Salem sump tube) to a small pediatric feeding tube, whenever possible. An NG tube promotes higher cuff pressures (mechanism discussed previously) and produces the inability to swallow when the cuff is overdistended. Gastric secretions may follow the NG tube to the hypopharynx, where, together with infected pharyngeal secretions, they are aspirated into the lungs. Keeping the head of the bed elevated may help prevent aspiration in the last case.

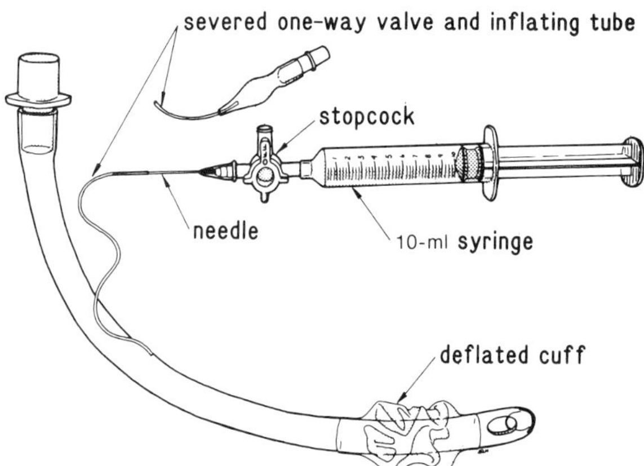

Figure 27–2. Attachments for emergency cuff inflation in case of a faulty inflating line. (Reproduced by permission from Sills, J. An emergency cuff inflation technique. *Respiratory care*, 31(3):200, 1986.)

Dealing with a Cuff Leak

One of the most difficult problems in cuff management is identifying and dealing with a cuff leak. A leak may exist around the cuff or within the inflation system, and which type of leak may be difficult to determine. A minimal leak around the cuff is normal when the minimal leak technique (MLT) is used for cuff inflation. If the leak's size increases and exhaled tidal volumes decrease, the leak may be eliminated by simply turning the head and shoulders slightly or by changing body position in some other way.

Sometimes damage to the cuff, inflation valve, or inflation tube produces a very slow leak. Over one or more days, the cuff requires more and more air for inflation, but the patient's respiratory status is unaffected. This problem is relatively easy to deal with. Replacement of the pilot balloon or insertion of a stopcock into a malfunctioning valve may stop the leak. If the leak persists, the leak is probably in the cuff itself. The physician is called, and the tube is replaced at a convenient time.

In the critical care setting, other signs may accompany the loss of inflation volume and demand immediate attention. A large air leak may be felt at the nose or mouth and around the stoma of a tracheostomy tube. The ventilator patient may exhibit low exhaled volumes—the exhaled tidal volume is less than the preset inspired volume by at least 100 cc. When a significant leak is present or when a patient shows signs of hypoxemia, the clinician disconnects the patient from the ventilator and performs manual bagging. Determination of the problem is postponed until the hypoxemia reverses. More air may be injected via the cuff's inflating tube to seal the trachea and permit adequate ventilation.

As the situation permits and before cuff inflation, the pharynx may be suctioned, and the cuff completely deflated. If the amount aspirated equals the amount previously instilled, the inflation system is patent, and other factors are responsible for the leak, such as change in body position, tracheal dilatation, and increased ventilator pressures applied to noncompliant lungs. This approach allows the clinician to rule out a defect in the inflation system. The physician is called if the leak reoccurs. Though the cuff may be patent, a tube with a larger internal diameter may be indicated to seal off the leak between the cuff and tracheal wall. Most important, *do not continue to add air into the cuff*!

TUBE STABILIZATION

During the intubation period, interventions focus on the prevention of unnecessary tube movement or external pressure to the tube. External forces applied to an endotracheal tube are readily transmitted from the lips or nares to the posterior pharynx, posterior rim of the glottis, and cuff site, causing further trauma to the mucosa. The same principle applies to a tracheostomy tube, except the mucosa may suffer more damage because the tube is short, and forces are not buffered by the upper airway.

Taping the Tube

After intubation, the endotracheal tube is taped securely to the face. Different techniques are used, but most clinicians first apply benzoin or a similar protective substance to the sides of the face and tube to make the tape stick better. A long strip of 1-in adhesive tape is used to encircle the neck and secure the tube as shown in Chapter 25. Care is taken to pull the nasal tube away from the alae to prevent ischemia. For an oral tube, the tape should leave the mouth accessible for mouth care and allow for full movement of the head. Since secretions tend to loosen the tape, the tape is changed every day, and the oral tube is moved from one side of the mouth to the other before retaping. This procedure provides an opportunity to carefully inspect the nose and mouth with a flashlight for signs of infection and pressure necrosis. Also, daily mouth care may be given at the same time (description to follow), and the oral airway, if present, changed or removed for cleaning.

Stabilization of the Ventilator Circuit

Stabilization of the ventilator circuit is another way to reduce leverage and traction on the airway. The tubing is suspended by an overhead or side support (Fig. 27–3). If necessary, a small towel is used to support the tubing's weight and to elevate the circuit off the patient's chest. In any case, the tubing is not elevated above the level of the tube's 15-mm adaptor. Such action promotes the drainage of water condensation in the tubing into the patient's lungs. Other actions to reduce leverage on the tube include utilization of the two-way swivel adaptor to decrease rotational forces and utilization of the elastic connectors on the ventilator circuit to act as shock absorbers.

Removing Water Condensation

When water condenses in the tubing, the circuit may be momentarily disconnected from the patient, and the water is drained into a separate bowl or an in-line water trap (Fig. 27–4). Keeping the tubing free of water condensation reduces the weight of the circuit, relieves the pressure on the artificial airway, and at the same time facilitates the laminar flow of gas. To prevent contamination of respiratory equipment, water is *never* drained backwards into a humidifier or nebulizer.

Eliciting Patient Cooperation

The alert patient is encouraged to hold the ventilator tubing during turning or moving in bed.

Anxious patients who repeatedly try to talk are reminded that the absence of vocalization is normal, since the tube passes through the vocal cords (i.e., endotracheal tube) or bypasses them (i.e., tracheostomy tube). Rather than allow attempts at vocalization, which may cause frustration and laryngeal damage, with endotracheal tube only, the nurse encourages the patient to use paper and pencil, magic slate, or another means to communicate concerns and wishes (see Table 17–5 for ways to establish a communication system).

Every effort is made to quickly control agitated or combative patients. If providing reassurance and support has no effect, such patients are sedated and

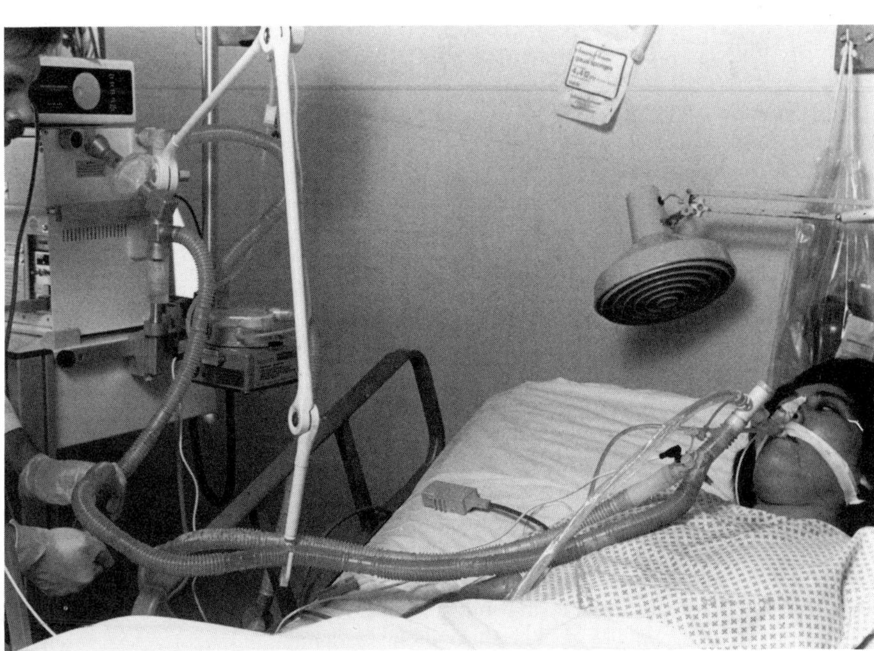

Figure 27–3. General setup for ventilator and breathing circuit.

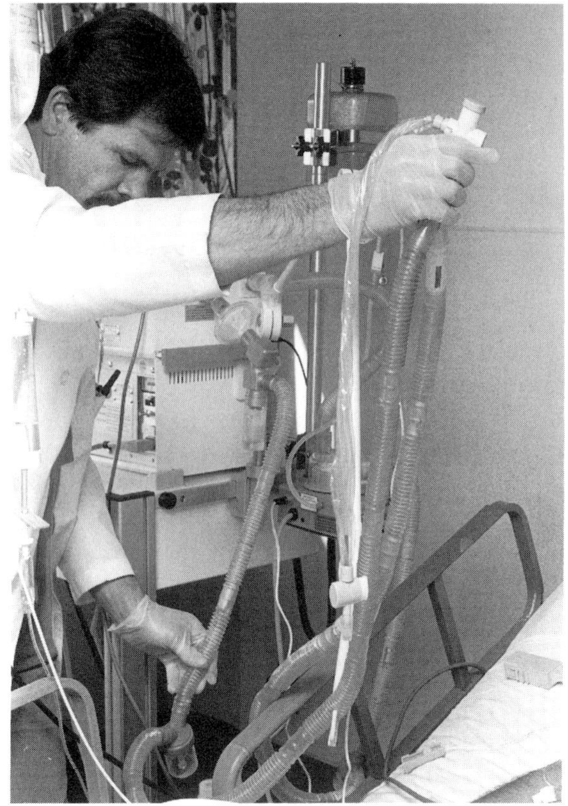

Figure 27–4. Draining water from a breathing circuit. Water is emptied into a small plastic jar (water trap) placed in-line, close to the ventilator.

restrained to prevent accidental extubation. Some intensive care units routinely apply loose restraints to the wrists for all patients with endotracheal tubes, because of the high incidence of accidental extubations. Though restraints may stimulate feelings of helplessness and hopelessness, most patients tolerate them if they are told that they serve to protect them from inadvertently pulling the tube out. Removing restraints during lucid moments during the day may be safe for some patients, as long as they are monitored closely. However, they should be ready to be applied again at times when sensorium is likely to change (e.g., at night and when hypoxemia or electrolyte disorders are present). Children or adults who react to restraints with aggressive behavior may tolerate wrapping the hands with gauze, without tying the wrists to the bed.

HUMIDIFICATION

When an endotracheal or tracheostomy tube bypasses the upper airway, the body has no way to warm and humidify air before it reaches the lungs. Without warming and humidification, dry, cold air passes down the trachea, impairing mucociliary clearance, drying secretions, and promoting formation of crusts. Crust formation in turn can obstruct both artificial and natural airways and contributes to atelectasis and pneumonia.

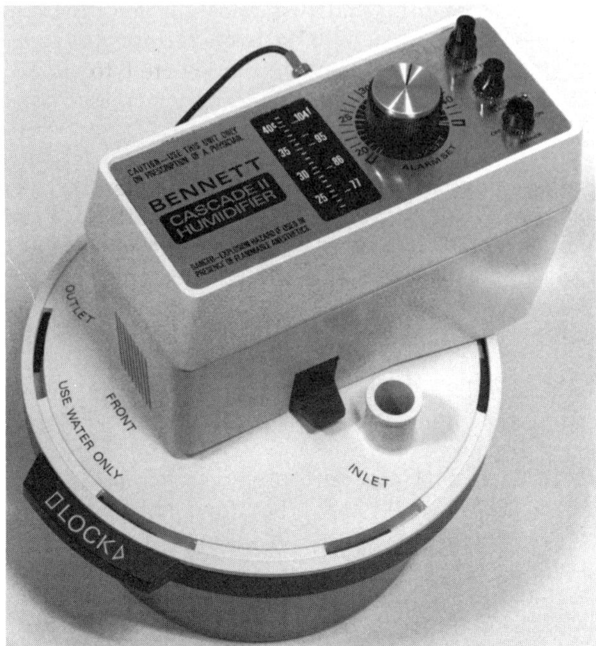

Figure 27–5. Bennett Cascade humidifier with immersion heater. (Courtesy of the Puritan-Bennet Corp., Lenexa, Kansas.)

A humidifier, such as the Bennett Cascade, is used to bring inspired gas to 100% relative humidity and warm gas to body temperature. The Bennett Cascade with its immersion heater is connected to many ventilators (Fig. 27–5). It is preferred over many other bubble diffusion type humidifiers because it produces more bubbles and smaller bubbles at higher gas flows.

The spontaneously breathing intubated patient may be connected to a humidifier or nebulizer via a *T-piece* or *T-tube* apparatus (Fig. 27–6). This apparatus has a 14-in reservoir tube on the expiratory side to prevent the patient from breathing in cool, dry, room air. If the patient inhales room air, more tubing may be added to the reservoir, and liter flow may be increased

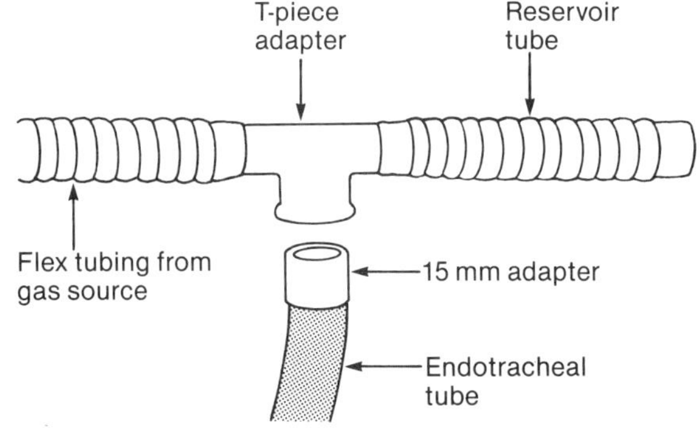

Figure 27–6. T-piece apparatus for attachment to an endotracheal tube.

so that it is greater than the patient's minute ventilation. For a patient with high minute ventilation, the Bennett Cascade humidifier is connected to a high capacity flow meter so that flow can be increased from 15 L/min, as in a conventional setup, to 40 or more. The setup is ordered as "high flow cascade," and FIO_2 is adjusted via an in-line oxygen blender. Unless secretions are thick, a humidifier is better than a nebulizer because humidification avoids the side effects associated with mist therapy (e.g., wheezing and increased shortness of breath).

The nurse and respiratory therapist are responsible for monitoring gas temperature in heated humidifers and nebulizers. Appropriate temperature for high humidity is usually between 37° and 38° C, and never above 40° C (104° F). Monitoring involves listening for activation of a temperature alarm (see Chapter 28), reading an in-line thermometer, or feeling breathing tubes during monitoring of vital signs. Gas temperatures over 38° C or tubes that are too hot to touch indicate gas overheating, a cause of airway burns, thin, watery secretions, and patient discomfort.

BRONCHIAL HYGIENE

Adequate humidification and fluid intake help to liquefy secretions and facilitate their removal. Combined with frequent repositioning of the patient, these interventions may prevent mucus retention and pneumonia.

Position changes every 1 to 2 hours promote ventilation to all lung segments and help to drain retained mucus into large airways and to stimulate deep breathing and coughing. While turning patients, the nurse may notice that some become more short of breath on one particular side. In patients with unilateral lung disease, such as atelectasis or pneumonia, a lower PaO_2 may occur when the diseased lung is dependent (Remolina et al, 1981). A ventilation and perfusion abnormality develops because the increased pulmonary blood flow to dependent diseased alveoli is mismatched with the decreased ventilation to the same area. If a preference for one side is noted, a blood gas is taken while the patient is on the opposite side; FIO_2 is increased, if hypoxemia exists.

The patient may require more aggressive therapy, including postural drainage (see Chapter 19) and aspiration of secretions from the lungs (discussed subsequently), if the bronchial hygiene measures presented fail to prevent or alleviate mucus retention.

MONITORING FOR COMPLICATIONS

The patient's nose, sinuses, ears, mouth, pharynx, neck, and chest are evaluated daily for the presence of infections and other complications.

Pneumonia is always a potential complication because the tube impairs coughing and the ability to swallow pharyngeal secretions. The presence of both respiratory disease and tracheal intubation predisposes the intensive care patient to colonization of the upper airway with gram-negative bacilli, which, when aspirated, may cause pneumonia.

Monitoring for pneumonia involves inspecting sputum (see Chapter 12) and sending a sputum sample to the laboratory for culture, sensitivity, and Gram's stain. For mucus-producing patients, a sample is sent every three days or when signs of infection appear. These signs include any change in the color or amount of sputum, fever, increased white blood cell (WBC) count, and radiologic evidence of a new or progressive pulmonary infiltrate. WBCs and intracellular bacteria in the sputum confirm the diagnosis of pneumonia and guide the physician in the choice of antibiotic.

The nurse monitors other signs and symptoms that may indicate complications (Table 27–1). Finally, the nurse consults with the physician daily to determine whether intubation is still indicated.

Table 27–1. SIGNS AND SYMPTOMS OF COMPLICATIONS DURING INTUBATION

Signs and Symptoms	Complications	Interventions
Persistent coughing	Tube misplacement if chest x-ray film indicates tube tip is at the carina. Stimulation of irritant receptors produces coughing. Bronchospasm if accompanied by decreased breath sounds or wheezing. Airway irritability if no significant change in lung sounds. Coughing should be controlled to minimize laryngotracheal injury.	Call physician to reposition tube 5 ± 2 cm above carina. Call physician. The patient needs bronchodilator therapy. Stabilize the tube to prevent unnecessary movement. Provide reassurance so patient is less likely to become agitated. Instill a few cc of liquid anesthetic down the tube to help reduce coughing.
Unilateral decreased breath sounds, usually of left lung Chest x-ray finding of right bronchial intubuation	Accidental intubation of right main stem bronchus.	Call physician to reposition tube 5 ± 2 cm above carina. Increase FIO_2, if signs of hypoxemia are present.
Wheezing Decreased breath sounds	Bronchospasm due to cardiopulmonary disease or intolerance to mist or ultrasonic therapy.	Call physician to evaluate need for more aggressive bronchodilator therapy or a change from a nebulizer to a humidifier.

Table continued on following page

Table 27–1. SIGNS AND SYMPTOMS OF COMPLICATIONS DURING INTUBATION *Continued*

Signs and Symptoms	Complications	Interventions
Change in the amount, consistency, color, or odor of sputum Rhonchi Fever Increased white blood cell count Infiltrate on chest x-ray film	Pulmonary infection.	Send a tracheal aspirate for culture, sensitivity test, and Gram's stain; continue to monitor changes in the mucus, when suctioning the patient. Consult physician and other health team members to evaluate entire bronchial hygiene program. If mucus is thick, increase humidification and hydration and try bronchial lavage before suctioning. Turn and deep breathe q1 to 2h. Implement postural drainage with percussion and vibration over area of infiltrate, as tolerated. Administer antibiotic therapy, as ordered by physician. Change from minimal leak to no-leak technique for cuff inflation, if aspiration is suspected or possible, given the patient's circumstances. Use careful handwashing and strict aseptic technique when indicated to prevent the spread of organisms. (Other preventive measures are described in Table 28–5).*
Agitation Self extubation attempts	Pain or discomfort from the tube or cuff, often exacerbated by accompanying anxiety and disorientation. ABG abnormalities.	Stabilize tube to prevent unnecessary movement. Provide sedation. Use cautiously for spontaneously breathing patients and hold medication, if respiratory rate or V_T decreases significantly. Provide reassurance. Encourage significant others to visit frequently. Apply loose restraints to wrists to prevent accidental extubation. Encourage use of pad and pencil or magic slate to communicate feelings or desires. Orient patient to time, place, and person, continually repeating key information, if necessary. Obtain ABG and medical evaluation, if agitation is not controlled.
Suctioning of food or gastric contents from tracheostomy or endotracheal tube	Pulmonary aspiration from incompetent glottis, cuff underinflation, leak in cuff, or (rare) tracheoesophageal fistula.	Inflate cuff to minimal occluding volume. Place patient NPO and call physician. Tracheoesophageal fistula may be confirmed by esophagoscopy or methylene blue dye challenge. Instillation of blue methylene dye into the stomach followed by suctioning blue-tinged secretions from the endotracheal tube confirm a TE fistula. The pilot balloon or entire tube may be changed, if malfunction of the cuff inflation system is suspected.
Pulsating tracheostomy tube	Cuff or shaft is resting against a major systemic artery.	Protect tube from movement. Call physician for immediate medical evaluation. If erosion into the artery occurs, exsanguination may follow.
Cuff requiring more and more air for inflation Air leak noted around stoma or over nose or mouth Low exhaled tidal volumes, i.e., greater than 100 cc discrepancy between exhaled V_T and preset inspiratory V_T	Leak in cuff inflation system. Leak around the cuff due to tracheal dilatation, increased ventilator pressures applied to noncompliant lungs, or both.	Manually bag the patient to reverse hypoxemia. Inject a few cc of extra air into cuff, if necessary, for a seal. Check the patency of the inflation system. Amount aspirated should equal amount of air instilled. Check cuff pressure. Call physician. Other possible interventions: replace pilot balloon in some tube designs, insert stopcock into malfunctioning inflation valve, change head or body position. (See text for discussion of air leaks and emergency cuff inflation techniques.)

Table 27–1. SIGNS AND SYMPTOMS OF COMPLICATIONS DURING INTUBATION *Continued*

Signs and Symptoms	Complications	Interventions
High cuff pressure of greater than 25 cmH_2O	Right or left main stem bronchial intubation.	Reposition tube in trachea, as previously described.
	Kinked tube.	Support ventilator tubing to avoid extra traction on the tube. For oral tube, reposition tube to the other side of the mouth, and try to insert an oral airway to stabilize tube more. As a last resort, the physician may extubate and reintubate with a nasal tube or a tube of a more kink-resistant material.
	Lumenal obstruction by secretions or blood. Usually occurs when secretions are thick, humidification inadequate, or intubation traumatic.	The tube must be changed. Call physician and prepare for extubation and reintubation.
	Malposition of tube's bevel against tracheal wall.	Manually bag the patient to try to establish airway patency. If necessary, the physician may reposition tube or replace it with a different tube with a different bevel angle.
	Associated with dramatic change in body position, e.g., supine to prone or far side lying position.	Withdraw air in cuff to achieve safe cuff pressure. For Lanz tube, insert syringe into inflation valve periodically to allow pressure equalization between cuff and pilot balloon.
	May be unavoidable, when high ventilator pressures or PEEP is used.	Monitor intracuff pressure and report any further rise in cuff pressure.
Bubbling of secretions in mouth *Sudden* ability to talk Low exhaled volumes Large discrepancy between exhaled V_T and preset inspiratory V_T	Cuff rupture.	Verify problem by deflating and reinflating cuff. Assume cuff rupture if unlimited air is aspirated; trachea does not seal (i.e., ventilator does not trigger) with injection of air into the cuff; or external inflating system seems patent. Manually bag the patient with 100% oxygen, call the physician, and prepare for extubation and reintubation.
Persistent hoarseness after extubation	Laryngeal ulceration, granuloma, synechia, or motor paresis.	Caution patient not to strain voice. Apply cool or heated aerosol or ultrasonic nebulization. Monitor for signs of upper airway obstruction
Days, weeks, or months after extubation: Dyspnea Cough Difficulty raising secretions Wheezing Stridor (i.e., a late sign—airway diameter less than 5 mm)	Laryngeal or tracheal stenosis.	Monitor patient for up to 6 months postextubation for increasing signs and symptoms of upper airway obstruction. Further medical evaluation may include laryngoscopy, fiberoptic endoscopy, tomograms, flow volume loops, or other tests.

*Adherence to new Universal Precaution (UP) guidelines recommended by Centers for Disease Control may indirectly decrease risk for pulmonary infection. Guidelines are currently implemented hospital-wide in many acute settings in an effort to reduce risk of blood exposure, particularly to AIDS and hepatitis pathogens, and to reduce risk of cross contamination between patients and health workers when infection status of patient is unknown. Replacing Blood and Body Fluid Precautions UP guidelines require the health worker to wear gloves when contact with any patient is anticipated.

Routine Tracheostomy Care

Most nursing interventions focus on keeping the stoma and tube clean and free of secretions and mucus encrustations in an effort to prevent infection and maintain airway patency. A procedure for routine cleaning is reviewed in the box on pages 676 and 677. Other pertinent information is summarized, as follows:

1. Routine cleaning is performed at least once a shift and PRN. When secretions are copious, the stoma is cleaned q4h, and the dressing is changed q1 to 2h, as needed.
2. Postintubation cleaning is performed q4h for the first 2 days. During this period, some surgeons prefer that the tape *not* be changed to avoid any possibility of excessive pressure to the tube and stoma.
3. Continual oozing of secretions around the stoma may indicate the need for more frequent pharyngeal suctioning to keep the stoma clean. Keep in mind that secretions around the stoma may come from two sources as follows:
   a. Oral or nasal secretions dripping down the pharynx, past incompetent vocal cords, and to immediately above the cuff.
   b. Mucus that is coughed up around the cuff or pushed upward by a large ventilator breath.
4. The stoma is a surgical wound requiring aseptic care. Sterile gloves are essential to prevent infection as well as cross contamination between patients.
5. Use of a tracheostomy care kit is essential for

cleaning tubes with an inner cannula because it provides a sterile pipe cleaner or brush. Otherwise, it is convenient but not absolutely necessary.

6. Disposable cannula tracheostomy tubes (e.g., Shiley) do not require cleaning of the inner cannula. Rather, the disposable inner cannula is discarded and another sterile one is inserted into the outer cannula.
7. The tracheostomy tape is tied loosely enough to allow one finger between tape and neck. If the fit is too tight, the stoma is covered and compressed, predisposing the patient to infection and subcutaneous emphysema; air cannot escape from under skin layers. If the fit is too loose, the tube moves in and out during respiration, predisposing the patient to stomal and tracheal injury as well as to unintentional extubation.
8. Tracheostomy buttons are *not* removed for cleaning. Cleaning around the stoma site is sufficient.

ROUTINE TRACHEOSTOMY CARE

EQUIPMENT

Needed items are provided in a prepackaged tracheostomy kit, except for those in the top row of the illustration.

Top row: hydrogen peroxide (H_2O_2); normal saline (NS); scissors.

Center row: containers for H_2O_2 and NS; sterile precut tracheostomy dressing (sterile 4 × 4 gauze without cotton filler is also acceptable); clean tracheostomy tape.

Bottom row: sterile gloves; cotton swabs (Q tips), brush or pipe cleaners, forceps, sterile 4 × 4s.

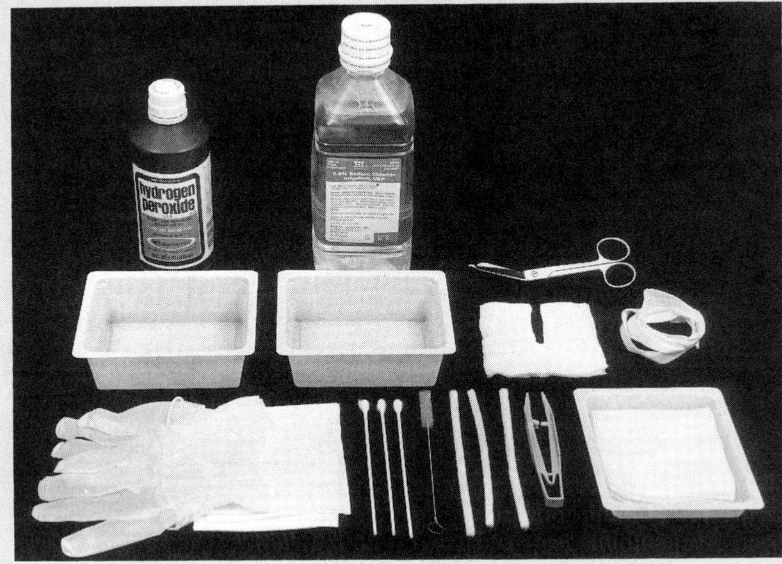

PROCEDURE

1. Wash hands.
2. Explain procedure to patient and provide reassurance.
3. Suction trachea and then the pharynx, if necessary. Remove the old tracheostomy dressing and wipe off excess mucus by the stoma with a sterile 4 × 4 gauze.
4. Put on sterile gloves.
5. Remove the inner cannula, if present (A). Place the cannula in a bowl of 1:1 solution of H_2O_2 and normal saline, and quickly brush the inside and outside of the cannula, with a pipe cleaner or brush provided in a tracheostomy care kit (B). Rinse the cannula in a bowl of normal saline, shake dry, and lock back into place, while stabilizing the flange (C, D).

FOR PATIENTS WITH BORDERLINE LOW Pa_{O_2}***s***

If possible, replace the inner cannula with an extra disposable one. Take your time during cleaning.

6. Dip Q tips or 4 × 4 gauze in H_2O_2 and thoroughly clean *first* the stoma and *then* the external portion of the tube, carefully removing encrusted secretions. Dry area with sterile 4 × 4 gauze.
7. Apply zinc oxide or antibiotic ointment to red or irritated skin around the stoma, if ordered.
8. Change the tracheostomy tape, if soiled. Use prepared tape in tracheostomy kit or cut a long (20-in) piece of tape in half. Make 1/8-in slits about 3/4 in from one end of each tape. Attach tapes to flange, as shown in E. Pull the strings tightly, extend them around the neck, and tie a secure square knot or knotted bow away from the flange and stoma area. Remove the old tape.

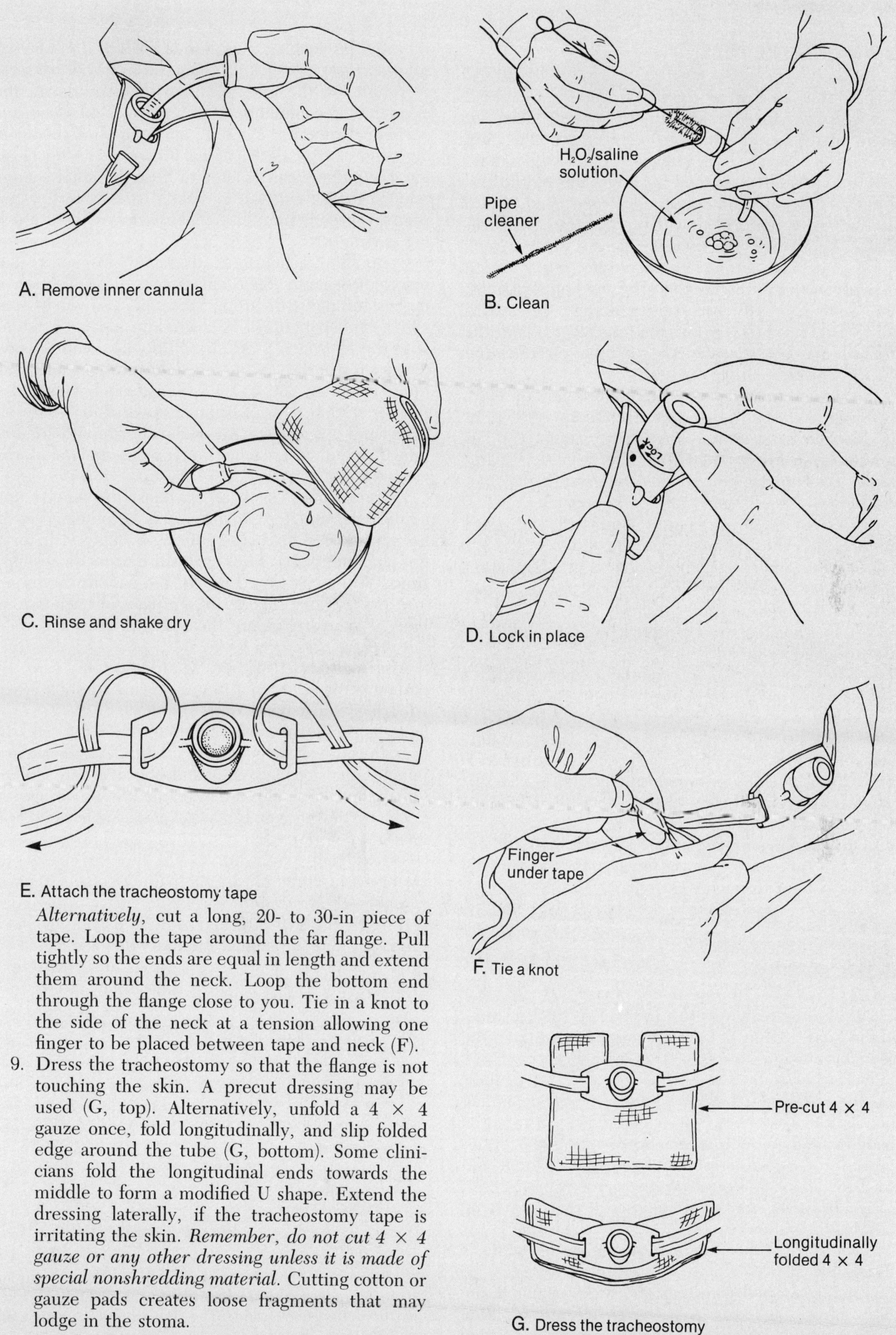

A. Remove inner cannula

B. Clean

C. Rinse and shake dry

D. Lock in place

E. Attach the tracheostomy tape

F. Tie a knot

G. Dress the tracheostomy

Alternatively, cut a long, 20- to 30-in piece of tape. Loop the tape around the far flange. Pull tightly so the ends are equal in length and extend them around the neck. Loop the bottom end through the flange close to you. Tie in a knot to the side of the neck at a tension allowing one finger to be placed between tape and neck (F).

9. Dress the tracheostomy so that the flange is not touching the skin. A precut dressing may be used (G, top). Alternatively, unfold a 4 × 4 gauze once, fold longitudinally, and slip folded edge around the tube (G, bottom). Some clinicians fold the longitudinal ends towards the middle to form a modified U shape. Extend the dressing laterally, if the tracheostomy tape is irritating the skin. *Remember, do not cut 4 × 4 gauze or any other dressing unless it is made of special nonshredding material.* Cutting cotton or gauze pads creates loose fragments that may lodge in the stoma.

CHANGING THE TUBE

The physician changes the first tracheostomy tube 2 to 7 days after surgery. This first change may require retention sutures or a hook to secure the trachea and prevent its slippage back into the wound before tube insertion. A well-established tract develops by the end of the first week, and subsequent tube changes are usually easily performed without the use of instruments. Thereafter, the tube is changed once a week in the acute care setting and about once every month or every two months for the clinic or home patient. The acute care patient is given nothing by mouth (NPO) for a few hours before the tube change, and the stomach may be evacuated via NG tube to reduce the chance of aspiration.

The tracheostomy tube's obturator and an extra tracheostomy tube of the same size are always kept at the bedside in case of accidental extubation or other problems. To insert a new tube after accidental extubation, the clinician puts on gloves, if readily available, and follows these steps as quickly as possible:

1. Remove the inner cannula, if present, and insert the obturator into the outer cannula.
2. Deflate the cuff. If the patient is in no apparent distress, inflate the cuff first to check for leaks and then deflate for insertion.
3. Lubricate the tip with sterile, water-soluble lubricant or lidocaine jelly.
4. Insert the new tube, carefully following the stomal tract to avoid the tip's displacement into surrounding tissue.
5. Hold the tube in place and remove the obturator.
6. Inflate the cuff and reattach tube to ventilator.
7. Check equality of breath sounds and peak inspiratory pressure on the ventilator, which should return to preextubation level.
8. If coughing or respiratory distress persists, remove the tube and try again or attempt to manually bag the patient through the stoma.
9. Call the physician.

HOME SETTING

Care for the patient with a permanent tracheostomy in the home setting is basically the same as that in the acute care setting, except for a few differences. First, since tracheostomy care is usually done by the patient, not the nurse or some other person, cross contamination is not a concern. Clean technique with careful handwashing initially is practiced during the entire procedure instead of sterile technique. Gloves and tracheostomy kits are an unnecessary expense in most cases. However, gloves are advised if another person besides the patient is cleaning the tracheostomy.

To clean the inner cannula, the patient has either a disposable paper cup or a glass dish that can be thoroughly washed with soap and water or put in the dishwasher afterwards. A preferred cleaning solution is a 1:1 ratio of hydrogen peroxide and tap or distilled water. After soaking the cannula for 2 or 3 minutes in solution, a pipe cleaner may be utilized to scrub secretions off the inner walls of the cannula. A pipe cleaner is recommended over a brush because it is cheaper over time, since all such supplies should be disposed of after the cleaning procedure. After cleaning, the patient is instructed to rinse the inner cannula under running tap water, shake excess water off, and reinsert directly into the tracheostomy, without touching any object.

Generally tracheostomy dressings are not recommended because they encourage the collection of mucus and moisture around the stoma (Hodgkin et al, 1984). The patient is instructed to clean the stoma with the hydrogen peroxide solution and cotton applicators once a day and as needed, while cleaning the inner cannula. The tracheostomy tape is changed at the same time. In addition, patient and family are instructed to report any signs of skin irritation or infection and any changes in mucus noticed during cleaning.

Extra supplies, such as tracheostomy tape, cotton applicators, and 4 × 4 gauze, may be obtained at the hospital before discharge, during a clinic visit, or in the community at a local drug store or medical supply store. When cost is a concern, the patient can improvise and use long shoe strings in place of tracheostomy tape, if shoe strings are washed with soap and water between uses.

After daily tracheostomy or laryngectomy care, the patient with an open tube may wish to stick a self-adhering stomashield onto the neck (Fig. 27–7). A foam flap covers the tube opening, filters dust and dirt from the air, and helps reduce sometimes embarrassing mucus expulsions into the atmosphere or onto clothes. Other types of shields are available that tie around the neck, or the patient can wear a washable neck scarf for the same purpose.

Patient and family are taught how to change the tracheostomy tube in case the patient coughs it out by mistake. The procedure is relatively easy in the home setting because the tracheostomy is usually of longer duration, and the stomal tract is well established. At home, as in the acute care setting, an extra tube is always kept. The procedure is basically the same as

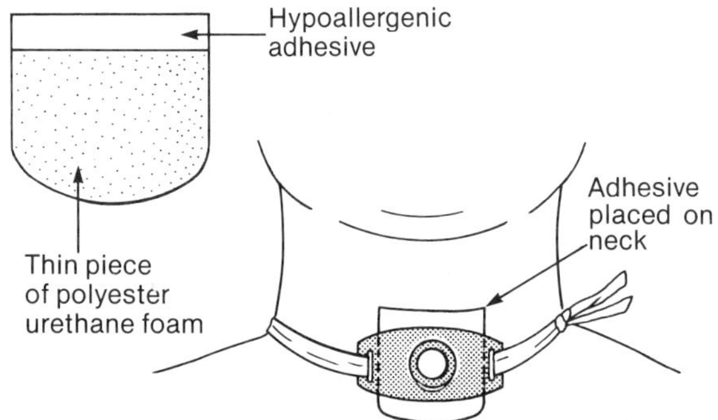

Figure 27–7. The stomashield (left) is placed on the neck so that it covers the tracheostomy tube opening, as shown by the dotted lines (right). The stomashield is manufactured by Medmart, Inc., Los Angeles, California.

previously described, except cuff inflation is usually unnecessary, since in most of these patients, the tracheostomy tubes are cuffless. After reinsertion, the patient is asked to take a few deep breaths and to notice how the tube feels in order to check for adequacy of ventilation and correct tube position.

Extubation (Decannulation)

Endotracheal tube removal is referred to as *extubation*, while tracheostomy tube removal is more specifically referred to as *decannulation*. Extubation (decannulation) occurs when indications for intubation are no longer present and when the patient is able to clear his own secretions and protect the airway from aspiration.

The procedure is explained to the patient and postextubation respiratory therapy is set up ahead of time to prevent oxygen desaturation immediately after the procedure. FIO_2 is usually set 0.10 higher than that provided immediately before extubation. If a nasal prong unit is ordered, it is applied beforehand.

The patient is preoxygenated, and the lungs and pharynx are thoroughly suctioned. At the peak of a deep breath, the cuff is deflated, and the tube is pulled out quickly as the patient exhales. Then, the patient is encouraged to deep breathe and cough. This procedure is about the same for decannulation, except the stoma is covered with an occlusive dressing.

POSTEXTUBATION MONITORING

Postextubation monitoring involves staying with the patient until he feels confident that he can breathe on his own without difficulty. Also, the nurse observes closely for stridor and other signs indicating laryngospasm and supraglottic or subglottic edema. Because 22 to 35% of patients have laryngeal incompetence following general anesthesia, such patients are monitored for signs of possible aspiration. Hoarseness is present in the majority of patients and is due to edema, ulceration, granulomata, synechia, or motor paresis. Sore throat and dysphagia develop in about half of extubated patients. Most complaints are minor and resolve within days, although hoarseness may persist for several weeks in some cases.

If stridor occurs, it is treated with corticosteroids and a topical aerosol vasoconstrictor (e.g., racemic epinephrine), and reintubation is performed, if the stridor still persists. Since stridor is a late and serious sign indicating airway narrowing to less than 5 mm, monitoring focuses on detecting earlier and more subtle signs of upper airway obstruction, such as mild dyspnea, cough, and difficulty raising secretions. Sometimes, signs are absent at first and then develop insidiously over 3 weeks to 5 months, as the result of glottic or subglottic stenosis. Most signs, however, appear within the first 3 weeks of extubation.

Patients with tracheostomy stomas are reassured that stomas will close on their own within 4 or 5 days. Until that time, coughing is performed with pressure to the stoma to prevent air leakage and a weak, ineffective cough.

In the weeks following decannulation, clinical problems may include presence of an unavoidable scar or a keloid formation, persistent open stoma, and dysphagia. Tracheal stenosis is the most common serious complication and is most frequent at the stomal level and less frequent at the cuff level or tip of the tube.

PSYCHOSOCIAL ADJUSTMENT

Patients who are concerned about the appearance of the residual stomal scar are reminded that the scar is a small price to pay for the tracheostomy, a life-

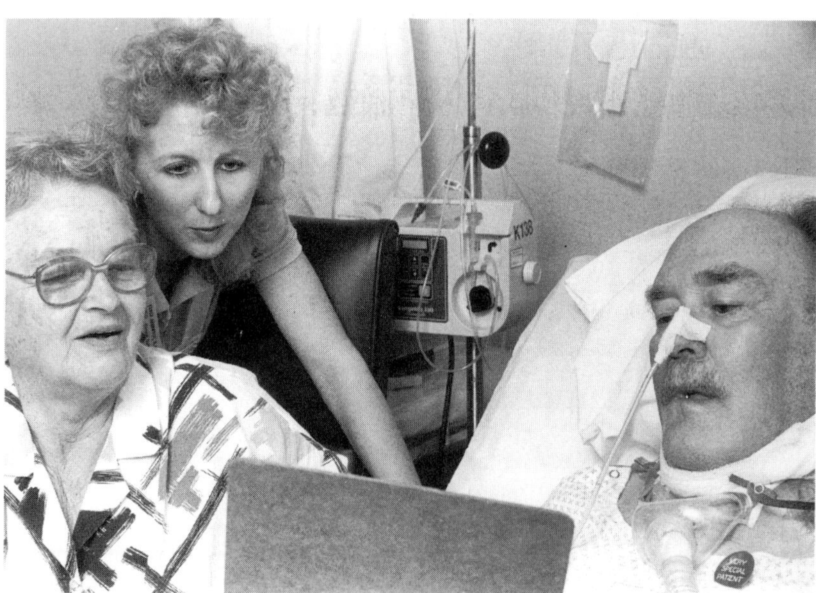

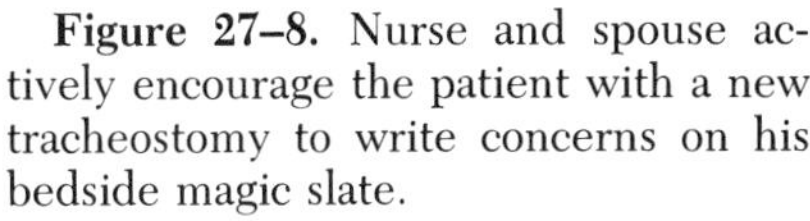

Figure 27–8. Nurse and spouse actively encourage the patient with a new tracheostomy to write concerns on his bedside magic slate.

saving measure. When a body image problem persists, the nurse encourages the patient to verbalize concerns related to the scar. In some cases, the nurse may encourage the self-conscious patient to wear a neck scarf or a top with a high neck (e.g., turtle neck style shirt), until the scar becomes less obvious to a casual observer.

This same basic approach may be used for the patient who is adapting to a new tracheostomy. Furthermore, in both cases, the nurse encourages the family to support the patient by actively listening to his concerns and by affirming either verbally or nonverbally that they care about the patient, regardless of any physical flaw (Fig. 27–8).

Simultaneously, the nurse and family work together to gradually refocus the patient's attention away from the tracheostomy or tracheostomy scar, and towards more participation in activities of daily living. (See information on self-care education, Chapter 17.) This approach facilitates the transition from the sick role to self care, thus helping the patient reconstruct a more positive body image.

Naso-oral and Tracheobronchial Suctioning

Intubated and nonintubated patients who cannot cough or expectorate respiratory secretions on their own may need naso-oral or tracheobronchial suctioning. In these cases, the nurse uses a suction catheter attached to a vacuum source to remove secretions from the mouth and lungs and to maintain airway patency (Fig. 27–9).

INDICATIONS

Indications for tracheobronchial suctioning include the presence of audible secretions, rhonchal fremitus, or rhonchi in the chest that persist in spite of the patient's efforts to cough.

Indications for naso-oral or oropharyngeal suctioning include the pooling of secretions in the nasal or oral pharynx, especially above the cuff of an endotracheal tube. The pharynx is routinely suctioned before cuff deflation of an artificial airway, to prevent the aspiration of secretions into the lungs. Also, pharyngeal suctioning is sometimes employed to stimulate coughing and deep breathing in the nonintubated patient, when other more conservative measures fail to do so.

CONTRAINDICATIONS

Contraindications include profund refractory hypoxemia and an irritable myocardium manifested by increased incidence of cardiac arrhythmias. Suctioning may be contraindicated or performed with caution in patients with severe hypertension or increased intracranial pressure, since the procedure is likely to exacerbate these conditions.

COMPLICATIONS

Because of the extent and severity of potential complications, suctioning is *not* a routine procedure. Suctioning is performed only when indicated, and it should be performed only by personnel trained in proper technique. Contrary to previous beliefs, mucosal trauma associated with the procedure is believed to be related more to suctioning technique—repetition, vigor, duration, and negative pressure—rather than to suction catheter design (Jung and Gottlieb, 1976).

Brief mention of complications helps the reader understand why emphasis is placed on the establishment of an unquestionable need for suctioning and why so much emphasis is placed on the specifics of a technique. Repeated suctioning may result in subatmospheric intrapulmonic pressure, resulting in microatelectasis around the catheter tip and, if severe, atelectasis of lung segments and lobes. Continuous negative suction causes the tip to adhere to the tracheal mucosa. Upon catheter withdrawal, the tip strips the trachea of its ciliated epithelium and impairs the mucociliary escalator, predisposing the patient to mucus stasis and secretion encrustation. These changes may be accompanied by mucosal hemorrhages and erosions immediately after the cessation of vacuum (Sackner et al, 1973).

In addition, failure to adequately aspirate the left lower lobe may occur. Each catheter blindly passed through an endotracheal tube has less than a 1 in 3 chance of entering the left main stem bronchus, owing to normal anatomy at the tracheal bifurcation (see Figure 2–10A). This point may explain the increased incidence of left lower lobe secretion retention and atelectasis noted in intubated patients (Freedman and Goodman, 1982).

In any case, suctioning of the tracheobronchial tree is considered a last resort in the management of tracheobronchial secretions. Every effort is made to turn, cough, deep breathe, and even admonish the patient to expectorate secretions on his own. Not only can suctioning be a frightful experience for the patient, but it is associated with other serious side effects and complications. The evacuation of large amounts of air in addition to secretions, combined with temporary disconnection from the ventilator, results in hypoxemia (Boutros, 1970). Repeated passage of the catheter past the upper respiratory tract and into the lungs promotes bacterial colonization in the lungs, which in turn sometimes leads to pneumonia. Mechanical stimulation by the suction catheter may initiate reflex bronchoconstriction. Combined with hypoxemia, such stimulation may contribute to life-threatening arrhythmias, including bradycardia, tachyarrhythmias, premature ventricular contractions, and even cardiac arrest (i.e., asystole).

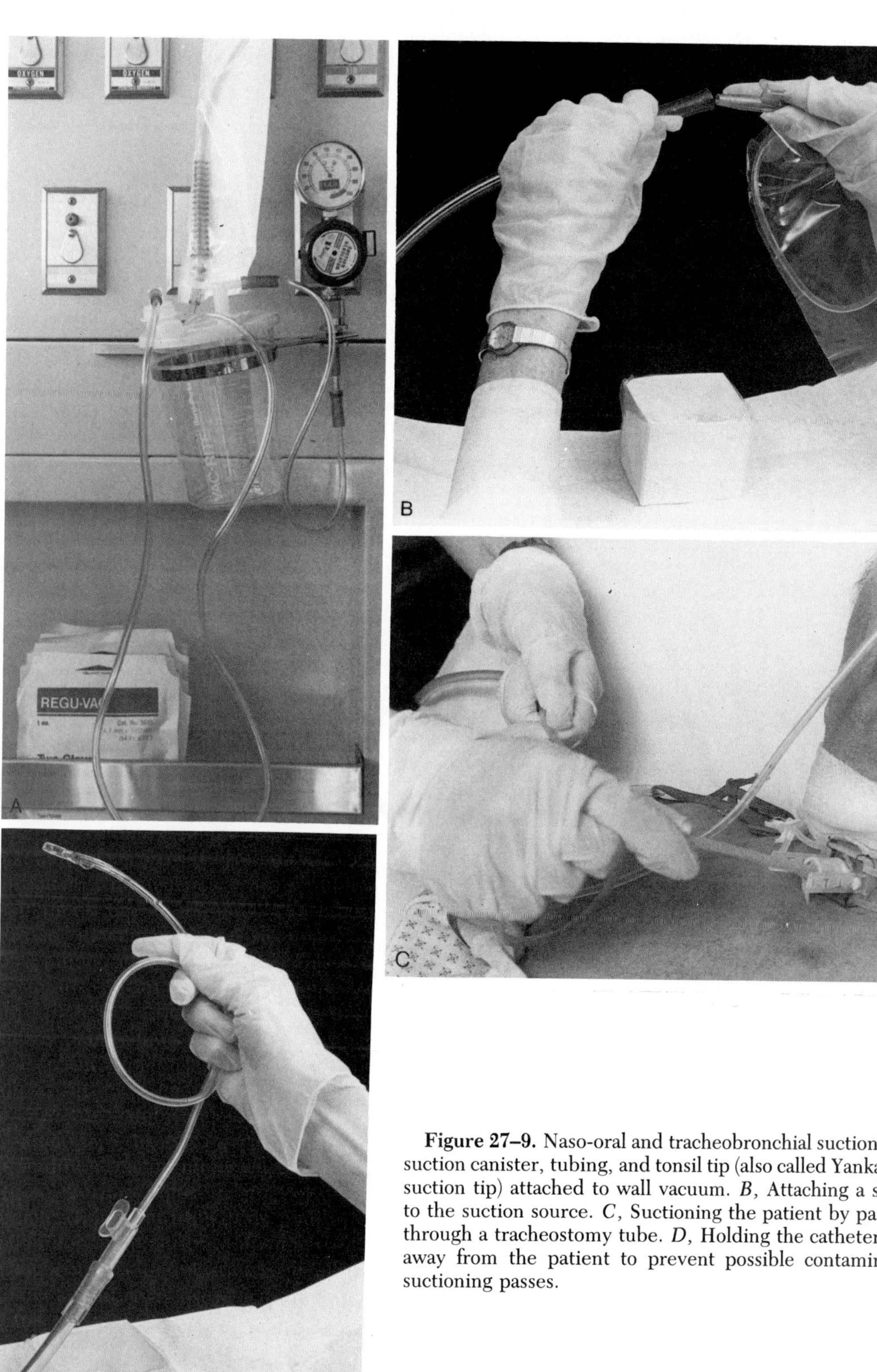

Figure 27–9. Naso-oral and tracheobronchial suctioning. *A*, Bedside suction canister, tubing, and tonsil tip (also called Yankauer pharyngeal suction tip) attached to wall vacuum. *B*, Attaching a suction catheter to the suction source. *C*, Suctioning the patient by passing a catheter through a tracheostomy tube. *D*, Holding the catheter with one hand away from the patient to prevent possible contamination between suctioning passes.

SUCTIONING PROCEDURES

Procedures for suctioning the upper and lower airways in the clinical setting are summarized in the next four boxes for quick reference. Key concepts and adaptations related to suction catheters and suctioning methods are discussed beginning on page 687.

PREPARATION FOR SUCTIONING

PROCEDURE	*RATIONALES AND PRECAUTIONS*
1. *Assemble the following equipment:* a. Portable or wall suction unit with connecting tube attached. b. Sterile suction catheters. c. Sterile gloves d. Sterile cup with 1 to 2 oz sterile water (optional). e. Towel. f. 30 cc (Lanz cuff) or 12 cc syringe. g. Water soluble lubricant. h. Clean cup or bottle of tap water for rinsing connecting tubing. i. Self-inflating resuscitator bag connected to O_2 flow meter at 15 L/min. j. Available in prepackaged kits.	Ready availability of equipment facilitates strict adherence to aseptic technique during the procedure. The cup of sterile water (or normal saline) may be used to clear the catheter of thick mucus between suctioning passes.
2. *Wash your hands.*	Handwashing with povidone-iodine (Betadine) or a similar solution is recommended in the hospital setting.
3. *Explain the procedure to the patient and provide reassurance.*	Information and reassurance helps to allay the patient's anxiety and elicit full cooperation.
4. *Check the vacuum.* a. With the connecting tubing unoccluded, the pressure gauge should read 80 to 100 mmHg.	Suctioning with inadequate or excess suction may cause severe hypoxemia. Amount of suction may vary between suction devices, even when pressure readings are the same.
b. Test the suction by briefly occluding the connecting tubing end and adjust, if necessary.	Greater than 100 mmHg pressure is not more effective in removing secretions and greatly increases trauma (Riegel and Forshee, 1985).
5. *Select an appropriate suction catheter.* a. Type: straight, angled b. Size: (French) size 14 for adults (French) size 10 for children	The straight catheter is appropriate in most cases. Use the angled catheter for left lower lobe atelectasis/consolidation. *Do not* use the Aero-flow catheter for suctioning through the nose, because the O-shaped tip may cause tissue trauma and nose bleeding.
Remember, catheter diameter should be no greater than half the internal diameter of the endotracheal or tracheostomy tube.	Too large a catheter increases the amount of negative pressure applied to the lungs and promotes atelectasis and hypoxemia. Too small a catheter increases airway resistance and requires more negative pressure to aspirate a given amount of secretions (Rindfleisch and Tyler, 1983).
6. *Place a towel over the patient's anterior chest area* (optional).	The towel protects the patient's gown from secretions that are coughed out through the artificial airway or from condensed water dripping from respiratory devices (e.g., tubing during ventilator disconnection).
7. *Put on sterile gloves.* (Use two gloves, not one glove.)	The two-glove technique protects against herpetic whitlow and cross contamination among patients, personnel, and equipment.
8. *Lubricate the catheter.* a. Place a small amount of sterile water soluble lubricant on a sterile towel or sterile glove packaging.	A water-soluble rather than an oil-based lubricant is used because the latter causes aspiration pneumonia.

PROCEDURE	*RATIONALES AND PRECAUTIONS*
b. Pick up the catheter and rub the tip and sides of the catheter in the lubricant.	Lubrication facilitates smooth catheter advancement through the upper airway or long endotracheal tube. It is rarely necessary for tracheostomy suctioning.
9. *To attach catheter to connecting tubing*	
a. Hold the catheter in the "sterile" hand and the connecting tubing in the other "clean" hand.	*Note*, Now the clean hand is available to manipulate the catheter's air vent (occlude it for suction) and to touch the patient or ventilator, as needed.
b. Attach catheter to connecting tubing.	
10. *Get ready to suction!* Carefully slide your hands towards the catheter tip.	Continuous contact with the catheter prevents loss of catheter control and inadvertent breaks in aseptic technique.

SUCTIONING THE UPPER AIRWAY

The nurse follows these steps any time nasal or oropharyneal suctioning is needed and *always* before deflating the cuff of an artificial airway. (See Chaper 24 for adaptations for suctioning through an oral or nasal artificial airway.)

PROCEDURE	*RATIONALES AND PRECAUTIONS*
1. Prepare to suction, as described on page 682.	
2. Leave the catheter air vent *open*.	
3. *For oropharyngeal suctioning*, gently insert the catheter into the mouth and advance the catheter tip about 3 to 4 inches to pooled secretions in the pharynx.	Suctioning (i.e., vent occlusion) during catheter advancement increases risk for panic reactions, tissue trauma, and hypoxemia.
a. Go deep, just above the glottis for the intubated patient.	Secretions may be pooled above the cuff of the artificial airway.
b. For supine patients in the side-lying position, concentrate on the dependent side of the oropharynx.	Secretions gravitate towards the dependent side.
Remember, when suctioning is limited to the upper airway, use the oral approach, if possible.	Suctioning through the mouth is usually less traumatic than suctioning through the nose.
4. *For nasopharyngeal suctioning*	
a. Choose a patent naris. Assessment of nasal patency involves *inspection* for the absence of nasal obstruction or recent trauma and *palpation*. Press each nostril closed separately, ask the patent to sniff each time, and choose the naris that conducts the most air.	Choosing the most patent airway reduces trauma and increases chance of successful catheter tip advancement into the pharynx. Avoid nares with nasal polyps, deviated septum towards chosen nares, swollen nasal mucosa, and history of nose bleeds.
b. Gently insert the catheter inferiorly and medially through one of the nostrils to reach pooled secretions in the pharynx.	The inferior medial direction of the tip keeps the catheter close to the nasal septum and away from conchae protruding into the passageway.
Remember, use the nasal approach when anticipating tracheobronchial suctioning in nonintubated patients or when the oral approach is impossible, e.g., clenched teeth, uncooperative patient, mouth trauma.	The nasal approach reduces sharp curves in catheter direction and facilitates entry of the catheter tip into the trachea of the nonintubated patient.
5. Slowly withdraw the catheter, while *intermittently* occluding the air vent and rotating the catheter. *Do not apply continuous suction!*	Continuous suction causes the catheter to grab the mucosa and strip the trachea unil suction is released. Also, it may cause severe hypoxemia and respiratory distress. Rotation prevents invagination of the mucosa into the catheter's tip and side ports.
6. Suction both sides of the mouth as well as the pharynx.	
a. If the patient coughs, withdraw the catheter tip, allow him to expectorate mucus to the mouth. Then, continue suctioning.	Keeping the patient involved in the procedure helps him to take at least some responsibility for self care and increases self worth. Also, PRN suctioning by

Box continued on following page

SUCTIONING THE UPPER AIRWAY Continued

PROCEDURE	*RATIONALES AND PRECAUTIONS*
b. When oropharyngeal secretions are excessive, use Yankauer suction tip attached to a separate suction source. Direct the alert patient to suction himself.	the patient reduces the amount of pooled pharyngeal secretions and, hence, risk for aspiration and mouth infection.
c. Suction through a nasopharyngeal airway, if repeated nasopharyngeal suctioning is anticipated. *Option*, suction through or next to an oral airway.	Use of an artificial airway facilitates catheter advancement, reduces tissue trauma, and maintains a patent airway.
7. Rinse the connecting tubing with tap water or a germicidal rinse.	After 8 hours, connecting tubing becomes significantly contaminated with organisms that colonize the patient's respiratory tract (Cunningham and Sergent, 1983). Most health agencies use a rinse to reduce colonization. Disposable suction cannisters and connecting tubing are discarded every 24 hours.
8. Dispose of catheter and gloves.	
a. Hold the coiled catheter in one hand. With the other hand, pull the glove off with the catheter inside.	Appropriate disposal of catheters and gloves helps prevent the spread of infection.
b. If the patient has pneumonia or is on secretion precautions, discard used supplies into a separate bag. Then, dispose of according to hospital isolation procedures.	

SUCTIONING THE LOWER AIRWAY—THE INTUBATED PATIENT

The nurse follows these steps for suctioning the tracheobronchial tree of an intubated patient. The tube's soft cuff remains inflated during the entire procedure.

PROCEDURE	*RATIONALES AND PROCEDURES*
1. Prepare to suction, as described on page 682.	
2. Preoxygenate the patient for 30 seconds to 2 minutes, as indicated by the situation.	
a. Bagging method (see page 689). Ask another person to bag while you suction.	Method and duration of preoxygenation depend on available respiratory equipment, mode of ventilation, and stability of PaO_2. Increasing FIO_2 to 1.0 or 0.40 more than resting FIO_2 is best accompanied by three to six hyperinflations.
b. Ventilator method (see page 689).	
3. Identify an entry port.	
a. Entry ports include the endotracheal or tracheostomy tube itself (disconnect the ventilator); capped swivel adaptor; or self-sealing adaptor.	
b. Whenever possible, utilize another person to stabilize the tube or adaptor during catheter advancement.	Pressure on the adaptor or tube is most likely to occur when one person performs the entire procedure. Traction on the tube in turn causes trauma to the mouth, nostril, and respiratory mucosa.
c. Two persons are usually necessary for ventilator disconnection or bagging.	Use of two persons facilitates quick, smooth, and aseptic passage of the catheter and prompt ventilator reconnection.
4. Quickly advance the catheter until resistance is met. Pull back 1 to 2 cm and suction *intermittently*, while slowly withdrawing the catheter. *Do not take longer than 10 to 15 seconds for each suctioning pass!*	If the nurse advances and withdraws the catheter smoothly and without stopping, she will be well within the 10 to 15-second time period. Do not use continuous suction. Avoid poking motions of the catheter.
5. Hyperinflate and postoxygenate for 1 to 5 minutes, as indicated by the situation.	Recovery to baseline PaO_2 takes 1 to 5 minutes.

PROCEDURE	RATIONALES AND PRECAUTIONS
6. Suction again (repeat step 4 and step 5), if secretions persist.	
a. If the patient coughs secretions up to the stoma or endotracheal tube, suction to that level.	Avoidance of deep suctioning reduces trauma and contamination.
b. Encourage tracheostomy patients to cough remaining secretions into a tissue.	
7. Suction the pharynx with the same catheter, if needed. *Remember, once you contaminate the catheter with oropharyngeal secretions, use a new sterile catheter and sterile gloves for subsequent tracheobronchial passes.*	Some patients have minimal tracheobronchial secretions and large amounts of oropharyngeal secretions. Lung hyperinflations and coughing tend to push secretions up around the cuff and into the pharynx during the procedure.
8. Rinse the connecting tubing in tap water or germicidal rinse. Dispose of catheter and gloves.	
9. Evaluate the effectiveness of the intervention and presence of side effects. Side effects include arrhythmias, hypoxemia, hypotension, hypertension, increased intracranial pressure, rapid or irregular pulse, tachypnea, cyanosis, dyspnea, and use of accessory muscles of respiration.	Signs of mucus retention indicate need for more suctioning; signs of hypoxemia indicate need for reevaluation of preoxygenation and postoxygenation methods.
10. Chart the intervention.	Charting provides documentation and guidelines for subsequent suction procedures.
a. Specify type: routine or individualized suctioning procedure.	
b. Time of intervention.	
c. Extent (i.e., number of passes).	
d. Secretions, color, consistency, amount, and odor.	
e. Patient reactions, problems, or adverse effects.	
f. Recommendations for future suctioning.	

SUCTIONING THE LOWER AIRWAY—THE NONINTUBATED PATIENT

The nurse suctions the nonintubated patient using the above procedure for the intubated patient (page 684), with only a few modifications, as described.

PROCEDURE	RATIONALES AND PRECAUTIONS
1. *Positioning*	
a. Place the patient in semi-Fowler's position.	Promotes general relaxation, oxygenation, and ventilation. Allows the catheter tip to curve anteriorly toward the trachea during catheter advancement
b. Remove pillow, and place head in neutral position.	Maintains airway patency as well as patient comfort.
c. Choose a patent nares for catheter insertion.	(See Suctioning the Upper Airway for description.)
2. *Preoxygenation and postoxygenation*	
a. Place an oxygen mask over the mouth, insert a nasal prong in the accessible nostril, or both.	
b. Ask the patient to take slow deep breaths during the entire procedure.	
c. Particularly for a patient with a borderline low PaO_2, ask another person to assist by holding the oxygen mask to the patient's mouth, and holding the patient's hand.	Deep suctioning is a frightful experience. Touching the patient or holding the hand provides reassurance and prevents the patient from grabbing at the suction catheter during the procedure.

Box continued on following page

PROCEDURE	*RATIONALES AND PRECAUTIONS*
3. *Catheter advancement to the pharynx*	
a. Advance a well-lubricated catheter through the nose, inferiorly and medially.	
b. Ask the patient to stick out his tongue, as you pass the catheter down the back of the nasopharynx.	Sticking the tongue out prevents the base of the tongue from falling back towards the posterior pharyngeal wall and narrowing the airway. Also, it helps avoid coiling of the catheter in the mouth (a common problem) and greatly facilitates catheter tip advancement past the oropharynx.
c. If catheter advancement into the pharynx stimulates a productive cough, withdraw the catheter and suction intermittently. Do not proceed to tracheal suctioning.	Tracheal suctioning is necessary, if coughing results in adequate mucus expectoration.
d. For repeated suctioning consider insertion of a nasopharyngeal airway. An oral airway may be inserted, if suctioning via the mouth is necessary (e.g., in comatose patients).	Avoids trauma to the nose. Oral airway guides the catheter to the hypopharynx.
e. Allow the patient to rest 1 to 2 minutes before proceeding to the lower airway.	A brief rest allows the patient to relax and prepare psychologically for the rest of the procedure. Also, providing additional reassurance at this time maximizes cooperation.
4. *Catheter advancement into the trachea* This is the most difficult part of the procedure.	The following method is used when easy tracheal entry is anticipated.
a. Pinch the connecting tubing to eliminate unnecessary suction.	Suction is minimal but may contribute to hypoxemia in patients with borderline low PaO_2s.
b. Instruct the patient to take a very deep breath in or to cough.	A deep breath or cough opens the glottis.
c. Quickly slide the catheter past the epiglottis and into the trachea until resistance is met or until the patient begins to cough vigorously.	Speed and timing are crucial. The catheter will not pass into the trachea unless catheter advancement coincides *exactly* with the brief opening of the glottis.
The alternative method is more reliable than the blind technique presented, because it allows the nurse to determine the location of the catheter tip near the glottis, as described next. Chances for successful tracheal entry are much greater.	
• Advance the catheter disconnected from the tubing.	Disconnection eliminates suction and allows the patient to breathe through and around the suction catheter.
• Listen at the opening of the air vent for the presence of breath sounds. Check to be sure the patient is still deep breathing and not holding his breath.	Presence of breath sounds indicates that the catheter tip is still in the upper airway and the patient is not holding his breath. Cessation of breath sounds indicates breath holding or passage of the tip into the esophagus.
• Advance the catheter 1 to 2 in during each inspiration. When the tip stimulates a cough, quickly slide the catheter into the trachea.	The glottis is open during inspiration.
• Otherwise, advance the tip until breath sounds cease; the tip is entering the esophagus. Withdraw it a few centimeters. Now it is above the epiglottis. Ask the patient to cough, while you quickly pass it into the trachea.	Remember, timing of catheter advancement with the cough is crucial to successful tracheal entry.
• Verify tracheal entry by listening briefly for breath sounds before hooking the catheter up to suction.	Breath sounds may be the only reliable sign of tracheal entry in patients without a cough reflex.

PROCEDURE	RATIONALES AND PRECAUTIONS
5. *Suctioning*	
a. When the catheter tip meets resistance on advancement, pull back 1 to 2 cm and apply intermittent suction during catheter withdrawal, as previously described.	
b. Encourage coughing and deep breathing during catheter withdrawal.	These techniques help mobilize secretions, increase the amount of mucus aspirated, and decrease need for further suctioning.
6. *Patient recovery*	
a. Allow the patient to rest and reoxygenate for at least 2 minutes between suctioning attempts.	
b. Some patients require complete catheter withdrawal between attempts to avoid hypoxemia and unbearable discomfort. Others tolerate resting with the suction catheter near the epiglottis.	Leaving the catheter near the epiglottis eliminates need for repeated advancements through the upper airway. Also, the catheter is ready for tracheal entry should the patient cough spontaneously.

Use of One or Two Gloves? In the hospital setting, suctioning is ideally performed while wearing two gloves. One gloved hand is kept sterile at all times for handling the sterile catheter; the other hand is kept sterile for preparation of the catheter. Thereafter, however, it is considered clean.

A two-glove technique is recommended over a one-glove technique because it helps to prevent cross contamination among patients, health care personnel, and respiratory equipment. Nurses are at high risk for *herpetic whitlow*, a herpes simplex virus (type 1) affecting the digits of the hands (Fig. 27–10). The high risk seems to be related to the following five factors: (1) direct contact with respiratory secretions through the catheter's suction control vent, (2) direct contact with oropharyngeal secretions, (3) susceptibility of skin to dermatitis and nosocomial infection due to repeated handwashing, (4) absent or poor handwashing technique between patients, and (5) lack of antibodies for herpes simplex virus (Greaves et al, 1980; Louis and Silva, 1979; Bohen, 1982).

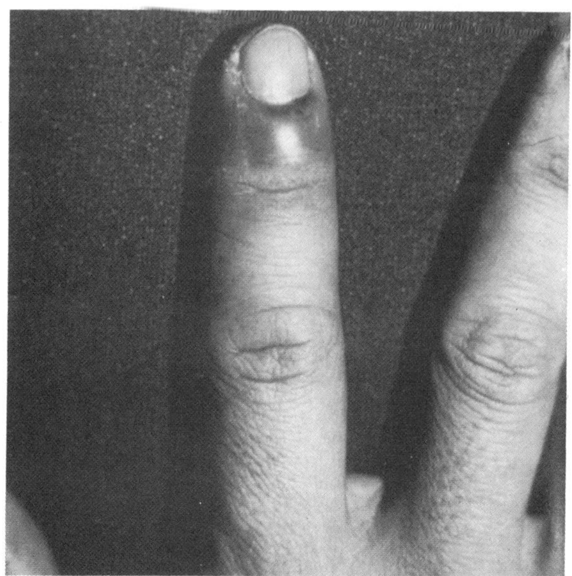

Figure 27–10. Herpetic whitlow affecting the right index finger in a 30-year-old health professional. Though in this case the erythema and finger discomfort were localized at the nail's edges, signs of disease may appear in the pulp of the finger as well. (Reproduced by permission from Louis, D. and Silva, J. Herpetic whitlow: herpetic infections of the digits. *The journal of hand surgery,* 4(1):90, 1979.)

A one-glove or no-glove technique may be indicated in certain situations. For example, a one-glove technique is used in most rehabilitation settings because it is easier for the patient to learn and perform correctly over a long period of time. The chronic respiratory patient's immunodefense system is relatively intact and hence able to fight infection, should contamination occur. Also, the patient's immediate environment is typically infection free. In another situation, a tracheostomy patient, preparing for home discharge, may concentrate on meticulous handwashing before and after suctioning and not wear gloves.

No-glove or Clean-glove Technique with a Closed Suction System. The no-glove technique is used for suctioning with a closed system, such as Cath 'N Sleeve by Davol, Inc., and Trach Care by Ballard Medical Products (Fig. 27–11). In these catheters in a sleeve arrangement, gloving with sterile gloves is not mandatory because catheter and sleeve are left attached to the patient's artificial airway. However, gloving and a separate suctioning setup are necessary for nasal and oral suctioning. Moreover, many intensive care units routinely use a clean-glove technique because of the increasing incidence of infectious diseases, including AIDS, among their patient populations.

Suctioning through a closed suction system has several advantages over the standard suctioning procedure presented in this text. First, it is quicker because suctioning involves fewer steps. Second, the catheter may be reintroduced into the trachea numer-

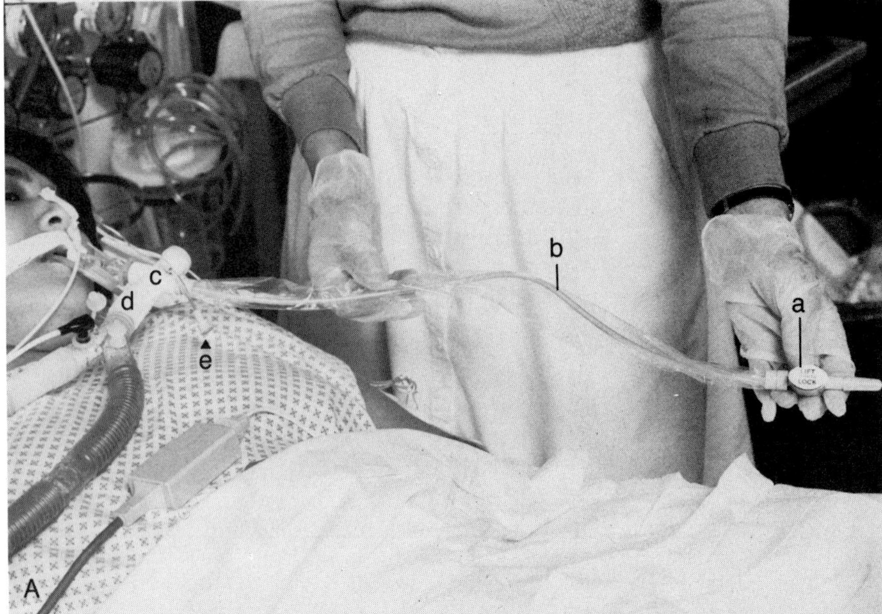

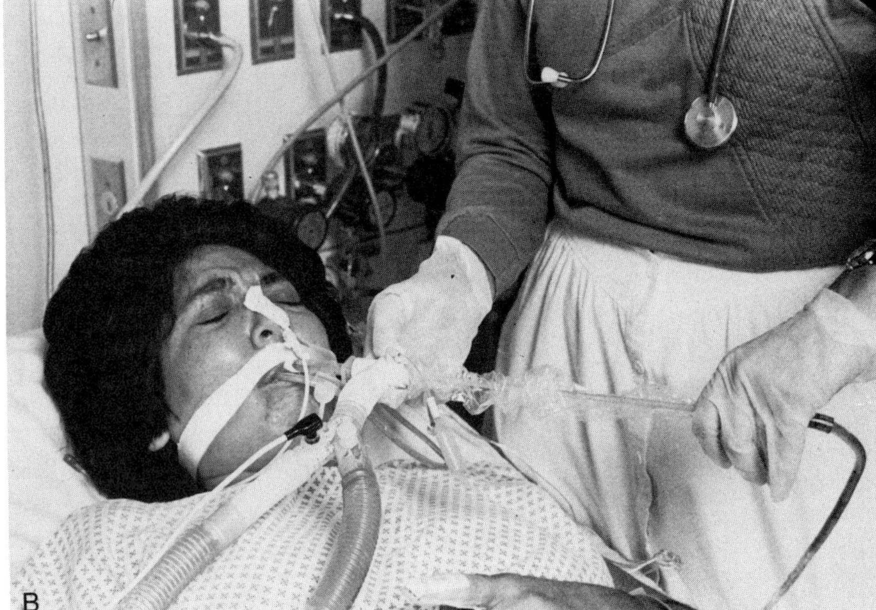

Figure 27–11. Closed suction system. *A*, TrachCare (Ballard Medical Products). a, Suction control valve; b, Sheathed 14-French suction catheter; c, Sealed T piece. The seal is located where the catheter enters the T piece. It serves to maintain PEEP during suctioning; d, Flex tubing to ventilator circuit; e, Irrigation port for tracheal lavage (described elsewhere). *B*, A nurse moves the catheter through the sheath and T-piece adapter to suction the patient. Multiple suctioning passes were necessary to clear this trauma patient's airways of copious secretions.

ous times without increasing the patient's risk of infection. Research indicates no significant differences in rate or magnitude of contamination between the multiple-use catheter of the closed suctioning system and the single-use catheter of the standard suctioning procedure (Ritz et al, 1986). Last, a special adapter placed between the endotracheal tube and ventilator permits suctioning without interruption of ventilations (Birdsall, 1986). The seal near the catheter tip maintains positive end expiratory pressure PEEP (see Chapter 28). These features help to prevent or reduce complications during suctioning, such as arterial oxygen desaturation, bradycardia, and hypotension.

Suction Catheter Type

Suction catheters are divided into *straight* and *angled* types (Fig. 27–12).

Straight suction catheters come in a variety of designs, e.g., Tri-flo, Aero-flo (Argyle), and whistle-tip (Link et al, 1976). Many clinicians favor the Aero-flo catheter for intubated patients because its O-shaped tip is designed to minimize mucosal contact and is less injurious to mucus transport than many conventional straight suction catheters (Sackner et al, 1973; Landa et al, 1980).

Chapman and colleagues (1986) indicate that the

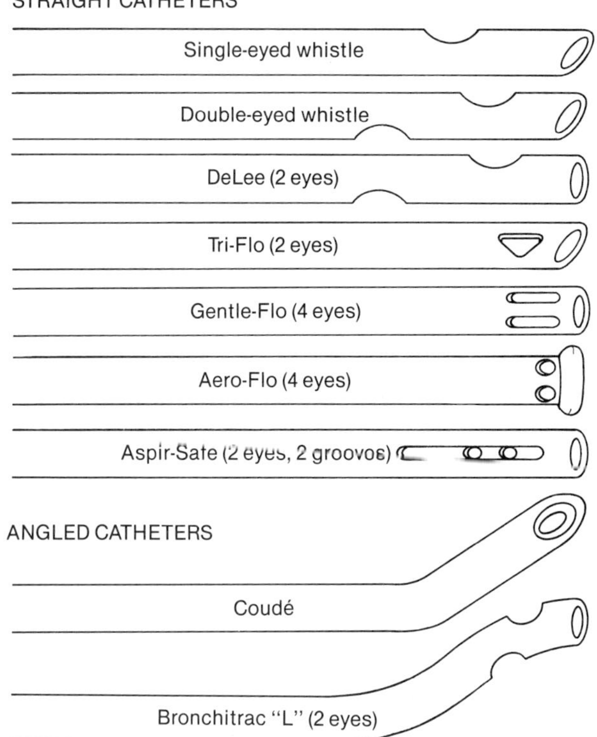

Figure 27–12. Distal tip configurations of straight and angled suction catheters.

Aspir-Safe catheter may be more efficient and safe than other catheters, such as the Aero-flo, Regu-vac, and Tri-flo. The Aspir-Safe catheter has an atraumatic tip based on principles of the Aero-flo design but without the Aero-flo O-shaped tip, which can impede nasal insertion. Other clinicians emphasize correct technique and do not prefer one design over another, except for insistence on at least one side port. Experts agree that multiple side ports may minimize the aspiration of pulmonic gas and reduce the frequency of catheter tip invagination of the bronchial mucosa (Link et al, 1976).

Many tracheostomy patients prefer soft rubber catheters (e.g., straight, red rubber, Robinson catheter) for suctioning, because the soft catheter tip produces less trauma during catheter advancement.

The *angled* or *coudé* suction catheter is used for patients with left lower lobe lung pathology to increase the chance of successful passes into the left main stem bronchus. Chances of doing this are best when suctioning through a tracheostomy rather than an endotracheal tube (Kubota et al, 1980) and when the angled suction catheter is prepackaged in a straight rather than a coiled configuration (Haberman et al, 1973).

The new *Bronchitrac "L"* angled catheter (see Fig. 27–12) is designed to automatically enter the left main stem bronchus, without the special manipulations required when using a standard angled or coudé catheter. Research is in progress to assess the efficacy of the Bronchitrac "L" catheter.

Suction Catheter Size

As a general rule, French size 14 is suitable for adults, and size 10 is suitable for children. In any case, the catheter diameter should be no greater than half the internal diameter of the endotracheal or tracheostomy tube. This provides room for ambient air to flow in a retrograde fashion within the tube's lumen to replace the volume aspirated by the catheter tip.

Preoxygenation

The nurse preoxygenates the patient for 30 seconds to 2 minutes before suctioning, as indicated by the situation. Preoxygenation is necessary to minimize hypoxemia during and after the suctioning procedure, though little agreement exists as to exactly how it should be done. As a guideline, the nurse uses one of the following two methods:

For the Ventilator Method

First, increase the FIO_2 to 1.00 or at least 0.40 more than the resting FIO_2. Second, wait 1 to 2 minutes for the FIO_2 to increase to the new level. Ventilator washout time may take up to 2 minutes for low intermittent mandatory ventilation (IMV) rates. Also, PaO_2 stabilization may take longer in patients with atelectasis or other ventilation perfusion (V/Q) abnormalities. Last, deliver 3 to 6 large breaths by pushing the manual tidal volume or preferably the sigh button on the ventilator. Preoxygenation delivered with hyperinflation provides better protection against hypoxemia than preoxygenation without hyperinflation (Goodnough, 1985).

For the Bagging Method

The nurse uses a manual resuscitator bag to deliver three to six large breaths. This method is used for ventilator patients as well as for patients breathing spontaneously on a T-tube.

When positive end-expiratory pressure (PEEP) is an adjunct to mechanical ventilation, a special PEEP adaptor may be attached to the resuscitator to maintain PEEP during bagging and avoid excessive hypoxemia (see Chapter 28 for definition and description of IMV, PEEP, and other modes of mechanical ventilation). Some research suggests, however, that PEEP adaptors may be unnecessary, even in the case of high levels of PEEP, provided the patient is hyperinflated and oxygenated with 100% oxygen before and after suctioning (Douglas and Larson, 1985).

Both ventilator and bagging methods have advantages and disadvantages. Utilization of the ventilator for preoxygenation is advantageous because it is convenient and allows delivery of a known tidal volume and peak pressure. However, the lag time required to achieve a high FIO_2 in the ventilator circuit delays suctioning.

Bagging is advantageous because the change to a new FIO_2 is immediate. Also, it avoids the inadvertent and prolonged administration of 100% oxygen via ventilator after the procedure

Bagging has several disadvantages, however. First, it is logistically difficult unless another person is available to bag in between suctioning passes. Second, it requires disconnection and reconnection to the ventilator several times for each suctioning procedure. Disconnection may result in loss of PEEP, hypoxemia, and frequent sounding of the ventilator alarm. The traditional 1-L self-inflating resuscitator bag is unsuitable for large patients. It does not permit adequate hyperinflation in patients with baseline tidal volumes of 800 ml or greater (Goodnough, 1985). Last, peak pressure delivered to the airways is unknown during bagging; it is relatively uncontrollable, unless the bag has a pop-off valve set appropriately at 40 to 50 cmH_2O (Riegel and Forshee, 1985).

Identification of an Entry Port

For an intubated patient on a ventilator, the current trend seems to be suctioning through the capped opening on the ventilator's *swivel adaptor* (Fig. 27–13, center), although some situations may require ventilator disconnection and entry directly down the artificial airway. Belling and associates (1978) found that PaO_2 decreased by 24% during suctioning on the ventilator through the adaptor, compared with a 67% drop in PaO_2 off the ventilator. Whenever suctioning is performed through the capped swivel adaptor, great care is taken to avoid contamination of the suction catheter—the adaptor cap tends to fall on the catheter during catheter advancement.

Another option for patients on high PEEP levels is to suction through a *self-sealing adaptor* (Fig. 27–13, right). This technique may significantly reduce hypoxemia, since PEEP is maintained during suctioning, and room air is not inspired into the lungs. However, high suction flow rates may exceed the volume of air delivered by the ventilator, causing negative airway pressure and atelectasis. Because of this potential complication, Brown and coworkers (1983) recommend this technique for high flow IMV setups and discourage its use for controlled or assisted ventilation. Moreover, some clinicians do not use self-sealing adaptors because of their concern over catheter tip contamination and difficulty advancing the catheter tip into the adaptor's rather stiff entry port.

Suctioning the Patient

The nurse quickly advances the catheter down the tube until resistance is met. After pulling back 1 to 2 cm, the nurse applies intermittent suction, while slowly withdrawing the catheter. These hints will help the nurse perfect this technique as follows:

1. *Never* apply suction during catheter advancement.
2. Do not apply continuous suction at any time.
3. Always avoid poking or prodding movements. Instead, use gentle twisting or circular motions during catheter withdrawal, keeping the catheter in constant motion so the tip does not impact against the mucosa. The circular motion, important for most catheters without torsional stiffness, involves rolling the catheter between the fingers, turning it 180 to 360 degrees, so that the catheter tip turns with the rest of the catheter.
4. *Do not take longer than 10 to 15 seconds for*

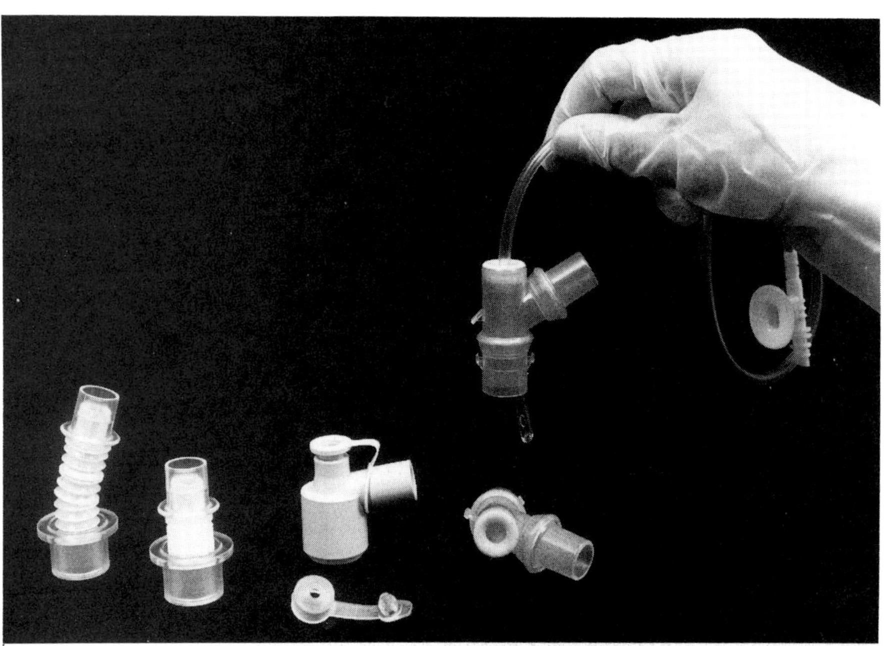

Figure 27–13. Ventilator connector and entry ports for tracheal suctioning. Left, Flex connector (Omniflex) in extended and collapsed positions. Center, Swivel adapter with capped suction port (Portex). The extra cap in the foreground is used during fiberoptic bronchoscopy. Right, Self-sealing adapter (Bodai swivel Y).

each suctioning pass. Longer periods may cause significant hypoxemia.

5. When using the standard coudé catheter, keep the head in the midline position, and point the catheter tip towards the left. To increase the chance of left bronchial intubation, do not rotate or twist the catheter during advancement. Placing a guidemark on one or both sides of the catheter along its longitudinal axis helps to prevent rotation, but such a catheter is not commercially available (Kubota et al, 1980).

6. Head and body position seems to make no difference in entering the left main stem bronchus, when a straight catheter is used. However, since success is unlikely, always use the coudé or Bronchitrac L catheter for attempted left bronchial passes.

Postoxygenation

The nurse hyperinflates and postoxygenates the lungs for 1 to 5 minutes, as indicated by the clinical situation. Hyperinflations serve to help increase FIO_2 and reverse microatelectasis during the procedure. Length of time required for postoxygenation varies among patients because each one experiences different degrees of hypoxemia. The lowest drop in SaO_2 commonly occurs more than 20 seconds for adults, 10 seconds for infants, after the conclusion of a suctioning pass (Brown et al, 1983). Recovery time is usually 1 to 3 minutes but may be as long as 5 minutes when high levels of PEEP are applied, before SaO_2 and PaO_2 return to baseline levels (Decampo and Civetta, 1979).

If the critical care patient is postoxygenated with an FIO_2 of 1.00, brief hyperinflation may be carried out at a lower FIO_2 (i.e., approximating the patient's baseline FIO_2) before ending the suctioning procedure. This measure helps to prevent or reverse absorption atelectasis, an adverse side effect of delivering a high FIO_2 (see Chapter 13). Moreover, supernormal PaO_2s are highly undesirable in COPD patients with hypoxic ventilatory drives, particularly during weaning from mechanical ventilation.

Collection of Sputum Samples

Collection of a sputum sample for laboratory analysis is relatively easy, if the patient is nonintubated. The patient is merely asked to cough up sputum directly into a sterile specimen container.

For the intubated patient, a sterile specimen container or *Leuken's trap* is attached between the sterile suction catheter and connecting tubing (Fig. 27–14). The best specimens are collected after aerosol treatments early in the morning. Normally, suction catheters are not rinsed with a solution to increase the amount trapped in the specimen container. However, if milking the container's tubing does not help aspirate thick mucus into the container, a very small amount of sterile saline, but not bacteriostatic saline, may be used to rinse the catheter.

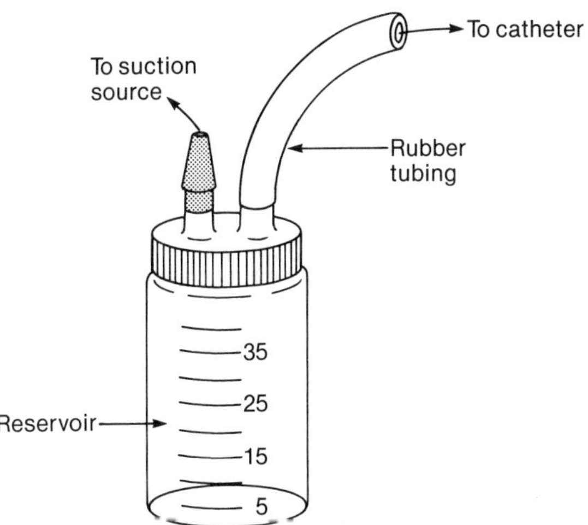

Figure 27–14. The Leuken's trap is a type of sputum specimen container. After the suctioning procedure, the catheter and contaminated suction connector (shaded gray) are discarded, and the rubber tubing is connected directly to the reservoir's top.

EVALUATION

Though evaluation is listed here for convenience towards the end of the suctioning procedure, in practice it begins earlier with preoxygenation of the patient and continues throughout the procedure. The most important monitoring involves that for signs of hypoxemia (e.g., cyanosis, tachypnea, arrhythmias) and patient discomfort. In the critical care unit, the nurse uses the cardiac monitor to watch for arrhythmias during and after suctioning. Similarly, she observes the arterial pressure tracing during hyperinflations for signs of extreme blood pressure changes. Remember that large lung inflations may cause bradycardias and hypotension, particularly in patients with unstable blood volumes.

Chest Assessment Findings

Between suctioning passes or after the conclusion of the procedure, the nurse palpates the chest for rhonchal fremitus and auscultates the lungs for rhonchi and breath sounds. Persistent rhonchi indicate the need for more suctioning. A decrease in the intensity of breath sounds without audible rhonchi may indicate that secretions are on the way up. The nurse waits until rhonchi become evident before suctioning again. When this is difficult to evaluate, ask the patient whether he feels the need for more suctioning. Most alert patients can indicate whether secretions are high enough to be aspirated by the suction catheter.

If suctioning stimulates wheezing and secretions are minimal, the patient may need more aggressve bronchodilator therapy to open airways, before secretions can be aspirated. Sometimes suctioning stimulates uncontrollable coughing. In this case, instilling a few cc of liquid anesthetic (lidocaine) may help to suppress the ineffective cough.

Sometimes secretions are minimal because they are too thick and tenacious to be aspirated. In these cases, the clinician encourages increased fluid intake, as tolerated, and reviews other means of liquefying secretions, e.g., increased humidification and aerosol therapy. Some clinicians use *tracheal lavage*, defined as the instillation of 2 to 5 cc of normal saline intratracheally, to liquefy secretions, produce a cough, and prevent encrustations along the sides of the artificial airway. After instillation, the patient is reconnected to assisted ventilation for a few deep breaths and then suctioned. For the patient with a closed suction system, normal saline is instilled into the irrigation port (Fig. 27–11,e) rather than directly down the endotracheal or tracheostomy tube. A similar procedure is followed for the nonintubated patient, except saline is instilled directly into the catheter, with the thumb occluding the air vent, when the catheter is fully advanced in the trachea.

Although tracheal lavage may benefit selected patients in stimulating a cough, most of the saline settles in central rather than peripheral airways and is not suctioned out of the lungs (Hanley et al, 1978). Repeated lavage may contribute to heart failure in patients on restricted fluid intake. Largely for these reasons, tracheal lavage has been stated to have little or no value in the thinning, mobilizing, and removal of dried secretions (Ackerman, 1985), and it may be dangerous for the borderline, heart failure patient. Tracheal lavage is best replaced with other bronchial hygiene techniques, such as increased airway humidification and increased oral fluid intake.

Psychologic Response

In addition to physiologic effects, the nurse evaluates psychologic response to the procedure. Some patients may demonstrate acute anxiety and refuse any further suctioning attempts because of fear of suffocation, associated loss of control, and inability to cope with yet another traumatic event. In this case, the nurse takes time to (1) encourage the patient to fully express feelings and concerns; (2) explain that the shortness of breath, though largely unavoidable during suctioning, should improve after catheter withdrawal and after mucus aspiration from the lungs; (3) repeat exactly why suctioning is needed; and (4) promise to gently advance the catheter only when the patient is ready. If the patient continues to refuse the procedure, the physician is called to discuss more fully the consequences of not being suctioned and the alternative ways to achieve the same results. In many cases, after one suctioning experience, the patient tries harder to turn, cough, and deep breathe regularly and fully cooperate in other bronchial hygiene measures that will either eliminate or greatly reduce suctioning frequency.

CHARTING

The nurse charts the specific suctioning procedure used for the patient as well as the effects and side effects of therapy. If cardiac arrhythmias or other signs of hypoxemia are present, the nurse documents the specific method used for preoxygenation and postoxygenation, e.g., six manual breaths with a resuscitator bag or 2 minutes of assisted ventilation with an FIO_2 of 1.00. In consultation with other health team members, a new plan is decided upon and documented in the chart for a more effective preoxygenation and postoxygenation method, e.g., 3 minutes of assisted ventilation with periodic sighs on an FIO_2 of 1.00, combined with suctioning through the aperture of a swivel adaptor. This approach insures modification of standardized methods to individual patient needs.

HOME SETTING

Most patients in the home setting dislike suctioning to such a degree that encouragement to stay well hydrated, take regular aerosol treatments, and use postural drainage may substantially reduce the need for suctioning. When they do need suctioning, however, it is performed applying the same principles as those described for the hospital setting, with the following adaptations in technique and equipment.

Three basic differences exist in suctioning techniques. First, as with tracheostomy care, the home patient uses a clean rather than a sterile technique during the entire procedure. Though a no-glove technique is usually adequate, a single-glove technique may be advised in certain situations, e.g., history of faulty handwashing technique, recent surgery, and immunosuppression. Second, in the home setting, deep breathing alone is usually sufficient for preoxygenation and postoxygenation in the spontaneously breathing patient with a permanent tracheostomy. Third, the person who performs the suctioning is more frequently the patient or a family member rather than a health professional. The patient or family member may need continual reassurance that some shortness of breath during suctioning is normal. At the first sign of shortness of breath, rather than stop breathing or withdraw the catheter, patients are encouraged to continue deep breathing and catheter advancement. Also, they are reminded that the shortness of breath will disappear after obstructive secretions are suctioned out of the lungs.

When the tracheostomy patient first learns how to suction himself, use of the disposable straight catheters provided in kits may be best, until family and patient feel comfortable with technique, and special equipment needs can be evaluated. The problem with disposable catheters is the expense of using and disposing of several catheters a day. To reduce expense, patients may utilize nondisposable red rubber catheters (Davol). After use, the patient rinses the catheter

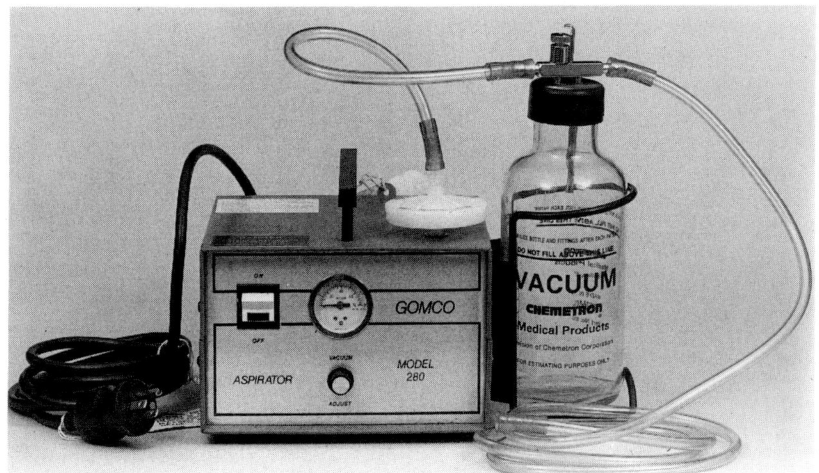

Figure 27–15. Portable suction machine used in the home setting. (Courtesy of National Medical Homecare, Sacramento, California.)

and tubing by suctioning tap water from a disposable paper cup. The catheter is disconnected and placed in a special pan of soapy water for soaking. At the end of the day, all catheters are washed in warm soapy water and boiled in water for 10 minutes for sterilization. After air drying, the catheters are stored in clean plastic bags or foil (Hodgkin et al, 1984).

In the home setting, suction is provided by a portable suction machine (Fig. 27–15). Since most portable suction machines plug into wall sockets with AC current, patients with mucus retention problems are advised to keep a battery operated portable unit in case of power failure.

Suction jar and tubing as well as the pan for soaking catheters are all cleaned daily, using the same soap and water cleaning technique recommended in Chapter 21. In addition, the cup of tap water and suction jar fluid are disposed of daily; emptying contents down the toilet is most convenient.

Mouth Care

After suctioning the lower airway and upper airway, the nurse provides mouth care for the intubated patient. Mouth care involves, first, assessing the oral mucosa to determine whether it is normal or abnormal (Table 27–2), and then, giving appropriate mouth care as shown in the box *Mouth Care for the Intubated Patient.*

The need for meticulous mouth care in respiratory patients, particularly intubated ones, cannot be overemphasized. The presence of an artificial airway in the mouth predisposes the patient to tissue trauma in the oral cavity. Moreover, respiratory patients tend to have other risk factors for stomatitis and infection. Some of these risk factors are dryness of the mouth; dehydration; decreased salivary flow due to decreased jaw movements; increased oral secretions, which are pooled above the inflated cuff, a medium for bacterial growth; poor nutrition; immunosuppression from steroids, acquired immune deficiency disease (AIDS), leukemia, or other secondary disease; and frequent mechanical stimulation with a suction catheter. When the patient is extubated, some of these risk factors are eliminated, but others remain or are accompanied by new risk factors. For example, extubation may eliminate pooled secretions and need for suctioning, but the patient's mouth may remain dry, owing to insensible fluid loss from mouth breathing and dehydration from antidiuretic medications.

The goals of mouth care are fourfold as follows: (1) to keep the lips and oral mucosa clean, soft, moist, and intact; (2) to prevent stomatitis, infection, caries, and peridontal disease by removing debris and plaque from around the teeth without damaging the mucosa; (3) to alleviate oral pain and discomfort, prevent halitosis, and leave a fresh feeling in the mouth; and (4) to promote increased appetite and oral intake.

Table 27–2. SIGNS OF NORMAL AND ABNORMAL ORAL MUCOSA

	Abnormal Oral Mucosa	
Normal Oral Mucosa	***Stomatitis (Mucositis)*** • ***Inflammation of the mucosa of the mouth***	***Oral Infection*** • ***Culture needed for diagnosis and medical treatment***
Pink, moist	Red, shiny, and edematous	Signs of stomatitis
Absence of lesions, crusts, and hard debris	Bleeding tendency	Coated or encrusted oral ulcerations
		Red, dry, and swollen tongue with white or brownish coating

MOUTH CARE FOR THE INTUBATED PATIENT

PROCEDURE	***RATIONALES AND PRECAUTIONS***
To Prepare	
1. Gather the following equipment: a. Hydrogen peroxide (U.S.P. 3%) b. Sterile normal saline or sterile water c. Mouthwash d. 2 clean cups e. Small soft toothbrush f. Denture brush, if available g. Toothette (sponge on a stick) h. Emesis basin i. Towel j. French size 14 catheter attached to suction k. Lip lubricant l. Cotton-tipped applicators	Ready availability of equipment facilitates quick implementation of the procedure.
2. Apply clean gloves.	Gloves protect both nurse and patient from possible infection.
3. Explain procedure to the patient and provide reassurance.	An explanation of procedure and purpose helps to elicit full cooperation and reduces anxiety during cleaning. Also, patients may not understand the need for frequent cleaning.
4. Place towel over upper chest area.	Protects gown and can be used to dry the mouth.
5. Mix 1:1 ratio of hydrogen peroxide saline solution in a clean cup. Add an equal portion of mouthwash to enhance taste, if desired (1:1:1 ratio). This is the cleaning solution.	Hydrogen peroxide is a readily available, effective germicidal agent. Though commercial mouthwash may be used to enhance taste, it is not effective as a sole cleaning agent. It may cause irritation and hypersensitivity stomatitis and, hence, is reserved for patients with normal or near normal oral mucosa. Normal saline aids in the formulation of granulation tissue and the promotion of local healing. It may have a slightly inhibitory effect on bacterial growth (Maurer, 1977).
6. Pour normal saline into a second clean cup. This is the rinsing solution.	A rinsing solution is needed to rinse away the taste and foaming bubbles of the peroxide and the excess debris after cleaning.
7. Remove the oral airway, if present. If the airway is needed for a bite block, leave it in place during cleaning and ask the respiratory therapist to help you change it after cleaning.	Removal of the airway will expose more mucosa for cleaning. The bite block of the airway will prevent you from being bitten by the comatose or agitated patient. Also, it will help keep the orotracheal-endotracheal tube stabilized
8. Check to be sure the patient does not have leak around the cuff of the tracheal tube. Minimal leak is OK, if the patient can handle oral secretions without difficulty.	A leak around the cuff predisposes to aspiration of cleaning or rinsing solution into the lungs.
9. If appropriate, ask the alert patient with a nasotracheal or tracheostomy tube to remove dentures or partial plates, if they are not already out of the mouth. a. To clean, brush off debris with denture brush or toothbrush and place in denture cup with self-cleaning solution. b. Replace in mouth later, after procedure.	Debris tends to stick to dental appliances. Also, appliance removal is necessary to inspect underlying mucosa for sores.
To Clean the Mouth	
1. Ask the alert patient to open the mouth.	
2. If the oral mucosa is normal, gently brush the teeth with the toothbrush and the peroxide:saline solution as follows:	

PROCEDURE	*RATIONALES AND PRECAUTIONS*
a. Place brush at the margin of the gums and make a sweeping motion towards the crowns of the teeth. b. Brush both back and front surfaces this way, frequently dipping the brush into the cleaning solution. Then, brush the top surfaces with a horizontal motion (Daeffler, 1981).	A toothbrush cleans debris off the teeth better than a toothette. However, if the patient does not tolerate the brush, do not hesitate to switch to a toothette. Discomfort may cause the anxious patient to refuse all forms of mouth care. An alternative to the toothette is gauze wrapped around a tongue depressor.
c. Gently brush the tongue, as tolerated.	Excess pressure on the tongue may cause nausea and retching.
d. Work around the tube and adhesive tape. *Be careful not to bump the tube!* If necessary, ask a second person to stabilize the tube during cleaning.	Bumping the tube may cause tissue trauma or laryngeal edema (endotracheal tube) and may stimulate coughing.
e. Switch to a toothette for hard-to-get areas and when gums begin to bleed.	Accessibility limits use of the toothbrush. Some patients without stomatitis may have sensitive gums and tend to bleed. Excessive pressure with a toothbrush may damage mucosal surfaces.
3. Use the following cleaning modifications if you note signs of severe stomatitis or oral infection, thrombocytopenia, and neutropenia:	
a. A toothette.	It is softer and less likely to damage the oral mucosa compared with a brush.
b. Sterile normal saline *without* hydrogen peroxide, as directed by the physician. *Exception*: Hydrogen peroxide solution may be used selectively to loosen debris and crusting of abnormal tongue coatings.	Hydrogen peroxide is not used when the patient has fresh granulation surfaces in the mouth because it tends to break down new tissue. Some authorities do not recommend routine use in stomatitis because it may irritate the tongue and buccal mucosa and predispose to superinfections (Daeffler, 1980).
c. Remember that culture and sensitivity specimens of ulcers should be done *before* any cleaning of the mouth.	The cleaning solution alters the flora of the ulcer and possibly, culture and sensitivity results. Reliable and valid results are needed to determine appropriate antibiotic or antifungal agent for the infection.
To Rinse the Mouth	
4. Help the alert patient rinse the mouth with rinsing solution, swishing the solution between the teeth, if possible, and spitting waste into the emesis basin. For patients with orotracheal tubes, those in comas, or those who cannot handle oral secretions:	Rinsing helps to loosen debris and irrigate tissues.
a. Rinse the teeth with a toothette and normal saline.	
b. Suction the mouth intermittently to prevent solution from pooling in the mouth and dripping into the pharynx.	Using suction helps prevent risk of aspiration and allows more effective rinsing with greater quantities of saline.
b. Use a toothette or cotton-tipped applicator to remove debris, as needed.	
To Massage the Gums	
5. Press the brush or toothette against the gums and move it towards the biting surfaces of the teeth. Do all accessible gum areas. a. Massaging is recommended for a few minutes, 2 to 3 times a day (Maurer, 1977).	In the absence of chewing, massaging produces intermittent pressure, which is transferred to the blood vessels and relieves vascular stasis. Also, it may stimulate salivary flow, allow for normal keratinization of the epithelium, and help protect against trauma.
b. Skip this step, if the patient has an orotracheal tube in place.	Gum areas are not fully accessible for massaging. Also, massaging may overly prolong the procedure and increase patient discomfort and agitation, with greater tension on the tube.

Box continued on following page

MOUTH CARE FOR THE INTUBATED PATIENT Continued

PROCEDURE	*RATIONALES AND PRECAUTIONS*
To Protect the Lips	
6. Apply lip lubricant to lips with cotton applicators.	Lubricant prevents evaporation of moisture and drying, cracking, and excoriation of the lips. Petroleum jelly is commonly used in the clinical setting because it effectively forms a thick occlusive barrier. However, it is associated with aspiration pneumonia and is flammable. Use of a water-soluble lubricant is preferable because it eliminates these risks.
7. Dispose of gloves, suction catheter, and other disposable supplies. Remove towel from patient's upper chest area.	

To achieve these goals, the nurse performs mouth care at least every 4 to 8 hours for intubated patients with normal or near normal oral mucosa, and more frequently when lips or mouth appear dry (Fig. 27–16). For patients with stomatitis or infection, mouth care may be needed every 1 to 2 hours. Failure to give mouth care over an extended period of 2 to 6 hours may nullify the benefits of past care (Daeffler, 1981).

Note that the same mouth care procedure and frequency guidelines apply to nonintubated respiratory patients with signs of stomatitis or mouth infection. Patients who use mouth breathing continuously and who are NPO usually need mouth care every 1 to 2 hours. Nonintubated patients with normal oral mucosa may use toothbrush and toothpaste as well as commercial mouthwash, as desired.

For intubated patients, mouth accessibility is a consideration in scheduling mouth care with other nursing and respiratory therapy duties. It is usually not a problem for a cooperative patient with a nasotracheal or tracheostomy tube. However, accessibility is a problem for a patient with an orotracheal tube. For this reason, if possible, mouth care is performed when the oral airway is removed for daily replacement, when the adhesive tape is changed and the tube switched to the opposite side of the mouth, or when a tube holder is repositioned. At these times, the respiratory therapist is usually available for help, and the oral cavity can be simultaneously and thoroughly assessed using a flashlight and tongue depressor.

Most of the recommendations on mouth care presented are based on clinical experience, limited respiratory research (Szlakiewicz, 1986) and oncology research reflected in mouth care literature (Daeffler, 1980; Daeffler, 1981; Mauer, 1977). Oncology research is relevant because oncology patients tend to have the same risk factors for stomatitis and infection as respiratory patients. Because of these limitations, recommendations here must be used as a guideline only, until further research clarifies the best protocol for oral hygiene in respiratory patients.

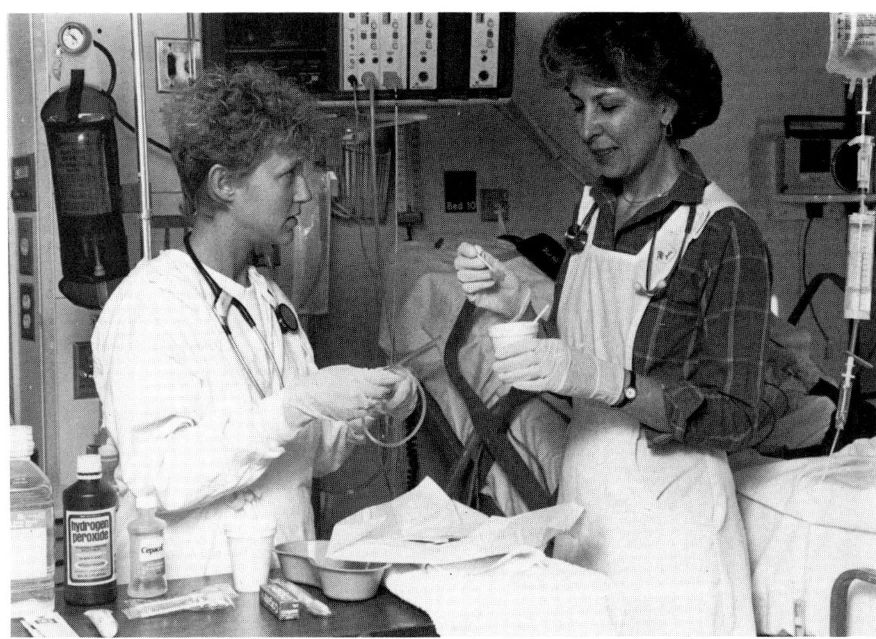

Figure 27–16. Two nurses prepare for a mouth care procedure for a comatose patient.

In addition, keep in mind that the nurse may need to drastically alter procedure, depending on individual circumstances. For example, the alert postsurgical patient with a nasotracheal tube may be willing and able to sit upright in bed and effectively brush his teeth with toothbrush and toothpaste on his own.

HOME SETTING

The same procedure for mouth care may be followed in the home setting with a few adaptations. Since the patient has a tracheostomy rather than an endotracheal tube and is in a stable medical condition, he tends to have a normal oral mucosa compared with the hospitalized intubated patient. Hence, use of a toothbrush and toothpaste followed by rinsing with water or mouthwash is acceptable and usually preferred by the patient. The procedure is done without use of clean gloves, unless the patient is immunosuppressed or unless a caregiver is doing the mouth care.

If signs of stomatitis or infection appear, the physician is notified. A 1:1 to 1:4 ratio of hydrogen peroxide:saline or water solution may be used with a soft toothbrush. The saline or water does not have to be sterile, unless the patient is immunosuppressed; an alternative is to mix 1 teaspoon of salt to 1 pint water.

Support of the Family

Since the patient is often a member of a larger family system, care of the intubated respiratory patient in-

Table 27–3. NURSING INTERVENTIONS FOR FAMILY SUPPORT

Interventions	Rationales
Assign a primary nurse to communicate daily with the family either in person or by telephone.	This continuity facilitates communication and establishment of a relationship of trust between family and health providers.
Encourage the family to verbalize fears, concerns, and feelings regarding the recent illness.	Family members have a need to relive the critical incident that led to intensive respiratory care or hospital admission, e.g., acute dyspnea leading to intubation. In the home, families need to talk about how they are coping with extra respiratory care duties and the COPD patient's psychologic coping mechanisms.
During the family's first visit with the intubated patient Explain the patient's diagnosis; current physical, emotional, mental status; and respiratory care provided. Explain physical surroundings, including equipment at the bedside.	This approach meets the family's informational needs, helps to relieve anxiety, and prepares them for participation in self-care education (see Chapter 17).
Tell the family that the patient cannot talk because of the endotracheal or tracheostomy tube. Explain why phonation is not possible. Explain how family members can best communicate with the patient. Encourage touching.	Avoids unnecessary anxiety associated with inability to speak. Patient and family need verbal reassurance that speech will return after tube removal or cuff deflation.
Emphasize small accomplishments or changes in condition that indicate favorable medical progress or adaptive coping ability.	Positive reinforcement for small accomplishments makes the family aware of progress and gives them hope that the patient's condition will continue to improve.
Provide relief for supportive family members. Encourage family at the hospital to go home for a good night's rest but to feel free to call for an update of the patient's condition.	Family members are often unable to assess their own need for physical and psychologic renewal. Sometimes they remain at the bedside because they do not know what else to do. Other times they feel guilty about going out and having a good time, while the patient is barely coping with his lung disease.
Help the family at home to schedule regular time off from home care responsibilities. Remind families that taking care of themselves indirectly benefits the patient. A well-rested and relaxed person can give more and better psychologic and physical support than a tired, stressed person.	They need permission to leave the patient's situation, while they attend to their own needs.
Ask the family to identify one member responsible for communicating information to other family members. Keep this person informed of the patient's physical, emotional, and mental status and the changes in medical treatment and nursing care.	Family members have a need for this information but are uncertain as to how to obtain it. Assignment of a family spokesperson relieves hospital staff of answering numerous calls from the family and assures a unified and consistent approach to the patient.
Utilize available human resources (e.g., medical social worker, psychologist, person trained in crisis intervention, hospital volunteers, community agencies) to establish communication with the family during crisis and to address common concerns, such as lack of finances, housing, meals, and so forth.	Families in disequilibrium are unable to seek available resources on their own. During hospital admission, volunteers can provide information regarding visiting hours, location and hours of the cafeteria, and physical arrangement of the unit or ward. Community agencies provide a variety of services, equipment loans, nutritious meals, and so forth.
Encourage the family to talk to the physician regarding the patient's medical condition.	The physician can answer medical questions that the nurse cannot answer. Further dialogue may help the family better understand and accept the patient's disease process. Also, the physician can deal with medication needs (e.g., sedatives and tranquilizers) for distressed family members.

volves support of the family as well as the patient. *Family* refers to a relative or anyone else who is significant to the patient.

Particularly when a family member is intubated upon hospital admission, the family may become disorganized and powerless to seek resources that might help them cope adaptively with such a crisis situation. Thereafter, the patient's acute illness imposes other stressors, such as role changes within the family, social isolation, financial concerns, transportation problems to and from the hospital, fear of loss of the loved one, and emotional turmoil while the family member is hospitalized (Hodovanic et al, 1984).

Some of these stressors may follow the family and the recently discharged tracheostomy patient to the home setting. The basic difference between the hospital and home situation is that in the hospital setting, the family may become *totally* disorganized, and thus more receptive to crisis intervention. In the home setting, family disorganization may be less, provided family members have participated in discharge planning. Yet, once the patient is home, he may revert to former coping patterns and remain unwilling to implement role changes or modify his belief system. As family members become more frustrated, maladaptive coping patterns add more stress to the lives of both the patient and these family members.

Furthermore, in the home setting, providing around-the-clock care for an intubated patient is a tremendous burden for family members. Usually, the magnitude of this burden is not fully appreciated until the family members actually start to perform the care at home.

With this background information in mind, the nurse may use the interventions in Table 27–3 to support the family and reduce stressors that render them seemingly powerless.

Conclusion

This chapter has presented care of the intubated patient. Discussion has covered many different topics, ranging from basic airway care, routine tracheostomy care, and psychologic support of patient and family, to the details of tracheal suctioning, mouth care, and monitoring for complications during intubation as well as postextubation. It is hoped that the depth of this chapter has prepared the clinician for the challenge of meeting the multidimensional needs of the intubated patient across the health care continuum. Moreover, though this content may help the nurse to make better clinical decisions, key questions still remain. For example, we still do not know the *best* technique for tracheal suctioning or for providing mouth care, even though a nurse may perform each of these procedures at least twelve times a day. Once respiratory research answers these basic questions, care of the intubated patient will become more effective, and attention may be more justifiably focused on other more technologic aspects of care.

REFERENCES

Ackerman, M.: The use of bolus normal saline instillations in artificial airways: Is it useful or necessary? *Heart and lung*, 14(5):505–506, 1985.

Baker, P., Baker, J., and Koen, P.: Endotracheal suctioning techniques in hypoxemic patients. *Respiratory care*, 28(12):1563–1568, 1983.

Barrocas, A., Tretola, R., and Alonso, A.: Nutrition and the critically ill pulmonary patient. *Respiratory care*, 28(1):50–61, 1983.

Belling, D., Kelley, R., and Simon, R.: Use of the swivel adaptor aperture during suctioning to prevent hypoxemia in the mechanically ventilated patient. *Heart and lung*, 7(2):320–322, 1978.

Bernhard, W., Yost, L., Joynes, D., Cothalis, S., and Turndorf, H.: Intracuff pressures in endotracheal and tracheostomy tubes—related cuff physical characteristics. *Chest*, 87(6):720–725, 1985.

Birdsall, C.: How do you use a closed suction adapter? *American journal of nursing*, 86(11):1222–1223, 1986.

Bodai, B.: A means of suctioning without cardiopulmonary depression. *Heart and lung*, 11(2):172–176, 1982.

Bohen, M.: Herpetic whitlow. *Journal of the operating room research institute*, 1(3):172–173, 1982.

Boutros, A. R.: Arterial blood oxygenation during and after endotracheal suctioning in the apneic patient. *Anesthesiology*, 32(2): 114–118, 1970.

Brown, S., Stansbury, D., et al: Prevention of suctioning-related arterial oxygen desaturation. *Chest*, 83(4):621–627, 1983.

Chapman, G., Kim, C., et al: Evaluation of the safety and efficiency of a new suction catheter design. *Respiratory care*, 31(10):889–895, 1986.

Cunningham, C. and Sergent, J.: A preliminary view of the contamination of suction apparatus. *Focus on critical care*, 10(4):10–14, 1983.

Daeffler, R.: Oral hygiene measures for patients with cancer. II. *Cancer nursing*, 3(6):427–432, 1980.

Daeffler, R.: Oral hygiene measures for patients with cancer. III. *Cancer nursing*, 4(1):29–35, 1981.

DeCampo, T. and Civetta, J.: The effect of short-term discontinuation of high level PEEP in patients with acute respiratory failure. *Critical care medicine*, 7(2):47–49, 1979.

Demers, R.: Complications of endotracheal suctioning procedures. *Respiratory care*, 27(4):453–457, 1982.

Douglas, S., Larson, E.: The effect of a positive end-expiratory pressure adapter on oxygenation during endotracheal suctioning. *Heart and lung*, 14(4): 396–400, 1985.

Freedman, A. and Goodman, L.: Suctioning the left bronchial tree in the intubated adult. *Critical care medicine*, 10(1): 43–45, 1982.

Goodnough, S.: The effects of oxygen and hyperinflation on arterial oxygen tension after endotracheal suctioning. *Heart and lung*, 14(1):11–17, 1985.

Greaves, W., Kaiser, A., et al: The problem of herpetic whitlow among hospital personnel. *Infection control*, 1(6):381–385, 1980.

Haberman, P., Green, H., et al: Determinants of successful selective tracheobronchial suctioning. *New england journal of medicine*, 289(20):1060–1063, 1973.

Hanley, M., Rudd, T., and Butler, J.: What happens to intratracheal saline instillations? *American review of respiratory disease*, 117(4):124S, 1978.

Hodgkin, J., Zorn, E., and Connors, G.: *Pulmonary Rehabilitation—Guidelines to Success*. Boston, Butterworth Publishers, 1984.

Hodovanic, B., Reardon, D., Reese, W., and Hedges, B.: Family crisis intervention program in the medical intensive care unit. *Heart and lung*, 13(3):243–249, 1984.

Jung, R. and Gottlieb, L.: Comparison of tracheobronchial suction catheters in humans. *Chest*, 69(2):179–181, 1976.

Kirilloff, L. and Maszkiewicz, R.: Guide to respiratory care in critically ill adults. *American journal of nursing*, 79(10): 2005–2012, 1979.

Kubota, Y., Magaribuchi, T., et al: Evaluation of selective bronchial suctioning in the adult. *Critical care medicine*, 8(12):748–749, 1980.

Kubota, Y., Magaribuchi, T., et al: Selective bronchial suctioning in the adult using a curve-tipped catheter with a guide mark. *Critical care medicine*, 10(11):767–769, 1982.

Landa, J., Kwoka, M., et al: Effects of suctioning on mucociliary transport. *Chest*, 77(2):202–207, 1980.

Leske, J.: Needs of relatives of critically ill patients: a follow-up. *Heart and lung*, 15(2):189–193, 1986.

Link, W., Spaeth, E., et al: The influence of suction catheter tip design on tracheobronchial trauma and fluid aspiration efficiency. *Anesthesia and analgesia . . . current researches*, 55(2):290–298, 1976.

Louis, D. and Silva, J.: Herpetic whitlow: herpetic infections of the digits. *Journal of hand surgery*, 4(1):90–93, 1979.

Maurer, J.: Providing optimal oral health. *Nursing clinics of north america*, 12(4):671–685, 1977.

Powaser, M., et al: The effectiveness of hourly cuff deflation in minimizing tracheal damage. *Heart and lung*, 5(5):734–741, 1976.

Remolina, C., Khan, A., Santiago, T., and Edelman, N.: Positional hypoxemia in unilateral lung disease. *New england journal of medicine*, 304(8):523–525, 1981.

Riegel, B. and Forshee, T.: A review and critique of the literature on preoxygenation for endotracheal suctioning. *Heart and lung*, 14(5):507–518, 1985.

Rindfleisch, S. and Tyler, M.: Points of view—duration of suctioning: an important variable. *Respiratory care*, 28(4):457–459, 1983.

Ritz, R., Scott, L., Coyle, M., and Pierson, D.: Contamination of multiple-use suction catheter in a closed-circuit system compared to contamination of a disposable, single-use suction catheter. *Respiratory care*, 31(11):1086–1091, 1986.

Sackner, M., Landa, J., Greeneltch, N., and Robinson, M.: Pathogenesis and prevention of tracheobronchial damage with suction procedures. *Chest*, 64(3):284–290, 1973.

Sills, J.: An emergency cuff inflation technique. *Respiratory care*, 31(3):199–201, 1986.

Stauffer, J. and Silvestri, R.: Complications of endotracheal intubation, tracheostomy, and artificial airways. *Respiratory care*, 27(4):417–434, 1982.

Szlakiewicz, R.: Prevention of Oral Deterioration in Endotracheally Intubated Patients. Los Angeles, University of California, 1986.

Mechanical Ventilation

28

Main Objectives

1. **Define the following terms: negative pressure ventilation, positive pressure ventilation, high frequency jet ventilation, iron lung, chest cuirass, body wrap, compressible volume loss, stacked breaths, super positive end expiratory pressure (PEEP), optimal PEEP, peak inspiratory pressure, sigh volume, sensitivity, expiratory retard, plateau pressure, low exhaled volume, oximetry PaO_2, and capnogram.**

2. **State the two main indications for mechanical ventilation and the role of pH in decision-making processes.**
3. **State the four goals of mechanical ventilation.**
4. **Compare and contrast the following:**
   a. **Negative and positive pressure ventilation.**
   b. **Pressure-cycled, volume-cycled, and time-cycled positive pressure ventilators.**
   c. **Mask CPAP and nasal CPAP.**
5. **Define and describe indications and complications for at least three of the following modes of ventilation: controlled, assist-control, intermittent mandatory ventilation (IMV), synchronized intermittent mandatory ventilation (SIMV), PEEP, CPAP, and pressure support ventilation.**
6. **Explain how the demand flow CPAP system may increase work of breathing.**
7. **Select a positive pressure ventilator in your clinical setting. Describe the indications for adjustment of each of the following settings: mode, FIO_2, tidal volume (V_T), sigh volume, sensitivity, inspiratory to expiratory (I:E) ratio, inspiratory flow rate, and peak inspiratory pressure.**
8. **List three common ventilator-related problems. Explain how to troubleshoot each problem.**
9. **List four patient complications of mechanical ventilation. For each complication, state the physiologic mechanism involved, signs and symptoms, and interventions to prevent or minimize adverse effects on the body.**
10. **Name the components of a basic ventilator check.**
11. **Describe how to monitor ABG results, effective and static compliance, oximetry PaO_2, transcutaneous PO_2 and PCO_2, and end-tidal PCO_2.**
12. **List weaning criteria that help assess mechanics of breathing, oxygenation, and ventilation.**
13. **Describe traditional and SIMV methods for weaning the patient off mechanical ventilation.**
14. **State the four phases of psychologic adjustment to mechanical ventilation. Describe nursing interventions to facilitate patient progress through these phases towards active participation in rehabilitative care.**
15. **Define long-term mechanical ventilation. Discuss goals, criteria for implementation, and nursing care.**
16. **Describe and state the indications for the following three alternatives to long-term mechanical ventilation: diaphragm pacing, rocking bed, and pneumobelt.**

This chapter discusses mechanical ventilation. When considered with Chapter 27 on care of the intubated patient, it prepares the reader for application of content in the case study at the end of the book.

Though most of the content in this chapter concerns respiratory care in acute care settings, basic concepts apply to mechanical ventilation in extended care and home settings as well. For example, negative pressure ventilators mentioned in this chapter may be used for patients in chronic ventilatory failure regardless of setting. The nurse's check for positive pressure ventilators explained here is basically the same regardless of the type or model of ventilator attached to the patient. The needs assessment and discharge checklist for ventilator-dependent patients may be used by home health nurses as well as by acute care nurses discharging the patient to the home setting.

Indications

The decision to use mechanical ventilation is separate from the decision to intubate. In emergency situations, however, mechanical ventilation nearly always follows intubation, at least until time permits a more thorough assessment of the patient's overall condition and respiratory status.

The two main indications for mechanical ventilation include *inadequate ventilation* and *hypoxemia.* In the first case, apnea or alveolar hypoventilation may cause a falling pH and a stable or rising $PaCO_2$. A gradually rising $PaCO_2$ usually signals an imminent need for ventilatory support, but it is not an entirely reliable indicator, especially in the presence of mixed ABG disorders. The pH is the most important indicator (see Chapter 13). Mechanical ventilation is usually needed for patients with respiratory acidosis with a pH of less than 7.2. However, the physician may decide to intubate at a higher pH, depending on individual circumstances. A patient in acute ventilatory failure that worsens over minutes or hours, in spite of vigorous therapy, nearly always requires intubation and mechanical ventilation, whether the pH is 7.2, 7.3, or some other value.

The second indication, hypoxemia, may be severe, requiring an FIO_2 beyond the level comfortably and reliably provided by a nonrebreathing, partial rebreathing, or other mask. Mechanical ventilation permits application of a high FIO_2 simply by turning a knob on a ventilator. In some cases, after initiation of mechanical ventilation, the change in ventilatory pattern substantially improves mechanics of breathing and oxygenation so that FIO_2 can be reduced to below 0.50.

Patients with either inadequate ventilation or hypoxemia invariably have one or more of the following other indications for mechanical ventilation: *inadequate lung expansion, respiratory muscle fatigue, excessive work of breathing, unstable ventilatory drive*, and early *postoperative prophylaxis* to prevent respiratory acidosis, poor lung expansion, or respiratory muscle fatigue in high risk patients.

In addition, a patient with a *closed head injury* may require mechanical ventilation to reduce $PaCO_2$ to values of 25 to 30 mmHg. The resulting alkalosis reduces brain swelling and intracranial pressure. When severe, traumatic *flail chest* is another indication for mechanical ventilation (Pierson, 1983a).

As discussed previously in this book, mechanical ventilation for the patient with chronic obstructive pulmonary disease (COPD) is deferred for as long as possible. This type of patient can tolerate a $PaCO_2$ of 60 mmHg or higher, and acute respiratory failure is likely to reverse with bronchodilator administration, vigorous respiratory therapy, and other measures. Intubation and mechanical ventilation become necessary only when consciousness becomes impaired, when acute respiratory acidosis becomes progressively worse, or when uncontrollable agitation makes sedation and mechanical ventilation mandatory.

Goals

The goals of mechanical ventilation include the following (Smith, 1983):

1. To adjust alveolar ventilation to a level determined as normal for each patient.
2. To improve V/Q relationships and oxygenation.
3. To decrease the work of breathing.
4. In high risk surgical patients, to provide prophylactic ventilation for 12 to 24 hours during the post-operative period.

Positive Pressure Ventilation

The type of mechanical ventilation in the acute care setting is positive pressure ventilation. A positive pressure ventilator is the power source that forces gas into the lungs. The positive intrathoracic pressure expands the lungs and chest wall (Fig. 28–1). The cessation of gas flow permits the chest and lungs to recoil to resting position and airway pressure to return towards normal.

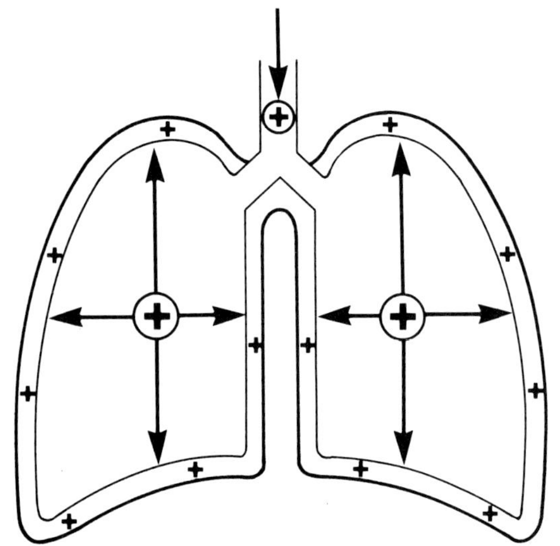

Figure 28–1. Diagrammatic representation of the effects of positive intrathoracic pressure. The positive pressure expands the lungs and chest wall.

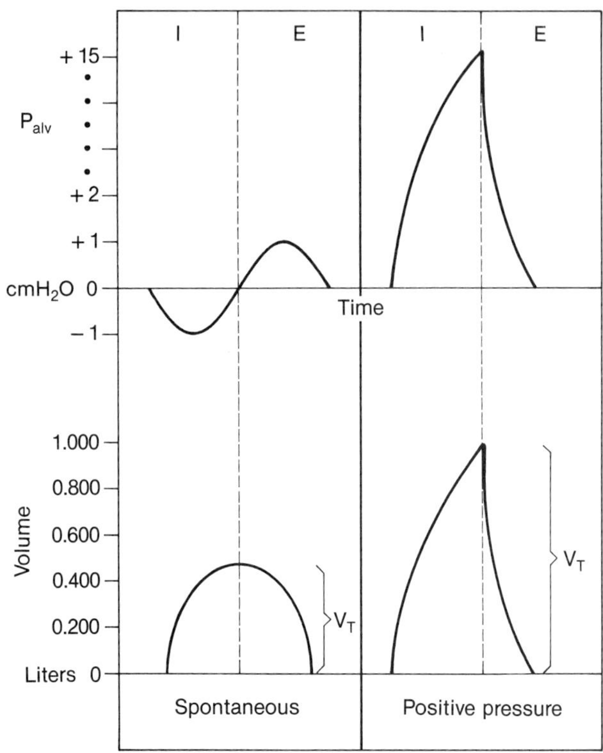

Figure 28–2. Alveolar pressure (top) and lung volume changes (bottom) during spontaneous and positive pressure breathing. (I = inspiration; E = expiration.)

A comparison of pressure and volume changes during spontaneous breathing and positive pressure breathing will help the nurse understand the adverse effects of positive pressure ventilation discussed subsequently in this chapter. First, note in Figure 28–2 that alveolar pressure changes are exactly the opposite during the two phases of the respiratory cycle. For example, during positive pressure breathing, alveolar and pleural pressures become more positive during inspiration (top, right) instead of more negative, as occurs during spontaneous breathing (top, left). Second, during positive pressure breathing, the alveolar pressure waveform is different, with pressures remaining positive throughout inspiration and expiration. Last, positive pressure breathing delivers greater volumes compared with spontaneous breathing. The current trend in ventilator volume adjustment is to deliver large tidal volumes at a slow respiratory rate to achieve an adequate minute ventilation.

TYPES OF POSITIVE PRESSURE VENTILATORS

Many different types of positive pressure ventilators are available for clinical use, some with as many as 20 controls. Some have built-in monitoring and alarm systems and numerous other features, including gas blenders, air filters, pressure pop-off valves, humidifiers and nebulizers, water traps, gas sampling ports, and thermometers.

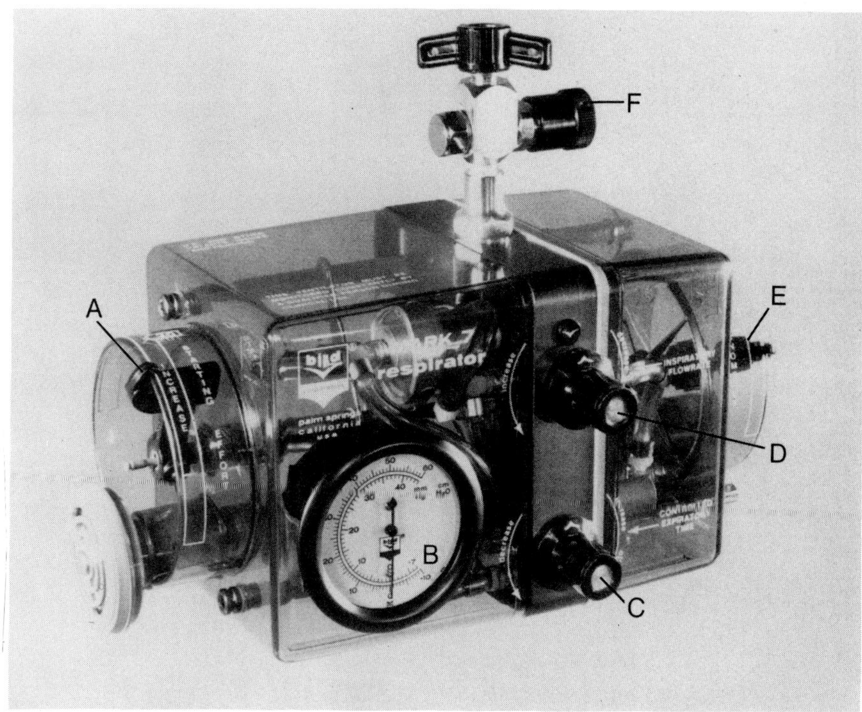

Figure 28–3. Bird Mark 7 pressure–cycled (limited) ventilator. (Courtesy of Bird Products Corporation, Palm Springs, California.) A, Sensitivity control. B, Airway pressure manometer. C, Expiratory time control. D, Inspiratory flow rate control. E, Pressure control. F, Rotary on/off switch.

This diverse group of ventilators may be classified in many different ways, e.g., by characteristic pressure and flow waveform, drive mechanism, single versus double circuitry, and presence of a computer or microprocessor. The most basic classification method is by *cycling mechanism*, defined as the method used to stop inspiration and start expiration. Ventilators are pressure-cycled, also called pressure-limited; volume-cycled; time-cycled; or some combination of these types.

Pressure-Cycled Ventilators

A *pressure-cycled ventilator*, such as the Bird Mark 7, 8, 10, or 14, allows air to flow into the lungs until a preset pressure is reached (Fig. 28–3). A valve then closes, and expiration begins. Though this type of machine is commonly used for intermittent positive pressure breathing (IPPB) treatments, it is no longer the ventilator of choice for continuous mechanical ventilation, except occasionally for comatose or drug-overdose patients with normal lungs that are easy to ventilate. The Bird series of ventilators are commonly used as back-up ventilators because they are pneumatically powered and not affected by power failure.

The biggest problem with a pressure-cycled ventilator is that the delivery of a desired tidal volume is not guaranteed but varies with changing airway resistance. Hence, the postoperative patient whose lung compliance and airway resistance change over a short period of time may become inadvertently overventilated (i.e., respiratory alkalosis), as improved lung mechanics permit delivery of more gas at the same preset pressure. Similarly, the COPD patient with bronchospasm or increased mucus retention may become underventilated (i.e., respiratory acidosis), as increasing airway resistance gradually reduces tidal volume.

Other problems exist with pressure-cycled ventilators. They have a limited pressure capability and cannot effectively and safely ventilate stiff noncompliant lungs that require high pressures over 50 to 60 cmH_2O. Also, FIO_2 cannot be controlled unless the machine is attached to an oxygen blender.

Although models used in the hospital setting, such as the Bird or Bennett PR series (Fig. 28–4), have a knob to adjust flow rate for patients who are difficult to ventilate, these pneumatically powered models require a 40 to 70 lb/in^2 gas source, or they must be attached to an electrically driven compressor. Many *electrically* powered pressure-cycled ventilators utilized in chronic care settings are convenient because they plug into an electric wall outlet, but they may lack the flow capabilities of ventilators designed for acute care settings.

Volume-Cycled Ventilators

A *volume-cycled ventilator* allows gas to flow into the lungs until a preset volume of gas has been delivered or expelled from the ventilator. Examples of volume-cycled ventilators include the Bear 1 and Bear 2 (Bear Medical Systems, Inc.) (Fig. 28–5), Puritan Bennett MA-1 (Fig. 28–6) and MA-2, Monaghan 225/SIMV, and Ohio CCV-2, SIMV. Because these ventilators are versatile and have a high pressure capability

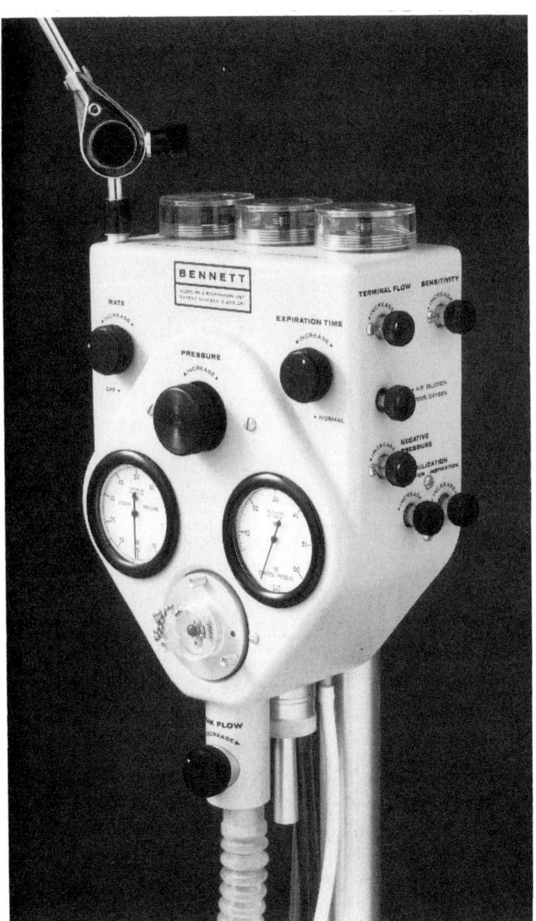

Figure 28–4. Puritan-Bennett PR-2 pressure limited ventilator. (Courtesy of Puritan-Bennett Corp., Lenexa, Kansas.)

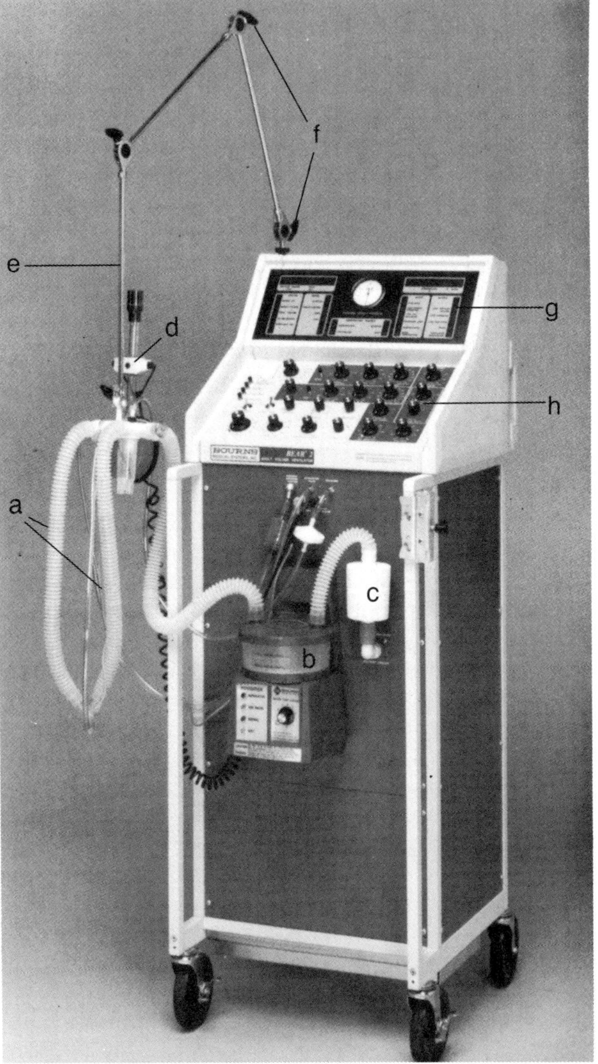

A

Figure 28–5. Bear 2 Adult Volume Ventilator. *A*, The ventilator system. a, Breathing circuit (nondisposable); b, Humidifier located in-line along the inspiratory side of the breathing circuit; c, Bacterial filter for main gas flow; d, Monitoring spirometer attached to expiratory side of breathing circuit; e, Support arm attached to plastic manifold; f, Retaining screws for adjustment of support arm; g, Display panel of signals and alarms; h, Control panel.

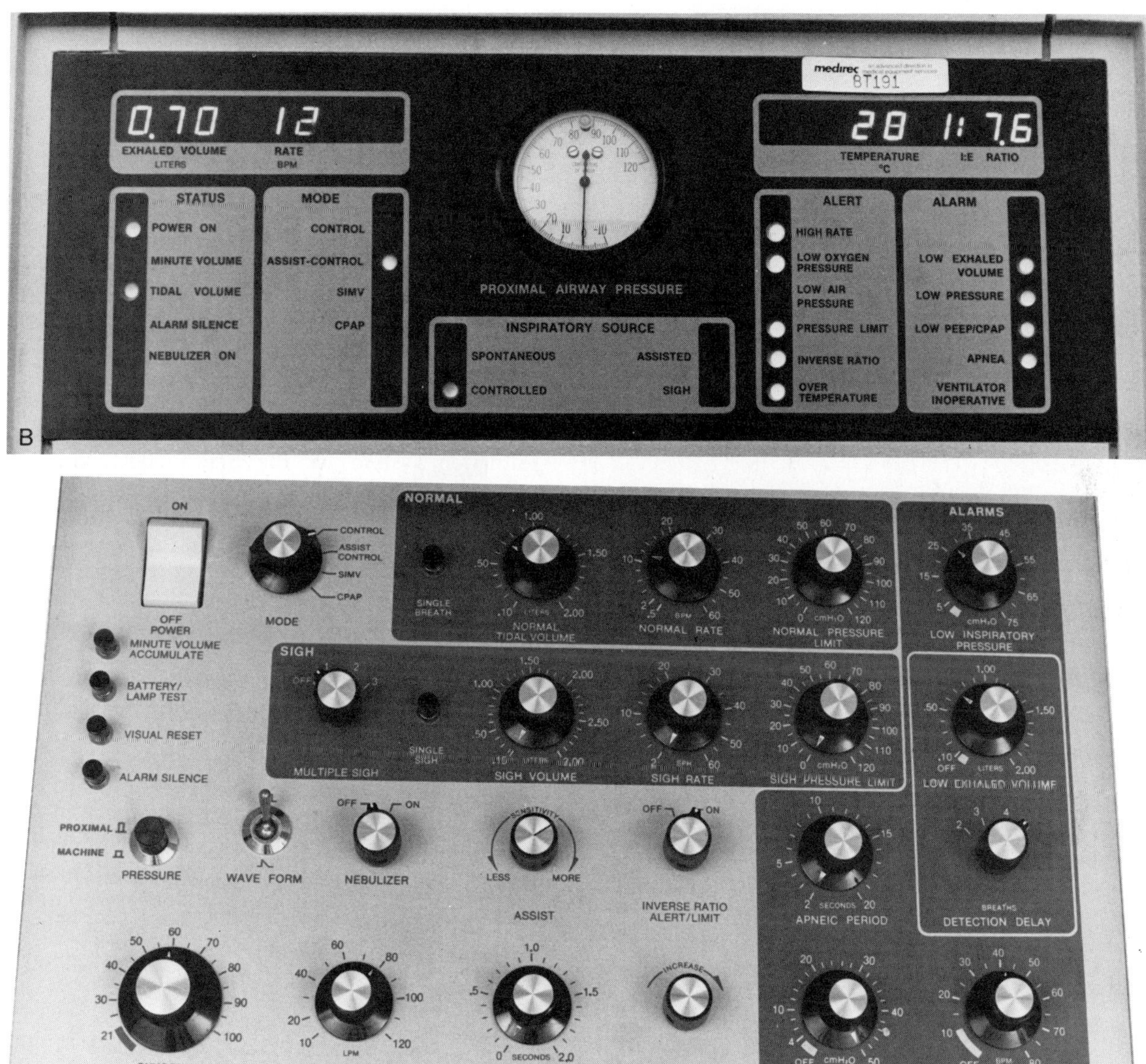

Figure 28–5 *Continued B,* Display signals and alarms. *C,* Control panel. (*A,* Courtesy of Bear Medical Systems, Inc., Riverside, California.)

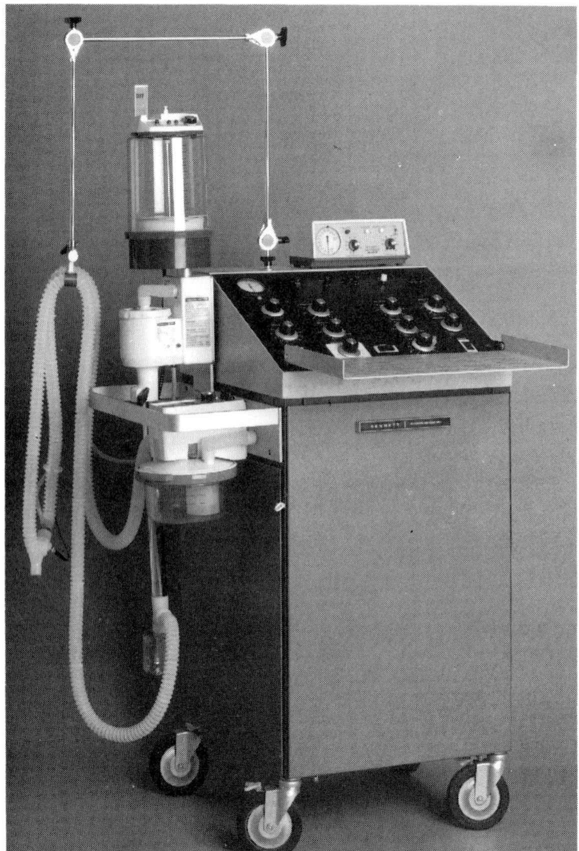

Figure 28–6. Puritan-Bennett MA-1 volume-limited ventilator. (Courtesy of Puritan-Bennett Corporation, Lenexa, Kansas.)

of up to 120 cmH_2O, they are suitable for use in the critical care setting, where acute chest disease and surgical intervention are likely to drastically alter lung mechanics. These ventilators deliver a constant tidal volume, regardless of changing compliance and airway resistance.

A small amount of each delivered volume, however, is compressed within the ventilator and connecting tubing circuit between the ventilator and patient. This *compressible volume loss* varies, depending on the distensibility of the ventilator's tubing, the amount of pressure and volume delivered, and the water level in the humidifier, but it usually averages about 3 to 4 cc/cmH_2O pressure, e.g., 3 cc × peak pressure (30 cmH_2O) = 60 cc compressible volume loss. The compressible volume loss is subtracted from the preset volume delivered, e.g., 800 cc, to yield the actual volume delivered to the patient's lungs, 800 cc − 60 cc = 740 cc.

Many of the older and more durable volume-cycled ventilators, such as the Puritan-Bennett MA-1 and Emerson 3-PV, are also used in chronic care settings. Some clinicians believe that, even for the acute care setting, use of the more sophisticated ventilators offers no clear advantage, when extra cost, maintenance, and training of personnel are considered.

Time-Cycled Ventilators

A *time-cycled ventilator* allows air to flow into the lungs until a preset length of time has elapsed. Delivered volume, pressure, and flow may vary, depending on ventilator characteristics and patient mechanics. Examples of ventilators that are primarily time-cycled include the Engstrom; the Emerson 3-PV and 3-MV; Siemens Servo 900, 900B, and 900C (Fig. 28–7); the Bourns BP200 (Bear Medical Systems, Inc.); and the Bird Babybird ventilators. Some pressure-cycled units, such as the Bennett PR series, can be either pressure- or time-cycled, depending on the control settings.

Computer- and Microprocessor-Controlled Ventilators

The most technologically sophisticated ventilator has a computer, a microprocessor system, or both either built into a volume- or time-cycled ventilator or attached to provide electronic memory, breath-by-breath automatic control of ventilator functions, monitoring alarms, and digital and message display systems. Examples of such ventilators are the Bear 5, Puritan-Bennett 7200, and Siemens Computer Aided Ventilation system for the Servo 900C and 900D models (Fig. 28–7B). Most of these ventilators do not fall into one classification. For example, the Puritan-Bennett 7200 ventilator is classified as an electrically powered, pneumatically driven, microprocessor-controlled volume ventilator. Though it is a volume ventilator, similar to other modern ventilators, it has a pressure support feature that allows the clinician to add positive pressure during the ventilator breath to decrease the work of breathing. Computer and microprocessor-controlled ventilators are most appropriate for patients with severe adult respiratory distress syndrome, burns, or multisystem failure. Such patients may have such high minute ventilation requirements and such low respiratory system compliances that older ventilators, such as the Bennett MA-1, are incapable of ventilating them (Pierson et al, 1986c).

HIGH FREQUENCY JET VENTILATION

Some volume ventilators, such as the Bear 1 or Bear 2 ventilator, may be supplemented with a *high frequency jet ventilator* to provide another mode of ventilation called *high frequency jet ventilation* (HFJV) (Fig. 28–8 and Fig. 28–9).

HFJV is one of three types of high frequency ventilation (HFV) listed in Table 28–1 and used most frequently in the clinical setting. Though the topic is beyond the scope of this text, a brief mention of two basic differences between HFV and conventional positive pressure ventilation will provide a foundation for understanding the purpose of the jet ventilator and specialized monitoring considerations discussed in other sources (Warren and Howell, 1983; Gruden,

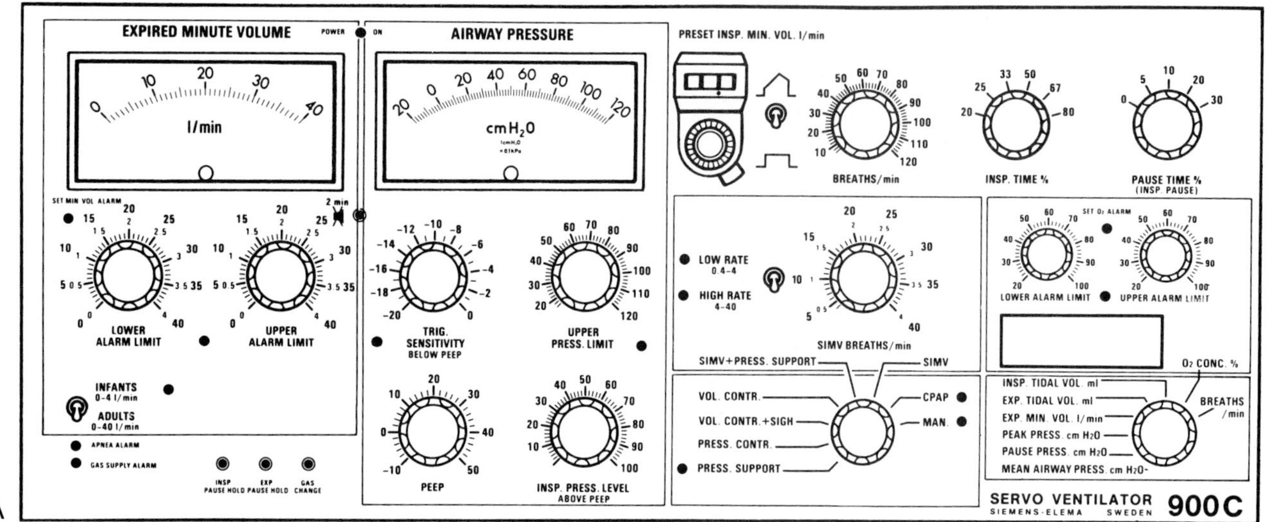

Figure 28–7. Siemens Servo 900C ventilator. *A*, Control panel.

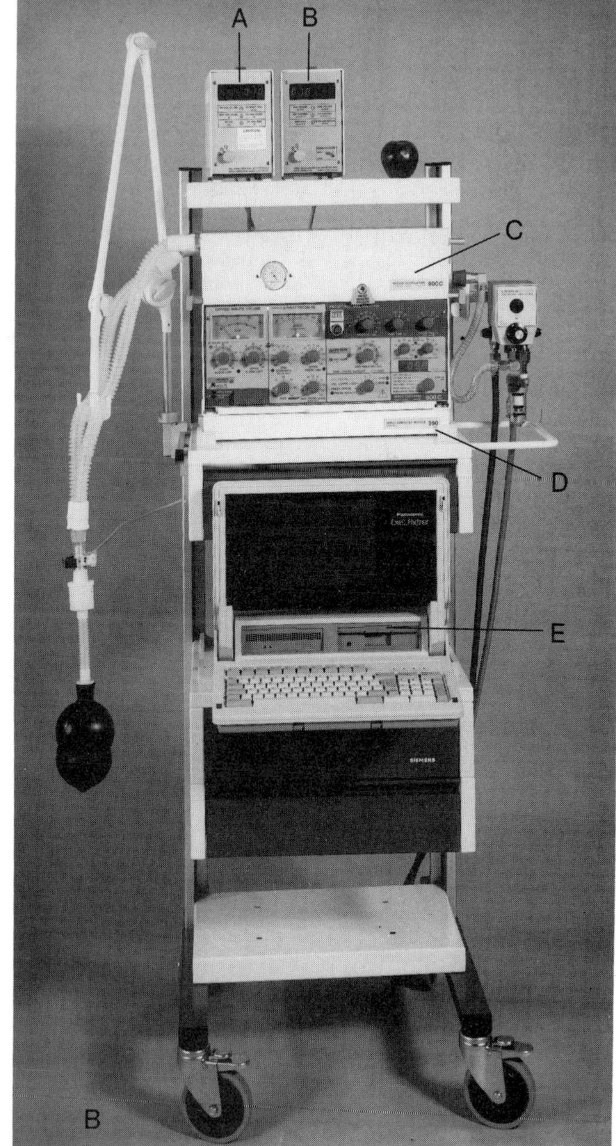

Figure 28–7 *B*, Ventilator integrated with a computer aided ventilation system. A = CO_2 analyzer; B = Lung mechanics calculator; C = Ventilator; D = Computer module; E = IBM compatible personal computer. (Courtesy of Siemens-Elma Ventilator Systems, Schaumburg, Illinois.)

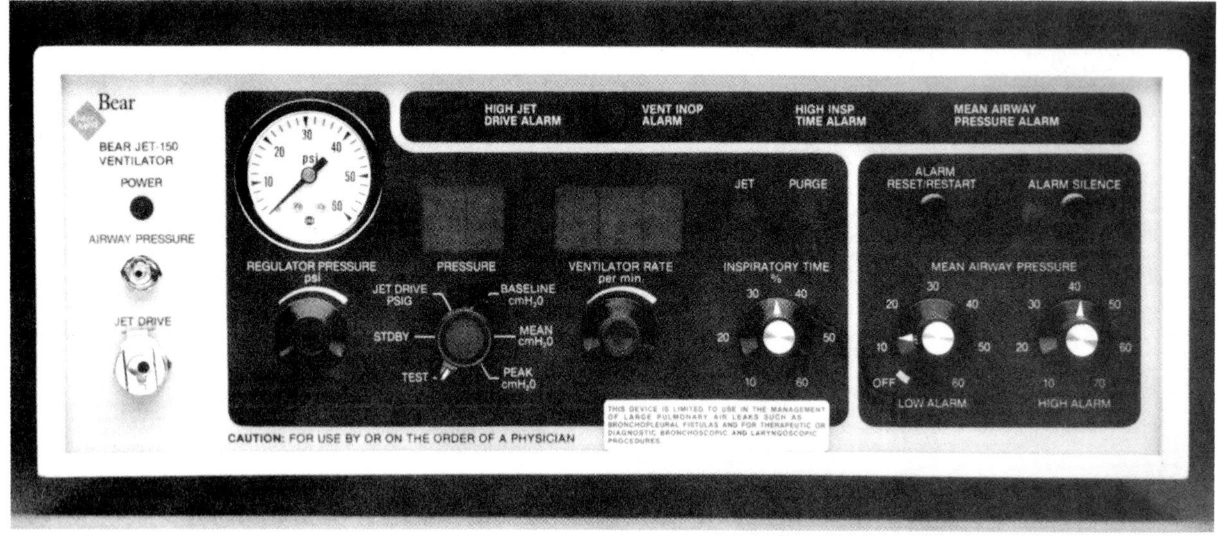

Figure 28–8. High frequency jet ventilator. This compact Bear Jet–150 model is used in conjunction with the Bear 1 or Bear 2 Adult Volume Ventilator. (Courtesy of Bear Medical Systems, Inc., Riverside, California.)

Table 28–1. TYPES OF HIGH FREQUENCY VENTILATION*

Type	Description	Rate	Tidal Volume
High frequency positive pressure ventilation (HFPPV)	Uses a volume ventilator with a low internal compressible volume and small tidal volumes.	60 to 100 breaths/min	3 to 6 ml/kg
High frequency jet ventilation (HFJV)	Uses a jet ventilator to deliver a jet of gas through a small cannula of a jet endotracheal tube. Entrainment of humidified gas enhances V_T.	100 to 400 (usually 100–200) breaths/min	200 to 400 ml
High frequency oscillation (HFO)	A high frequency pulse generator (i.e., loudspeaker or piston pump) generates oscillations during both inspiration and expiration, with exceptionally small tidal volumes resulting.	900 to 3000 vibrations/min	50 to 150 ml

*Data from Hudson, L. High frequency ventilation. *Pulmonary perspectives* [American College of Chest Physicians], 1(4): 1–2, 1984.

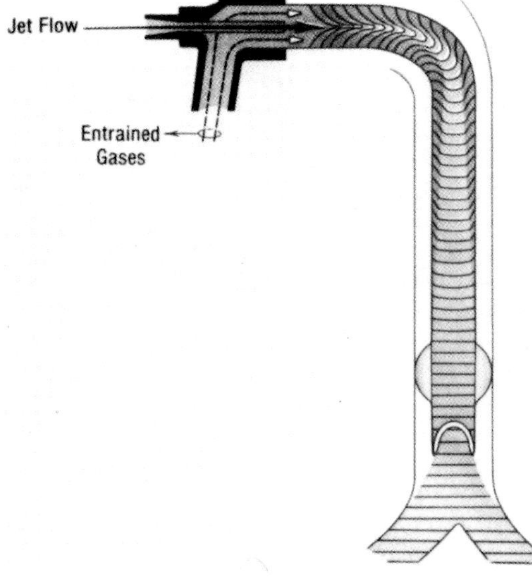

Figure 28–9. Conceptual drawing of the jet flow of gases. The jet flow moves down airways as a progressively broadening wave of decreasing pressure. (Reproduced by permission from Carlon, G., Kahn, R. et al. Clinical experience with high frequency jet ventilation. *Critical care medicine,* 9(1):2, 1981.)

Table 28–2. POTENTIAL ADVANTAGES AND DISADVANTAGES OF HIGH FREQUENCY VENTILATION (HFV) COMPARED WITH CONVENTIONAL VENTILATION

Advantages/Disadvantages	Clinical Implications
Advantages	
Lower peak intratracheal, alveolar, and intrathoracic pressures, since HFV delivers less positive pressure to the lungs.	Reduced incidence of barotrauma. Promotion of bronchopleural fistula closure. Absent or reduced *fluid retention,* a problem associated with positive pressure ventilation.
Less cardiac depression—lower peak airway pressures reduce interference with venous return to the heart.	Reduced incidence of hypotension and low cardiac output.
Fewer fluctuations in intracranial pressure, although mean intracranial pressure (ICP) may not decrease (Quan et al, 1983).	Creates a "quiet" surgical field for brain microsurgery. May help stabilize intracranial pressure (ICP) for critically ill neurologic patient.
Decreased need for sedation, analgesics, and paralyzing agents. HFV suppresses spontaneous breathing and decreases thoracoabdominal movements.	Improvement in alveolar ventilation and oxygenation. Agitation and abnormal ABGs may return if the patient is returned to conventional positive pressure breathing.
Reduction in ventilator circuitry by the airway during anesthesia for rigid bronchoscopy and laryngoscopy.	Reduces competition between anesthesiologist and surgeon for the airway and may provide a better view down the trachea during partial or complete ventilatory support.
Disadvantages	
Mean alveolar pressure may be equal to or greater than P_{alv} during conventional ventilation. When the patient is ventilated at a high FRC, HFV may not be more beneficial than conventional ventilation.	HFV may make a bronchopleural fistula larger, not smaller. Risk for barotrauma may be increased in some cases.
In HFJV, gas humidification is via a constant drip of fluid into the jet.	Potential for fluid overload, unless fluid administration is carefully monitored.
Requires specially trained personnel who can constantly and appropriately monitor the patient and special HFV equipment.	Experience, availability of trained personnel, and cost factors limit use of HFV to medical centers where HFV is under clinical investigation.
Remains an experimental technique! Mechanisms of action and clinical uses are not well defined. Lack of standardization in equipment and ventilator circuits makes monitoring difficult.	Clinical response of the patient is unpredictable and may be worse than the response with conventional ventilation. Long-term effects of HFV are unknown.

1985). First, HFV is different from conventional ventilation in that it ventilates the patient using relatively small tidal volumes at exceedingly high respiratory rates. Second, ventilation and oxygenation are accomplished by gas diffusion and convection, rather than the bulk flow of gas, as with conventional ventilation.

The main advantages and disadvantages of HFV are summarized in Table 28–2. The major advantage is that the small tidal volumes result in lower intratracheal pressures and a potential reduction in many complications associated with the delivery of positive pressure ventilation to the lungs, e.g., barotrauma and hypotension. The major disadvantage is that this relatively new ventilatory technique is still considered experimental. Clinical use is limited to patients with large pulmonary leaks (e.g., bronchopleural fistulas, tracheoesophageal fistulas), patients requiring ventilatory support during bronchoscopy and laryngoscopy, and clinically deteriorating patients in acute respiratory failure, e.g., adult respiratory distress syndrome (ARDS), who cannot be adequately ventilated with conventional ventilation (Hudson, 1984; MacIntyre, 1985).

Ventilator Setup and Settings

Knowledge of the basic ventilator setup and settings prepares the nurse to appropriately monitor the patient receiving conventional positive pressure ventilation. The importance of this knowledge cannot be overemphasized. As ventilators become more sophisticated, clinicians increasingly rely on the respiratory therapist to set up the ventilator, to periodically monitor ventilator settings, and to suggest adjustments to correct ventilatory problems that arise during mechanical ventilation. In spite of the respiratory therapist's vital role, however, the provision of a comfortable pressure waveform and an optimal alveolar ventilation requires the efforts of all members of the health care team. The nurse's role is crucial because, as the provider of continuous and total patient care for at least an 8-hour period, he or she is most available and best equipped to readily observe and evaluate the effects of therapy in light of the overall condition of the patient. Moreover, close monitoring is required, not simply because of patient ventilator dependency, but also because the efficacy and patient tolerance of different modes of ventilation used in the critical care setting are largely unproven and unpredictable. Weaning the patient from a ventilator is still considered more of an art than a science. Hence, comprehensive respiratory care requires a knowledgeable and experienced nurse who can evaluate the beneficial as well as adverse effects of therapy and work with the physician and respiratory therapist to adapt ventilatory settings to patient requirements. Only then will clinicians be better able to fit the ventilator to the patient instead of vice versa.

VENTILATOR CIRCUIT

The ventilator circuit used in mechanical ventilation is basically the same as that used in intermittent positive pressure breathing (IPPB) treatments (see Fig. 22–15), except that an exhalation tube is usually attached to a spirometer or other device that senses flow and visually displays the volume of each exhaled breath. A humidifier is placed in line between the manifold and ventilator to humidify and warm inspiratory gas to slightly higher than 37°C (see Fig. 27–5). Other ventilator attachments, including a thermometer for checking gas temperature, a small nebulizer for aerosol treatments, and a probe for gas sampling and airway pressure measurements, may lie along the inspiratory tube (Fig. 28–10).

MODES OF VENTILATION

Modern ventilators have one or more knobs that allow the clinician to dial in the desired mode of ventilation (see Fig. 28–5C and Fig. 28–7A). Basic terminology to define or describe modes is summarized in Table 28–3. Since many different abbreviations often exist for the same mode, familiarization with the content of Table 28–3 will enhance comprehension of respiratory literature as well as communication among health team members in clinical and research settings.

Controlled

The patient receiving continuous mechanical support or inspiratory positive pressure ventilation (IPPV) is usually in the *control mode* or *assist-control mode* (Fig. 28–11A). To achieve *controlled* mechanical ventilation (CMV), the sensitivity knob is turned off, and the ventilator is adjusted to deliver a fixed number of breaths/min, regardless of patient effort to alter frequency. This mode is used only when the patient's ventilatory drive to breathe is depressed, e.g., drug overdose, postanesthesia, central nervous system (CNS) injury, and sedation for uncontrollable agitation. Also, it is used for the rare occasion when respiratory paralysis makes it necessary to ventilate the patient, e.g., status epilepticus and tetany.

Assisted

Assisted ventilation is achieved by increasing sensitivity until the patient triggers his own respirations (Fig. 28–11B). Although tidal volume and flow rate may be altered, frequency is determined solely by the patient and may be quite variable, depending on the respiratory pattern. This mode is never used in the clinical setting; if the patient suddenly becomes apneic or hypoventilates, the ventilator is not set to deliver back-up mechanical breaths.

Assist-Control

Most patients receiving continuous ventilatory support are in the *assist-control* mode. Essentially, this is the mode with a preset automatic back-up rate (control mode) should the patient's respiratory rate significantly decrease, as illustrated in Figure 28–11C. The assist mode allows the patient to exercise respiratory muscles while triggering each inspiration.

Intermittent Mandatory Ventilation (IMV) and Synchronized Intermittent Mandatory Ventilation (SIMV)

The intermittent mandatory ventilation (IMV) mode allows the patient to breathe spontaneously and provides a preset number of ventilator breaths to insure

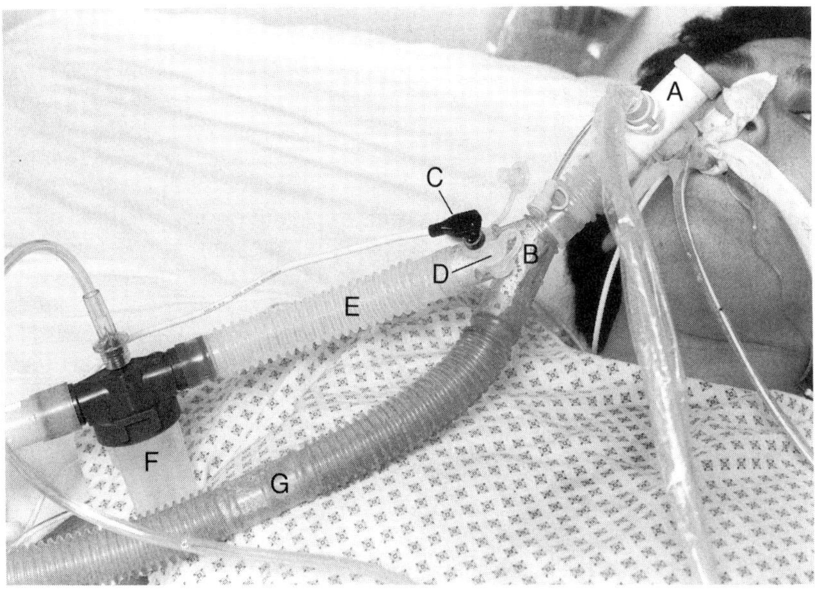

Figure 28–10. A disposable ventilator breathing circuit. A, Closed suction system; B, Y connector; C, Temperature probe for monitoring gas temperature; D, Proximal airway pressure port for proximal airway pressure monitoring (not used here); E, Inspiratory tube; F, In-line nebulizer; G, Expiratory tube.

Table 28–3. TERMINOLOGY FOR MODES OF MECHANICAL VENTILATION

Abbreviation	Term	Definition
A/C	assist-control mode	Combination of AMV and CMV for the back-up rate.
AMV	assisted mechanical ventilation	The patient triggers his own breaths at his own respiratory rate.
CDP	continuous distending pressure	Same as CPAP.
CMV	controlled mechanical ventilation	Ventilator delivers positive pressure breaths at fixed time intervals.
CPAP	continuous positive airway pressure	Spontaneous tidal breathing with a fixed amount of positive pressure (PEEP) applied to the airway throughout the respiratory cycle.
CPPB	continuous positive pressure breathing	Same as CPAP.
CPPV	continuous positive pressure ventilation	AMV or CMV with PEEP.
EPAP	expiratory positive airway pressure	Spontaneous breathing with positive pressure (PEEP) applied to the airway only during expiration. Airway pressure becomes ambient or subambient during inspiration.
IAV	intermittent assisted ventilation	Same as SIMV.
IDV	intermittent demand ventilation	Same as SIMV.
IMV	intermittent mandatory ventilation	Delivery of a preset number of ventilator breaths to a spontaneously breathing patient.
IPPB	intermittent (inspiratory) positive pressure breathing	A short 10- to 20-minute positive pressure treatment to deliver aerosol or hyperinflate the lungs. Do not confuse with IPPV.
IPPV	inspiratory positive pressure ventilation	A general term referring to continuous mechanical support of a patient.
NEEP	negative end expiratory pressure	Application of subatmospheric pressure to the airways during expiration.
PEEP	positive end expiratory pressure	Application of positive pressure to the airways at the end of expiration.
PSV	pressure support ventilation	Application of a preset amount of positive pressure to the airways during inspiration.
SIMV	synchronized intermittent mandatory ventilation	Same as IMV, except ventilator breaths are synchronized to the patient's inspiratory phase of respiration.
ZEEP	zero end expiratory pressure	PEEP of zero.

adequate alveolar ventilation without respiratory fatigue. Because the mandatory ventilator breaths are not synchronized with the patient's breaths, they may become *stacked* on top of spontaneous breaths, as illustrated in Figure 28–11D. Although stacked breaths may significantly increase airway pressure, recent evidence indicates that they do not cause major changes in cardiac output or pleural pressure, and they do not increase the incidence of barotrauma (Pucket et al, 1982). The major disadvantage of the IMV mode is that it requires the addition of a second circuit with low resistance, one-way valves, and continuous gas flow to prevent the rebreathing of expired gas. Compared with continuous mechanical ventilation, however, this mode (and SIMV described subsequently) has many potential advantages, as follows (Weisman et al, 1983):

1. Decreased tendency to hyperventilate the patient. Fewer mechanical breaths are delivered. The patient is allowed to determine his own Pa_{CO_2} level.

2. Decreased need for sedatives, narcotics, and muscle relaxants to synchronize the patient's breathing with the ventilator. IMV is an alternative for patients in the assist-control mode who hyperventilate and breathe out of phase with the ventilator. Similarly, it may avert implementation of controlled ventilation and use of heavy sedation or muscle paralysis to control agitated patients.

3. Lower mean airway pressure, resulting in fewer complications.

4. More uniform distribution of ventilation and perfusion. Spontaneous breaths are preferentially distributed to dependent regions, whereas positive pressure breaths are distributed to more compliant, nondependent regions.

5. Facilitation of the weaning process. It may be particularly helpful for the patient who appears to be psychologically dependent on the ventilator.

6. Prevention of respiratory muscle atrophy and incoordination. The mode is thought to minimize disuse atrophy and promote synchrony between the diaphragm and chest wall muscles.

7. Decreased likelihood of cardiac decompensation during weaning. The gradual transition to spontaneous breathing avoids rapid falls in intrathoracic pressure.

In spite of these advantages, as Weisman and associates (1983) point out, little experimental or clinical data either prove or disprove theoretic advantages and disadvantages of IMV. In some cases, the change from CMV to IMV may produce cardiac decompensation,

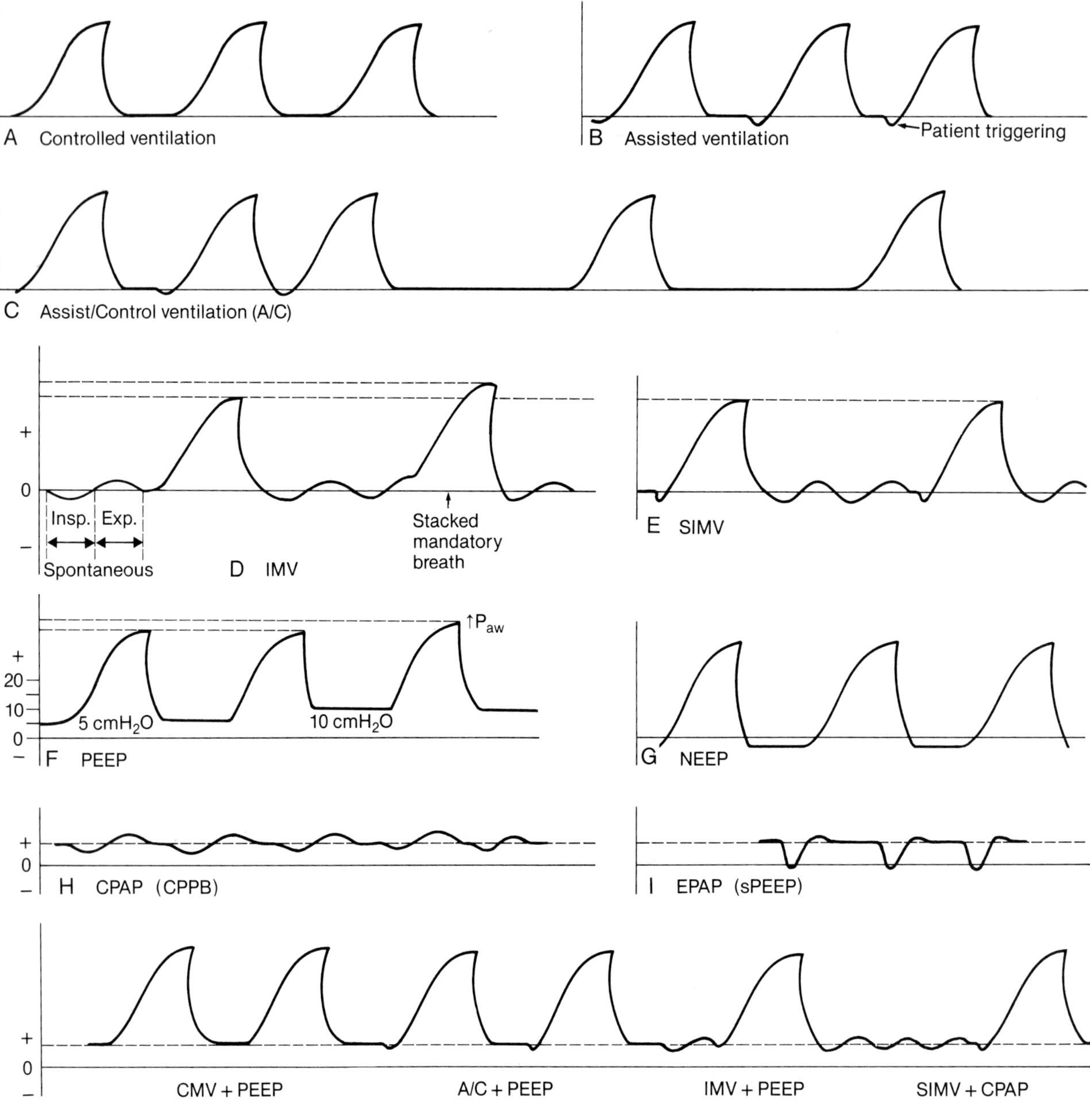

Figure 28–11. Modes of mechanical ventilation.

as in the patient with left ventricular failure. For this reason, the use of IMV and SIMV remains a controversial subject.

Synchronized intermittent mandatory ventilation (SIMV) is the same as IMV, except each mandatory breath is activated by the patient's own inspiratory effort and, hence, is always synchronized with his breathing pattern, as illustrated in Figure 28–11E. Stacking does not occur. SIMV is built into the most recently manufactured ventilators and is easily attained by dialing in the mode. However, synchronization of IMV breaths offers no proven physiologic advantage, and some clinicians believe it may not be worth the expense of purchasing a new ventilator that provides this mode or an IMV controller to incorporate into an older ventilator.

Positive End Expiratory Pressure (PEEP)

Positive end expiratory pressure (PEEP) is achieved when the ventilator's expiratory valve is adjusted to provide back pressure in the lungs of up to 15 cmH_2O (Fig. 28–11F) and, in severe ARDS, up to 15 to 45 cmH_2O. The latter parameter is referred to as *super PEEP* and is only occasionally utilized because of the increased incidence of complications. PEEP is a supplement to the control, assist-control, or IMV mode of ventilation. It is used to increase Pao_2 and tissue oxygen delivery in patients with acute respiratory failure and to prevent alveolar and airway collapse during expiration. For the patient who is already on a high FIo_2, PEEP permits reduction of the FIo_2 to a safer level, thus lessening the likelihood of lung damage from oxygen toxicity. Exactly how PEEP improves pulmonary function and gas exchange is not well understood, but the main mechanism involved relates to an increase in functional residual capacity (FRC) (Shapiro et al, 1983). Previously inflated alveoli are further inflated, and previously collapsed alveoli are recruited to increase gas volume. By recruiting alveoli and redistributing pulmonary perfusion, PEEP effectively combats refractory hypoxemia and reduced lung compliance, the hallmarks of ARDS, the disorder routinely requiring PEEP. More specifically, PEEP changes unventilated/perfused shunt lung units into acceptable lung units with a normal to high V/Q ratio. Beyond 10 to 15 cmH_2O of PEEP, however, acceptable lung units may be converted to dead space units, and the extra back pressure in the lungs may reduce cardiac output. These events worsen pulmonary perfusion, increase intrapulmonary shunting, and increase V/Q ratios to well over 10.0. Since the degree of shunt reduction with PEEP is influenced by hemodynamic changes, careful monitoring is required to find the optimal PEEP level for each patient. *Optimal* or *best PEEP* is defined as *a* Pao_2 *greater than 60 mmHg with an* FIo_2 *less than or equal to 0.50, while maintaining an adequate cardiac output* (Shapiro et al, 1983).

PEEP and Continuous Positive Airway Pressure (CPAP) Adjustment. To add PEEP to a modern ventilator, the clinician turns the *PEEP/CPAP knob* until the end-expiratory pressure on the pressure gauge matches the prescribed level of PEEP. An alternative is to add a PEEP valve to the expiratory side of the ventilator circuit. Individual situations may require sensitivity, inspiratory flow, or other minor adjustments.

Negative End Expiratory Pressure (NEEP)

Negative end expiratory pressure (NEEP) is achieved by applying up to 5 cmH_2O of subatmospheric pressure to the airway during the expiratory phase (Fig. 28–11G). This mode was originally developed with the control or assist-control mode to lower mean airway pressure and increase venous return during positive pressure ventilation, but it is rarely used today. NEEP is associated with serious complications, such as premature airway collapse leading to air trapping and increased venous return leading to pulmonary edema, and other methods are now available to more safely ventilate and treat the patient with imminent peripheral cardiovascular collapse.

Continuous Positive Airway Pressure (CPAP)

Continuous positive airway pressure (CPAP) is achieved by the application of PEEP to spontaneous breathing, as shown in Figure 28–11H. It was originally used in 1936 to treat hypoxemia associated with pulmonary edema and in 1971 to decrease mean airway pressure and increase survival rate of infants with respiratory distress syndrome. The literature currently supports the use of CPAP in adults to increase Pao_2 in the perioperative period and early stages of acute respiratory failure (George, 1983). In addition, it is utilized as a primary mode of ventilation to help reexpand atelectatic lung tissue or as a final step before endotracheal extubation. Its advantages include keeping airway pressure to within more acceptable limits and of depressing cardiac output less than that achieved with controlled mechanical ventilation (CMV) or assisted mechanical ventilation (AMV) with PEEP or IMV with PEEP.

The goals of CPAP are to increase functional residual capacity (FRC) with an accompanying improvement in Pao_2 and to decrease intrapulmonary shunt, work of breathing, and oxygen consumption. Finer and Kelly (1983) define *optimal CPAP as the level of distending pressure that results in the lowest A-*ao_2 *gradient without markedly increasing* $Paco_2$*, decreasing pH, or adversely affecting circulatory status.*

CPAP requires the same type of ventilator circuitry as the IMV mode. Airway pressures up to about +10 to +15 cmH_2O are maintained by a *continuous* or *demand flow* system of CPAP.

In a *continuous flow CPAP system*, e.g., Emerson IMV or Puritan-Bennett MA-1 ventilator, a constant flow of gas passes through the breathing circuit and is available for spontaneous breathing between ventilator-delivered breaths. This system does not utilize a valve in the breathing circuit.

The *demand flow CPAP system* utilizes a one-way valve within the circuitry of the ventilator. This demand valve opens when the patient generates sufficient negative pressure during a spontaneous inspiratory effort. Demand flow systems are built into several ventilator models, such as the Puritan-Bennett MA-2, Bear 1 or 2, and Siemens Servo 900B. New ventilators, such as the Bear 5, may have both the demand and continuous flow options for use with IMV/SIMV.

The major disadvantage of the CPAP mode of mechanical ventilation pertains to the demand flow system. The increased inspiratory effort required to open the ventilator's demand valve may cause increased work of breathing and respiratory muscle fatigue (Gibney et al, 1982). A demand valve may require generation of an inspiratory force of -3 to -6 cmH_2O for activation (Christopher et al, 1985). This effort is significantly greater than that required to trigger a normal spontaneous breath or a breath by any other mode of mechanical ventilation. In addition, the CPAP mode may decrease rather than increase $Pa{O_2}$, if the lower airway pressure permits a rise in cardiac output and better perfusion of poorly ventilated lung segments.

Mask CPAP. CPAP may be delivered via mask to avoid tracheal intubation and mechanical ventilation and to prevent the need for reintubation after extubation (Branson et al, 1985) (Fig. 28–12). In the postoperative patient, continuous or periodic CPAP is used to prevent and treat postoperative atelectasis, increase $Pa{O_2}$, and help remove respiratory secretions. Periodic CPAP is defined as hourly CPAP treatments for 25 to 35 consecutive breaths at the highest tolerated pressure, most often 15 cmH_2O.

The main advantages and disadvantages of mask CPAP are summarized in Table 28–4, along with clinical implications for monitoring the patient. Contraindications may include facial or laryngeal trauma, recent tracheal or esophageal anastomosis, gastric resection, and increased risk for vomiting, e.g., gastrointestinal bleeding or ileus.

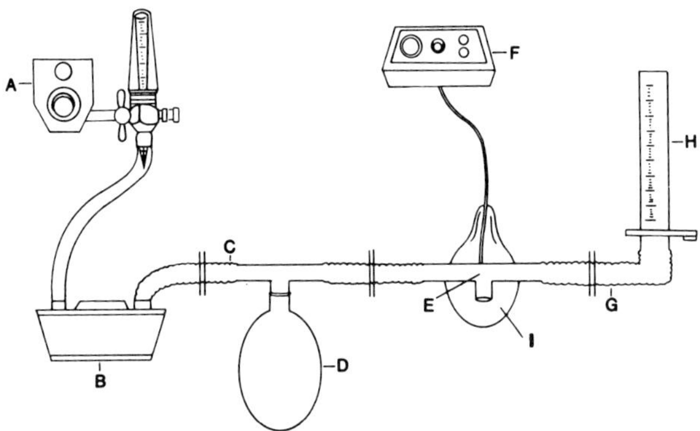

Figure 28–12. A continuous flow mask, CPAP system. A, oxygen blender; B, large-volume, low resistance humidifier; C, inspiratory limb; D, reservoir bag (3 to 5 L); E, T-piece to patient; F, airway pressure manometer and high-low pressure alarm; G, expiratory limb; H, threshold resistor (PEEP valve); I, mask. (Reproduced by permission from Branson, R., Hurst, J., and DeHaven, C. Mask CPAP: state of the art. *Respiratory care,* 30(10):849, 1985.

Expiratory Positive Airway Pressure (EPAP)

EPAP, sometimes called *spontaneous PEEP* (sPEEP), is similar to CPAP except that airway pressure is permitted to become ambient or subambient during inspiration, as shown in Figure 28–11I. CPAP is clinically preferred over EPAP because, for incompletely understood physiologic reasons, it causes less variation in FRC, and its effects are more predictable (Wilson, 1983).

Some clinicians, however, prefer EPAP by mask over CPAP by mask because the former requires lower flow rates, resulting in less likelihood of air swallowing, abdominal distention, and possible perforation. Also, EPAP results in lower mean intrathoracic pressure and may be better tolerated by patients with compromised cardiovascular function (Schmidt et al, 1977).

Pressure Support Ventilation (PSV)

PSV is the application of a preset amount of positive pressure to the airway during inspiration. It is applied to spontaneous breaths to reduce the patient's effort to breathe and thereby decrease work of breathing and oxygen demands on ventilatory muscles.

There are two basic approaches to using PSV (MacIntyre, 1986). First, a low level of PSV, e.g., 5 to 10 cmH_2O, may be applied to assist spontaneous breaths during another mode of ventilation, such as SIMV. Second, PSV may be used as a separate ventilatory mode. For example, in postoperative patients, inspiratory positive pressure is added to spontaneous breathing to achieve a tidal volume of 10 to 12 mg/kg (Prakash and Meij, 1985). This amount of pressure is enough to compensate for the resistance of the ventilator tubes and humidification system. This method may replace assist-control, IMV, and SIMV modes of ventilation used during weaning from mechanical ventilation. It has the advantage of substantially improving patient comfort, since the patient controls the depth and timing of inspiration, while potentially increasing endurance conditioning of ventilatory muscles and promoting a shorter weaning period.

Combinations

All the major modes of mechanical ventilation have been presented. Commonly used combinations are illustrated in Figure 28–11J. In addition, PSV may be applied to SIMV, AMV, and CPAP demand modes of mechanical ventilation.

OTHER SETTINGS

The previous text has presented all major modes of mechanical ventilation to facilitate collaboration with other health team members in the critical care setting.

Table 28–4. ADVANTAGES AND DISADVANTAGES OF MASK CPAP

Advantages/Disadvantages*	Clinical Implications
Advantages	
Can be comfortably applied without patient cooperation.	May be more effective at lung expansion and secretion removal than other interventions that require patient cooperation, e.g., incentive spirometry, coughing and deep breathing, postural drainage.
Works by passive inflation of the lungs, as opposed to active inflation required during incentive spirometry.	Passive mechanics of breathing helps to control postoperative pain and splinting respirations. The patient may need less pain medication.
Positive airway pressure is less than that during any positive pressure therapy.	Risk for barotrauma is low. Cardiovascular depression is unlikely in patients with adequate volume status.
May avoid endotracheal intubation or reintubation and mechanical ventilation in selected patients with mild to moderate acute respiratory failure. Continuous mask CPAP is insitituted before Pa_{O_2}/FI_{O_2} is less than 250.	Spontaneous breathing is better than mechanical ventilation because it avoids the numerous complications associated with tube placement and positive pressure ventilation. However, since the patient's condition is unstable or potentially unstable, close monitoring is required.
Disadvantages	
The increase in FRC achieved during CPAP is lost within 10 minutes after mask removal.	Nurses should monitor CPAP pressure with vital signs to insure delivery of the prescribed CPAP and an adequate FRC.
	Check to be sure the mask is properly applied to the face. If necessary, apply water-soluble jelly to the mask to maintain a more effective seal. Remember that an effective seal is not necessarily a tight one. Air leaks around the mask are permissible as long as the pressure in the system is maintained.
Hypoventilation may occur with excessive levels of CPAP—alveolar overdistention increases V_D/V_T and results in CO_2 retention.	Monitor the patient for signs of alveolar hypoventilation, CO_2 narcosis, increasing hypoxemia, and incoordinated breathing pattern.
Wearing the CPAP mask may cause complications, most commonly nasal bridge pain, erythema at the site of application, and patient intolerance.	Use a lightweight, soft, and pliable CPAP mask to reduce facial trauma and promote comfort. Adjust seal as described.
	Carefully inspect the face q4h and PRN for skin rash and tissue trauma.
	Provide emotional support. Explain the purpose and procedure for mask CPAP, emphasizing the overwhelming advantages over intubation and mechanical ventilation.
Increased risk for air swallowing and pulmonary aspiration.	Use a transparent mask to allow visualization of airway for secretions and vomitus. Periodically remove the mask, help the patient expectorate mucus into tissue, and promptly reapply mask to face.
	Monitor for signs of gastric distention. Check with physician for nasogastric tube order for patients with high levels (over 10 cmH_2O) of CPAP and for postoperative and trauma patients who have a tendency toward gastric atony and altered mental status.

*Data from Branson, R., Hurst, J. and DeHaven, C. Mask CPAP: State of the art. *Respiratory care*, 30(10): 846–857, 1985.

The list of modes and other ventilator settings may be reduced to basic parameters relevant to working with patients on either technologically advanced ventilators or simpler ventilators in the home or extended care facility. Basic ventilator parameters are listed in the following box.

BASIC VENTILATOR PARAMETERS

MODES OF VENTILATION
Controlled
Assist-control
IMV and SIMV
PEEP
CPAP
Pressure support

OTHER SETTINGS
FIO_2
V_T and f (minute ventilation)
Sigh volume
I:E ratio
Inspiratory flow rate
Pressure waveform settings

ALARM SYSTEMS
Airway pressure
Exhaled volume
Gas temperature
FIO_2

Fractional Inspired Oxygen Concentration (FIO_2)

In critical situations, FIO_2 is set at 1.00 to prevent hypoxemia and then lowered to keep PaO_2 greater than 60 mmHg. For accuracy, each new setting is checked with an oxygen analyzer (Fig. 28–13), and the FIO_2 knob is adjusted to give the precise amount of prescribed oxygen. When an oxygen blender is added to a ventilator setup (e.g., IMV on the Puritan-Bennett MA-1), the FIO_2 knob on the ventilator is set at 1.00 and the desired FIO_2 is dialed in on the oxygen blender.

Tidal Volume and Respiratory Rate (Minute Ventilation)

Tidal volume is set at 10 to 15 cc/kg of ideal body weight, usually 500 to 1000 cc. Respiratory rate is usually 10 to 14 breaths/min in the control mode. In the assist-control mode, the patient determines rate, and the back-up rate is set to provide 70 to 80% of the patient's usual minute ventilation. These values are periodically adjusted to maintain an acceptable minute ventilation, PaO_2, and pH. For many ventilators that are primarily time-cycled (e.g., Servo series), tidal volume cannot be set directly but must be set indirectly by altering other parameters, such as respiratory rate and minute ventilation.

Sigh Volume

A *sigh* is a ventilator breath that is about 1½ times the patient's tidal volume. The use of sighs at preset intervals was once thought to combat atelectasis and shunting associated with fixed low tidal volumes. Now it is established that high tidal volumes and slow respiratory rates without sighs will avoid these adverse effects (Fairley, 1976). Nevertheless, some physicians still order sighs. Others regard them as relatively unimportant and order them only when tidal volume is low (i.e., less than 7 cc/kg).

Most ventilators provide a means for *manually* delivering a tidal volume or sigh. Volume ventilators

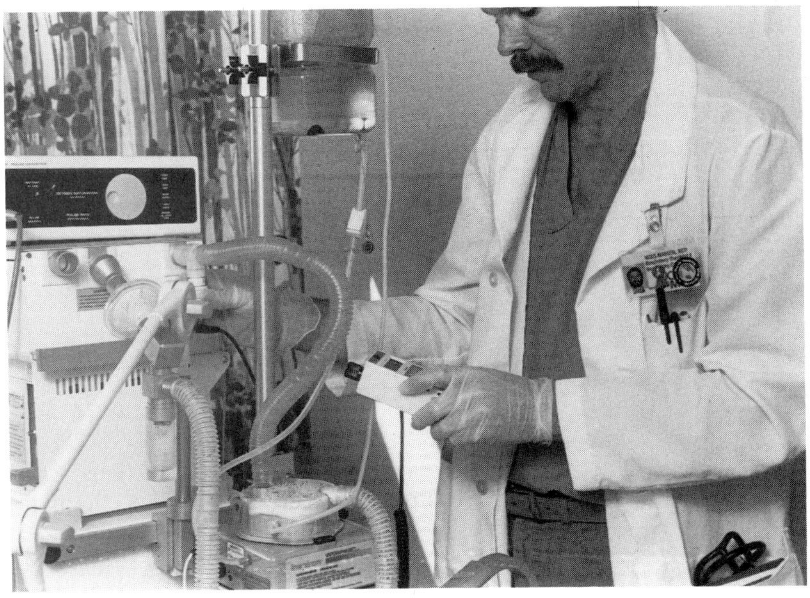

Figure 28–13. A respiratory therapist checks FIO_2 by attaching an oxygen analyzer in-line, on the inspiratory side of the breathing circuit.

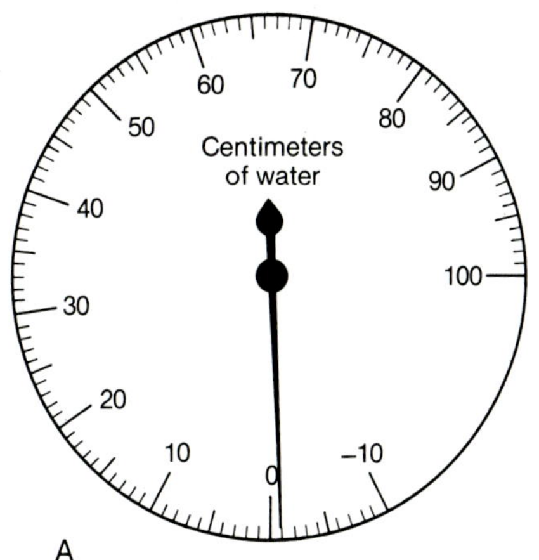

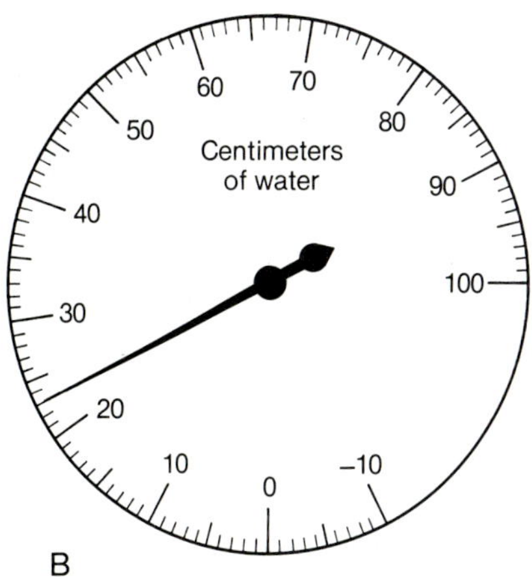

Figure 28–14. Reading the pressure manometer. During assisted breathing, the maximum negative pressure reading of −1.0 cm H_2O in *A* represents ventilator sensitivity. In *B*, the maximum positive number of 23 cm H_2O is the peak inspiratory pressure.

provide a sigh button to push to deliver hyperinflations before and after suctioning.

Sensitivity

The sensitivity knob determines the patient effort required to initiate assisted breathing. It is *off* in the control mode. For assisted breathing, it is gradually increased until the needle on the pressure gauge moves to −0.5 to −1.5 cmH_2O to trigger each breath (Fig. 28–14A). If sensitivity is too high (i.e., −0.25 to −0.50), self-cycling or chattering will occur. If it is too low (i.e., below −1.5 to −2.0 cmH_2O), the increased work of breathing may prompt the patient to hypoventilate.

Inspiratory:Expiratory (I:E) Ratio

On some ventilators, inspiratory and expiratory times are set in seconds. Normal inspiratory time is 0.5 to 1.5 seconds. It rarely exceeds 1.5 to 2.0 seconds because of patient discomfort and the adverse effects of positive pressure on cardiovascular function. Expiratory time may be set so that the I:E ratio is 1:2. The COPD patient requires a ratio of 1.3 to 1.5 to facilitate alveolar emptying on expiration. Inspiratory time may be prolonged and the I:E ratio reversed in an attempt to prevent atelectasis in the critically ill neonate or adult. However, the short expiratory time resulting from this practice may produce inadvertent PEEP and stacked breaths.

On other ventilators, inspiratory time and I:E ratio cannot be dialed in but are obtained by adjusting other parameters, such as inspiratory flow rate, airway pressure, and respiratory rate.

Inspiratory Flow Rate

Flow is the volume of gas that passes a given point in a unit of time. Inspiratory flow is controlled by a calibrated knob (20 to 120 L/min). The average inspiratory flow rate is 40 to 60 L/min. Higher flow rates of up to 100 L/min may be required to ventilate patients with severe lung disease and a high minute ventilation. In COPD, high flow rates improve gas exchange because more gas redistributes to underventilated alveoli, and these and other alveoli empty more completely since more time is allowed for the expiratory phase of respiration (Connors et al, 1981). However, if inspiratory flow is too high and inspiratory time too short, increased airway turbulence may offset the advantages of a high flow rate, and alveolar ventilation ($\dot{V}_A$) may decrease rather than increase.

In the adjustment of flow rate, perhaps the most important relationship to remember is the higher the flow rate, the shorter the inspiratory time, and vice versa, i.e., the lower the flow rate, the longer the inspiratory time. In addition, a higher flow rate increases peak inspiratory pressure, whereas a lower flow rate decreases peak inspiratory pressure.

Peak Inspiratory Pressure

This parameter is determined by watching the needle on the airway pressure gauge swing up during a normal inspiration. The highest pressure attained is the *peak inspiratory pressure* (PIP) (Fig. 28–14B). Ideally, it is a proximal reading taken via a probe close to the patient's airway rather than a machine system pressure reading. Although airway pressure is not set for a volume ventilator and varies with changing airway resistance and compliance, separate knobs exist to set pressure limits. The *low pressure limit* is set slightly below the patient's usual PIP. When the pressure needle fails to reach PIP, activation of the low pressure alarm usually indicates improved lung mechanics, hypoventilation, or ventilator disconnection. The *high pressure limit* is set about 10 to 20 cmH_2O above peak inspiratory pressure. It is routinely used to help detect worsening lung mechanics and to protect against barotrauma, hypotension, and other complications associated with excessive airway pressure. When the high pressure limit is reached, an alarm is activated and excess gas is vented to the atmosphere via a pop-off valve.

Settings to Alter Pressure Waveform

Other settings exist to modify the positive pressure waveform. Some ventilators provide *sine wave contouring* to facilitate simulation of the normal respiratory cycle.

The *expiratory retard* may be adjusted to provide resistance to expiratory gas flow and prolong expiration. The resulting waveform (Fig. 28–15A) helps prevent airway collapse in COPD, thus serving the same function as pursed-lip breathing.

The *inspiratory hold* or *plateau* knob may be adjusted to produce a *pressure hold* or *volume hold* waveform (Fig. 28–15B). These modifications are sometimes used to help expand atelectatic lung segments, prevent premature alveolar collapse, and facilitate aerosol delivery to more distal lung regions. Also, the volume hold (Fig. 28–15C) creates a *plateau pressure* that is used to calculate lung compliance (described subsequently).

ALARM SYSTEMS

Pressure-cycled ventilators may monitor only one or two parameters, e.g., low exhaled volume and temperature control, whereas other ventilators have a sophisticated visual and audible alarm system that monitors many parameters, including airway pressure; gas temperature; exhaled volume; FIO_2; I:E ratio to guarantee an I:E of at least 1:1; low PEEP-CPAP; apnea; and total gas, electronic, or AC power failure (see Fig. 28–5B). In any case, the nurse must be familiar with each ventilator's monitoring system and the clinical implications of each audible and visual alarm. Respiratory nurses, respiratory therapists, procedure books, equipment manuals, and product represenţives can help provide the details of individual alarm systems and better prepare the staff nurse to respond appropriately when an alarm is activated.

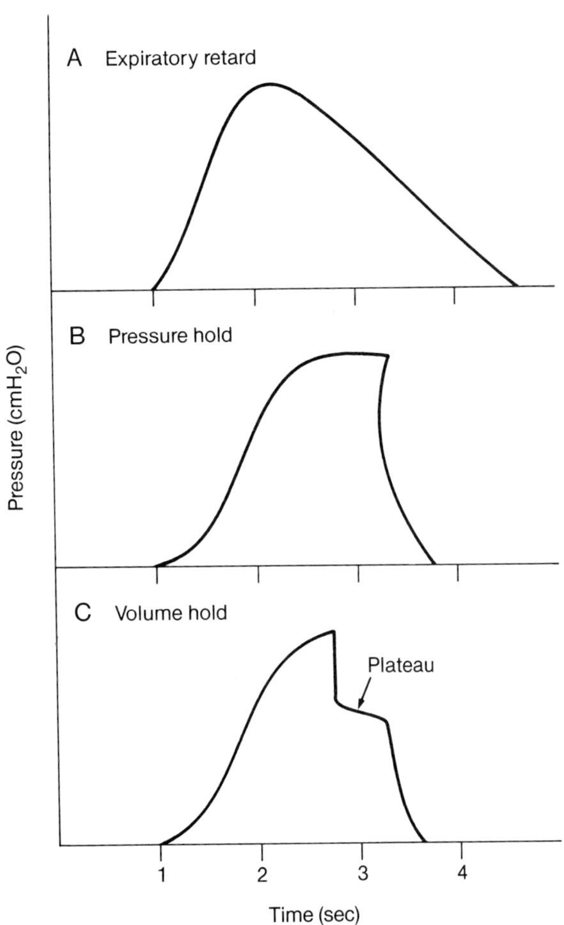

Figure 28–15. Pressure waveforms.

Complications During Mechanical Ventilation

Care of the patient on mechanical ventilation largely focuses on the detection, treatment, and prevention of complications of intubation (see Table 27–1) and mechanical ventilation.

Complications of mechanical ventilation relate to either a ventilator problem or an actual patient problem, such as pulmonary infection or malnutrition.

COMMON VENTILATOR-RELATED PROBLEMS

Respiratory nursing care includes monitoring the patient-ventilator system for *low exhaled volume, gas under- or overheating,* and *high peak inspiratory pressure.* As mentioned previously, modern ventilators have built-in alarm systems that sound when these and other ventilator-related problems arise. Yet, reliance on alarms can create a false sense of security. They can malfunction or be set inappropriately by mistake; alarms are intended only as back-ups for close observation of the patient. Hence, the nurse must actively monitor for at least the three previously mentioned common ventilator-related problems.

Low Exhaled Volume

The patient has *low exhaled volume* when tidal volume is more than 50 to 100 cc lower than the patient's current baseline tidal volume on the ventilator. This situation activates the ventilator's low exhaled volume or low pressure alarm. Causes of low exhaled volume include patient disconnection from coughing, movement, an inadequately positioned ventilator circuit, a leak in the ventilator system, and a malfunctioning spirometer. Interventions are summarized as follows:

1. When the patient becomes disconnected, quickly reconnect him to the ventilator circuit, reset the alarm system if not automatic, and rearrange tubing, support arm, or body position to help prevent disconnection.

Restrain the patient's arms if necessary.

2. After suctioning, *firmly* attach the ventilator circuit to the endotracheal or tracheostomy tube to prevent disconnection.

3. Place a folded towel on the patient's chest or shoulder to support the weight of the breathing circuit and eliminate unnecessary traction on the airway.

4. *For a leak*, check the entire ventilator circuit for patency, beginning at the airway and ending at the ventilator itself. Be sure the thermometer, gas probe, and extra O_2 bleed-in line are not loose and have not fallen off. Check to be sure the humidifier reservoir is tightly screwed on.

5. Check the spirometer for moisture that might be interfering with volume accuracy. Dry or change the bellows (Bennett) or electronic sensing device (Bear series).

Gas Under- or Overheating

Humidified gas is warmed to body temperature. Gas below 36°C may cause mucosal drying and irritation, mucus thickening, and impairment of the mucociliary escalator, all leading to mucus retention and possibly pneumonia. Gas over 38°C may cause airway burns; increase in thin, watery secretions; and patient discomfort.

Monitoring gas temperature is introduced in Chapter 27. Three other basic interventions follow:

1. Appropriately increase or decrease the gas temperature and humidity by adjusting the dial on the ventilator's humidifier.

2. Check the heating device for malfunction. Call the respiratory therapist, if necessary.

3. Keep distilled water in the humidifier up to the "filled" level to help prevent gas overheating.

High Peak Inspiratory Pressure

High peak inspiratory pressure activates the high pressure alarm. It may indicate a ventilator-related problem, such as a kinked breathing tube; increased obstruction in the patient-ventilator system; or a patient-related problem, such as increased pulmonary restriction, as in pneumothorax or ARDS. Table 28–5 explains how to differentiate between patient- and ventilator-related problems and how to intervene appropriately.

PATIENT PROBLEMS

The remainder of this section on complications during mechanical ventilation focuses on patient-related rather than ventilator-related problems. Mechanisms responsible for each problem are summarized here in the text, whereas clinical manifestations and nursing interventions are listed in Table 28–5 for quick reference in the clinical setting. Most complications discussed here relate to the application of positive pressure to the lungs.

Cardiovascular Impairment

Cardiovascular impairment is caused by application of positive pressure to the lungs. Positive pressure increases lung volume, which in turn increases P_{pl} and P_{tp}, decreases venous return to the right side of the heart, and decreases cardiac output, as explained in Chapter 4. The most immediate and readily observable effect of the decreased cardiac output is hypotension.

Factors that influence the degree of cardiac depression include the following:

1. *Mean or peak inspiratory pressure*: high PIP (30 to 60 cmH_2O) decreases cardiac output more than low PIP (12 to 30 cmH_2O).

2. *Mode of mechanical ventilation*: cardiac depression is greatest with CMV, less with IMV + PEEP, and even less with CPAP.

3. *Lung and chest wall compliance*: depression is greatest with healthy compliant lungs and much less with diseased noncompliant lungs, because diseased lung tissue buffers the transmission of airway pressure to the pleural space.

4. *Preload of the right ventricle*: when end-diastolic cardiac pressures are elevated, and high levels of PEEP are applied, right heart distention is likely to flatten and shift the interventricular septum to the left. Compression of the left ventricle decreases stroke volume and cardiac output to levels that are refractory to fluid challenges (Pick et al, 1982).

5. *Pulmonary vascular resistance (PVR)*: super PEEP may increase PVR, and thus right ventricular afterload, making it more difficult for the right ventricle to maintain stroke volume.

6. *Hypoxia, acidosis, hypovolemia, pharmacologic depression, and vasopressor or vasodilator therapy*: these factors may increase the rate or magnitude of cardiovascular changes.

Barotrauma

As with cardiovascular impairment, barotrauma is related to application of positive pressure to the lungs. High mean airway pressure causes alveolar rupture. Gas moves along perivascular sheaths towards the mediastinum to produce pneumomediastinum and along tissue planes to produce subcutaneous emphysema. Gas rupturing the mediastinal pleura produces a pneumothorax.

Barotrauma is believed to be more likely in the patient with severe COPD or bullous lung disease who receives large tidal volumes or high levels of PEEP. However, statistical correlation between PEEP levels, mortality, and incidence of pneumothorax is not well established. Barotrauma in ARDS appears to be related to the severity of disease rather than the level of applied airway pressure (Shapiro et al, 1983).

Pulmonary Oxygen Toxicity

The mechanism responsible for pulmonary oxygen toxicity is discussed in Chapter 13.

Text continued on page 726

Table 28–5. COMPLICATIONS DURING MECHANICAL VENTILATION*

Complication	Signs and Symptoms	Interventions	Rationale
Cardiovascular impairment	↓ blood pressure (B/P) ↓ cardiac output (Q) ↑ pulse Arrhythmias ↑ PCWP (pulmonary capillary wedge pressure) ↑ CVP (central venous pressure) Normal, ↑, or ↓ PaO_2, depending on the magnitude of the decreased cardiac output and degree of tissue O_2 extraction Mental confusion ↓ urine output ↓ $P\bar{v}O_2$ ↓ tissue O_2 delivery (calculated by multiplying cardiac output by O_2 content of arterial blood). Note that with PEEP, a fall in O_2 delivery may occur despite an increasing PaO_2	Check B/P, heart rate and rhythm, sensorium, and peripheral perfusion after any increase in PEEP/CPAP or other change in ventilatory mode. If hemodynamic monitoring is available, monitor cardiac output (Q), cardiac index (CI), pulmonary vascular resistance (PVR), pulmonary capillary wedge pressure (PCWP), and tissue O_2 delivery.	Small increases in mean airway pressure or as little as 5 cmH_2O PEEP may result in hypotension and up to a 25 to 50 % reduction in cardiac output. A different mode of ventilation may alter mean airway pressure and, hence, B/P and Q. These parameters help determine whether the therapy causing the increased airway pressures (e.g., increased V_T, increased PEEP, switch from CPAP to IMV, and increase in mandatory ventilator breaths) is actually increasing oxygenation. The nurse withholds any ventilatory change that significantly decreases Q and fails to increase PaO_2 to an acceptable level.
		Closely monitor patients with acute myocardial infarction or limited myocardial function, particularly those with high levels of PEEP or low PCWP.	Cardiac depression is likely if PEEP is greater than 10 cmH_2O or left ventricular filling pressure (PCWP) is less than 18 mmHg (Grace and Greenbaum, 1982; Nikki et al, 1982).
		Closely monitor COPD patients for increased lung hyperinflation.	Lung hyperinflation is likely to worsen the hypotension. Incomplete alveolar emptying increases intrathoracic pressure, impedes venous return, and decreases cardiac output. This *auto-PEEP* phenomenon may occur any time the ventilator cycles before the lung returns to normal resting volume.
		Give a fluid challenge as ordered by the physician if PEEP decreases cardiac output.	A fluid challenge will increase intravascular volume, increase venous return, and restore cardiac output. It is effective in most cases. However, if a low cardiac output persists, ventricular dysfunction is likely to exist (Shapiro et al, 1983).
		Provide reassurance.	Reassurance helps to relieve anxiety, promote bronchial relaxation, and decrease airway resistance and alveolar pressures.
		Use bronchodilators, PRN suctioning, and other bronchial hygiene measures as indicated by the situation.	These measures improve lung compliance, increase PaO_2, and reduce the need for high inspiratory pressure to ventilate the patient.
		Promptly call the respiratory therapist to help assess ventilator settings whenever the patient breathes out of phase with the ventilator or repeatedly activates the high pressure alarm.	A ventilator adjustment may prevent fighting the ventilator, further increases in airway pressure, and cardiovascular impairment.

Table 28–5. COMPLICATIONS DURING MECHANICAL VENTILATION* *Continued*

Complication	Signs and Symptoms	Interventions	Rationale
Barotrauma	Sudden increase in peak inspiratory pressure (i.e., over 5 cmH_2O greater than the patient's usual PIP) Sudden patient agitation or coughing with frequent activation of high pressure alarm ↓ static and effective compliance Palpable subcutaneous emphysema over neck and anterior chest areas Deterioration in ABGs or B/P Decreased to absent breath sounds, hyperresonant percussion note (pneumothorax) Chest x-ray: subcutaneous emphysema, pneumomediastium, pneumoperitoneum, pneumothorax	Call the physician for immediate medical evaluation. Prepare for chest tube insertion if a large pneumothorax is suspected.	A severe oxygenation and ventilatory problem may be present. One or more chest tubes may be necessary to eliminate air in the pleural or mediastinal space, allow full lung expansion, and normalize blood gases.
		Avoid high pressure settings for patients with severe COPD, ARDS, or a history of pneumothorax.	These patients are at high risk to develop barotrauma.
		When PEEP is added, collaborate with the respiratory therapist to reduce V_T, increase f, and adjust peak flow to keep peak pressure within tolerable limits. Reduce or eliminate sigh volume.	PEEP increases peak pressures. The listed interventions reduce peak pressures and the likelihood of barotrauma.
		If a fresh tracheostomy is present, avoid tying the tracheostomy tape too tightly around the neck.	A large pneumomediastinum and subcutaneous emphysema may resolve without complications and further treatment if gas is permitted to escape out to the atmosphere via stomal tissue planes.
Pulmonary oxygen toxicity	FIO_2 over 0.50 Substernal distress (early) Nonproductive cough (early) Paresthesias General malaise Fatigue Vomiting Decreasing vital capacity ↑ peak inspiratory pressure ↓ lung compliance ↑ $P(A\text{-}a)O_2$ ↓ diffusion capacity Alveolar pattern on the chest x-ray	Implement measures to decrease FIO_2 to below 0.50 and maintain a PaO_2 greater than or equal to 70 mmHg (60 mmHg in COPD).	The patient will not develop toxicity when FIO_2 is below 0.50. The disorder occurs when FIO_2 is greater than 0.50 for more than 24–48 hours. The longer the exposure time, the more extensive the pathologic changes in the lungs.
		Closely monitor blood gases, VC, peak inspiratory pressure, and compliance.	VC decreases after 6 hours on an FIO_2 of 1.00. PaO_2 is particularly important to monitor, because a sudden drop in PaO_2 is an early sign of ARDS. An increased PIP and decreased lung compliance (C_L) may indicate increased lung restriction and impending pulmonary oxygen toxicity.
		Stabilize the patient's general condition as soon as possible, especially fluid and electrolyte balance, nutrition, and cardiovascular status.	An optimal physical condition may decrease susceptibility to acute lung injury.
Positive fluid balance	↑ body weight or failure to lose weight with starvation Fluid intake exceeding output ↓ VC, ↓ effective compliance Low hematocrit and low serum sodium from hemodilution Peripheral edema Lung crackles or decreased breath sounds	Monitor daily weight, peripheral edema, intake and output, and lung sounds.	Signs of positive fluid balance (e.g., weight gain, increasing peripheral edema, fluid intake greater than output, and lung crackles) indicate a need for diuretic medication.
		Limit salt intake and give diuretics.	Salt causes fluid retention. Diuretics will help prevent or treat heart failure.
		Provide for meticulous skin care and range of motion (ROM) exercise to immobile extremities.	These interventions lessen the extent and adverse effects of peripheral edema, e.g., increased susceptibility to skin breakdown.
		Monitor vital signs as mechanical ventilation is withdrawn.	Fluid returning to central vessels may precipitate cardiac decompensation in patients with poor cardiopulmonary reserve.

Table continued on following page

Table 28–5. COMPLICATIONS DURING MECHANICAL VENTILATION* *Continued*

Complication	Signs and Symptoms	Interventions	Rationale
Gastric distention and ileus	Abdominal distention Large gastric air bubble on chest x-ray or on percussion over stomach ↓ V_T and ↑ respiratory rate Abdomen tender to palpation or complaint of an uncomfortable stomach Sudden decrease in amount of gastric drainage in suction canister over last few hours	For a gastric air bubble, place your hand on the stomach and apply firm pressure in an attempt to burp the patient. *Note,* try this only if you are sure the stomach is empty and the head of the bed is elevated. If unsuccessful, call the physician for an order to pass an nasogastric (NG) tube into the stomach.	This intervention decompresses the stomach. An empty stomach and elevated head of the bed prevent aspiration of gastric contents that might escape with the burp.
		Monitor abdominal girth and bowel sounds.	Increased abdominal girth and absent bowel sounds indicate decreased to absent gastric motility. An NG tube may be needed. If an NG tube is already in place, hold all tube feedings and call the physician.
		Check with the physician regarding insertion of a rectal tube if needed for ileus.	A rectal tube drains air from the lower gastrointestinal tract.
		To initiate oral or NG feedings, give small amounts and increased feedings as tolerated. Dilute formula with water or normal saline if serum sodium is low when the patient complains of abdominal cramping, distention, or diarrhea. Aspirate from the NG tube before each feeding. If the aspirate is greater than half the previous feeding, omit the feeding and reinstill aspirate to avoid fluid and electrolyte loss. Monitor serum electrolyte levels.	The gradual introduction of nutrients to the gastrointestinal tract promotes patient tolerance and prevents complications, such as electrolyte disorders and diarrhea.
		If an NG tube is connected to suction, check the tube's position by instilling a small amount (about 30 cc) of air while auscultating over the stomach. If air is heard, the tube is correctly positioned in the stomach, and the nurse may irrigate with 30 cc of normal saline to promote tube patency. Sometimes injecting air down the sump of a Salem tube will promote drainage and eliminate the need to disconnect the tube for irrigation.	Routinely checking for NG tube patency is one way to quickly identify blocked NG tubes, patient intolerance to tube feedings, and other situations leading to gastric distention.
Gastrointestinal (GI) bleeding	Guaiac-positive stools or NG aspirate Decreased gastric pH (less than 3.0) Dark red or bloody stools or NG aspirate Decreased hematocrit	Guaiac stools and NG aspirate.	Stool or aspirate that looks normal may have traces of blood in it.
		Give antacids or H_2 blocker (Cimetidine or Ranitidine). Monitor gastric pH to evaluate drug effectiveness.	GI bleeding is less likely to occur when these medications raise gastric pH over 3.5.
		Carefully monitor patients on steroids or antibiotics and patients with hypoxemia, hypercarbia, low platelet counts, or clotting disorders.	These patients are at increased risk to develop GI bleeding.
		Begin tube feedings as soon as possible after onset of acute illness.	Food or formula in the stomach decreases risk of GI bleeding.

Table 28–5. COMPLICATIONS DURING MECHANICAL VENTILATION* *Continued*

Complication	Signs and Symptoms	Interventions	Rationale
Gastrointestinal (GI) bleeding *(Continued)*		Transfuse with blood as needed. Monitor hematocrit, stools, and NG aspirate.	Blood transfusions elevate hemoglobin and hematocrit to normal and improve oxygen-carrying capacity of hemoglobin. Monitoring is necessary to detect further signs of bleeding.
		Give psychologic support.	Support helps to reduce stress associated with acute illness. Stress may exacerbate the GI bleeding.
Increased restriction or obstruction versus a ventilator-related problem	High peak inspiratory pressure Frequent activation of high pressure alarm ↑ respiratory rate Breathing out of phase with the ventilator (fighting the ventilator) Agitation, anxiety, ↑ B/P, ↑ pulse, diaphoresis Audible rhonchi (without a stethoscope) Symptoms range from complaint of an uncomfortable breathing pattern to acute shortness of breath or sensation of choking or suffocation	Suction the patient.	In most cases, suctioning relieves airway obstruction (from mucus) and PIP returns to normal. Also, passage of a suction catheter will help determine whether the airway is patent or has become obstructed by mucus or an overinflated cuff.
		Provide verbal reassurance, elevate the head of the bed, and further question the patient about his symptoms.	Reassurance calms the patient, promotes bronchial relaxation, and may decrease airway resistance. Sometimes an uncomfortable body position, bladder distention, or pain causes the patient to become anxious, agitated, and fight the ventilator.
		Monitor ventilator tubing q1–2h for condensed water. To empty excess water, disconnect the circuit at the airway and drain the water into a basin. Reconnect and manually sigh the patient. Then, disconnect at the humidifier and drain again into a basin or waste basket.	Water in the tubing causes increased airway resistance and airflow limitation.
		Check the entire circuit for a leak, beginning at the airway and ending at the ventilator.	A small leak may allow the ventilator to cycle but may reduce V_T, FIO_2, and PaO_2. Increased demand for ventilation from hypoxemia and agitation may cause a ventilator-related problem.
		Check for the presence of other activated alarms.	Other problems, such as inappropriate I:E ratio, may be causing the patient to activate alarms.
		Double check ordered settings for V_T, f, and FIO_2. Take a minute ventilation reading and check the value with that obtained during the last ventilator check. If it has changed significantly, call the physician and check blood gases.	Checking orders assures correct settings and guards against inadvertent errors. A decreased $\dot{V}_E$ suggests decreased alveolar ventilation. Blood gases are needed to assess oxygenation and ventilation.
		For agitation or asynchronous breathing, manually bag the patient with a resuscitator bag for a few minutes.	Manual bagging may correct the abnormal breathing pattern and help the patient readjust to mechanical ventilation without further agitation.
Pulmonary infection	Change in amount, consistency, or color of sputum Rhonchi and crackles Fever Increased total white blood cell (WBC) count Increased number of immature WBCs (left shift) Infiltrate on chest x-ray	See Table 27–1 for basic interventions. Preventive measures are reviewed here.	
		Optimize airway and body defenses, e.g., optimal nutrition; attention to unresolved medical problems; adequate hydration; humidity to inspired gas; meticulous mouth, skin, and wound care.	Optimal airway care helps to keep the mucociliary escalator intact and prevent problems associated with pulmonary infection, e.g., mucus retention, contamination, colonization. Meticulous mouth care helps maintain normal oral flora; optimal skin and wound care helps prevent cross contamination.

Table continued on following page

Table 28–5. COMPLICATIONS DURING MECHANICAL VENTILATION* *Continued*

Complication	Signs and Symptoms	Interventions	Rationale
Pulmonary infection (*Continued*)		Carefully wash your hands after draining water out of ventilator tubings and after any other direct contact with the patient or equipment. Remember *never* to drain water backward into a humidifier or nebulizer.	Hand contamination of hospital personnel is the most common source of cross infection in patients using respiratory therapy devices (Christopher et al, 1983). Draining water into a reservoir may contaminate the reservoir.
		Follow *strict* aseptic technique during suctioning and tracheostomy stomal care. Adhere to the "clean" to "dirty" principle during patient care.	These interventions prevent contamination of the lower respiratory tract.
		Send a tracheal aspirate to the laboratory for culture and sensitivity, Gram's stain every 3 days.	Sputum sample results detect bacterial colonization or infection and possible cross infection between patients on the same ward.
		Use unit-dose vials or small multiple-dose vials for aerosol medication or normal saline lavage. Refrigerate multiple-dose vials as recommended by the manufacturer.	These interventions prevent contamination by diluent or medication routes.
		Discard unused sterile water containers within 24 hours after opening.	Opened water containers are a possible source of infection after 24 hours, particularly in warm environments.
		Follow hospital guidelines for surveillance, disinfection, and sterilization of ventilatory equipment (usually a respiratory therapy department responsibility). (1) Change ventilator circuits every 24 to 48 hours and inspiratory line filters every week. (2) Empty water in humidifier or nebulizer reservoirs every 8 to 24 hours and fill with fresh distilled water. (3) Take periodic bacteriologic samples at key ventilator sites. (4) Use disposable circuits if cost is not prohibitive.	Bacteria is exhaled or expectorated in mucus. They extend along the ventilator circuit's expiratory limb within 2 to 4 days. Routine changing of ventilator circuits halts this process and prevents additional airway contamination from bacteria *(Pseudomonas, Acinetobacter, Flavobacterium, Alcaligenes)* that grow in water droplets in tubings and humidifier reservoir.
Malnutrition	***General*** Weight loss Easily pluckable hair Peripheral edema Total lymphocyte count less than 1200 Serum albumin less than 3.4 gm/100 ml Transferrin less than 300 mg % Muscle atrophy Anergic reaction to skin tests Negative nitrogen balance ***Respiratory*** Prolonged period of mechanical ventilation with stress, hypermetabolism, or limited dietary intake Fatigue Poor cough Decreased VC and V_T Recurrent pulmonary infections Increased atelectasis	Monitor for decreasing weight, VC, poor dietary intake, and presence of a stressed state.	These signs indicate possible malnutrition. Stress increases caloric needs. Body weight and VC are good gauges of the effects of starvation on the respiratory system. The decrease in diaphagmatic muscle mass is proportional to the decrease in body weight. VC progressively decreases in semistarvation (Askanazi et al, 1982). Close monitoring is necessary because some starving patients show no to few signs of respiratory difficulty until general signs of malnutrition are readily observable (Barrocas et al, 1983).
		Assemble the health care team to evaluate nutritional status.	A collaborative approach is needed to set goals for the replenishment of muscle and visceral protein, promotion of wound healing, return of weight to normal, restoration of immunocompetence, and normalization of nitrogen balance.

Table 28–5. COMPLICATIONS DURING MECHANICAL VENTILATION* *Continued*

Complication	Signs and Symptoms	Interventions	Rationale
Malnutrition (*Continued*)		If swallowing is impaired, pass a small feeding tube and start enteral feedings within 24 hours after intubation.	Nutrition prevents the immediate onset of starvation, provides calories for energy, and decreases the incidence of GI bleeding, as previously mentioned.
		Monitor for diarrhea and adjust tube feedings to maximize absorption and digestion: (1) use diluted feedings or small frequent feedings to decrease nutrient osmolarity; (2) add pancreatic enzymes for malabsorption; (3) use opiates to decrease bowel mobility; or (4) change the type of formula or try PULMOCARE (Ross Laboratories).	Formulas are administered according to individual patient tolerance and nutritional needs. PULMOCARE is a special nutritional formula for pulmonary patients.
		Use total parenteral nutrition (TPN) for stressed, malnourished patients with nonfunctional GI tracts.	Such patients cannot digest regular food or that provided in tube feedings.
		Give a mixture of glucose and fat rather than glucose alone.	A glucose-induced increase in CO_2 production and O_2 consumption may precipitate respiratory failure; the extra CO_2 must be excreted by the lungs.
		Give fat separate from the patient's basic TPN solution. It usually consists of a 10 or 20 % solution of emulsified fat infused IV 2 to 3 times a week. An oral form, MCT oil (15 ml TID or QID) is available for chronic cases.	Intravenous fat is compatible with TPN solution. However, it is given periodically rather than continuously for optimal nutrition and simplification of administration.
		Monitor $\dot{V}_E$, $PaCO_2$, respiratory quotient, weight, intake and output, and levels of electrolytes, serum glucose, urinary glucose and acetone, and other parameters as indicated by the situation.	These parameters help to adjust TPN calories, dextrose (glucose), fat, protein (amino acids), electrolytes, and trace elements to individual situations. Daily or more frequent evaluation may be necessary to provide only enough calories to meet acute demands and to prevent a glucose-induced increase in CO_2 production.
Respiratory muscle fatigue	***Signs of inspiratory muscle fatigue*** (in order of likely occurrence, according to Cohen et al, 1982) Change in electromyographic power spectrum of the diaphragm to a decrease in high frequency power (150 to 350 hertz) and an increase in low frequency power (20 to 40 hertz). The *high/low ratio* falls during fatiguing work to about 60 %. ↑ f and ↑ $\dot{V}_E$ Incoordinated respiratory movements: inspiratory abdominal paradox and respiratory alternans ↑ $PaCO_2$ and ↓ pH ↓ f and ↓ $\dot{V}_E$ leading to apnea or respiratory arrest (see Figs. 13–10 and 13–11 for explanation of ABG changes)	Monitor for signs of respiratory muscle fatigue, e.g., increased f and V_E, decreased VC and PIP.	The patient on mechanical ventilation is at risk for respiratory muscle fatigue, particularly in the presence of malnutrition. Keep in mind than nutritional replenishment may take 2 to 6 weeks. Decreased PIP indicates decreased inspiratory muscle strength. Ventilatory failure may occur when inspiratory muscle strength is less than 30 % of normal.
		Correct fluid and electrolyte disorders and provide nutritional support.	Fluid and electrolyte imbalance and malnutrition promote inspiratory muscle fatigue.
		Avoid use of paralyzing agents, e.g., curare, pancuronium.	Such agents promote respiratory muscle disuse and atrophy.
		Consider use of assist-control (A/C) mode or high IMV rates during nutritional replenishment.	This approach assures excretion of excess CO_2 (from glucose in the TPN) without excess fatigue. It prepares the patient for successful weaning from mechanical ventilation.

Table continued on following page

Table 28–5. COMPLICATIONS DURING MECHANICAL VENTILATION* *Continued*

Complication	Signs and Symptoms	Interventions	Rationale
Respiratory muscle fatigue (*Continued*)	***Other signs*** ↓ maximum inspiratory pressure ↓ VC Presence of a primary neuromuscular disorder Tachycardia Diaphoresis Use of inspiratory and expiratory muscles of respiration Complaint of fatigue and shortness of breath	When signs of fatigue appear, assess medication utilized for primary lung disorder, e.g., corticosteroids and anticholinergics for myasthenia gravis.	Fatigue may be due to a recent change in medication or a change in medication need.
		Continue theophylline preparation.	Theophylline improves diaphragmatic contractility and increases respiratory muscle endurance.
		Once ventilator weaning starts 1. Provide rest between weaning trials and at night.	Rest prevents excess fatigue, increases the likelihood of successful weaning trials, and builds patient confidence.
		2. Provide *undisturbed* sleep by closing the curtains around the patient, restricting visitors, eliminating unnecessary noises, and reducing monitoring functions during sleeping hours.	Undisturbed sleep promotes a deeper sleep pattern and more complete rest compared with disturbed sleep.
		3. Promptly return the patient to the A/C mode should physical status deteriorate.	Weaning is contraindicated when the patient's condition deteriorates.
		Implement passive/active ROM exercises to all extremities. Encourage ambulation with portable O_2 tank and resuscitator bag.	ROM exercises improves overall muscle endurance. Ambulation increases endurance, exercises the diaphragm, and provides external stimuli to the sensory-deprived patient.
		Use an inspiratory muscle trainer 5 to 10 min/day, working up to longer and more frequent periods (see Chapter 20).	Inspiratory muscle training increases respiratory muscle strength and endurance and helps prevent fatigue.

*See text for explanation of physiologic mechanisms.

Positive Fluid Balance

The etiology of positive fluid balance is poorly understood, but several mechanisms seem to be involved. As positive pressure decreases blood pressure, it also causes the inappropriate release of antidiuretic hormone and the decrease of renal blood flow and glomerular filtration. The kidneys conserve water, and the lungs cannot eliminate it because the ventilator circuit saturates inspired gas and may add as much as 300 to 500 ml of extra water to the body every 24 hours if a nebulizer is used. Moreover, the lymphatics cannot readily eliminate excess fluid from the lung because high intrathoracic pressure interferes with drainage, probably by compressing the vessels.

Gastric Distention and Ileus

Possible mechanisms for this complication include swallowed air, usually in the dyspneic or postresuscitation patient; decreased to absent gastric motility from recent abdominal surgery, coma, or brain stem lesion or other acute illness; and nonfunctioning nasogastric (NG) tube.

Gastrointestinal Bleeding

About 25 % of patients on mechanical ventilation develop guaiac-positive stools, and about 15 % lose enough blood to require a transfusion (Morrison, 1979).

Increased Restriction/Obstruction Versus a Ventilator-Related Problem

This is a common complication in the clinical setting. Initial interventions focus on determining the etiology of the problem, i.e., the patient, the airway, or the ventilator.

Patient problems include excess secretions, atelectasis, bronchoconstriction, pneumothorax, and anxiety.

Airway problems causing increased obstruction include a kinked or malpositioned endotracheal or tracheostomy tube, an overinflated cuff, and a mucus crusting along the tube's sides or over the tube's lumen.

Ventilator problems include the accumulation of condensed water in circuit tubing, which increases airway resistance and can cause inadvertent expiratory retard or PEEP. Other possibilities are a small leak in the system, a low FIO_2, or an inappropriate I:E ratio.

Pulmonary Infection

Placement of an airway past the larynx *always* results in contamination of the lower airway with gram-positive bacteria. This normal flora changes to primarily gram-negative bacteria during hospitalization, especially with antibiotic therapy or debilitation or the intensive care unit (ICU) environment. (Review Table 8–4 for microorganisms causing pneumonia.) Bacterial colonization can lead to infection by airway surfaces and eventually pneumonia. Most tracheal tubes become infected after nine days of mechanical ventilation (Comhaire and Lamy, 1981).

Factors contributing to the spread of organisms include (1) contaminated respiratory equipment; (2) inadequate handwashing; (3) prolonged close contact with patients; (4) adverse environmental factors, including ICUs with poor room ventilation, high traffic flow, and absent or inaccessible sinks for handwashing; and (5) decreased ability of the patient to cough and clear secretions.

Malnutrition

Many patients on mechanical ventilation experience progressive malnutrition, occasionally complicated by hypercatabolism for sepsis, fever, or the requirements of postoperative wound healing. Starvation is an immediate response whenever nutritional support is withheld. Glycogen stores become depleted after 12 to 16 hours. When protein and caloric intake are restricted for one to several weeks, abnormalities develop in pulmonary defense mechanisms, pulmonary structure and function, control of breathing, and respiratory muscle contractility (Rochester and Esau, 1984). Specific physiologic changes include visceral and muscle protein depletion, intercostal and diaphragmatic muscle cannibalization to meet energy needs, depressed hypoxic ventilatory response, delayed wound healing, impaired immunocompetence, decreased surfactant production, emphysematous lung changes, and pulmonary infarcts with cavitation. Medical complications may lead to respiratory failure, unsuccessful weaning from mechanical ventilation, and death.

Perhaps the most striking effect of malnutrition is the patient's inability to sustain adequate levels of ventilation. The COPD patient in particular is highly susceptible to respiratory muscle fatigue (defined hereafter) because malnutrition weakens respiratory muscles and because the COPD patient is already at a mechanical disadvantage from lung hyperinflation. Malnutrition predisposes COPD patients to ventilatory failure and death.

Furthermore, physiologic changes and signs and symptoms of malnutrition are more severe in any patient with preexisting chronic illness who is already in a state of protein-calorie malnutrition before the onset of acute illness.

Respiratory Muscle Fatigue

Respiratory muscle fatigue is defined as the *inability to maintain a normal* Pa_{CO_2} *in the absence of CNS depression* or *failure of a muscle to maintain or reattain required or expected force with continued or repeated contractions* (Pratter et al, 1982).

Fatigue is caused by *increased demand for ventilation* or *increased work of breathing. Increased demand for ventilation* is due to increased CO_2 production brought on by dextrose in total parenteral nutrition (TPN), sepsis, infection, fever, shivering, or agitation. Interventions focus on decreasing the demand for ventilation by altering TPN to patient needs, treating infection, controlling body temperature, and reducing agitation.

Increased work of breathing is due to a deteriorating cardiopulmonary condition or an inappropriate ventilator setting. Interventions focus on decreasing the work of breathing by decreasing bronchospasm; treating pulmonary edema; reversing atelectasis and mucus retention; and adjusting ventilator settings to achieve a comfortable, synchronous breathing pattern, as lung compliance changes.

Other factors that promote muscle weakness, deconditioning, and fatigue include malnutrition, hypophosphatemia, hypomagnesemia, and hypokalemia. Also, relaxant or paralyzing drugs and the controlled mode of ventilation may cause severe muscle disuse and atrophy.

When the patient cannot tolerate increased work of breathing, the high ventilatory load may produce muscle damage and fiber splitting unless the work is reduced and the muscles are allowed to rest. Rest usually reverses most fatigue experienced by patients and allows repletion of metabolic stores. However, the exact amount of rest needed to relieve different degrees of fatigue is not well established.

Other Complications

Other complications of mechanical ventilation include increased intracranial pressure, impaired hepatic function, anxiety reaction, and problems related to immobility, physical isolation, and sensory deprivation.

Basic Monitoring Parameters

Basic monitoring parameters include vital signs, chest assessment findings, rate and rhythm of the ECG, basic ventilator check, ABGs, and others as indicated by the situation.

VENTILATOR CHECK

The nurse checks the basic ventilator settings listed in the following box before, during, or after the quick chest examination (see Chapter 12).

COMPONENTS OF THE BASIC VENTILATOR CHECK

1. **Ventilator mode**
2. **FIO_2**
3. **Respiratory rate per minute** (f): there should be one chest excursion and one breath sound for each breath delivered by the ventilator. Note any significant change in the ratio of assisted breaths to machine-triggered controlled breaths. Try to differentiate between fighting the ventilator, e.g., breathing asynchrony, and "breathing around" the ventilator, defined as ineffective attempts to trigger additional breaths during exhalation. The former is a serious complication requiring intervention. The latter is usually innocuous as long as sensitivity is set appropriately, the patient is not in distress, and gas exchange remains uncompromised. For the IMV or SIMV mode, obtain the following parameters: (1) total number of breaths for patient and ventilator and (2) number of mandatory ventilator breaths.
4. **V_T**: preset tidal volume should equal measured exhaled tidal volume ± 50 cc unless otherwise specified.
5. **Peak inspiratory pressure**: note and record with each set of vital signs.
6. **PEEP**: how much?
7. **Alarm system**: is it on?

ARTERIAL BLOOD GAS (ABG) RESULTS

An ABG result may indicate a need to change ventilator settings to provide optimal ventilation and oxygenation. Basic ventilator changes to alter $PaCO_2$ and PaO_2 are described hereafter. For patients with multiple problems, ventilator changes are best made one at a time to better assess the effects of each change.

Changes to Increase $PaCO_2$

Respiratory alkalosis (i.e., alveolar hyperventilation) requires a ventilator adjustment to *decrease* minute ventilation. This change is accomplished by decreasing respiratory rate or tidal volume or some combination of the two. Changes in tidal volume are made in increments of 50 to 100 cc, and changes in respiratory rate are best limited to 2 to 4 breaths/min to allow gradual physiologic adjustment.

Another way to increase $PaCO_2$ is to add mechanical deadspace (see Fig. 5–4). Adding a flextube between the airway and ventilator circuit increases the mixing of exhaled CO_2 with inhaled gas from the ventilator, thus increasing PA_{CO_2} and $PaCO_2$. Deadspace is added in increments of no more than 50 to 60 cc, about one 4- to 6-in long flextube. Sometimes, the addition will normalize $PaCO_2$ and pH, but the higher $PaCO_2$ level stimulates the ventilatory drive to breathe, resulting in increased minute ventilation, signs of increased work of breathing, and patient demands to remove the extra tubing. Hence, mechanical deadspace may normalize ABGs and favorably stimulate ventilatory drive, but some patients will not tolerate the change.

Changes to Decrease $PaCO_2$

Respiratory acidosis (i.e., alveolar hypoventilation) requires a ventilatory adjustment to *increase* minute ventilation. The first step is gradually to eliminate any previously applied mechanical deadspace. Then, minute ventilation is increased by increasing *total* respiratory rate or tidal volume or a combination of these two actions. The increased rate is effective for patients receiving controlled breaths or a set number of IMV breaths. In the assist-control mode, however, tidal volume rather than rate is changed. Increasing respiratory rate is ineffective because the patient establishes his own rate and rarely relies on the controlled backup rate, except perhaps during sleep. Also, a high assist-control or controlled rate will override the patient's rate, making it difficult for him to trigger the ventilator and exercise respiratory muscles.

These ventilatory changes may be supplemented with other actions to decrease $PaCO_2$. Efforts focus on *decreasing CO_2 production* ($\dot{V}CO_2$), e.g., changing TPN solution, decreasing the work of breathing, reducing fever, and *decreasing deadspace ventilation.* The last usually involves improving Q in the V/Q ratio, e.g., correcting hypovolemia; treating left ventricular failure or pulmonary emboli; eliminating super PEEP; and reducing the use of drugs, such as norepinephrine and phenylephrine, that cause constriction of precapillary pulmonary vessels (Hotchkiss and Wilson, 1983).

Changes to Increase PaO_2

Hypoxemia is treated by increasing FIO_2 or PEEP or some combination of the two. FIO_2 is changed in increments of 0.10 to 0.20 (10 to 20% O_2 concentration). PEEP is added in increments of 2.5 to 5 cmH_2O when FIO_2 reaches 0.50 or when hypoxemia remains refractory to an increase in FIO_2.

These ventilatory changes may be supplemented with other methods to improve blood oxygenation and oxygen delivery to tissues. For example, increasing cardiac output by the use of vasopressor, vasodilator, or other unloading agents may improve the lungs' overall V/Q ratio and permit reduction of the FIO_2 to acceptable levels. A blood transfusion to maintain hemoglobin at 12 to 15 gm/dl will improve the oxygen-carrying capacity of arterial blood. Correction of alkalosis and hypophosphatemia will make the unloading of oxygen to tissues much easier (review content related to Figure 3–7 and the oxyhemoglobin dissociation curve). Oxygen consumption may be reduced by sedation, paralysis, or hypothermia.

Changes to Decrease PaO_2

FIO_2 is decreased in increments of 0.10 to 0.20 until an FIO_2 of 0.50 or less is reached. Then, PEEP may be withdrawn in 2.5 to 5.0 cmH_2O increments, as long as SaO_2 remains greater than 90 %, blood pressure changes by less than 20 mmHg, and cardiac rate and rhythm remain relatively stable.

pH and HCO_3^-

Other interventions may be necessary to bring PaO_2 and $PaCO_2$ within the patient's baseline levels before hospitalization and to normalize pH and HCO_3^-. See Table 13–4 for interventions to correct accompanying metabolic disorders.

COMPLIANCE

Three indicators exist to estimate compliance as follows: peak inspiratory pressure (PIP), dynamic or effective compliance, and static compliance. These parameters and their clinical interpretations are discussed in detail in Chapter 8.

Nursing interventions always incorporate PIP because an instantaneous value is obtained merely by glancing at the ventilator's pressure gauge when taking vital signs or implementing other aspects of care. No calculations are necessary. An increase in PIP signals increasing airway or ventilator circuit resistance or decreasing lung compliance, as long as ventilator setting (e.g., tidal volume) remain constant. If tidal volume has been adjusted, a new baseline PIP is recorded on the bedside chart for comparison with future PIP readings. This approach enables the nurse to detect most trends and major changes in lung mechanics.

Effective compliance is measured q2 to 4h to estimate the magnitude of a change in mechanics. The patient should be resting calmly, preferably in the supine position. Cuff pressure is adjusted to prevent air leaks, and, ideally, inspiratory flow rate is kept constant. PIP and tidal volume are noted, and a calculation performed as follows:

Effective Compliance

$$\frac{\text{Volume}}{\text{Pressure}} = \frac{\text{tidal volume}}{\text{peak inspiratory pressure (or PIP} - \text{PEEP)}}$$

Normal value = 100 ml/cmH_2O (0.10 L/cmH_2O) or about 10 ml/cmH_2O higher than static compliance

For accuracy, some clinicians determine tidal volume (V_T) by subtracting ventilator tubing compliance (3 cc/cmH_2O) from the exhaled tidal volume.

Static pressure is measured with dynamic compliance to more accurately assess pathologic processes under "no flow" conditions. At the peak of inspiration, expiration is momentarily delayed by using the "inflation hold" or "expiratory retard" dial on the ventilator or by pinching closed the expiratory line of the ventilator circuit. This delay allows equalization of lung pressures and minimization of airway resistance from rapid breathing and the airway and ventilator circuit. As the pressure needle starts to fall and pauses for a second or two, the clinician reads the plateau pressure before the needle quickly falls to complete exhalation. Then, static compliance is determined as follows:

Static Compliance

$$\frac{V}{P} = \frac{\text{tidal volume}}{\text{plateau pressure (PP) (or PP} - \text{PEEP)}}$$

Normal value = 70–100 ml/cmH_2O (0.07–0.10 L/cmH_2O) or about 10 ml/cmH_2O lower than effective compliance

In some settings, clinicians measure static and dynamic compliance at multiple tidal volumes and at a constant flow rate (i.e., usually 1 L/sec) and then plot static and dynamic pressure-volume curves. Changes in slope, contour, location, and distance between the two curves help the physician evaluate restrictive and obstructive processes and determine the optimal PEEP level that maximizes lung compliance without significantly reducing cardiac output.

NONINVASIVE MEASUREMENTS OF PaO_2 AND $PaCO_2$

An ABG measurement remains mandatory to accurately assess gas exchange. Yet, it is expensive, patients may suffer discomfort and complications associated with the arterial puncture or arterial cannula, and a lag time always exists before clinicians can receive and act on results. Hence, as new noninvasive methods to measure ABGs are developed, clinicians are gradually incorporating them into respiratory care and relying on them to more continuously monitor gas exchange and facilitate the weaning process.

Current technology is limited to noninvasive measurements of PaO_2 and $PaCO_2$. When a noninvasive measurement is initiated, the nurse notes the correlation between the noninvasive value and the arterial value. When the noninvasive measurement is significantly higher or lower than the patient's baseline value, the physician is notified, and an ABG may be ordered to validate results and obtain more data.

Oximetry Pao_2

Ear or finger oximetry is the most commonly used noninvasive measurement of Pao_2 in the adult patient. It is described in Chapter 23 in relation to the evaluation of oxygen therapy.

Transcutaneous Po_2 and Pco_2

Transcutaneous gas monitoring was introduced into neonatal ICUs over 10 years ago and is now used occasionally in adult ICUs, the operating room, and stress test laboratories. A *transcutaneous* PO_2 ($P_{tc}O_2$) reliably assesses Pao_2 in children and young adults as long as circulation is not grossly impaired (Yahav et al, 1981). The correlation between the two values falls during periods of peripheral vasoconstriction, shock, or surgery due to interference from some anesthetic gases. A *transcutaneous* PCO_2 ($P_{tc}CO_2$) measures arterial Pco_2 to an accuracy of ± 3 mmHg in any patient (Severinghaus, 1982).

Transcutaneous readings are taken via one or two heated electrodes placed on the surface of the skin where perfusion is good and fat deposits are minimal, e.g., anterior chest area just below the clavicle or upper arm . The machine is calibrated, the skin surface is rubbed thoroughly with alcohol, and a special solution is applied to the electrode's surface before application to the chest. A 10- to 20-minute stabilization period is necessary before a reading is taken from a digital display (Fig. 28–16). Once the system is operating correctly, continuous monitoring is possible, and high and low limit alarms may be set to alert health care personnel to a change in the patient's condition.

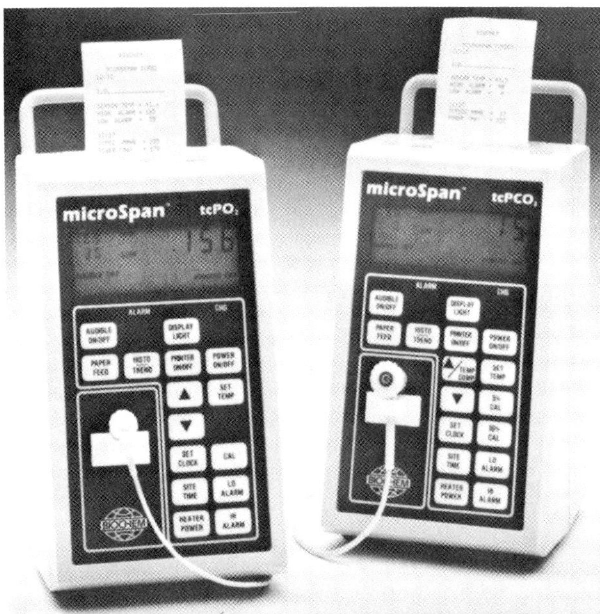

Figure 28–16. Transcutaneous Pco_2/Po_2 monitors with visual and graphic displays. The skin sensor is attached to the front panel of each of these portable monitors. (Courtesy of Biochem International Inc., Waukesha, Wisconsin.)

However, extra care is needed to follow specified calibration procedures, to wait for reading stabilization, and to rotate electrode sites every 2 to 6 hours to minimize the chance of skin burns (Knights, 1983).

End-Tidal Pco_2

End-tidal Pco_2 ($P_{ET}CO_2$), along with oximetry Pao_2, is routinely used to monitor adults on mechanical ventilation and others with acute respiratory problems. In some cases, it allows the rapid titration of PEEP without the need for a pulmonary artery catheter (Murray et al, 1985).

The $P_{ET}CO_2$ is measured with an infrared CO_2 analyzer built into a capnograph monitor (Fig. 28–17). In other cases, a sensor (e.g., pneumotachometer sensing device) is placed in the ventilator circuit as close as possible to the patient. A gas sample is delivered via long capillary tubing to a *mass spectrometer* for processing. If the mass spectrometer is connected to a respiratory monitoring system, such as the one in Figure 28–18, a computer makes calculations, and a monitor displays $P_{ET}CO_2$, the exhaled CO_2 waveform, and other pulmonary function measurements taken and calculated at the same time.

A normal expired CO_2 waveform, called a *capnogram*, is shown in Figure 28–19. At the beginning of exhalation, exhaled CO_2 (P_ECO_2) rises dramatically as the patient's anatomic deadspace is exhaled (1 in Fig. 28–19). A gently sloping alveolar plateau is reached as gas leaves alveolar units, and CO_2 concentration in the lung equilibrates (3). The peak expired CO_2 concentration at point 4 is referred to as the end-tidal pressure of CO_2 or $P_{ET}CO_2$.

Mechanical ventilation tends to prolong the alveolar plateau phase, as shown in the capnogram tracing in Figure 28–19B. The extra time for gas equilibration may greatly improve blood gas results.

In persons with normal lungs, $P_{ET}CO_2$ is about 1 to 4 mmHg below arterial Pco_2. Patients on mechanical ventilation have varying regional V/Q ratios and, hence, usually show more variation between $P_{ET}CO_2$ and $Paco_2$ levels. Because this *arterial end-tidal* Pco_2 *gradient* may vary from −6 to +20 mmHg, $P_{ET}CO_2$ is used to detect a change in the patient's condition (Kinasewitz, 1982). Trends are more important than absolute numbers.

A *high* $P_{ET}CO_2$ may indicate alveolar hypoventilation, V/Q mismatch, or marked reduction in cardiac output. In some patients, it indicates an improved condition; hence, when deadspace ventilation (V_D) is reduced and V_D/V_T decreases, the patient is able to exhale more CO_2.

A *low* $P_{ET}CO_2$ may indicate alveolar hyperventilation, improved V/Q ratio in a patient who is clinically improving, or increased alveolar deadspace (e.g., from a pulmonary embolus or large right-to-left cardiac shunt) in an acutely ill patient.

The shape of the capnogram gives additional clinical information. For example, the steep ascent of the

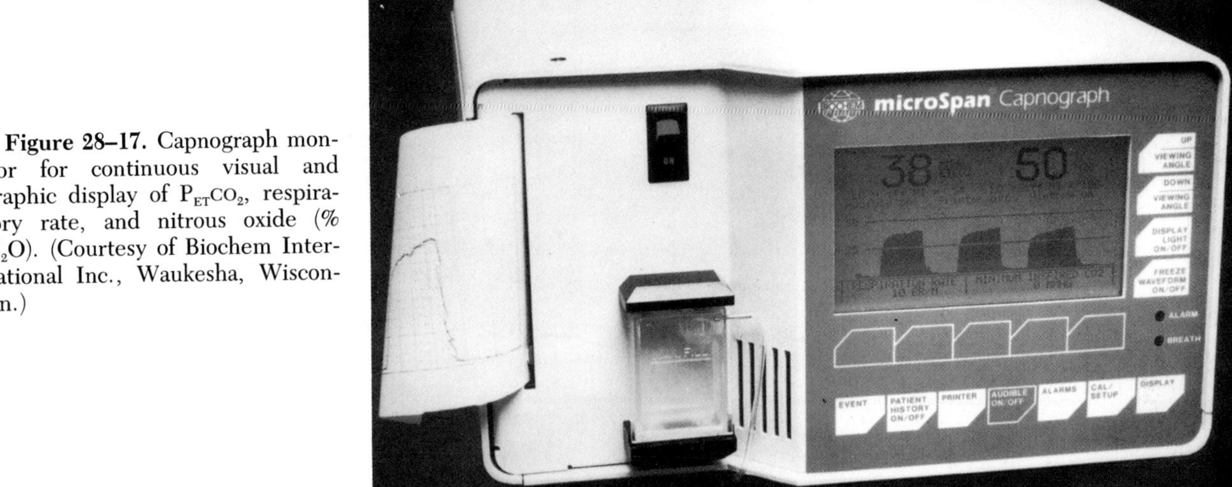

Figure 28–17. Capnograph monitor for continuous visual and graphic display of $P_{ET}CO_2$, respiratory rate, and nitrous oxide (% N_2O). (Courtesy of Biochem International Inc., Waukesha, Wisconsin.)

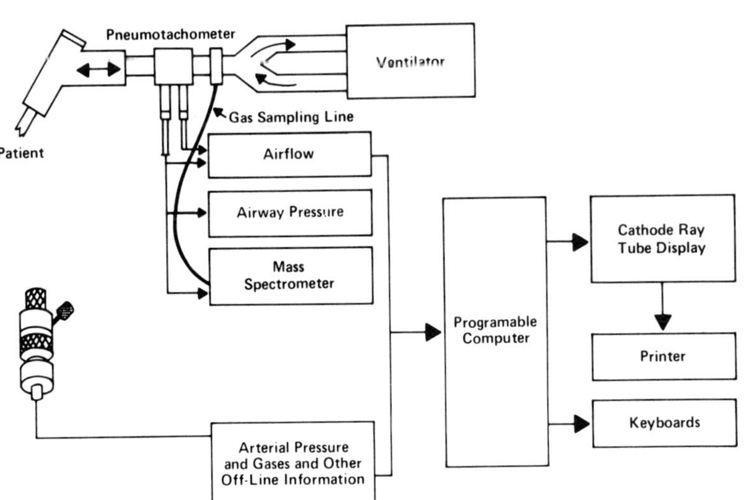

Figure 28–18. Respiratory monitoring system. Airflow and pressure and gas concentrations are measured simultaneously. Calculations are made by a computer utilizing these signals and off-line information. (Reproduced by permission from Bone, R. Monitoring patients in acute respiratory failure. *Respiratory care*, 27(6): 700–701, 1982.)

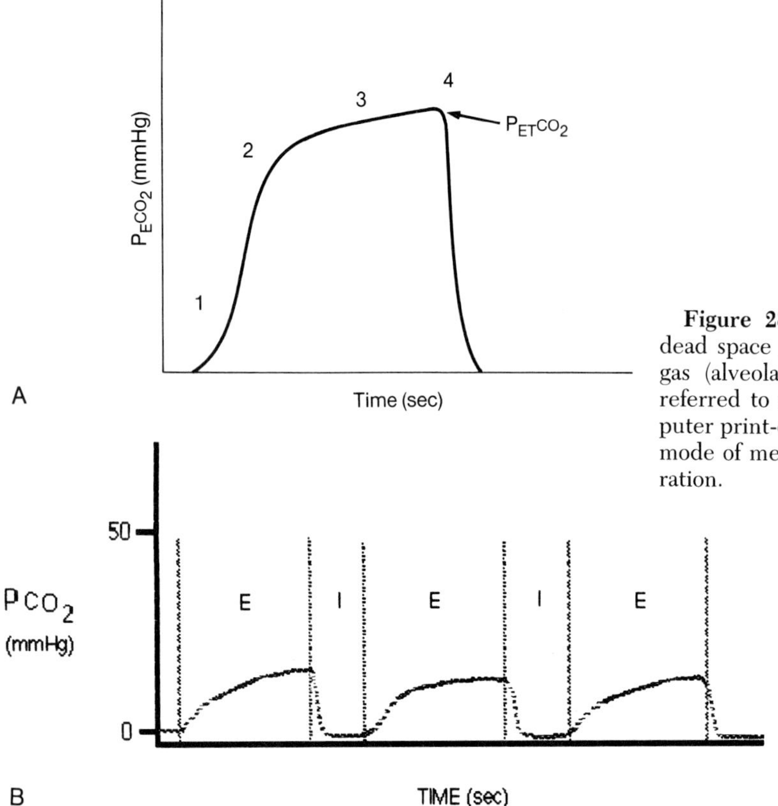

Figure 28–19. Capnograms. *A*, Normal capnogram. 1, dead space gas; 2, dead space and alveolar gas; 3, alveolar gas (alveolar plateau); 4, peak expired pressure of CO_2, referred to as the end-tidal CO_2 pressure $P_{ET}CO_2$. *B*, Computer print-out of capnogram waveforms in the assist-control mode of mechanical ventilation. E = expiration; I = inspiration.

second curve in Figure 28–20 reflects the severe COPD patient's mismatching and altered rate of alveolar emptying during exhalation. Other clinical applications include alteration in minute ventilation settings on the ventilator, detection of ineffective spontaneous breaths during IMV, and detection of rises in $Paco_2$ that correlate with increases in intracranial pressure.

Weaning the Patient from Mechanical Ventilation

Weaning, the process of withdrawing mechanical ventilatory support, is an art that depends on blood gas monitoring and, in particular, optimal nursing care because results are largely unpredictable, and ongoing psychologic support is crucial.

READINESS TO WEAN

A person's normal response to the withdrawal of mechanical support includes (1) decreased V_T and increased respiratory rate with $\dot{V}_E$ about the same or slightly reduced; (2) slight drop in Pao_2 due to atelectasis or, rarely, a drop in cardiac output; and (3) decreased alveolar ventilation and increasing V_D/V_T that cause $Paco_2$ to rise slightly and pH to drop slightly (Quan and Hasan, 1980). Though these changes may cause patient discomfort, they are minimal and require no intervention. However, they may become marked,

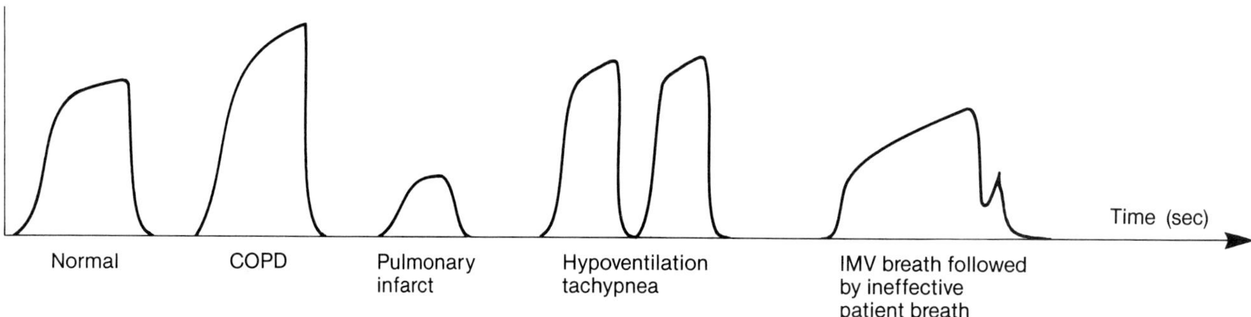

Figure 28–20. Abnormal capnograms.

Table 28–6. WEANING CRITERIA

Mechanics	
*Vital capacity (VC)	> 10 to 15 cc/kg (usually 1000 cc)
Tidal volume (V_T)	> 5 cc/kg (usually 200 cc)
Minute ventilation ($\dot{V}_E$)	< 10 L/min indicates that a high ventilatory requirement has been reduced.
Maximum voluntary ventilation (MVV)	≥ twice the $\dot{V}_E$
Maximum inspiratory pressure (MIP)	> −20 cmH_2O†
Respiratory rate (f)	< 35/min
Oxygenation	
*PaO_2	60 to 70 mmHg (50–60 mmHg for COPD) with $FIO_2 \leq 0.40$
$P(A\text{-}a)O_2$	< 300 to 350 mmHg with FIO_2 = 1.00
PaO_2/PA_{O_2}	> 0.15 or PaO_2/FIO_2 > 200 mmHg
Qs/Qt	< 20 to 25%
Ventilation	
*$PaCO_2$	< 45 mmHg or equal to the patient's baseline $PaCO_2$
V_D/V_T	< 0.60 except for some young patients who can sustain high ratios.

*Key criteria.
†In the clinical setting, a −30 value is actually more than a −20.

leading to failure of the weaning process, if the patient is not prepared in advance for the weaning process. Weaning does not begin until the patient is alert, oriented, and clinically stable with adequate circulation, absence of sepsis, and normal metabolic state. Complications listed in Table 28–5 should be resolved or at least under control. Specific weaning criteria are listed in Table 28–6. However, these criteria are only guidelines, since strict adherence to them may actually delay the weaning process. In a few cases, the use of vasopressors or aortic balloon counterpulsation may improve cardiac output and facilitate the weaning process.

Whichever method is used, the patient is first weaned to a reduced FIO_2, then weaned off mechanical ventilation, and finally weaned off the endotracheal or tracheostomy tube by extubation or decannulation (described previously).

WEANING TO A REDUCED FIO_2

FIO_2 is gradually reduced to 0.40 or less, and PEEP is gradually decreased to zero. This process begins as soon as possible after intubation but may take hours, days, or weeks to complete, depending on the situation. In some cases, PEEP is left at 2 to 5 cmH_2O rather than completely discontinued, and the patient is extubated on low PEEP levels to prevent the deterioration in PaO_2 associated with weaning (Quan and Hasan, 1980).

When PEEP is discontinued or substantially reduced, a 15 to 20 % increase in cardiac output and blood pressure may occur within the first few minutes. These parameters usually return to baseline levels within 20 minutes (Ellman and Dembirn, 1982). This rebound phenomenon is due to sudden hypervolemia or a change in catecholamine levels. To detect volume overload, cardiac decompensation, or other adverse effects, the nurse checks vital signs, cardiac rhythm, and hemodynamic measurements (pulmonary capillary wedge pressure) immediately after PEEP withdrawal, in 15 to 20 minutes, and then every 1 to 2 hours and PRN. Such close monitoring is also necessary after the change from the assist-control mode to IMV or from IMV to CPAP, because the patient with poor cardiopulmonary reserves may become volume overloaded, as positive pressure is withdrawn from the lungs. To prevent a rise in PCWP and a drop in cardiac output, PEEP is usually ordered. Inotropic or venodilator therapy may be used temporarily if weaning difficulties arise.

WEANING OFF THE VENTILATOR

No one best way exists to wean a patient off the ventilator. Methods vary, depending on physician preferences, unit protocol, and available equipment and health care personnel for monitoring. Familiarity with the traditional and IMV methods described hereafter enable the nurse to wean most patients off the ventilator.

Traditional Method

The traditional method involves switching from the assist-control or IMV mode to one or more T-piece trials. The patient with adequate cardiopulmonary reserves may require a short (i.e., 30 to 60 minutes) T-piece trial (method 1 in Fig. 28–21) or may be extubated without trial if he is awake and alert, breathing without difficulty (i.e., triggering the ventilator), and demonstrating good gag and cough reflexes. The patient with limited cardiopulmonary reserves usually requires longer periods on the T-piece before extubation. He is initially placed on the T-piece for 5 to 10 minutes, returned to the ventilator for 50 minutes, and gradually permitted longer periods on the T-piece during each hour as tolerated. If he is not extubated during the day, he is placed back on the ventilator at night, and the process continues in the morning after a good night's sleep (method 2 in Fig. 28–21).

Synchronized Intermittent Mandatory Ventilation (SIMV) Method

Whereas the traditional method begins when the patient is ready, the IMV method begins before the patient meets weaning criteria and proceeds according to changes in pH (Pierson, 1983a). In some patients, ventilator mandatory breaths are rapidly reduced to zero over a few hours, and the patient is promptly extubated (method 3 in Figure 28–21). Patients with limited cardiopulmonary reserves require a more grad-

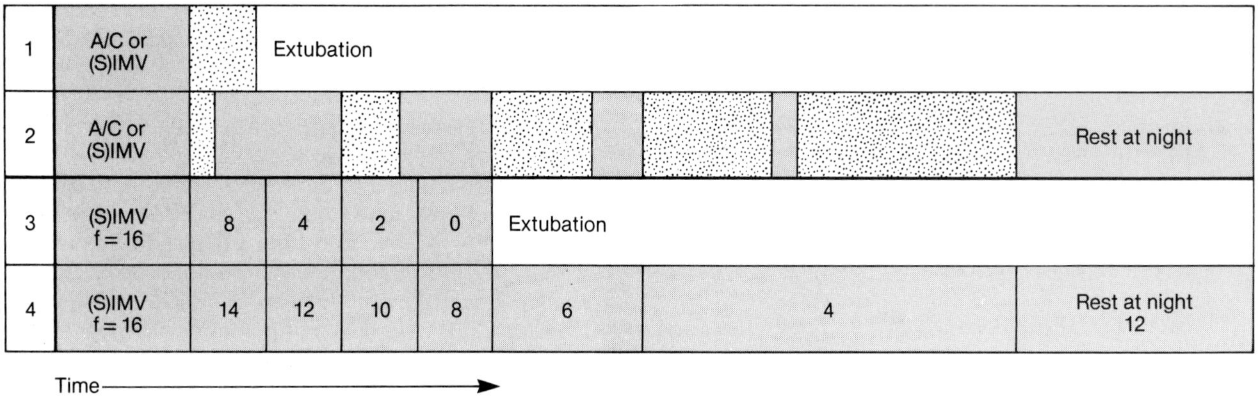

1	A/C or (S)IMV		Extubation					
2	A/C or (S)IMV							Rest at night
3	(S)IMV f=16	8	4	2	0	Extubation		
4	(S)IMV f=16	14	12	10	8	6	4	Rest at night 12

Time ⟶

Figure 28–21. Conceptual representation of traditional (1 and 2) and IMV (3 and 4) weaning methods. The dotted areas represent spontaneous breathing via T piece; the shaded areas represent periods of mechanical ventilation.

ual reduction in mandatory breaths, as exemplified by method 4 in Figure 28–21. Mandatory breaths are decreased by 1 to 2/min as tolerated. The patient's rate is increased at night to allow rest and reduced again in the morning to the lowest rate used the previous day.

With the IMV method, three problems may arise. First, clinicians may delay the weaning process by rigidly following a stepwise reduction in IMV breaths. As Pierson (1983b) emphasizes, weaning should proceed as far and as fast as pH allows.

Second, patients tend to remain at an IMV of 2 to 4/min, and further efforts to reduce the rate fail. In some cases, more time is needed before a further reduction in IMV rate is possible. Sometimes, however, the problem relates to the increased resistance associated with some modern ventilator IMV-CPAP circuitries (e.g., Bear 1 and 2) or a small diameter endotracheal tube. In this case, the only way to complete weaning may be to switch to a ventilator with lower resistance circuitry (e.g., MA-1), or switch to a T-piece, or extubate.

Third, confusion exists regarding (S)IMV as a primary mode of ventilation and (S)IMV as a weaning technique. The two may become confused, particularly when weaning takes place intermittently over days to weeks. For example, when clinical instability occurs at low IMV rates, further weaning is postponed, but increasing the IMV rate or switching to the assist-control mode is inadvertently overlooked until further clinical deterioration makes the change mandatory. This problem is less likely to happen when all health team members clearly understand the ventilatory goals for the patient.

A Basic Weaning Procedure

The following steps describe a basic weaning procedure. It is written for the T-piece method, but the same principles apply to the IMV method, except that monitoring occurs after each reduction in IMV rate, and the cuff is left inflated.

1. Always start weaning in the morning, when the patient is rested and better able to cope with stress.
2. Withhold all sedatives and other drugs that might decrease ventilatory drive.
3. Explain the procedure to the patient, emphasizing the following points:
   a. Spontaneous periods of breathing are necessary to retrain respiratory muscles, build endurance, and help the body adapt to a new breathing pattern.
   b. Some shortness of breath, discomfort, and fatigue are to be expected.
   c. A nurse or respiratory therapist will be in constant attendance or close by.
   d. If symptoms become intolerable, the patient will be returned to the ventilator.
4. Make the patient comfortable in an upright position, with a call light within reach. Suction the tracheal tube as well as above the cuff. Take baseline vital signs (B/P, heart rate and rhythm, respirations) and basic weaning PFT parameters (VC, V_T, MIP) if they have not already been taken.
5. Deflate the cuff to minimize air flow resistance and increase ventilation provided the swallow reflex is intact.
6. Put on the T piece and remain at the bedside, giving words of encouragement and noting any signs of hypoxemia or hypercarbia.
7. Return the patient to mechanical ventilation if signs of distress or respiratory muscle fatigue appear (see the box that follows). Remember that some patients may feel intense dyspnea despite adequate ABGs, as the respiratory center resets to a different $Pa{CO_2}$ level and lung stretch receptors and chest wall receptors adapt to a lower tidal volume.
8. At the end of a T-piece trial (i.e., after 5 to 10 minutes for the initial trial), assess ABG, vital signs, and PFT parameters before returning the patient to mechanical ventilation.
9. During weaning, take vital signs q5–10min for 30 minutes, q30min for 1 h, and then q1–2h.

SIGNS OF RESPIRATORY MUSCLE FATIGUE

Increased respiratory rate (> 35/min)
Tachycardia (> 120/min)
20 mmHg or more increase or decrease in B/P
Arrhythmias
Angina
Cyanosis
Abdominal paradox or respiratory alternans
pH < 7.3
Pao_2 < 55 mmHg or < 80 % of the preweaning value
Great decreases in V_T (< 200 cc)
Agitation or deteriorating mental status

10. Draw an ABG sample after extubation to establish new baseline values and to verify adequate oxygenation and ventilation.

USE OF NONINVASIVE RESPIRATORY MONITORING SYSTEMS

Monitoring the patient immediately postextubation may be easier with a noninvasive respiratory monitoring system that detects subtle or sudden changes in breathing pattern before a blood gas abnormality can be diagnosed. This type of system may be used routinely for any critically ill respiratory patient or for any spontaneously breathing individual at risk for an alteration in breathing pattern, e.g., history of apnea, upper airway obstruction, and laryngeal trauma from an endotracheal tube.

There are two types of systems as follows: (1) apnea monitoring systems that primarily monitor respiratory rate, and (2) more complex systems, including respiratory-inductive plethysmography, that monitor breathing patterns as well as other ventilatory parameters (see Respiratory-inductive Plethysmography).

Apnea Monitoring Systems

Many respiratory care units adapt the standard ECG lead monitoring system to serve as an apnea monitoring system. In addition to monitoring cardiac rate and rhythm, the ECG leads on the chest wall sense and record chest wall movements during each breath. The resulting waveform or graphic display of the breathing pattern is referred to as a measure of *respiratory impedance*. The waveform represents change in rib cage movement and may be displayed next to the ECG to facilitate continuous monitoring of breathing pattern in the acute care unit (Fig. 28–22, top). In addition, respiratory rate per minute may be displayed digitally. An alarm sounds when the respiratory rate rises above

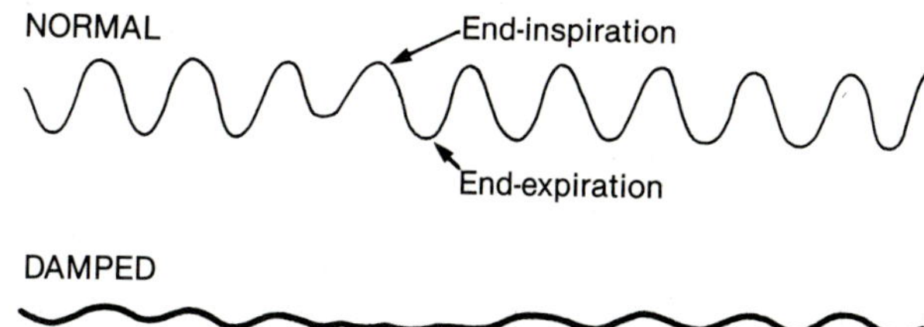

Figure 28–22. Normal and damped respiratory impedance tracings. Waveforms change configuration as rib cage movement varies slightly from breath to breath (normal tracing), and if chest electrodes intermittently lose adequate contact with the skin (damped tracing).

or falls below preset rates and when the waveform becomes overly damped (Fig. 28–22, bottom). In the last case, one or more chest sensors do not pick up adequate chest wall expansion. The waveform may return to normal when size or sensitivity is increased on the monitor, when chest leads are changed, or when a chest lead is moved more laterally to improve sensitivity.

In an acute or a chronic care setting, ECG lead system adaptation is sometimes not possible or applicable, and display of both respiratory impedance and respiratory rate is not crucial. In this case, a separate apnea monitoring system with separate chest leads, a digital display, and an alarm system may be used to monitor respiratory rate alone.

Respiratory-inductive Plethysmography

Respiratory-inductive plethysmography is a widely accepted method of assessing breathing pattern and ventilation noninvasively (Nochomovitz and Cherniack, 1986). The RESPIGRAPH system (Non-Invasive Monitoring Systems, Inc.) is an example of a plethysmograph that may be used in acute and ambulatory care settings. It is also an alternative to clinical polysomnography or long-term noninvasive respiratory monitoring in the diagnosis of breathing disorders during sleep.

An expandable cloth band is placed around the chest (Fig. 28–23). This band senses and records abdominal and rib cage movements and their sum continuously. The sum waveform on the polygraph recording is equated with tidal volume as shown by SUM (V_T) in Figure 28–24A. The system can monitor f, V_T, and $\dot{V}_E$ in addition to other parameters, such as oximetry Pao_2, that can be added to the digital and graphic displays. Also, this system has the special advantage of differentiating between central, obstructive, and mixed apneas by the analysis of the chest movement polygraph recordings (Fig. 28–24B and C). Moreover, Sackner (1986) reports that use of the RESPIGRAPH may save nearly two patient days on mechanical ventilation, because alarms allow the nursing staff to closely monitor the patient and facilitate safe extubation on weekends, late in the day, or *whenever* the patient meets extubation criteria.

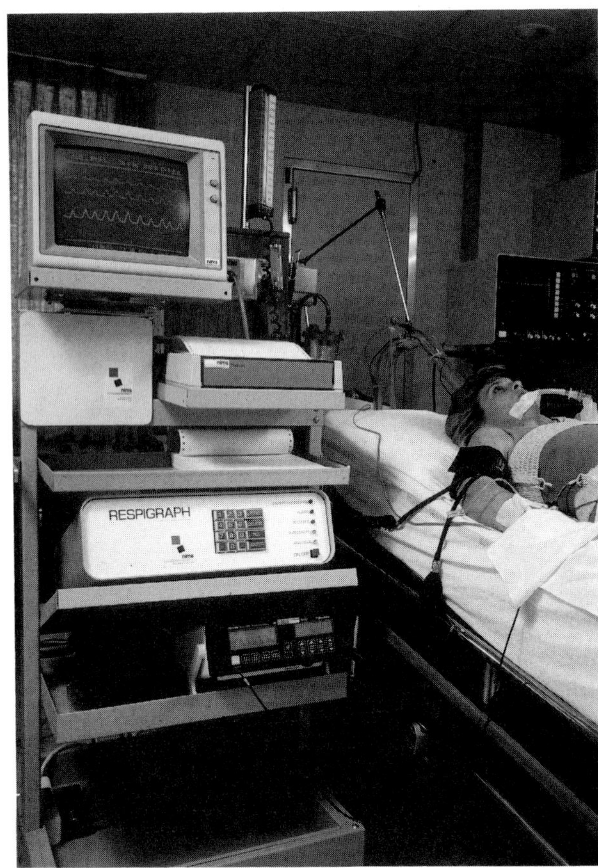

Figure 28–23. RESPIGRAPH system for noninvasive monitoring of breathing pattern. Equipment includes a monitor (top), printer, RESPIGRAPH control module, and pulse oximeter (bottom). The patient is wearing RESPIBANDS around the chest and abdomen to monitor chest and abdominal wall movements. (Courtesy of Non-Invasive Monitoring Systems, Inc., Miami Beach, Florida.)

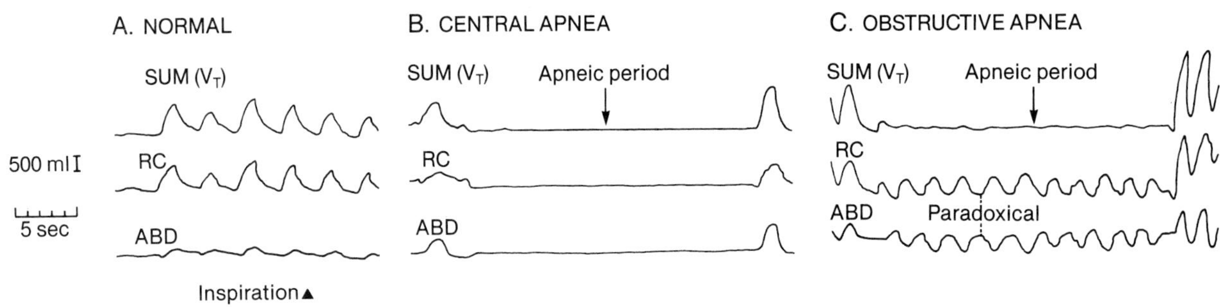

Figure 28–24. *A*, The normal RESPIGRAPH recording consists of abdominal displacement or movement (ABD), rib cage displacement (RC), and the sum of ABD and RC, or SUM (V_T). All wave patterns are clearly visible and in the same direction during each breath. *B*, In central apnea, no movement appears on ABD, RC, and SUM (V_T) tracings. The respiratory center fails to signal the respiratory muscles to contract, and the patient exerts no effort to breathe. *C*, Large ABD and RC movements are in equal and opposite directions. This paradoxical movement produced minimal oscillations of SUM (V_T). In contrast, the respiratory impedance tracing (not shown here) demonstrates large changes in rib cage motion, as the patient exerts effort to breathe.

Psychologic Support

Psychologic support is a key intervention during long-term mechanical ventilation as well as weaning from the oxygen, the ventilator, and the endotracheal tube. Without it patients may be continually plagued by intense anxiety, helplessness, aloneness, and continuing doubts about whether spontaneous ventilation and independence will ever be possible. These feelings are intensified by the inability to communicate verbally, the sensory overload in a busy ICU environment, and the clinically unstable physical condition.

Familiarity with the four phases of adjustment to mechanical ventilation prepares the nurse and others to provide appropriate psychologic support to any patient on ventilatory support. First described by Prugh and Taguiri (1954) in relation to polio patients, the four phases are (1) *preoccupation with survival;* (2) *denial and fantasy*, a regressive coping mechanism; (3) *depression and gradual accommodation to reality;* and (4) *active participation in rehabilitative care.* Patients move through these phases at different rates, and some may skip one or more phases. For example, patients with adequate cardiopulmonary reserves and strong psychosocial coping mechanisms may move from phase 1 directly to phase 4 as their physical condition rapidly improves, and they successfully meet each weaning goal proposed by the health care team. Alternately, patients with limited cardiopulmonary reserves or poor psychosocial assets are continuing challenges. They may move back and forth through these phases, depending on physical progress. Many times, the patient with underlying chronic disease actively participates in care until weaning begins. Then, as weaning imposes respiratory instability, he reverts to phase 1 or 2 and more thoroughly deals with the dilemmas and feelings associated with each phase. In the process, demanding and noncompliant behavior may prompt staff and family to feel ineffective and bewildered, wondering how to best deal with the situation.

The four adjustment phases are described hereafter with a focus on the difficult-to-wean patient and interventions to facilitate movement through the phases.

PREOCCUPATION WITH SURVIVAL

The patient is in a state of shock and disbelief at not being able to breathe on his own (Gibbons and Myler, 1981). He expresses concern regarding the possibility of mechanical failure or survival in general. In spite of increasing anxiety and feelings of dependency and helplessness, he remains cooperative with most forms of therapy.

Interventions

1. When intubation is planned, inform the patient of all details ahead of time, especially before surgery for the patient who will need mechanical ventilation after surgery. Emphasize the inability to talk since the cuff is inflated, and the need to develop nonverbal means of communication, such as writing with pad and pencil, squeezing hands, or using flashcards. Similarly, before weaning begins, fully inform the patient of the weaning procedure and answer his questions in a straightforward manner. Do not withhold information. Providing this information helps reduce the threat of ventilator dependency and associated anxiety.
2. During care, provide simple options to increase the patient's sense of control over the situation, e.g., turning to the right or the left.
3. Use touch—hold the patient's hand—to help relieve the anxiety and the sense of aloneness (Fig. 28–25A).
4. Familiarize significant others with weaning specifics and the bedside equipment so they feel comfortable staying with the patient and giving words of encouragement.
5. Eliminate unnecessary noises, e.g., promptly reset monitor alarms when they activate, to reduce stress and extraneous sensory input.

DENIAL AND FANTASY

The patient uses repression and denial to deal with threats to survival, and he fantasizes that he will eventually become independent from the ventilator. This is the most difficult stage to deal with because, in spite of superficial optimism, the patient exhibits ambivalent feelings, ranging from gratefulness for care given to accusations of staff incompetency and insensitivity. Much of this ambivalence is derived from mixed feelings towards ventilatory support; although the ventilator is seen as a life-saving friend, it is also seen as an intruder, an oppressor that perpetuates hopelessness and loss of control. If the patient remains in this stage, feelings of worthlessness may prompt him either to withdraw from efforts to help him or to react in anger by becoming more demanding and asking for proof that staff and family really care about his well being. Unless staff understand these psychodynamics, they may tend to label an angry patient as manipulative and react by firmly refuting accusations rather than analyzing the underlying cause of the patient's behavior.

Interventions

1. Explain to staff and significant others that displacement of ambivalent feelings onto them is occurring and that it is a normal response to mechanical ventilation and withdrawal of ventilatory support.
2. Encourage the patient to express his fears and doubts. Actively listen without attempting to complete sentences or thoughts for the patient. Utilize a social worker, psychiatrist, or chaplain to help with this process.
3. Allow the patient to have as much control as possible over his environment and care (Fig. 28–25B).

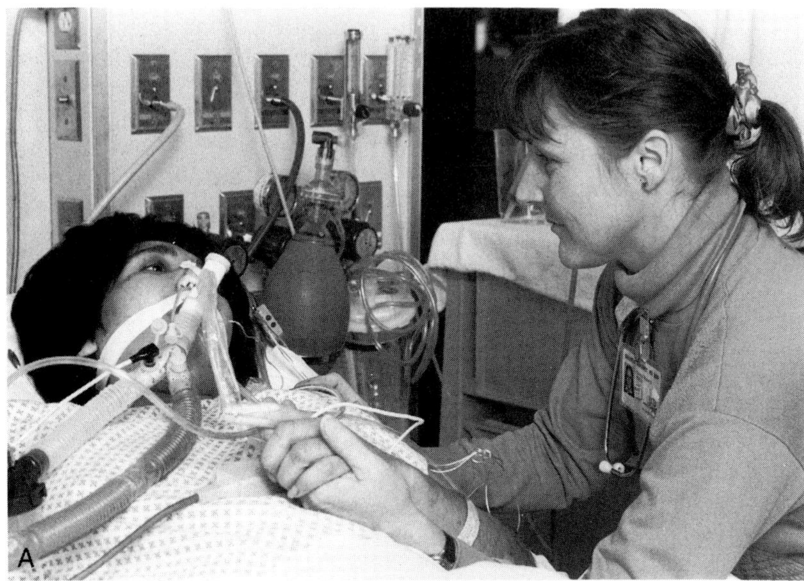

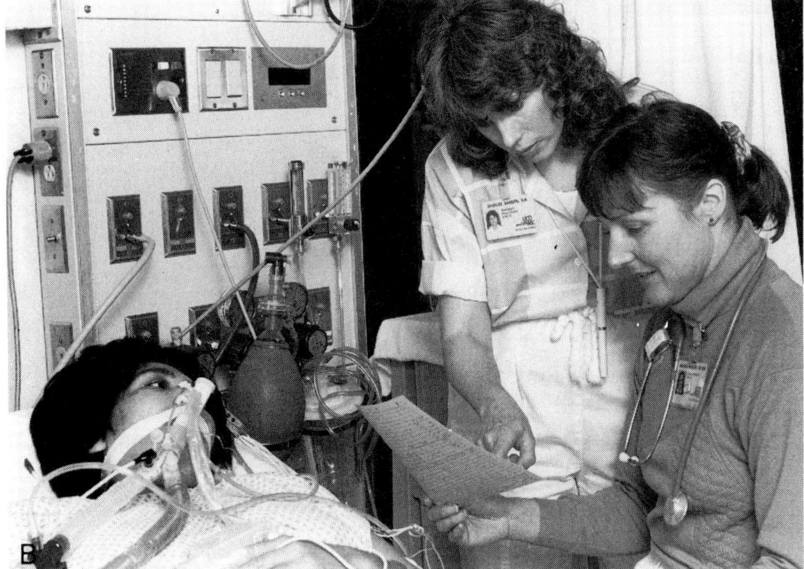

Figure 28–25. Nursing care of the ventilator-dependent patient. *A*, Touch is a powerful intervention for relief of anxiety. *B*, Nurses promote the self-care concept by including this alert patient in the decision-making related to general nursing care and weaning procedures for the day.

4. Project an image of dependability and predictability. Follow a set routine for monitoring and daily care so that care appears orderly. Deviations from the routine should be avoided, since they may be interpreted as incompetent care. Assign the same staff to the patient each day so that continuity is maintained and a relationship of trust can develop. When the patient expresses a preference, write it on the Nursing Kardex to insure staff compliance.

5. Arrange meetings with family and staff for planning consistent approaches to care and for mutual support. These meetings enable all concerned to maintain positive supportive roles throughout a long weaning process, and they prevent inappropriate displacement of staff frustrations onto the patient and other staff members.

6. Provide distractions for the patient to decrease the intensity of frustration, e.g., television, surprise visits by relatives, and ambulation outside the ICU.

DEPRESSION AND GRADUAL ACCOMMODATION TO REALITY

Particularly after a weaning attempt fails, the patient begins to face the reality of his situation and expresses grief over his many losses. Becoming depressed or irritable, he frequently asks "Will I live? Am I dying? What is the point of life if I cannot breathe without a ventilator? Why me?" As the patient reorders the values in his life, he becomes more cooperative and more ready and able to act on staff suggestions. In this stage, some patients request a do not resuscitate (DNR) status should their physical condition deteriorate, and weaning appears impossible.

Interventions

1. Do not react negatively to the patient's depression; it is an encouraging sign that the patient is coping adaptively. Instead, allow the patient to communicate distress and fear in an atmosphere of acceptance and understanding. Once fears are verbalized and ethical decisions made, the patient often develops internal resources to complete the weaning process.

2. Make available legal counsel and a nurse ethicist, or a member of the hospital's ethics committee, to help the patient, family, and staff face ethical decisions. Utilize a chaplain to attend to spiritual needs and strengthen the patient's will to live.

ACTIVE PARTICIPATION IN REHABILITATIVE CARE

With ethical decisions more or less resolved, the patient cooperates fully in all aspects of care and strives to make himself more independent. Once he reaches this stage and weaning criteria are met, weaning is likely to proceed without complication. Interventions focus on the setting of small goals with the patient, utilizing the principles covered in Chapter 16 to develop motivation, and the facilitation of self-care strategies to build confidence and restore health.

The Home Setting

Most of the basic principles of mechanical ventilation presented thus far apply to the home setting as well as to any setting outside the hospital, including nursing homes and community living centers. This last section of the chapter discusses two home applications as follows: nasal continuous positive airway pressure (CPAP) and long-term mechanical ventilation.

NASAL CONTINUOUS POSITIVE AIRWAY PRESSURE (CPAP)

Nasal CPAP is similar to mask CPAP (previously described) except a small mask fits over the nose rather than the mouth. It is a definitive treatment for mixed and obstructive sleep apneas, replacing tracheostomy as the most readily available alternative for relief of upper airway obstruction during sleep. In other cases it represents temporary treatment until the patient loses weight or obtains surgical correction by a uvulopalatopharyngoplasty operation. Also, nasal CPAP may be used to facilitate closure of a tracheostomy (Stocks, 1986).

Examples of a nasal CPAP system are the SleepEasy II (Respironics Inc.) and the Vitalfow series (Systems 2000 Inc.). The SleepEasy model in Figure 28–26 allows application of 5 to 15 cmH_2O positive pressure to the airway through a fixed level CPAP valve. Special prerequisites for use of a CPAP system include the following:

1. Documented effectiveness of the prescribed pressure in a laboratory
2. Patient cooperation
3. Nasal patency
4. Hypersomnolence during the day

Though the majority of patients who try nasal CPAP improve oxygenation during sleep and show objective and subjective improvement in daytime sleepiness, up to 33 % of patients do not benefit from the treatment. Treatment failure is usually due to nasal discomfort from the pressure sensation, excessive airway drying (decongestants or saline spray may be recommended), machine noise, and secondary social or intimacy problems with spouse or significant other (Sobers et al, 1986).

Nursing care involves monitoring for possible side effects including nasal drying and congestion, epistaxis, conjunctivitis, and skin rash or tissue trauma from poor mask fit. Patient and significant other are instructed to monitor airway pressure on the pressure gauge before going to sleep. Since maintenance of adequate airway pressure is the main problem at home, they are encouraged to report signs of increasing airway

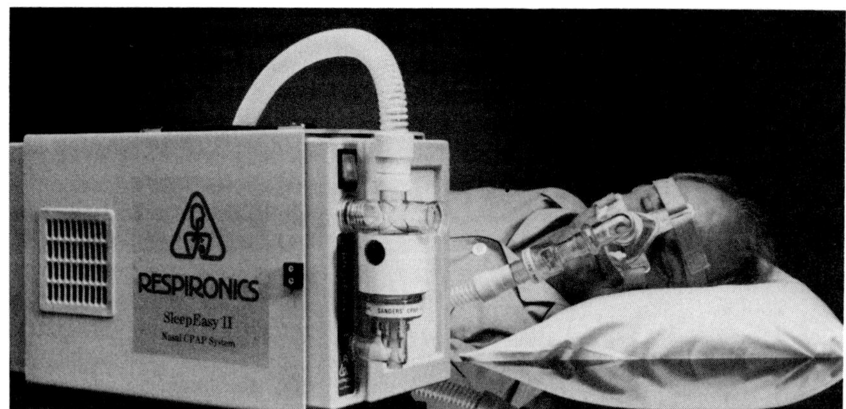

Figure 28–26. Nasal CPAP system used for mixed and obstructive sleep apneas. (Courtesy of Respironics Inc., Monroeville, Pennsylvania.)

obstruction at night, e.g., low CPAP pressure, snoring, and thrashing about in bed, and to report daytime hypersomnolence. To avoid acceptance problems, health team members should thoroughly discuss common problems with patient and family so they have a chance to prepare themselves physically and emotionally for the sensation and sound of nasal CPAP and possible personal inconveniences at home. Last, equipment care is similar to that of other durable medical equipment in the home (see Chapter 21).

LONG-TERM MECHANICAL VENTILATION

Long-term mechanical ventilation refers to mechanical ventilation out of the hospital setting either continuously or for predetermined periods of time during the day, night, or both. It is used for selected patients in chronic ventilatory failure or those who cannot maintain acceptable ABGs without current ventilatory support.

The goals of long-term ventilation are similar to those of pulmonary rehabilitation (presented in Chapter 18) as follows: reduce mortality, extend life span, improve physical and emotional functioning, improve quality of life, and maintain cost effectiveness (O'Donohue et al, 1986).

Cost effectiveness is a key issue because the current prospective payment system for health care reimbursement favors early hospital discharge of all patients, especially ventilator patients. Since these patients tend to have long and costly hospital stays, they are viewed as "financial losers." This trend towards home ventilator care has presented an increasing challenge to nurses and other health team members to provide home ventilator care that is more cost effective than hospital care and simultaneously comprehensive and continuing in nature.

Criteria for Implementation

Patients who benefit the most from long-term ventilatory support and those who adapt with fewer obstacles are those with ventilatory muscle dysfunction or central hypoventilation. These patients have normal lungs and do not require the complicated bronchial hygiene programs of the COPD patient, including suctioning, postural drainage, and other secretion control measures. Patients with pulmonary restrictive disease (e.g., interstitial fibrosis) are rarely candidates because by the time signs of chronic respiratory failure appear, the disease is far advanced, and mechanical ventilation may not significantly improve dyspnea, comfort, or physical function.

Though clinical experience and research data have shown which patients do well on long-term ventilation, criteria for implementation are not clear cut. Patient, family, and health team members must consider many factors before making a final decision. Moreover, the nurse as a primary care provider is in the best position to facilitate collaboration among all involved, so that the final decision is based on patient, family, and situational factors in addition to the medical factors listed in the box that follows.

CRITERIA FAVORING LONG-TERM MECHANICAL VENTILATION*

MEDICAL CRITERIA

Ventilatory muscle dysfunction, e.g., neuromuscular disorders
Central hypoventilation syndromes
Rapidly progressive diseases, e.g., amyotrophic lateral sclerosis (ALS)
Failure to wean from mechanical ventilation after many attempts by a skilled respiratory care team
Clinical stability
Stable pulmonary system and other body organ systems

*Data from O'Donohue, W. et al. Long-term mechanical ventilation—guidelines for management in the home and at alternate community sites (Report of the American College of Chest Physicians). *Chest* [Supplement], 90(1): 1S–16S, 1986.

Major diagnostic studies or therapeutic decisions are not anticipated for at least 1 month
Absence of aggressive bronchial hygiene requirements, e.g., suctioning, postural drainage, and so forth

PATIENT AND FAMILY CRITERIA

Patient and family understand the advantages and disadvantages of therapy, participate in decision-making processes, and still desire therapy *after* clinical stabilization of acute illness.

Patient, family member, significant other, home attendant, or some combination thereof is willing and able to participate extensively in discharge planning and home care.

SITUATIONAL CRITERIA

Financial and social costs of mechanical ventilation in the home are less than costs in the hospital.
Nurse, social worker, durable medical equipment (DME) vendor, and respiratory therapist can help in the evaluation of cost effectiveness for individual situations.

Physical environment of the home favors adaptation to the limitations of the home setting.
A home visit may be necessary to assess mobility between rooms and to the outside, presence of sufficient electric outlets for equipment, and home alarm or communication systems, e.g., intercom, bell, buzzer.

Access to a primary care physician and consulting specialist in respiratory care.

Financial coverage for home care follow-up.

Ideally, the decision-making process is initiated *immediately* after stabilization of acute illness, to allow as much time as possible for patient and family to assess ethical, personal, and situational factors. At the same time, health team members provide extensive explanations of the logistics of ventilatory support at home so that the patient's final decision is an informed one. Without a clear understanding of logistics, patients may feel overwhelmed and anxious about their ability to cope with a ventilator at home. Ultimately, they may refuse to further consider the possibility. In other cases, an uninformed patient may push for early home discharge, only to become overwhelmed and anxious upon arrival at home. These discussions on logistics also serve to reassure the patient that help is available for adaptation in the home setting and that home ventilation might be a viable option.

Alternatives to Mechanical Ventilation

Before suggesting a home ventilator, the physician may decide to try an alternative to mechanical ventilation. The alternatives listed in Table 28–7 may eliminate inconveniences and potential complications associated with tracheostomy tube placement and mechanical ventilation.

Positive Pressure Ventilation

In the home setting, mechanical ventilation may involve either positive or negative pressure ventilation. However, positive pressure ventilation is used most frequently. Positive pressure ventilators are usually either pressure-cycled (e.g., Thompson Bantam, Lifecare RBL) or volume-cycled (e.g., Lifeproducts LP 3, LP 4, LP 5, LP 6, Portable Volume Ventilator PVV). Most ventilators are small enought to fit on a bedside table at home or on the back of a wheelchair for portability (Fig. 28–27). Though the technology may include modern features, such as the microprocessor control feature, operation of a home ventilator is much simpler than operation of a ventilator in the acute care setting. For example, the LP 6 volume ventilator in Figure 28–28 has only three modes of ventilation (control, assist/control, and SIMV); a pressure limit feature; a pressure manometer; and a few alarms, including low pressure, high pressure, power failure, and low voltage alarms. It can operate from an AC power source or from an external or internal battery. Other positive pressure ventilators are simpler than the LP 6 and may be limited to high and low pressure alarms (Gilmartin and Make, 1986).

Negative Pressure Ventilation

Application of negative pressure to the chest sets up a pressure gradient, causing air to be pulled or sucked into the chest on inspiration (Fig. 28–29). Release of the negative pressure allows the lungs to passively recoil on expiration.

Negative pressure ventilation is used primarily for neuromuscular patients with mild respiratory failure. Some forms of negative pressure ventilation, such as the Pulmowrap, may be used for COPD patients to prevent hypoventilation at night and to rest the respiratory muscles, but the efficacy of this therapy is still under clinical investigation.

The three types of negative pressure ventilator systems are the tank (iron lung), cuirass (chest shell), and body wrap (Pulmowrap), as described in Table 28–8 and shown in Figures 28–30, 28–31, and 28–32.

Negative pressure ventilators have the advantages of being noninvasive, durable, and relatively easy to operate; they may avoid the need for tracheostomy completely. Yet their large cumbersome design, their imposition of limited mobility and limited accessibility, and their inability to regulate inspiratory air flow have restricted their use to a selected patient population without chronic airway disease and with relatively normal lungs. Nevertheless, many patients with diseases such as poliomyelitis or kyphoscoliosis have lived comfortably for years within the confines of the tank ventilator.

Table 28–7. ALTERNATIVES TO LONG-TERM MECHANICAL VENTILATION

Alternative	Description	Indications
Diaphragm pacing	A transmitter sends radiofrequency energy via an external antenna (coiled wire taped to skin) to a receiver implanted under the skin. The receiver has electrodes that stimulate the phrenic nerve and cause diaphragmatic contraction.	Central alveolar hypoventilation. Cervical cord injury or disease, with lesions above the C3 level of the spinal cord. Pacing may not be effective in lesions between C3 and C5 because all or some of the phrenic nerve cell bodies and lower motor neurons may be destroyed. The ideal candidate has normal phrenic nerves, diaphragm, and lungs.
Rocking bed	Bed and patient rock back and forth from foot-down to head-down positions. The rocking motion and gravity facilitate diaphragmatic excursions. Rocking to the foot-down position moves abdominal contents and diaphragm downward, thus allowing air to enter the lungs. Similarly, the head-down position allows the diaphragm to move downward to push air out of the lungs for expiration.	Neuromuscular disease with mild respiratory failure. Need for ventilatory assistance at night or when in a reclined position.
Pneumobelt	An inflatable bladder within a corset is placed around the patient's abdomen and under the clothes. Inflation with 30 to 50 cmH_2O pressure compresses abdomen and diaphragm upward for expiration. Passive deflation of the bladder allows the diaphragm to fall downward for inspiration, as long as the patient's head is elevated.	Neuromuscular disease with mild to moderate respiratory failure. Need for increased daytime mobility.

Table 28–8. NEGATIVE PRESSURE VENTILATORS

Ventilator	Description	Type of Ventilatory Support
Tank (iron lung) (see Fig. 28–30)	Metal airtight cylinder that encloses the patient up to the neck. Application of negative pressure creates a gradient, which in turn initiates air flow into the lungs. Adjustments are made to control respiratory rate and amount of negative pressure, determining V_T.	Continuous and nocturnal
Cuirass (chest shell) (see Fig. 28–31)	A dome-shaped shell that fits over the anterior chest area and abdomen and connects to a ventilator unit, e.g., Thompson 170-C, Thompson Multi-Vent. Negative pressure results in thoracic expansion. Custom-made shells are available for patients with severe chest deformities who have difficulties maintaining comfortable and effective seals.	Nocturnal
Body wrap (Pulmowrap) (see Fig. 28–32)	The patient sleeps in a poncho-style garment attached to a ventilator unit. The poncho is supported away from the patient by a hard grid that rests on a backplate or any firm surface. Like the cuirass, negative pressure expands the chest cage for inspiration. The body wrap is more comfortable than the cuirass because the grid has no direct contact with the skin, making pressure sores less likely.	Nocturnal

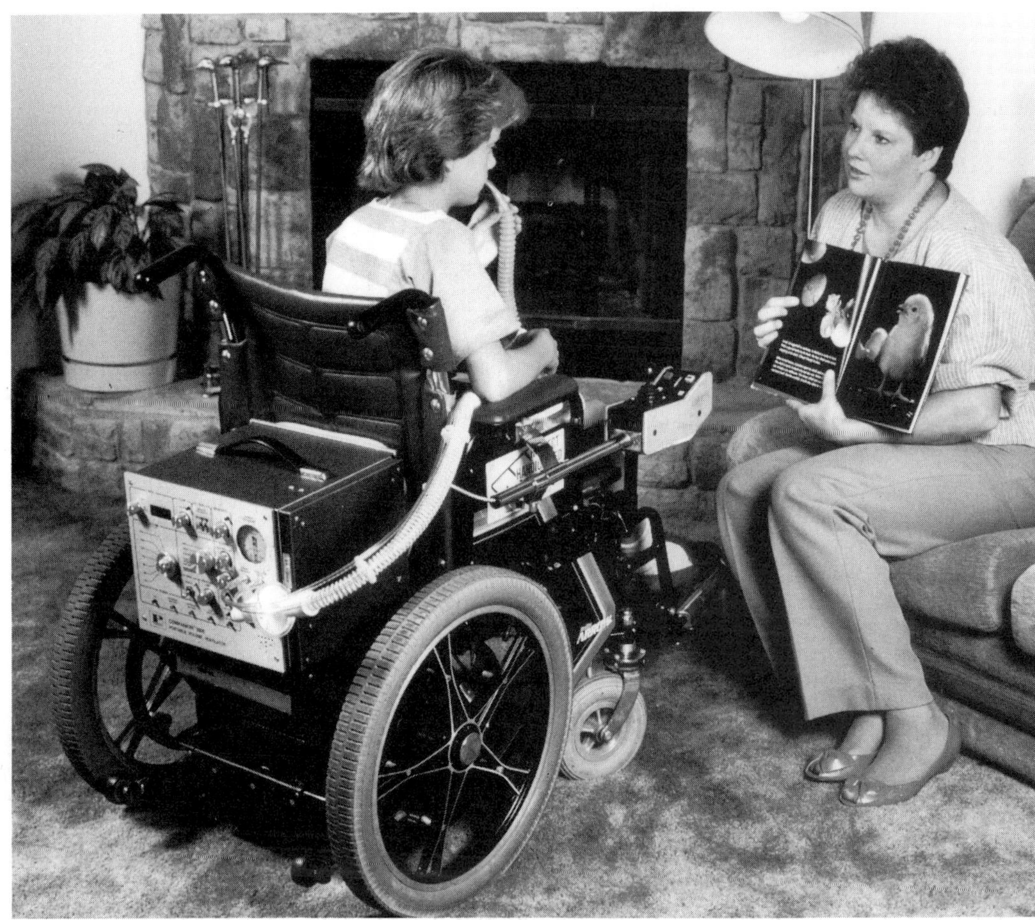

Figure 28–27. Portable volume ventilator positioned on the back of a wheelchair. (Courtesy of the Puritan-Bennett Corporation, Lenexa, Kansas.)

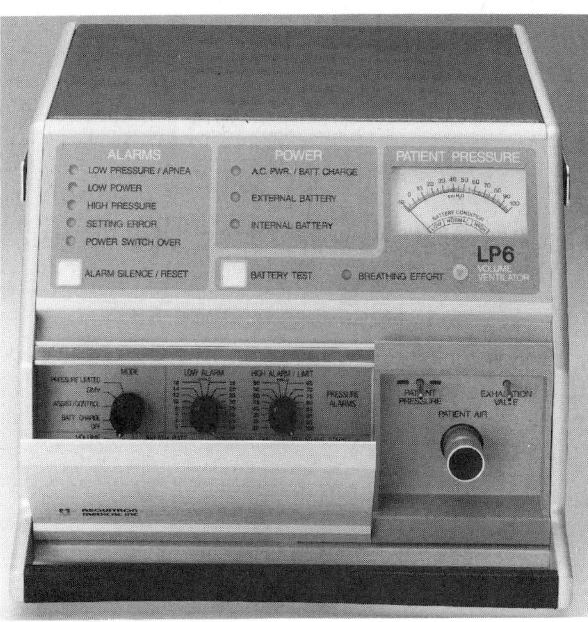

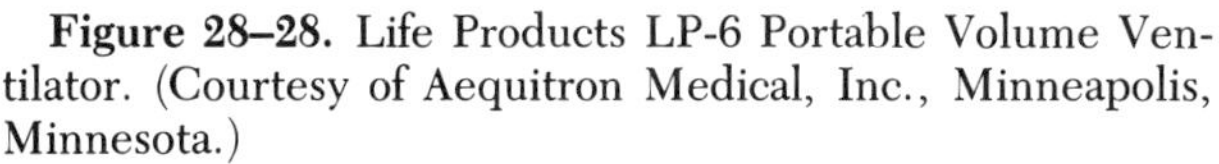

Figure 28–28. Life Products LP-6 Portable Volume Ventilator. (Courtesy of Aequitron Medical, Inc., Minneapolis, Minnesota.)

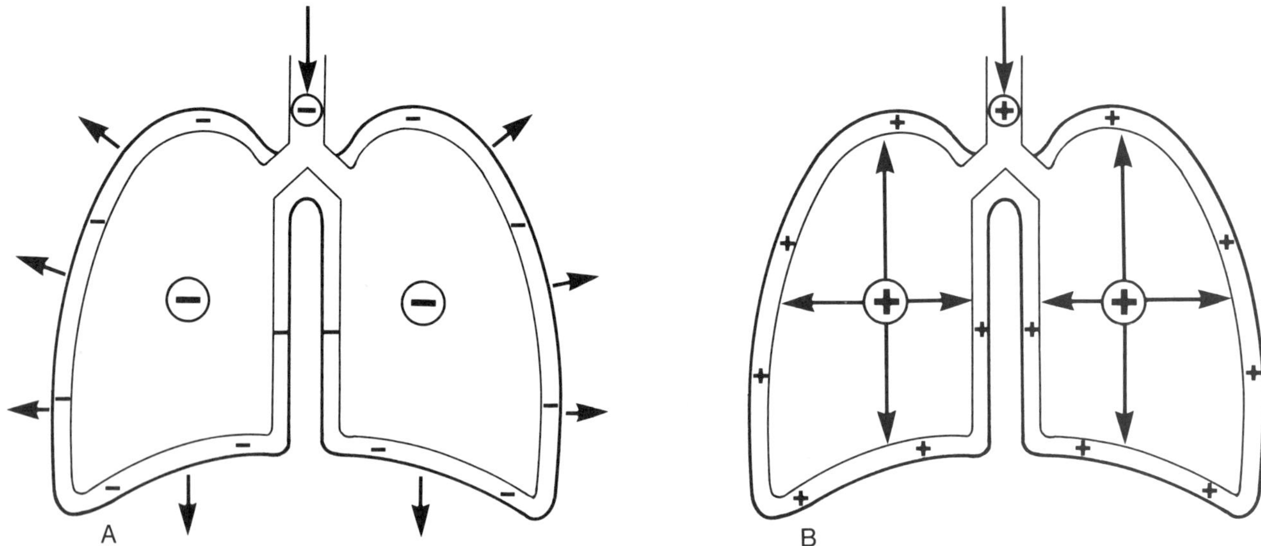

Figure 28–29. Comparison of negative (A) and positive (B) pressure ventilation.

Figure 28–30. Emerson Iron Lung. (Courtesy of J. H. Emerson Co, Cambridge, Massachusetts.)

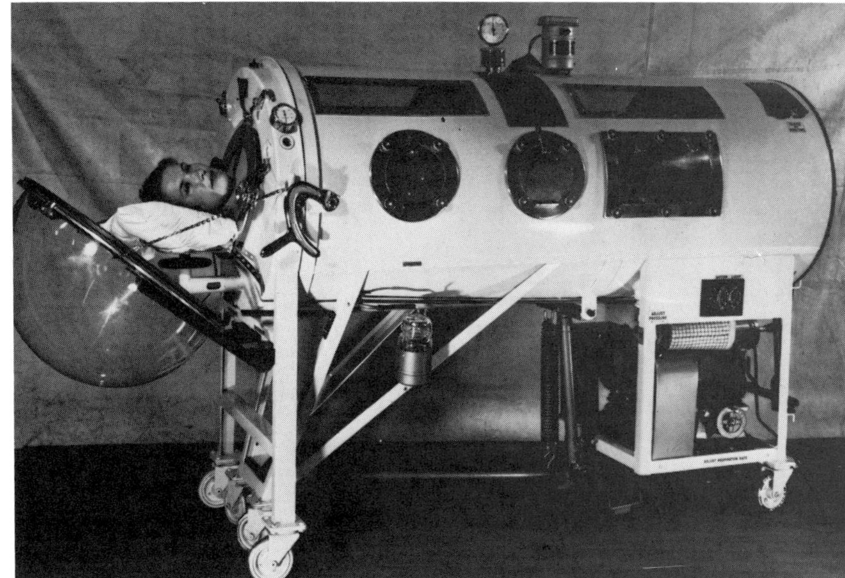

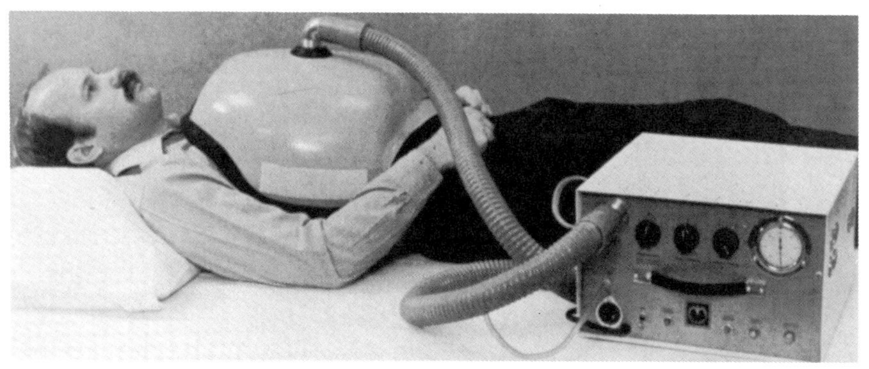

Figure 28–31. Chest shell (Lifecare) fitted over the anterior chest area and abdomen and attached to a negative pressure ventilator. (Reproduced by permission from Hill, N. Clinical applications of body ventilators. *Chest,* 90(6):900, 1986.)

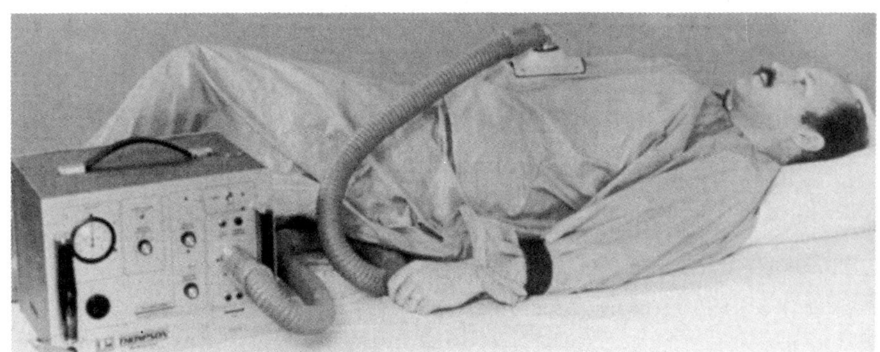

Figure 28–32. The body wrap (Pulmowrap) attached to a negative pressure ventilator. The form of the rigid plastic chest piece is visible underneath the impervious nylon jacket. This chest piece prevents collapse of the jacket onto the anterior chest area and abdomen during generation of negative pressure. The straps around the neck, arms, and feet prevent air leakage. (Reproduced by permission from Hill, N. Clinical applications of body ventilators. *Chest*, 90(6):900, 1986.)

The most serious complication of negative pressure ventilation is *tank shock*. Though mostly associated with the tank, the phenomenon may be observed to a lesser extent with other similar forms of negative pressure ventilation. In tank shock, the application of negative pressure to the abdominal cavity causes venous pooling in this area, resulting in a decreased venous return to the right atrium and, ultimately, a decreased cardiac output.

Use of a chest cuirass may cause pressure sores, if the contact between the shell's rim and the patient's skin is loose. Also, without a proper shell fitting (i.e., a custom shell may be necessary) and proper application by trained personnel, the cuirass may ineffectively ventilate the patient and fail to prevent significant alveolar hypoventilation during sleep.

Alternative to Negative Pressure Ventilation

Because of the aforementioned problems with negative pressure ventilation devices, research is in progress to develop other alternatives for the patient with relatively normal lungs. Kerby and associates (1987) recommend positive pressure ventilation via nasal mask over negative pressure ventilation for neuromuscular patients in chronic respiratory failure who require ventilation at night. They state that the delivery of positive pressure through a CPAP-type nasal mask has several advantages, including more nocturnal patient mobility, ease of application, patient synchronization of tidal volume, and absence of upper airway obstruction during sleep.

Nursing Care

Nursing care for the patient on long-term ventilation is essentially the same as that already described in this chapter, in Chapter 21, and in Chapter 27 on care of the intubated patient. Since long-term ventilation has rehabilitative aspects, the basic interventions related to self care and other topics in Part Four of this book also apply.

While delivering care, the nurse places major emphasis on collaboration with other health team members and completion of a needs assessment. A checklist may be used to guide discharge planning in the hospital and assessment and intervention in the home setting (Table 28–9).

Whenever possible, instruction regarding home care should take place in the hospital setting. The exact ventilator to be placed in the home should be tested for electric safety and mechanical function and should be used by the patient for at least 72 hours before hospital discharge (O'Donohue et al, 1986). During this time, trial periods off the ventilator may be implemented for prescription of free time off the ventilator at home.

After hospital discharge, the visiting nurse reinforces key content already taught (e.g., cleaning of equipment). The last two steps of the teaching-learning process, i.e., evaluation of outcomes and reteaching and relearning educational content, are emphasized.

Conclusion

This chapter has prepared the nurse for decision-making related to mechanical ventilation across the health care continuum. Basic information has been presented on positive and negative pressure ventilation, the ventilator setup, and basic monitoring parameters, such as the ventilator check, ABG results, and compliance measurements. In addition, detailed information has been presented on such topics as how to facilitate the weaning process, provide emotional support, and help the patient carefully consider long-term mechanical ventilation in the home setting.

The reader may be impressed with recent technologic advances in respiratory care, including new computer-aided ventilators, high frequency jet ventilators, and respiratory monitoring systems. Certainly these advances have improved the efficiency and, in some cases, the effectiveness of respiratory care. From another perspective, they have placed more responsibility on the nurse for the largely unpredictable effects of therapy and for prompt intervention if the new intervention fails to achieve the intended results.

Table 28–9. NEEDS ASSESSMENT/DISCHARGE CHECKLIST FOR THE VENTILATOR-DEPENDENT PATIENT*

Directions *For initial assessment* rate the patient or caregiver using the rating scale below. Write the score in the first column. Fill in other information as indicated. 0 = Unable to perform; no understanding 1 = Poor coordination and technique; minimal understanding 2 = Barely passable technique; basic understanding 3 = Good technique with intermittent coaching; good understanding 4 = Good to excellent technique without supervision; excellent understanding *For discharge planning* check appropriate columns and fill in information as indicated. *Date and initial* all evaluations and equipment orders.					**Comments** Date and initial all evaluations and equipment orders. Note special needs, response to instructions, and concerns in this section.
I. Ventilator Checklist (for training) Patient's name: Caregiver's name: Type of ventilation: positive, negative Specific times on and off the ventilator:	***Initial Assessment Score***	***Demonstration (Verbal Explanation)***	***Return Demonstration***	***Written Instructions Provided***	
Operation Set/adjust: Oxygen concentration Connect oxygen to ventilator circuit Mode: control, assist/control, SIMV Tidal volume Respiratory rate Peak pressure Humidifier temperature High pressure alarm Low pressure alarm Exhaled volume alarm Sensitivity					
Monitor peak inspiratory pressure					
Check for leaks in ventilator circuit and humidifier					
Maintenance Drain tubing of excess water Connect battery to ventilator Check and maintain battery Change ventilator filters and times:					
Cleaning the Ventilator Circuit Times:					
Disinfection solution:					
Change tubing With patient on ventilator With patient off ventilator					
Change humidifier With patient on ventilator With patient off ventilator					
Disassemble Tubing Humidifier					
Clean Tubing Humidifier					

Table 28–9. NEEDS ASSESSMENT/DISCHARGE CHECKLIST *Continued*

Dry Tubing Exhalation valve Humidifier					
Reassemble Tubing Humidifier: Fill with distilled water Attach to ventilator Verify appropriate temperature setting					
Test for leaks					
Clean manual resuscitator					
II. Emergency Procedures (knowing what to do for) Machine failure Power failure Obstructed airway Answering alarms, e.g., high pressure alarm, low pressure alarm Accidental extubation Use of manual resuscitator					
III. Supportive Respiratory Care Coughing and deep breathing Standard Manual cough in neuromuscular patients					
Frequent change in body position Side to side turning Transfers, e.g., bed to chair					
Postural drainage Percussion Vibration					
Tracheostomy care Tube and stoma care Tube change Cuff inflation and deflation Monitoring cuff pressure Speaking tube/attachment operation					
Tracheal suctioning Technique: gloved or ungloved Use of suction machine					
Pulmonary medications Names/dosages/schedules: Purposes Side effects Refill information					
Adequate fluid intake					
Diet instructions:					
Muscle conditioning exercises Range of motion Other:					

Table continued on following page

Table 28–9. NEEDS ASSESSMENT/DISCHARGE CHECKLIST *Continued*

Use of manual alarms and call systems Intercom Physical sound (bell or siren) Telephone or beeper system					
Introduction of equipment vendor to patient or caregiver					
Training of another caregiver for relief of primary caregiver					
IV. Equipment Checklist (for ordering)	***Equipment Vendor (Name)***	***Date Ordered***	***Delivery Date***	***Written Instructions Provided***	
Ventilator Equipment Ventilator (type/brand):					
Back-up ventilator (type/brand):					
Manual resuscitator with flex hose and tracheostomy tube adaptor					
Humidifier, heating element, mounting bracket (2 sets)					
15-inch tube (from ventilator to cascade humidifier) (3)					
Ventilator circuit tubing (3 sets)					
Exhalation valves (3)					
Flex hoses (3)					
Tracheostomy tube adaptor (3)					
Compressor with in-line nebulizer (for aerosol treatments)					
Disinfective solution					
Oxygen Stationary unit: Portable unit:					
Bleed-in connector for oxygen					
12-volt battery with cable					
Tracheostomy and Suctioning Equipment/Supplies Tracheostomy tubes (two extra) Type: Size: Cuffed or uncuffed, fenestrated Single or double cannula					
Tracheostomy care kits or Cotton tip applicators Pipe cleaners or brush Stoma dressings (optional) Tracheostomy tape					
Hydrogen peroxide					

Table 28–9. NEEDS ASSESSMENT/DISCHARGE CHECKLIST *Continued*

Suction catheters Type: Size:						
Gloves (optional)						
Suction machine AC/DC						
General Equipment Hospital bed Wheelchair with ventilator tray Walker with ventilator tray Ramp for home entrance Commode Patient lifter with slings Bedpan or urinal						
Other:						

*Adapted from Prentice, W. Ventilator dependent patient discharge checklist, teaching needs. In: Recommended Minimum Care Standards for Home Ventilators. Statement by the American Lung Association of San Diego and Imperial Counties, Quality Assurance Subcommittee, June, 1984.

Most important, though advanced technology helps, it is no substitute for a nurse who is thoroughly familiar with the patient's situation. A knowledgeable and experienced nurse is needed to help make basic and timely decisions, such as when to return the dyspneic patient to the ventilator during weaning to rest the ventilatory muscles and when to challenge the patient to wait a few more minutes to improve ventilatory muscle endurance.

REFERENCES

Askanazi, J., Weissman, C., et al: Nutrition and the respiratory system. *Critical care medicine,* 10(3):163–172, 1982.

Barrocas, A., Tretola, R., and Alonso, A.: Nutrition and the critically ill pulmonary patient. *Respiratory care,* 28(1):50–61, 1983.

Bone, R.: Complications of mechanical ventilation and positive end-expiratory pressure. *Respiratory care,* 27(4):402–407, 1982.

Bone, R.: Monitoring patients in acute respiratory failure. *Respiratory care,* 27(6):700–701, 1982.

Branson, R., Hurst, J., and DeHaven, C.: Mask CPAP: state of the art. *Respiratory care,* 30(10):846–857, 1985.

Christopher, K., Neff, T., et al: Demand and continuous flow intermittent mandatory ventilation systems. *Chest,* 87(5):625–630, 1985.

Christopher, K., Saravolatz, L., Bush, T., and Conway, W.: The potential role of respiratory therapy equipment in cross contamination. *American review of respiratory disease,* 128(2):271–275, 1983.

Cohen, C., Zagelbaum, G., et al: Clinical manifestations of inspiratory muscle fatigue. *The american journal of medicine,* 73(3):308–316, 1982.

Comhaire, A. and Lamy, M.: Contamination rate of sterilized ventilators in an ICU. *Critical care medicine,* 9(7):546–548, 1981.

Connors, A., McCaffree, D., and Gray, B.: Effect of inspiratory flow rate on gas exchange during mechanical ventilation. *American review of respiratory disease,* 124(5):537–543, 1981.

Covelli, H., Weled, B., and Beekman, J.: Efficacy of continuous positive pressure administered by face mask. *Chest,* 81(2):147–150, 1982.

DeCampo, T. and Civetta, J.: Effect of short term discontinuation of high-level PEEP in patients with acute respiratory failure. *Critical care medicine,* 7(2):47–49, 1979.

Demers R.: Methods of increasing airway pressure in acute respiratory failure. *Respiratory care,* 28(5): 592–595, 1983.

Driver, A., McAlevy, M., and Smith, J.: Nutritional assessment of patient with COPD and acute respiratory failure. *Chest,* 82(5):568–570, 1982.

Dupuis, Y.: Ventilators—Theory and Clinical Application. St. Louis, C.V. Mosby Co., 1986.

Ellman, H. and Dembin, H.: Lack of adverse hemodynamic effects of PEEP in patients with acute respiratory failure. *Critical care medicine,* 10(11):706–710, 1982.

Fairley, H.: The mechanical ventilation sigh is a dodo. *Respiratory care,* 21(11):1127–1130, 1976.

Finer, M. and Kelly, M.: Optimal ventilation for the neonate. Part I. Continuous positive airway pressure. *Respiratory therapy,* 13(1):43–48, 1983.

Gale, J. and O'Shanick, G.: Psychiatric aspects of respirator treatment and pulmonary intensive care. *Advances in psychosomatic medicine,* 14:93–108, 1985.

George, R.: Prevention of postoperative atelectasis. *Respiratory care,* 28(1):33–34, 1983.

Gibbons, J. and Myler, D.: Human care of the ventilator patient. In: Clinical Use of Mechanical Ventilation. (Rattenborg, C. and Via-reque, E.–Eds.). Chicago, Year Book Medical Publishers, Inc., 329–339, 1981.

Gibney, R., Wilson, R., and Pontoppidan, H.: Comparison of work of breathing on high gas flow and demand valve CPAP systems. *Chest,* 82(6):692–696. 1982.

Gilmartin, M. and Make, B.: Mechanical ventilation in the home: a new mandate. *Respiratory care,* 31(5):406–412, 1986.

Grace, M. and Greenbaum, D.: Cardiac performance in response to PEEP in patients with cardiac dysfunction. *Critical care medicine,* 10(6):358–360, 1982.

Gruden, M.: High frequency ventilation: an overview. *Critical care nurse,* 5(1):36–40, 1985.

Hill, N.: Clinical applications of body ventilators. *Chest,* 90(6):897–905, 1986.

Hotlackers, T., Loosbrock, L., and Gracey, D.: The use of the chest cuirass in respiratory failure of neurologic origin. *Respiratory care,* 27(3):271–275, 1982.

Hotchkiss, R. and Wilson, R.: Mechanical ventilatory support. *Surgical clinics of north america,* 63(2):417–439, 1983.

Hudson, L.: High frequency ventilation. *Pulmonary perspectives* (American College of Chest Physicians), 1(4):1–2, 1984.

Jenkinson, S.: Nutritional problems during mechanical ventilation in acute respiratory failure. *Respiratory care,* 28(5):641–645, 1983.

Kerby, G., Mayer, L., and Pingleton, S.: Nocturnal positive pressure ventilation via nasal mask. *American review of respiratory disease,* 135(3):738–740, 1987.

Johnson, D., Giovannoni, R., and Driscoll, S.: Ventilator-assisted Patient Care—Planning for Hospital Discharge and Home Care. Rockville, Maryland, Aspen Publishers, Inc., 1986.

Kinasewitz, G.: Use of end-tidal capnography during mechanical ventilation. *Respiratory care*, 27(2):169–171, 1982.
Knights, C.: Practical aspects of transcutaneous gas monitoring. *Respiratory therapy*, 13(3):53–54, 1983.
MacIntyre, N.: Jet Ventilation in the Adult with Breathing Rates Up to 150 BPM. Riverside, California, Bear Medical Systems, Inc., 1985.
MacIntyre, N.: Pressure support ventilation (editorial). *Respiratory care*, 31(3):189–190, 1986.
Morrison, M.: Respiratory Intensive Care Nursing, 2nd ed. Boston, Little, Brown, & Co., 1979.
Murray, I., Modell, J., Gallagher, T., and Banner, M.: Titration of PEEP by the arterial minus end-tidal carbon dioxide gradient. *Chest*, 85(1):100–104, 1984.
Nikki, P. et al: Ventilatory pattern in respiratory failure arising from acute myocardial infarction. *Critical care medicine*, 10(2):75–78, 1982.
Nochomovitz, M. and Cherniack, N.: Noninvasive Respiratory Monitoring. New York, Churchill Livingstone, 1986.
O'Donohue, W. et al: Long-term mechanical ventilation—guidelines for management in the home and at alternate community sites (Report of the American College of Chest Physicians). *Chest*, 90(1):1S–16S, 1986.
Pick, R., Handler, J., Murata, G., and Friedman, A.: The cardiovascular effects of PEEP. *Chest*, 82(3):345–350, 1982.
Pierson, D.: Indications for mechanical ventilation. *Respiratory care*, 28(5):570–578, 1983a.
Pierson, D.: Weaning from mechanical ventilation in acute respiratory failure: concepts, indications, and techniques. *Respiratory care*, 28(5):646–662, 1983b.
Pierson, D., Capps, J., and Hudson, J.: Maximum ventilatory capabilities of four current-generation mechanical ventilators. *Respiratory care*, 31(11):1054–1058, 1986c.
Podjasek, J.: Respiratory infection in the mechanically ventilated patient—an overview. *Heart and Lung*, 12(1):5–10, 1983.
Prakash, O. and Meij, S.: Cardiopulmonary response to inspiratory pressure support during spontaneous ventilation vs. conventional ventilation. *Chest*, 88(3):403–408, 1985.
Pratter, M., Corwin, W., and Irwin, R.: An integrated analysis of lung and respiratory muscle dysfunction in the pathogenesis of hypercapneic respiratory failure. *Respiratory care*, 27(1):55–61, 1982.
Prentice, W.: Ventilator dependent patient discharge checklist, teaching needs. In: Recommended Minimum Care Standards for Home Ventilators. Statement by the American Lung Association of San Diego and Imperial Counties, Quality Assurance Subcommittee, June, 1984.
Prentice, W., Wilms, D., and Harrison, L.: Outpatient management of ventilator-dependent patients. In: Pulmonary Rehabilitation—Guidelines for Success. (Hodgkin, J., Zorn, E., and Connors, G.–eds.). Boston, Butterworth Publishers, 1984.
Prugh, D. and Taguiri, C.: Emotional aspects of respirator care of patients with poliomyelitis. *Psychosomatic medicine*, 16(2):104–128, 1954.
Puckett, J., Smith, J., and Smith, R.: Synchronized versus nonsynchronized IMV and high frequency ventilation for IMV. *Respiratory care*, 27(3):289–291, 1982.
Quan, S. and Hasan, F.: Difficulties in weaning from mechanical ventilation. *Arizona medicine*, 37(9):622–625, 1980.
Quan, S., Otto, C., et al: High frequency ventilation—a promising new method of ventilation. *Heart and lung*, 12(2):152–155, 1983.
Rochester, D. and Esau, S.: Malnutrition and the respiratory system. *Chest*, 85(3):411–415, 1984.
Sackner, M.: From oxygen therapy to respiratory care: a perspective. *Respinews* (Series No. 1). Miami Beach, Florida, Noninvasive Monitoring Systems, Inc., 1986.
Schmidt, G., Parulkar, D., Brennan, T., and Feder, J.: EPAP without intubation. *Critical care medicine*, 5(4):207–209, 1977.
Severinghaus, J.: Transcutaneous blood gas analysis. *Respiratory care*, 27(2):152–159, 1982.
Shapiro, B., Cane, R., and Harrison, R.: Positive end-expiratory pressure in acute lung injury. *Chest*, 83(3):558–563, 1983.
Smith, J.: Application of mechanical ventilation in acute respiratory failure. *Respiratory care*, 28(5):579, 1983.
Sobers, M., Mitler, M., Butierrez, F., and Timms, R.: Acceptance of nasal CPAP in patients with obstructive sleep apnea. *American review of respiratory disease*, 133(4):A234, 1986.
Stocks, J.: Home nasal CPAP in adult obstructive sleep apnea. Symposium on home-management of the technology-dependent patient. Paper presented at the annual meeting of the American Lung Association and American Thoracic Society, 1986.
Warren, T. and Howell, C.: High frequency jet ventilation: a nursing perspective. *Heart and lung*, 12(4):432–439, 1983.
Watts, C.: Carbon dioxide elimination and capnography. *Respiratory therapy*, 10(6):107–112, 1980.
Weisman, I., Rinaldo, J., Rogers, R., and Sanders, M.: State of the art—intermittent mandatory ventilation. *American review of respiratory disease*, 127(5):641–647, 1983.
Wilson, R.: Intermittent CPAP to prevent atelectasis in postoperative patients. *Respiratory care*. 28(1):71–73, 1983.
Yahav, J., Mindorff, C., and Levison, H.: The validity of the transcutaneous oxygen tension method in children with cardiorespiratory problems. *American review of respiratory disease*, 124(5):586, 1981.

Hemodynamic Monitoring—Respiratory Applications

29

Main Objectives

1. State three main uses and at least four clinical indications for insertion of a pulmonary artery catheter.
2. In brief, describe how the physician inserts the catheter and positions the tip in a branch of the pulmonary artery.
3. Name at least six complications of pulmonary artery cathether insertion and hemodynamic monitoring.
4. Describe how hemodynamic readings are used to assess cardiopulmonary status.
5. Define and state normal values for the following parameters: pulmonary artery systolic and diastolic pressures, mean pulmonary artery (PA) pressure, pulmonary capillary wedge pressure (PCWP), PA diastolic pressure-PCWP gradient, pulmonary vascular resistance, and percent saturation of hemoglobin with oxygen in mixed venous blood ($S\bar{v}O_2$).
6. Explain why PA diastolic pressure cannot be used to estimate PCWP in pulmonary patients.
7. Describe how to analyze PCWP tracings at end-expiration during spontaneous breathing and during different modes of mechanical ventilation.
8. Explain changes in hemodynamic measurements that result from pulmonary disease or mechanical ventilation with positive end expiratory pressure (PEEP).

9. **Define and state the significance of transmural PCWP. Explain how it is estimated in the clinical setting.**
10. **State the significance and signs of lung zone 1 or 2 conditions.**
11. **State exactly when during the respiratory cycle the nurse injects the solution for determination of cardiac output.**
12. **Describe how to draw mixed venous blood from a patient's PA catheter.**

This chapter reviews basic respiratory applications of hemodynamic monitoring. The first part presents basic information to familiarize primarily the noncritical care nurse with the general use of the pulmonary artery (PA) catheter. This information complements the information contained in other chapters with hemodynamic aspects, specifically Chapters 4, 9, 13, and 28. Review of the glossary of vascular terms in Chapter 4 will facilitate comprehension of the interpretation of normal and abnormal hemodynamic values.

The last half of this chapter presents basic monitoring considerations primarily for the acute care nurse responsible for critically ill pulmonary patients. Emphasis is placed on the logistics of obtaining accurate pressure readings, a major consideration in monitoring the pulmonary patient.

Since hemodynamic monitoring as a separate topic is beyond the scope of this book and extensively covered elsewhere in the literature, the reader is referred to other sources for basic nursing care and technical aspects, e.g., Daily and Schroeder, 1985; Darovic, 1987; Guzzetta and Dossey, 1984; Osgood et al, 1984; and Wilkins et al, 1985.

Basic Information About Hemodynamic Monitoring

Hemodynamic monitoring refers to placement of a PA catheter (Fig. 29–1), sometimes called a *Swan-Ganz catheter*, in a branch of the PA and measurement of numerous hemodynamic parameters. Parameters include PA systolic and diastolic pressures, right atrial pressure (RAP), pulmonary capillary wedge pressure (PCWP), cardiac output, and others (e.g., mean PA pressure, pulmonary vascular resistance (PVR), systemic vascular resistance (SVR), cardiac index (CI)), derived by simple mathematic calculations. In addition, hemodynamic monitoring may include *arterial pressure monitoring*, defined as the use of an arterial catheter for the monitoring of systemic arterial pressure relationships.

USES AND CLINICAL INDICATIONS

In pulmonary patients, the PA catheter has three main uses. First, it is utilized to obtain a PCWP reading, also called a wedge pressure in the clinical setting, for assessment of LV preload and fluid status in the lungs. Second, the PA catheter provides a direct

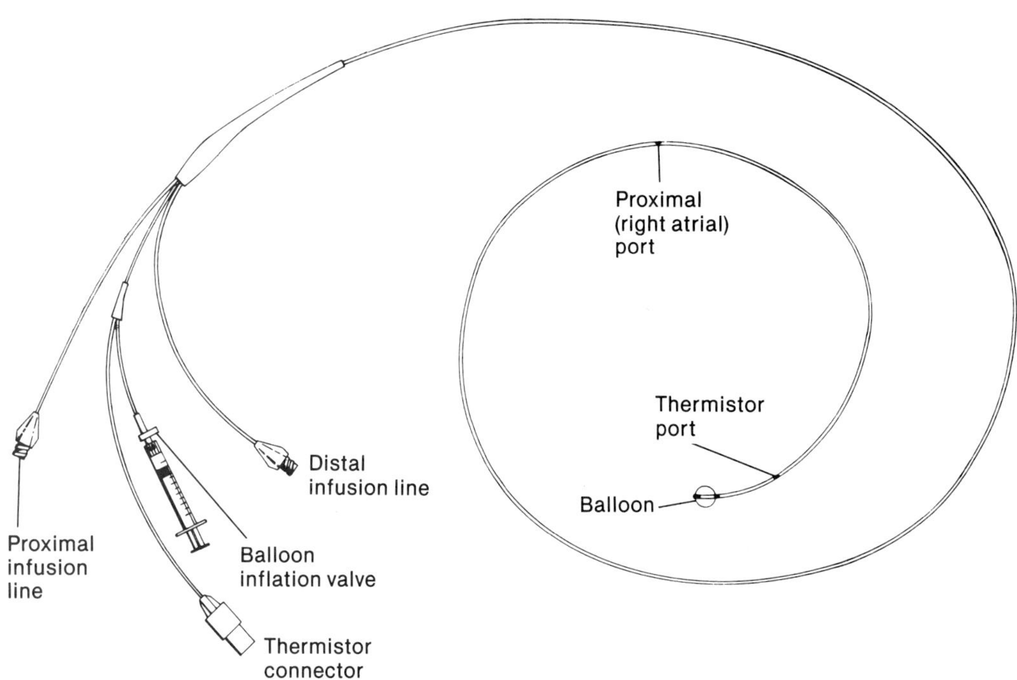

Figure 29–1. The #7 French quadruple lumen, thermodilution pulmonary artery catheter. (Reproduced and adapted by permission from Darovic, G. Hemodynamic Monitoring—Invasive and Noninvasive Clinical Application. Philadelphia, W. B. Saunders Co., 1987.)

cardiac output measurement in L/min, a much more reliable measurement compared with indirect measurements of cardiac output, such as blood pressure, pulse, and sensorium. Third, blood sampling through the catheter allows measurement and calculation of mixed venous oxygen pressure and arterial-venous oxygen content difference ($P\bar{v}O_2$ and $C(a\text{-}\bar{v})O_2$. These measurements allow thorough assessment of blood oxygen transport and tissue extraction in peripheral body tissues.

PA catheter placement is indicated in numerous clinical situations, as shown in the box. Familiarization with these indications is important because it helps the nurse anticipate those situations that might require PA catheterization for hemodynamic monitoring. Also, when one or more indications are no longer present, the nurse inquires about justification for continued use or requests prompt removal of the PA catheter. Removal eliminates risk for infection and other complications associated with the PA catheter. Also, continued use may not reduce mortality, though it facilitates the implementation of therapeutic interventions, such as fluid administration and afterload reduction in the critically ill (Brandstetter and Gitler, 1986). If hemodynamic monitoring is still needed, the nurse checks to be sure the PA catheter is changed every 3 days to help prevent infection.

INDICATIONS FOR PULMONARY ARTERY CATHETER PLACEMENT

- Fluid management:
  - Postoperative states
  - Circulatory shock
  - Adult respiratory distress syndrome (ARDS)
  - Acute renal failure
  - Myocardial infarction
- Assessment of cardiac output and oxygen tissue extraction in patients on mechanical ventilation with PEEP
- Detection of LV failure in patients with cor pulmonale
- Afterload manipulation (e.g., sodium nitroprusside infusion) in patients with LV failure
- Detection of pulmonary hypertension during oxygen administration and exercise
- Preoperative assessment of high risk candidates for pulmonary resection
- Detection of impending myocardial ischemia during anesthesia induction and the perioperative period (Snow, 1983)
- Diagnosis and differentiation of various cardiac diseases:
  - Acute ventricular septal defect
  - Acute mitral insufficiency
  - Cardiac tamponade
  - Restrictive and constrictive heart failure
  - Cardiac versus noncardiac pulmonary edema

CATHETER INSERTION

Catheterization is performed in a special procedures room under fluoroscopy. At the bedside, it is performed with continuous pressure and cardiac monitoring and portable fluoroscopy when available. The catheter is inserted by percutaneous venous puncture or by venotomy, using the subclavian, internal jugular, femoral, basilic, or proximal cephalic vein. The PA catheter is advanced to the right atrium and quickly floated, with the balloon at the tip inflated, through the right side of the heart to a branch of a pulmonary artery (Fig. 29–2A). Advancement is always performed quickly because the presence of the catheter in the right side of the heart can cause cardiac irritability and fatal arrhythmias.

When the catheter enters the PA, as evidenced by a PA tracing on the monitor display, the balloon is deflated, and the catheter is advanced into final position in a branch of the PA. Then, the balloon is inflated to obtain a PCWP tracing (Fig. 29–2B).

Immediately after catheter placement in the PA, infusion lines are connected to a pressurized, heparinized solution that permits slow intravenous (IV) infusion (2 to 3 ml/hr) to insure catheter patency (Fig. 29–3). Connection to a bedside pressure transducer setup allows continuous visualization of the PA waveform on the cardiac monitor after the procedure is over.

COMPLICATIONS

The complication rate ranges from 15 to 24% while only 3 to 4% of patients experience serious complications (Boyd et al, 1983; Keefer and Barash, 1983). Complications include hematoma, wound infection, multiple sticks during insertion, inability to wedge from balloon rupture, catheter misplacement in the RV or too distally in the PA, and premature atrial or ventricular contractions. Serious complications may include ventricular tachycardia or fibrillation; pulmonary hemorrhage; pulmonary infiltrate distal to the catheter tip, sometimes a pulmonary infarction; septicemia; air embolism; and valve rupture.

NORMAL AND ABNORMAL HEMODYNAMIC VALUES

Hemodynamic monitoring largely involves monitoring a few basic vascular pressures and interpreting them in relation to other hemodynamic parameters, when available. Normal ranges for basic vascular pressures are listed at the top of Table 29–1. (Other hemodynamic parameters are listed in the same table.)

The RAP is essentially a central venous pressure reading. A *high RAP* occurs in volume overload, in RV failure, occasionally in pulmonary hypertension, in chronic LV failure, in constrictive pericarditis, and in

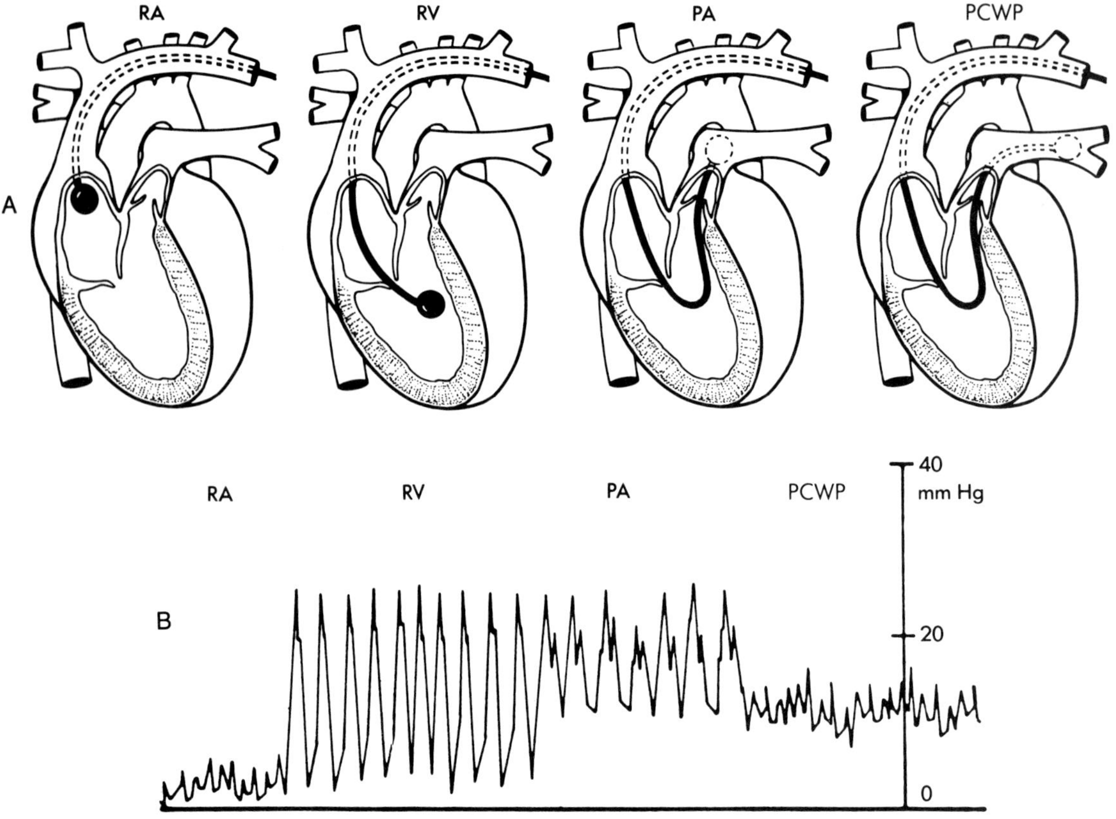

Figure 29–2. Insertion of the pulmonary artery catheter. *A*, Catheter position in the right atrium (RA), right ventricle (RV), main pulmonary artery (PA), and a branch of the PA for the pulmonary capillary wedge pressure (PCWP) reading. *B*, Corresponding pressure tracings during catheter insertion. (Reproduced by permission from Martin, L. Pulmonary Physiology in Clinical Practice. St. Louis, The C. V. Mosby Co., 1987.)

tricuspid stenosis and regurgitation. A *low RAP* may indicate hypovolemia and dehydration.

High PA systolic and diastolic pressures suggest one or more of the following conditions: (1) increased pulmonary blood flow (left-to-right cardiac shunts); (2) increased pulmonary venous pressure, as in mitral stenosis or LV failure; and (3) increased pulmonary vascular resistance from pulmonary disease, pulmonary hypertension, pulmonary embolism, vasopressors, hypoxemia, acidosis, or polycythemia. Further evaluation includes calculation of PVR to estimate the extent and severity of pulmonary disease and hypoxic vasoconstriction. Remember that normal PVR is about 60 to 100 dynes/sec/cm^{-5} (see Chapter 4).

Low PA pressures and *low PVR* may occur in response to overly aggressive vasodilator therapy.

A *high PCWP* develops with volume overload, impending myocardial ischemia, extremely high SVR, LV failure, mitral stenosis or insufficiency, and constrictive pericarditis.

A *low PCWP* suggests volume depletion; as with a low RAP, however, it may be a normal finding in the individual without cardiopulmonary disease.

In addition to absolute values, the nurse analyzes directional changes to assess hemodynamic status and response to specific interventions. Interventions may include fluid challenges to increase PCWP or fluid restriction to decrease PCWP; diuretics or vasodilators to decrease SVR, PCWP, and PVR; vasopressors to increase SVR; or high FIO_2 to relieve hypoxic vasoconstriction and decrease PA pressures. Generally, a 3- to 4-mmHg or greater change in pressure is considered significant, since measurements normally may fluctuate 1 to 3 mmHg.

Respiratory Applications

Principles of hemodynamic monitoring in the pulmonary patient are the same as those described for the cardiac patient (Guzzetta and Dossey, 1984), with a few specific respiratory applications. These applications consist of basic monitoring considerations (explained subsequently) and logistics necessary to accommodate large respiratory variations in pressure waveforms during spontaneous breathing and mechanical ventilation.

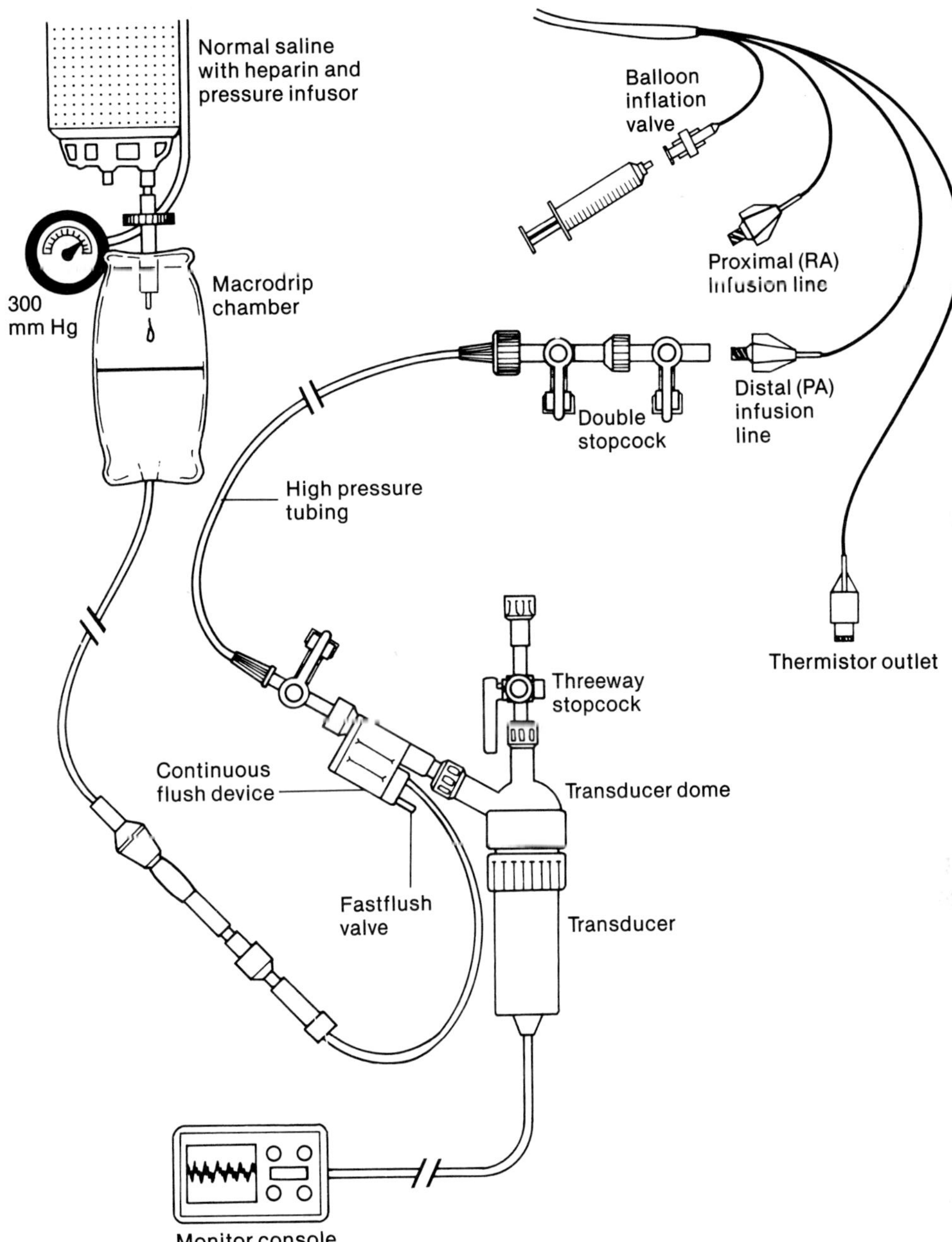

Figure 29–3. Components of the pulmonary artery catheter monitoring system. (Reproduced by permission from Darovic, G. Hemodynamic Monitoring—Invasive and Noninvasive Clinical Application. Philadelphia, W. B. Saunders Co., 1987, and adapted from Smith, R. Invasive pressure monitoring. American journal of nursing, 9:1514–1521, 1978.)

Table 29–1. COMMONLY USED PARAMETERS IN HEMODYNAMIC MONITORING*

Parameters	Normal Range
PA Catheter Vascular Pressures	
Right atrial (RA)	2 to 6 mmHg (mean)
Right ventricular (RV)	$\frac{\text{20 to 30 mmHg}}{\text{0 to 5 mmHg}}$
Pulmonary artery (PA)	$\frac{\text{20 to 30 mmHg}}{\text{5 to 15 mmHg}}$ or $\frac{25}{8}$
Pulmonary capillary wedge pressure (PCWP)	5 to 15 mmHg Equals diastolic PA in the absence of pulmonary disease.
Other Hemodynamic Parameters	
Cardiac output (Q)	5 to 8 L/min
Central venous pressure (CVP)	Less than 6 mmHg or 12 cmH_2O
Arterial pressure (BP)	$\frac{\text{90 to 120 mmHg}}{\text{60 to 80 mmHg}}$
Left atrial pressure (LAP)	4 to 12 mmHg
Left ventricular pressure (LVP)	$\frac{\text{100 to 140 mmHg}}{\text{0 to 5 mmHg}}$
Left ventricular end-diastolic pressure (LVEDP)	5 to 12 mmHg
Right ventricular end-diastolic pressure (RVEDP)	2 to 6 mmHg
Common Calculated Parameters	
Cardiac index $CI = \frac{\text{Q L/min}}{\text{BSA (body surface area)† in } M^2}$	2.5 to 4.0 L/min/m^2
Stroke volume $SV = \frac{Q}{\text{HR (heart rate)}}$	60 to 130 ml/beat (resting)
Mean PA pressure $\overline{PAP} = \frac{\text{systolic PAP} + (\text{diastolic PAP} \times 2)}{3}$	10 to 20 mmHg
Pulmonary vascular resistance $PVR = \frac{\overline{PAP} - PCWP}{Q} \times 80$	Less than 100 dynes/sec/cm^{-5} (1.0 mmHg/L/min) or 1/6 of SVR or less
Mean arterial pressure $\overline{BP} = \frac{\text{systolic BP} + (\text{diastolic BP} \times 2)}{3}$	80 to 100 mmHg
Systemic vascular resistance $SVR = \frac{\overline{BP} - RAP}{Q} \times 80$	800 to 1200 dynes/sec/cm

*Data from Osgood et al, 1984, and Daily and Schroeder, 1985. Normal range varies, depending on body size and other pressure relationships.

†Refer to Figure 29–14 to determine BSA.

Table 29–2. HEMODYNAMIC MEASUREMENTS IN PULMONARY DISEASE

Measurements	Vascular Pressure/Change in Value	Mechanism
RAP (or CVP)	Normal to ↑	Increased right ventricular preload due to fluid overload, heart failure, cor pulmonale.
PA systolic PA diastolic PAP	↑	Increased PVR and increased right ventricular afterload due to hypoxemia, acidosis, pulmonary hypertension.
PCWP (or LAP)	Normal to ↓	Left heart pressures are typically normal in the absence of heart disease. A low normal PCWP or LAP may be due to low cardiac output from emphysema. Noncompliant lungs (e.g., fibrosis) may prevent the transmission of a high LAP to the PA catheter tip, resulting in a low PCWP reading.
PA diastolic pressure–PCWP gradient	5 to 20 mmHg or greater	PA diastolic pressure is higher than PCWP due to high PVR from pulmonary disease. In normal persons, PA diastolic pressure is only 0 to 2 mmHg higher than PCWP.
Arterial pressure	Variable	Depends on alterations in cardiac output. Paradoxical pulse may be observed in patients with severe lung hyperinflation.
Cardiac output (Q)	Normal to ↓	Seen in emphysema or other diseases associated with extensive destruction of lung tissue. Heart failure further decreases Q.
	Normal to ↑; then ↓	Seen in chronic bronchitis or other conditions associated with hypoxemia, polycythemia, and hypervolemia. The onset of heart failure decreases Q.

BASIC CONSIDERATIONS FOR MONITORING THE PULMONARY PATIENT

High PA Pressures

One of the most characteristic hemodynamic signs in a pulmonary patient is high pulmonary artery pressures. PA systolic, PA diastolic, and mean PA pressures tend to be above the normal range listed in Table 29–1. High readings are due to severe ventilation/perfusion (V/Q) mismatching, lung hyperinflation, and high PVR. In a patient with chronic obstructive pulmonary disease (COPD), high pleural pressures alter transmural pressure differences across the heart to create high readings. The readings become even higher during shortness of breath or any kind of forced expiratory maneuver, because of the increased air trapping in the lungs at this time.

Normal to Reduced PCWP

Though PA pressures are high, PCWP remains normal to reduced, as shown in Table 29–2. Note in Table 29–1 that *15 mmHg* rather than the traditional 12 mmHg is the high limit for normal PCWP. Bone and coworkers (1977) point out that pulmonary patients with PCWPs of less than 15 mmHg have normal LV function and are not in LV failure.

The PCWP provides crucial information for clinical decision-making. Particularly in patients with RV failure and chronic cor pulmonale, a PCWP may be the *only* way to detect or rule out LV failure, when other more indirect signs are absent or inconclusive.

When the balloon is inflated (Fig. 29–4), the catheter tip is wedged, as shown in Figure 29–5, and blood flow stops distal to the tip. Because of venous stasis and absence of a pressure gradient, the mean pressure recorded from the catheter tip reflects the mean left atrial pressure (LAP). LAP roughly estimates LV end diastolic pressure (LVEDP), unless significant mitral disease, hypovolemia, or altered myocardial compliance or performance disturbs the relationship.

PA Diastolic Pressure—PCWP Gradient

Persons with normal pulmonary vasculature and normal cardiac function have little or no pressure gradient between PA diastolic pressure and PCWP readings. PA diastolic pressure is about equal to or 1 mmHg higher than the wedge pressure. Because of this correlation, the diastolic pressure is sometimes

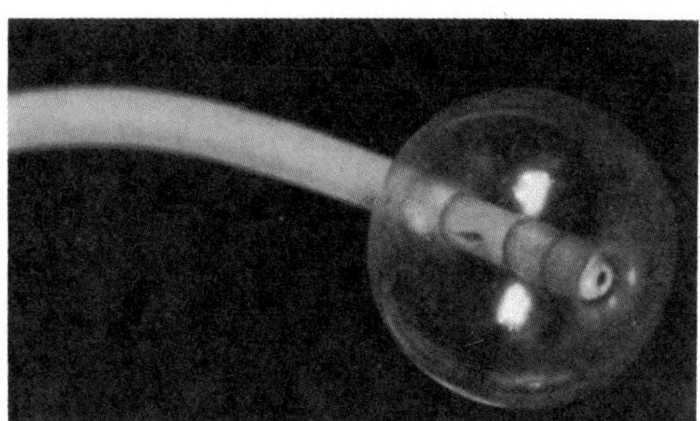

Figure 29–4. The #7 French thermodilution PA catheter balloon inflated with the recommended volume of 1.5 ml. The balloon protrudes over and cushions, but does not cover, the sensing tip. (Reproduced by permission from Darovic, G. Hemodynamic Monitoring—Invasive and Noninvasive Clinical Application. Philadelphia, W. B. Saunders Co., 1987.)

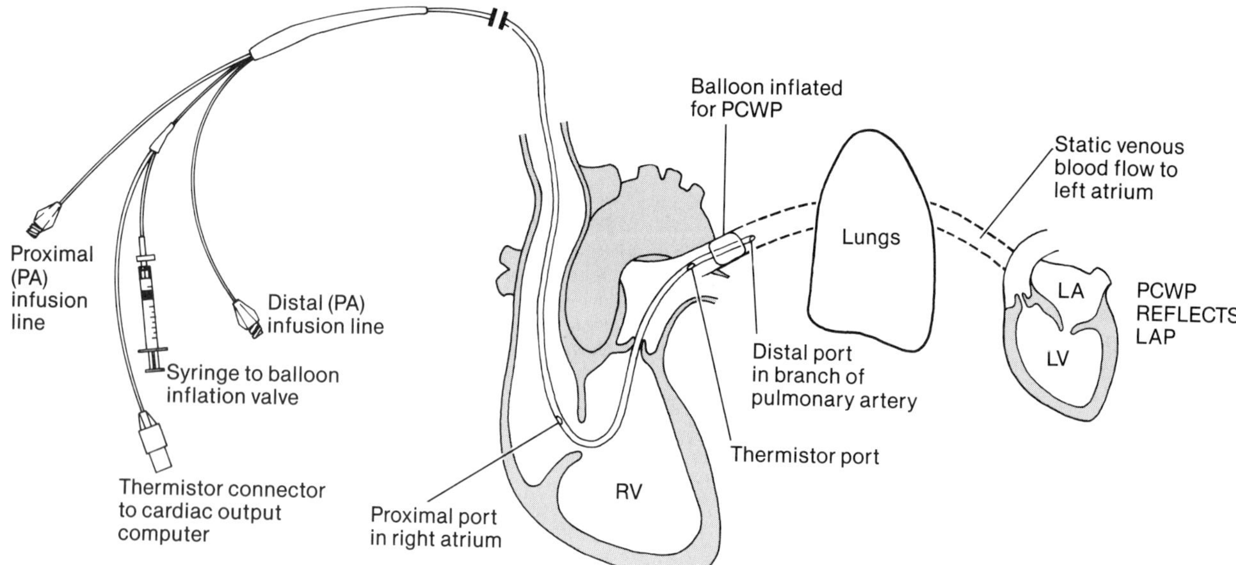

Figure 29–5. Pulmonary artery catheter (four-lumen model) in a branch of a pulmonary artery with the balloon inflated; the wedge pressure (PCWP) reflects left atrial pressure (LAP).

utilized to estimate PCWP and LAP, when a PCWP is not obtainable for some reason (e.g., balloon rupture).

However, in patients with pulmonary hypertension, these two measurements are not equal, and one cannot be used to estimate the other. PA diastolic pressure is about 5 to 20 mmHg higher than the wedge pressure owing to high PVR from severe parenchymal disease and other factors that increase PA pressures. The discrepancy may become more marked in the presence of tachycardia over 120 to 125 beats/min. In tachycardia, the brief cardiac diastole and high cardiac output through the pulmonary vascular bed widen the pressure gradient between the catheter tip and left atrium, even though the balloon is inflated and even though the PVR is normal (O'Quin and Marini, 1983).

Waiting for Stabilization of PCWP

During PCWP measurement, the nurse inflates the catheter balloon and waits several seconds for the PCWP to fall and stabilize before taking a reading. When PVR is greatly increased, the retrograde transmission of LAP through the pulmonary vasculature may be delayed. Waiting for stabilization of readings accommodates this delay and helps avoid measurement error.

Consistent RA Reference Point for Equipment Calibration

Maintaining a consistent RA reference point for equipment calibration is a basic monitoring consideration. To avoid measurement error, the nurse positions the setup's transducer at the level of the RA (i.e., midchest position), calibrates equipment at this level, and maintains a consistent RA reference point during subsequent pressure readings. Following this procedure is not a problem while monitoring either the comatose or cooperative patient. However, two problems commonly arise while monitoring pulmonary patients, particularly those who are hypoxemic, restless, and mentally confused and those who either slip down towards the foot of the bed in the supine position or insist on sitting bolt upright to avoid dyspnea.

First, nurses may use inconsistent RA reference points on the lateral chest area because of a COPD patient's increased AP diameter. To avoid this problem, the nurse is careful to abduct the arm, assess an accurate midchest position, and mark the position with a felt pen for future reference.

A second problem pertains to the patient's changing body position in bed. Though the nurse may use an appropriate RA reference point on the chest, a change in the position of the head of the bed or in general body position may cause unequal vertical levelling between the RA reference point and transducer. These two points must remain level (i.e., at the same vertical height) during pressure measurements. Unequal levelling introduces measurement error. To avoid this mistake, the nurse checks transducer placement every shift and PRN, before equipment calibration and with a reliable instrument, such as a carpenter's level (Fig. 29–6). Bed position, patient position, or vertical transducer placement is altered to keep the transducer even with the RA reference point. Moreover, the most reliable PA measurements are taken with the head of the bed elevated up to 45 degrees, with the patient in the supine position (Keating et al, 1986).

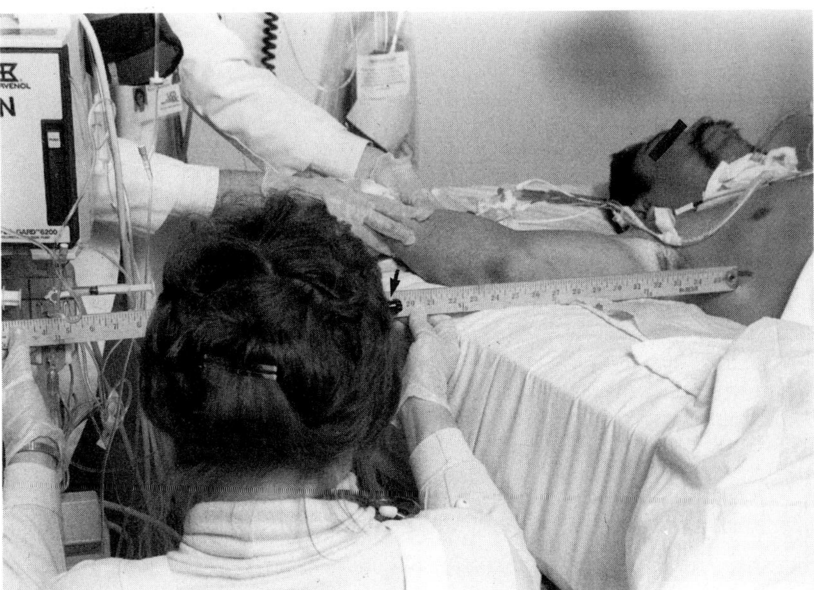

Figure 29–6. Proper leveling of the pressure transducer at the right atrial level of the chest. The nurse adjusts the level of the pressure transducer (by left hand) until the carpenter level's indicator bubble (by black arrow) reads a level position.

ACCOMMODATION OF RESPIRATORY VARIATIONS IN PRESSURE WAVEFORMS

Obtaining reliable PA catheter pressure readings largely depends on the nurse's ability to understand and accommodate respiratory variations in pressure waveforms. Accommodation involves reading pressures at end-expiration, using pressure tracings rather than digital displays for readings, and analyzing tracings appropriately in relation to spontaneous breathing and mode of mechanical ventilation.

Reading Pressures at End-Expiration

Pulmonary patients may demonstrate marked variations in pleural pressures and pressure waveform excursions during respirations, sometimes causing as much as a 10- to 20-mmHg variation in PCWP. Hence, it is crucial that the nurse read pressures at the end of a passive exhalation (Riedinger et al, 1981), when the patient appears calm (e.g., not agitated, not moving in bed, and not dyspneic from suctioning). At end-expiration, pressure in the intrathoracic cavity is constant, and changes in airway pressure during mechanical ventilation are at a minimum. The observed pressure is most likely to represent a true transmural vascular pressure rather than an increased intrapleural pressure.

To take readings at end-expiration, the nurse asks the alert, spontaneously breathing patient to briefly stop breathing after exhaling fully, while keeping the throat (i.e., glottis) open. This method helps to prolong the end-expiratory phase of respiration and stabilize pressures. However, it is not always effective and may create even more inaccuracy—some patients are too dyspneic to cooperate fully or they inadvertently close the glottis during breath holding, thus increasing intrathoracic and intrapleural pressures.

The most reliable method for taking end-expiratory pressure measurements involves the recording of pressure waveforms along with the ECG and careful analysis of the tracings. A 10- to 20-second long tracing of each waveform is usually required. Digital displays are limited in their ability to correct for respiratory varia-

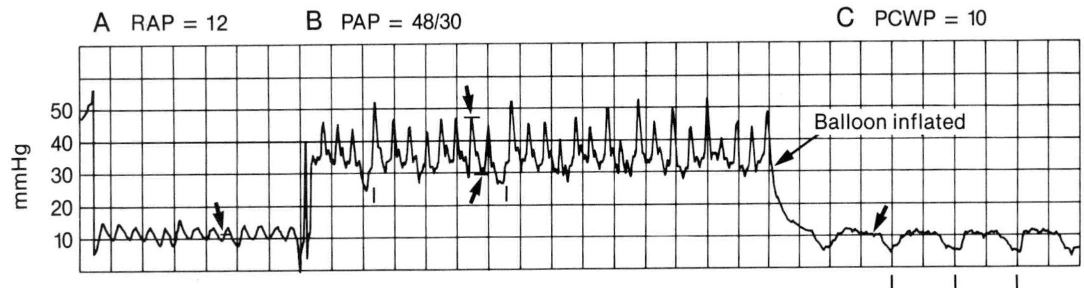

Figure 29–7. Pulmonary artery catheter tracings in a spontaneously breathing patient admitted for possible pneumonia. *A*, Right atrial pressure (RAP) tracing with no respiratory variation. The point for reading RA pressure is easy to find (see arrow). *B*, Pulmonary artery pressure (PAP) tracing with only two distinct inspiratory valleys labelled I at bottom of tracing. PA systolic and diastolic pressure readings are taken at an end-expiratory point (arrows). *C*, Pulmonary capillary wedge (PCWP) tracing with readily visible respiratory variation. PCWP is read at an end-expiratory point (arrow).

tions and artifacts. Periodic correlations should be made between digital and graphic readings to check accuracy of digital displays.

Pressure Tracings During Spontaneous Breathing

During spontaneous breathing, high excursions occur during expiration, as shown most clearly in Figure 29–7C. Periodic dips or valleys occur during inspiration, as negative pleural pressure causes lung inflation. Note that the inspiratory valleys are very short, since the normal inspiratory:expiratory (I:E) ratio is 1:2, and expiration is normally much longer than inspiration. When the patient is resting comfortably, the inspiratory valleys may be barely visible or may be absent in some sections of the tracing (Fig. 29–7A and B). Respiratory variation in C is greater than in A and B because the PCWP most directly reflects pressures in the lungs.

For tachypnea, Cheyne-Stokes respiration, or other irregular breathing patterns, the nurse takes a long pressure tracing, selects 2 to 3 waveforms that occur most frequently at end-expiration (immediately before the inspiratory valleys), and determines average pressure for the final reading. When analysis is difficult, a faster paper speed (e.g., 25 mm/sec) expands the waveform and may make analysis easier.

Pressure Tracings During Mechanical Ventilation

Application of positive pressure to the lungs increases intrapleural and intrathoracic pressures and results in increased RAP, PA pressures, and PCWP on the tracing. The amount of pressure increase depends on ventilator variables, such as the amount of positive pressure applied, I:E ratio, amount of airway resistance in the ventilator circuit, and mode of mechanical ventilation. In addition, the pressure increase depends on patient factors, such as resting PVR before application of positive pressure, lung compliance, activity level, and amount of active versus passive breathing.

The patient most likely to demonstrate high vascular pressures is critically ill with underlying chronic disease, who is on continuous mechanical ventilation with high levels of PEEP. Table 29–3 summarizes hemodynamic measurements during mechanical ventilation with PEEP. The discussion that follows explains pressure tracings during PEEP and other modes of mechanical ventilation as well as techniques for finding the correct end-expiratory point.

Effect of Different Modes of Ventilation. In the continuous positive airway pressure (CPAP) mode, PCWP and PA pressure fluctuations are the same as those described for spontaneous breathing.

In the control mode, fluctuations are exactly the

Table 29–3. HEMODYNAMIC MEASUREMENTS DURING MECHANICAL VENTILATION WITH PEEP

Measurement	Change in Value	Mechanism
RA pressure (or CVP)	↑ (transmural RAP may ↓)	Positive pressure increases intrathoracic, intrapleural, and RA pressures. The accompanying decrease in venous return to the heart decreases actual RA transmural pressure.
PA pressures	↑	Positive pressure increases PA systolic, diastolic, and mean pressures. Greater airway pressure increases PVR and RV afterload, while decreasing the RV preload of filling (Daily and Schroeder, 1985).
PCW pressure (or LAP)	↑ (transmural PCWP may ↓)	High PCWP reflects increased intrapleural pressure in reference to the atmosphere, not in reference to the heart LA chamber (i.e., transmural pressure). As PEEP increases airway and intrapleural pressures, the decrease in venous return to the heart and diastolic filling volume causes actual LA filling pressures to decrease. Hence, transmural PCWP decreases, as more positive pressure is added.
PA diastolic pressure-PCWP gradient	↓ (PA diastolic pressure-transmural PCWP gradient ↑)	Positive pressure further increases PVR and risk for falsely high readings, especially the PCWP reading. Also, catheter tip misplacement above the level of the left atrium, hypovolemia, and deviation of the intraventricular septum to the left from increased PVR may cause overestimation of PCW pressure. In this case, the PA diastolic pressure-PCWP gradient decreases. If the clinician can obtain a true transmural PCWP (i.e., a low value), then a large gradient exists.
Cardiac output (Q)	unchanged to ↓	PEEP decreases venous return (i.e., right ventricular filling), increases RV afterload, and decreases LV distensibility. All these factors contribute to a fall in cardiac output (Dorinsky and Whitcomb, 1983). The patient may require a fluid or medication adjustment after initiation or discontinuation of PEEP to compensate for the change in Q (see Chapter 28).
Arterial pressure	unchanged to ↓	Correlates with the decrease in cardiac output, which in turn is associated with increasing levels of intrapleural pressure.

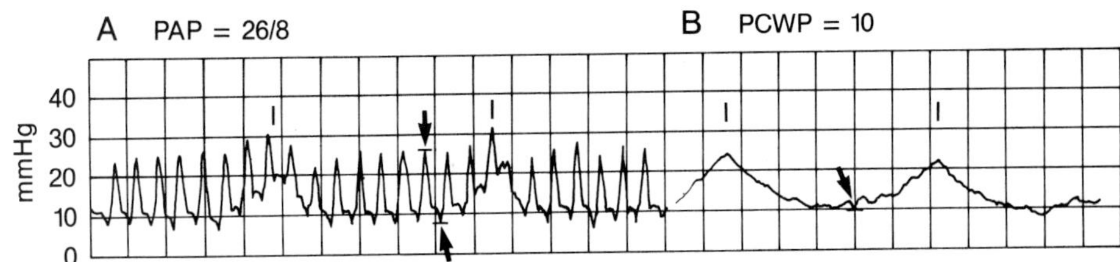

Figure 29–8. Pulmonary artery catheter tracings in the control mode of mechanical ventilation. The inspiratory peak (I) represents positive pressure from a ventilator breath. PAP and PCWP readings are taken at end-expiratory points (arrows). Note that respiratory variation is opposite that in the spontaneously breathing patient (see Fig. 29–7).

opposite of those for spontaneous breathing. PCWP rises during inspiration as the ventilator delivers a positive pressure breath and falls during expiration (Fig. 29–8).

For assist-control and synchronized intermittent mandatory ventilation (SIMV) modes, pressure fluctuations depend on whether the ventilator or the patient performs most of the work of breathing. In assist-control, even though the patient generates −1 to −2 cmH_2O to initiate assisted breaths, PCWP still rises during inspiration and falls during expiration provided the ventilator performs most of the work of breathing. However, if the patient performs most of the work, as in patients with strong ventilatory drives and high minute ventilations, PCWP will fall during inspiration and rise during expiration. These situations are extreme cases, however. Often the positive pressure delivered by the ventilator is balanced by the negative intrathoracic pressures of spontaneous efforts, and the PCWP and other pressures remain relatively stable throughout the respiratory cycle. If the patient is ventilated by the back-up control rate, then waveform excursions will be the same as those for the described control mode.

In the SIMV mode, waveform excursions are some combination of those for spontaneous, assisted, and controlled breathing. They may vary greatly within and between patients, and hence no concrete rules can be made about anticipated wave patterns. In Figure 29–9, the patient was performing most of the work of breathing with a set SIMV rate of 12/min and a total respiratory rate of 26/min. Inspiratory effort is represented by the valleys in the wave pattern. Ventilator breaths are not evident.

Techniques for Taking Pressure Readings. Techniques for taking pressure readings with the patient on mechanical ventilation are basically the same as those for spontaneous breathing. Emphasis is placed on careful observation of the patient's breathing pattern during pressure recordings to help in tracing analysis and on recording at a time when the patient is calm and not fighting the ventilator.

The main difference lies in the identification of the end-expiratory point on pressure waveforms for various modes of ventilation, as previously described. Identification of inspiration and expiration and end-expiratory point is fairly simple for CPAP and control modes, because their waveforms are predictable and easy to recognize. In contrast, finding end-expiration is difficult and largely unpredictable in other modes because of their different effects on the patient's breathing pattern and work of breathing. It is most difficult in IMV (SIMV) or combinations of modes, particularly when the patient cannot appropriately prolong expiration to facilitate pressure stabilization before recording. Several techniques may help the nurse find end-expiration.

Some modern ventilators, such as the Bear 2, provide a way to record proximal airway pressure and expiratory flow along with PA pressures, as shown in Figure 29–10 (Bellamy and Mercurio, 1986). End-expiration lies just after the expiratory flow and before the inspiratory pressure waveform.

Another aid to finding end-expiration is to record respiratory breathing pattern (i.e., respiratory impedance), as described in Chapter 28. Each rise in wave pattern represents chest expansion during inspiration. Each decending waveform represents expiration. The

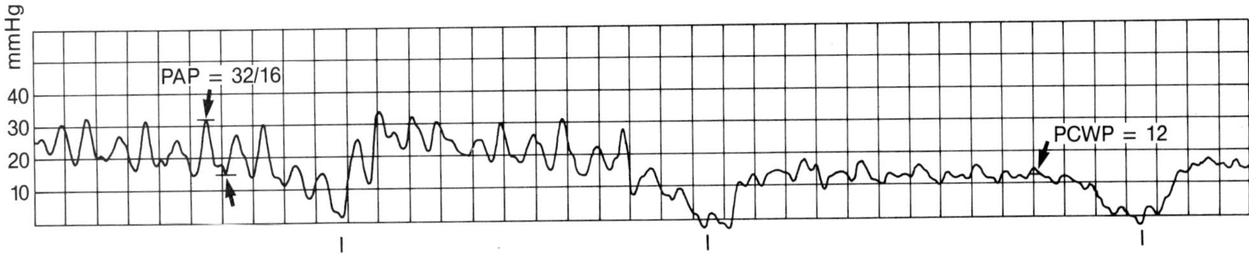

Figure 29–9. Pulmonary artery catheter tracings in the synchronized intermittent mandatory ventilation (SIMV) mode of mechanical ventilation, with the patient performing most of the work. I = inspiratory valley.

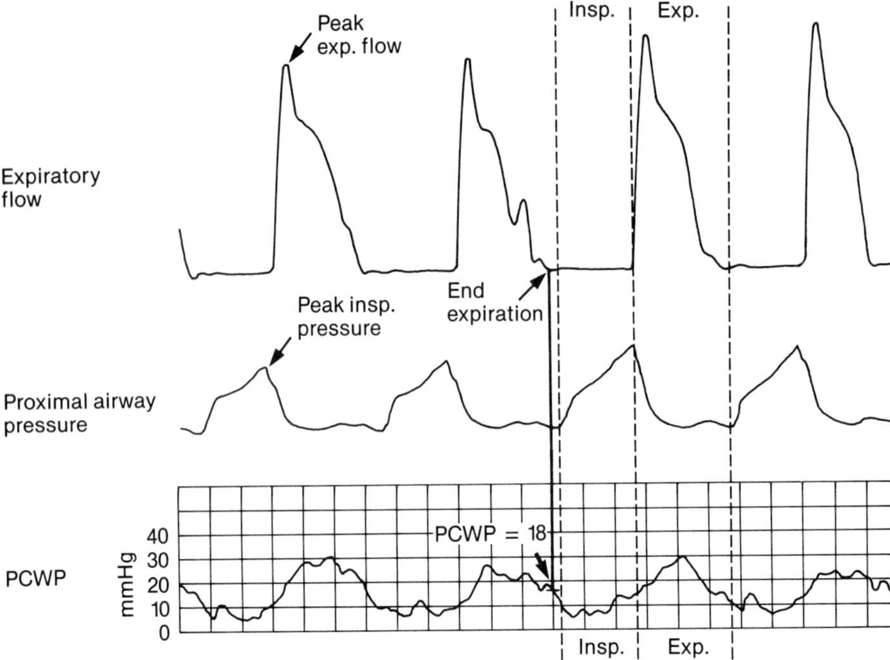

Figure 29–10. Use of expiratory flow and proximal airway pressure waveforms to determine pulmonary capillary wedge pressure (PCWP). The nurse draws a line from end-expiration (top) to the PCWP tracing (bottom). The intersection of the solid line with the PCWP waveform marks the correct place to read PCWP. The patient was in the assist-control mode of mechanical ventilation, with assisted breaths responsible for most of the minute ventilation.

end-expiratory point is located in the trough of the waveform. Though inspection of respiratory impedance tracings may help in the identification of the end expiratory point, these tracings are not always reliable guides. They may be of poor quality, and waveforms do not always correlate exactly with the respiratory cycle.

When hemodynamic aids are not available, the nurse marks inspiration and expiration on the pressure tracing, while watching the patient's chest as well as the ventilator's pressure manometer. If necessary, two representative high and low pressures are averaged for the final determination.

When used consistently, the hemodynamic monitoring techniques described result in more accurate pressure readings. Even though techniques may be refined, during severe bronchospasm end-expiratory PCWP may remain excessively high and will not reflect true transmural pressure on the left side of the heart.

Measurement On or Off the Ventilator? Because the application of positive pressure to the lungs may greatly increase intrapleural pressure and create false high PCWP and PA pressures, the question arises as to whether readings should be taken with the patient on or off the ventilator. Measurements taken on the ventilator may be 5 to 10 mmHg higher than those taken during spontaneous breathing off the ventilator. The difference is most noticeable when PEEP is applied or when the auto-PEEP effect is observed (see Table 28–5).

Most clinicians recommend taking measurements while the patient remains on the ventilator to determine the effects of mechanical ventilation and PEEP, to establish baseline measurements for monitoring trends, and to avoid unnecessary hypoxemia and forced expirations during spontaneous breathing off the venilator. Moreover, the discontinuation of PEEP may cause sudden increased venous return, hypervolemia within central vessels, and potential alveolar flooding. In selected circumstances, the physician may disconnect the patient from the ventilator every 8 to 12 hours to note any discrepancies between PCWPs on and off mechanical ventilation and PEEP.

MEASUREMENT OF TRANSMURAL PRESSURES

To reduce the discrepancy between observed PCWPs and actual transmural pressures filling the left atrium and ventricle, the physician may request measurement of the transmural pressures. These pressures are nearly equivalent to intracardiac pressures at end-expiration and, hence, are more accurate than the vascular pressures read from the pressure tracing.

The box on the opposite page contains an explanation of the inaccuracy of the PCWP reading during mchanical ventilation and shows how to calculate transmural PCWP. A mean intrapleural pressure of −3 mmHg is used for P_{pl} in the example of normal spontaneous breathing on the left. Intrapleural pressure is more positive in the example on the right due to the effects of positive pressure.

Transmural PCWP may be measured or estimated three ways in the clinical setting (Smucker, 1986). First, measured alveolar pressure may be subtracted from the wedge pressure. Alveolar pressure (P_{alv}) is obtained by manually occluding the ventilator's exhalation port late in expiration and reading the pressure on the ventilator's gauge. This method is relatively easy, but it assumes that the measured airway pressure reflects alveolar pressure, which is not always the case.

A second method involves measurement of intrapleural pressure with an intrapleural or esophageal balloon and subtraction of this pressure from intracardiac pressure. Though this method is relatively accurate, it is rarely done because, even in normal individuals, it is technically difficult.

A third method is to completely eliminate unpredictable respiratory waveform fluctuations by respiratory paralysis with a drug, such as pancuronium. Paralysis and return to a controlled mode of mechanical ventilation eliminate forced exhalations, air trapping in the lungs, and excessively high intrapleural pressures. The clinician then either can utilize the first method for calculation of transmural PCWP or can analyze trends in regular PCWP tracings for decision-making.

When elimination of large respiratory variations is undesirable (e.g., muscle atrophy associated with prolonged respiratory paralysis) or unavoidable (e.g., auto-PEEP effect), the clinician must not rely on the PCWP reading for decision-making. Decisions are made based on data from numerous respiratory assessment parameters. Moreover, decisions are usually incremental in nature.

For example, the administration of small fluid challenges combined with close monitoring of chest assessment and hemodynamic findings may be necessary to assess the patient's ability to accept fluid without experiencing right-sided heart failure and pulmonary edema. The decision to continue fluid challenges as ordered by the physician is made over time, after evaluation of each response to therapy.

TRANSMURAL PULMONARY CAPILLARY WEDGE PRESSURE (PCWP)

DEFINITION

Difference between intravascular pressure (PCWP reading) and extravascular pressure represented by alveolar or intrapleural pressure.

FORMULA

Transmural PCWP = PCWP − P_{pl} (or P_{alv})

EXAMPLES

End-Expiration during Normal Breathing

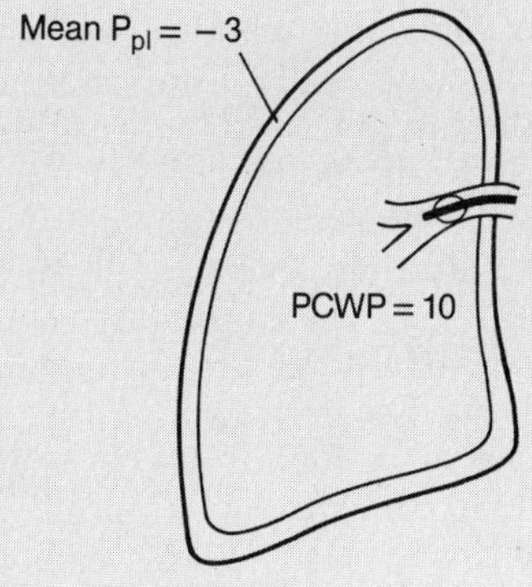

Transmural PCWP = 10 − (−3) = 13 mmHg

End-Expiration during Mechanical Ventilation

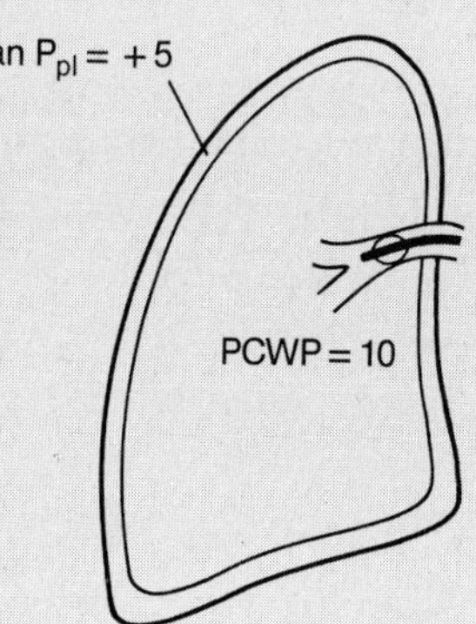

Transmural PCWP = 10 − (+5) = 5 mmHg

CONCLUSION

The PCWP reading is an overestimation of transmural PCWP in the patient on mechanical ventilation.

INACCURATE PCWP DURING ZONE 1 OR ZONE 2 LUNG CONDITIONS

In addition to the problem of positive pressure, another problem of the pulmonary patient is the one of inaccurate pressure readings related to the PA catheter position in the lungs and the V/Q ratios in the surrounding lung zone. To better understand this potential problem, review the zones in the normal lung in Figure 5–8.

During catheterization, the PA catheter tip normally floats into lung zone 3, where blood flow is greatest and vessels are easily entered. A postcatheterization AP, PA, or cross-table, lateral chest x-ray film confirms correct placement below the left atrium. If the catheter tip rests in zone 1 above the LA or zone 2 at the LA, where P_{alv} is consistently higher than venous pressure (P_{ven}), the wedged catheter tip is subject to P_{alv} rather than a true PCWP or LAP. The PCWP reading is likely to be inaccurate. Inaccuracy is greatest when the patient is on mechanical ventilation with greater than 10 cmH_2O PEEP.

Most important, inaccuracies occur in a correctly placed catheter *anytime* altered V/Q ratios by the catheter tip produce a P_{alv} that is greater than P_{ven}. For example, diuresis, hemorrhage, hypovolemia, or PEEP may convert a zone 3 region to zone 1 or 2 conditions, as P_{ven} is decreased, P_{alv} is increased, or both.

The nurse notifies the physician when signs of zone 1 or 2 conditions appear. These signs include (1) damped PCWP waveform, as shown in Figure 29–11; (2) great respiratory variations; (3) PCWP greater than PA diastolic, or *overwedging*; and (4) an increase in PCWP by more than half the applied increment of PEEP during passive exhalation (O'Quin and Marini, 1983).

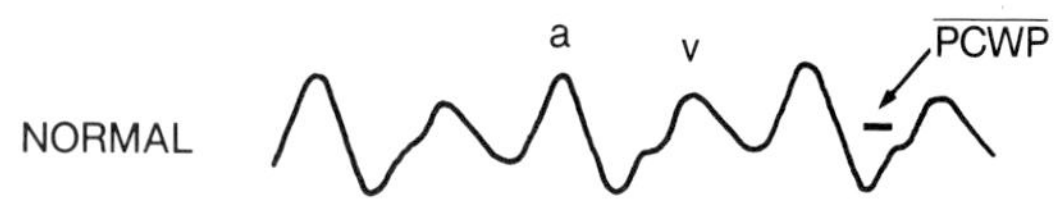

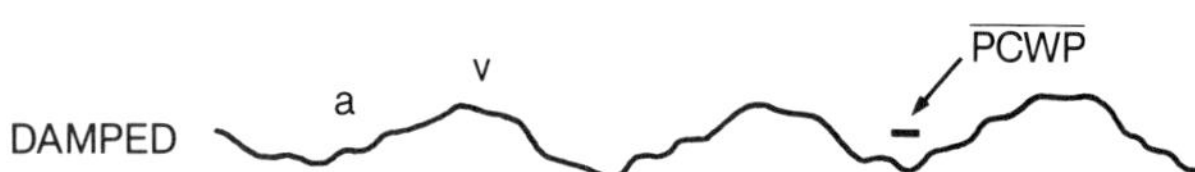

Figure 29–11. Normal and damped pulmonary capillary wedge pressure tracings. *In a normal tracing,* the *a wave* reflects left atrial systole and correlates with the P wave on the ECG (not shown here). The *v wave* reflects the mitral valve bulging back into the left atrium during left ventricular systole; it correlates with the T wave on the ECG. The *c wave* represents mitral valve closure; it may be normally absent or barely visible between the a and v wave. *In a damped tracing,* a and v waves are distorted.

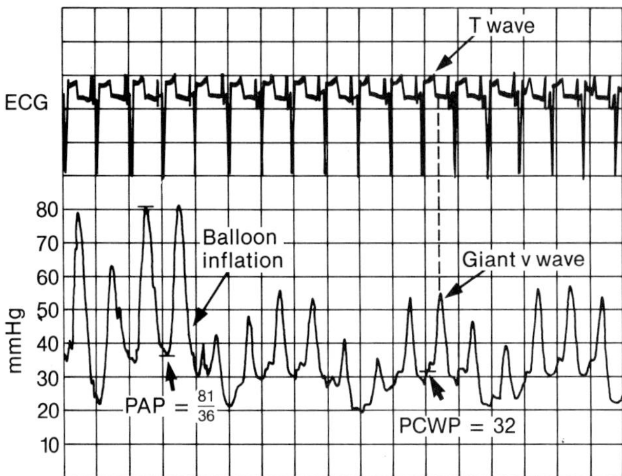

Figure 29–12. The ECG tracing (top) and the pulmonary capillary wedge pressure (PCWP) tracing (bottom) in a spontaneously breathing patient with status/postmyocardial infarction and left ventricular failure. The giant v waves reflect the regurgitation of blood into a dilated, noncompliant left ventricle. *Note* the following: (1) the v wave correlates approximately with the T wave on the ECG and (2) the giant v waves were disregarded in obtaining the mean PCWP reading because they do not accurately reflect LV end-diastolic pressure.

Efforts to Assure a Clear PCWP Tracing and Zone 3 Lung Conditions

In the evaluation of a damped waveform, the nurse must keep in mind that many PA waveforms are likely to look damped compared with a waveform recorded under more controlled conditions in a special procedures room during catheter insertion. The damped appearance may be associated with a need to flush the infusion line, use of a slow speed to conserve paper during frequent bedside readings, and use of a small calibration scale to accommodate the pulmonary patient's high PA systolic and diastolic pressure readings. Therefore, to determine whether undesirable zone 1 or 2 conditions have really occurred, the nurse may try flushing the infusion line, increasing paper speed, or changing the calibration scale to obtain a clearer PCWP tracing. Moreover, continual efforts to assure a clear PCWP tracing, even in the midst of large respiratory variations, are important because the nurse may more effectively monitor components of the PCWP waveform. For example, identification of large v waves, as shown in Figure 29–12, may be the key finding leading to confirmation of mitral regurgitation.

Overwedging may occur as a PA catheter tip spontaneously floats further into a branch of the PA during coughing, turning, deep breathing, or other daily activities. A classic sign of overwedging is an upward sloping PCWP tracing, as shown in Figure 29–13. Overwedging may indicate a conversion of zone 3 conditions to zone 2 conditions and a need for catheter respositioning by the physician as well as better securing of the catheter at the insertion site. However, overwedging may also be due to inadvertent overinfla-

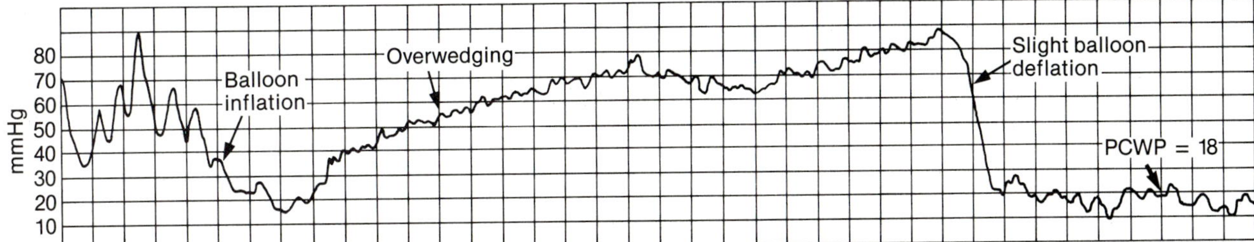

Figure 29–13. Overwedging due to inadvertent overinflation of the PA catheter's balloon.

tion of the balloon. In Figure 29–13, the nurse over-inflated the balloon by mistake. To correct the error, she slowly aspirated a minuscule amount of air until the normal PCWP waveform appeared. In subsequent PCWP readings, nurses caring for this extremely dyspneic patient were particularly careful to inject *only* enough air, and no more, to produce the change in waveform from PAP to PCWP. The amount of air required varied between readings largely because of changes in breathing pattern; intrapulmonary pressures; and, possibly, catheter tip position.

CARDIAC OUTPUT (Q)

Cardiac output (Q) is a major determinant of oxygen transport to the periphery. Changes in Q in pulmonary disease are described in Chapter 4 and are summarized in Table 29–2. Mechanisms responsible for the fall in Q associated with mechanical ventilation and PEEP are described in Chapter 28 and summarized in Table 29–3.

Q is measured utilizing the thermodilution method (Darovic, 1987). With the patient in the supine position, the nurse injects 3 to 10 ml of 5% dextrose or 0.9% saline at room temperature or iced through the RA port of the PA catheter. The rate and degree of temperature change sensed by a thermistor at the catheter tip is related to blood flow across the tip. A cardiac computer attached to the catheter calculates the Q in seconds and displays it digitally in L/min.

To reduce inaccuracy, the nurse takes the average of readings from three separate injections. If one reading is inconsistent with the other two readings, it is discarded; the two remaining readings are averaged. An inconsistent reading is one that varies by more than 10% from the other two readings (Kadota, 1985).

Emphasis is placed on the administration of each injection at the end of expiration, and as fast as possible, optimally over 1 to 3 seeconds. For tachypneic patients, the nurse may start the injection at the beginning of expiration, to insure injection completion at end-expiration. In spite of attention to optimal technique, however, if the patient is breathing spontaneously and out of phase with the ventilator, Q will vary unpredictably. In these cases, some clinicians recommend at least three determinations initiated at evenly spaced intervals during the respiratory cycle (Snyder and Powner, 1982).

Another way to reduce inaccuracy in readings in pulmonary patients is to use the iced injectate (0° to 4° C) rather than the room temperature injectate (19° to 25° C), whenever the patient's Q is extremely low (e.g., less than 3 L/min) and whenever the patient is hypothermic (e.g., postsurgery and during sepsis). These situations increase the probability of inaccurate readings, particularly when standard technique involves use of room temperature injectate. Use of iced injectate insures the required minimum of 10° difference between patient temperature and injectate temperature. It also improves accuracy when a closed injectate delivery system is used, rather than a prefilled syringe (Barcelona et al, 1985).

In patients in shock or with cardiomegaly and low stroke volume, the nurse may check the manufacturer's instructions for a special "delay start" injection technique to improve accuracy. This technique compensates for delayed injectant circulatory time in the body.

Cardiac Index (CI). Cardiac index is a more sensitive index of cardiac output (Q) because it takes into consideration differences in body size. CI is defined mathematically as *Q divided by body surface area* (BSA). The BSA is in m^2 and is taken from a nomogram (Fig. 29–14). Normal CI is 2.5 to 4.0 L/min/m^2. Abnormal readings lie outside this range. Increased and decreased CI values are interpreted in the same way as those for the increased and decreased Q values.

MIXED VENOUS OXYGEN PRESSURE AND ARTERIAL-VENOUS OXYGEN CONTENT DIFFERENCE ($P\bar{v}O_2$ and $C(a\text{-}\bar{v})O_2$)

The PA catheter allows sampling of mixed venous blood for the determination of $P\bar{v}O_2$ and $C(a\text{-}\bar{v})O_2$. As explained in Chapter 13, these parameters are important because they help the clinician assess the tissue oxygen extraction and the balance between total oxygen supply and demand at the tissue level.

The nurse draws the mixed venous blood sample from the PA catheter's distal port, as described in the box on page 767. The procedure for preparing a sample for laboratory analysis is the same as for any other ABG (see Chapter 13).

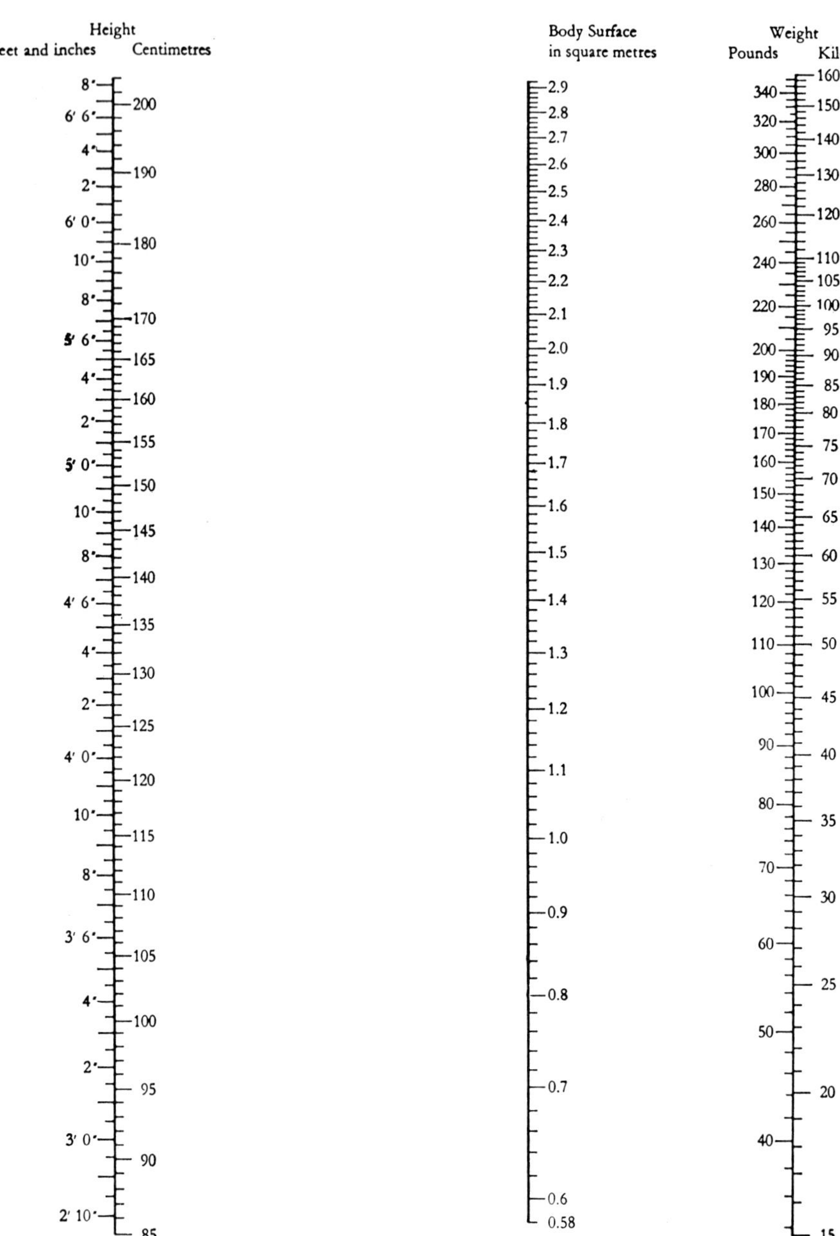

Figure 29–14. A body surface chart. *To determine a patient's body surface area* (1) locate height in feet and inches, or in centimeters, on the height scale (left); (2) locate weight in pounds or kilograms on the weight scale (right); (3) connect these two points with a straight edge; and (4) the point of intersection of the straight edge with the middle scale is the patient's body surface area in square meters. (Reproduced by permission from Meschan, I., Ott, D.: Introduction to Diagnostic Imaging. Philadelphia, W. B. Saunders Co., 1984.)

PROCEDURE FOR DRAWING MIXED VENOUS BLOOD FROM A PULMONARY ARTERY CATHETER

1. Gently aspirate the inflation valve to be sure the catheter balloon is deflated. Check to be sure a PA waveform, not a PCWP waveform, is on the monitor.
2. Locate an access point (i.e., stopcock) along the PA infusion line. The sample is never drawn from the proximal RA port because small veins continue to empty into the right side of the heart, and venous mixing is incomplete.
3. Aspirate 3 to 6 ml of blood or enough blood to clear the dead space of the tubing and catheter. Discard this sample.
4. Use a 3- to 5-cc heparinized syringe and slowly aspirate 2 to 3 ml of mixed venous blood. Slow and gentle aspiration prevents vessel walls from collapsing around the catheter and insures the acquisition of free flowing venous blood rather than arterial blood.
5. The $P\bar{v}CO_2$ result should be at least 2 mmHg greater than a simultaneously drawn $PaCO_2$ result. If this is not the case, assume the sample is arterial blood and carefully redraw another sample.

When arterial and mixed venous blood samples are drawn simultaneously, the arterial-venous oxygen content difference ($C(a\text{-}\bar{v})O_2$) is calculated (see Chapter 13). When considered together, PaO_2, $P\bar{v}O_2$, and $C(a\text{-}\bar{v})O_2$ help the clinician find the PEEP level that optimizes arterial and tissue oxygenation and reduces intrapulmonary shunting.

CONTINUOUS MONITORING OF $S\bar{v}O_2$

A special PA catheter made by Oximetrix (Mountain View, California) permits the monitoring of PA pressures, PCWP, RA pressure (CVP), and Q, as well as the continuous monitoring of $S\bar{v}O_2$. $S\bar{v}O_2$ is defined as *the percent saturation of hemoglobin with oxygen in mixed venous blood.* It is measured at the catheter tip utilizing the fiberoptics built into the catheter. A microprocessor averages the computed $S\bar{v}O_2$ values over a 5-second interval and continuously reports the value on a digital display and on a slow (4 in/hr) trend recorder. Examples of a $S\bar{v}O_2$ recording are shown in Figures 29–15 and 29–16. In Figure 29–15, note how giving packed red blood cells significantly increases $S\bar{v}O_2$. In Figure 29–16, note how the effects of therapy are readily observable on the tracing. Continuous monitoring of the critically ill patient in this way provides immediately available information for medical and nursing decision-making. Also, it reduces the number of blood samples the nurse must draw from the PA catheter and send to the laboratory for analysis. The reliability of $S\bar{v}O_2$ values is checked initially and periodically, as needed, by comparing the graphic display $S\bar{v}O_2$ with a laboratory $S\bar{v}O_2$ value obtained at the same time. Otherwise, blood sampling for laboratory analysis is unnecessary.

The normal $S\bar{v}O_2$ is between 60 and 80% (Paulus, 1987). Changes in value reflect changes in oxygen utilization at the tissue level (see Chapter 13). Though $S\bar{v}O_2$ may be employed primarily as a reflection of SaO_2, it is best employed with other parameters, such as PaO_2, SaO_2, $C(a\text{-}\bar{v})O_2$, and cardiac output, to assess oxygenation.

Conclusion

This chapter provides a general overview of hemodynamic monitoring to enhance comprehension of con-

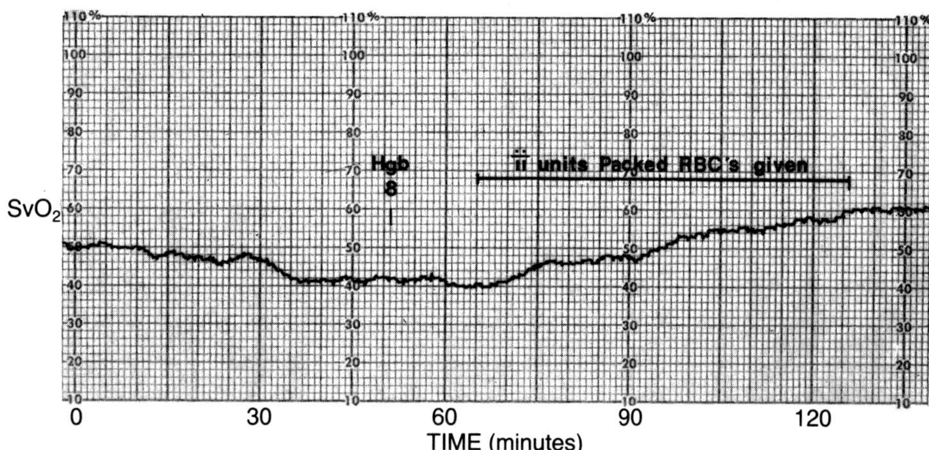

Figure 29–15. $S\bar{v}O_2$ as a reflection of change in hemoglobin. (Reproduced by permission from Darovic, G. Hemodynamic Monitoring—Invasive and Noninvasive Clinical Applications. Philadelphia, W. B. Saunders Co., 1987.)

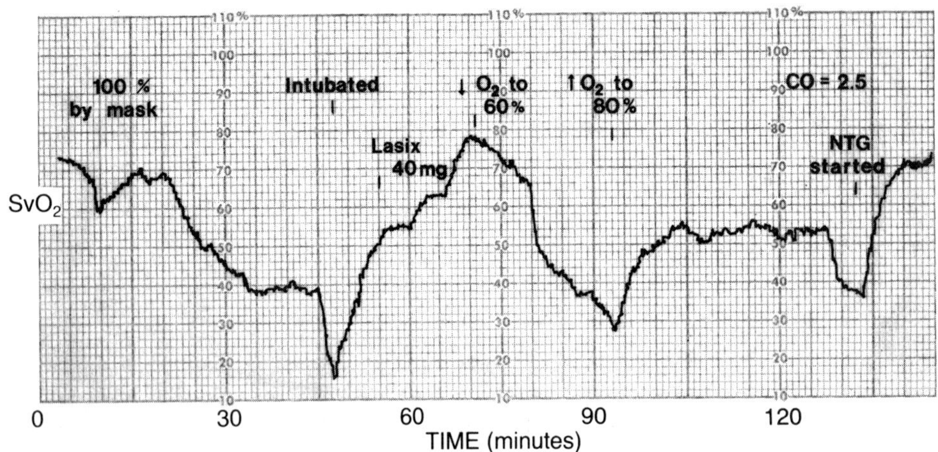

Figure 29–16. Wide fluctuations in $S\bar{v}O_2$ bar that reflect the patient's response to treatment for hypoxemia and cardiac pump failure. NTG = nitroglycerin; CO = cardiac output (Q). (Reproduced by permission from Darovic, G. Hemodynamic Monitoring—Invasive and Noninvasive Clinical Applications. Philadelphia, W. B. Saunders Co., 1987.)

tent in other chapters of this book. In addition, it provides basic respiratory applications to complement existing cardiovascular literature on the topic.

Monitoring the pulmonary patient with a PA catheter remains a nursing challenge because it is the nurse who takes pressure tracings, finds end-expiratory points, and averages values for final determinations. It is the nurse who calms the combative patient who is on mechanical ventilation, works to overcome technical problems, and questions the continued use of the PA catheter in uncomplicated cases of ARDS, postcoronary artery bypass surgery, and myocardial infarction. Most important, when the accuracy of pressure readings is limited by COPD or hemorrhagic shock, it is the nurse who must utilize other assessment parameters besides the PCWP for the safe administration of fluids or medications.

The nurse is now prepared to meet these challenges and provide reliable measurements for decision-making in spite of great fluctuations in respiratory pressure waveforms. However, when unreliable measurements are unavoidable or when indications for catheter placement are no longer present, the nurse's duty is to encourage catheter discontinuation. Such invasive technology is appropriate only when benefits clearly outweigh risks of complications.

REFERENCES

American Edwards Laboratories: Understanding Hemodynamic Measurements Made with the Swan-Ganz Catheter. Santa Ana, California, American Edwards Laboratories, Division of American Hospital Supply Co.

Barcelona, M., Patague, L., et al: Cardiac output determination by the thermodilution method: comparison of ice-temperature injectate versus room-temperature injectate contained in prefilled syringes or a closed injectate delivery system. *Heart and lung*, 14(3):232–235, 1985.

Bellamy, P. and Mercurio, P.: An alternative method for coordinating pulmonary capillary wedge pressure measurements with the respiratory cycle. *Critical care medicine*, 14(8):733–734, 1984.

Bodai, B.: Use of the pulmonary arterial catheter in the critically ill patient. *Heart and lung*, 11(5):406–416, 1982.

Bone, R., Goheen, J., and Ruth, W.: Radiographic, hemodynamic and clinical comparison of pulmonary venous hypertension complicating acute respiratory failure in severe chronic airway obstruction. *Chest*, 71(2):284–287, 1977.

Boyd, K., Thomas, S., Gold, J., and Boyd, A.: A prospective study of complications of pulmonary artery catheterizations in 500 consecutive patients. *Chest*, 84(3):245–248, 1983.

Brandstetter, R. and Gitler, B.: Thoughts on the Swan-Ganz catheter. *Chest*, 89(1):5–6, 1986.

Cengiz, M., Crapo, R., and Gardner, R.: The effect of ventilation on the accuracy of pulmonary artery and wedge pressure measurements. *Critical care medicine*, 11(7):502–507, 1983.

Daily, E. and Schroeder, J.: Hemodynamic Waveforms—Exercises in Identification and Analysis. St. Louis, C.V. Mosby Co., 1983.

Daily, E. and Schroeder, J.: Techniques in Bedside Hemodynamic Monitoring, 3rd ed. St. Louis, C.V. Mosby Co., 1985.

Darovic, G.: Hemodynamic Monitoring—Invasive and Noninvasive Clinical Applications. Philadelphia, W.B. Saunders Co., 1987.

Dorinsky, P. and Whitcomb, M.: The effect of PEEP on cardiac output. *Chest*, 84(2):210–216, 1983.

Gershan, J.: Effect of PEEP on pulmonary capillary wedge pressure. *Heart and lung*, 12(2):143–148, 1983.

Guzzetta, C. and Dossey, B. (eds.): Cardiovascular Nursing—Bodymind Tapestry. St. Louis, C.V. Mosby Co., 1984.

Kadota, L.: Theory and application of thermodilution cardiac output measurement: a review. *Heart and lung*, 14(6):605–614, 1985.

Keating, D., Bolyard, K., Eichler, E., and Reed, J.: Effect of side lying positions on pulmonary artery pressures. *Heart and lung*, 15(6):605–610, 1986.

Keefer, J. and Barash, P.: Pulmonary artery catheterization—a decade of clinical progress? *Chest*, 84(3):241–242, 1983.

O'Quin, R. and Marini, J.: Pulmonary artery occlusion pressure: clinical physiology, measurement, and interpretation. *American review of respiratory disease*, 128(2):319–326, 1983.

Osgood, C., Watson, M., Slaughter, M., and MacIntyre, N.: Hemodynamic monitoring in respiratory care. *Respiratory care*, 29(1):25–34, 1984.

Palmer, P.: Advanced hemodynamic assessment. *Dimensions of critical care nursing*, 1(3):139–144, 1982.

Paulus, D.: Invasive monitoring of respiratory gas exchange: continuous measurement of mixed venous oxygen saturation. *Respiratory care*, 32(7):535–541, 1987.

Raper, R. and Sibbald, W.: Misled by the wedge? The Swan-Ganz catheter and left ventricular preload. *Chest*, 89(3):427–434, 1986.

Riedinger, M., Shellock, F., and Swan, H.: Reading pulmonary artery and pulmonary capillary wedge pressure waveforms with respiratory variations. *Heart and lung*, 10(4):675–678, 1981.

Smucker, M.: Cardiovascular monitoring of patients with pulmonary disease. *Heart and lung*, 15(3):244–250, 1986.

Snow, N.: Preinduction use of pulmonary artery catheters during cardiac surgery. *Chest*, 83(3):587, 1983.

Snyder, J. and Powner, D.: Effects of mechanical ventilation on the measurement of cardiac output by thermodilution. *Critical care medicine*, 10(10):677–681, 1982.

Wilkins, R., Sheldon, R., and Krider, S.: Clinical Assessment in Respiratory Care. St. Louis, The C.V. Mosby Co., 1985.

Chest Tube Drainage Systems and Post-thoracotomy Care

30

Main Objectives

1. Define the following terms: thoracostomy, thoracotomy, pleural tube, mediastinal tube, Heimlich's one-way valve, thoracentesis, vented sump tube, straight and right-angled tubes, waterseal, tidalling, chest tube stripping, and pleurodesis.
2. State the indications for and purpose of a chest tube drainage system.
3. Explain the difference between an intrapleural and mediastinal tube in terms of anatomic location and danger to the patient during accidental disconnection.
4. Describe and state implications for monitoring one-, two-, three-, and four-bottle chest tube drainage systems.
5. Discuss the following aspects of post-thoracotomy care: optimal patient positioning in bed; arm and shoulder range of motion exercises; pain relief; body position and incisional support during deep breathing exercises; and monitoring of chest tube drainage, tube patency, amount of suction, breath sounds, and chest tube dressing.
6. Differentiate between milking and stripping a chest tube. Explain why stripping is now rarely used in the clinical setting.
7. State the significance of the absence of bubbling in the waterseal chamber of a patient with a mediastinal sump tube.

8. **Describe the use of chest tube clamps for a patient with a chest tube drainage system.**
9. **State six interventions for reducing the size of a bronchopleural fistula (i.e., air leak) in a patient on mechanical ventilation.**
10. **State indications and techniques for chest tube removal.**
11. **Explain why the pulmonary patient is at increased risk for postoperative pulmonary complications.**
12. **Describe the role of general anesthetics, opiates, and barbiturates in postoperative complications. State at least four interventions for reducing or eliminating adverse effects involving the respiratory, cardiovascular, and central nervous systems.**

The main body of this chapter discusses chest tube drainage systems and related post-thoracotomy care. The content prepares the nurse to care for any patient with a chest tube or chest tube drainage system.

The last section of the chapter focuses solely on the post-thoracotomy patient and the prevention of postoperative complications related to the administration of general anesthetics. These agents play a major role in postoperative complications in any pulmonary patient receiving general anesthesia.

Indications

A drainage system is required after chest tube placement for surgery involving the thorax (i.e., thoracotomy procedures), pneumothorax, pleural effusion, and other disorders listed in the box.

The purpose of the chest tube drainage system is threefold as follows: (1) to drain air, fluid, or both from the chest cavity; (2) to prevent drainage from reentering the chest; and (3) to restore and maintain normal pleural and intrathoracic pressures throughout the respiratory cycle.

INDICATIONS FOR CHEST TUBE PLACEMENT

Thoracotomy surgical procedure
Pneumothorax
- Spontaneous pneumothorax: large (20 to 25% or greater); symptomatic patient; presence of underlying lung disease
- Tension pneumothorax with dyspnea and mediastinal shift
- Progressive iatrogenic pneumothorax

Pleural effusion
Hemothorax
Pneumohemothorax
Chylothorax
Empyema
Sucking wound from penetrating chest trauma
Bronchopleural fistula

Chest Tube Insertion

One or two chest tubes are inserted in surgery, in the emergency room, or in a hospital ward. In the last case, most instruments and supplies are on the emergency thoracostomy tray. *Thoracostomy* is defined as insertion of a tube through a closed chest, whereas the term *thoracotomy* refers to the incision itself.

The physician may use one of a variety of straight and right-angled chest tubes. Most tubes are made of vinyl, Silastic, or latex nonthrombogenic material and are multifenestrated to prevent tip occlusion from clots and adjacent tissue. Commonly used tubes are the straight type (Fig. 30–1). They are usually transparent and may have distance markers to guide correct positioning in the pleural space. Sizes depend on the internal diameter of the tube. Large tubes (i.e., 20 to 36 French or 5 to 11 mm internal diameter) are used

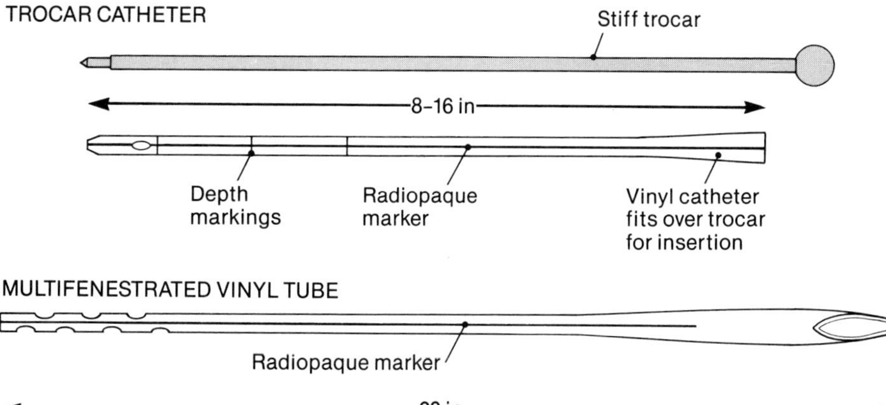

Figure 30–1. Straight chest tubes.

to drain blood or thick pleural debris. Smaller tubes (i.e., 16 to 20 French) are used for pneumothorax and most pleural effusions. Similar to endotracheal tubes, chest tubes have radiopaque markers to assess their position within the chest on the chest x-ray film.

To insert a tube, the physician infiltrates a local anesthetic under the skin and uses one of two surgical methods as follows: (1) the trocar method, which involves chest penetration with a pointed metal trocar, and removal of the trocar, leaving the catheter in place (Fig. 30–1A) and (2) the blunt dissection method, which involves use of forceps for blunt dissection into the pleural space for tube insertion (Fig. 30–2). After chest tube insertion, the external end of the chest tube is connected to a chest drainage unit (Fig. 30–3). To prevent tube displacement, the physician sutures skin next to the tube, wraps the ends of the suture around the tube, and ties off the ends, thus anchoring the tube to the chest wall. Bacteriostatic ointment may be applied to the incisional site. Though some physicians may prefer to cover the site with petroleum gauze to prevent air leaks, dry gauze is recommended because petroleum gauze may macerate the skin and predispose the patient to infection (Miller and Sahn, 1987). A 4 × 4 square of gauze is cut down the center, split over the tube, and taped occlusively to the chest. Also, the tube is taped to the chest to prevent tension on the tube and sutures during movement (Fig. 30–4).

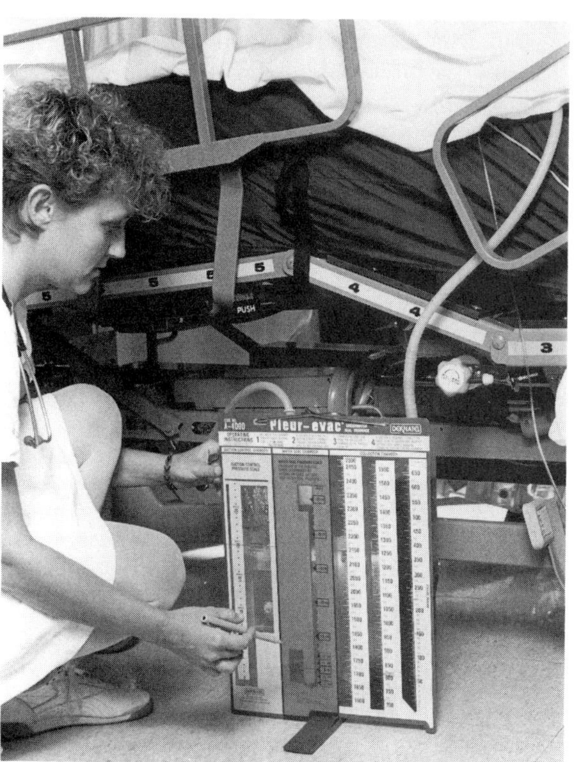

Figure 30–3. A nurse marks the level of fluid drainage in a Pleur-evac chest tube drainage system.

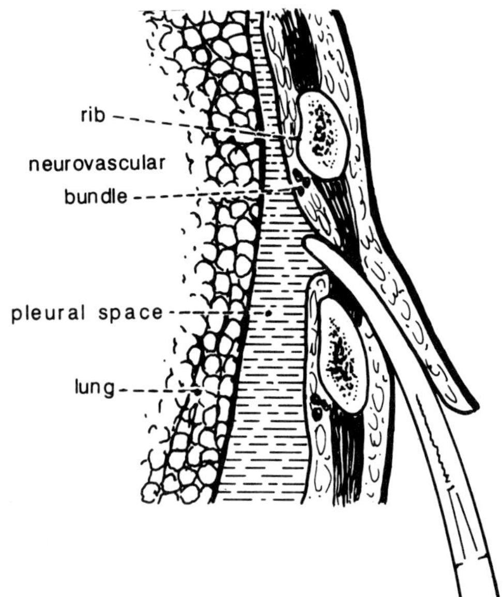

Figure 30–2. Blunt dissection method of chest tube insertion. The skin incision is made with a scalpel, and the forceps penetrates the pleural space as shown. After dilatation of the tract with a finger, the chest tube is clamped at the proximal end with the forceps and inserted into the pleural space. (Reproduced by permission from Miller, K. and Sahn, S. Chest tubes: indications, technique, management and complications. *Chest*, 91(2):260, 1987.)

PLEURAL AND MEDIASTINAL CHEST TUBES

Chest tubes are classified as pleural or mediastinal tubes, depending on the intrapleural versus mediastinal location of the tube's tip.

Pleural chest tubes are always inserted into the anterior chest area, preferably anterior to the midaxillary line to prevent the patient from lying on the tube. To drain air, an intrapleural tube is placed in

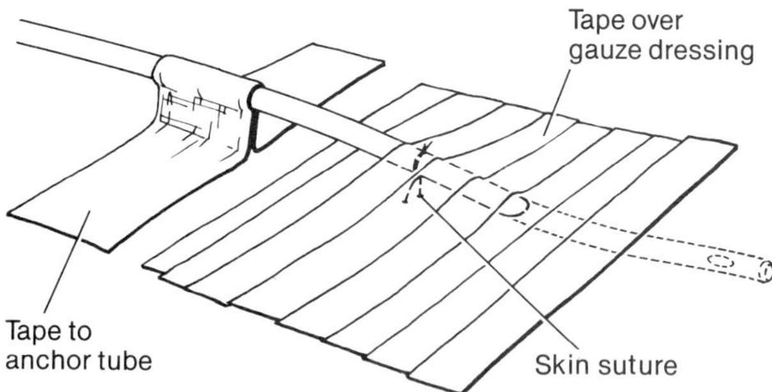

Figure 30–4. Occlusive chest tube dressing with the tube properly anchored to the chest. The dotted lines represent the tube under the dressing, sutured to the skin, and draining the chest. Tape anchors and suture anchors prevent side-to-side movement and outward movement of the tube, respectively.

the lung apex at the second or third intercostal space, midclavicular line (ICS, MCL). To drain fluid, the tube is placed in the lateral chest area at the fourth or fifth ICS, anterior axillary line (AAL) and sometimes as low as the eighth or ninth ICS, midaxillary line (MAL). The tube's tip is advanced several inches into the pleural space along the surface of the lung.

Tubes inserted just before chest closure during cardiac surgery are usually mediastinal, not pleural space tubes. One tube is positioned in the anterior mediastinum beneath the sternum, exiting the chest at the epigastrium. In addition, a right-angled tube may be placed more inferiorly between the diaphragm and the inferior pericardium.

Chest tubes inserted in a trauma patient may be pleural, mediastinal, or both depending on the extent of pathology. Similarly, some mediastinal tubes inserted during cardiac surgery may also be pleural tubes, if surgery either intentionally or unintentionally extended into the lung's pleura. Although a true mediastinal tube differs from a pleural tube (negative inspiratory pressures are not as great, and lung collapse does not occur with accidental disconnection), *all* chest tubes are treated as if they were intrapleural tubes. The following discussion pertains to an intrapleural chest tube unless otherwise stated.

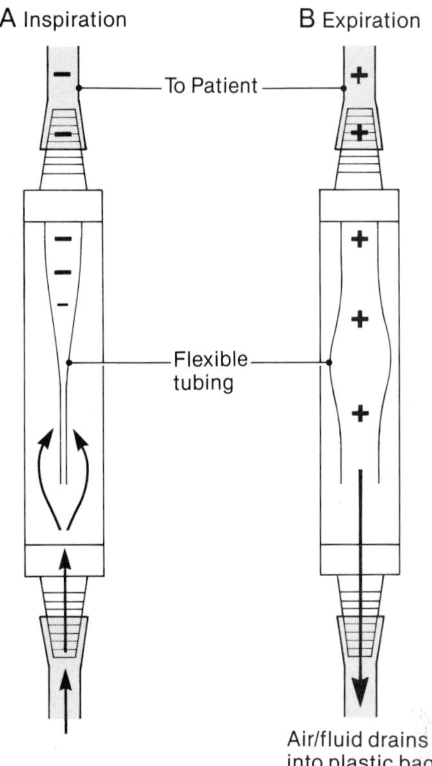

Figure 30–5. Heimlich's one-way valve. *A*, During inspiration, negative intrapleural pressure collapses the flexible tubing and prevents outside air from entering the thorax. *B*, During expiration, positive pressure opens the flexible tubing and allows air and fluid to drain into an attached plastic bag.

ATTACHMENT TO DRAINAGE SYSTEM OR ONE-WAY VALVE

Usually, chest tubes are attached to a drainage system. However, if interhospital transport is anticipated, a tube may be attached to Heimlich's one-way valve instead (Fig. 30–5). This valve permits air and fluid to drain out, without allowing the same air to travel back into the chest and enter the lungs during inspiration. A sterile dressing or glove is taped over the end of the tube. Sometimes, this valve is used in the hospitalized patient for pneumothorax that is taking days to weeks to resolve.

THORACENTESIS

Occasionally, the evacuation of fluid from the pleural space is needed, but insertion of a chest tube is not indicated. For example, the physician may need only a small amount of pleural fluid for the medical diagnosis, or a pleural fluid evacuation is desired to relieve dyspnea and discomfort in the patient with recurring pleural effusions.

In these cases, the physician performs a *thoracentesis* procedure, defined as insertion of a needle into the pleural space to drain air and fluid. For this procedure, the patient sits on the edge of the bed with arms resting across the bedside table. While the nurse helps the patient maintain this position, the physician injects local anesthetic into the posterior chest area above the diaphragm. An 18-gauge spinal needle attached to a three-way stopcock is introduced over the top of a lower rib and into the pleural space. A small amount of pleural fluid for laboratory analysis is removed via a syringe attached to the stopcock. The rest of the fluid is drained into a plasma vacuum bottle.

Alternatively, thoracentesis is performed in the recumbent position with the patient's arm resting behind his head or away from the side. The recumbent position is associated with improved patient comfort, a reduced incidence of nausea and lightheadedness, and a reduced need for pain medication (Fishman, 1983). A 14-gauge needle (e.g., Intracath) is used for chest penetration, and a plastic needle catheter is used for drainage into a vacuum bottle (Fig. 30–6).

Penetration into the pleural space is commonly called a *tap*. When a tap is unproductive of air or fluid, it is termed *dry*. A *traumatic* tap occurs when blood is aspirated by a syringe after initial chest penetration, as in an inadvertent puncture of the liver or spleen.

When large amounts of pleural fluid are anticipated, a chest tube drainage system is used for fluid evacuation. After needle withdrawal from the chest, the puncture site is dressed with an antiseptic and occlusive dressing.

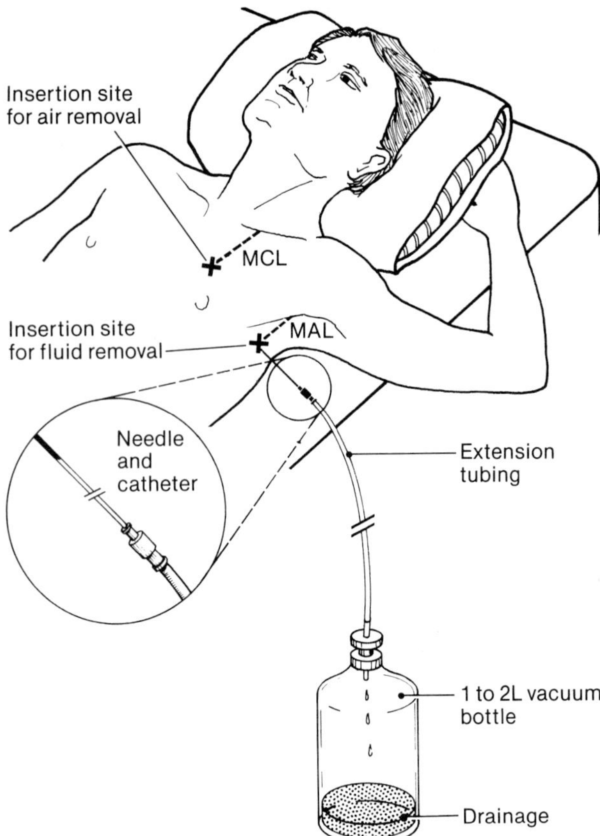

Figure 30–6. Recumbent body position and insertion sites for thoracentesis. The insertion site for air removal is the second or third intercostal space (ICS), midclavicular line (MCL). The site for fluid removal is typically the fourth or fifth ICS, midaxillary line (MAL).

The complication rate of thoracentesis is relatively high. Seneff and associates (1986) found that about 46% of thoracentesis procedures are complicated with at least one adverse occurrence. Major complications compose 14% of cases, and minor complications compose 33%. The most commonly occurring major complication is pneumothorax. Minor complications include pain, persistent cough, dry taps, and subcutaneous fluid collections.

Types of Drainage Systems

The availability of numerous types of commercial chest tube drainage systems as well as the limited knowledge and experience of health care professionals working with the different types often decrease the efficiency and effectiveness of clinical problem solving. To reduce confusion, to prepare clinicians to deliver optimal patient care, and to promote critical analysis of more recently developed drainage systems, this text focuses on establishing a baseline knowledge of the one-, two-, three-, and four-bottle drainage systems. Though packaged in different forms, most modern drainage units are one of these systems.

ONE-BOTTLE SYSTEM

This system works best when used to drain air or a small amount of fluid from the chest (Fig. 30–7). The single bottle serves as a collection chamber, as drainage flows by gravity 2 to 3 feet below the level of the patient's chest into the empty bottle. It also serves as a *waterseal*. Before connection to the patient, the bottle is filled with sterile normal saline so that the tip of the long waterseal tube lies 2 cm underneath the water. This waterseal then seals the chest, thus maintaining negative pressures during breathing and preventing the retrograde movement of air back into the chest. If for some reason the waterseal is lost (e.g., evaporation or accidental tipping of the bottle on its side) and the tube's tip communicates with the atmosphere, negative pleural pressures will pull air into the chest to create a pneumothorax.

During normal respiration, the fluid in the waterseal tube moves up towards the chest during inspiration and down during expiration, since pleural pressure becomes more negative during inspiration and more positive during expiration. This so-called *tidalling* is exactly reversed during mechanical ventilation. Positive pressure pushes the waterseal fluid level down on inspiration and allows the level to fluctuate upwards during passive expiration. Normal tidalling is from 2 to 12 cmH_2O, depending on the patient's activity and the diameter of the tube; it may increase to over 20 cmH_2O during vigorous coughing, upper airway obstruction, or respiratory distress.

When setting up the one-bottle system, the nurse is careful to fill the bottle to no more than 2 cm above the waterseal tube tip. A higher fluid level may significantly increase work of breathing, since the patient has a longer column of fluid to move during respiration, and more positive pressure is required to push drainage out through the waterseal.

Bubbling is normally absent in the waterseal of a properly functioning chest tube drainage system. However, immediately after chest tube insertion and occasionally thereafter, bubbling is seen as air and fluid drain from the pleural cavity. The rate of bubbling correlates with the rate of drainage.

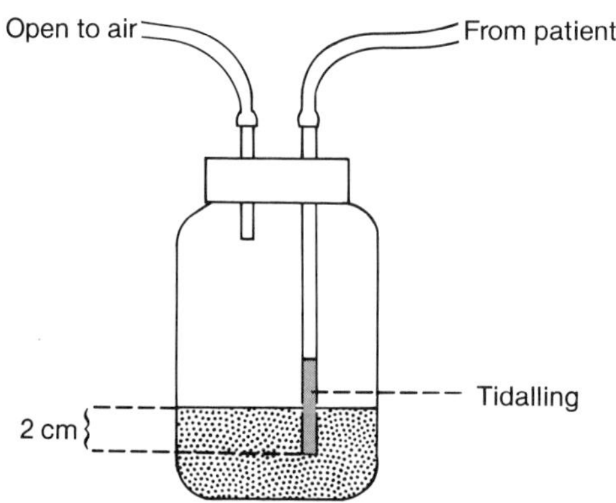

Figure 30–7. One-bottle chest drainage system for gravity drainage.

In Figure 30–7, as drainage accumulates in the bottle, air is displaced to the atmosphere via the short tube open to air. Most important, the vent or tube open to air is *never* clamped or occluded. Clamping suppresses drainage and may result in a pneumothorax.

TWO-BOTTLE SYSTEM

A variety of two-bottle systems are used in the clinical setting. The system in Figure 30–8A functions in the same manner as the one-bottle system, except drainage and waterseal components are separate. This arrangement facilitates the monitoring of drainage output and avoids the previously described situation in which drainage accumulation increases the work of breathing.

The system in Figure 30–8B is essentially a one-bottle system with a dead-space bottle attached for connection to suction. Some machines are supplied with this extra bottle to protect the suction source from inadvertent siphoning of fluid into the machinery. A dead-space bottle may be added to a three-bottle system as well.

The physician may order suctioning for more effective drainage, particularly when the chest x-ray film shows incomplete evacuation of air or fluid from the pleural space. The simplest way to add suction to a two-bottle system is to attach it directly to a machine, such as the Emerson or Sorenson pump. It is quieter than wall suction, uses an electrical source of power, and permits the selection of precise levels of negative suction of up to at least 50 cmH_2O.

Figure 30–8C is a one-bottle system attached to a suction control bottle, which in turn is connected to wall suction. When fluid drainage becomes excessive, the physician may switch to a three-bottle system.

THREE-BOTTLE SYSTEM

This system consists of the standard two-bottle system illustrated in Figure 30–8A, with the addition of a suction control bottle (Fig. 30–9A).

Suction facilitates evacuation of a large volume of air or fluid. In addition, it is used to compensate for a small diameter chest tube and to keep the lung expanded when a continuous air leak or bronchopleural

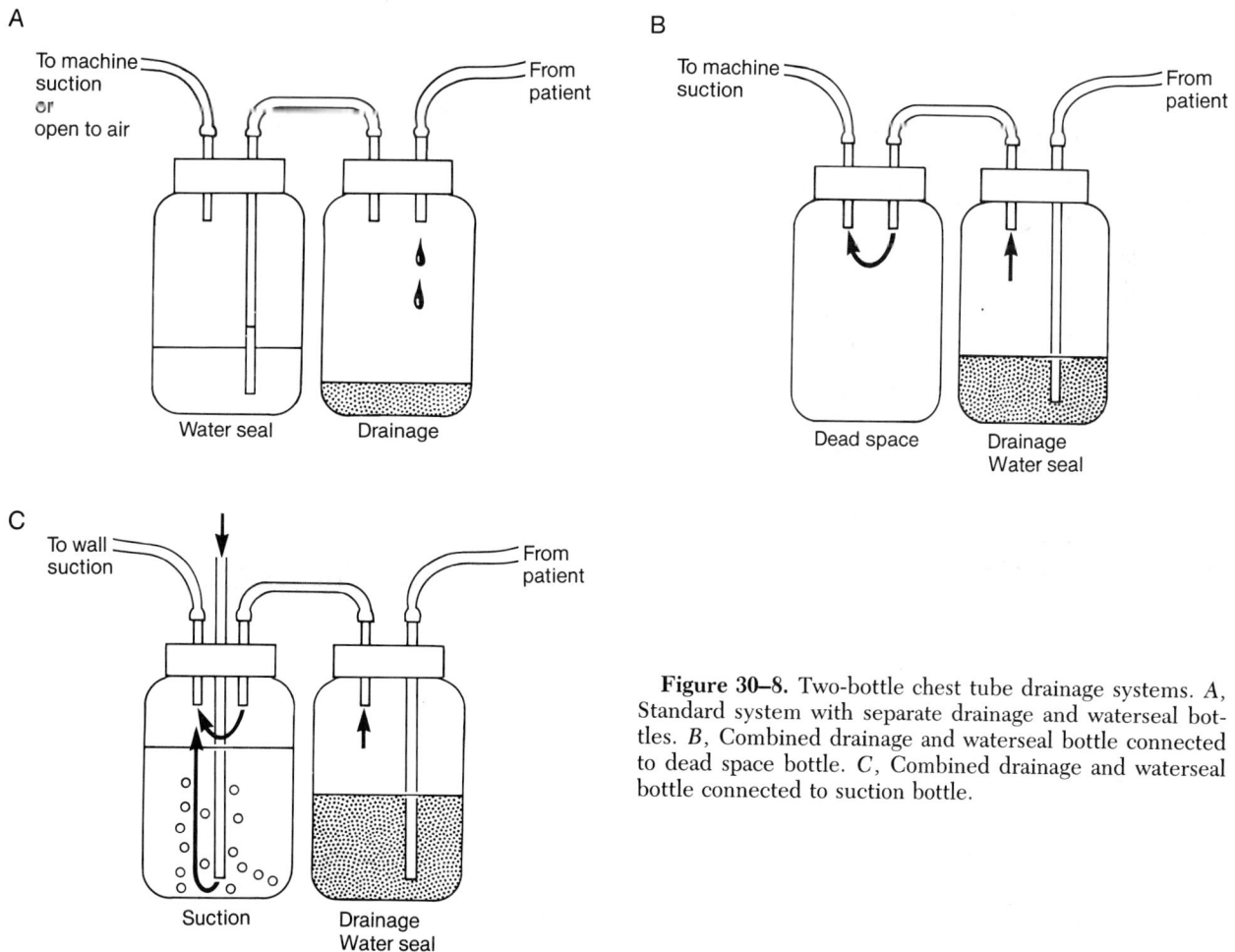

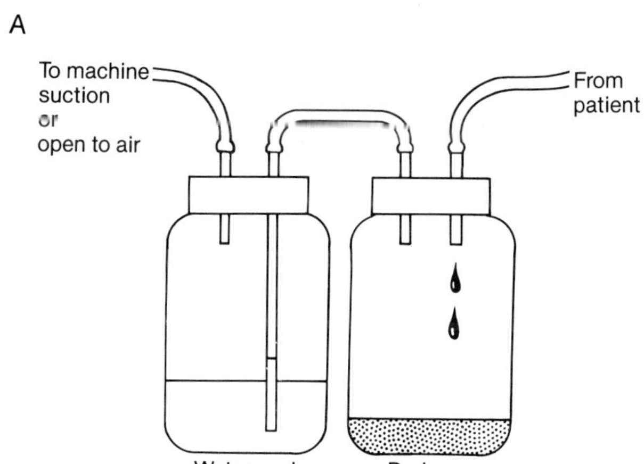

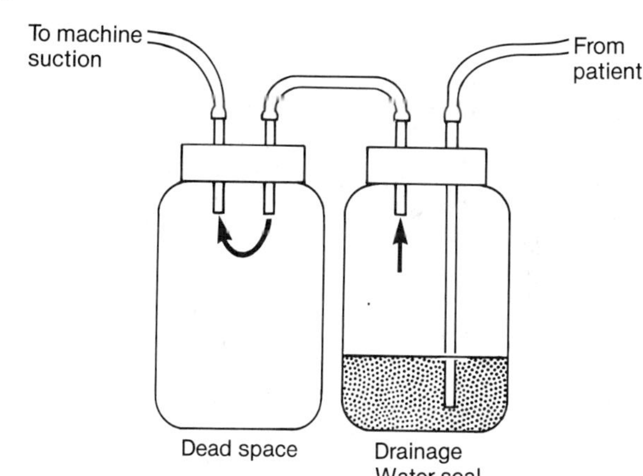

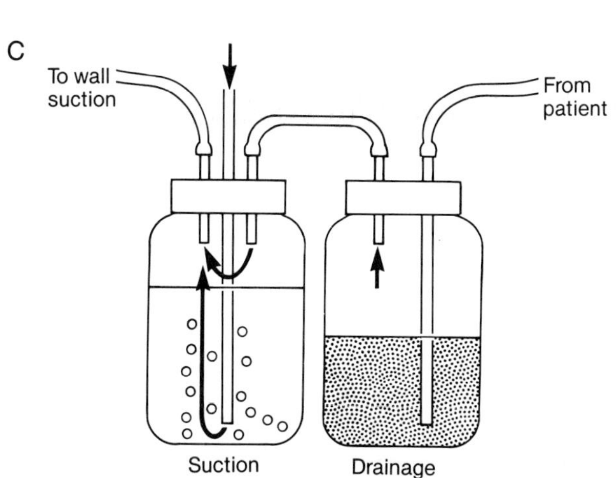

Figure 30–8. Two-bottle chest tube drainage systems. *A*, Standard system with separate drainage and waterseal bottles. *B*, Combined drainage and waterseal bottle connected to dead space bottle. *C*, Combined drainage and waterseal bottle connected to suction bottle.

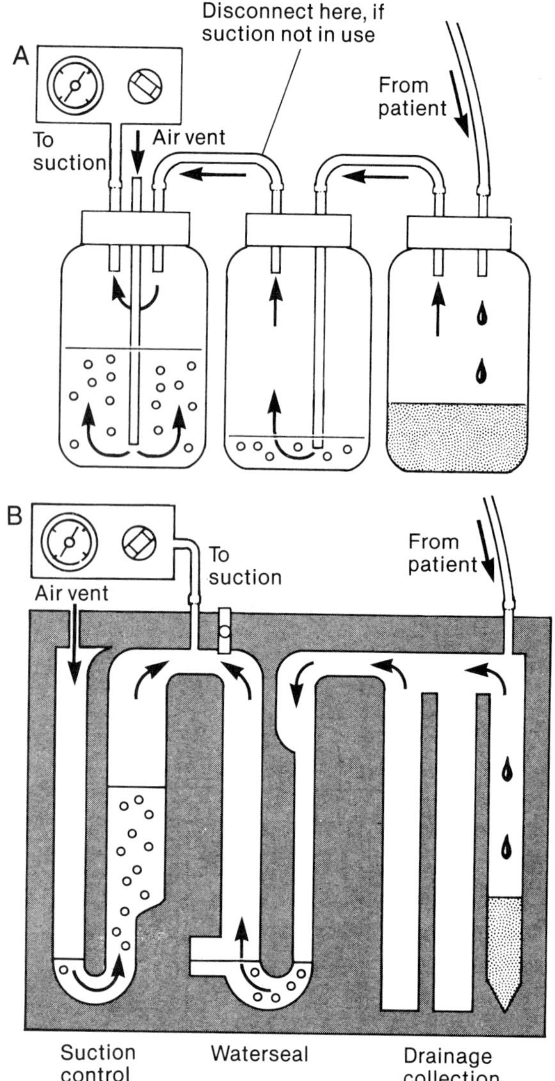

Figure 30–9. Three bottle (chamber) chest tube drainage systems. *A*, Standard three-bottle system. *B*, Pleur-evac system. (Reproduced and adapted by permission from Luce, J., Tyler, M., and Pierson, D. Intensive Respiratory Care. Philadelphia, W. B. Saunders Co., 1984.)

fistula is present. Most thoracic surgeries, including routine thoracotomies, open heart procedures, lung resections, and diaphragmatic or esophageal operations require at least 10 to 20 cmH_2O of suction. Although suction is needed to drain clots, debris, and fresh blood from the chest, it may also increase an air leak. For example, a small air leak manifested by intermittent bubbling in the waterseal bottle is not uncommon in the postsurgical patient, but it usually seals off spontaneously within 1 or 2 days. Suction may draw lung tissue and chest wall surfaces together to promote healing, but excessive early suction applied to an inelastic lung may further open a leak.

The drainage of fluid and subsequent displacement of air towards the source of suction is summarized in Figure 30–9A. As in the one- and two-bottle setups, tidalling is observed in the waterseal tube, but fluctuations are reduced because of the application of continuous suction. In this system, *it is the depth of the long suction tube under water or normal saline and not the amount of wall suction that determines the amount of suction delivered to the patient.* As wall suction is gradually increased, air is first sucked up from the waterseal bottle. Additional suction pulls atmospheric air down through the suction tube. The air bubbles through the waterseal and exits via the wall suction. As the suction tube is placed deeper in the water, the wall suction must be increased to overcome the extra water pressure necessary to pull in atmospheric air through the suction tube. Suction is increased to achieve gentle continuous bubbling. Vigorous bubbling is unnecessary and potentially dangerous, since it promotes evaporation and variation in the amount of suction delivered.

The popular Pleur-evac system (by Deknatel) is essentially a three-bottle drainage system assembled in one plastic unit (Fig. 30–9B), with only a few modifications. For example, the drainage chamber—three columns in a series—is calibrated to facilitate the monitoring of volume (Fig. 30–10). The waterseal chamber has three important features as follows: (1) a positive pressure release valve that vents excess pressure to the room (not visible in Fig. 30–10); (2) a float valve that maintains the waterseal during periods of high negative intrapleural pressure, e.g., maximal inspiration during vigorous coughing; and (3) a well indicator located just below the float valve. The well fills with fluid when high negative pressure pulls water up from the waterseal. Note that the suction control chamber can only be filled to 25 to 29 cmH_2O. Its air vent (located on the top, back side of the same chamber in Fig. 30–10) may be covered with a muffler that is sometimes mistaken for a plug.

FOUR-BOTTLE SYSTEM

The four-bottle system is a three-bottle system plus a safety valve and manometer bottle attached next to the drainage chamber, as shown in Figure 30–11A. The Double Seal plastic unit by Argyle (Fig. 30–11B) has the same basic design as the Pleur-evac system (see Fig. 30–10), except the sequence of the chambers is reversed and the pathway through the waterseal to the suction source is more tortuous. The fourth chamber serves as a positive pressure safety release valve should the suction become disconnected or obstructed. Also, it is a second waterseal and manometer, estimating negative pressure in the drainage chamber and pleural space.

OTHER TYPES OF DRAINAGE SYSTEMS AND ADDITIONAL FEATURES

Other drainage systems incorporate other combinations of the aforementioned bottle arrangements.

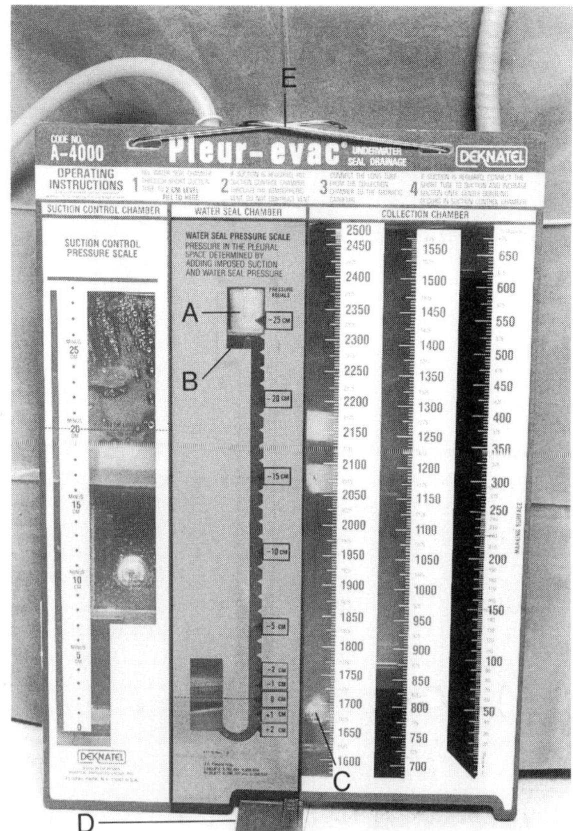

Figure 30–10. Pleur-evac chest drainage unit in operation. *A*, Float valve; *B*, Well indicator; *C*, Self-sealing diaphragm for drainage sampling (located on back side); *D*, Floor stand; *E*, Metal hooks to hang the unit on the side of the bed.

Additional features may include bedside stands, self-sealing diaphragms for specimens or water level adjustments, positive and negative pressure release valves, or suction control dials to replace the suction control bottles, e.g., Thora-Klex (Davol) (Fig. 30–12).

Pediatric units and some adult units incorporate an air flow meter underneath the waterseal to estimate the size of an air leak in L/min. Pediatric and infant units have drainage chambers calibrated in ½- to 1-ml increments.

Post-thoracotomy Nursing Care

Nursing care involves the monitoring of patient positioning, coughing, and deep breathing technique, pain medication, and other parameters discussed subsequently.

PATIENT POSITIONING

The head of the bed is elevated 20 to 30 degrees, and the patient is turned from side to side (as indicated by the situation) to promote chest drainage and prevent tube occlusion and atelectasis.

Note that the pneumonectomy patient usually has no chest tube because the hemithorax is expected to fill up with fluid and fibrose. If he has a tube, it may be clamped, connected to gravity drainage without suction, or connected to a special pneumonectomy drainage unit (e.g., Pleur-evac A-4301) that regulates pleural pressure to minimize the possibility of mediastinal shift. The physician may order that this type of patient be turned from the supine position to the affected operative side only. Lying on the operative side promotes fluid accumulation within the hemithorax and relieves pressure on the bronchial stump.

In addition to turning, arm and shoulder range of motion exercises may be performed to help prevent shoulder ankylosis, to minimize pain and chest discomfort, and to promote full lung expansion postoperatively. Initially, the nurse provides pain medication and performs passive arm exercises TID for the patient, slowly abducting the arm laterally and above the head, as tolerated. Then the patient may be taught to use a towel to put the affected arm and shoulder through range of motion exercises (Fig. 30–13). As the arm becomes stronger, the patient may use some of the active arm exercises described in Chapter 20. When chest trauma or surgery is extensive or recovery is slow, the nurse and physician consult the physical therapist to help establish an appropriate arm exercise regimen. The regimen may include gravity resistance exercises and arm weights to increase muscular strength and pulleys to reduce the effect of gravity on motion, thereby facilitating a greater range of motion for the shoulder joint (MacKenzie, 1981).

COUGHING AND DEEP BREATHING

A coughing and deep breathing technique is described in Chapter 19. Incentive spirometry (Chapter 19) or, in select cases, intermittent positive pressure breathing (IPPB) (Chapter 22) may be necessary to promote deep breathing every 1 to 2 hours. In addition huffing, called forced exhalation technique, may be used in conjunction with deep breathing to help loosen secretions before coughing.

Chapter 19 presents evaluation criteria to guide patient monitoring during coughing and deep breathing. Attention to the following parameters will facilitate the monitoring of post-thoracotomy patients who are trying to deep breathe effectively.

Pain Medication

Is the patient given adequate pain medication before deep breathing and coughing procedures? Before arm and shoulder range of motion exericises? Splinting and decreased breath sounds indicate poor lung expansion and a need for more pain medication. Effective deep breathing and coughing and full range of motion are difficult, if not impossible to achieve, if the patient is suffering from pain.

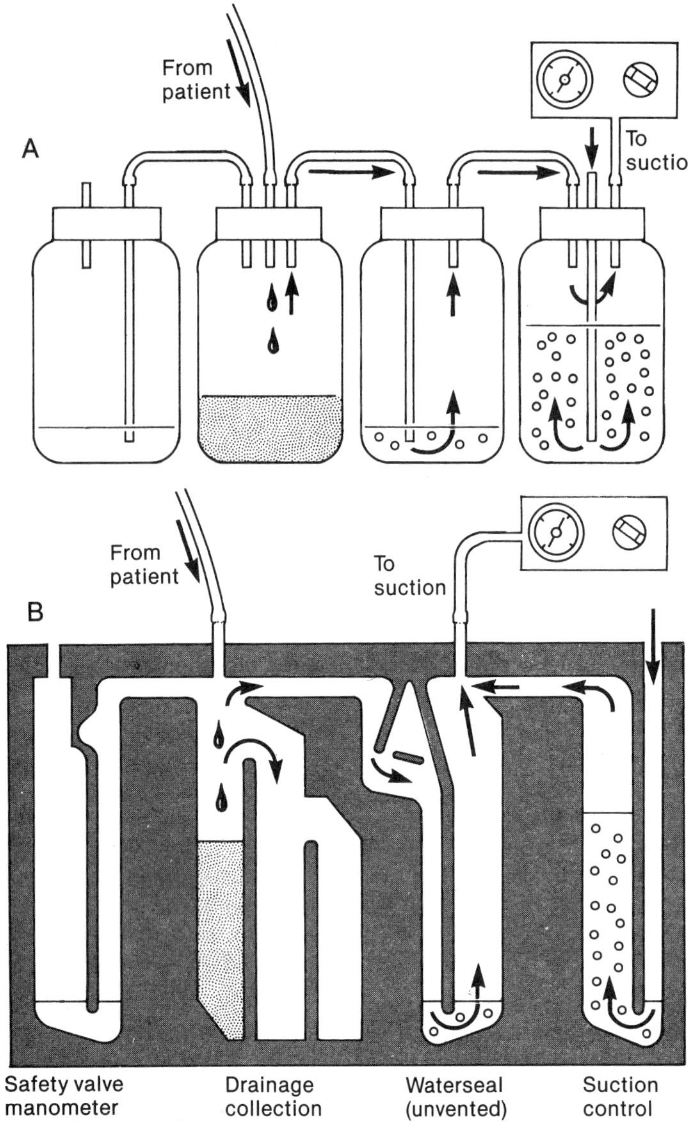

Figure 30–11. Four-bottle (chamber) chest tube drainage systems. *A*, Standard four-bottle system. *B*, Argyle Double-Seal drainage system. (Reproduced and adapted by permission from Luce, J., Tyler, M., and Pierson, D. Intensive Respiratory Care. Philadelphia, W. B. Saunders Co., 1984.)

Proper Body Position

For effective coughing and deep breathing, the patient sits upright in bed, over the edge of the bed, leaning over the bedside table for additional support, or in a chair. The upright position significantly increases functional residual capacity (FRC) and facilitates posterior excursions of the chest. In addition, activity to achieve the proper body alignment and the upright position helps mobilize respiratory secretions. For critically ill patients unable to achieve the upright position, elevate the head of the bed 30 to 40 degrees and flex the knees slightly.

Incisional Support

Does the patient know how to support his incision to reduce pain and discomfort? In the immediate postoperative period, the application of firm pressure over the incisional area with a pillow or folded bath blanket provides support (Fig. 30–14A). When the patient can lean forward or when chest tubes are removed, the nurse may use the method of supporting a lateral thoracotomy incision shown in Figure 30–14B. Anterior and posterior pressure is applied just below the incision. In addition, the patient is taught how to support his own lateral incision as shown in Figure 30–14C. The arm of the unaffected side is placed across the chest with the hand applying pressure just below the incision. The arm and elbow of the affected side apply pressure against the chest wall to further support the incisional site. As in method A, additional support may be gained in methods B and C by placing a small folded towel over the incision before the application of inward pressure.

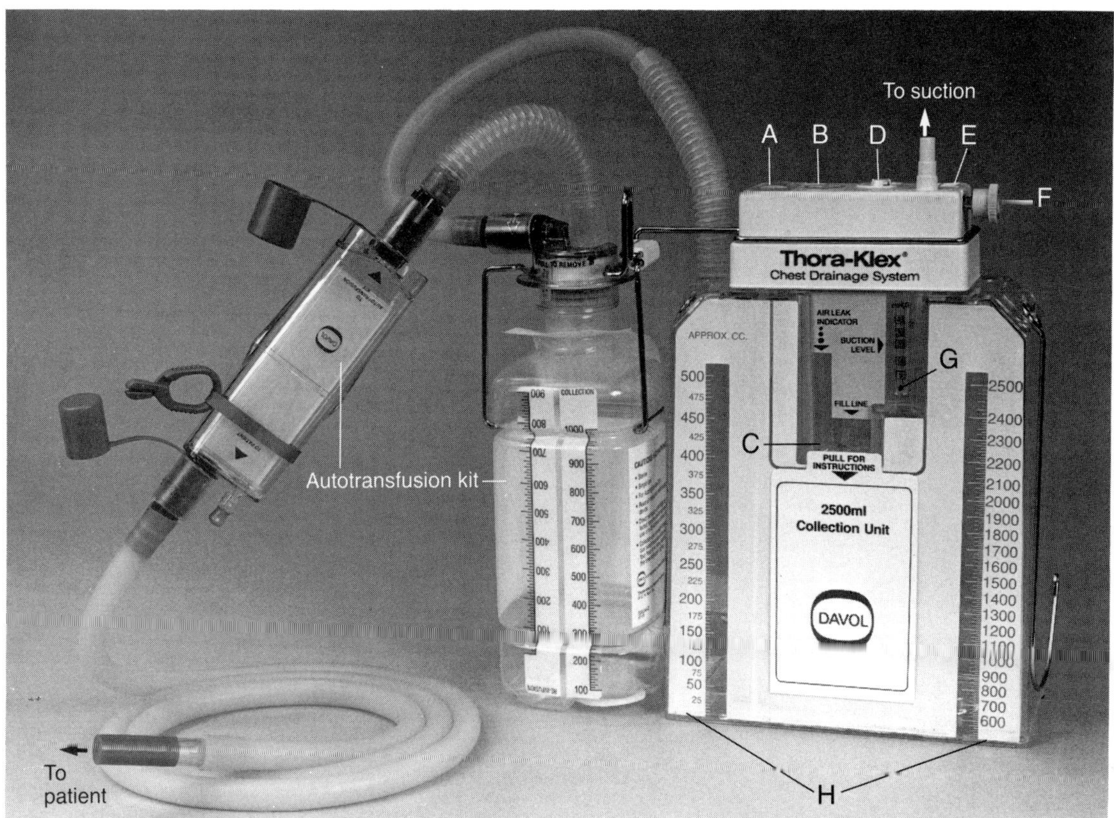

Figure 30–12. Thora-Klex "waterless" chest drainage unit. The adjustable suction control feature at the top of the unit substitutes for the waterseal chamber of a standard three-chamber unit. The autotransfusion kit is an accessory feature that provides postoperative blood collection and reinfusion. (Courtesy of Davol Inc., Cranston, Rhode Island.)

A, Negative pressure indicator. It reads YES when negative pressure is maintained.
B, Injection port. This port permits the injection of 15 cc of normal saline into the air leak indicator chamber.
C, Air leak indicator chamber used to monitor an air leak. *It does not serve as the waterseal.*
D, Negative pressure relief valve. It vents excess pressure over -50 cmH_2O.
E, Positive pressure relief valve.
F, Suction control dial. Turn counterclockwise to increase suction.
G, Suction level indicator (float ball).
H, Drainage chamber.

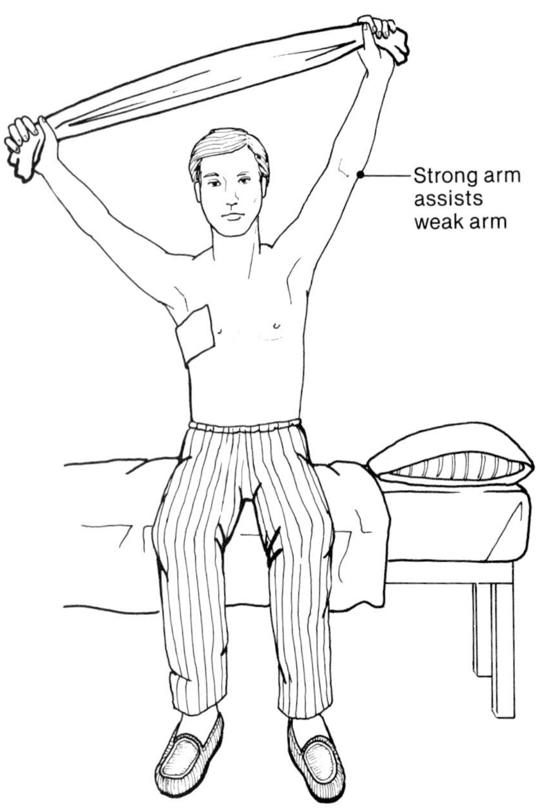

Figure 30–13. Post-thoracotomy arm and shoulder mobility exercises using a towel.

A. Recumbent position, mid-sternal incision

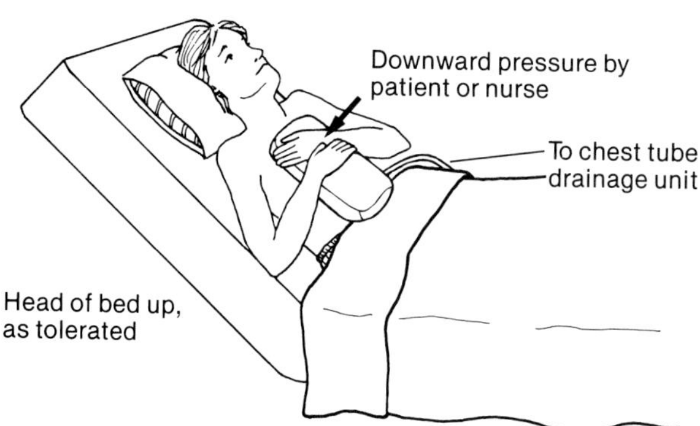

Figure 30–14. Providing incisional support during deep breathing and coughing.

B. Upright position, lateral incision supported by nurse

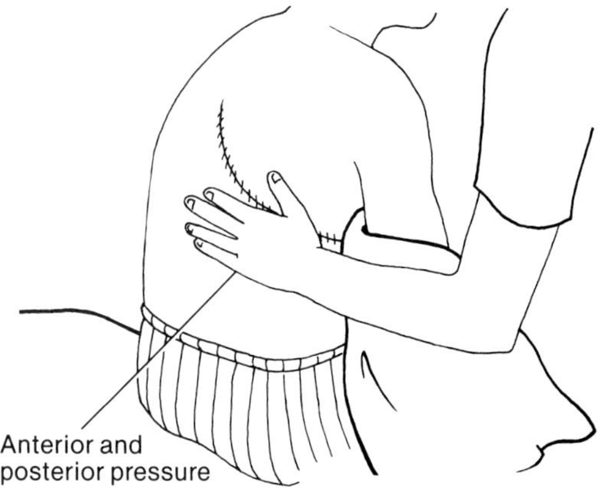

C. Upright position, lateral incision supported by patient

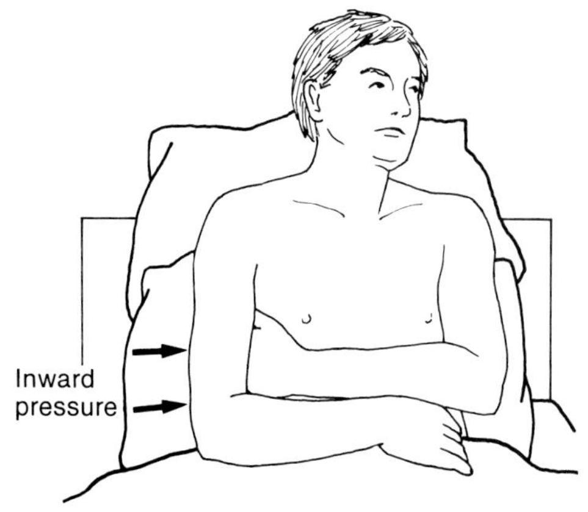

DRAINAGE

Note the color, consistency, and amount of chest tube drainage. Use a pen to mark the drainage level at the end of each shift, and calculate the total output in the bedside notes. Always monitor output during each set of vital signs. A *sudden increase* in drainage indicates hemorrhage or sudden patency of a kinked or obstructed tube. A *sudden decrease* in drainage indicates chest tube obstruction, tube malpositioning in the chest, or malfunctioning of the drainage system, e.g., loss of suction and excessive fluid accumulation in dependent loops of tubing.

To insure proper drainage, the nurse checks that the tubing is neither too short nor too long. Short tubing restricts patient movement and causes excessive traction on the tube. When fluid accumulates in coiled loops or long dependent loops, suction may become ineffective. Ideally, the tubing lies horizontally on the bed, extending 2 to 3 feet towards the foot and then *directly* down to the drainage system below (see Fig. 30–3).

For fluid drainage, the nurse lifts portions of tubing off the bed until the fluid drips into the drainage chamber. For bloody or thick drainage, squeezing the chest tube between fingers and palm and promptly releasing it helps to loosen clots from the tip and sides of the tubing (Fig. 30–15). This squeezing technique may be utilized along the length of the chest tube q15 to 30 minutes to insure tube patency after cardiac surgery. If tube obstruction is suspected, the physician may order chest tube *stripping* (described subsequently).

If fluid does not drain in spite of meticulous nursing care, the physician may order a chest x-ray film to check for proper tube placement in the pleural space. Repositioning the tube's tip by pockets of fluid through guidance of the x-ray film may relieve tube obstruction and facilitate drainage. If drainage remains minimal, the physician may irrigate the tube or insert a new chest tube to insure tube patency and to reach fluid or air pockets from a slightly different angle.

Chest Tube Milking and Stripping

The technique of *milking* involves pinching and stabilizing the tube distally with one hand, while fingers of the other hand compress the tube and move proximally toward the patient (von Hippel, 1970). Clots at the tube's tip move back into the chest, where they are gradually absorbed. More recently, however, milking has become a general term referring to squeezing, twisting, or rolling the tube over a clamp to break up clots and work them down into the drainage chamber. Milking is usually unnecessary when a tube is inserted to drain air rather than fluid. Moreover, the squeezing technique shown in Figure 30–15 is alway safer and usually sufficient to promote the drainage of fluid.

Chest tube *stripping* may be used when a chest tube remains blocked, in spite of milking efforts. To strip a tube, the nurse occludes and stabilizes the chest tube proximally with one hand, while the thumb and forefinger of the other hand pinch and pull the rubber tubing distally. The proximal hand (i.e., closest to the patient's chest) is released first, causing a suction effect within the tube and chest. This technique may be repeated along sequential segments of tubing. An alternative method is to use a hand tube stripper (i.e., roller) (Fig. 30–16).

Chest tube stripping is a controversial topic. Many hospitals require a physician's order; many clinicians recommend the technique only as a last resort, since stripping can produce negative pressures exceeding -200 to -400 cmH_2O (Duncan and Erickson, 1982). Since lung entrapment in tube eyelets and persistent air leaks can occur with as little as -15 to -20 cmH_2O suction (Stahly and Tench, 1977), many clinicians fear that the excessive negative pressures associated with

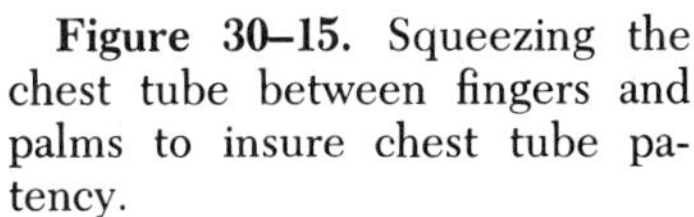

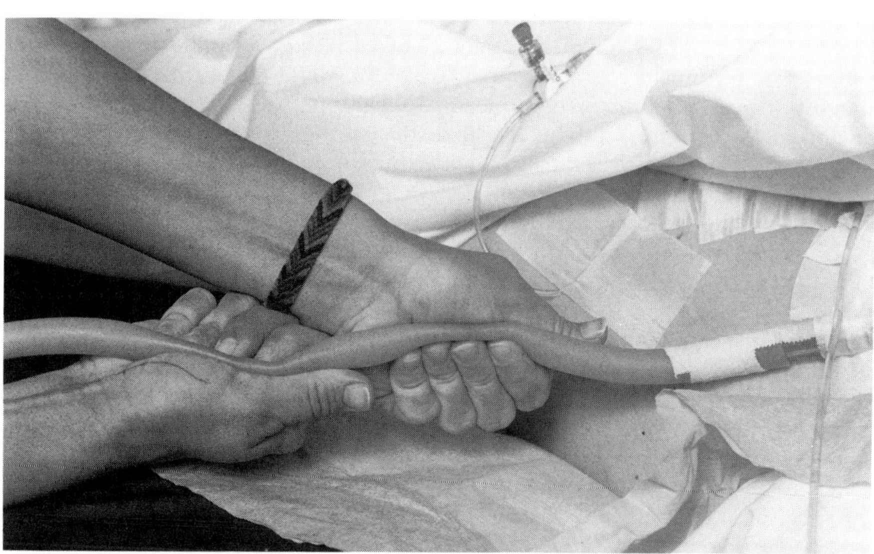

Figure 30–15. Squeezing the chest tube between fingers and palms to insure chest tube patency.

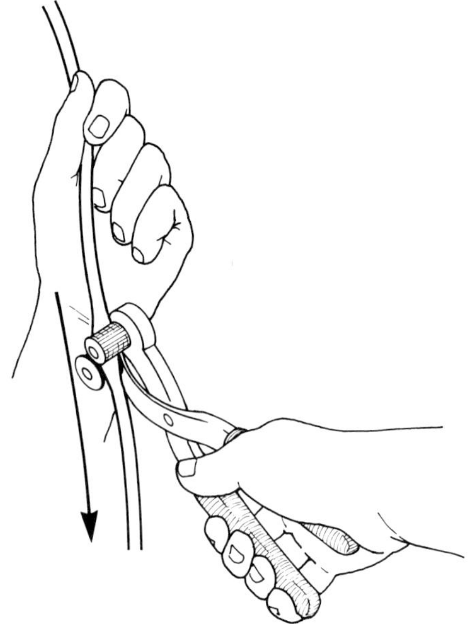

Figure 30–16. Use of a hand tube stripper as a last resort to clear a blocked chest tube.

stripping will stimulate new bleeding, prevent closure of air leaks, or inflict unnecessary trauma to lung tissue.

Manufacturers concerned with possible complications have developed chest drainage units with pressure release valves. However, research involving postcardiac surgery patients with mediastinal tubes indicates that venting negative pressure through a valve does not make a difference in amount of drainage produced (Duncan et al., 1987). A pressure release valve may unnecessarily complicate the design and operation of drainage units, without significantly reducing complications associated with excess negative pressure.

Until future research provides clearer guidelines, nurses must become familiar with techniques and variables that contribute to negative pressure and adapt nursing interventions accordingly (Isaacson et al., 1986). Generally, milking is safer than stripping because it produces less negative pressure. The amount of negative pressure produced by stripping is related to the length of tubing stripped, the method, and the type of chest tube. Negative pressure is greatest when stripping the entire length of tubing, when using the hand tube stripper (i.e., roller), and when stripping the pleural rather than the mediastinal tube (Knauss, 1985).

Whereas squeezing or milking is most appropriate for a pulmonary patient with an intrapleural tube and small to moderate amounts of drainage, both milking and occasional stripping may be needed to keep a tube patent in the postcardiac surgery patient with large amounts of thick, bloody drainage. Lim-Levy and colleagues (1986) discourage the use of stripping within the first 16 hours after cardiac surgery because it leads to a higher volume of drainage compared with the volume from patients whose tubes were neither milked nor stripped.

WATERSEAL

Monitoring the waterseal chamber is just as important as monitoring drainage. First, check to be sure the waterseal is filled to the 2-cm fill line. Second, check for tidalling—it insures a patent system. Last, check for an air leak (i.e., bubbling in the waterseal).

Absent Tidalling

Absent tidalling indicates reexpansion of the lung or chest tube obstruction. The nurse always assumes obstruction, until proved otherwise, because obstruction may cause pneumothorax or hemothorax. First, check for kinked tubing. Inspect connection sites for clots, and milk the tubing. Connections should be tightened with thin Parham bands or properly taped with nonstretchable adhesive tape to permit inspection. One inch adhesive tape is placed horizontally across rather than completely around the connector. The tape may be reinforced with encircling tape at both ends of the connector (Fig. 30–17). This technique permits the continuous inspection of the connector for clots.

In addition, note that the clear, plastic serrated connector in Figure 30–17 is a large bore, straight type, not the type with small bore, tapered ends, e.g., five-in-one connector. Straight connectors may be less likely to become plugged with clots compared with connectors with tapered ends (Besson and Saegesser, 1983).

Air Leak Assessment

When an air leak is present, the nurse notes its size and occurrence during respiration. Size is estimated in two ways. First, if the patient's drainage system (e.g., Pleur-evac A-4005) has an air leak meter, the nurse reads the flow rate (i.e., L/min) registered on the meter. Second, the nurse observes the extent of bubbling during inspiration and expiration, e.g., small inspiratory leak, large expiratory leak, and large continuous leak. Both methods of estimating air leak size are used because the accuracy rate for meter readings may be as low as 67% (Tyler et al., 1985).

A small air leak is likely to disappear after 1 or 2 days. When a moderate to large leak suddenly appears, the nurse follows this procedure to diagnose the problem:

1. Apply pressure to the skin around the chest tube insertion site. If the leak stops, a few stitches to the site may stop atmospheric air from being sucked into the chest from around the chest tube.
2. *Momentarily* (i.e., 1 to 3 seconds) clamp the chest tube close to the patient.
   a. If the leak persists, the leak is in the tubing, at

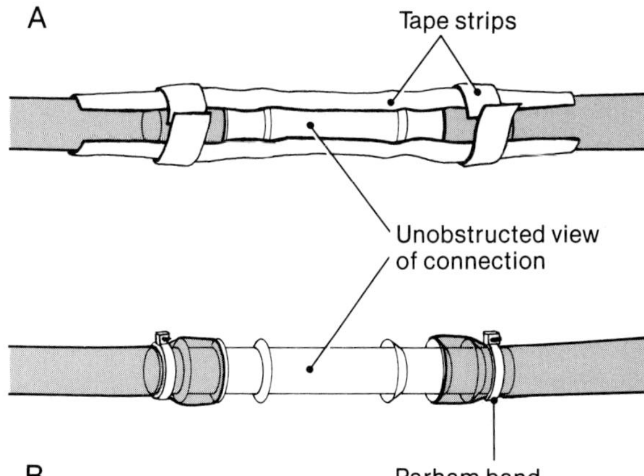

Figure 30–17. The securing of chest tube connections with strips of cloth adhesive tape (A) or Parham bands (B).

a loose connection, or in a faulty or cracked drainage unit. Clamping at intervals along the length of tubing will determine the exact location of the leak.

b. If the leak stops, the leak is in the patient. A larger chest tube or more suction may be needed to evacuate air at the same rate as leakage into the pleura.

Continuous vigorous bubbling in the waterseal may be due to accidental tube disconnection or removal. In the case of disconnection, the nurse immediately reconnects the tube to the drainage system. If the patient does *not* have an air leak, the tube may be temporarily pinched shut or clamped until it can be readily connected to the drainage unit. In the case of accidental tube removal, the nurse applies direct pressure to the chest tube site, preferably with a sterile dressing and calls the physician. If the patient is known to have a large air leak and symptoms of pneumothorax become worse, leave the chest tube site open to air until the physician arrives.

Bronchopleural Fistula

Intermittent or continuous bubbling in the waterseal 24 hours after chest tube insertion and evacuation of a pneumothorax indicates the presence of a bronchopleural fistula. If the leak is large and gas exchange compromised, measures are taken to reduce the size of the leak. Appropriate measures may include using intermittent mandatory ventilation (IMV) instead of continuous ventilation, decreasing IMV mandatory breaths, decreasing or eliminating positive end expiratory pressure (PEEP) or continuous positive airway pressure (CPAP) levels, decreasing inspiratory time, decreasing tidal and sigh volumes, avoiding expiratory retard, and employing the lowest level of suction that maintains lung inflation (Pierson, 1982). Moreover, staffs of medical centers who have clinical experience with high frequency ventilation may use this mode of mechanical ventilation to promote air leak closure and to avoid barotrauma and other complications associated with conventional positive pressure ventilation.

One problem that may arise in a patient with a bronchopleural fistula is the accumulation of bubbling foam in the drainage chamber. The foam may spill over into other chambers or make drainage monitoring difficult. To eliminate or reduce this problem, the nurse may follow one or more of these suggestions: (1) promptly change the drainage chamber system when almost full; (2) use systems with separate drainage and waterseal chambers; and (3) ask the physician about the addition of an antiflatulent agent, such as simethicone (Mylicon), 40 mg, to the drainage chamber.

Vented Sump Tubes

Continuous bubbling in the waterseal always indicates abnormality, except in the case of the vented sump chest tube. Some surgeons use a sump tube for mediastinal postcardiotomy drainage. It has one or two filtered vents that extend the length of the tube and open into the main lumen at the tube's tip (Fig. 30–18). With the application of suction, atmospheric air is sucked down the side sump tube to the tube's tip and out via the chest tube's main lumen and drainage system. The continuous flow of air keeps the tube patent and results in more complete drainage without having to milk or strip the tube (Fishman, 1983). In this case, continuous bubbling in the waterseal is normal. Bubbling does not indicate the presence of an air leak. The cessation of bubbling is a danger signal indicating tube occlusion or a faulty drainage system.

SUCTION CONTROL

The nurse checks for the correct amount of suction. If necessary, the water level in the suction control chamber is adjusted by either adding normal saline or aspirating excess fluid with a sterile suction catheter. Continuous gentle bubbling should be present, and the air vent should remain open at all times. If suction is discontinued, the tubing between the waterseal and the suction control bottle is opened to air; in plastic units, the suction tubing is disconnected, thus opening the waterseal to air.

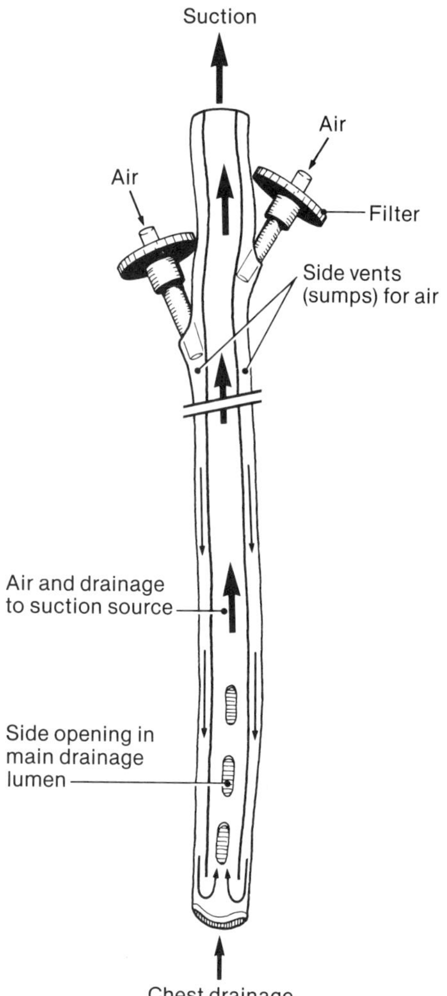

Figure 30–18. Vented sump tube. This soft, flat silicone tube has two side vents and a main drainage lumen. The arrows indicate the direction of air and drainage movement when the tube is positioned in the mediastinum.

When high suction is required (i.e., over −20 to −30 cmH_2O), chest tube bottles connected to a high suction source, such as the Emerson or Sorenson pump, are preferred over most plastic disposal units. However, Fishman (1983) reports that adding mercury to the control chamber is one way to increase suction in a plastic unit. One centimeter of mercury in the suction control chamber creates 13.6 cmH_2O pressure rather than 1 cmH_2O pressure.

Maintaining Suction During Transport

When transport is anticipated between hospital locations, the nurse has two options to maintain adequate suction for the patient. First, the nurse may temporarily discontinue the suctioning process and open the waterseal to air until the patient returns to the unit. This option is most appropriate for patients with low suction (10 to 20 cmH_2O), minimal anticipated drainage, and no air leak. The second option is a special portable suction device attached to a compressed air source (Pickard and Beall, 1983).

OTHER PARAMETERS

Other parameters that the nurse monitors in the patient with a chest tube include breath sounds and dressings. The presence of chest tube clamps at the bedside is also checked.

Breath Sounds

Breath sounds should be equal on both sides of the anterior chest area (i.e., of the mediastinal tube) or slightly decreased around a pleural chest tube site. When breath sounds become more diminished or absent and crackles are heard peripherally, check for other signs of pneumothorax and atelectasis.

Chest Tube Dressing

Check to be sure the dressing is dry and intact. Reinforce with tape PRN. Check surrounding chest and neck areas for subcutaneous emphysema, and mark these areas with a felt-tipped pen to monitor for the possible spread of air in tissue planes.

Chest Tube Clamps

Two rubber shod chest tube clamps are kept at the bedside for emergency use, for diagnostic purposes (e.g., air leak assessment), and for changing drainage systems. Sometimes, a chest tube is clamped, and a chest x-ray film is taken to determine whether the lung is likely to collapse when the tube is removed. Most important, remember never to clamp the chest tube of a patient with an air leak. When transferring a patient, open the waterseal to air or use portable suction, as described, but do not clamp the chest tube. The clamps are to accompany the patient during transport for emergencies only.

Chest Tube Removal

Chest tubes are removed when the indication for tube thoracostomy is no longer present or the tube becomes nonfunctional. More specifically, they may be removed at least 1 day after air leak cessation or when less than 50 to 100 ml of fluid drains per day; 1 to 3 days postcardiac surgery, 2 to 6 days post-thoracotomy surgery, and about 2 weeks post-thoracoabdominal surgery due to expected prolonged pleural drainage. A tube for empyema is removed when drainage slows, and the infected space is obliterated. In other cases, the tube is removed when dark or serous fluid oozes from around the chest tube, indicating that the tip is no longer in communication with a fluid pocket. In a simple pneumothorax, the appearance of a small amount of serosanguineous fluid in the previously clear tubing or the empty drainage chamber is indication for tube removal. This drainage commonly occurs as an air leak seals off, and it represents an inflammatory response of surrounding tissues near the tip of the chest tube.

To remove a chest tube, the physician pulls it out in one quick motion at the peak of inspiration during Valsalva's maneuver or during the expiratory phase of crying in children. Simultaneously, the slip stitch at the site is tightened. Additional sutures, skin clips, and an occlusive dressing may be necessary to seal the tract. These items are removed within 3 to 5 days. A chest x-ray is ordered 12 to 24 hours after tube removal to check for residual air and fluid.

The procedure may vary slightly, depending on the situation. For example, if two chest tubes are interconnected by a Y connector, the remaining chest tube is always clamped before the other one is removed to prevent air from being sucked into the remaining tube and pleural space. Also, some physicians coordinate repeated patient Valsalva's maneuvers and manual compression of the tube tract to express residual air or fluid from the pleural space before tightening the slip stitch and closing the tract.

To prevent recurrence of pneumothorax, the physician may use pleurodesis before chest tube removal. *Pleurodesis* is the instillation of an irritating substance, such as tetracycline, talc, or kaolin, to promote adhesions between visceral and parietal pleurae. These adhesions serve to seal off the air leak and help prevent the inward collapse of the lung. When pleurodesis or other measures fail to prevent spontaneous pneumothorax, a thoracotomy may be necessary to suture or staple the air leak, to produce pleural abrasions, to resect defective lung tissue, or all three.

Immediately after chest tube removal, the patient with spontaneous pneumothorax is warned that the risk for another pneumothorax is greater for a person with a history of pneumothorax, compared with a person without such a history. Therefore, key signs to immediately report to their physician include chest or shoulder pain especially on inspiration, shortness of breath, or vague chest discomfort and dry cough.

Pleurodesis is also performed before chest tube removal in patients with large malignant pleural effusions. Tetracycline (20 mg/kg) is instilled into the pleural space and the tube is clamped for 1 to 2 hours. After unclamping, suction is applied to promote fluid removal and apposition of pleural surfaces. The chest tube is removed when the drainage is minimal (50 to 100 ml/24 hr) and the chest x-ray shows full lung expansion (Miller and Sahn, 1987).

Prevention of Pulmonary Complications

The information presented thus far has focused on caring for the patient with a chest tube drainage system, whether the patient is on the ward with a single chest tube for pleural effusion or pneumothorax or in the critical care unit recovering from lung resection, cardiac surgery, or some other major thoracotomy operation. Whatever the case, the prevention of pulmonary complications, such as atelectasis, pneumonia, and pneumothorax, largely depends on the nurse's skill at monitoring the key parameters described in previous sections.

Interventions may be adequate to prevent pulmonary complications and promote full recovery to health in patients with relatively normal lungs or with routine chest tube insertions. However, the challenge of avoiding pulmonary complications is much greater for chronically ill patients undergoing thoracotomy because they have many if not all of the risk factors for postoperative complications (see Table 8–3). In these high risk patients, respiratory interventions must be intense and well integrated with other nursing functions, such as vital signs, hemodynamic measurements when applicable, and personal hygiene care.

Many other factors account for the need for intensive respiratory care in post-thoracotomy patients, including the stress of surgery, immobility, anxiety, and high pain levels due to large surgical incisions. One factor not emphasized is the role of general anesthetics.

ROLE OF GENERAL ANESTHETICS IN POSTOPERATIVE COMPLICATIONS

The general anesthetics listed in the following box contribute to the postoperative pulmonary complications of atelectasis, mucus retention, pneumonia, and pulmonary aspiration (Table 30–1).

GENERAL ANESTHETICS (INHALATIONAL AGENTS)

Halogenated hydrocarbons
- Halothane (Fluothane)

Halogenated ethers
- Methoxyflurane (Penthrane)
- Enflurane (Ethrane)
- Isoflurane (Forane)

Nitrous oxide

The nursing interventions listed in Table 30–1 serve to reduce the incidence or intensity of the adverse effects.

Table 30–1. ADVERSE EFFECTS AND COMPLICATIONS OF GENERAL ANESTHETICS IN THE POSTOPERATIVE PERIOD*

Body System	Adverse Effects and Complications with Implicated Anesthetics	Nursing Interventions
Central nervous system (CNS)	Delirium Headache Drowsiness Anorexia Emergence excitement Prolonged emergence	Check sensorium with vital signs. Check for airway patency and proper body positioning. Maintain a quiet environment. Provide reassurance that the operation is over and that recovery is in progress. Provide medication for headache.
Respiratory system	Atelectasis Mucus retention Pneumonia Pulmonary aspiration	Implement deep breathing exercises q1 to 2h, utilizing pain medication, proper body positioning, and incisional support to promote full lung expansion and mucus expectoration during coughing. Check for the chest tube's patency and properly functioning drainage system. Promptly treat nausea and vomiting with slow deep breathing, antiemetic medication nasogastric suction, or all three. Elevate head and turn patient to side to help prevent aspiration. Closely monitor patients with preexisting cardiopulmonary disease, since they are at high risk for complications.
Cardiovascular system	Myocardial depression Arrhythmias with halothane and enflurane Myocardial infarction	Carefully monitor cardiac rate and rhythm, blood pressure, and chest assessment findings postoperatively. Monitor hemodynamics during and after surgery in patients with histories of infarction or other cardiac problems. Suspect infarction with onset of arrhythmias, LV failure, hypotension, and serum isoenzyme elevation. Note that cardiac symptoms may be masked by operative pain or postoperative medication. Provide adequate oxygenation, and promptly treat arrhythmias with appropriate medication.
Gastrointestinal system	Nausea and vomiting Possible hepatotoxicity with halothane	Use nasogastric suctioning for patients with delayed gastric emptying, e.g., abdominal surgery. Maintain comfort by providing pain medication when needed. Encourage use of preoperative antiemetic medication for a patient at high risk for vomiting (i.e., history of postoperative emesis) and for a patient for whom vomiting would be dangerous (i.e., ocular or middle ear surgery). Watch for the following first signs of halothane-associated hepatitis: fever; anorexia; vomiting; malaise; and tender liver, 2 to 3 days after surgery.
Renal system	Decreased renal function	Monitor urine output q1 to 2h postoperatively. Renal blood flow, glomerular filtration rate, and urine output should return to normal within a few hours after anesthetic discontinuation. Watch for signs of renal failure in a patient receiving a fluorinated anesthetic. This type of agent is not a primary one because of increased risk of nephrotoxicity.
Immune system	Possible immunosuppression that may not be clinically significant. Possible mutagenicity, carcinogenicity, and teratogenicity.	Monitor for postoperative neutropenia. Inhalational anesthetics are avoided during pregnancy because of their teratogenic potential and their effects on the uterus (e.g., decreased uterine blood flow and tone).

*Adapted from Boucher, B., Witt, W., and Foster, T.: The postoperative effects of inhalational anesthetics. *Heart and lung*, 15(1):63–69, 1986.

A role of the nurse caring for the post-thoracotomy patient, or any other surgical patient recovering from general anesthesia, is to monitor for nonrespiratory as well as respiratory adverse effects of general anesthetics. Most of the nonrespiratory effects provided in Table 30–1 directly or indirectly affect airway patency, oxygenation, and ventilation.

The overall incidence of postoperative anesthetic complications is reported to be as high as 78% (Boucher et al., 1986). Though the rate is high, current use of inhalational anesthetic agents with a variety of analgesic, amnesic, and muscle relaxing agents during anesthesia, makes detection of many adverse effects difficult. Moreover, because of the intensity of the nursing care as well as the patient's altered mental status from pain medication, postoperative complications may go unnoticed.

When reviewing Table 30–1, keep in mind that some adverse effects, such as mild myocardial depression (e.g., fall in blood pressure) and drowsiness, normally occur whenever a general anesthetic is administered. When severe, the adverse effects may lead to serious complications, such as pneumonia and myocardial infarction, particularly in patients with preexisting pulmonary disease and heart disease, respectively.

Certain adverse effects, such as prolonged emergence from anesthesia, depend on the type of agent, length of administration, dosage, and pharmacologic interactions with other medications. For example, a highly lipid soluble agent, such as methoxyflurane, results in slower emergence from anesthesia than a moderately soluble agent, such as halothane, particularly in obese patients. Prolonged administration time is a common cause of prolonged emergence. High doses of a general anesthetic agent may result in prolonged emergence. When used with another agent, such as an opiate, a barbiturate, or a benzodiazepine, general anesthetic agents may cause significant hypoventilation, hypotension, and CNS depression. Furthermore, accompanying use of a muscle relaxant or paralyzing agent, such as pancuronium, predisposes the patient to apnea and respiratory arrest, unless paralysis reverses spontaneously or pharmacologically with administration of an antagonist.

Conclusion

This chapter presents chest tube drainage systems and related post-thoracotomy care. When the nursing care described is integrated with other measures such as aggressive bronchial hygiene measures, airway care, and hemodynamic monitoring, to prevent postoperative pulmonary complications, the critically ill patient may receive the best care possible. The patient with underlying chronic pulmonary disease has a better chance of full recovery from either routine chest tube insertion or thoracostomy during a major surgical operation.

Though this chapter and other chapters in this part of the book prepare the nurse to implement specialized interventions, the interventions may be inappropriate in individual situations, unless they are applied within a broad problem-solving framework. The next part of this book describes the integration of assessment and intervention within the nursing process.

REFERENCES

Besson, A. and Saegesser, F.: Intrathoracic fluid collections. Color Atlas of Chest Trauma and Associated Injuries, vol. 1. Oradell, New Jersey, Medical Economics Co., Inc., 1983.

Boucher, B., Witt, W., and Foster, T.: The postoperative adverse effects of inhalational anesthetics. *Heart and lung,* 15(1):63–69, 1986.

Brenner, B.: Comprehensive Management of Respiratory Emergencies. Rockville, Maryland, Aspen Systems Corporation, 1985.

Cohen, S. and Stack, M.: How to work with chest tubes. *American journal of nursing,* 80(4):685–712, 1980.

Duncan, C. and Erickson, R.: Pressures associated with chest tube stripping. *Heart and lung,* 11(2):166–171, 1982.

Duncan, C., Erickson, R., and Weigel, R.: Effect of chest tube management on drainage after cardiac surgery. *Heart and lung,* 16(1):1–9, 1987.

Fishman, N.: Thoracic Drainage: A Manual of Procedures. Chicago, Year Book Medical Publishers, Inc., 1983.

Fuchs, C.: The ins and outs of chest drainage systems. *Nursing 86,* 16(12):26–33, 1986.

Isaacson, J., George, L., and Brewer, M.: The effect of chest tube manipulation on mediastinal drainage. *Heart and lung,* 15(6):601–605, 1986.

Kersten, L.: Chest Tube Drainage System. (Intensive Care Unit Nursing Procedure). San Francisco, Moffitt Hospital, University of California, 1973.

Kersten, L.: Chest-tube drainage system—indications and principles of operation. *Heart and lung,* 3(1):97–101, 1974.

Knauss, P.: Chest tube stripping: is it necessary? *Focus on critical care,* 12(6):41–43, 1985.

Lim-Levy, F., Babler, S., et al.: Is milking and stripping chest tubes really necessary? *Annals of thoracic surgery,* 42(1):77–80, 1986.

MacKenzie, C. (ed.): Chest Physiotherapy in the Intensive Care Unit. Baltimore, Williams & Wilkins, 1981.

Miller, K. and Sahn, S.: Chest tubes—indications, technique, management and complications. *Chest,* 91(2):258–264, 1987.

Munnell, E. and Thomas, E.: Current concepts in thoracic drainage systems. *The annals of thoracic surgery,* 19(3):261–268, 1975.

Pickard, L. and Beall, A.: Portable suction device for use in patients with postoperative pleural air leaks. *The annals of thoracic surgery,* 36(1):103–104, 1983.

Pierson, D.: Persistent bronchopleural air leak during mechanical ventilation: a review. *Respiratory care,* 27(4):408–416, 1982.

Seneff, M., Corwin, R., Gold, L., and Irwin, R.: Complications associated with thoracocentesis. *Chest,* 90(1):97–100, 1986.

Stahly, T. and Tench, W.: Lung entrapment and infarction by chest tube suction. *Radiology,* 122(2):307–309, 1977.

Tyler, M., Capps, J., Pierson, D., and Rusch, V.: Accuracy of the Pleur-evac A-4005 patient air leak meter under steady flow conditions. *Heart and lung,* 14(3):307–308, 1985.

von Hippel, A.: Chest Tubes and Chest Bottles. Springfield, Illinois, Charles C Thomas, 1970.

CLINICAL APPLICATION

Part Six

Previous chapters establish an extensive theory base for decision-making in respiratory nursing care. This theory base is incomplete, however, without showing how it relates to the nursing process and how application of the nursing process leads to goal attainment.

A respiratory theory base is of no value unless the nurse uses decision-making skills to selectively apply knowledge to the nursing process. To understand this principle, consider the conceptualization of respiratory nursing care shown in Figure P6–1. The respiratory theory base provides the theory for data-based decisions; the nursing process provides a problem-solving framework for application of the theory base. Yet, goal attainment depends neither on theory alone nor on the nursing process alone, but on the ability of the nurse to selectively merge the two components through clinical diagnostic reasoning. Ultimately, goal attainment depends on decision-making skill. In Figure P6–1, decision-making skill is placed between theory base and nursing process, because it is central to the appropriate merging of the two components. From another perspective, theory related to respiratory assessment and intervention is filtered through decision-making processes, as it is applied to the nursing process. The lines linking the theory base to the nursing process are dotted rather than solid to represent that decision-making processes are fluid and as yet relatively, poorly defined in the literature.

The result of applying theory to nursing process is goal attainment, specifically the reduction of respiratory illness, the optimization of wellness, and the provision of comprehensive and continuing respiratory care, as shown at the bottom of Figure P6–1.

With this background in mind, Chapter 31 (*Nursing Diagnosis and Intervention*) presents the nursing process applied to pulmonary patients. The emphasis on assessment is designed to further develop decision-making skills, thus facilitating the merging of theory and practice. Chapter 32, *The Case Study,* is an example of how to implement decision-making skills in the clinical setting.

Though clinical application is the most important part of this book, its description is relatively short in length and incompletely developed. Its incompleteness reflects the state of the art of respiratory nursing diagnosis and diagnostic clinical reasoning in collaborative practice. These areas of inquiry are still in their infancy and are evolving very slowly amidst professional practice issues. This text, it is hoped, will prompt others to further develop a collaborative theory base for refinement of decision-making skills in respiratory nursing care.

Terms commonly used to describe the process of decision-making in respiratory nursing care are listed in the glossary.

Glossary of Commonly Used Terms in The Process of Decision-making

categoric decision—a decision based on a few defining criteria, regardless of other data.

clustering of information—grouping of related signs and symptoms around a cue.

collaborative diagnosis—clinical judgment that requires collaboration with other health team members for assessment or intervention.

cue—distinguishing sign or symptom for a diagnostic category.

data base—systematic compilation of patient information.

decision-making skill—ability to use clinical reasoning to deliver comprehensive and continuing respiratory care.

decision rule—guideline or criterion for choosing the best respiratory intervention.

decision tree—a branching, line diagram used to illustrate reasoning processes leading to a diagnosis. The diagram begins with a cue or information cluster, representing the root of the tree. The branches represent decision and observation contingencies.

deduction—problem solving that begins with generalization. It works backwards through a systematic proof, leading to a precise statement of truth or falsity.

diagnostic reasoning process—complex mental process used to identify and classify phenomena in presenting clinical situations.

diagnostic statement—health problem written in standard nursing diagnosis format.

evaluation criterion—statement of expected outcomes.

goal—standard for measuring the success or failure of a respiratory intervention.

health need—condition requiring action to reduce or eliminate a health problem.

health problem—deficit or potential deficit in the health status of an individual, a family, or a community. It may be an *actual* problem, a *potential* problem (i.e., high risk for development), or a *possible* problem (i.e., not enough information to rule in or rule out).

heuristics—art or science of using practical guides or intuitive judgments to determine choices in problem-solving situations.

incremental decision—variable or reversible decision that depends on data assessed at the moment. It is usually associated with a series of mental decision-making processes, eventually leading to a correct diagnosis and intervention

induction—process of discovering general laws by observation and combination of specific instances.

inference—judgments imposed on data from a set of preexisting categories (i.e., diagnoses).

intervening variable—variable that affects the acuity, etiology, or treatment of a health problem.

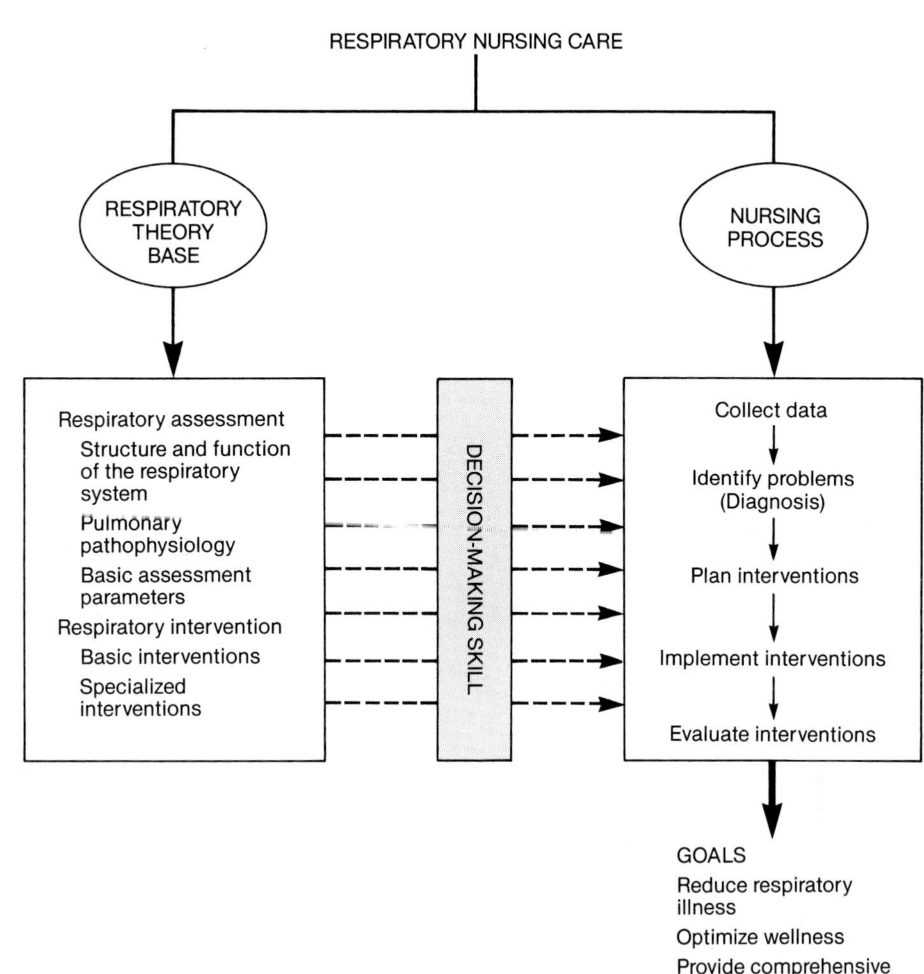

Figure P6–1. Respiratory nursing care. Decision-making skill (gray area) is central to the merging of theory with components of the nursing process.

invalid data clustering—assuming a relationship between data, when no relationship exists; leads to diagnostic errors.

lack of closure—failure to diagnose a problem from an adequate data base; leads to diagnostic errors.

North American Nursing Diagnosis Association (NANDA)—association dedicated to the development and use of nursing diagnoses.

nursing diagnosis—clinical judgment about an individual, a family, or a community that provides the basis for prescriptions for therapy that the nurse is accountable (see Introduction for complete definition). A collaborative diagnosis is considered a nursing diagnosis, if the nurse is accountable for the related nursing care.

nursing process—problem-solving framework for nursing care comprised of five components as follows: (1) data collection, (2) diagnosis (i.e., problem definition), (3) planning of the intervention, (4) implementation of the intervention, and (5) evaluation of the intervention.

objective data—observable signs, e.g., physical finding, laboratory data, hemodynamic reading.

outcome statement—written form of a goal or evaluation criterion.

premature closure—diagnosis in the presence of an inadequate data base; leads to diagnostic errors.

Problem Oriented Record (POR)—system for charting patient care; includes data base, problem list, initial and revised care plans, and progress notes.

SOAP charting—a format for narrative charting that includes *s*ubjective data, *o*bjective data, *a*nalysis, and *p*lan for intervention.

subjective data—historical data reported by a patient.

validation—collection of additional data to shape, refine, rank, verify, or eliminate hypotheses in the diagnostic process.

Nursing Diagnosis and Intervention

31

Main Objectives

1. Describe the key role of assessment in the nursing process. Include the following in your answer:
   a. The five components of the nursing process.
   b. Three places where assessment blends into intervention, making assessment central to comprehensive respiratory care.
2. Name three criteria for selection of an appropriate nursing model or assessment tool for populations with respiratory problems.
3. Define the following terms: data base; patient profile; nursing diagnosis; actual, potential, and possible health problems; health need; clinical inference; and validation.
4. Define and describe the diagnostic process. Include the following in your answer:
   a. How diagnosis blends with data collection.
   b. How to interpret a cluster of respiratory signs and symptoms.
   c. How respiratory diagnosis leads directly to identification of health needs.
5. Name and describe three common patterns of diagnostic error.
6. Define the term heuristics. Discuss the key role of heuristics in cue interpretation, respiratory diagnosis, and development of a taxonomy of respiratory nursing diagnoses for collaborative practice.
7. Name at least three diagnoses for each of these respiratory disorders: bronchial asthma, chronic bronchitis, emphysema, upper airway obstruction, chronic restrictive disease, acute pneumo-

nia, cardiogenic pulmonary edema, acute atelectasis, and cor pulmonale.

8. Explain how to write a diagnostic statement.
9. Describe how to plan and evaluate respiratory interventions.
10. Discuss seven intervening variables that affect the acuity, etiology, and treatment of physiologic and psychosocial respiratory problems.
11. Select a respiratory patient in your clinical setting. Write an overall goal as well as evaluation criteria for anticipated respiratory interventions.
12. Discuss how to implement and refine decision-making skills in the clinical setting.

Nursing diagnosis, whether solely cognitive or in written form, is the responsibility of all nurses who strive to help deliver comprehensive respiratory care.

This chapter elaborates on basic principles presented in the introduction of this book. Its purpose is threefold as follows: (1) to review the components of the nursing process as they apply to the pulmonary patient, with emphasis on the diagnostic process; (2) to put respiratory content in this book within a process framework; and (3) to serve as a guide for the implementation of decision-making skills in the clinical setting.

The components of the nursing process are shown in Figure 31–1. The illustration is the same as that in the Introduction with only a few additions. The additions emphasize the interrelationships between assessment and intervention. As mentioned in the Introduction, components of the nursing process are not necessarily sequential. As the nurse alternates between assessment and intervention, assessment becomes central to intervention and each component of the nursing process, as described throughout this chapter.

Data Collection

Assessment begins with data collection. The purpose of data collection is threefold as follows: (1) it provides a complete data base, (2) it provides a patient profile, and (3) it facilitates respiratory diagnosis (problem definition).

THE DATA BASE

A *data base* is a systematic compilation of patient information. In the clinical setting, it might be referred to as *nursing history, admission interview, assessment interview format,* or *initial nursing assessment.*

Finding a framework that facilitates respiratory data collection and analysis has always been a problem for

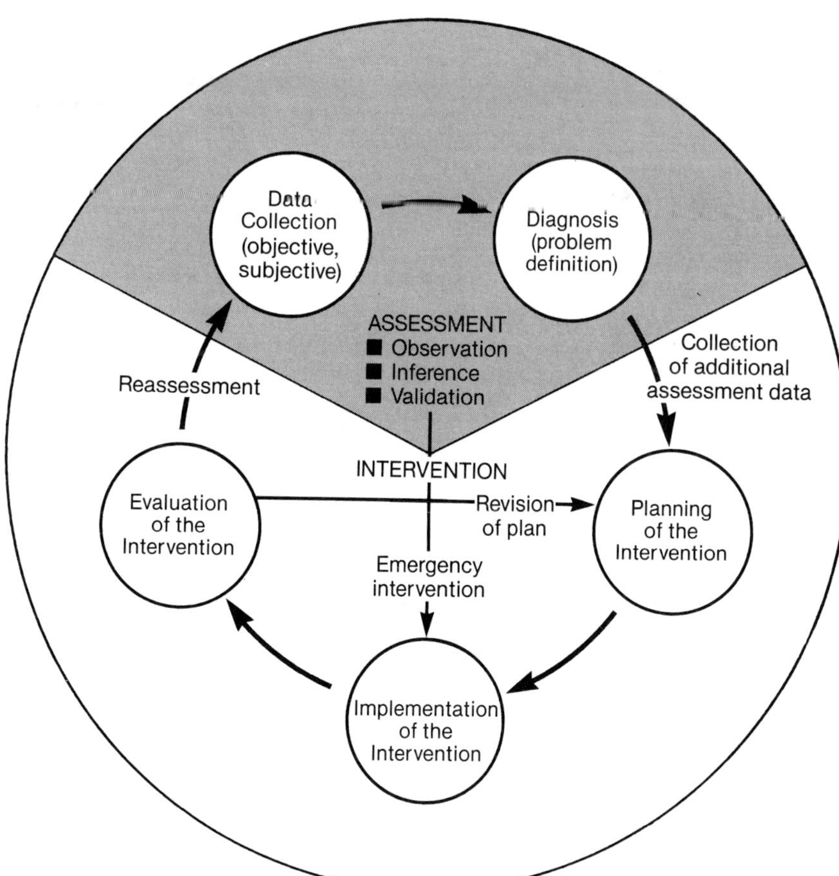

Figure 31–1. Components of the nursing process. Assessment is shaded because of its key role in the nursing process.

clinicians. In the past, graduate students of respiratory nursing at the University of California at Los Angeles employed the Systems-in-Change Model for Nursing Practice (Chrisman and Fowler, 1980) because it permits the gathering of a comprehensive data base for pulmonary patients. Yet, similar to most models, this model has its limitations. It is theoretically weak in helping the nurse process the gathered information and arrive at correct diagnoses.

Many nurses use a conceptual nursing model, such as the Roy Adaptation Model, the Johnson Behavioral Nursing Model, or the Newman Health Care Systems Model, to collect data, identify problems, and intervene appropriately. These models are helpful in the analyses of patient problems (Fawcett, 1984). However, their data collection categories are oriented more towards the general medical-surgical patient rather than towards the respiratory patient. In addition, categories are broad and oriented to only a few selected problems, such as oxygenation (e.g., the "oxygen and circulation" category in the Roy Adaptation Model). Owing to this limitation, nurses must develop their own subcategories to facilitate the collection of data specific to respiratory problems. In some cases, gross modification of general categories to include basic respiratory parameters is necessary to avoid missing crucial information and making an incorrect or incomplete set of nursing diagnoses.

Criteria for Respiratory Assessment Tools

Whatever the nursing model chosen, the assessment tool developed must meet three criteria. First, the assessment tool must facilitate data collection for a broad range of problems as follows:

Types of problems	Rationale
Acute and chronic	Respiratory patients commonly have coexisting acute and chronic problems, e.g., the COPD patient in acute ventilatory failure.
Mild, moderate, and severe	Problems occur with different degrees of severity. Though not always having top priority, mild problems are important, because health enhancing interventions, such as moving to a smog-free environment, may reduce illness and prevent the progression of pulmonary disease.
Psychosocial and biophysical (physiologic)	Chapter 16 shows how biophysical problems are meshed with psychosocial problems.
Respiratory and nonrespiratory	Pulmonary patients may present with signs and symptoms suggesting problems involving other body systems. For example, the patient with cystic fibrosis may present with pancreatic insufficiency, vitamin K deficiency, gastrointestinal problems, and sexual dysfunction related to sterility.

The second criterion for an assessment tool is that it must facilitate the identification of risk factors for the development of respiratory diseases or problems. Examples of risk factors include history of cigarette smoking (increased risk for chronic obstructive pulmonary disease [COPD] and lung cancer), exposure to potential allergens (increased risk for airway irritability or bronchospasm), and exposure to asbestos (increased risk for asbestosis and asbestos-related diseases).

Last, each assessment tool must be adaptable to clinical circumstances. The length varies, depending on the nurse's time allotted for assessment, e.g., one to two pages for short admission inteviews. Content may vary slightly, depending on the specific patient population, e.g., young asthmatic patients versus elderly COPD patients with cor pulmonale, ambulatory patients versus ventilator-dependent patients. The assessment format may vary, depending on the expertise of the nurse, e.g., specific fill-in-the-blank questions for beginners, broad open-ended questions for experts.

THE PATIENT PROFILE

The second purpose of data collection is to provide a *patient profile,* an overall view of the patient that presents enough personal, social, environmental, and economic information to identify basic health needs and the effect of illness on the patient's life and family. After acute illness, a patient profile helps health care professionals identify adaptive and maladaptive behaviors and longstanding untreated problems that have led to acute exacerbation and repeated hospitalizations. Depending on the extent and nature of the patient's contact with health care professionals, it may take several days, weeks, or months to develop a profile.

Diagnosis (Problem Definition)

Data collection helps the nurse identify health problems.

TYPES OF PROBLEMS

Health problems or nursing diagnoses are divided into three types: *actual, potential,* and *possible.*

An *actual problem* is a difficulty or concern that does in fact exist based upon the data gathered at the time of assessment. When stated in writing, an actual problem is *not* prefaced by the word "actual." All problems are assumed to be actual unless labelled "potential" or "possible." Many problems are diagnosed on the basis of history alone. For example, mucus production is an actual problem if a normally healthy patient known as a provider of a reliable history reports the coughing up of large amounts of mucus. Similarly, as Chapter 13 points out. an arterial blood gas (ABG) result, such as SaO_2 and $PaCO_2$, may be the only piece of data supporting an oxygenation and ventilatory problem, respectively.

A *potential problem* is a difficulty or a concern that a patient has an unusually high risk of developing or experiencing (Mayers, 1983). Gathered data do not indicate that a problem is in fact present, but it is likely to develop if the patient continues his present life style and practices. For example, the history of occasional smoking may not indicate a ventilatory problem, but with continued smoking airway obstruction and other ventilatory problems are likely to develop. Risk factors, such as smoking and exposure to lung irritants or occupational hazards, usually indicate potential problems.

A *possible problem* is a situation requiring more information before a particular difficulty or concern can be confirmed or ruled out as a problem (Mayers, 1983). A problem may remain categorized as a possible problem until additional objective information confirms its presence. For example, although complaints of chest tightness suggest possible bronchoconstriction, objective findings, e.g., wheezing on auscultation or improvements in postbronchodilator values on the pulmonary function test, are needed to diagnose *actual* bronchoconstriction. Similarly, a patient's signs and symptoms are sometimes so vague that the nurse suspects a problem, but the clinical situation or the standing orders do not permit the gathering of other crucial data to confirm or rule out the diagnosis. An asthmatic without any change in condition except for decreased breath sounds might have a nursing diagnosis of possible bronchoconstriction until the physician examines the patient, orders appropriate tests, and makes the actual diagnosis. Possible problems are important in nursing because they alert others to the possibility of actual or potential problems. In addition, this category allows the nurse without experience or knowledge of respiratory disease to label and report a problem without worrying about legal repercussions, if the diagnosis turns out to be partially or completely incorrect.

THE NATURE OF THE DIAGNOSTIC PROCESS

Definition

The diagnostic reasoning process is a "complex, sometimes unconscious, integration of critical-thinking and data-collecting processes that clinicians use to identify and classify phenomena in presenting clinical situations" (Carnevali, 1984). The process is the foundation for treatment decisions.

The Blending of Diagnosis with Data Collection

In clinical and educational settings, the step between data collection and nursing diagnosis is made to seem clear-cut and almost automatic. For example, a nurse is asked to collect a complete data base and then list problems, using a provided format, though no guidance is given as to how to identify the main problems. The nurse may spend up to 1 hour collecting data and still may find herself at a loss, because she does not know how to organize or interpret the overwhelming amount of information. When she seeks help, she discovers that she has neglected to collect details crucial to the identification and further analysis of respiratory problems. Her lack of diagnostic reasoning skills prevented task completion.

Though diagnosis is conceptualized as the second step in the nursing process, in practice it is an ongoing nursing process that begins the moment the nurse approaches the patient for the initial nursing assessment. Unless it begins at this time, the nurse will not be able to mentally sift through data obtained during the interview, zero in on critical problem areas that need detailed assessment, and arrive at a tentative problem list within a reasonable amount of time. Unless key information is collected, the nurse will not be able to analyze problems, plan care, and evaluate outcomes.

DIAGNOSTIC TOOLS

The diagnostic process involves use of three diagnostic tools as follows: *observation, inference,* and *validation.*

Observation

The nurse cannot collect pertinent data without first knowing *what* to observe. Florence Nightingale most aptly stated, "The most important practical lesson that can be given to nurses is to teach them what to observe—how to observe—what symptoms indicate improvement—what the reverse—which are of importance—which are of none—which are the evidence of neglect—and what kind of neglect" (1969).

In respiratory nursing, the nurse must have a firm knowledge base in pulmonary disease, normal versus abnormal assessment findings, common respiratory problems, and respiratory interventions. This knowledge assures a nurse's readiness to observe. More specifically, it increases the nurse's perceptual acuity to respiratory *cues* or key clinical findings. With this knowledge, the nurse can readily perceive and interpret the patient's appearance, age, medical diagnosis, dress, manner, and movements and formulate an initial impression. When the patient coughs productively during the initial encounter, it serves as a cue, prompting the nurse to automatically think "possible mucus retention problem." If the chart documents severe obstructive disease and the patient's initial statement is, "There is nothing wrong with me," the nurse thinks "possible denial of disease process, a common coping mechanism in this type of patient."

Inference

The nurse's two previous statements are examples of *clinical inferences,* judgments imposed on subjective and objective data from a preexisting set of categories (i.e., diagnoses). Although the basics of making an inference may be obtained through instruction, clinical experience is required to refine this skill.

After initial observations, the nurse *immediately* begins to generate two to five possible diagnoses in her mind. These serve as hypotheses. To help in their formulation, the nurse mentally searches for the following:

- Abnormal findings
- Absence of expected findings
- Changes in baseline signs and symptoms
- Clustering of signs and symptoms around significant cues

Clustering Information Around Cues. Cues are important because they help define diagnostic categories, such as bronchoconstriction and mucus retention. Consider the following cluster of symptoms:

dyspnea }
wheeze* } bronchoconstriction, bronchospasm

By itself, dyspnea indicates a broad diagnostic category, such as alteration in respiratory function, though pathologically the dyspnea may be of respiratory or nonrespiratory origin. When clustered with wheeze, dyspnea is interpreted differently. Wheeze is followed by an asterisk because it is a defining cue for the two following problems: *bronchoconstriction and bronchospasm.* Bronchoconstriction is a broad category for airway narrowing from bronchial tumor, mucus plug, asthma, or some other pathologic lesion. Bronchospasm refers specifically to the airway narrowing as seen in asthma, i.e., the muscle around the airway contracts.

The presence of wheeze in the previous cluster diagnoses one or both of these problems. However, the absence of wheeze does not rule them out. Rather, the clinician must collect more data (e.g., pulmonary function test results) for further analysis.

Study this cluster of information:

dyspnea }
severe wheeze* }
history of asthma* } bronchospasm
fatigue }

Wheeze is a cue for both bronchoconstriction and bronchospasm. When it is combined with a documented history of asthma, the nurse narrows the diagnosis to bronchospasm.

Some cues are highly specific and in turn always lead to a specific diagnosis regardless of other data. For example, a Pa_{O_2} of 40 mmHg always indicates hypoxemia, since the specific cue for hypoxemia is a Pa_{O_2} of less than 60 mmHg, and since 40 mmHg is well below the 60 mmHg limit. Similarly, inspiratory stridor always indicates upper airway obstruction. The nurse may cluster other signs around the original cue, e.g., generalized decreased breath sounds, high pitched cough, and snoring. But identification of the one critical cue is sufficient for diagnosis and prompt intervention, particularly in acute situations.

While searching for cues, the nurse must not forget to look at clusters of information as a whole. Some clusters will not have a critical cue to facilitate diagnosis. Consider the following cluster:

normal PFTs }
18-pack-year history of cigarette smoking } potential airway obstruction (airflow limitation)

Both findings help diagnose potential airway obstruction. The 18-pack-year history of cigarette smoking is a high risk factor for COPD and lung cancer. It suggests potential airway obstruction. The normal PFT is objective evidence for the absence of obstructive disease at this time. It indicates that the problem is a potential, not an actual, one.

The following cluster emphasizes the point that a cue may have no meaning in and of itself. The items that accompany it make it a cue.

hacking cough* }
denial of other cardiopulmonary symptoms }
history of asthmatic attack } bronchospasm

Though wheeze is the typical cue for bronchospasm, in this case the patient presented with cough in the absence of wheeze and other cardiopulmonary symptoms. The history of asthmatic attack and the nurse's recalling that not all asthmatics wheeze prompted her to think of bronchospasm. In the absence of this history, the nurse might think of another problem, such as airway hyperirritability.

In summary, the nurse keeps in mind the following five points to guide the collecting and clustering of pulmonary signs and symptoms:

1. Look for cues for likely problems or problems that require immediate intervention, e.g., hypoxemia, upper airway obstruction.
2. Cluster other findings around these cues. Table 31–1 provides more examples of how to cluster information around cues. Likely problems are investigated by further data collection and interpretation.
3. When cues are absent or when a cluster lacks a cue, collect more information or look at the cluster as a whole.
4. Be on the alert for etiologies of possible problems. Often an etiology or risk factor suggests or confirms a diagnosis, e.g., failure to clean respiratory equipment suggests a possible chest infection (Table 31–2).
5. Begin to look for health needs, as described hereafter.

Identification of Health Needs. Once a tentative problem is identified, the nurse begins to search for a health need. Related to but not synonymous with a health problem, a *health need* refers to action neces-

Table 31–1. EXAMPLES OF CLUSTERING OF SIGNS AND SYMPTOMS AROUND CUES

Signs and Symptoms	Diagnosis
Denies wheezing, dyspnea Chest tightness* ↑ B/P, ↑ P, ↑ RR Wheezing on auscultation* Cough	Bronchoconstriction Possible mucus retention
Recent history of asthmatic attacks* Wheezing heard without stethoscope* Acute dyspnea Overuse of aerosol inhaler Statements of impending death	Bronchospasm Potential respiratory arrest Possible panic reaction
Coughing up ¼ cup sputum per day* Diagnosis of chronic bronchitis Lungs clear except for occasional expiratory rhonchi in lung bases* No change in PFTs Chest x-ray film clear Sputum C & S, Gram's stain negative	Mucus production (not a problem if controlled by bronchial hygiene measures) Potential mucus retention, chest infection
Increased sputum production in the last 24 hr No change in other signs and symptoms Scattered rhonchi throughout chest*	Mucus retention Potential chest infection
Thick viscous sputum* Decreased sputum production Complaints that respiratory treatments do not help expectoration No change in breath sounds	Thick mucus Possible increased mucus retention Possible dehydration
↓ breath sounds and end inspiratory crackles right lower lobe (RLL)* Chest film negative Complaints of (c/o) general fatigue No ABGs available	Impaired ventilation RLL
Lungs clear except rhonchi with morning cough Dyspnea on exertion* Use of accessory muscles of respiration* Abnormal breathing pattern Lung hyperinflation on chest film	Increased work of breathing Activity intolerance
Diaphoresis, lethargy, slow response to verbal questioning Acute dyspnea* Use of accessory muscles of respiration Monitor-sinus tachycardia 130/min	Respiratory distress Potential respiratory and cardiac arrest
4 hr postendotracheal extubation Hoarse voice Inspiratory stridor* Vital signs stable except for ↑ pulse Use of inspiratory accessory muscles of respiration	Upper airway obstruction Potential respiratory and cardiac arrest
Panic reaction at onset of dyspnea* History of COPD Failure to take PRN bronchodilator at appropriate times Sedentary life style	Inability to control dyspnea Possible decreased exercise tolerance, knowledge deficit
Decreased breath sounds throughout chest; a few expiratory wheezes heard anteriorly Receiving 400 mg/day anhydrous theophylline* c/o difficulty in expectoration PFTs unavailable	Possible bronchodilator undermedication
PaO_2 = 80 mmHg in a 15-year-old asthmatic*	Hypoxemia
$PaCO_2$ = 47 mmHg in a 55-year-old male with COPD*	Alveolar hypoventilation
$PaCO_2$ = 53 mmHg in a 55-year-old male with COPD*	Ventilatory failure
Vital signs and chest assessment findings stable Frequent expressions of feelings of loss regarding job, friends, physical capabilities. Comments such as "No one understands how I feel."* c/o insomnia, decreased appetite, difficulty concentrating on simple tasks Reluctance to socialize	Depression Possible social isolation

Table continued on following page

Table 31–1. EXAMPLES OF CLUSTERING OF SIGNS AND SYMPTOMS AROUND CUES *Continued*

Signs and Symptoms	Diagnosis
c/o dyspnea after climbing one flight of stairs Denial of other complaints FEV_1 900 cc on PFT* Barrel chest on physical examination	Severe airway obstruction (chronic airflow limitation)
Increase in wheezing in COPD patient Decrease in breath sounds RLL and left lower lobe (LLL) c/o chest discomfort, dyspnea Cough and sputum production Chest x-ray film shows increase in areas of consolidation RLL and LLL (There are many key cues in this group of findings. See if you can find a cue for each subdiagnosis.)	Increased airway obstruction Subdiagnoses: bronchoconstriction, impaired ventilation RLL and LLL, mucus retention, possible chest infection
Lungs clear Vital signs stable Slight pedal edema* Nocturia* Difficulty putting on shoes	Fluid retention possibly due to right ventricular failure
5 hr post myocardial infarction Denial of chest pain Monitor-sinus tachycardia 104/min B/P increase from 140/80 to 150/90 mmHg Upon admission, lungs clear except for a few fine inspiratory crackles RLL laterally. Now, lungs clear except for coarse inspiratory crackles entire RLL and LLL.*	Impaired ventilation Fluid retention possibly due to left ventricular failure or pulmonary edema Actual or potential decreased cardiac output
Concern with weight gain and moonface-appearance associated with use of oral steroids Reluctance to socialize; if on oxygen therapy, reluctance to wear nasal cannula and use ambulatory oxygen set up outside home* Barrel chest and finger clubbing on physical examination Comments such as "I just don't look like I used to. Who wants to visit a decrepit old woman?"	Alteration in body image Social isolation Possible decreased self esteem
Recent hospital admission Repeated expressions of concern regarding disease state and level of functioning* Hyperactive body movements and gestures Altered speech pattern, e.g., accelerated rate and volume or pinched, feeble speech Slight dyspnea, diaphoresis, nervousness	Anxiety
Recent hospitalization of 65-year-old male with severe bronchial asthma, hypoxemia, ventilatory failure Patient states intention to fly to a resort in 2 wk against medical advice Patient insists sputum is clear; nurse viewing same specimen states it is yellow* When physician discusses prognosis and limitations of disease, patient jokes about condition and changes subject	Denial of disease process and its implications
Patient expresses reluctance to take theophylline (Theobid) pills because he already feels 100% better* History of self discontinuation of medication after recovery from acute exacerbations of COPD Absence of posthospitalization follow-up care by visiting nurses trained in respiratory care	Noncompliance due to knowledge deficit, denial of disease process, or both

*Key cue.

Table 31–2. EXAMPLES OF AN ETIOLOGY SUGGESTING A DIAGNOSIS

Etiology	Possible Diagnosis
Failure to clean and dry respiratory equipment daily before reuse Persistent mucus retention problem	Chest infection
Faulty technique during delivery of aerosol bronchodilator Bronchodilator undermedication An environment with numerous potential allergens and lung irritants	Bronchoconstriction
Inadequate fluid intake	Thick mucus
Noncompliance with ordered oxygen therapy Removal of oxygen mask during meals Failure to preoxygenate before tracheal suctioning	Hypoxemia
Bronchoconstriction problem Thick mucus Ineffective coughing or deep breathing Faulty or suboptimal technique during use of incentive spirometry and postural drainage with percussion and vibration	Mucus retention
Physiologic changes associated with COPD, e.g., barrel chest, finger clubbing	Alteration in body image
Fear of respiratory symptoms during intercourse Sterility as occurs in chronic bronchitis, cystic fibrosis, long-term steroid therapy	Sexual dysfunction

sary to solve a problem. A problem is solved by meeting a need (Bloch, 1974).

Ideally, diagnosis leads directly to identification of the health need. For example, the nurse assumes that the patient in bronchospasm needs bronchodilator medication and possibly steroids. When diagnoses are this specific, health needs are usually readily evident and interventions naturally follow. When diagnoses are broad, appropriate interventions are not readily apparent, and further data collection lacks focus.

Many nurses are fairly adept at identifying health needs and sometimes do so without diagnosing actual problems. If a patient appears cyanotic and dyspneic, the acute care nurse readily identifies the need for oxygen. A subsequent ABG result confirms or rules out the diagnosis of hypoxemia. In contrast, health needs of patients with chronic lung disease may not become apparent until the end of data collection or during the planning stage of intervention, when the nurse has a more complete patient profile. From this perspective, since consideration of health needs occurs to varying degrees during assessment, nurses must know about respiratory intervention *before* initiation of data collection. This is a good example of the blending of intervention with assessment.

Validation

After the initial generation of hypotheses, the nurse collects data to shape, refine, rank, verify, or eliminate hypotheses. This is the process of *validation*. To sort out possible causes of problems, questioning may deviate considerably from the established interview format. Whenever a line of questioning ceases to yield pertinent information, the nurse reverts back to the neutral general categories of the chosen assessment tool. Through experience, each clinician develops tactics to reduce the number of steps necessary to validate hypotheses. Again, familiarity with significant cues facilitates the switch to new hypotheses and the search for new data to validate revised hypotheses.

There is another aspect of validation that is key to motivational assessment (see Chapter 16). Not only does the nurse validate information for her own purposes, she also corroborates the patient's hypotheses about his illness with her own. When a discrepancy between the two occurs, she strives to attain mutual agreement (Carrieri and Sitzman, 1979). The nurse may need to delay validation of some hypotheses, depending on time limitations and the COPD patient's state of action or nonaction (see Chapter 16). In the latter case, the patient's psychologic coping mechanisms may hinder collaboration.

THE END OF DATA COLLECTION

The nurse ends data collection when all the needed or available data for diagnosis are collected, when further data collection is likely to yield little significant return, or when a problem is urgent and requires immediate care. By this time, *one* to *three* top-priority problems should already be identified with a relatively high degree of certainty. If the nurse has doubts or specific concerns about possible diagnoses, she may return to the bedside to further develop the patient profile, identify needs for selection of interventions, or explore the patient's attitudes towards the health care team.

Most important, during this whole process, skill does not depend upon a comprehensive inventory but upon hypothetico-deductive reasoning (Barrows and Tamblyn, 1980) combined with accommodation of the patient's psychologic defense mechanisms.

PATTERNS OF DIAGNOSTIC ERROR

Diagnostic errors occur in clinical practice unless the nurse consciously tries to avoid them. Three common patterns of diagnostic errors are *premature closure, lack of closure,* and *invalid data clustering* (Bruce and Snyder, 1982).

Premature closure is a diagnosis made with an inadequate data base. For example, the nurse who notes a smoking history may diagnose airway obstruction without gathering PFTs and other assessment data for validation. Similarly, the acute care nurse might assume mucus retention without assessment of lung sounds or chest x-ray findings.

Lack of closure occurs when an adequate data base is present, but the nurse fails to diagnose a problem. The reason relates to an inadequate knowledge base, a limited interpretation skill, or a failure to consult other health team members.

As in most diagnostic errors, consultation helps prevent lack of closure. The rationale for consultation is twofold. First, it provides expertise for diagnosis of many interrelated problems. Second, consultation provides an unbiased view of the clinical situation. When nurses work intensely or for long periods with the same patient and family, the close relationship may bias the nurses' mental processing of information and lead to diagnostic errors.

Invalid data clustering refers to a false assumption of a relationship between data when no relationship exists. For example, the nurse mistakenly assumes a relationship between a positive fluid balance (i.e., signs of fluid retention) and early inspiratory crackle when, in fact, this type of crackle is related to chronic bronchitis not fluid retention from left ventricular failure. This error is unlikely to occur if the nurse is more thoroughly educated and experienced in respiratory diagnosis.

HEURISTICS FOR DIAGNOSIS

Thus far, this chapter has presented the process of diagnosis in detail. The question remains, however, how does the nurse implement this large and rather ill-defined body of knowledge in clinical practice? What practical guides are available to facilitate hypothetico-deductive reasoning in the clinical setting?

Unfortunately, no theoretic framework exists to help the nurse mentally process assessment data and arrive at correct diagnoses. Several investigators have proposed flow charts and other models to aid in clinical decision-making (Lane et al, 1983; Harper, 1981). However, current models are impractical for changing clinical situations and fail to teach the overall process of hypothetico-deductive reasoning.

Heuristics for Cue Interpretation

Until appropriate models are formulated, nurses must develop their own practical guides or heuristics for data collection, cue interpretation, and problem identification. Cue interpretation is most important because research indicates that use of refined hypothetico-deductive reasoning skills does not lead to correct diagnosis, if the clinician interprets the data incorrectly (Elstein et al, 1978). If nurses cannot correctly interpret cues, they are not ready for problem-solving situations.

Detailed respiratory content presented in this book may be generalized and recategorized into practical tabulated form (Table 31–3 through Table 31–7).

Table 31–3. OBSTRUCTIVE AND RESTRICTIVE PULMONARY DISEASE

	Obstructive Disease	Restrictive Disease
Definition	Increased resistance to air flow	Decrease in lung volume
Pathologic features	Luminal obstruction Intrinsic airway narrowing Peribronchial obstruction	Loss of lung tissue Loss of functioning alveoli Decreased lung and chest wall compliance
Respiratory problems	Bronchoconstriction, airway obstruction, or airflow limitation* Impaired ventilation Thick mucus Increased sputum production Mucus retention Potential chest infection Decreased exercise tolerance Inability to control dyspnea Sleep pattern disturbance	Problems may be absent with mild to moderate disease Hypoxemia* Impaired ventilation Potential mucus retention or chest infection Other problems associated with superimposed obstructive disease
Implications for intervention	Bronchodilators, antibiotics, bronchial hygiene program, dyspnea control, breathing retraining with PLB	Oxygen, bronchial hygiene program (less intense since mucus retention is not a problem), dyspnea control, breathing retraining
Goals	Decrease in bronchoconstriction, airway obstruction, or airflow limitation Absent to minimal mucus production and retention	Normal oxygenation Patent airways and inflated alveoli

*Characteristic.

Table 31–4. KEY CLINICAL FINDINGS IN OBSTRUCTIVE AND RESTRICTIVE DISEASE

Assessment Parameter	Obstructive Disease	Restrictive Disease
History	Dyspnea Cough Sputum production Wheeze	Dyspnea Dry cough Fatigue Chest discomfort or pain
Pulmonary medications	Bronchodilators Antibiotics Oxygen Diuretics Potassium chloride	Oxygen Corticosteroids Diuretics Potassium chloride
Chest examination	Tachypnea 1:4 I:E ratio PLB Increased AP diameter ↓ chest expansion (bilateral) Crackles, rhonchi, wheeze Generalized decreased breath sounds Decreased tactile fremitus Hyperresonance to percussion	Tachypnea 1:1 I:E ratio Rapid, shallow breathing Chest cage deformity or postoperative chest ↓ chest expansion often unilateral or asymmetric Crackles Localized bronchial breath sounds with egophony and bronchophony Increased tactile fremitus Dullness to percussion
ABGs	Pa_{O_2} normal to ↓ Pa_{CO_2} normal to ↓ (early) ↑ (late) Acidemia with ↑ Pa_{CO_2}	Pa_{O_2} normal to ↓ Pa_{CO_2} normal to ↓ (early) ↑ (late) Alkalemia with ↓ Pa_{CO_2}
PFTs	VC ↓ RV and TLC ↑ FEV_1/FVC (%) ↓ Response to bronchodilator	VC ↓ All lung volumes ↓ FEV_1/FVC (%) ↑ No response to bronchodilator
Chest x-ray	Lung hyperinflation: flat diaphragms, widened ICS, increased AP diameter, lung hyperlucency (oligemia), and so forth Increased bronchovascular markings Bullae	Loss of lung volume: plate-like atelectasis, fissure displacement, crowded bronchovascular markings, elevated diaphragms, narrowed ICS, mediastinal shift, and so forth. Interstitial pattern Alveolar pattern
Motivation (low, medium, high)	Low due to denial, depression, anxiety, repression, social isolation, fear of suffocation, knowledge deficit	Variable
Self-care education (low, medium, high)	Low: pulmonary symptoms and age limit the patient's ADLs and muscle coordination for respiratory techniques (e.g., inhaler); patient demonstrates lack of knowledge regarding preventive measures.	Medium: fewer respiratory interventions are required to control symptoms; patient resumes most ADLs but demonstrates lack of knowledge regarding preventive measures

Table 31–5. KEY CLINICAL FINDINGS IN COPD

	Asthma	Bronchitis	Emphysema
Pulmonary symptoms	Dyspnea preceded by cough and wheeze Chest tightness or sense of suffocation	Cough Sputum production	Dsypnea Cough
Age of onset	Childhood Adulthood	25 to 40 years of age	50 to 60 years of age
Disease course	Variable	Variable	Persistent downhill course once symptoms appear
Work of breathing	↑	↑	↑ ↑
Chest examination	Use of accessory muscles ↑ I:E ratio Lung hyperinflation during attacks Wheezing Decreased breath sounds (late)	Use of accessory muscles ↑ I:E ratio Cyanosis Peripheral edema Crackles, rhonchi	Excessive use of accessory muscles ↑ I:E ratio Lung hyperinflation Weight loss Decreased breath sounds
Pao_2	↓ during attacks	↓	Near normal until end-stage disease
$Paco_2$	↓ slightly ↑ with severe acute disease	↑	Normal to slightly ↓
PFTs	↓ expiratory flow rates ↑ TLC (FRC) during attacks Great response to bronchodilator Normal diffusing capacity (DL) between attacks	↓ expiratory flow rates Near normal TLC Small response to bronchodilator Normal DL	↓ expiratory flow rates ↑ TLC No response to bronchodilator ↓ DL
Pulmonary artery pressures	↑ during attacks	↑ ↑ from hypoxic vasoconstriction	↑ with moderate loss of pulmonary vessels
Cardiac output	Normal ↑ during attacks	Normal to ↑	↓

Table 31–6. RESPIRATORY PROBLEMS ASSOCIATED WITH PULMONARY DISEASES

Diseases	Respiratory Problems
Obstructive	
Upper airway obstruction	Potential respiratory arrest Airway obstruction* Hypoxemia Alveolar hypoventilation
Bronchial asthma	Bronchospasm* Mucus retention (mucus plugs)* Hypoxemia Alveolar hypoventilation Uncontrolled coughing Uncontrolled acute dyspnea Postnasal drip (allergic rhinitis)
Chronic bronchitis	Mucus production* Mucus retention* Hypoxemia Alveolar hypoventilation Fluid retention
Emphysema	Increased work of breathing* Potential mucus retention
Restrictive	
Chronic disease, e.g. diffuse interstitial fibrosis	Problems may be absent in mild to moderate disease Hypoxemia* Impaired ventilation Decreased exercise tolerance Potential mucus retention/chest infection
Acute pneumonia	Chest infection* Thick mucus* Mucus retention* Pleuritic chest pain Infective coughing or deep breathing Impaired ventilation in pathologic areas Hypoxemia Alveolar hyperventilation (early disease) Alveolar hypoventilation (late disease)
Acute cardiogenic pulmonary edema	*Early:* Impaired ventilation Absent to mild hypoxemia Fluid overload or fluid retention *Late:* Fluid overload or fluid retention Ventilatory failure Severe hypoxemia Increased work of breathing Problems associated with obstructive disease may be present in patients with mixed chest pathology
Acute atelectasis	*Early:* Impaired ventilation* Ineffective coughing or deep breathing Absent to mild hypoxemia* *Late:* Mucus production or retention Severe hypoxemia Alveolar hypoventilation Potential or actual chest infection Problems associated with pneumonia and obstructive disease may develop, if airways and alveoli remain collapsed or obstructed with secretions

*Key problem.

Table 31–7. PROBLEMS ASSOCIATED WITH ADVANCED PULMONARY DISEASE (COR PULMONALE)

Biophysical Problems	Psychosocial Problems
Fluid retention Hypoxemia Inability to control dyspnea Inability to perform ADL Ineffective breathing pattern Muscle weakness or deconditioning Poor nutritional status Sleep pattern disturbance Ventilatory failure Weight gain from steroids, heart failure Weight loss from terminal illness	Alteration in body image Anxiety Decreased self-esteem Denial of disease process and its implications Depression Dysfunctional grieving Fear of suffocation Impaired verbal communication Inadequate situational support systems Ineffective family coping Knowledge deficit Noncompliance (nonadherence) Role disturbance Sensory deprivation Sexual dysfunction Social isolation

These tables serve as a set of heuristics to guide the mental storage and retrieval of information for the identification and interpretation of cues and respiratory problems. Though these tables help the nurse initiate respiratory assessment, validation of hypotheses may require more specific assessment tools, such as those presented in the assessment chapters of this book (see Chapters 10 through 17)

Similarly, decision trees may guide cue interpretation and hypothesis generation. From a conceptual viewpoint, the task of the diagnostician is to identify cues, mentally process them, and propose one or more problems (Fig. 31–2).

The expert nurse gathers a few crucial cues, subconsciously makes several deductions, and proposes problems in a matter of minutes. Most clinicians, however, need more time for assessment. They gather more data to consciously decide whether the patient has obstructive or restrictive disease (first branch in the decision tree in Figure 31–2), where the disease is located (second branch), and what type of pulmonary disease is present (third branch). Determination of obstructive versus restrictive disease is important, because patients with each type have different sets of problems, requiring different therapies and different therapeutic goals, as reviewed in Table 31–3. The location of pathology is important, because this information guides the search for assessment data to confirm or rule out problems. Specific medical diagnoses are important because they often serve as critical cues in the clustering of information for respiratory diagnoses. Also, interventions, and hence data collection for their evaluation, differ for various pulmonary diseases. The goal of therapy is important because the nurse continuously gathers information to assess appropriate goal attainment for patients with restrictive and obstructive disease.

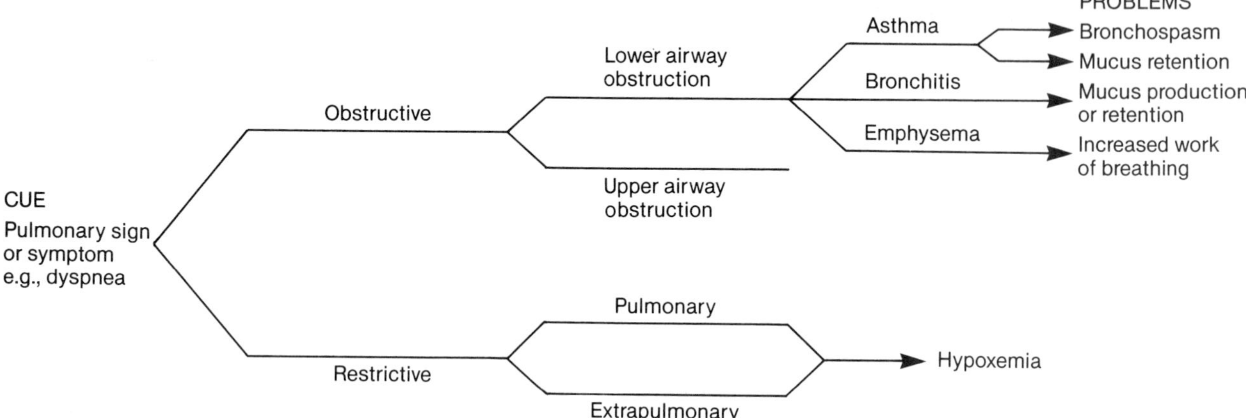

Figure 31–2. Example of a decision tree for respiratory diagnosis. Clinical reasoning begins with a cue, e.g., dyspnea (to the left), and ends with a problem identification (to the right). Distinguishing problems are listed for COPD and restrictive lung diseases.

The nurse may utilize Table 31–4 to help collect and interpret assessment data relating to restrictive and obstructive disease. Key clinical findings in asthma, bronchitis, and emphysema (the classic obstructive diseases) are summarized in Table 31–5.

Respiratory problems found in specific obstructive and restrictive diseases are summarized in Table 31–6. Decision-making is easier when the medical diagnosis is known, because most diseases have characteristic problems.

Problems associated with advanced pulmonary disease (cor pulmonale) are reviewed in Table 31–7. In cor pulmonale, decision-making is usually a complex and time-consuming process because of the numerous actual, potential, and possible problems requiring assessment.

Heuristics and Intuition

Though heuristics are commonly known as "rules of thumb" or "practical guides," a more precise definition is *the art or science of using practical guides or intuitive judgments to guide choice in problem-solving situations.*

Previous discussion has focused on the "practical guides" of the definition, without attention to the intuitive judgment aspect. Intuition is perhaps the most important aspect, as evidenced by the true meaning of the word. The term heuristics is derived from the ancient Greek verb *heuriskein*, meaning "to discover" or "to find."

With the discovery notion in mind, heuristics help the nurse intuit to generate hypotheses and identify problems correctly. More specifically, heuristics allow the nurse to have an "Aha!" experience. They provoke a "bright idea" towards problem solution that involves a sudden reorganization of one's mode of problem conception. When assessing the multiproblem respiratory patient, several "Aha!" experiences may be necessary to eventually identify the correct respiratory problem.

While mentally scanning clinical findings, the nurse may use the diagnostic heuristics in Table 31–8 to provoke insight and validate hypotheses. These heuristics are oriented towards incremental decision-making, the difficult type of decision-making described in the Introduction. Note that implications for theory development have been included in Table 31–8 to guide the development of a needed taxonomy of respiratory nursing diagnoses for collaborative practice.

THE DIAGNOSTIC STATEMENT

Once validated by diagnostic reasoning processes, respiratory problems are communicated in the form of a diagnostic statement. The diagostic statement has two parts: the *health problem* and the *etiology of the problem.* Each part is stated clearly and concisely, ideally in two or three words. The whole statement should be specific enough to be clinically useful and understandable to other members of the health care team. Additional guidelines for the formulation and writing of respiratory diagnoses follow:

1. *Limit each diagnostic statement to one actual, potential, or possible problem.* Be careful not to confuse a health problem with a health need. Nursing diagnoses from the Seventh Conference on the Classification of Nursing Diagnoses are listed in Table 31–9 to use as a guide. The nurse may need to modify suggested diagnoses or make up new ones for application to respiratory patients.
2. *Remember that a health problem indicates the presence of a health need. It requires a plan; otherwise it is not a problem.* Depending on baseline findings, abnormal findings (e.g., low PaO_2 of 58 mmHg) may not pose a problem for the patient.

Table 31–8. DIAGNOSTIC HEURISTICS

Heuristic	Description	Clinical Implications	Implications for Theory Development
Planning	There should be a plan and a well-defined purpose behind every question.	The clinician must know assessment and intervention aspects of each problem before approaching the patient and interpreting data.	Develop a taxonomy of respiratory diagnoses to serve as a guide for planning. Remember that it cannot substitute for cue interpretation skills.
Hypothesis specificity	No hypothesis should be more specific or more general than evidence on hand justifies.	Look for broad (nonspecific) defining characteristics for general (broad) problems and specific characteristics for specific problems, e.g., decreased breath sounds and impaired lung ventilation match because both are nonspecific (broad).	Develop broad diagnoses with subcategories. Match the level of specificity (generality) between cues and hypotheses.
Competing hypothesis	Consider at least two or three competing hypotheses. Consider each piece of information in relation to each of these hypotheses.	Do not restrict choice to only one hypothesis, even if all data seem to confirm the choice. Be systematic about assessing each competing hypothesis.	Develop numerous categories and subcategories to facilitate differential diagnosis in the multiproblem respiratory patient.
Reinterpretation	Review all information again in relation to the new hypothesis. Categorize findings as tending to either confirm or rule out the new hypothesis.	Reinterpret clinical findings in this way whenever clinical findings change. In stressful or incremental decision-making situations, collaborate with physicians and others to reinterpret data. Skipping this heuristic leads to misdiagnosis by omission.	Develop a methodology for teaching nurses how to process information in relation to each hypothesis. Many nurses tend to omit this process. Study ways to reduce the memory burden imposed upon nurses by this heuristic, e.g., separate decisions into categoric and incremental levels, use computers to facilitate data analysis.
Negative inference	When high cost assessment is under consideration to confirm a diagnosis, consider low cost assessment as well. *High cost assessment* refers to any diagnostic maneuver that is expensive, uncomfortable, or risky for the patient. *Low cost assessment* might rule out one or more hypotheses to make high cost assessment unnecessary. Also, it might increase the probability that the high cost assessment will yield definitive treatment.	Do not forget to consider cost. For example, the nurse might consider using finger oximetry to measure SaO_2 rather than obtaining a PRN ABG, an invasive procedure. A high oximetry SaO_2 reading may rule out hypoxemia and make the ABG unnecessary.	Consider cost factors in the development of assessment and intervention aspects of each problem.

Typology adapted from Elstein, A., Shulman, L., Sprafka, S., et al. Medical Problem Solving—An Analysis of Clinical Reasoning. Cambridge, MA: Harvard University Press, 1978.

Table 31–9. APPROVED NURSING DIAGNOSES LISTED BY CODE NUMBER AND HUMAN RESPONSE PATTERN*

Pattern 1: Exchanging—A human response pattern involving mutual giving and receiving

1.1.2.1	Nutrition, altered: More than body requirements
1.1.2.2	Nutrition, altered: Less than body requirements
1.1.2.3	Nutrition, altered: Potential for more than body requirements
1.2.1.1	+ Infection: Potential for
1.2.2.1	+ Body temperature, altered: Potential
1.2.2.2	+ Hypothermia
1.2.2.3	+ Hyperthermia
1.2.2.4	+ Thermoregulation, ineffective
1.3.1.1	Bowel elimination, altered: Constipation
1.3.1.2	Bowel elimination, altered: Diarrhea
1.3.1.3	Bowel elimination, altered: Incontinence
1.3.2	Urinary elimination, altered patterns
1.3.2.1.1	+ Incontinence, stress
1.3.2.1.2	+ Incontinence, reflex
1.3.2.1.3	+ Incontinence, urge
1.3.2.1.4	+ Incontinence, functional
1.3.2.1.5	+ Incontinence, total
1.3.2.2	+ Urinary retention
1.4.1.1.	Tissue perfusion, altered: renal, cerebral, cardiopulmonary, gastrointestinal, peripheral + +
1.4.1.2.1	Fluid volume excess
1.4.1.2.2.1	Fluid volume deficit: Actual (1)
1.4.1.2.2.1	Fluid volume deficit: Actual (2)
1.4.1.2.2.2	Fluid volume deficit: Potential
1.4.2.1	Cardiac output, altered: Decreased
1.5.1.1	Gas exchange, impaired
1.5.1.2	Airway clearance, ineffective
1.5.1.3	Breathing pattern, ineffective
1.6.1	Injury, potential for
1.6.1.1	Injury, potential for: Suffocating
1.6.1.2	Injury, potential for: Poisoning
1.6.1.3	Injury, potential for: Trauma
1.6.2.1.1	Skin integrity, impaired: Actual
1.6.2.1.2	Skin integrity, impaired: Potential
1.6.2.2	+ Tissue integrity, impaired
1.6.2.2.1	Tissue integrity, impaired: oral mucous membrane

Pattern 2: Communicating—A human response pattern involving sending messages

2.1.1.1	Communication, impaired: Verbal

Pattern 3: Relating—A human response pattern involving establishing bonds.

3.1.1	+ Social interaction, impaired
3.1.2	Social isolation
3.2.1	Role performance, altered
3.2.1.1.1	Parenting, altered: Actual
3.2.1.1.2	Parenting, altered: Potential
3.2.1.2.1	Sexual dysfunction
3.2.2	Family processes, altered
3.3	+ Sexuality, altered patterns

Pattern 4: Valuing—A human response pattern involving the assigning of relative worth

4.1.1	Spiritual distress (distress of the human spirit)

Pattern 5: Choosing—A human response pattern involving the selection of alternatives

5.1.1.1	Coping, ineffective individual
5.1.1.1.1	+ Adjustment, impaired
5.1.2.1.1	Coping, ineffective family: Disabled
5.1.2.1.2	Coping, ineffective family: Compromised
5.1.2.2	Coping, family: Potential for growth
5.2.1.1	Noncompliance (specify)

Pattern 6: Moving—A human response pattern involving activity

6.1.1.1	Mobility, impaired physical
6.1.1.2	Activity intolerance
6.1.1.3	Activity intolerance: Potential
6.2.1	Sleep pattern disturbance
6.3.1.1	Diversional activity, deficit
6.4.1.1	Home maintenance management, impaired
6.4.2	Health maintenance, altered
6.5.1	Self-care deficit: Feeding
6.5.1.1	+ Swallowing, impaired
6.5.2	Self-care deficit: Bathing/hygiene
6.5.3	Self-care deficit: Dressing/grooming
6.5.4	Self-care deficit: Toileting
6.6	+ Growth and development, altered

Pattern 7: Perceiving—A human response pattern involving the reception of information

7.1.1	Self-concept, disturbance in: Body image
7.1.2	Self-concept, disturbance in: Self-esteem
7.1.3	Self-concept, disturbance in: Personal identity
7.2	Sensory/perceptual alterations: Visual, auditory, kinesthetic, gustatory, tacile, olfactory + + +
7.2.1.1	+ Unilateral neglect
7.3.1	+ Hopelessness
7.3.2	Powerlessness

Pattern 8: Knowing—A human response pattern involving the meaning associated with information

8.1.1	Knowledge deficit (specify)
8.3	Thought processes, altered

Pattern 9: Feeling—A human response pattern involving the subjective awareness of information.

9.1.1	Comfort, altered: Pain
9.1.1.1	+ Comfort, altered: Chronic pain
9.2.1	Anxiety
9.2.2.1	Grieving, dysfunctional
9.2.2.2	Grieving, anticipatory
9.2.3	Violence, potential for: Self-directed or directed at others
9.2.4	Fear
9.2.5	+ Post-trauma response
9.2.5.1.1	Rape-trauma syndrome
9.2.5.1.2	Rape-trauma syndrome: Compound reaction
9.2.5.1.3	Rape-trauma syndrome: Silent reaction

*Reproduced and adapted by permission from McLane, A. (ed.). Classification of Nursing Diagnoses—Proceedings of the Seventh Conference, North American Nursing Diagnosis Association. St. Louis, C. V. Mosby Co., 1987.

+ = New diagnosis approved 1986.

+ + = See NANDA Taxonomy I for numerical code to designate specific tissue (McLane, 1987).

+ + + = See NANDA Taxonomy I for numerical code to designate specific senses (McLane, 1987).

3. *Note the severity or extent of the problem.* The following qualifiers help the nurse prioritize problems and plan interventions:
   a. *Mild, moderate, severe* (use PFT guidelines in Chapter 14, when appropriate), e.g., severe bronchoconstriction.
   b. *Acute, chronic,* e.g., acute upper airway obstruction.
   c. *Situational* (associated with specific situations), e.g., situational depression related to recent death of spouse.
4. *Identify the etiology or cause of the problem.* Since etiology suggests possible solutions to the problem, it is a major consideration in the next step of the nursing process—the planning of interventions.
   a. Use "due to" as a link whenever you are sure of an etiology, e.g., acute situational anxiety due to financial problems.
   b. Use "related to" whenever the exact cause-and-effect relationship is uncertain or vague, e.g., severe bronchospasm related to exposure to allergens in the home.
   c. List all etiologies. Respiratory diagnoses commonly have more than one etiology, e.g., mucus retention due to bronchospasm, dehydration, and ineffective coughing.
   d. Change etiology as the patient's condition changes. *Initial diagnosis,* bronchoconstriction due to airway hyperirritability and possible allergic reaction. After onset of pulmonary edema, bronchoconstriction related to pulmonary edema.
   e. Whenever etiology is unknown or insufficient time or expertise (or both) is available to determine etiology, use "of unknown or undetermined etiology," e.g., acute upper airway obstruction of undetermined etiology. Another way to deal with this circumstance is to omit etiology from the diagnostic statement until further assessment reveals the probable cause of the problem.
   f. Whenever a similar or identical etiology appears in a list of problems, consider adding the etiology as a separate diagnosis. An example follows:

      To this list:
      Medication noncompliance related to exercise intolerance and inaccessible pharmacy location. Inadequate cleaning of home respiratory equipment due to dyspnea on exertion.
      Add:
      Exercise intolerance related to cor pulmonale and muscle deconditioning.
   g. Make sure etiology is not a restatement of the problem.

      Wrong: Bronchospasm related to increased bronchomotor tone.

      Right: Bronchospasm related to aspirin ingestion.
   h. Do not confuse etiology with the overall problem. Ask yourself, "Which came first?" and put your answer (etiology) in the second clause.

      Wrong: Knowledge deficit related to inability to control shortness of breath.

      Right: Inability to control shortness of breath related to knowledge deficit.
5. *State both problem and etiology components as specifically as possible.* When having difficulty determining labelling problems, however, use *broad* titles, such as impaired ventilation or alteration in respiratory function.
6. *Remember, a patient can have a constellation of related problems that are treated together as well as separately,* e.g., impaired ventilation, hypoxemia, bronchoconstriction, mucus retention. Narrowing down problems in this way is essential to comprehensive care, because each problem requires a specific approach for assessment and intervention. For example, impaired ventilation might require assisted ventilation; hypoxemia, oxygen; bronchoconstriction, mainly bronchodilators; and mucus retention, increased fluid intake with coughing and deep breathing.
7. *Scrutinize your list of diagnoses.* Are diagnoses clearly written? Are labels consistent with standard respiratory terminology and those used in your practice setting? Is the list complete?

Labelling and charting specific respiratory diagnoses may be problems in practice settings allowing only a few standardized broad categories. To adapt broad North American Nursing Diagnosis Association (NANDA) categories, the nurse may use the following format: *impaired gas exchange: hypoxemia related to V/Q abnormality.* Though institutional rules may emphasize use of broad categories, the nurse in collaborative practice must remember to consider *all* of the patient's specific respiratory diagnoses during assessment and intervention. The more specific the diagnosis, the more appropriate the intervention is likely to be.

Intervention

Intervention refers to the planning, implementation, and evaluation of respiratory care. Decision-making in this phase of the nursing process tends to be incremental rather than categoric because of different clinical manifestations of the same problem and because no *one* best solution exists for common problems. Because of the incremental nature and uncertainty of decision-making, careful planning is necessary to determine appropriate interventions and facilitate favorable patient outcomes.

PLANNING OF THE INTERVENTION

Planning involves several processes as follows: identifying top-priority problems, initiating further data collection and analysis, setting goals, deciding on appropriate interventions, and writing evaluation criteria.

Identification of Top-Priority Problems

The nurse identifies one to three top-priority problems, if not already done during the assessment phase. When priorities are set at the very beginning of the planning stage, the nurse is better able to decide what to do first for the multiproblem patient.

The following three questions help in the identification and ranking of top-priority problems:

1. *What are the patient's acute health needs?* Nursing diagnoses may be mentally converted back into health needs and divided into acute, preventive, and maintenance categories. These categories are defined in Table 17–7. Acute needs reflect top-priority problems.

2. *What is the patient's overall health status?* Better? Worse? Status quo? Problems often change in urgency and priority, depending upon changes in health status.

3. *Which health problem is most important to patient and family?* This problem must be one of the top-priority problems.

Collection of Additional Data

In most cases, the nurse collects enough data during assessment to identify acute problems and needs. However, because of limited time, energy, and other situational constraints, the nurse may be unable to identify preventive and maintenance teaching-learning needs associated with chronic problems. Sometimes, the nurse identifies an acute problem, such as acute bronchospasm due to exposure to allergens in the home. But the need for immediate intervention takes precedence over further data collection to assess etiology, in this case allergens in the home. After stabilization of acute illness, the nurse employs a specific assessment tool, such as the interview form for home assessment of potential allergens or lung irritants (Table 10–7), to further analyze problems and plan interventions. Again, the blending of assessment with intervention in the nursing process becomes evident.

Analysis of Intervening Variables

In pulmonary disease, seven main intervening variables affect the acuity, etiology, or treatment of physiologic and psychosocial problems. Consideration of these variables is essential before deciding upon a general approach to the patient and a specific plan.

Level of Wellness or Severity of Physiologic Dysfunction. Use PFTs and blood gases to identify the severity of physiologic problems (e.g., acute exacerbation? life-threatening? chronic?) as well as plan an approach to management of psychosocial problems.

Psychosocial Coping Mechanisms. How much intervention will the patient tolerate? Remember that the severe COPD patient in his emotional straitjacket cannot tolerate interventions that cause extreme states of action or nonaction. This is especially important when considering grief and loss or body image problems. For example, in helping the COPD patient face the irreversibility of his disease and the loss of prior level of functioning, the nurse cannot realistically expect all patients to pass through all of Engle's following four phases of the grieving process: shock and disbelief, developing awareness, restitution, and resolution (Engle, 1964). The patient's psychologic coping mechanisms of denial, repression, and isolation, which allow him to adapt physiologically, do not encourage development of awareness. Development of awareness or restitution might be a realistic goal. Development of the last phase, resolution of the loss and acceptance of a new life pattern, however, is a realistic initial goal only for patients with excellent psychosocial assets, not the typical severe COPD patient. In addition, resolution of losses may not be realistic for many disabled pulmonary patients because, unlike an amputated limb, shortness of breath (SOB) is ill defined and impossible to touch or see directly to facilitate its incorporation into a new set of body boundaries. These factors are important to consider in the assessment of psychosocial problems *as well as* psychosocial aspects of pathophysiologic problems.

Chest Pathology. Identification of restrictive versus obstructive disease processes as well as the components of mixed pathology (e.g., asthmatic or bronchitic components, anatomic emphysema, upper airway obstruction) helps the nurse identify appropriate goals and nursing interventions, as discussed in Chapters 7, 8, and 9.

Potential for Recovery. This variable has two aspects. First, input from the physician regarding *medical prognosis* is necessary before the nature and extent of interventions can be planned. Second, *level of motivation* determines the degree to which the patient is able or willing to participate in decision-making and the probability of successful outcomes. If the patient has not developed the first two components of the motivational model discussed in Chapter 16, planning of respiratory interventions is premature.

Situational Support Systems. This variable includes the availability of family and friends for psychologic support and the monitoring or performance of various aspects of care; financial assistance, a crucial variable for the individual with a critical or disabling illness; availability of respiratory equipment; and availability of basic follow-up care.

Efficiency of the Plan. Proposed interventions must be efficient in terms of time, energy, and money spent by the patient, nurse, other health care providers, and community. As an example, consider a patient scheduled for 10 sustained maximal inspirations every hour in the immediate postoperative period. The plan is efficient when treatments are timed around vital sign assessments and other activities, thus allowing for adequate periods of uninterrupted sleep or rest. The plan is inefficient and undesirable when treatments are scheduled at varied times within the hour because of the unnecessary waste of time and energy. The patient suffers shortened sleep periods. The nurse takes extra time and energy to encourage the tired, sleep deprived, and anxious patient to take treatments regularly and with correct technique.

Setting Goals

A goal is a standard for measuring the success or failure of interventions in solving problems. It is a statement of what the nurse expects to observe, hear, or see demonstrated at a given point in time. Although the nurse usually sets one goal for each problem analyzed in problem-oriented charting, emphasis is placed on the identification of one or two overall goals. An overall goal is oriented towards the *total* patient situation or a whole constellation of related problems responsible for illness.

Chapter 16 discusses how to develop mutually satisfying goals with the patient. Once developed, rephrasing may be necessary to facilitate monitoring by health professionals. The following points help the nurse write appropriate goals:

1. A goal must be generally stated to give direction to a plan but must be specifically stated in behavioral objective form, e.g., in 1 month the patient will report performing ADL* without any increase in SOB.
2. A goal must be congruent with the problem statement. For example, if the diagnosis is severe dyspnea on exertion, the goal must concern controlling dyspnea rather than some other related problem.
3. A goal must take into consideration individual manifestations of pathology as well as sensitive indicators of improvement for each situation, e.g., in 24 hours, the patient will demonstrate on auscultation an increase in breath sounds in the RLL.

Deciding on Appropriate Interventions

The nurse considers a range of alternative interventions and then decides on one to three interventions for each problem. Numerous alternative interventions may be generated from different resources, including respiratory textbooks, protocols, procedure books, and memory recall. The selection of one to three interventions is more difficult because it requires the consideration of individual patient need and the numerous intervening variables that affect patient outcome.

To facilitate selection, the nurse uses decision rules as guides. Main decision rules are listed here, but these may need alteration, depending on clinical circumstances and patient preferences.

DECISION RULES FOR RESPIRATORY INTERVENTIONS

1. Select the alternative with the greatest probability for goal attainment.
2. Select the alternative with the lowest risk to patient, family, health care providers, or any combination of these.
3. Select the alternative that meets a mutually satisfying goal set by patient and providers. Not applicable in some cases, e.g., comatose patient, respiratory distress patient.

The best intervention is one that rates high in probability for goal attainment and low in risk and is designed to meet a mutually satisfying goal. When an intervention does not meet all criteria, the nurse generates other alternatives or selects a suboptimal or risky intervention. In the case of a risky intervention, plans then focus on reducing risk.

The Importance of Risk Reduction. To better understand the importance of risk reduction, consider the following clinical situation. A critical care nurse needs to aspirate through the endotracheal tube of a ventilator patient to alleviate an airway obstruction problem (i.e., mucus plugs). The goal of therapy is relief of airway obstruction, as evidenced by decreased rhonchi on chest examination, decreased peak inspiratory pressures on the ventilator's pressure manometer, and no signs of respiratory distress. Though mucus is present, the decision to suction is not a clear-cut one because the patient is on high PEEP with a low PaO_2, and he will not tolerate hypoxemic episodes during suctioning.

Applying the first decision rule, the nurse rates suctioning *high* for probability of goal attainment. Suctioning is likely to remove mucus and relieve airway obstruction, since rhonchi are readily audible over the anterior chest.

Applying the second decision rule, the nurse rates risk *high* for hypoxemia, cardiac arrhythmias, and other complications, since the patient already has a borderline low PaO_2 on a high FIO_2.

If assessment parameters remain stable, the nurse decides that the benefits of suctioning will outweigh the risks of complications. She plans to aspirate through the patient's tube but with special attention to the particulars of intervention, i.e., adequate preoxygenation and postoxygenation and quick passage of the suction catheter through a self-sealing adaptor.

In this case, detailed planning reduced risk to an acceptable level. Planning helped the nurse decide with confidence that suctioning was reasonably safe, as long as certain provisions were carried out to reduce the risk of hypoxemia. In addition, it validated the original premise that benefits will outweigh risks.

*Activities of daily living.

From this perspective, *consideration of the way an intervention is carried out is equally as important as the intervention itself* when planning respiratory care.

Other Points. After problem analysis, the nurse may still have insufficient information for determing appropriate interventions. In this case, the nurse returns to data collection or collaborates with other health team members in problem analysis. When patient and family do not provide needed information, the nurse emphasizes the importance of their role in problem-solving and encourages them to provide the information as soon as possible.

When the solution to a health problem depends more on medical rather than nursing intervention, the nurse acts as a patient advocate and calls crucial data to the attention of the physician.

The planning of interventions may take place over days to weeks after a few initial interventions have been implemented and evaluated. Planning is most efficiently done when input from patient, family, and all health team members is considered simultaneously. Ideally, major decisions are made during clinical rounds or team conferences. Whenever possible, the introduction of each intervention is spaced over time to allow adequate intervals for self-care education and rallying of internal and external resources to cope with complicated treatment regimens.

Writing Evaluation Criteria

The nurse writes evaluation criteria for each intervention proposed. Similar to goals, evaluation criteria are statements of expected outcomes, but they tend to be more specific.

Example: In 1 week, the patient will report to the nurse that he can get himself out of bed, walk to the bathroom to attend to personal hygiene needs, and get dressed for the day without significant dsypnea.

In some cases, an evaluation criterion might be the same as an overall goal.

Example: Within 5 days, the patient's Pa_{CO_2} level will return to 38 to 42 mmHg.

Chapter 17 describes how to write evaluation criteria for basic respiratory interventions (see section entitled "Learning Objectives and Evaluation Criteria"). The same principles apply to the writing objectives for specialized interventions. Table 31–10 may be used as an additional guide in the formulation of evaluation criteria for the overall nursing care plan.

Once an evaluation criterion is in written form, read it over and make sure it is logical and as concise as possible. Verify that it actually measures the success or failure of the intervention.

Table 31–10. GUIDELINES FOR NURSING OUTCOME STATEMENTS (GOALS AND EVALUATION CRITERIA)*

An outcome statement includes	Common categories of nursing outcomes include
Subject who is to perform the expected behavior (patient)	Patient verbalizations about what they know, understand, or feel about a situation
Conditions under which the behavior will occur	Patient behavior patterns relating to specific situations (demonstration)
Criteria for determining acceptable performance	Patient traits, behaviors, or symptoms related to illness, disease process, or emotional disability, e.g., laboratory tests or signs and symptoms
A statement phrased in positive rather than negative terms (if possible)	Patient environment: those circumstances in the patient's environment that have significance, e.g., housekeeping
Description of terminal behavior (action verb)	
Projected deadline	

*After Mayers, M. A Systematic Approach to the Nursing Care Plan, 3rd edition. New York: Appleton-Century-Crofts, 1983.

IMPLEMENTATION OF THE INTERVENTION

Once a plan is formulated, the nurse begins to implement the intervention. Nursing actions in this treatment stage of the nursing process strive to maximize patient and family participation and to restore, maintain, and promote health (American Nurses Association, 1973). In its pure form, however, this stage is rather short lived because evaluation of interventions begins immediately or shortly after implementation and continues until treatment ends.

EVALUATION OF THE INTERVENTION

If theorists were to identify the next weakest link in the nursing process (after diagnosis), it probably would be evaluation of the intervention. Because evaluation requires use of assessment skills, a nurse weak in diagnosis is likely to be weak in evaluation as well. A study by Grossbach-Landis and McLane (1979) documents the inadequate or inappropriate use of nursing assessment skills during respiratory intervention. The investigators assessed the learning needs of 30 registered acute care nurses who regularly suctioned patients through an endotracheal or tracheostomy tube. They found that only 62% suctioned according to correct procedure. Examples of incorrect technique included excessively high suction pressures, failure to encourage coughing before suctioning, failure to hyperventilate or preoxygenate before and after suctioning, and suctioning over the 15-second deadline. Only 17 of 30 nurses observed (57%) provided psychologic support by alerting patients about to be suctioned and explaining their intention. In spite of these alarmingly low scores on intervention, the most deficient category in the study was assessment. Only 38% of nurses received correct ratings for assessment during intervention (evaluation). "Evaluation of the effectiveness of the nursing intervention was clearly lacking in 90 percent of subjects observed, a reflection of the task-oriented nature of nursing practice in the setting studied." Only three nurses auscultated the chest after suctioning. Other nurses aspirated patients routinely, regardless of need or presence of observable side effects. Some assumed the presence of secretions. Others suctioned patients without adequate knowledge of their vital signs.

Until nurses become more knowledgeable in respiratory health problems and needs and more proficient at complex respiratory interventions, a resource person (e.g., in-service educator, clinical nurse specialist, respiratory therapist) should be available to help staff nurses evaluate the success or failure of interventions. Evaluation of one respiratory intervention, such as suctioning, may be easy; when evaluated with other respiratory interventions in progress, such as postural drainage, aerosol therapy, and incentive spirometry, only an experienced clinician can determine whether an evaluation criterion is optimal for the patient in question.

Once treatment is in progress, evaluation is ongoing. Criteria written in the planning stage usually need modification based on the initial response to treatment and the identification of more sensitive indicators. For example, after teaching a patient pursed-lip breathing (PLB) the nurse might write the following evaluation criteria:

1. The patient states PLB feels comfortable and that it helps him control dyspnea.
2. The patient's respiratory rate decreases from 26 to 20/min during use of PLB.

If the nurse notes during a practice session that a certain faulty technique (e.g., I:E ratio of 1:1) invariably causes the patient to abandon PLB and become more dyspneic, an I:E ratio of 1:2 might be added as an additional criterion that will also help other nurses monitor technique during practice.

In essence, criteria must be brief and selective to be useful. For this purpose, the nurse might develop criteria from those listed under *For Overall Improvement in Condition* in Part 4 of this book. Then, to gain specificity, the nurse modifies or adds one or two criteria listed under *For Correct Technique.* Because evaluation criteria require constant modification, the nurse must become familiar with all criteria for basic respiratory interventions. Only then will ready recall of select criteria be possible for application in the clinical setting.

Revision of the Plan

During implementation and evaluation of the intervention, the nurse collects assessment data that relate to overall goals and evaluation criteria. If criteria for a specific intervention are met, the intervention or combination of related interventions is labelled beneficial to the patient. If criteria are *easily* met (with plenty of leeway), the intervention may be discontinued or the overall treatment plan may be adjusted to reduce time, energy, and money channelled into respiratory procedures. If criteria are *not* met, the intervention or technique may be inappropriate, its timing in relation to other interventions may be suboptimal, or the patient's disease process might have changed enough to require an alteration in the nature or intensity of the intervention.

Plan revision is relatively easy when criteria are based either on observable technique such as I:E ratio during PLB, or on clear-cut sensitive indicators, such as PaO_2. In these cases, the nurse usually moves from evaluation directly to plan revision, as illustrated by the arrow between the two steps in Figure 31–1. Reassessment is unnecessary. In the first case, the nurse revises the original plans to achieve a breathing pattern closer to the target I:E ratio. In the second case, the nurse revises plans to achieve an acceptable PaO_2, thus saving the patient from further hypoxemia and ventilatory failure. Such plan revisions automatically occur when the nurse is thoroughly familiar with teaching-learning needs or when standing orders indicate what to do for abnormal ABGs or PFTs.

Reassessment

Sometimes, plan revisions save the patient's life without actually solving pulmonary problems. Since pulmonary problems are usually interrelated and evaluation criteria for main interventions tend to be similar or identical, failure to meet criteria on any *one* intervention commonly calls for *total* reassessment of the situation to determine how different segments of the plan should be revised. For example, a drop in PaO_2 might require reassessment of hypoxemia, ventilatory failure, and mucus retention problems. If PaO_2 drops while rhonchi in the chest increase, interventions might call for an increased FIO_2 as well as adjustments on the mechanical ventilator to compensate for the change in lung compliance and airway resistance and increased emphasis on bronchial hygiene interventions.

Hence, particularly in pulmonary disease, one cannot short circuit the nursing process for long periods without eventually reassessing the total patient situation. The pulmonary nurse temporarily moves directly from evaluation to plan revision; when problems persist, all problems must be considered together and recycled simultaneously back through data collection and diagnosis (see Fig. 31–1). Failure to regularly reassess problems leads to fragmented care, temporary improvement in clinical status, and repeated hospitalizations.

The Key Role of Assessment in the Nursing Process

This chapter has shown that assessment conceptually consists of only data collection and diagnosis. In practice, however, it blends into intervention at three points. First, planning interventions often requires additional data collection and diagnosis. Second, implementation of the intervention requires ongoing evaluation and utilization of assessment skills. Third, evaluation blends into the data collection phase whenever persistent problems must be recycled for reassessment and whenever data collection is initiated on a new patient already receiving some form of respiratory therapy. Comprehensive assessment always includes evaluation of current therapy.

Clearly, assessment has a key role in the nursing process (see Fig. 13–1). When this concept is implemented in the clinical setting, the beginner quickly becomes an expert in respiratory nursing care. A characteristic of an expert is the ability to appropriately move back and forth between assessment and intervention, relying on assessment data and decision-making skills to guide intervention. In the process, the nurse always focuses on assessment rather than intervention, on respiratory problems rather than respiratory procedures. Once a problem is understood and diagnosed, intervention naturally follows, as described throughout this book. A procedure book may be used as a guide. However, the strict application of respiratory procedures is replaced with modification of interventions, according to the constant flow of assessment data.

Briefly, the expert relies on decision-making skills rather than on "cookbook recipes." Cookbook recipes may help initiate diagnostic reasoning processes, emergency procedures, or routine procedures, such as changing a tracheostomy dressing. Yet implementation eventually requires decision-making skills to individualize care. Consider the following emergency situation: upon observing prolonged apnea in a patient, the expert nurse moves directly from assessment to implementation of the intervention (vertical arrow in Figure 31–1), from the respiratory arrest diagnosis to resuscitation procedures, with little to no mental cognition and planning. Eventually, however, reassessment is necessary to deal with implementation problems and to modify the problem list. In both acute and long-term care settings, reassessment demands the constant recycling of old problems and the diagnosing of new ones. The current challenge is to prevent the forgetting of old and less urgent problems during the reassessment phase.

Thus far, this chapter describes all components of the nursing process, with emphasis on assessment. How to implement decision-making skills is described next.

Implementation of Decision-making Skills

Attention to the following points will help the nurse implement decision-making skills in the clinical setting.

Allow the diagnosis to arise from the data. The nurse will encounter variations in diagnostic labels and charting guidelines among clinical settings. Largely because of these variations and terminology problems, the nurse may try to "fit" a diagnosis into one of a few approved categories and, as a result, arrive at a more nonspecific and inaccurate diagnosis. To avoid this pitfall, remember to *allow the diagnosis to arise from the data.* First, make the diagnosis; then, put a label on it, using the guidelines in this chapter.

Collaborate with other health team members. Most respiratory diagnoses are collaborative in nature. Clinical rounds, multidisciplinary care conferences, and informal consultations with physicians, respiratory therapists, physical therapists, and others caring for the patient will improve the efficiency and effectiveness of diagnosis and intervention.

Find a mentor. Written guidelines are poor substitutes for observing an expert make categoric and incremental decisions in respiratory care. When diagnostic reasoning is unclear, always ask for an explanation of assessment and intervention.

Practice making respiratory decisions. Experience facilitates recognition of cue clusters suggesting a diagnosis. Rather than delegate decisions to others, make a diagnosis yourself and ask the physician, respiratory nurse specialist, or others for validation.

Support research on respiratory diagnoses. Research is needed to describe reliable and valid respiratory diagnoses so that two professionals assessing the same patient will arrive at an identical and accurate diagnosis. Decision-making will become easier once all concerned health professionals collaborate and develop a taxonomy for respiratory diagnoses. Collaborative efforts may be coordinated through NANDA.*

Establish a charting structure that reinforces decision-making processes. The charting system must document the nursing process in terms of patient problems, not nursing tasks completed. The most widely used charting system that has this advantage is the *problem-oriented record (POR) system.* The structure and organization of this system force the nurse to consider assessment and problem identification before the formulation of interventions.

Make changes to reinforce the focus on problems. Multiple institutional changes are usually necessary to alter the way nurses conceptualize patient care. For example, to reinforce the focus on problems, administrators can encourage staff nurses to communicate nursing reports in terms of patient problems. Nursing education departments can focus in-service programs on respiratory diagnoses commonly used in practice, such as hypoxemia, bronchoconstriction, and ventilatory failure.

*NANDA, St. Louis University School of Nursing, 3525 Caroline St., St. Louis, Missouri 63014.

THE PROBLEM-ORIENTED RECORD SYSTEM

A complete explanation of the POR system is beyond the scope of this text. However, a brief summary of selected components will help the nurse adapt the system to respiratory patients and understand the case study in Chapter 32. The four parts of the POR system correspond closely with the steps of the nursing process, as shown in Table 31–11.

The Problem List

After data collection, health team members collaborate and write out active problems on the interdisciplinary problem list on the front of the chart or in the bedside notes. In the example in Table 31–12, the physician enters the medical diagnosis of asthmatic bronchitis and the main problem of bronchospasm. Several hours later, the nurse adds problems 3 and 4, based on signs of mucus retention and a history of COPD. Two days later, the nurse adds problem 5 when the patient continually demonstrates an inability to carry out personal hygiene measures.

In health agencies where separate medical and nursing problem lists are kept, the nurse writes collaborative nursing diagnoses (problems 2 through 5) on the separate list for nursing problems. The diagnoses are written in accepted nursing diagnosis format, as shown in Table 31–13. As with interdisciplinary problem lists, problems on the nursing diagnosis list are either crossed out or labelled "resolved" and dated and initialed, once the problem is resolved. Similarly, diagnoses are updated daily, according to the changing clinical situation.

The Nursing Care Plan

The nurse follows agency guidelines for writing the nursing care plan.

To facilitate the thinking of appropriate goals, interventions, and evaluation criteria, the nurse keeps in mind the following three categories:

1. Reassessment—What additional data are needed to refine diagnosis and plan care?
2. Treatment—What therapeutic interventions will solve the problem?
3. Education—What self-care education is needed to prevent recurrence of the problem?

Table 31–11. PROBLEM-ORIENTED RECORDS AND THE NURSING PROCESS

Parts of Problem-Oriented Records	Steps of the Nursing Process
Data base (admission interview)	Data collection
Problem list	Diagnosis (problem definition)
Initial and revised care plans	Planning of intervention
Progress notes	Implementation and evaluation of interventions

Table 31–12. INTERDISCIPLINARY PROBLEM LIST

Problem	Active Problems	Date Entered, Initials	Date Resolved, Initials
1	Asthmatic bronchitis	1/27 O.P.	
2	Bronchospasm	1/27 O.P.	2/2 E.K.
3	Mucus retention	1/27 E.K.	
4	Potential chest infection	1/27 E.K.	
5	Activity intolerance	1/29 E.K.	

Progress Notes

Progress notes have three forms as follows:

1. **Narrative in *SOAP* form:**
   *S*ubjective data
   *O*bjective data
   *A*nalysis
   *P*lan
2. **Flow sheets:**
   Routine or daily care
   Cumulative data
   Assessment data for trend analysis
3. **Final summary or discharge notes:**
   Discussion of each problem
   Progress in the attainment of goals
   Identification of future goals

SOAP Charting

SOAP components in narrative charting are summarized in outline form.

1. Subjective data (Historical data)
   a. Pulmonary symptoms: shortness of breath, wheeze, pleuritic chest pain, cough, sputum production, hemoptysis, voice change.
   b. What the patient said he did, e.g., walked 5 blocks without shortness of breath.
   c. Patient's perception of the problem, e.g., "I have emphysema and I'm going to die."
2. Objective data
   a. Physical findings
      (1) Chest assessment findings
      (2) Vital signs

Table 31–13. NURSING DIAGNOSIS (PROBLEM) LIST

Problem	Nursing Diagnosis (Problems)	Date Entered, Initials	Date Resolved, Initials
1	Acute severe bronchospasm related to asthma	1/27 E.K.	2/2 E.K.
2	Mucus retention related to bronchospasm and chest cold	1/27 E.K.	
3	Potential chest infection related to mucus retention	1/27 E.K.	
4	Activity intolerance related to asthma and muscle deconditioning	1/29 E.K.	

(3) Hemodynamic readings
b. Data personally observed
(1) Activities
(2) Medications
(3) Respiratory treatments
c. Laboratory data
(1) Chest x-ray film
(2) Pulmonary function tests
(3) Blood gas results
(4) Blood hematocrit, hemoglobin, theophylline level, and so forth.

3. Analysis (analysis ot subjectıve and objective data)
   a. Problem identification or change in problem status
   b. Interpretation of findings. May include discussion of variables affecting acuity, causality, or management of the problem.
   c. Impression of progress. Is the patient better? Worse? Status quo?
   d. Implication for intervention. What does the patient need now?
4. Plan (respiratory interventions to resolve problem and attain goal)
   a. Reassessment plan
   b. Treatment plan
   c. Self-care education plan

An example of a community health nurse's *SOAP* charting on a COPD patient follows:

Problem 1: Mucus retention related to bronchoconstriction and chronic bronchitis.

S: c/o chest tightness and dyspnea on exertion. Woke up twice last night with cough and mucus production. Coughing up 2 tbs mucus per day.

O: Appears comfortable, in no apparent distress. Afebrile. No cyanosis or use of accessory muscles of respiration. Lungs on auscultation: diffuse wheezing throughout lung fields. Decreased breath sounds in lung bases. Mucus slightly yellow in appearance. Wife reports that the patient is taking tetracycline 250 mg QID, without missed doses.

A: The mucus retention problem is unchanged from last week. The chest tightness and wheezing are new findings, indicating a bronchoconstriction problem. To resolve both problems, the patient needs medical treatment with bronchodilators to open airways and permit increased mucus expectoration. The tetracycline should help prevent pneumonia, provided the patient does not develop drug resistance.

P:
1. Encourage patient to see physician immediately for medical evaluation.
2. Consult physician regarding patient's condition and need for bronchodilatation.
3. Encourage patient to drink at least 2 to 3 quarts of liquid per day to liquefy mucus and facilitate expectoration.
4. Continue self-care education plan, beginning with how to evaluate sputum.
5. Monitor for change in temperature, lung sounds, sputum, and signs of chest infection.
6. Call patient tomorrow to evaluate progress and provide psychologic support.

In this example, the nurse records only subjective and objective data that are most pertinent to the individual patient situation. If the nurse returns and teaches the patient how to monitor his own sputum, the intervention and the patient's response to it are recorded under objective data. Whenever possible, reference is made to the updated nursing care plan to avoid repeating information.

Conclusion

This chapter has presented the five components of the nursing process applied to pulmonary patients. In addition, it has thoroughly discussed respiratory diagnosis, the weakest link in the nursing process. It is hoped that this emphasis on process will help the nurse mentally organize and selectively utilize knowledge in this book for diagnostic and treatment decisions. The benefits of this approach to care are innumerable. The clinician is prepared to take full responsibility for total respiratory care, collaborating on a regular basis with the physician and other members of the health care team. As clinicians refine their decision-making skills, researchers can collect descriptive data towards the task of developing a taxonomy of respiratory diagnoses and a theoretic framework to facilitate decision-making processes. As the efficiency and effectiveness of respiratory nursing care increase, the patient is more likely to receive comprehensive and continuing respiratory care at a reasonable cost.

Currently, perhaps the best and most practical way to learn how to merge respiratory content with the nursing process is through a case study. The case study in Chapter 32 helps the nurse implement decision-making skills in the clinical setting.

REFERENCES

American Nurses Association: Standards of Nursing Practice. Kansas City, American Nurses Association, 1973.

Aspinall, M.: Nursing diagnosis—the weak link. *Nursing outlook*, 24(7):433–437, 1976.

Aspinall, M. and Tanner, C.: Decision Making for Patient Care—Applying the Nursing Process. New York, Appleton-Century-Crofts, 1981.

Barrows, H. and Tamblyn, A.: Problem-Based Learning—An Approach to Medical Education. New York, Springer Publishing Co., 1980.

Bloch, D.: Some crucial terms in nursing—what do they really mean? *Nursing outlook*, 22(11):689–694, 1974.

Bruce, J. and Snyder, M.: The right and responsibility to diagnose. *American journal of nursing*, 82(4):645–646, 1982.

California Thoracic Society, Pulmonary Nurse Specialist Subcommittee: Guidelines for Nursing Care of the Pulmonary Patient. Oakland, California, California Thoracic Society, 1984.

Carlson, J., Craft, C., and McGuire, A.: Nursing Diagnosis. Philadelphia, W. B. Saunders Co., 1982.

Carnevali, D.: Nursing Care Planning: Diagnosis and Management, 3rd ed. Philadelphia, J. B. Lippincott, Co., 1983.

Carnevali, D., Mitchell, P., Woods, N., and Tanner, C.: Diagnostic Reasoning in Nursing. Philadelphia, J. B. Lippincott Co., 1984.

Carpenito, L.: Handbook of Nursing Diagnosis. Philadelphia, J. B. Lippincott Co., 1984.

Carpenito, L.: Nursing diagnosis in critical care: impact on practice and outcomes. *Heart and lung,* 16(6):595–605, 1987.

Carrieri, V. and Sitzman, J.: Components of the nursing process. In The Nursing Process—A Humanistic Approach (LaMonica, E.–ed.). Menlo Park, California, Addison Wesley Publishers Ltd., 1979.

Chrisman, M. and Fowler, M.: The Systems-in-Change Model for Nursing Practice. In Conceptual Models for Nursing Practice, 2nd ed. (Riehl, J. and Roy, S. C.–eds.). Norwalk, Connecticut, Appleton-Century-Crofts, 1980.

Dalton, J.: Nursing diagnosis in a community health setting. *Nursing clinics of north america,* 14(3):525–531, 1979.

Elstein, A., Shulman, L., Sprafka, S., et al: Medical Problem Solving—An Analysis of Clinical Reasoning. Cambridge, Massachusetts, Harvard University Press, 1978.

Engle, G.: Grief and grieving. *American journal of nursing,* 64(9):93–98, 1964.

Fawcett, J.: Analysis and Evaluation of Conceptual Models of Nursing. Philadelphia, F. A. Davis Co., 1984.

Field, L.: The implementation of nursing diagnosis in clinical practice. *Nursing clinics of north america,* 14(3):497–508, 1979.

Fortin, J.: Legal implications of nursing diagnosis. *Nursing clinics of north america,* 14(3):553–561, 1979.

Fraher, J.: Nursing diagnoses and care plans in critical care. *Critical care nurse,* 3(6):94–98, 1983.

Gebbie, K. and Lavin, M.: Classifying nursing diagnoses. *American journal of nursing,* 74(2):250–253, 1974.

Gordon, M.: Nursing Diagnosis—Process and Application. New York, McGraw-Hill Book Co., 1982.

Grossbach-Landis, I. and McLane, A.: Tracheal suctioning: a tool for evaluation and learning needs assessment. *Nursing research,* 28(4):237–242, 1979.

Guzzetta, C.: A holistic approach to nursing diagnosis. In Cardiovascular Nursing—Bodymind Tapestry (Guzzetta, C. and Dossey, B.–eds.). St. Louis, C. V. Mosby Co., 1984.

Guzzetta, C. and Dossey, B.: Nursing diagnosis: framework, process, and problems. *Heart and lung,* 12(3):281–291, 1983.

Harper, R.: A Guide to Respiratory Care—Physiology and Clinical Applications. Philadelphia, J. B. Lippincott Co., 1981.

Hickey, M.: Nursing diagnosis in the critical care unit. *Dimensions of critical care nursing,* 3(2):91–97, 1984.

Jacox, A.: Theory construction in nursing. *Nursing research,* 23(1):4–13, 1974.

Johnson, D.: State of the art of theory development in nursing. In Theory Development: What, Why, How? (15–1708). New York, National League for Nursing, 1978.

Kersten, L.: Heuristics and heuristic knowledge (unpublished paper). School of Public Administration, University of Southern California, Los Angeles, 1985.

Kim, M., McFarland, G., and McLane, A.: Classification of Nursing Diagnoses—Proceedings of the Fifth National Conference. St. Louis, C. V. Mosby Co., 1984.

Lane, G., Cronin, K., and Peirce, A.: Flow Charts—Clinical Decision Making in Nursing. Philadelphia, J. B. Lippincott, Co., 1983.

Mayers, M.: A Systematic Approach to the Nursing Care Plan, 3rd Ed. New York, Appleton-Century-Crofts, 1983.

McCloskey, J.: How to make the most of body image theory in nursing practice. *Nursing 76,* 6(5):68–72, 1976.

Mundinger, M. and Jauron, G.: Developing a nursing diagnosis. *Nursing outlook,* 23(2):95–98, 1975.

Nightingale, F.: Notes on Nursing—What it is, and What it is not. New York, Dover Publications, Inc., 1969.

Putzier, D., Padrick, K., Westfall, U., and Tanner, C.: Diagnostic reasoning in critical care nursing. *Heart and lung,* 14(5):430–437, 1985.

Sjoberg, E.: Nursing diagnosis and the COPD patient. *American journal of nursing,* 83(2):245–248, 1983.

Soares, C.: Nursing and medical diagnoses: a comparison of variant and essential features. In The Nursing Professions: Views Through the Mist (Chaska, N.–ed.). New York: McGraw-Hill Book Co., 1978.

Stevens, B.: ANA's standards of nursing practice: what they tell us about the state of the art (editorial). *Journal of nursing administrtion,* 4(5):16–18, 1974.

The Case Study

32

Main Objectives

1. Select a patient in your clinical area that has pulmonary problems.
   a. After a brief nursing report, cluster assessment data appropriately and formulate a tentative problem list.
   b. Assess the patient, using at least five assessment parameters discussed in this book.
   c. Write a list of nursing diagnoses.
   d. Identify three top priority nursing diagnoses.
   e. Analyze one nursing diagnosis, using the SOAP format.

2. Describe the clinical course of Mr. K. in this case study, from the onset of acute illness to adaptation to chronic pulmonary disease.

3. Name at least four problems (i.e., nursing diagnoses) Mr. K. experienced during pulmonary rehabilitation. Describe nursing interventions for these problems.

4. Discuss how knowledge of respiratory nursing care in acute and rehabilitative settings can help you individualize care to your own patient population.

This case study applies nursing diagnosis and intervention to an actual patient situation. In addition, the study provides a total view of the patient, Mr. K., and his tribulations as he moves through the health care continuum.

The first part of the chapter focuses on decision-making skills in the intensive care unit (ICU) and implementation of basic respiratory assessment parameters presented in this book. The second part describes Mr. K.'s clinical course, beginning with his acute restrictive pulmonary disease in the ICU and ending with his adaptation to chronic illness in the home setting. The third and last part focuses on the pulmonary problems he encounters during pulmonary rehabilitation.

Decision-making in the Intensive Care Unit (ICU)

The blending of assessment with intervention depends on decision-making skills, particularly clinical diagnostic reasoning. In most ICUs, nursing assessment and, hence, clinical diagnostic reasoning begins while listening to a nursing report about the patient's condition. Afterwards, the nurse goes to the bedside, reviews the respiratory assessment parameters, and formulates the nursing diagnoses to guide intervention.

NURSING REPORT

The following nursing report provides an initial data base for Mr. K. The report itself is reproduced to the left. Cues to possible problems are indicated in italics. Cue interpretation is explained to the right. Though the report was sketchy, the nurse was able to use her respiratory knowledge base to identify cues, cluster information, and formulate a tentative list of top priority problems before actually going to the bedside for the initial nursing assessment.

Nursing Report for Mr. K.	**Cue Interpretation**
Mr. K. is a 43-year-old male *precision metal grinder* admitted on 4/9 to the respiratory ICU in acute respiratory failure. The admission is an inter-hospital transfer for the purpose of further medical evaluation and *weaning from mechanical ventilation.*	Pulmonary problems may relate to an occupational lung disease. Environmental assessment of the home or workplace may be needed in the future to determine the nature and extent of exposure to metal grindings. The patient may be anxious, stressed, and depressed from past unsuccessful weaning attempts.
Medical diagnoses *Diffuse interstitial lung disease* of unknown etiology.	Interstitial fibrosis—a pulmonary restrictive disease with decreased lung compliance. Possible problems include hypoxemia, impaired ventilation, potential mucus retention, and chest infection. Watch for signs of underlying obstruction disease.
Acute respiratory failure with *ventilator dependence.* Status post (S/P) open lung biopsy on 3/25.	Mechanical ventilation—watch for common problems associated with therapy, such as hypotension, barotrauma, oxygen toxicity, positive fluid balance, gastric distention and ileus, gastrointestinal bleeding, malnutrition, respiratory muscle fatigue, and so forth.
Status post *tracheostomy on 4/5* with insertion of # 8.5 mm nonfenestrated Shiley tracheostomy tube.	The tracheostomy is only 3 to 4 days old. Watch for stomal infection, hemorrhage, excessive cuff pressure, and subcutaneous emphysema. Has the tube's inner cannula been cleaned recently? The decreased anatomic deadspace (VD_{ANAT}) from the tracheostomy may facilitate weaning from mechanical ventilation.
Admission weight *72.5 k*	72 kg is an average weight for an adult male, suggesting adequate nutritional status, a criterion for weaning. Also, the patient's weight is needed to determine ventilator V_T, medication dosages (e.g., antibiotics, vasopressors), fluid balance, and cardiac index used in hemodynamic monitoring.
Vital signs *Temperature 37° C*	The patient is afebrile. However, infection is *not* ruled out, since infection may be present in the absence of fever.
Heart rate and rhythm 101 beats/min, *sinus tachycardia* without ectopy	The tachycardia indicates that the workload of the heart is increased.
Respirations 43/min	The tachypnea indicates high VD_{ANAT} and high alveolar deadspace or VD_{ALV} (i.e., deadspace effect). Analysis of V_E and ABGs are needed for further assessment of ventilation and oxygenation.
Blood pressure (B/P) 150/90	Borderline hypertension is present.

NURSING REPORT *Continued*

Neurologic signs The patient is *restless and lethargic*, slow to respond to physical and verbal stimulation. When awakened, he appropriately obeys simple commands. He moves all extremities spontaneously and to command. *Pupils are 2 mm in diameter bilaterally*, with brisk response to light.	The restlessness and questionable mental orientation indicate possible self extubation. Application of soft restraints to wrists is a top priority intervention. The pupils may be slightly constricted from narcotics to control agitation.
Right lateral chest tube attached to Pleur-evac chest tube drainage system with 20 cmH_2O pressure.	Why does the patient have a chest tube? Post open lung biopsy pneumothorax? Bronchopleural fistula? Empyema? Consult the physician. Check for chest tube patency and signs of barotrauma.
Foley catheter to gravity drainage. *Output measures 90 ml/hr* of clear yellow urine.	Foley catheter predisposes the patient to urinary tract infection. Urine output over 30 ml/hr indicates adequate kidney perfusion. Check other indicators of normal kidney function as follows: blood urea nitrogen level (BUN, normal is 7 to 20 mg/dl) and blood creatinine level (CR, normal is 0.7 to 1.3 mg/dl).
Normal saline infusing at 100 ml/hr.	Intake and output are nearly balanced. Check the patient's blood sodium level. Normal saline may be indicated to treat hyponatremia, or it may be causing hypernatremia. Check for history of cardiac disease and heart failure. High intravenous infusion rates may contribute to fluid retention and precipitate right or left ventricular heart failure.
Enteroflex nasogastric tube in place.	Check for nasogastric tube patency. Enteroflex tube adjustment or replacement is an expensive intervention. It is performed by a physician and usually requires a postinsertion chest x-ray film to verify correct tube placement in the stomach. Check orders for nutritional support, e.g., continuous tube feedings to avoid malnutrition and respiratory muscle fatigue.
Ventilator (Bear 2 volume ventilator). Assist-control mode, $FIO_2 = 0.40$, $PEEP = 8\ cmH_2O$, $f = 12/min$, $V_T = 900\ cc$.	Pulmonary oxygen toxicity is not likely, since the FIO_2 is well below 0.50 to 0.60. Watch for adverse effects of PEEP, including hypotension and barotrauma. The patient's spontaneous respiratory rate of 40 breaths/min is overriding the ventilator's back-up rate of 12 breaths/min. V_T is appropriate. Normal V_T = 10 to 15 cc/kg body weight. The patient's estimated $V_T = 73 \times 15 = 1095$ cc. At this point, the most immediate need is bedside assessment of cardiopulmonry status, including an ABG for objective assessment of oxygenation and ventilation. Does the patient have an indwelling arterial catheter for blood sampling? Is an oximeter available for noninvasive blood gas measurements?

Information Clusters

The information from this limited data base may be rearranged into clusters, as shown hereafter. Critical cues are indicated by an asterisk. At this point, all problems are possible or potential rather than actual. The one exception is increased work of breathing, diagnosed from the high respiratory rate. A respiratory diagnosis, such as impaired gas exchange, is likely but not assumed until arterial blood gas results or chest assessment findings indicate an actual problem.

Information Clusters	Problems
precision metal grinder* interstitial disease of unknown etiology	occupational lung disease
respiratory rate 40/min* tachycardia restlessness lethargy questionable mental orientation	increased work of breathing hypoxemia alveolar hypo- or hyperventilation anxiety respiratory muscle fatigue
rt lateral chest tube to Pleuro-evac status post open lung biopsy mechanical ventilation probably high peak inspiratory pressures	barotrauma chest infection
normal saline at 100 ml/hr* history of heart failure ?? critically ill patient	fluid overload
absence of nutritional supplement* mechanical ventilation increased work of breathing	malnutrition

The Tentative Problem List

Next, the nurse formulates a tentative problem list, ranking the previously listed problems from highest to lowest in priority, with greatest importance placed on acute needs.

TENTATIVE PROBLEMS IDENTIFIED DURING THE NURSING REPORT

Hypoxemia
Alveolar hypo- or hyperventilation
Anxiety
Increased work of breathing
Respiratory muscle fatigue
Barotrauma, chest infection, or both
Fluid overload
Malnutrition
Occupational lung disease

This list helps the nurse decide which problems to thoroughly cover during assessment and which areas to superficially cover. Moreover, particularly in the acute setting, the ranking of these problems is never fixed. For example, hypoxemia is a top priority problem now, but in 4 hours it may be ranked lower on the list, as respiratory intervention (e.g., increasing FIO_2) occurs during the assessment process. The important point to remember is to always have a tentative problem list to guide assessment.

REVIEW OF RESPIRATORY ASSESSMENT PARAMETERS

Based on the nursing report, two interventions were mandatory before the nurse proceeded with respiratory assessment. First, the nurse placed soft restraints around Mr. K.'s wrists, explaining that the restraints were for his protection to prevent self extubation during periods of restlessness or disorientation. Second, the nurse drew an ABG sample.

Respiratory assessment occurred in two ways. First, the nurse performed a brief initial nursing assessment, with emphasis on vital signs, neurologic signs, chest assessment findings, and the ventilator check. Simultaneously, the nurse began a comprehensive review of respiratory assessment parameters, including the pulmonary history, chest examination, blood gas results, chest x-ray films, and others. Over 24 to 48 hours, data collected from the medical chart, family members, Mr. K.'s physicians, and Mr. K. himself helped the nurse understand the circumstances surrounding the illness. Also, the data helped rule out, identify, and prioritize the many clinical problems that arose from the growing data base.

Pulmonary History

Chief Complaints. *Dyspnea at rest* for the last 3 weeks with cough and sputum production. *Fever* up to 101° F.

Present History. Mr. K. was in his usual state of good health until 3 weeks ago. At this time, he developed a cough productive of scant amounts of watery sputum, followed by increasing dyspnea at rest.

In early March, he went to an industrial clinic; a chest x-ray film taken at the clinic showed an interstitial and alveolar pattern consistent with severe pneumoconiosis. *A few days later,* Mr. K. saw a pulmonologist who recommended an open lung biopsy. Reluctant to have surgery, Mr. K. went back to his private physician, who first suspected pneumoconiosis. This physician prescribed tetracycline. However, Mr. K. discontinued the antibiotic after 5 days because he developed a skin rash over his chest, abdomen, back, and arms. He was then given a course of penicillin.

On 3/19, 3 days before admission to his local hospital, Mr. K. borrowed a small oxygen cylinder from a friend for use while moving about his apartment. On 3/21, 1 day before admission, he experienced ten brief periods of dyspnea while talking that left him pale, diaphoretic, and gasping for air for about 10 seconds. Silence and rest in an upright position gradually relieved the dyspnea. His girlfriend stated that he required 15 minutes to climb one flight of stairs and "he looked like he wasn't going to make it."

On 3/22, Mr. K. was admitted to a local hospital with tachypnea, cyanosis, use of accessory muscles of respiration, and profound hypoxemia. *Three days later (3/25),* an open lung biopsy was performed for diagnostic purposes. The results confirmed the diagnosis of acute interstitial pneumonia with extensive interstitial fibrosis. The silica level in the tissue was 41 mcg/gm of tissue. Following the biopsy, Mr. K.'s chest tube was removed but reinserted because of the recurrent pneumothorax with bronchopleural fistula. He was treated with penicillin and high dose methylprednisolone with no improvement in clinical condition. A tracheostomy was performed on 4/5 because of the inability to wean from mechanical ventilation. Over his clinical course, the white blood cell (WBCs) count gradually increased from 17,000 to 32,000 with a left shift due to increasing numbers of immature WBCs. His hematocrit value fell from 46 to 35%.

Past History. Mr. K. had the usual childhood diseases and intussusception at the age of 5 years, requiring surgery and incidental appendectomy. He had hepatitis in Germany in 1960. His history is negative for cardiopulmonary problems, gastrointestinal disease, renal disease, epilepsy, diabetes, venereal diseases, and gout.

Family History. His father died of unknown causes at age 77. His mother died in her late 40s of breast cancer. His family history is negative for tuberculosis and other pulmonary diseases, diabetes, and cardiovascular disease.

Residence and Recent Travel. The patient is divorced and lives alone in an apartment in a large city. He has no pets at home. He has not traveled out of town in the past 2 years. He states that the smog in the city has not caused breathing difficulties except during the past 3 weeks.

Smoking. He smoked one pack of cigarettes a day for 20 years until January 1. Since January, he has smoked no more than a total of three packs of cigarettes.

Alcohol. Mr. K. drinks alcoholic beverages occasionally (frequency not specified).

Immunizations. None are documented in the chart.

Allergies. He reports a skin rash with tetracycline, as described. He denies allergy to food, pollen, and dusts.

Occupational History. Mr. K.'s occupations include hospital clerk during service in the U. S. Army in Germany, salesman for aqueduct parts, and owner of a bar. Seven years ago, he opened his own metal grinding business. He is the only worker in his small, 2000 ft^2 workroom; however, his brother recently began working there in his absence. The shop has never been inspected by the Occupational Safety and Health Administration (OSHA) to assess safety standards. Mr. K. states that the walls and surfaces are typically covered with black dust. In the absence of an adequate exhaust system, he attempts to clear the air during grinding by using fans, but dust persists in the air during work hours. He does not use a respirator, but 1 month ago he started wearing a disposable mask purchased in a hardware store. He grinds mostly ferrous materials from a local foundry, though sometimes he works on steel or stainless steel. He is not sure of the composition of his grinding stone. In the past, many grinding wheels were made of sandstone, producing high levels of airborne silica dust during grinding. However, such stones have recently been replaced by aluminum oxide or silicon carbide stones. He denies working with beryllium, asbestos, or chrome; in addition, he denies pulmonary symptoms on exposure to the workplace.

Review of Systems. General signs and symptoms include fever and general fatigue associated with the present illness. Mr. K. reports no chills or night sweats, anxiety, depression, or anorexia. His usual weight is 215 lb (97.7 kg), and height is 5 ft 11 in.

Review of specific body systems reveals only recent insomnia at night due to dyspnea.

Discussion. Data from the pulmonary history introduces new information clusters:

Information Clusters	Problems
insomnia restlessness dyspnea	sleep pattern disturbance
history of dyspnea with interrupted speech pattern cuffed tracheostomy tube	impaired communication
history of fever 101° F.* increased white blood cell count with left shift*	infection, etiology?
20-pack-year history of cigarette smoking	chronic airway obstruction
reduced hematocrit* fatigue	anemia
healthy until 3 weeks ago only 43 years old 25-kg weight loss over 5 weeks temporarily unemployed on bedrest with arms restrained unable to talk	powerlessness disturbance in body image, self-esteem, role performance, or all three
work as metal grinder possible exposure to silica, iron oxides, aluminum, hard metals no exhaust system in workplace no protective mask or respirator black dust in air	acute accelerated occupational lung disease unsafe work environment
brother now working in shop	brother at risk for the development of occupational lung disease

Several factors, such as clinical circumstances, organization of nursing care, and division of labor among health care professionals, determine what cues the nurse identifies and follows up. In the beginning of this case study, data from the "change-of-shift" report allowed the nurse to identify top priority problems, i.e., problems that needed immediate nursing bedside assessment. In contrast, data from the pulmonary history revealed problems that were important but were of lower priority for the nurse at that moment. For example, impaired communication is important, but as long as the patient is resting comfortably, further assessment is postponed until after ventilation and oxygenation are thoroughly evaluated. Similarly, the infection problem is important, but as long as the patient does not need immediate temperature-reducing interventions, this problem is of lower priority for nursing. Infection remained a top priority problem for the physicians, who soon ordered a "fever work up" (urine, sputum, pleural fluid for culture and sensitivity and Gram's stain, and blood cultures) and antibiotics.

Hence, problems suggested by the pulmonary history did not greatly alter the list of top priority problems identified earlier. However, two new pieces of information could help the nurse in her approach to the patient and his family. First, the acute illness changed Mr. K. from a healthy middle-aged man to a ventilator-dependent patient in a matter of weeks. This devastating blow to his physical and psychologic well being may reinforce feelings of helplessness and hopelessness, making it even more difficult to wean him from the ventilator.

Implications for intervention include the immediate identification of at least one family member or significant other, probably the brother or girlfriend or both in this case, to serve as a support person for Mr. K. If the critical care nurse has insufficient time to speak with these people, the head nurse, clinical specialist, clinical psychologist, or social worker is called upon to help communicate information to them and to support them in any way possible so that they, in turn, can support the patient.

The pulmonary history indicates that Mr. K. may have been exposed to high levels of silica, placing him at risk for *silicoproteinosis*, an accelerated form of acute silicosis that has a high mortality rate. Early identification of silica exposure is important because medical treatment includes whole lung lavage. This procedure is accomplished by inserting a special endotracheal tube down the right and left main stem branches and washing the lungs with normal saline.

Mr. K.'s physicians immediately requested an occupational medicine consultation to try to determine more precisely the nature and extent of Mr. K.'s exposure to silica and other substances. Though Mr. K. is currently a poor candidate for whole lung lavage because of his unstable ventilatory status, silica exposure is important to establish in case the ventilatory status stabilizes and lavage becomes possible.

In the occupational medical consultation, the role of the nurse is to facilitate communication between Mr. K.'s brother and the physician so that Mr. K.'s lung irritant exposure is determined and the brother understands his own high risk for occupational lung disease unless appropriate safety standards are instituted.

Pulmonary Medications

On the day of admission, Mr. K.'s medications included the following:

1. Tobramycin, 110 mg intravenous piggy-back medication (IVPB) loading dose, followed by 75 mg IVPB q8h maintenance dose.
2. Cefoxitin, 2 gm, IVPB q6h.
3. Methylprednisolone (Solu-Medrol), 60mg, qd.
4. Morphine sulfate, 4 mg, q2h PRN agitation if systolic B/P greater than 130.
5. Lorazepam (Ativan) STAT doses PRN agitation. Methylcellulose eyedrops, 2 gtts OU q2h if not blinking.

Discussion. Tobramycin and cefoxitin are antibiotics used to treat suspected infections. Tobramycin was ordered for coverage of gram-negative rods; cefoxitin was ordered for coverage of gram-positive microbes, *Enterobacter* sp., and anaerobes from oral flora in case of pulmonary aspiration. Subsequently, examination results of body fluids came back from the laboratory as positive.

4/9. Urinalysis showed slight pyuria (pus in urine), 3+ bacteriuria, gram-negative rods.

4/11. Sputum and pleural exudate cultured *Enterobacter,* sensitive to tobramycin.

4/15. Sputum cultured *Enterobacter* and *Acinetobacter,* sensitive to moxalactam and piperacillin.

Interventions to reduce and prevent further infection included (1) broader spectrum of antibiotic coverage; (2) daily Foley catheter care and daily dressing changes at other catheter sites; and (3) discontinuation of indwelling lines as soon as the patient's condition stabilizes, beginning with Foley catheter. Erythromycin, 1 gm IVPB q6h, was added to Mr. K.'s antibiotic therapy. Cefoxitin, a cephalosporin, was changed to piperacillin, a broad spectrum, third generation penicillin.

Methylprednisolone (Solu-Medrol), an intravenous corticosteroid was given to Mr. K. in the other hospital to treat the acute interstitial disease process, was continued.

Morphine sulfate was given initially to control agitation but thereafter was given sparingly to avoid respiratory depression. Instead, lorazepam, a benzodiazepine with antianxiety and sedative effects, was administered. When Mr. K. became combative, haloperidol (Haldol), a tranquilizer used for psychotic behavior, was given instead. It does not produce respiratory depression and has few side effects other than extrapyramidal reactions, tachycardia, and changes in blood pressure.

Mr. K. never required the methylcellulose eyedrops for lubrication because he never became comatose and never lost the blinking reflex.

Chest Examination

General Appearance. Mr. K. is a well-developed white male, lying supine in bed with soft restraints to upper extremities. He is ventilator dependent and has a chest tube, tracheostomy tube, radial arterial line, Foley catheter, and ECG leads in place. He remains tachypneic and restless on an FIO_2 of 0.40.

Inspection. No extrathoracic signs of respiratory distress except for cyanosis of the mucous membranes of the lips and a slight grimace. Chest and other body skin surfaces are pale and without petechiae, ecchymoses, rashes, or scars except for a well-healed, small, linear right lower quadrant abdominal scar.

A # 8.5-mm cuffed Shiley tracheostomy is in place. The stoma looks dry and without redness or other signs of irritation or infection.

A right lateral chest tube is connected to an adult Pleur-evac chest tube drainage unit, with 20 cmH_2O suction. The dressing around the insertion site is dry and intact. The patient has an intermittent, large inspiratory air leak manifested by vigorous bubbling in the waterseal chamber during inspiration. Tidalling in the waterseal chamber is about 4 cmH_2O. The chest tube is draining small amounts (20 ml since admission) of straw-colored foamy fluid.

The chest is symmetric and normal in configuration. Respiratory rate is 40/min, with 100% assisted ventilator breaths. The patient does not appear to be fighting the ventilator. I:E (inspiratory:expiratory) ratio is about 1:1. The patient is using mostly neck, intercostal, and shoulder muscles for breathing, with suprasternal notch retractions and very little diaphragmatic movement.

Palpation. The trachea is in the midline position. No crepitus is evident around the tracheostomy, neck, anterior chest area, or chest tube site. Skin surfaces are warm and diaphoretic. Rhonchal fremitus is palpable over the anterior chest, disappearing after coughing and tracheal suctioning. Estimated central venous pressure (CVP) is 10 cmH_2O.

Percussion. Deferred.

Auscultation. Normal breath sounds throughout all lung fields, except bronchovesicular breath sounds around the chest tube site. Inspiratory crackles right and left lower lobes (RLL and LLL) to T4 level. Scattered rhonchi throughout the chest, clearing after the patient is suctioned for small to moderate amounts of white mucus. No wheezing or pleural rubs.

Cor. PMI of cardiac impulse is palpated in the fifth intercostal space, midcostal line (ICS, MCL). The pulse is forceful but not sustained, about 2 cm in diameter in the supine position. The patient has a split S_2 with a loud P_2 component heard in the second ICS, left sternal border (LSB). No S_3, S_4, murmurs, or pericardial friction rubs were auscultated. The cardiac monitor shows sinus tachycardia 100 to 110/min without ectopy.

Extremities. The extremities are without clubbing, edema, or cyanosis. However, the nail beds of the

Information Clusters	Problems
cyanotic mucous membranes* grimace tachypnea restlessness use of accessory muscles of respiration poor capillary refill of nail beds	hypoxemia
bubbles in waterseal chamber of Pleur-evac* bronchovesicular breath sounds around chest tube site	chest tube air leak pneumothorax atelectasis or early pulmonary consolidation
crackles to T4* scattered rhonchi white mucus normal CVP no S_3 gallop history of fibrosis no history of cardiovascular disease	mucus production or retention interstitial lung disease atelectasis
loud P_2 signs of hypoxemia	pulmonary hypertension

fingers show poor capillary refill. Dorsal pedalis and posterior tibial pulses are 1 to 2+ on a scale of 0 to 4+.

Discussion. Data from the chest examination introduced new clusters of information, as shown in the table. (The critical clues indicated with an asterisk.

Identification of cyanotic mucous membranes clustered with other signs of respiratory distress makes hypoxemia an actual diagnosis. In collaboration with the physician, the nurse obtains an ABG sample to measure the severity of the hypoxemia and the increase of FIO_2.

The bubbling in the Pleur-evac's waterseal chamber indicates a chest tube air leak due to PEEP, high suction, bronchopleural fistula, or some combination thereof. The bronchovesicular breath sounds may be from compression of lung tissue from a pneumothorax; air in the pleural space might be compressing adjacent lung tissue, atelectasis from inadequate lung expansion, or consolidated alveoli from pneumonia. These processes cannot be assessed without a chest x-ray film.

Rhonchi on auscultation and suctioning of white mucus indicates a mucus production and retention problem. This problem is likely for any intubated patient, since the endotracheal tube slows functioning of the mucociliary escalator. Inspiratory crackles and a history of fibrosis indicate interstitial lung disease, particularly since signs of heart failure (e.g., elevated CVP, S_3 gallop, history of cor pulmonale and cardiovascular disease) are absent. However, at least some of the crackles may be due to acute atelectasis or mucus retention. Differentiation between these processes may be impossible, since Mr. K.'s condition does not permit a complete chest examination at this time and since his chest was clear to auscultation before this present illness. Again, a chest x-ray film is needed to assess findings.

Vital Signs and Hemodynamic Readings

One hour after admission, Mr. K.'s vital signs were as follows: B/P 80/50, temperature 37° C., heart rate 105/min, and respirations 33/min. Hypotension responded to Trendelenburg's position and fluid challenge with normal saline solution. Two hours later, a pulmonary artery catheter was inserted to assess overall fluid status and to monitor pulmonary artery (PA) wedge pressures during fluid administration. By this time, Mr. K.'s B/P increased to 135/58 (mean 84 mmHg). Hemodynamic readings are as follows:

PA systolic	40 mmHg
PA diastolic	22 mmHg
PA mean	28 mmHg (calculated)
PA wedge (PCWP)	17 mmHg
RA mean	9 mmHg
Cardiac output (Q)	11.4 L/min
Cardiac index (CI)	6.35 L/min/m^2 calculated using body surface area (BSA) = 1.77
Systemic vascular resistance (SVR)	533 dynes/sec/cm^{-5} (calculated)
Pulmonary vascular resistance (PVR)	77 dynes/sec/cm^{-5} (calculated)

Vital signs and hemodynamic readings prompted the nurse to think of the following information clusters:

low systemic vascular resistance (SVR)* hypotension* normal body temperature high Q and CI*	sepsis, source of infection?
elevated PA wedge* crackles in lungs recent bolus of normal saline	fluid overload
high PA readings* signs of hypoxemia intestitial fibrosis	pulmonary hypertension

Discussion. The first information cluster has all the classic signs of septic shock except for the normal body temperature. Hypothermia typically occurs in septic shock.

In assessing a list of hemodynamic readings, the nurse checks to see whether readings were taken from a digital or graphic display. Since Mr. K. is tachypneic and using accessory muscles of respiration, the nurse can expect great respiratory variation in hemodynamic wave patterns. Hence, graphic analysis is essential for accuracy. Even with graphic analysis, PA pressures may be elevated because of the increased intrathoracic pressures and increased airway resistance associated with mechanical ventilation and increased work of breathing. The graphic displays in Figure 32–1 show how the nurse determined hemodynamic readings, after 20 mg of furosemide (Lasix) was given to diurese the patient. Ventilator expiratory flow (Fig. 32–1A) was used to determine the PA reading (Fig. 32–1B). In Figure 32–1C and 32–1D, the dips below baseline correspond with inspiratory chest movement.

Mr. K.'s systolic, diastolic, and mean pulmonary artery readings are elevated, suggesting pulmonary hypertension from interstitial fibrosis, hypoxic vasoconstriction, or both. The lack of correlation between the PA diastolic reading (22 mmHg) and the PA wedge reading (17 mmHg) is consistent with pulmonary hypertension. However, the normal PVR of 77 dynes/sec/cm^{-5} is inconsistent. PVR should be elevated in light of the patient's acute pulmonary disease and signs of severe hypoxemia. Later PVR values were more credible. They were in the range of 150 to 200 dynes/sec/cm^{-5}. The discrepancy may be due to measurement error. When an inaccurate hemodynamic reading (PA mean, PCWP, or Q) is applied to the PVR formula, the calculated PVR will not reflect the patient's clinical state.

Blood Gases and Pulmonary Function Tests

Preoperative pulmonary function tests (PFTs) from the other hospital confirmed severe restrictive disease, with a reduced vital capacity of 1.2 L. Prior to transfer, Mr. K.'s PaO_2 and $PaCO_2$ were 64 and 57, respectively, on an FIO_2 of 0.40. No other baseline measurements were recorded in the chart.

ABGs and PFTs are always analyzed in relation to ventilator settings. In Table 32–1, Mr. K.'s blood gas values are correlated with other important measurements recorded at the time of blood sampling.

PFTs and Ventilator Settings. First, look at assessment data collected at 1000 on 4/9 (see Table 32–1), the day of admission. Two measurements provide important information about mechanics of breathing as follows: minute ventilation ($\dot{V}_E$) and peak inspiratory pressure (PIP). $\dot{V}_E$ is 35 L/min, a grossly elevated value. Now turn to Figure 5–6, and plot the $PaCO_2$ of 45 mmHg on the x axis of the graph, with the $\dot{V}_E$ of 35 L/min on the y axis. The intersecting point lies at the top of the graph. Mr. K.'s V_D/V_T is well over both the normal V_D/V_T (0.33) and the maximum value (0.60) used as a weaning criterion. Mr. K.'s deadspace ventilation is largely responsible for the increased work of breathing.

Second, note that Mr. K.'s peak inspiratory pressure is well over 30 cmH_2O. It is 40 to 70 cmH_2O, even after the respiratory therapist made adjustments to reduce airway turbulence and promote laminar flow

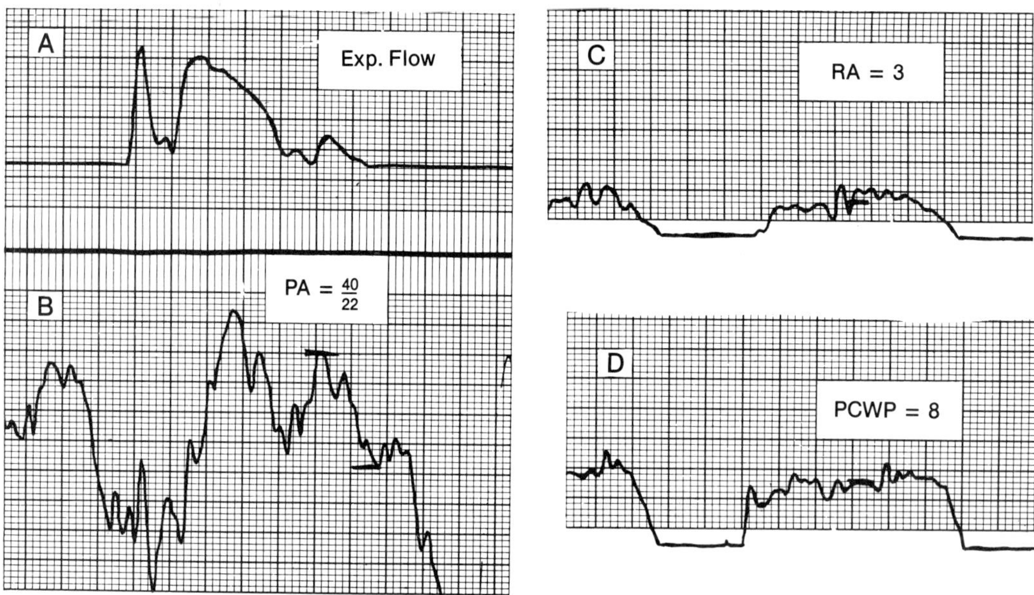

Figure 32–1. Mr. K.'s hemodynamic wave patterns. The nurse used the expiratory flow wave pattern in A to help locate an end-expiratory point for pulmonary artery systolic and diastolic readings in B. End-expiration is easier to identify for the right atrial pressure in C and pulmonary artery wedge pressure in D. Each large box on the graph paper represents 5 mmHg.

Table 32–1. RESPIRATORY ASSESSMENT DATA FOR MR. K.

Date: 4/9	Time:					
Assessment Parameter	*1000*	*1200*	*1300*	*1500*	*1500*	*1900*
PFTs and Ventilator Settings						
Ventilator mode	A/C	A/C	A/C	SIMV	Same	SIMV
FIO_2	0.40	0.75	0.60	0.50		0.50
PEEP cmH_2O	8	8	8	6		6
Set f	12	20	20	25		25
Total f	32 to 40	30 to 40	38 to 42	38 to 50		48
V_T (set) ml	900	700	600	600		600
V_T (spontaneous)	300	375				600
$\dot{V}_E$ L/min	35	29.8	28.4	30.8		33.1
PIP cmH_2O	40 to 70	40 to 55	32 to 48	30		25 to 35
CL_{dyn} L/cmH_2O	0.017	0.014	0.015	0.013		0.022
Blood Gases						
pH	7.47	7.45	7.43	7.43	7.41*	7.43
$PaCO_2$ mmHg	45	44	45	49	53*	48
PaO_2 mmHg	49	207	152	70	36*	67
HCO_3^- mEq/L	33	31	30	33	34*	32
Base excess	+9.1	+7.2	+5.2	+7.6	+8.3*	+7.2
SO_2 %	86	99	99	94	69*	94
Others						
$A\text{-}aO_2$ gradient mmHg	180	272	220	226		230
a/A ratio	0.21	0.43	0.40	0.24		0.22
$C(a-\bar{v})O_2$ ml/100 ml (assume hemoglobin = 10 gm%)					3.54	

*Mixed venous blood.

into the lungs. These high pressures combined with the 8 cmH_2O PEEP may prevent closure of the bronchopleural fistula or may make the fistula even larger. Mr. K.'s risk for barotrauma gradually became less throughout the day, as the ventilator mode was switched from assist-control to synchronized intermittent mandatory ventilation (SIMV), as V_T was reduced, and as sedation was given to control agitation. Moreover, to promote air leak closure, Mr. K.'s physicians considered but did not implement utilization of the relatively new mode of mechanical ventilation, i.e., high frequency jet ventilation.

Because of the time constraints placed upon the nurse, PIP rather than static or dynamic compliance measurements were made to monitor lung compliance. Increasing PIP suggests decreasing compliance from fluid or mucus in the lungs, air in the pleural space, or water condensation in the ventilator circuit: decreasing PIP suggests increasing compliance from an improved pulmonary status or decreased resistance in the patient, ventilator circuit, or both. Later, the nurse calculated dynamic compliance (CL_{dyn}) at 0.017 L/cmH_2O (normal CL_{dyn} = 0.05 L/cmH_2O). Mr. K.'s lung compliance is greatly reduced, a typical finding in interstitial fibrosis.

After gathering and analyzing these PFT data, the nurse realized that the size of the chest tube air leak was not consistently noted and charted. If the pleural leak was small during PFT measurements, then the measurements and calculations probably reflect true mechanics of breathing. If the leak was large, and as much as one third of $\dot{V}_E$ was going out through the chest tube drainage system, PFT determinations are distorted. However, general trends may be useful. V_D/V_T is more accurately determined by collection and analysis of exhaled gas rather than by using Figure 5–6, as described previously.

Blood Gases. An important collaborative goal for the health care team was to adjust the ventilator to maintain normal oxygenation (e.g., PaO_2 greater than 60 to 65 mmHg, and SaO_2 greater than 90 to 94 %) and normal ventilation (e.g., $PaCO_2$ 50 mmHg, a value close to preadmission $PaCO_2$). These goals were not always met owing to the patient's cardiopulmonary instability and labile V/Q relationships in the lungs.

Mr. K.'s 1000 ABG value showed moderately severe hypoxemia, primary metabolic alkalosis, and secondary respiratory acidosis (i.e., alveolar hypoventilation).

The hypoxemia is moderately severe because the PaO_2 is below 60 mmHg. The value lies well within the oxyhemoglobin dissociation curve's critical zone. The hypoxemia was treated by maintaining PEEP at 8 cmH_2O, increasing FIO_2 to 0.75, and slowly infusing two units of packed red blood cells (PRBCs). The PRBCs served to improve the anemia and simultaneously to increase the oxygen-carrying capacity of the blood. The 1200 ABG value showed that PaO_2 increased to 207 mmHg. FIO_2 was gradually reduced to 0.50 to reduce the risk of oxygen toxicity. PEEP was decreased to 6 cmH_2O, maintaining SaO_2 at 94 % as shown on the 1500 ABG result.

Mr. K. has a primary rather than a secondary metabolic alkalosis because a pH of 7.47 lies on the alkaline not acid side of 7.4. The metabolic alkalosis was believed to be due to past nasogastric suction or hypokalemic alkalosis from high dose steroids. Some of the metabolic alkalosis may be compensating for the chronic respiratory acidosis, but no preadmission serial ABGs or electrolyte measurement results were available to further assess the cause of the alkalosis.

The $Paco_2$ of 45 mmHg is interpreted as alveolar hypoventilation. V_T was gradually decreased from 900 to 600 cc to increase $Paco_2$ to near 50 mmHg. This maneuver had little effect, however, as Mr. K. increased respiratory rate to 50/min to try to compensate for smaller tidal volumes. $Paco_2$ never reached 50 mmHg until later, when Mr. K. was given lorazepam (Ativan), 4 mg, intravenously for sedation.

Other Parameters. The high A-ao_2 gradient in the 200 mmHg range indicates the presence of primary pulmonary disease and, in this case, possibly superimposed mild pulmonary edema from fluid overload (normal A-aDo_2 = 5–20 mmHg).

Comparison of the 226 mmHg gradient at 1500 with the 230 mmHg gradient at 1900 indicates that intrapulmonary shunting is remaining relatively constant. The other gradients in Table 32–1 are measured at different FIo_2 levels and on different modes of mechanical ventilation. Hence, they cannot be used for comparison because changing FIo_2 and the mode of mechanical ventilation alters V/Q relationships in the lungs unpredictably.

The 1200 a/A ratio of 0.43 is less than normal (0.80). This finding confirms intrapulmonary shunting. Remember that intrapulmonary shunting is associated with a rising A-ao_2 gradient and a falling a/A ratio.

At 1500, note the circumstances surrounding the reduction in a/A ratio from 0.40 to 0.24. The increase in shunting may be due to increased tachypnea and increased deadspace ventilation associated with the change in ventilation modes from the assist-control mode to the SIMV mode. The tachypnea on SIMV did not significantly increase $Paco_2$ (49 mmHg is acceptable), but the accompanying increased work of breathing promoted fatigue and physical decompensation. In Mr. K.'s case, ventilation was switched back to the assist-control mode during the night.

At 1500, the nurse simultaneously drew an ABG sample from the arterial line and a mixed venous blood gas sample from the pulmonary artery catheter. The $P\bar{v}o_2$, a measure of tissue oxygenation, is within the normal range of 35 to 40 mmHg. However, this measurement probably does not accurately reflect changes in cardiac output or tissue oxygenation because the patient has an abnormally low SVR, and septic shock is suspected. In septic shock, $P\bar{v}o_2$ is normal to elevated due to arteriovenous shunting in the systemic capillary bed.

The arteriovenous oxygen content difference of 3.54 ml/100 ml represents a decrease or narrowing of the $C(a\text{-}\bar{v})o_2$ (normal $C(a\text{-}\bar{v})o_2$ = 5 ml/100 ml). This sign is consistent with septic shock.

Chest X-ray Film

Mr. K.'s admission chest x-ray film is shown in Figure 32–2. It is a supine anterior-posterior (AP) film that demonstrates a diffuse alveolar-interstitial process in all lung fields. Radiopaque confluent densities and air bronchogram signs confirm the alveolar pattern. The fine network of thickened interstitium and small cystic spaces forms the interstitial or reticular pattern. Since no previous films are available for comparison and since the film is a hazy supine one, the clinician cannot determine exactly how much of the alveolar-interstitial markings is due to a chronic process and how much is due to an acute process. Markings may be caused by the presence of pulmonary fibrosis, fluid, mucus, or some combination thereof (e.g., fluid overload, interstitial pneumonia). Other findings from this chest x-ray film include the following:

1. Cardiac silhouette at the upper limits of normal to slightly enlarged.
2. Tracheostomy.
3. Feeding tube with its tip in the left upper abdominal quadrant just medial to the gastric air bubble. Later, the physician extended the tip into the gastric air bubble.
4. Pulmonary artery catheter with its tip at the level of the right main PA.

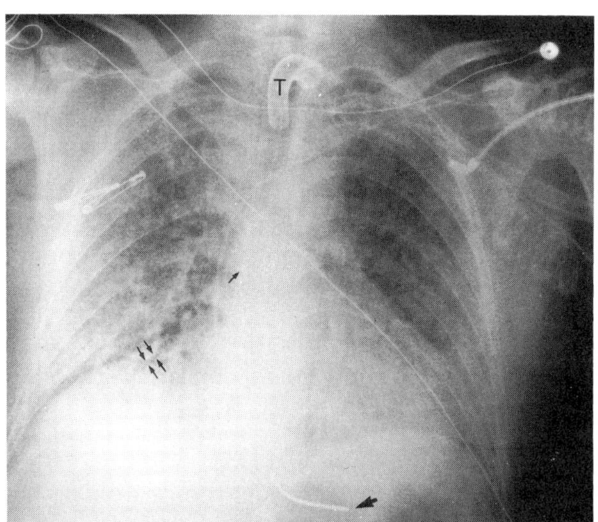

Figure 32–2. Mr. K.'s chest x-ray film on hospital admission. This anteroposterior view shows a diffuse alveolar-interstitial pattern throughout all lung fields. The group of small arrows mark the borders of an air bronchogram. The single small arrow marks the PA catheter tip in the right PA (barely visible here). The large arrow marks the tip of the feeding tube in the stomach. The T identifies the tracheostomy tube.

5. Safety pins by the right clavicle. (The nurse forgot to check for artifacts before the film was taken.)

Motivation

In the first few hours after admission, assessment of biophysical problems took precedence over assessment of motivational state. Based on limited data, Mr. K.'s motivational state seemed appropriate for his clinical circumstances. He remained cooperative and oriented to person and place but not to time. He communicated appropriately by nodding his head to questions answered with yes or no, using bedside communications charts, and writing with pad and pencil.

Over the next 24 to 48 hours, he became gradually more disoriented to time, place, and person, particularly at night. The night nurses reported his inappropriate smiling, obscene gestures, paranoid behavior, hallucinations, and attempts to get out of bed. These periods of agitation were accompanied by respiratory instability; manifested by increased tachypnea; minute ventilations of up to 40 L/min; and abnormal ABGs, requiring frequent ventilator adjustments to maintain satisfactory oxygenation and ventilation. During the day, when the patient was more oriented, he claimed that his panic reactions at night were related to morphine sulfate administration. The health care team obtained a psychiatric consultation and concluded that the patient's agitation was probably related to ICU psychosis or adverse reactions to medications (e.g., sedatives or high dose steroids), reinforced by feelings of anxiety and powerlessness. At this time, the physicians discontinued the morphine sulfate and switched from lorazepam to haloperidol (Haldol) for control of agitation.

Three nursing interventions were most helpful in relieving Mr. K.'s panic reactions. First, the nurse used continual reality orientation. During vital sign assessments, the nurse stated, "Mr. K., I'm the nurse. It is 10:00 at night, and I'm going to take your blood pressure." Explaining procedures before implementation helped to reduce Mr. K.'s anxiety about what was going to happen to him.

Second, the nurses kept distracting noises, such as monitor and ventilator alarms, to a minimum to avoid excess sensory stimulation. This intervention also permitted more complete rest between vital sign assessments.

Third and last, the nursing staff allowed his girlfriend, Alice, to remain at the patient's side at night. Her interventions—holding hands; stroking his hair; reorienting him to time, place, and person; and reminding him of their future together—proved more effective than sedation or other interventions implemented by health team members.

With constant reality orientation and psychologic support, Mr. K. gradually developed a present awareness context, the first element of the motivational model discussed in this book. Sometimes, his perception of reality was distorted, but it did not seem to affect his determination to get well because he had a strong personal goal—"to get well and feel normal." Thus, though in critical condition, Mr. K. was able to build a future awareness context early in his clinical course; Alice was the critical factor. Not only did she help Mr. K. focus on the goal, but she became knowledgeable about the details of Mr. K.'s condition so that she could repeatedly point out his progress to him on a daily basis. Becoming aware of his progress, in turn, helped Mr. K. to develop incentive motivation to strive yet another day toward his goal.

Self-Care Education

Self-care education was inappropriate for Mr. K.'s high acuity level upon hospital admission. Most of the time he was not ready to learn because hypoxemia, acid-base disorders, sleep deprivation, and hemodynamic instability hindered his mental functioning. Also, tracheal intubation made communication difficult. Therefore, patient education was used.

In the first hour after admission, the nurse oriented Mr. K. to the bedside unit, including the nurse's call light, the sounds of the monitor and ventilator alarms, and the equipment within the patient's sight. This knowledge served to reduce anxiety related to the ICU setting.

Though self-care education per se was impossible, the nurse maintained a self-care orientation by providing simple choices related to routine care, e.g., turning to the right or the left, suctioning once versus twice. This approach helped to counter Mr. K.'s feelings of powerlessness. In addition, it kept him involved in his care, preparing him to take more and more responsibility for respiratory interventions as his condition improved.

Simultaneously, Alice was encouraged to participate in care. At Mr. K.'s request, she helped the nurse with personal hygiene measures, including tracheostomy care. Later, when Mr. K. began to sleep through the night without panic episodes, Alice spent more time at the hospital during the day, giving psychologic support during the process of weaning from mechanical ventilation.

CONSOLIDATION OF ASSESSMENT DATA

Thus far, the nurse has formed numerous information clusters during respiratory assessment. Towards the end of assessment, the nurse mentally consolidates data into updated information clusters. These clusters are shown hereafter. As in previous examples, cues in each cluster are indicated with asterisk. Note that the larger data base has permitted identification of only one problem for each information cluster. In some cases cues have become more specific, e.g., high V_D/V_T for increased work of breathing. In other cases no cues are identified, because all pieces of information are of equal specificity, and the cluster as a whole identifies the problem.

Information Clusters	Problems
unstable low PaO_2 cyanotic mucous membranes at times altered mental status	hypoxemia
signs of sepsis* multiple indwelling catheters microorganisms in urine, sputum, and pleural exudate* elevated WBC with left shift yellow mucus	infection
high peak inspiratory pressures PEEP 8 cmH_2O chest tube air leak* history of recurrent pneumothorax	barotrauma
tachypnea elevated V_E high V_D/V_T* diaphoresis tachycardia use of accessory muscles of respiration	increased work of breathing
limited ability to communicate bedrest with arm restraints no privacy mental disorientation aggressive behavior history of failure to wean from mechanical ventilation	powerlessness
suctioning of mucus rhonchi on auscultation bronchovesicular breath sounds acute interstitial and alveolar pattern on chest x-ray film	mucus retention
life-threatening illness poor medical prognosis powerlessness fear of unknown restlessness diaphoresis repeatedly asking, "Am I getting better?"	anxiety
critical illness bedrest with arm restraints ICU setting nothing by mouth (NPO) (tube feedings) inability to communicate verbally sleep deprivation anxiety	sensory-perceptual alteration
brother working in metal grinding shop unsafe work environment	occupational lung disease (brother)

The Problem List

In consultation with other members of the health care team, the nurse groups related problems and ranks them from highest to lowest priority, as shown hereafter.

GROUPS OF PROBLEMS

Hypoxemia, increased work of breathing
Infection, barotrauma
Anxiety, powerlessness, sensory-perceptual alteration
Mucus retention
Occupational lung disease (brother)

Keep in mind that this list focuses mostly on actual problems that require an immediate plan. Assessment of other problems, such as unsafe workplace, is postponed until after disease stabilization.

NURSING DIAGNOSIS AND INTERVENTION

After validation of Mr. K.'s problems, the nurse writes each problem in nursing diagnosis format. The list of acute nursing diagnoses is presented in the box.

INITIAL NURSING DIAGNOSES IDENTIFIED IN THE ICU

Hypoxemia due to V/Q mismatching in the lungs
Increased work of breathing related to increased V_D/V_T and increased demand for ventilation
Infection related to sepsis, multiple indwelling catheters, and pneumonitis
Barotrauma related to high ventilator pressures and poor healing of pulmonary tissues
Situational anxiety related to life-threatening illness
Powerlessness related to limitations imposed by critical illness and mechanical ventilation
Sensory-perceptual alteration related to critical illness and the ICU setting
Possible occupational lung disease (brother) related to inhalation of lung irritants

Analysis of Increased Work of Breathing

After nursing diagnoses are identified, the nurse further analyzes each problem to determine respiratory intervention. One of Mr. K.'s top priority diagnoses—increased work of breathing (WOB)—is analyzed hereafter to show how assessment leads into intervention. The basic format for analysis is the SOAP format described in the previous chapter. After reading this example, the reader is encouraged to analyze Mr. K.'s other nursing diagnoses using the SOAP format, applying information in this book to Mr. K.'s data base.

Problem: Increased work of breathing related to increased V_D/V_T and increased demand for ventilation.
Date: 4/9
Time: 1900

Subjective Data. Complaints of (c/o) general fatigue and shortness of breath when respiratory rate greater than 40 breaths/min. Patient denies other cardiopulmonary symptoms.

Objective Data. *Vital signs*: stable, except respiratory rate 35 to 48/min. Monitor: sinus tachycardia 110/min. *Ventilator settings*: SIMV 12/min, FIO_2 0.50, PEEP 6 cmH_2O, V_T 600 cc. The patient's $\dot{V}_E$ is 33 L/min. Peak inspiratory pressures have decreased to 25 to 35 cmH_2O. Dynamic compliance has increased to 0.22. *Chest assessment findings*: maximal chest excursions, with patient using neck, intercostal, and shoulder accessory muscles for breathing. No breathing asynchrony. I:E ratio 1:1. Skin warm, diaphoretic, without cyanosis. On auscultation: bronchovesicular breath sounds around chest tube site, and scattered rhonchi clearing after suctioning. *Chest x-ray*: alveolar-interstitial pattern remains unchanged. *ABGs:* pH 7.43, $PaCO_2$ 48, PaO_2 67, HCO_3^- 32, and SaO_2 94 %. *Activity:* agitated at times; attempting to climb out of bed despite restraints and verbal reassurance.

Analysis. Mr. K. still has increased work of breathing (WOB). Some signs have improved, e.g., PIP has decreased and CL_{dyn} has increased slightly, suggesting improved compliance of the lungs. $\dot{V}_E$ has decreased from 40 to 33 L/min, suggesting that the patient is using less energy and less oxygen for breathing. However, he remains fatigued. His agitation is dramatically increasing the WOB. The chest x-ray film findings have not improved. Other signs of increased WOB, such as use of accessory muscles of respiration, tachycardia, and diaphoresis, are also indicators of respiratory distress and respiratory muscle fatigue. Estimated V_D/V_T remains more than 0.85, a grossly elevated value suggesting that a large percentage of total body oxygen consumption is being used for breathing.

Thus far, Mr. K. seems to be compensating for the increased WOB. Blood pH is normal. He has adequate cardiac reserve as evidenced by his ability to increase cardiac output on demand. He has normal kidney function to allow adjustments in HCO_3^- as needed. However, his ventilatory reserve is nearly gone, and respiratory muscle fatigue is imminent. Hence, intervention should remain focused on immediate reduction of WOB.

Plan. *Overall goal* is to decrease the WOB, as evidenced by estimated V_D/V_T less than 0.66, $\dot{V}_E$ less than 20 L/min, and no signs of respiratory muscle fatigue.

Intervention 1. Control agitation as follows: (1) give PRN haloperidol (Haldol) medication, (2) encourage patient to express his concerns and feelings in writing, and (3) allow Alice to remain at bedside to provide continual reassurance, reality orientation, and psychologic support.

Rationale: Agitation causes increased tachypnea, increased V_D/V_T, and increased WOB. In some cases, ventilator adjustments are unable to correct ABGs and compensate for respiratory instability. Encouraging communication will reduce frustration and agitation due to communication problems. Alice was successful in the past in helping to reduce his agitation.

Intervention 2. Treat infection with ordered antibiotics.

Rationale: Infection, similar to agitation and fever, increases demand for ventilation. If this demand is eliminated, WOB will decrease.

Intervention 3. Provide for rest at night as follows: (1) switch to assist-control mode as ordered, (2) provide for a quiet environment, and (3) control agitation.

Rationale: Resting respiratory muscles allows repletion of metabolic stores and more efficient respiration. It prevents asynchronous breathing patterns that result in increased WOB.

Intervention 4. Promptly call respiratory therapist to adjust ventilator whenever airway turbulence persists, as evidenced by sounding of high pressure alarm, high PIP, uneven rise of pressure needle, and abnormal I:E ratio.

Rationale: Airway turbulence will worsen alveolar hypoventilation and hypoxemia, thus increasing demand for ventilation and, ultimately, WOB.

Intervention 5. Call the physician if WOB increases, as evidenced by increasing tachypnea and minute ventilation.

Rationale: If sedation does not reduce WOB, a paralyzing drug, such as pancuronium, may be indicated.

Mr. K.'s Clinical Course

This part of the chapter moves away from the nursing process and focuses on Mr. K. and his clinical course in the ICU, on the ward, and at home. The description serves three purposes. First, it familiarizes nurses in all settings with the tribulations of a respiratory patient as he moves through the health care continuum. Understanding the patient's experience helps to individualize care in specific settings. Second, examination of Mr. K.'s clinical course clarifies expected disease progression and procedures for basic interventions, such as weaning from mechanical ventilation, discontinuation of chest tubes, and tapering of oral steroids. Third and last, this case shows how emphasis on certain assessment parameters changes as the patient's condition improves and how basic assessment findings (e.g., lung sounds, PFTs) reach a new equilibrium in the home setting.

IN THE ICU

Mr. K. remained in the ICU for 3 weeks. During this time, gas exchange gradually improved. On the day of admission, he was returned to the assist-control mode of ventilation to decrease WOB. Pa_{O_2} gradually increased to 80 to 90 mmHg. The A-a_{O_2} gradient decreased after diuresis with furosemide (Lasix). Pa_{CO_2} stabilized at 45 to 50 mmHg as respiratory rate decreased to 26 to 30/min, and $\dot{V}_E$ decreased to 25 L/min.

Mr. K.'s sensorium and overall condition also improved. He experienced fewer periods of disorientation at night. When he became agitated, he responded to words of reassurance and haloperidol (Haldol) medication. He cooperated in range of motion exercises to prevent muscle deconditioning. Most invasive lines and catheters were discontinued after the first 2 days of intensive care. Blood culture results remained negative. The urinary tract infection, empyema, and pneumonia were successfully treated with antibiotics over several weeks. WBCs gradually declined to normal numbers, and the patient remained afebrile for the rest of his hospital stay.

Within 2 days after admission, the health care team had implemented plans for all the problems on Mr. K.'s initial nursing diagnosis list. Malnutrition was added to the list because the patient had a low serum albumin level, low caloric intake, and weight loss. Nutritional stores were repleted by tube feedings, starting with half-strength Isocal and gradually working up to 2000 cal/day of full-strength Isocal. (The patient was gradually switched to solid food after weaning from mechanical ventilation.)

Though most parameters improved, Mr. K. had two persistent problems as follows: (1) bronchopleural fistula and (2) difficulty in weaning from mechanical ventilation. The bronchopleural fistula never closed because of delayed wound healing from steroids. When the leak became bigger, suction was increased to 60 cmH_2O to eliminate air from the pleural space as fast as it leaked out from the lung. Thereafter, the air leak remained unchanged. Yet Mr. K. experienced several pneumothoraces requiring chest tube repositioning or insertion of another chest tube.

Weaning from Mechanical Ventilation

Weaning from mechanical ventilation began on 4/12, the third day of admission, after Mr. K.'s critical condition began to stabilize. He was switched from the assist-control mode of ventilation to the SIMV mode at 26 breaths/min. F_{IO_2} was decreased to 0.45; PEEP was decreased to 3 cmH_2O. Thereafter, the SIMV rate was gradually decreased over several days to 4 breaths/min on 4/20. Simultaneously, Mr. K.'s activity level was gradually increased, as tolerated, starting with dangling his legs over the edge of the bed BID, then sitting in a chair BID.

After each change in ventilator setting, a blood sample was drawn from a radial arterial line. ABGs were monitored to assure adequate gas exchange and to guide decision-making regarding the next step in the weaning process. In addition, daily PFTs (e.g., V_T, spontaneous VC, PF, MIP, MEP) were followed to aid in respiratory assessment.

On 4/21, rather than decrease SIMV breaths to 2/min, the physicians decided to switch respiratory set ups and use CPAP with FIO_2 at 0.45 and 3 cmH_2O positive pressure. They determined that breathing through the demand valve of the Bear 2 volume ventilator at the low SIMV rate was increasing Mr. K.'s WOB and prolonging the weaning process. (Extra effort is required to open the demand valve on inspiration.)

Mr. K. did well on the new CPAP set up. The positive pressure helped to keep his right lung expanded. SaO_2 remained greater than 95 %, and $PaCO_2$ was 50 mmHg. During the night he was returned to the Bear 2 volume ventilator, SIMV 4 breaths/min, to allow respiratory muscles to rest and to guard against atelectasis and mucus retention.

After 1 day of CPAP, Mr. K. was placed on a T piece and then on a tracheostomy collar with FIO_2 at 0.40. ABGs remained satisfactory during these changes.

By this time, the arterial line had already been discontinued. An arterial stick was necessary to draw blood for an ABG. Such invasive measures were kept to a minimum by use of noninvasive measures of SaO_2 and CaO_2 whenever possible. For example, the nurse monitored SaO_2 during the night q2 to 4h by oximeter to be sure SaO_2 did not fall below 90% during sleep. End-tidal PCO_2 was monitored by capnography to detect excessive alveolar hypoventilation. In Mr. K.'s case, end-tidal PCO_2 was consistently 13 to 15 mmHg lower than the arterial PCO_2. The nurse called the physician whenever the end-tidal PCO_2 increased to 37 to 40 mmHg.

On 4/25, the physician changed Mr. K.'s tracheostomy tube to a fenestrated Shiley tube. The physician deflated the cuff and capped the end of the tube so that Mr. K. was breathing solely through his own upper airway. The tube's fenestration served to decrease resistance to air flow within the trachea.

On 4/27, Mr. K. began to ambulate at the bedside. Again, the nurses used oximetry to check SaO_2 periodically. Whenever SaO_2 decreased below 90%, the nurses increased FIO_2 as ordered to correct the oxygen desaturation.

Psychologic Adjustment. Chapter 28 explains the four phases of psychologic adjustment that a patient goes through during the weaning process. With the support of health team members and his girlfriend, Alice, Mr. K. moved through the first three phases of adjustment while in the ICU. At the time of transfer to the ward, he was somewhere between phase 3 (depression and gradual accommodation to reality) and phase 4 (active participation in rehabilitative care). His inability to deal with reality was related to the presence of the tracheostomy tube and the unresolved ethical issues related to his guarded medical prognosis. Also, when respiratory instability interrupted or slowed the weaning process for days at a time, he doubted the possibility of extubation in the future.

Nursing intervention focused on the following four interventions:

1. Encouraging Mr. K. to verbalize his feelings.
2. Reassuring him that a slow weaning process is normal for a person with his disease process.
3. Providing positive reinforcement for daily progress.
4. Asking the physician to again discuss Mr. K.'s condition with him. Mr. K. could not remember previous medical explanations, owing to altered mental status.

ON THE WARD

On 4/28, Mr. K. was transferred to the ward with a tracheostomy and two chest tubes to 40 cmH_2O suction. By this time, the main medical diagnosis was changed to idiopathic pulmonary fibrosis. Silicosis was ruled out because of the very small amounts of silica found in the lung biopsy specimen.

Mr. K.'s clinical course on the ward is summarized hereafter.

4/30 The suction to the chest tube drainage system is gradually decreased to 20 cmH_2O, as the bronchopleural fistula becomes smaller. Two days later suction is discontinued, and the drainage system is left at 10 cmH_2O pressure. Intravenous methylprednisolone sodium succinate (Solu-Medrol) is switched to oral prednisone, 60 mg daily, to treat the pulmonary fibrosis.

5/3 The tracheostomy was removed and an Olympic tracheostomy button inserted to maintain the stoma. A small pneumothorax persists at the right lung base with the chest tube to waterseal, but pleural adhesions are preventing further lung collapse. The plan is to leave the chest tubes in for slow granulation of the pleural space.

5/6 A consulting thoracic surgeon decides against surgery to close the bronchopleural fistula. The chest tubes are repositioned again owing to recurrent right upper and lower lobe (RUL and RLL) pneumothoraces (Fig. 32–3A and B). The surgeon cut the chest tubes off close to the chest and inserted Heimlich valves to facilitate ambulation. The one-way Heimlich valves provided for the continuous escape of air from the pleural space without chance of pneumothorax. Rubber gloves were wrapped around the end of the tubes to collect the minimal amounts of pleural drainage.

5/8 The patient is markedly dyspneic with minimal exertion. He is weak but in good spirits. Dry crackles

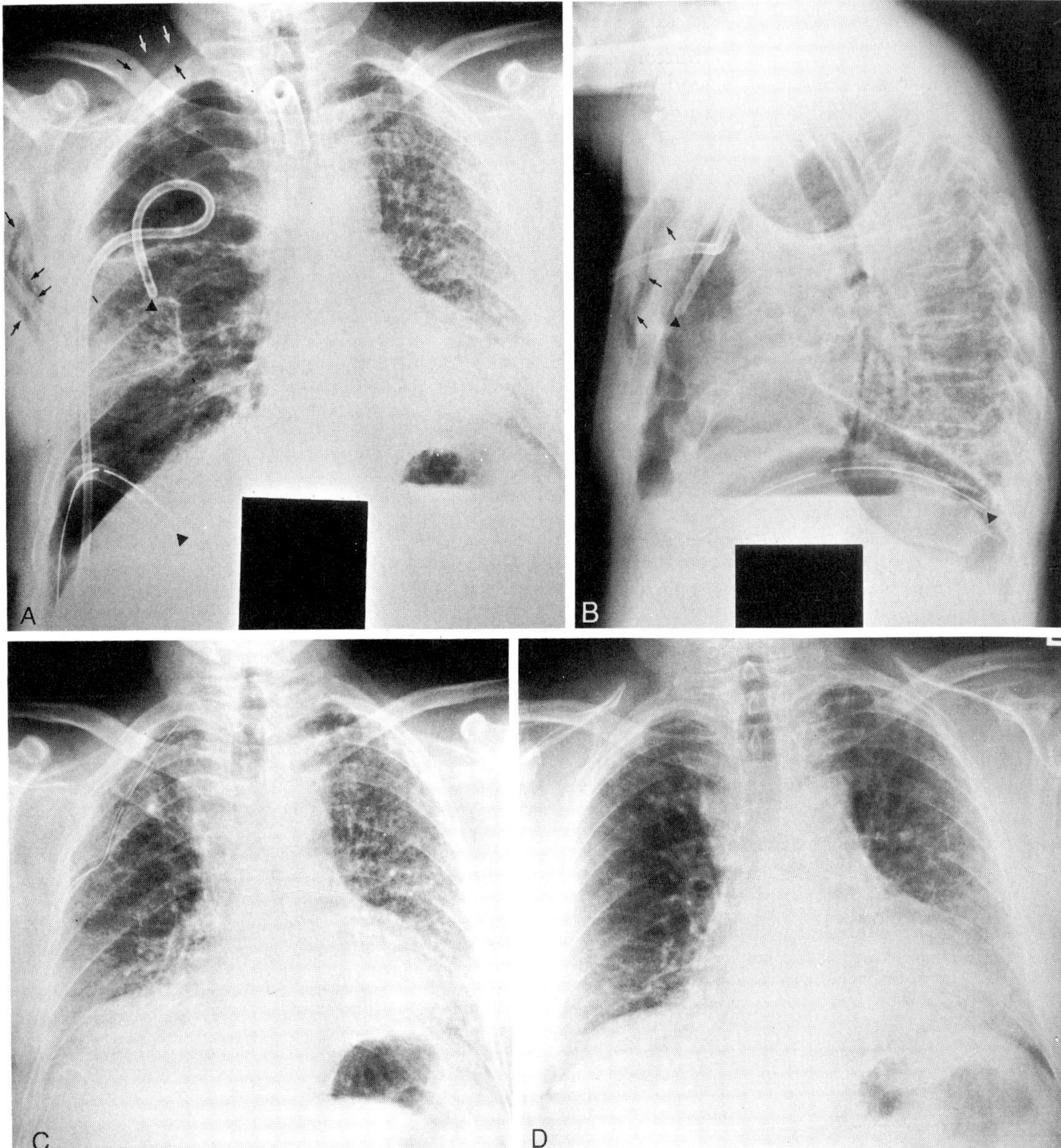

Figure 32–3. Mr. K.'s serial chest x-ray films over a 7-week period. *A* and *B*, Frontal and lateral views of the chest taken on 5/6. A chest tube is seen in the RUL and in the RLL for pneumothoraces, manifested by areas of hyperlucency in the lung fields. Extensive interstitial disease and loss of lung volume are seen in the left lung field. The small arrows mark locations of subcutaneous emphysema in the soft tissues of the right shoulder, right axilla, and anterior chest area (lateral film). The arrowheads mark distal chest tube tips. *C*, Frontal view taken on 5/9. The tracheostomy tube and subcutaneous emphysema are gone. The right pneumothoraces are also gone, except for a minimal pneumothorax evident on a lateral film not shown here. The right heart border and left diaphragm are obscured (silhouette signs), because of pneumonia. *D*, Frontal view taken on 6/30. The pneumothoraces, chest tubes, and silhouette signs are gone. The interstitial pattern in the lung fields is less prominent compared with the pattern in C. These findings are consistent with resolving pneumonia and improvement in the interstitial disease.

from fibrosis are auscultated throughout all lung fields. Decreased breath sounds in the RLL persist near the chest tube site. Sao_2 is 93 % on nasal cannula at 5 L/min.

5/9 The chest x-ray film shows nearly complete resorption of the pneumothoraces (Fig. 32–3C). ABGs continue to improve. The tracheostomy button is removed, and an occlusive dressing is placed over the stoma. The health care team meets with Mr. K. to discuss his hospital discharge.

5/10 Resting ABGs on 1 L/min cannula are pH 7.45, Pao_2 61 mmHg, $Paco_2$ 42 mmHg, and Sao_2 92%. To determine oxygen prescription during exercise, the respiratory nurse specialist and the respiratory therapist use a portable O_2 set up and exercise Mr. K. on the ward while monitoring Sao_2 with a finger oximeter. This study determined that Mr. K. needs 3 L/min oxygen flow during exercise.

5/11 Mr. K. is discharged. His orders include the following:

1. Prednisone, 60 mg, PO daily.
2. Home oxygen, 1 L/min at rest, 3 L/min with exercise.
3. Diphenhydramine hydrochloride (Benadryl), 50 mg, PO q HS PRN insomnia.
4. Acetaminophen (Tylenol) No. 3, 1 to 2 tablets, PO q4h PRN pain.
5. Clean chest tube insertion site with hydrogen peroxide BID.

AT HOME

Mr. K.'s clinical course at home is summarized hereafter, as related by health professionals caring for him in the chest clinic and in the home setting.

6/6 Mr. K. fatigues easily with exertion at home but denies dyspnea at rest, even off oxygen. He is starting to go out to restaurants and movies, using a small portable liquid oxygen system. The chest tubes were discontinued 1 week ago without complications. The lungs have the same decreased breath sounds over the RLL and crackles over all lung fields, most prominent over the LLL. Mr. K. has a "buffalo hump" and is gaining weight (190 lb), probably because of his steroid medication and voracious appetite.

6/28 A PFT is orderd to assess Mr. K.'s baseline lung function. Test results shown in Table 32–2 indicate the presence of moderately severe restrictive lung disease, with severe diffusion impairment. The low DL explains why the patient needs oxygen with activities of daily living. Furthermore, even though he has a 20-pack-year history of cigarette smoking, Mr. K. has no signs of airway obstruction on this PFT. (See page 845, Appendix II, for a detailed interpretation of this PFT.)

6/30 Results from a complete exercise study indicate that Mr. K.'s decreased exercise tolerance is primarily due to gas exchange abnormalities rather than to mechanical or ventilatory limitation. The exercise

Table 32–2. MR. K.'S PULMONARY FUNCTION TEST

Lung Volumes BTPS		*Predicted*	*Observed*	*% Predicted*	*After Bronchodilator*	*% Predicted*
Vital capacity (VC)	(L)	4.87	2.81	58		
Inspiratory capacity (IC)	(L)					
Exp. res. vol. (ERV)	(L)					
Residual volume (RV)	(L)	2.01	1.52	76		
Total lung cap. (TLC)	(L)	6.65	4.33	65		
Residual vol./TLC	(%)	< 33	35			
Funct. resid. cap. (FRC)	(L)	3.77	2.30	61		
Mechanics of Breathing						
Forced expir. vol. (1 sec) (FEV_1)	(L)	3.70	2.48	67	2.46	67
% Expir. in 1 sec (FEV_1/FVC)	(%)	> 70	88		88	
Forced vital capacity (FVC)	(L)	4.87	2.81	58	2.81	58
Forced mid exp flow	(L/sec)	3.82	4.53	119	4.36	114
Max. vol. vent (MVV)	(L/min)	159	166	104	166	104
Peak exp flow	(L/sec)	8.95	7.43	83	7.56	84
Peak inspir flow	(L/sec)	5.20	6.36	122	7.21	139
Diffusion (Transfer Factor)						
Pulm. diffusing cap (DL_{CO}) (Single breath CO) (ml/min/mmHg)		30.7	6.6	22		
Pulm. diffusing cap (DL_{CO}) corrected for Hgb (ml/min/mmHg)		30.7	8.0	26		
Alveolar volume (single breath) (L) = 3.78						
Hemoglobin (Hgb) gm % = 11.8						

Table 32–3. EXERCISE STUDY FOR OXYGEN PRESCRIPTION

Heart Rate (HR) and Blood Gases	At Rest	During Exercise	
HR	78	115	*Name:* Mr. K.
pH	7.46	7.48	*Oxygen:* 1 L/min via Linde walker
$Paco_2$	34.5	32.4	*Predicted maximum heart rate:* 182
Pao_2	110.5	58.2	*Treadmill setting:* 1 mph, 0 grade
HCO_3	24.3	24.1	*Exercise time:* 8 min
B.E.	+1.8	+2.2	*Comments or reason for stopping:* shortness of breath and "feet hurt."
Sao_2	98.3	92.2	
Finger oximetry			*Results:* The patient's oxygen saturation (Sao_2) remained adequate during exercise, i.e., greater than 90 %. This suggests that the patient does not need increased supplemental oxygen at this time.
Pao_2	97	93	

study for oxygen prescription indicated that oxygen at 1 L/min is sufficient during exercise (Table 32–3). Oxygen at rest is discontinued after results from a resting ABG on room air indicated adequate oxygenation. The chest x-ray film in Figure 32–3D shows a slight improvement in parenchymal densities and no change in heart enlargement when compared with the chest x-ray film of 5/9 in Figure 32–3C. Note that the right pneumothorax is gone. The right heart border and left diaphragm are now visible (absent silhouette sign), indicating resolution of RML and LLL pneumonia.

7/7 Mr. K. complains of dyspnea on exertion during hot summer days in smoggy Los Angeles. He is working in his metal grinding shop using an appropriate breathing mask for protection from lung irritants. He complains of lack of libido, but this problem resolved spontaneously after prednisone was tapered below 30 mg daily.

8/4 A gallium lung scan is performed on Mr. K. in the nuclear medicine department to help assess disease activity. The test result was negative. When considered with the other tests performed thus far, the result indicates that Mr. K.'s pulmonary fibrosis is inactive. Hence, the physicians continued to taper the prednisone as long as Mr. K. continued to improve clinically. The prednisone was tapered as follows:

5/23 50 mg daily
6/6 40 mg daily
7/7 40 mg daily (it was not reduced because of increasing pulmonary symptoms).
8/4 30 mg daily for 2 weeks, followed by 20 mg daily for 1 week, and 17.5 mg daily for 1 week.
9/1 15 mg daily
11/17 10 mg daily

12/1 Mr. K. still has dyspnea on exertion, but with the help of his girlfriend and visiting nurses, he learns how to live within the limitations of his disease. Though all problems are not resolved, respiratory care is discontinued because Mr. K. moved to another state, Oklahoma, to live with a relative.

Pulmonary Rehabilitation

The rehabilitative process began early in Mr. K.'s clinical course, when the critical care nurse approached him with a self-care orientation in the ICU. This step prepared Mr. K. for more intensive rehabilitative measures on the ward and in the home setting.

Though Mr. K. never attended a formal rehabilitation program, nursing diagnosis and intervention described in this last part of the case study helped Mr. K. to achieve the main goal of pulmonary rehabilitation, i.e., the highest level of functional activity that a person is capable of.

NURSING DIAGNOSIS AND INTERVENTION

Nursing diagnoses for acute respiratory nursing care have been described. Nursing diagnoses for pulmonary rehabilitation are listed in Table 32–4. The reader is encouraged to compare these diagnoses with those identified in the ICU. These diagnoses are made using the same decision-making processes described in the previous section.

Hypoxemia

Note that hypoxemia, the primary problem associated with restrictive pulmonary disease, spans all three settings.

Nursing intervention focused on administration of appropriate amounts of oxygen and relief and preven-

Table 32–4. NURSING DIAGNOSES FOR PULMONARY REHABILITATION

On the Ward	At Home
Hypoxemia due to V/Q mismatching and recurrent pneumothoraces*	Hypoxemia due to V/Q mismatching and diffusion impairment*
Inability to perform ADL due to pulmonary disease, muscle deconditioning, and lack of knowledge about energy conservation techniques*	Decreased exercise tolerance due to pulmonary disease and muscle deconditioning*
Self-care deficit related to overdependency on girlfriend*	Potential disease exacerbation related to tapering of prednisone*
Altered body image related to tracheostomy	Potential mucus retention related to pulmonary disease and hot smoggy climate
Anxiety related to guarded medical prognosis	Decreased libido related to steroids and possible psychosocial problems
Mucus retention related to resolving pneumonia	Obesity related to steroids and increased food intake

*Top priority problems.

tion of V/Q mismatching. Specific interventions included the following:

1. Maintenance of a bronchial hygiene program, including coughing, deep breathing, and gradual increase in activity.
2. Monitoring dyspnea, chest assessment findings, and air leak in the chest tube drainage system for possible extension of the pneumothoraces.
3. Instruction in the proper use of oxygen at rest and during exercise.
4. Instruction in the use and maintenance of liquid oxygen systems at home.

Inability to Perform Activities of Daily Living

Inability to perform activities of daily living (ADL) was another top priority problem. The nurses and physical therapist on the ward implemented a few basic relaxation and muscle conditioning exercises. Moreover, during ambulation Mr. K. was encouraged to walk slowly and pace himself to reduce dyspnea on exertion. Later, in the home situation, Mr. K. was able to perform most ADL by himself, but he still had decreased exercise tolerance related to ambulation and climbing beyond one flight of stairs. The visiting nurse prepared a daily walking program for Mr. K. He recorded accomplishment of daily goals on a wall chart (e.g., in city blocks walked and flights of stairs climbed without significant dyspnea). The nurse also taught him diaphragmatic breathing to help him decrease respiratory rate and normalize breathing pattern during activity.

Self-Care Deficit

After transfer from the respiratory ICU, Mr. K. became more and more dependent on Alice until the ward nurses finally insisted that he begin to care for himself, e.g., learn tracheostomy care, perform his own personal hygiene measures. Part of this self-care deficit was the natural result of allowing his girlfriend to play a strong supportive role in the ICU. Her strong participant role was adaptive in the ICU because of Mr. K.'s critical condition. However, her role had become maladaptive in the ward setting because it prevented Mr. K. from practicing self-care strategies, building self-confidence, and taking full responsibility for his own care.

Nursing intervention focused on the following:

1. Teaching Alice how to give back this responsibility to Mr. K.
2. Providing positive reinforcement whenever Mr. K. practiced self-care.

Mr. K. gradually learned to perform tracheostomy care and ADL on his own on the ward. In retrospect, however, the transition to independence might have been smoother had the ICU nurses further reinforced the self-care concept before the patient left the ICU.

Altered Body Image

The nurses identified a body image problem because of Mr. K.'s ambivalent feelings towards his tracheostomy. Most of the time, Mr. K. expressed thankfulness for his tracheostomy because it saved his life in the ICU and now allowed him to breathe without mechanical assistance. Sometimes, however, he saw it as an intruder, a "nuisance" that made him feel self conscious in front of visitors. Though he said he wanted to get rid of it, he feared the risk of physical decompensation associated with extubation.

Nursing intervention included the following:

1. Helping Mr. K. to verbalize feelings related to the tracheostsomy, possible extubation, and self consciousness in front of visitors.
2. Reassuring him that the tracheostomy is a temporary measure and that the hole will gradually close after extubation.
3. Providing a mirror so that Mr. K. could view his tracheostomy during tracheostomy care. Visualization facilitates the cleaning precedure and helps the patient incorporate the tracheostomy into his body image.

The body image problem was resolved immediately after extubation.

Anxiety

Mr. K.'s anxiety was related mostly to his guarded medical diagnosis, though some of it was related to his tracheostomy and anticipated extubation.

The physician discussed his disease and prognosis with him at length. Essentially, Mr. K. was told that, although the disease was somewhat unpredictable, it tended to be progressive, and his long-term prognosis was guarded.

Nursing intervention focused on the following:

1. Encouraging Mr. K. to express fears related to this medical prognosis.
2. Providing continued positive reinforcement for small improvements in condition.
3. Helping Mr. K. to express ambivalent feelings about working in his metal grinding shop for a living.

As with his body image problem, signs of Mr. K.'s anxiety gradually disappeared after tracheal extubation. In Mr. K.'s case, tracheal extubation represented a major turning point in rehabilitative care. It gave him the confidence he needed to complete the weaning process started in the ICU and to fully participate in rehabilitative care.

Mucus Retention

Mr. K. had some mucus retention in the ICU and on the ward, though it never became a problem until after extubation. When the nurses identified increased coughing, complaints of difficulty raising mucus, and rhonchi in the chest, they gave a PRN aerosol treatment with isoetharine (Bronkosol) via a hand-held nebulizer. After the treatment, deep breathing and coughing facilitated mucus expectoration. In one instance, the nurse removed the tracheostomy button and suctioned directly into the trachea. The sputum remained clear, and the mucus retention problem was resolved before hospital discharge.

In the home setting, the visiting nurse identified a potential mucus retention problem whenever Mr. K. complained of dyspnea and sputum production during hot or smoggy weather. Intervention included the following:

1. Encouraging increased fluid intake to 2 L/day to keep secretions liquefied.
2. Teaching Mr. K. what to do (e.g., stay inside, avoid exertional activities) in case of a smog alert.
3. Encouraging him to call his doctor if his sputum increased in amount or changed from white to yellow in color.

Potential Disease Exacerbation

Potential disease exacerbation related to tapering of prednisone was never a problem on the ward because the prednisone was not tapered until after hospital discharge. In the home setting, however, this was a top priority problem. Several interventions helped prevent disease exacerbation. First, the information on steroids given to Mr. K. in the hospital was reinforced, with emphasis on the need for *gradual* rather than sudden reduction of dosage to avoid both disease exacerbation and signs of steroid withdrawal.

Second, the nurse carefully monitored pulmonary symptoms and chest assessment findings each week to detect possible signs of decompensation, as the prednisone was gradually reduced. She advised Mr. K. to remain on the same dosage and to see his physician whenever breath sounds became more distant or whenever dyspnea, sputum production, and general fatigue increased. She advised him to continue the ordered tapering schedule whenever chest assessment findings remained baseline normal and signs of steroid withdrawal were absent or limited to general fatigue.

Last, the nurse checked to be sure Mr. K. was taking his daily prednisone early in the morning, the time that coincides with the body's normal high output of steroids.

Decreased Libido

Steroids contributed to two other problems of decreased libido and obesity.

A decreased sexual drive is sometimes seen in patients on high dose steroids. In this case, Mr. K. was reluctant to discuss with the nurse his sexual problem. When the nurse learned of it from the physician in the chest clinic, she tactfully encouraged discussion of the topic without success. Then she moved on to other topics, respecting the patient's desire to keep this problem between his physician and himself. As mentioned previously, this problem was resolved after the prednisone was tapered to a lower dose.

Obesity

Mr. K.'s obesity was related to sodium retention from steroids as well as frequent snacks and soft drinks between meals. Both the obesity and slight buffalo hump on his back might have caused an accompanying body image problem. However, the nurse never identified this problem because Mr. K. always spoke favorably of himself and his relationship with his friends.

The visiting nurse, physician, and Mr. K. agreed to the following plan to resolve the obesity problem:

1. A reduction in snacks between meals.
2. The switch from soft drinks to water or a sugar-free drink.
3. A no-added-salt diet to avoid fluid retention.
4. Use of high protein foods, protein additives, and a balanced diet to assure intake of vitamins and trace elements.
5. Weekly weighing of himself at home and monitoring of values.
6. Use of a contingency contract. Alice agreed to clean Mr. K.'s apartment every week if he in turn continued to lose 1 to 2 lb/week, to a weight of 190 lb. Then they would reevaluate the situation.

Though this plan was agreed upon by all persons involved, Mr. K. preferred to postpone its implementation until after hypoxemia and decreased exercise tolerance began to improve. He could not cope with working on too many problems at once. Later, after the visiting nurse discontinued services, he finally acknowledged that his obesity was probably contributing to his decreased exercise tolerance, and he began the weight-reducing program on his own. Though he now had motivation to resolve the problem, intervention was interrupted by his move to Oklahoma.

The Final Medical Diagnosis

Mr. K.'s final medical diagnosis was usual interstitial pneumonitis (UIP) in remission. Though past silica exposure was documented and exposure to iron oxides aluminum, hard metals, and aluminum remained a possibility, occupational lung disease was never formally diagnosed. After Mr. K.'s medical records were forwarded to Oklahoma for follow up at another medical facility, the nurse and other health team members never heard from the patient and girlfriend again.

Conclusion

Nurses collaborated with other health professionals over an 8-month period to reduce Mr. K.'s respiratory illness, optimize wellness, and provide comprehensive and continuing respiratory care.

In retrospect, the nursing staff identified one neglected problem, i.e., potential or possible occupational lung disease (OLD) related to exposure to lung irritants in the workplace. Even though OLD was medically ruled out, Mr. K.'s metal grinding shop was never examined to be sure his working environment was safe. Moreover, though this problem was identified upon hospital admission, it became lost among the numerous acute problems that took precedence. This error of omission illustrates two points. First, nurses in all settings must collaborate to prevent the loss of old problems during reassessment. Second, nurses need to develop new ways to increase access to nurse consultants, such as the respiratory nurse specialist and occupational health nurse, who regularly deal with specific respiratory problems in the workplace.

In spite of this neglected problem, most of Mr. K.'s pulmonary problems were either resolved or controlled by self-care strategies. His adaptation to acute and then chronic illness was facilitated by problem-centered nursing care. Nurses used refined respiratory decision-making skills to move back and forth between assessment and intervention, constantly confirming, ruling out, or modifying diagnoses, such as hypoxemia, alveolar hypoventilation, and self-care deficit, as Mr. K. became better or worse and as he moved from the ICU to the ward and finally to the home setting.

This case study shows how decision-making processes across the health care continuum can lead to excellence in respiratory nursing care and thus enrich the lives of respiratory patients and their families.

APPENDIX

Appendix I—Pulmonary Abbreviations and Symbols*

General

$\downarrow$—decrease.
$\uparrow$—increase.
$<$—less than.
$>$—greater than.
Δ—change.
$\dot{X}$—a dot above any symbol indicates a time derivative, e.g., per minute.
$\bar{X}$—a dash above any symbol indicates a mean value.
%X—a percent sign *preceding* a symbol indicates percentage of the predicted normal value.
X/Y%—a percent sign *after* a symbol indicates a ratio function with the ratio expressed as a percentage, e.g., $FEV_1/FVC\% = 100 \times FEV_1/FVC$.

Large Capital Letters

C—concentration in blood phase; also a general symbol for compliance.
F—fractional concentration of a gas.
P—partial pressure or tension.
Q—volume of blood.
S—percent saturation in blood phase.
V—gas volume. Also a general term for ventilation.

Small Capital Letters

A—alveolar
ALV—alveolar
ANAT—anatomic
B—barometric
D—dead space
E—expired
ET—end tidal
I—inspired
L—lung
T—tidal
STPD—standard temperature and pressure, dry. Temperature of 0° C; pressure of 760 mmHg, and no water vapor.
BTPS—body condition as follows: body temperature (37°C), ambient pressure (760 mmHg at sea level), and saturated with water vapor.
ATPD—ambient temperature and pressure, dry.
ATPS—ambient temperature and pressure, saturated with water vapor.

Lower Case Letters

a—arterial blood
c—capillary blood
c′—pulmonary end-capillary blood
v—venous blood
$\bar{v}$—mixed venous blood
an—anatomic
anat—anatomic
f—frequency of respirations per minute
max—maximum
t—time

Others

ABG—arterial blood gas.
AIDS—acquired immune deficiency syndrome.
AP—anteroposterior.
ARC—AIDS-related complex.
ARDS—adult respiratory distress syndrome.
$AaDO_2$—alveolar-arterial oxygen pressure difference. Same as $P(A\text{-}a)O_2$.
a/A—arterial/alveolar ratio.
BPD—bronchopulmonary dysplasia.
$C(a\text{-}v)O_2$—arteriovenous oxygen content difference. Same as $Ca_{O2} - Cv_{O2}$.

*Adapted from American College of Chest Physicians. American Thoracic Society pulmonary terms and symbols. *Chest*, 67(5):583–593, 1975.

CI—cardiac index.
Cdyn—dynamic compliance.
C_L—lung compliance.
Cst—static compliance.
COPD—chronic obstructive pulmonary disease.
CPAP—continuous positive airway pressure.
$D_{L_{CO}}$—diffusion capacity of the lung (measured with carbon monoxide).
D_L/V_A—diffusion per unit of alveolar volume.
ERV—expiratory reserve volume.
$FEF_{25-75\%}$—forced expiratory flow over the middle half of the forced vital capacity.
FEV_t—forced expiratory volume, timed; e.g., air exhaled at 1, 2, 3 seconds.
FI_{O_2}—fractional inspired oxygen concentration.
FRC—functional residual capacity.
FVC—forced vital capacity.
GPB—glossopharyngeal breathing.
HFV—high frequency ventilation.
IC—inspiratory capacity.
IMV—intermittent mandatory ventilation.
IRV—inspiratory reserve volume.
I:E—inspiratory:expiratory ratio.
IPPB—intermittent positive pressure breathing.
LLL—left lower lobe of the lung.
LUL—left upper lobe of the lung.
MBC—maximum breathing capacity. Same as MVV.
MIFR—maximum inspiratory flow rate.
MMFR—maximum mid expiratory flow rate. Old term for $FEF_{25-75\%}$.
MVV—maximum voluntary ventilation. Same as MBC.
P_{aw}—pressure in the airway, level to be specified.
PA—pulmonary artery or posteroanterior.
$P(A\text{-}a)O_2$—alveolar-arterial oxygen pressure difference. Previously referred to as $A\text{-}aD_{O_2}$.
PCWP—pulmonary capillary wedge pressure.
PEEP—positive end-expiratory pressure.
PEF—peak expiratory flow.
PFT—pulmonary function test.
PIF—peak inspiratory flow.
P_{pl}—pleural pressure.
PSV—pressure support ventilation.
P_{tc}—transcutaneous partial pressure.
P_{tm}—transmural pressure of an airway or blood vessel.
P_{tp}—transpulmonary pressure.
P_L—transpulmonary pressure.
PT—physical therapy.
PVR—pulmonary vascular resistance.
$\dot{Q}$—cardiac output per minute.
$\dot{Q}_s/\dot{Q}_t$—percent intrapulmonary shunt.
R—respiratory exchange ratio. Also a general symbol for resistance.
RLL—right lower lobe of the lung.
RML—right middle lobe of the lung.
RUL—right upper lobe of the lung.
RQ—respiratory quotient.
RV—residual volume.
SIMV—synchronized intermittent mandatory ventilation.
SVC—slow vital capacity.
SVR—systemic vascular resistance.
TB—tuberculosis.
TLC—total lung capacity.
$\dot{V}_{maxXX\%}$—maximum expiratory flow (i.e., instantaneous) measured at a specified volume; e.g., $\dot{V}_{max75\%}$ is the maximum expiratory flow after 75% of FVC has been exhaled.
$\dot{V}$—minute ventilation.
V_E—minute ventilation.
VC—vital capacity.
V_D—dead space ventilation.
V_D/V_T—dead space to tidal volume ratio.
V/Q—ventilation/perfusion ratio.
V_T—tidal volume.
TV—tidal volume.
$\dot{V}CO_2$—carbon dioxide production per minute (STPD).
$\dot{V}O_2$—oxygen consumption per minute (STPD).
$\dot{V}CO/\dot{V}O_2$—respiratory exchange ratio.
W—general term for mechanical work of breathing.
WOB—general term for mechanical work of breathing.
Z—airway generation, e.g., Z = 1 (trachea) to Z = 23 (alveolar sacs).

Appendix II—Answers to Study Questions

Pharmacology Case Study Answers (Chapter 11)*

A

All the pulmonary medications are appropriately prescribed. *Aminophylline* is a methylxanthine bronchodilator with about 80% theophylline anhydrous content. *Tetracycline* is a bacteriostatic antibiotic effective against a broad range of gram-negative and gram-positive organisms. *Solu-Medrol* (methylprednisolone) is an intravenous corticosteroid preparation. *Bronkosol (Isoetharine)* is an adrenergic autonomic active agent with beta-1 and beta-2 activity. *Oxygen* is a respiratory depressant and not considered.

B

The patient probably has severe lung disease because he is on bronchodilators from three different drug groups, each with a different pharmacologic action. These drugs create an additive bronchodilating effect to relieve the problem of bronchoconstriction manifested by wheezing. Also, Solu-Medrol acts synergistically to increase responsiveness to Bronkosol, the beta-2 drug.

The patient has a mucus production problem (retention) because he is coughing up sputum. The tetracycline guards against a possible chest infection. Sputum culture and sensitivity (C & S) and Gram's stain results are not available to confirm infection, but yellow sputum and acute pulmonary symptoms suggest its presence, even though the patient is afebrile.

C

Theophylline

The patient's daily aminophylline dose is 960 mg. This amount equals 768 mg theophylline anhydrous (960 mg × 0.80). It is well below the 900 mg/day theophylline limit, the rule of thumb described in Chapter 11.

The patient is probably not undermedicated because the blood theophylline level is within the 10 to 20 mcg/ml therapeutic range. Also, normal rather than decreased breath sounds were reported over all lung lobes, indicating adequate lung ventilation. However, theophylline toxicity is still a possibility, since patients may become toxic at normal theophylline levels.

Key Interventions

1. Monitor the patient for side effects and clinical signs of toxicity. (Review Table 11–14.)
2. Check theophylline levels every 24 to 48 hours. (Review Table 11–16 for interpretations.)

Bronkosol (Isoetharine)

The patient may develop arrhythmias and other beta-1 related side effects, because the heart rate is elevated to 120 beats/min, and hourly treatments are ordered. Bronkosol is relatively short acting, but may act for up to 3 hours.

Key Interventions

1. Monitor for tachycardia, arrhythmias, chest pain, hypertension, and nervousness.
2. As wheezing improves, encourage decreasing Bronkosol IPPB treatments to every 2 to 4 hours to lessen side effects and risk of tachyphylaxis and to allow more time for rest.
3. Recommend changing to metaproterenol (Alupent) or albuterol (Proventil, Ventolin) aerosol via hand-held nebulizer, once acute dyspnea is relieved. These drugs are longer acting, permitting longer dosing intervals. Though the patient may feel more secure with IPPB, the hand-held nebulizer is just as effective as IPPB for aerosol delivery.

Tetracycline

The dosage is appropriate. *Side effects* may include stomach discomfort, anorexia, nausea, vomiting, diar-

*See page 250.

rhea, skin rashes, depressed prothrombin activity, photosensitivity, anemia, thrombocytopenia, neutropenia, and eosinophilia. *Other problems* may include drug resistance, superinfection (particularly in a compromised host), and poor systemic absorption.

Key Interventions

1. Monitor for aforementioned side effects.
2. Monitor sputum changes. If signs of infection persist, the antibiotic should be changed or another one added to cover more microorganisms.
3. Do not give milk products, antacids, or iron preparations within 1 hour of tetracycline administration. These agents decrease absorption. Absorption is increased when tetracycline is taken at least 1 hour before meals or 2 hours after, but this is not an absolute requirement. In fact, small amounts of food with oral administration may decrease stomach discomfort and improve drug tolerance.

Solu-Medrol

The dosage is appropriate. The normal dosage for this 72-kg man is 5 mg/kg or 360 mg daily. He is curently receiving 240 mg/24 hours. Signs of steroid dependency are unlikely, in the absence of previous steroid therapy. Other side effects should not be a problem unless the patient develops heart failure or other complications.

Key Interventions

1. Monitor for routine steroid side effects. (See Chapter 11.)
2. After acute disease stabilization, encourage the rapid tapering of Solu-Medrol to 30 mg q 12 hours and the conversion to oral prednisone, 40 mg daily (given at 8:00 am), followed by alternate-day steroids, as indicated by the specific situation.

COMMENT

In this case study, clinical improvement depends on the simultaneous implementation of pulmonary drugs and more basic bronchial hygiene measures, including adequate hydration, deep breathing, coughing, and postural drainage, if necessary. Both types of therapies must be aggressive, so that once bronchodilators begin to dilate airways, the patient can promptly expectorate retained secretions.

Arterial Blood Gas Interpretations (Chapter 13)*

The numbers 1 to 6 under problems IA and IB correlate with questions 1 through 6 in the Guide to Arterial Blood Gas (ABG) Interpretation. These more detailed answers clarify methodology for arriving at a final interpretation. The answers for problems II through IV are in summary form.

*See page 365.

PROBLEM IA

1. No—Pa_{O_2} and O_2 sat. are below normal, indicating hypoxemia. The hypoxemia is moderately severe, since it is less than 60 mmHg, the upper limit of the oxyhemoglobin dissociation curve's critical zone.

2a. No—pH is well below the normal range of 7.38 to 7.42, indicating that the disorder is acute and little to no compensation has taken place.

2b. The pH is on the acidic side of 7.40, indicating that the primary disorder is acidosis.

3. Pa_{CO_2} is high (respiratory acidosis or alveolar hypoventilation).

4. HCO_3^- is normal, indicating that the kidneys have not yet compensated for the respiratory acidosis. Compensation takes 2 days.

5. The primary disorder is respiratory acidosis. Metabolic (renal) compensation is not present. In addition, the patient is in ventilatory failure, since Pa_{CO_2} is greater than 50 mmHg.

6. The final interpretation is acute respiratory acidosis with ventilatory failure and hypoxemia.

PROBLEM IB

1. No—Pa_{O_2} and O_2 sat. are below normal. A Pa_{O_2} of 55 indicates moderate hypoxemia. This is severe for a young adult.

2a. Yes—the pH is within normal limits, indicating that the ABG values are normal, or full compensation has occurred for an acid-base disorder.

2b. The pH is on the acidic side of 7.40. If a disorder exists, the primary process must be acidosis.

3. Pa_{CO_2} is high (respiratory acidosis or alveolar hypoventilation).

4. HCO_3^- is also high (metabolic alkalosis).

5. Primary respiratory acidosis (alveolar hypoventilation) with a compensatory metabolic alkalosis. Renal compensation is complete, since pH is normal. Also, the patient is in chronic ventilatory failure, since the Pa_{CO_2} is over 50, and the disorder is at least 2 days old (enough time for renal compensation).

6. The final interpretation is chronic, *fully* compensated respiratory acidosis, with ventilatory failure and hypoxemia. Unrelated primary metabolic alkalosis is also present.

PROBLEM IIA

Hypoxemia (severe).

Primary respiratory alkalosis (alveolar hyperventilation).

An acute process without renal compensation.

The final interpretation is acute respiratory alkalosis with hypoxemia.

PROBLEM IIB

Hypoxemia (severe).

Primary respiratory alkalosis with compensatory metabolic acidosis.

A chronic process with full renal compensation.

The final interpretation is chronic *fully* compensated respiratory alkalosis, with hypoxemia.

PROBLEM IIIA

Mild hypoxemia, since O_2 sat. is less than 95%. However, accurate interpretation requires the patient's age. A PaO_2 of 80 mmHg is high for an elderly person but may be low for a young person.

From another perspective, note that PaO_2 is artificially elevated to 80 mmHg, owing to alveolar hyperventilation. Without hyperventilation, $PaCO_2$ would increase to normal (40 mmHg), and the patient's PaO_2 would decrease to a lower level (75 mmHg). Remember that on room air, a change in $PaCO_2$ is accompanied by a change in PaO_2 by an equal amount.

Primary metabolic acidosis with a compensatory respiratory alkalosis.

An acute process with partial respiratory compensation. A clinical history is needed to determine how long respiratory compensation has been going on.

The final interpretation is *partially compensated* metabolic acidosis, with hypoxemia.

PROBLEM IIIB

Normal oxygenation.

Primary metabolic acidosis with compensatory respiratory alkalosis.

Full respiratory compensation is present.

The final interpretation is *fully compensated* metabolic acidosis, with normal oxygenation.

PROBLEM IVA

Hypoxemia (mild).

Primary metabolic alkalosis.

An acute process.

Strictly speaking, no respiratory compensation is present; yet, one might say that there is some compensation, if the patient's $PaCO_2$ is normally 38 or 39 mmHg.

The final interpretation is acute metabolic alkalosis, with hypoxemia.

PROBLEM IVB

Hypoxemia (worse compared with the PaO_2 in Problem IVA).

Primary metabolic alkalosis with compensatory respiratory acidosis.

Compensation is nearly complete.

The final interpretation is *almost fully* compensated metabolic alkalosis, with hypoxemia.

Pulmonary Function Test (PFT) Interpretations

The following PFT interpretations follow the format summarized in the PFT guide in Chapter 14..

PFT#1—MR. R. (CHAPTER 14)*

Lung Volumes

A. Vital capacity (VC) is at the lower limit of normal (86% predicted).

B. RV/TLC is elevated (52%) because RV is elevated while TLC remains normal. The increased RV, increased FRC, and increased RV/TLC are all signs of air trapping in the lungs, an obstructive process.

Mechanics of Breathing

A. FEV_1 is greatly reduced (28% predicted).

B. FEV_1/FVC is less than 70%, a sign of an obstructive process. A *severe* obstructive disease is present because FEV_1 is under 1.0 L. Restrictive disease is absent because the TLC value is normal.

C. FVC is mildly reduced.

D. Air flow is reduced everywhere, especially in small airways, since $FEV_{25-75\%}$ is only 5% predicted.

E. The FVC is less than the slow VC (420 cc difference), a finding consistent with obstructive disease.

F. The patient demonstrates significant improvement in postbronchodilator values, a sign of reversible airway disease (bronchospasm). Upon quick determination, all three indicators—FEV_1, FVC, and $FEF_{25-75\%}$—show more than a 15% change in postbronchodilator values. Calculations confirm this conclusion:

	improvement in ml	*% change*
FEV_1	170	$\frac{0.170}{0.700} = 0.24$ or 24%
FVC	600	$\frac{0.600}{2.660} = 0.22$ or 22%
$FEF_{25-75\%}$	5	$\frac{5}{9} = 0.55$ or 55%

G. Flow volume loop—the marked reduction in flow rates and scooping along the expiratory curve indicate obstructive disease.

Diffusing Capacity

DL is at the lower limits of normal (84% predicted). If a previous PFT were available, the clinician would determine whether the present value is less than that previous PFT value. If the value has decreased, then at least some loss in alveolar capillary surface is probable. The *alveolar volume* measurement has not been discussed in Chapter 14. It is a measure of total lung capacity (TLC) made on a single breath maneuver. In

*See page 396.

this case, alveolar volume (4.23 L) is much less than the TLC by the rebreathing method (6.43 L). This discrepancy indicates air trapping in the lungs.

Arterial Blood Gases

Normal oxygenation, ventilation, and acid-base balance.

Conclusion

Severe obstructive pulmonary disease with marked air trapping in the lungs and significant improvement with aerosol bronchodilator.

Comments

The patient, Mr. R., has a long history of chronic asthma. The PFT was taken after recovery from an episode of acute asthmatic bronchitis. Current pulmonary medications have not yet maximally bronchodilated his airways, because prebronchodilator values do not equal postbronchodilator values. Reevaluation of his pulmonary medications may be necessary to determine how to further dilate the airways without producing or increasing side effects.

PFT #2—MR. W. (CHAPTER 14)*

Lung Volumes

A. Vital capacity is reduced.
B. RV/TLC is normal—no air trapping is present. However, TLC is reduced to 60% predicted, a diagnostic sign of restrictive disease.

Mechanics of Breathing

A. FEV_1 is normal.
B. and C. FEV_1/FVC is increased over 80% because the total volume or forced vital capacity (FVC) is reduced proportionally more than the FEV_1. This change is typical in restrictive disease.
D. $FEF_{25-75\%}$ is elevated, indicating supranormal flow rates in small airways, a finding in mild to moderate restrictive disease.
E. FVC is less than the slow VC, but the difference is only 130 cc and could be due to varying effort rather than obstruction.
F. Postbronchodilator studies were not ordered on this patient.
G. Flow volume loop—the pattern is restrictive. The loop looks like a small, normal flow volume loop.

Diffusing Capacity

Without a previous PFT value, the DL of 89% predicted is interpreted as normal, suggesting an intact alveolar-capillary surface available for gas exchange. However, the 89% predicted is actually reduced from the 114% predicted on a past PFT value not presented here. This finding confirms a loss of alveolar-capillary surface area.

*See page 397.

Arterial Blood Gases

There is mild hypoxemia on room air with normal ventilation and normal acid-base balance.

Conclusion

Moderately severe restrictive disease with mild hypoxemia.

Comments

Mr. W.'s medical diagnosis is idiopathic interstitial fibrosis. He has classic clinical findings of fibrosis, including dry sounding crackles throughout most lung regions on auscultation, a reduced diffusing capacity on PFT, and hypoxemia.

MR. K. (CHAPTER 32)*

Lung Volumes

A. Vital capacity (VC) is reduced.
B. RV/TLC is about normal. No air trapping is present. TLC is reduced to 65% predicted, indicating moderately severe restrictive disease.

Mechanics of Breathing

A. FEV_1 is reduced.
B. and C. FEV_1/FVC is increased to nearly 90%, a sign indicating restrictive lung disease. Note that the total volume forced vital capacity (FVC) is reduced proportionally more than the FEV_1.
D. $FEF_{25-75\%}$ is on the high side of normal. Remember that supranormal flow rates in small airways are seen in restrictive lung disease due to decreased lung compliance.
E. The slow VC and FVC are identical. No air trapping is present.
F. Postbronchodilator PFT values show no significant improvement, when compared with prebronchodilator values. No airway obstruction is evident.

Diffusing Capacity

DL is severely reduced, even when the hemoglobin level is taken into account.

Conclusion

Moderately severe restrictive ventilatory defect with severe diffusion impairment. Signs of airway obstruction are absent. These results are consistent with a diffuse interstitial disease.

*See page 833.

EPILOGUE

The goal of this book has been to provide an extensive collaborative theory base for decision-making in respiratory nursing. The reader might wonder why nursing diagnoses were not integrated throughout the book. Admittedly, integration would help make the conceptual link between assessment and intervention clearer for individual lung diseases and procedures. However, the reason for this intentional omission is simple. The state of the art of collaborative respiratory diagnosis is still in its infancy because of the following:

1. Respiratory diagnoses are by nature collaborative and must be developed collaboratively, a situation only now emerging.
2. Existing diagnoses are considered tentative because they lack confirming support of clinical research. More specifically, they lack reliable defining criteria that are conceptually congruent with other diagnoses.

So, the main unanswered question is, how can the development of nursing diagnoses in collaborative practice be facilitated?

One way to advance the state of the art of respiratory nursing is to promote interdependence and collaboration between disciplines. From this perspective, it is not enough for nursing to develop independently a taxonomy of respiratory diagnoses or to interface unilaterally nursing diagnoses with collaborative problems, a concept introduced in the literature only recently. Simultaneous communication with those in medical subspecialties and other disciplines is necessary to establish and clarify defining criteria, to discuss role ambiguity in specific clinical situations, and to further interdisciplinary efforts in general. With a focus on interdependence rather than on independence, on complementary roles rather than on competing roles, health team members may more successfully integrate decision-making processes and avoid piecemeal approaches to theory building that limit the number of fruitful research questions.

Another way to promote the development of respiratory diagnoses is for nurses to think of themselves as reflective practitioners. A reflective practitioner believes that clinical practice *is* research. The two are inseparable and ongoing. The nurse formulates and continually revises intuitive understandings of clinical situations while providing care. This reflection-in-action may yield a new set of nursing diagnoses for other researchers to test systematically and empirically. Most important, this approach may be the only way to narrow substantially the gap between theory and practice. By strengthening interdependence at the professional level and reflection-in-action at the personal level, nurses will be better prepared to shape the future of nursing in a relevant and meaningful way.

Index

Note: Page numbers in *italics* refer to illustrations; page numbers followed by t refer to tables.

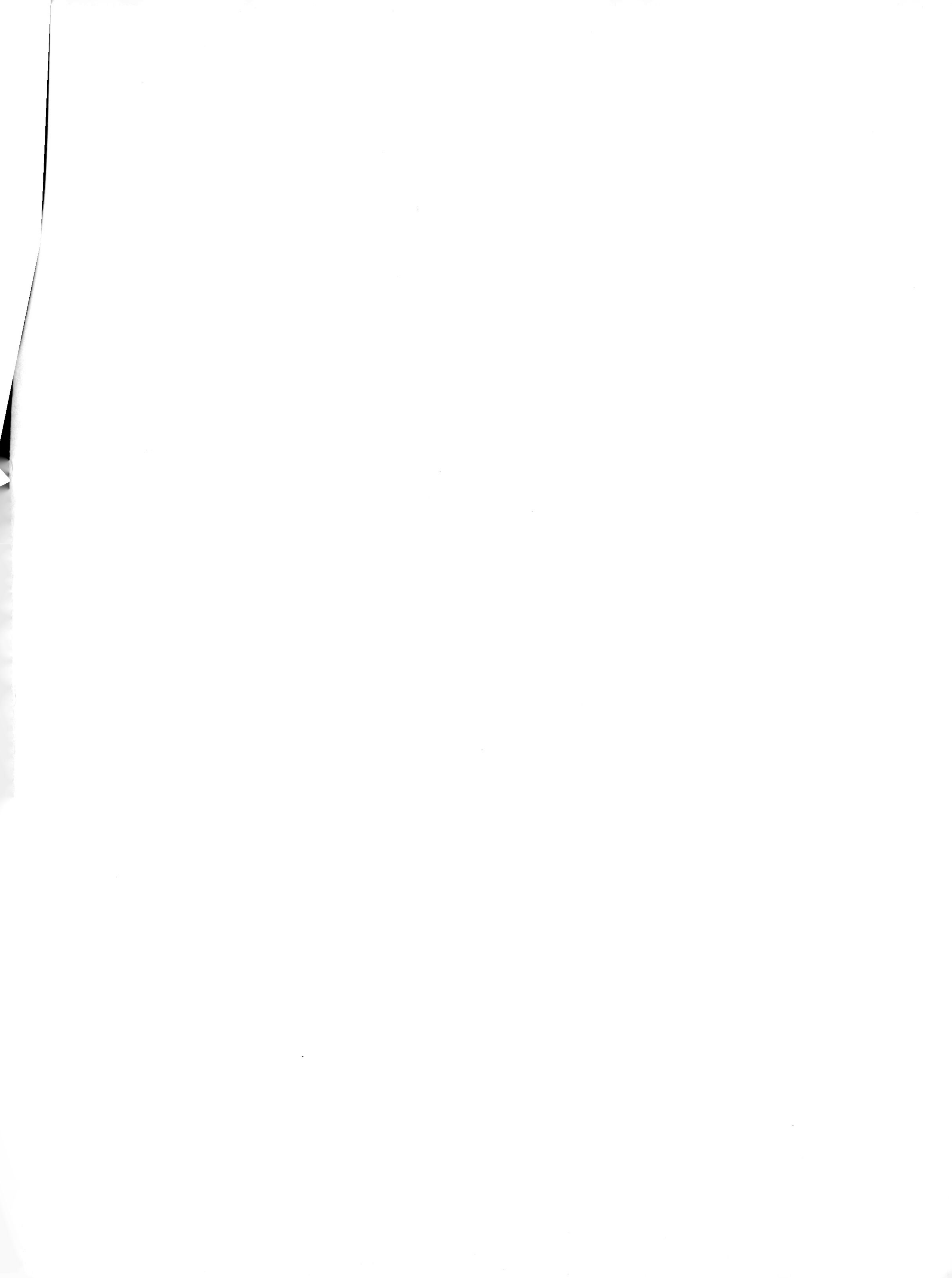